N

POCKE'

of Nursing, Medicine and
Professions Allied to Medicine

UK Edition

MOSBY'S
POCKET
DICTIONARY
of Nursing, Medicine
and Professions Allied
to Medicine

UK Edition

Kenneth N. Anderson

Lois E. Anderson

ᴎᴀ Mosby

LONDON • BALTIMORE • BOGOTÁ • BOSTON • BUENOS AIRES
CARACAS • CARLSBAD, CA • CHICAGO • MADRID
MEXICO CITY • MILAN • NAPLES, FL • NEW YORK
PHILADELPHIA • ST LOUIS • SYDNEY • TOKYO
TORONTO • WIESBADEN

Copyright © 1995 Times Mirror International Publishers Limited

Published in 1995 by Mosby, an imprint of Times Mirror International Publishers Limited

Printed in England by Clays Ltd, St Ives plc

ISBN 0 7234 2006 8

For full details of all Times Mirror International Publishers Limited titles, please write to Times Mirror International Publishers Limited, Lynton House, 7–12 Tavistock Square, London WC1H 9LB, England.

A CIP catalogue record for this book is available from the British Library.

Contents

Preface

The first UK edition of *Mosby's Pocket Dictionary of Nursing, Medicine and Professions Allied to Medicine* is a **comprehensive, succinct** and **portable** reference book. The terms and definitions included in this edition embrace a variety of health science fields, including **nursing, midwifery, physiotherapy, radiography, occupational therapy, dentistry, pharmacy, podiatry, psychiatry, dietetics, medicine,** and **complementary therapies**, making this book appropriate for **students** and **practitioners** in these fields. It is an abridgement of *Mosby's Medical Nursing and Allied Health Dictionary* (now in its fourth edition).

This UK edition features:

- Up-to-date terms and definitions that reflect current UK practice, terminology and spellings.

- More than 60,000 entries which provide the breadth and depth of coverage required for diploma and degree level education.
- Comprehensive definitions which include terminology from many fields of health care.

In the complex and changing world of health care, *Mosby's Pocket Dictionary of Nursing, Medicine and Professions Allied to Medicine* provides an affordable, compact, but thorough and usable resource that will enhance your knowledge of health care terminology and facilitate communication with professionals from other fields of health care.

UK Contributors

Mary Brewin, MSc, TDip COT, Senior Lecturer, School of Health and Social Sciences, Coventry University, and Research Worker Occupational Therapy Clinical Terms Project.

David Evans, MD, FRCP, FRCPath. Formerly Consultant Pathologist, South Glamorgan Health Authority.

Jill Gregson, Formerly Senior Education Manager, Faculty of Nursing Studies, The North West College of Nursing and Midwifery.

Janet Griffiths, LDS, BA, Hospital Dental Surgeon/Care of Adult Special Needs, Cardiff Dental Hospital and School.

Joanna Husbands, SRN, RM, ADM, PGCEA, Midwifery Lecturer, Queen Charlotte's College of Health and Science.

Mandy Langford, Formerly Chair, British Complementary Medicines Association, St Charles Hospital.

Sue Ritter, Lecturer in Psychiatric Nursing, Institute of Psychiatry, University of London.

Mel Stewart, MEd MCSP, DipTP, School of Physiotherapy, Queen Elizabeth Medical Centre.

Maxwell Summerhayes, BPharm, PhD, MRPharmS, ICRF Principal Oncology Pharmacist, Guy's Hospital.

Vera Todorovic, MSc, SRD, Manager, Department of Dietetics and Nutrition, Bassetlaw General Hospital, Worksop.

Sally Waddington, Senior Tutor, Department of Radiographic Education, Avon & Gloucestershire College of Health.

Steve West, BSc, DPodM, FChS, SRCh, Head of Department & Dean, Department of Podiatry, School of Human & Health Sciences, University of Huddersfield.

Acknowledgements

To bring a concise and reliable abridgement into print takes the effort of many people. We would like to thank Richenda Milton-Thompson and Helen Bowen for the detailed editorial work they undertook to ensure this dictionary reflected UK terminology and spellings.

We also acknowledge and appreciate the work of all who participated in the development of the original US edition of this dictionary, particularly Kenneth N. Anderson and Lois E. Anderson, who wrote and edited the work.

The following consultants assisted in the development of the US edition of this dictionary:

Donna C Aguilera, PhD, FAAN
Kathleen G Andreoli, DNS, FAAN
Miriam G Austrin, RN, BA
Diane M Billings, RN, EdD
Violet A Breckbill, RN, PhD
Carolyn H Brose, EdD, RN
Charlene D Coco, RN, MN
Bruce Colbert, MS, RRT
Mary H Conover, RN, BS
Helen Cox
Joyce E Dains, RN, DrPH
Rene A Day, RN, MSc
Claire M Fagin, PhD, FAAN
A Jolayne Farrell, RN, MPH
William F Finney, MA, RT
Marilyn E Flood, RN, PhD
Catherine Ingram Fogel, RNC, MS
Carol P Fray, RN, BA, BSN, MA
Anne Gray, MEd, BA, DipNEd
Janet Gray, BSN, MA
Susan Grobe, RN, PhD
Maureen W Groër, RN, PhD
James Randall Hansbrough, PhD, MD
Lorrie N Hegstad, RN, PhD
Jane Hirsch, RN, MS
Eugene M Johnson, Jr, PhD
Virginia Burke Karb, RN, PhD
Judith Belliveau Krauss, RN, MSN
Mavis E Kyle, RN, MHSA
Linda Armstrong Lazure, RN, MSN
Maxine E Loomis, RN, PhD, FAAN
Jannetta MacPhail, RN, PhD, FAAN
Ann Marriner-Tomey, RN, PhD, FAAN
Tink Delker Martin, MACT, PT
Edwina A McConnell, RN, PhD
Janice M Messick, RN, MS, FAAN
B B Michniak, PhD, MPS, MI Biol
Patricia A Mickelsen, PhD
Susan I Molde, RN, MSN
Mary N Moore, PhD, RN
Helen K Mussallem, OC, BN, MA, EdD, OStJ, LLD, DSc, FRCN, MRSH
Susan Jenkinson Neuman, RN, BA
Jeanmaire R Offner, MD
Marie L O'Koren, RN, EdD, FAAN
Kathleen Deska Pagana, PhD, RN
Ann M Pagliaro, RN, MSN
Anne G Perry, RN, MSN
Susan Foley Pierce, RN, MSN
Patricia A Potter, RN, MSN
Jack D Preston, DDS
Malvin E Ring, DDS, MLS, FACD
Ginette Rodger, RN, BScN, MNAdm
Charlotte Searle, DPhil, RN
Kay See-Lasley, MS, RPh
Susan Budassi Sheehy, RN, MSN, CEN
Dan Shock, BS, RT (R)
Sandra L Siehl, RN, MSN
Margretta M Styles, RN, EdD, FAAN
June M Thompson, RN, MS
Catherine A Trombly, MA, OTR, FAOTA
Diana M Uhler, RN
Lerma Ung
Lucille Whaley, RN, MS
Bethany L Wise, MS, MT (ASCP), CLS

Guide to the dictionary

- Entries are alphabetized letter by letter, disregarding spaces or hypens between words; for example:

analgesic   **artificial lung**
anal membrane   **artificially acquired**
analogue   **immunity**
artificial nutrition

- Alphabetization is alphanumeric; words and numbers from a single list with numbers positioned as though they were spelled-out numerals; for example: **Nikolsky's sign/90-90 traction/ninth nerve**.

- Small subscript and superscript numbers are disregarded in alphabetizing; for example: **No/N$_2$O/nobelium**.

- Headwords: "headword" refers to any alphabetized and nonindented definition, be it a single word-term or a compound term. Compound headwords are given in their natural word order; for example: **abdominal surgery**, not **surgery, abdominal**; **achondroplastic dwarf**, not **dwarf, achondroplastic**. (There are few exceptions to this natural word order, most of which concern formal classifications, for example "comfort, alteration in: pain, ...'').

- Terms that are synonymous with a headword or derived from a headword that immediately precede or follow the definition, are not included as a separate entry. Therefore, if a term is not listed at the expected place, you might find it among the boldface terms of the immediately preceding or immediately following entry.

a, symbol for arterial blood.

A, 1. abbreviation for **atomic weight. 2.** symbol for **mass number.**

A68, symbol for a protein found in the brain tissue of Alzheimer's disease patients. It is also found in the developing normal brains of fetuses and infants but begins to disappear by the age of 2 years.

Å, symbol for **angstrom.**

AA, 1. abbreviation for **achievement age. 2.** abbreviation for **Alcoholics Anonymous.**

aa, (in prescriptions) abbreviation for ana, indicating an equal amount of each ingredient to be compounded.

Ab, abbreviation for **antibody.**

abacterial, any atmosphere or condition free of bacteria; literally, without bacteria.

abaissement, a falling or depressing; in ophthalmology, the displacement of a lens.

abalienation, 1. a state of physical deterioration or mental decay. **2.** a state of insanity. **abalienate,** *v.,* **abalienated,** *adj.*

A band, the area between two I bands of a sarcomere, marked by partial overlapping of actin and myosin filaments.

abarthrosis. See **synovial joint.**

abarticular, 1. of or pertaining to a condition that does not affect a joint. **2.** of or pertaining to a site or structure remote from a joint.

abarticulation, 1. dislocation of a joint. **2.** a synovial joint.

abasia, the inability to walk, as in paralytic abasia that paralyses the leg muscles. **abasic, abatic,** *adj.*

abaxial, 1. of or pertaining to a position outside the axis of a body or structure. **2.** of or pertaining to a position at the opposite extremity of a structure.

Abbé-Estlander operation {Robert Abbé, American surgeon, b. 1851; Jakob A. Estlander, Finnish surgeon, b. 1831}, a surgical procedure that transfers a full-thickness section of one oral lip to the other lip.

Abbot pump, a small portable pump that can be adjusted and finely calibrated to deliver precise amounts of medication in solution through an intravenous infusion set.

ABC, abbreviation for **aspiration biopsy cytology.**

abdomen, the portion of the body between the thorax and the pelvis. The abdominal cavity contains the lower portion of the oesophagus, the stomach, the intestines, the liver, the spleen, the pancreas, and other visceral organs. The abdominal cavity is lined with two layers of peritoneum, a serous membrane. **abdominal,** *adj.*

abdominal actinomycosis. See **actinomycosis.**

abdominal aorta, the portion of the descending aorta that passes from the aortic hiatus of the diaphragm into the abdomen. It supplies many different parts of the body, such as the testes, ovaries, kidneys, and stomach. Its branches are the coeliac, superior mesenteric, inferior mesenteric, middle suprarenal, renal, testicular, ovarian, inferior phrenic, lumbar, middle sacral, and common iliac arteries.

abdominal aortography, the process of producing a radiograph of the abdominal aorta using a radiopaque contrast medium.

abdominal aponeurosis, the conjoined tendons of the oblique and transverse muscles of the abdomen.

abdominal bandage, a broad supportive bandage commonly used after abdominal surgery.

abdominal binder, a bandage or elasticized wrap that is applied around the lower part of the torso to support the abdomen, sometimes applied after abdominal surgery to decrease discomfort.

abdominal breathing, breathing in which the majority of respiratory work is done by the diaphragm and abdominal muscles.

abdominal delivery, the delivery of a child through a surgical incision in the abdomen. The procedure performed may be any of the several kinds of caesarean section.

abdominal-diaphragmatic breathing, respiration in which the abdomen moves out while the diaphragm descends during inspiration.

abdominal fistula, an abnormal passage from an abdominal organ to the surface of the body. In a colostomy, a passage from the bowel to an opening on the surface of the abdomen is created surgically.

abdominal girth, the circumference of the abdomen, usually measured at the umbilicus.

abdominal hernia, a hernia in which a loop of bowel protrudes through the abdominal musculature, often through the site of an old surgical scar.

abdominal hysterectomy, the excision of the uterus through the abdominal wall.

abdominal pain, acute or chronic localized or diffuse pain in the abdominal cavity. Abdominal pain is a significant symptom because its cause may require immediate surgical or medical intervention. The most common causes of severe abdominal pain are inflammation, perforation of an intraabdominal structure, circulatory obstruction, intestinal or ureteral obstruction, or rupture of an organ located within the abdomen. Specific conditions include appendicitis, perforated gastric ulcer, strangulated hernia, superior mesenteric arterial thrombosis, and small and large bowel obstruction. Conditions producing acute abdominal pain that may require surgery include appendicitis, acute or severe and chronic diverticulitis, acute and chronic cholecystitis, cholelithiasis, acute pancreatitis, perforation of a peptic ulcer, various intestinal obstructions, abdominal aortic aneurysms, and trauma affecting any of the abdominal organs. Gynaecological causes of acute abdominal pain that may require surgery include acute pelvic inflammatory disease, ruptured ovarian cyst, and ectopic pregnancy. Abdominal pain associated with pregnancy may be caused by the weight of the enlarged uterus; rotation, stretching, or compression of the round ligament; or squeezing or displacement of the bowel. Chronic abdominal pain may be functional or the result of overeating or aerophagy. Organic sources of abdominal pain include peptic ulcer, hiatus hernia, gastritis, chronic cholecystitis and cholelithiasis, chronic pancreatitis, pancreatic carcinoma, chronic diverticulitis, intermittent low-grade intestinal obstruction, and functional indigestion.

abdominal pulse, the pulse of the abdominal aorta.

abdominal quadrant, any of four topographical areas of the abdomen divided by two imaginary vertical and horizontal lines intersecting at the umbilicus. The divisions are the left upper quadrant (LUQ), the left lower quadrant (LLQ), the right upper quadrant (RUQ), and the right lower quadrant (RLQ).

abdominal reflex, a superficial neurological reflex obtained by firmly stroking the skin of the abdomen, normally resulting in a brisk contraction of abdominal muscles in which the umbilicus moves toward the site of the stimulus. This reflex is lost in diseases of the pyramidal tract.

abdominal regions, the nine topographical subdivisions of the abdomen, determined by four imaginary lines, in a 'noughts and crosses' grid pattern, imposed over the anterior surface. The upper horizontal line passes along the level of the cartilages of the nine ribs; the lower along the iliac crests. The two vertical lines extend on each side of the body from the cartilage of the eighth rib to the centre of the inguinal ligament. The lines divide the abdomen into three upper, three middle, and three lower zones: right hypochondriac, epigastric, and left hypo-

chondriac regions (upper zones); right lateral, umbilical, and left lateral regions (middle zones); right inguinal, pubic, and left inguinal regions (lower zones).

abdominal splinting, a rigid contraction of the muscles of the abdominal wall. It may result in hypoventilation and respiratory complications.

abdominal surgery, any operation that involves an incision into the abdomen, usually performed under general anaesthesia. Some kinds of abdominal surgery are **appendectomy, cholecystectomy, colostomy, gastrectomy, herniorrhaphy,** and **laparotomy.**

abdominal tenaculum. See **tenaculum.**

abdominocentesis. See **paracentesis.**

abdominocyesis. See **ectopic pregnancy.**

abdominoscopy, a procedure for examining the contents of the peritoneum in which an electrically illuminated tubular device is passed through a trocar into the abdominal cavity.

abducens nerve, the sixth cranial nerve. It controls the external rectus muscle, turning the eye outward.

abduction, movement of a limb away from the body.

abduction boots, a pair of orthopaedic casts for the lower extremities, available in both short-leg and long-leg configurations, with a bar incorporated at ankle level to provide hip abduction.

abductor, a muscle that draws a body part away from the midline, or one part from another.

Abernethy's sarcoma a malignant neoplasm of fat cells, usually occurring on the trunk.

aberrancy. See **aberrant ventricular conduction.**

aberrant, 1. of or pertaining to a wandering from the usual or expected course, such as various ducts, nerves, and vessels in the body. **2.** (in botany and zoology) of or pertaining to an abnormal individual, such as certain atypical members of a species.

aberrant goitre, an enlargement of a supernumerary or ectopic thyroid gland.

aberrant ventricular conduction (AVC), the temporary abnormal intraventricular conduction of a supraventricular impulse, usually associated with a change in cycle length.

aberration, 1. any departure from the usual course or normal condition. **2.** abnormal growth or development. **3.** (in psychology) an illogical and unreasonable thought or belief, often leading to an unsound mental state. **4.** (in genetics) any change in the number or structure of the chromosomes. **5.** (in optics) any imperfect image formation caused by unequal refraction or focalization of light rays through a lens.

abetalipoproteinaemia, a rare inherited disorder of fat metabolism, characterized by acanthocytosis, low or absent serum betalipoproteins, and hypocholesterolaemia.

abient, characterized by a tendency to move away from stimuli.　　**abience,** *n.*

ability, the capacity to act in a specified way because of the possession of appropriate skills and mental or physical fitness.

abiogenesis, spontaneous generation; the theory that organic life can originate from inanimate matter.　　**abiogenetic,** *adj.*

abiosis, a nonviable condition or a situation that is incompatible with life.　　**abiotic,** *adj.*

abiotrophy, a premature depletion of vitality or the deterioration of certain cells and tissues, especially those involved in genetic degenerative diseases.　　**abiotrophic,** *adj.*

ablation, an amputation, an excision of any part of the body, or a removal of a growth or harmful substance.

ablepsia, the condition of being blind.

abnerval current, an electric current that passes from a nerve to and through muscle.

abnormal behaviour, maladaptive acts or activities detrimental to the individual and to society.

abnormal psychology, the study of mental disorders and maladaptive behavior, including neuroses and psychoses, and of normal phenomena that are not completely understood, such as dreams and altered states of consciousness.

ABO blood groups, the most important of several systems for classifying human blood based on the antigenic components of the red blood cell. The ABO blood group is identified by the presence or absence of two different antigens, A or B, on the surface of the erythrocyte. The four blood types in this grouping, A, B, AB, and O, are determined by and named after these antigens. Type AB indicates the presence of both antigens; type O the absence of both.

aboiement an involuntary making of abnormal, animal-like sounds, such as barking. Aboiement may be a clinical sign of Gilles de la Tourette's syndrome.

abort, 1. to deliver a nonviable fetus; to miscarry. **2.** to terminate a pregnancy before the fetus has developed enough to survive ex utero. **3.** to terminate in the early stages or to discontinue before completion, as to arrest the usual course of a disease, to stop growth and development, or to halt a project.

aborted systole, a contraction of the heart that is usually weak and is not associated with a radial pulse.

abortifacient 1. producing abortion. **2.** an agent that causes abortion.

abortion, the spontaneous or induced termination of pregnancy before the fetus has developed enough to be expected to live if born. Kinds of abortion include **habitual abortion, infected abortion, septic abortion, threatened abortion,** and **voluntary abortion.**

abortive infection, an infection in which some or all viral components have been synthesized, but no infective virus is produced.

abortus, any incompletely developed fetus that results from an abortion, particularly one that weighs less than 500 g.

abortus fever, a form of brucellosis, the only one endemic to North America. It is caused by *Brucella abortus,* an organism so named because it causes abortion in cows. Infection in humans results from contact with cows infected with *B. abortus.*

abouchement, the junction of a small blood vessel with a large blood vessel.

aboulia. See **abulia.**

ABPN, abbreviation for **Association of British Paediatric Nurses.**

abrachia, the absence of arms.　　**abrachial,** *adj.*

abrade, to remove the epidermis or other skin layers, usually by scraping or rubbing.

abrasion, a scraping, or rubbing away of a surface by friction. Abrasion may be the result of trauma, such as a skinned knee; of therapy, as in dermabrasion of the skin for removal of scar tissue; or of normal function, such as the wearing down of a tooth by mastication. **abrade,** *v.,*, abrasive, *adj.*

abreaction, an emotional release resulting from mentally reliving or from bringing into consciousness, through the process of catharsis, a long-repressed, painful experience.

abrosia, a condition caused by fasting or abstaining from food. See **anorexia.**

abruptio placentae, separation of the placenta implanted in normal position in a pregnancy of 20 weeks or more or during labour before delivery of the fetus. It occurs approximately once in 200 births, and, because it often results in severe haemorrhage, it is a significant cause of maternal and fetal mortality.

abscess, a cavity containing pus and surrounded by inflamed tissue, formed as a result of suppuration in a localized infection (characteristically, a staphylococcal infection). Healing usually occurs when an abscess drains or is incised.

absence seizure. See **petit mal seizure.**

absenteeism, (for health or related reasons) absence from work. The most common causes of absenteeism include influenza and lower back pain.

absent without leave (AWOL), describing a patient who leaves a psychiatric facility without authorization.

absolute alcohol. See **dehydrated alcohol.**

absolute discharge, a final and complete termination of the patient's relationship with a hospital.

absolute growth, the total increase in size of an organism or a particular organ or part, such as the limbs, head, or trunk.

absolute humidity, the actual weight or content of water in a measured volume of air. It is usually expressed in grams per cubic metre or pounds per cubic foot or cubic yard.

absolute refractory period. See **refractory period.**

absolute temperature, temperature that is measured from a base of absolute zero on either the Kelvin scale or the Rankine scale.

absolute values (red cell indices), these are: mean corpuscular haemoglobin concentration (MCHC), mean corpuscular diameter (MCD), mean corpuscular volume (MCV) and mean corpuscular haemoglobin (MCH).

absolute zero, the temperature at which all molecular activity ceases. On the Kelvin scale, absolute zero is estimated to be equal to -273° C.

absorb, 1. the act of taking up various substances; for example, the tissues of the intestines absorb fluids. **2.** the energy transferred to tissues by radiation, such as an absorbed dose of radioactivity.

absorbable gauze, a gauzelike material, produced from oxidized cellulose, that can be absorbed. It is applied directly to bleeding tissue for haemostasis.

absorbance, the degree of absorption of light or other radiant energy by a medium through which the radiant energy passes.

absorbed diphtheria and tetanus vaccine, a toxoid preparation used for active immunization against diphtheria and tetanus.

absorbed diphtheria, tetanus and pertussis vaccine, an active immunizing agent used for the routine immunization of children against these conditions.

absorbed dose, (in radiation dosimetry) the energy imparted by ionizing radiation per unit mass of irradiated material at the point of interest. The SI unit of absorbed dose is the gray (Gy), equivalent to 1 joule per kilogram.

absorbent dressing, a dressing of any material applied to a wound or incision to absorb secretions.

absorbent gauze, a gauze for absorbing fluids. The form, weight, and use vary. Gauze may be a fine fabric in rolled single layers for spiral bandages, or it may be a thick, many-layered pad for a sterile pressure dressing.

absorbifacient, 1. any agent that promotes or enhances absorption. **2.** causing or enhancing absorption.

absorption, 1. the incorporation of matter by other matter through chemical, molecular, or physical action, as the dissolving of a gas in a liquid or the taking up of a liquid by a porous solid. **2.** (in physiology) the passage of substances across and into tissues, such as the passage of digested food molecules into intestinal cells or the passage of liquids into kidney tubules. Kinds of absorption are **agglutinin absorption, cutaneous absorption, external absorption, interstitial absorption, intestinal absorption, parenteral absorption, and pathological absorption. 3.** (in radiation dosimetry) the transfer of energy from a beam of ionizing radiation to the matter with which it interacts.

absorption coefficient, (in radiology) the fractional loss in intensity of radioactive energy as it interacts with an absorbing material. It is usually expressed per unit of thickness or per unit mass.

absorption rate constant, a value describing how much drug is absorbed per unit of time.

absorption spectrum, the range of electromagnetic energy that is used for spectroanalysis, including both visible light and ultraviolet radiation; also, a graph of spectrum for a specific compound.

absorptivity, absorbance divided by the product of the concentration of a substance and the sample path length.

abstinence, voluntary avoidance of any substance or the performance of any act for which the person has an appetite.

abstract a condensed summary of a scientific article, literary piece, or address.

abstraction, a condition in which the teeth or other maxillary and mandibular structures are below their normal position or away from the occlusal plane.

abstract thinking, the final stage in the development of the cognitive thought processes in the child. During this phase, thought is characterized by adaptability, flexibility, and the use of concepts and generalizations.

abulia, a loss of the ability or a reduced capacity to function voluntarily or to make decisions. Also spelled **aboulia.**

abuse, 1. improper use of equipment, a substance, or a service, such as a drug or programme, either intentionally or unintentionally. **2.** to attack or injure. A kind of abuse is child abuse.

abuse of the elderly, physical, psychological, sexual or material abuse, as well as violation of the rights of safety, security, and adequate health care of older adults. The victim of such abuse is generally an older woman with physical or mental impairment who lives with an adult child or another relative.

abutment, a tooth, root, or implant for the support and retention of a fixed or movable prosthesis.

abutment tooth, a tooth selected to support a prosthesis.

ABVD, an anticancer drug combination of doxorubicin, bleomycin, vinblastine, and dacarbazine.

Ac, symbol for actinium.

A-C, abbreviation for alveolar-capillary.

a.c., (in prescriptions) abbreviation for *ante cibum,* a Latin phrase meaning "before meals." The times of administration are commonly 7 AM, 11 AM, and 5 AM.

acacia gum, a dried, gummy exudate of the

African sleeping sickness. See **African trypanosomiasis**.

African tick fever. See **relapsing fever**.

African tick typhus, a rickettsial infection transmitted by ixodid ticks and characterized by fever, maculopapular rash, and swollen lymph nodes.

African trypanosomiasis, a disease caused by the parasites *Trypanosoma brucei gambiense* or *Trypanosoma brucei rhodesiense*, transmitted to humans by the bite of the tsetse fly. The disease is fatal unless treated. Kinds of African trypanosomiasis are **Gambian trypanosomiasis** and **Rhodesian trypanosomiasis**.

afterbirth, the placenta, the amnion and the chorion, and some amniotic fluid, blood, and blood clots expelled from the uterus after childbirth.

aftercare, health care offered a patient after discharge from a hospital or other medical facility.

afterdepolarization, a slow channel depolarization that follows in the wake of an action potential. It is thought to be responsible for atrial and ventricular ectopic beats, especially in the setting of digitalis toxicity.

afterload, the load, or resistance, against which the left ventricle must eject its volume of blood during contraction.

afterloading, (in radiotherapy) a brachytherapy technique in which an unloaded applicator is placed in or close to the lesion to be irradiated and subsequently loaded with the radioactive source. It allows accurate positioning of the applicator with no radiation exposure to the health care team. Afterloading may be manual afterloading or remote afterloading.

aftermovement, an involuntary muscle contraction that causes a continued movement of a limb after a strong exertion against resistance has stopped.

afterpains, contractions of the uterus common during the first days postpartum. They tend to be strongest in breast-feeding mothers and multiparae, resolves spontaneously, and may require analgesia.

afterpotential wave, either of two smaller waves, positive or negative, that follow the main spike potential wave of a nerve impulse, as recorded on an oscillograph tracing.

Ag, symbol for silver.

AGA, abbreviation for appropriate for gestational age.

agalactia, the failure of the mother to secrete enough milk to breast-feed an infant after childbirth.

agamete, 1. any of the unicellular organisms that reproduce asexually by multiple fission, such as bacteria and protozoa. **2.** any asexual reproductive cell, such as a spore or merozoite, that forms a new organism without fusion with another cell.

agametic, asexual; without recognizable sex organs or gametes. Also **agamous**.

agamic, reproducing asexually, without the union of gametes; asexual.

agammaglobulinaemia, a rare disorder characterized by the absence of the serum immunoglobulin, gamma globulin, associated with an increased susceptibility to infection. The condition may be transient, congenital, or acquired.

agamogenesis, asexual reproduction, as by budding or simple fission of cells; parthenogenesis. **agamocytogenic, agamogenetic, agamogenic, agamogonic** *adj.*

agamont. See **schizont**.

agamous. See **agametic**.

aganglionic megacolon. See **Hirschsprung's disease**.

agar-agar, a dried hydrophilic, colloidal product obtained from certain species of red algae. It is widely used as the basic ingredient in solid culture media in bacteriology.

ageing, the process of growing resulting in part from a failure of body cells to function normally or produce new body cells to replace those that are dead or malfunctioning. See also **assessment of the ageing patient, senile**.

ageism, an attitude that discriminates, separates, stigmatizes, or otherwise disadvantages older adults on the basis of chronological age.

agency, (in law) a relationship between two parties in which one authorizes the other to act in his behalf as his agent.

agenesia corticalis, the failure of the cortical cells of the brain, especially the pyramidal cells, to develop in the embryo, resulting in infantile cerebral paralysis and severe mental retardation.

agenesis, 1. congenital absence of an organ or part, usually caused by a lack of primordial tissue and failure of development in the embryo. **2.** impotence or sterility. **agenic,** *adj.*

agenetic fracture, a spontaneous fracture caused by an imperfect osteogenesis.

ageniocephaly, a form of otocephaly in which the brain, cranial vault, and sense organs are intact but the lower jaw is malformed. **ageniocephalic, ageniocephalous,** *adj.*

agenitalism, a condition caused by the lack of sex hormones and the absence or malfunction of the ovaries or testes.

agenosomia, a congenital malformation characterized by the absence or defective formation of the genitals and protrusion of the intestines through an incompletely developed abdominal wall.

agenosomus, a fetus with agenosomia.

agent, (in law) a party authorized to act on behalf of another and to give the other an account of such actions.

Agent Orange, a U.S. military code name for a mixture of two herbicides, 2,4-D and 2,4,5-T, used as a defoliant in South East Asia during the 1960s war in Vietnam. The herbicides were unintentionally contaminated with the highly toxic chemical dioxin, a cause of cancer and birth defects in animals and of chloracne and porphyria cutanea tarda in humans. See **dioxin.**

age of majority, the age at which a person is considered to be an adult in the eyes of the law.

agglutination, the aggregation or clumping together of cells as a result of their interaction with specific antibodies called agglutinins, commonly used in blood typing and in identifying or estimating the strength of immunoglobulins or immune sera.

agglutination-inhibition test, a serological technique useful in testing for certain unknown soluble antigens.

agglutinin, a specific kind of antibody whose interaction with antigens is manifested as agglutination.

agglutinin absorption, the removal from immune serum of antibody by treatment with homologous antigen, followed by centrifugation and separation of the antigen-antibody complex.

agglutinogen, any antigenic substance that causes agglutination by the production of agglutinin.

aggregate, the total of a group of substances or components making up a mass or complex.

aggregate anaphylaxis, an exaggerated reaction of hypersensitivity rapidly induced by the injection of an antigen that forms a soluble antigen-antibody complex.

aggression, a forceful, self-assertive action or attitude that is expressed physically, verbally, or symbolically. Kinds of aggression are constructive aggression, destructive aggression, and inward aggression.

aggressive personality, a personality with behaviour patterns characterized by irritability, tantrums, destructiveness, or violence in response to frustration.

aggressive-radical therapy, (in psychiatry) a form of therapy that introduces the political and social viewpoints of the therapist into the therapeutic process.

agitated, describing a condition of psychomotor excitement characterized by purposeless, restless activity. Pacing, crying, and laughing without apparent cause are often seen and may serve to release nervous tension associated with anxiety, fear, or other mental stress. **agitate,** *v.,* **agitation,** *n.*

agitated depression, a form of depression characterized by severe anxiety accompanied by continuous physical restlessness.

agitation, a state of chronic restlessness, generally observed as a psychomotor expression of emotional tension.

agitographia a condition characterized by abnormally rapid writing in which words or parts of words are unconsciously omitted.

agitophasia,, a condition characterized by abnormally rapid speech in which words, sounds, or syllables are unconsciously omitted, slurred, or distorted. The condition is commonly associated with agitographia.

agnathia, a developmental defect characterized by total or partial absence of the lower jaw. **agnathous,** *adj.*

agnathocephalus, a fetus with agnathocephaly.

agnathocephaly, a congenital malformation characterized by the absence of the lower jaw, defective formation of the mouth, and placement of the eyes low on the face with fusion or approximation of the zygomas and the ears. **agnathocephalic, agnathocephalous,** *adj.*

agnathus, a fetus with agnathia.

agnathy. See **agnathia.**

agnogenic myeloid metaplasia. See **myeloid metaplasia.**

agnosia, total or partial loss of the ability to recognize familiar objects or persons through sensory stimuli as a result of organic brain damage.

agonal respiration, a type of breathing that usually follows a pattern of gasping succeeded by apnoea. It generally indicates the onset of respiratory arrest.

agonal thrombus, an aggregation of blood platelets, fibrin, clotting factors, and cellular elements that forms in the heart in the process of dying.

agonist, 1. a contracting muscle whose contraction is opposed by another muscle (an antagonist). **2.** a drug or other substance having a specific cellular affinity that produces a predictable response.

agoraphobia, an anxiety disorder characterized by a fear of being in an open, crowded, or public place, such as a field, tunnel, bridge, congested street, or busy department store, where escape may be difficult or help not available in case of sudden incapacitation.

agranular endoplasmic reticulum. See **endoplasmic reticulum.**

agranulocyte, any leukocyte that does not contain cytoplasmic granules, such as a monocyte or lymphocyte.

agranulocytosis, an abnormal condition of the blood, characterized by a severe reduction in the number of granulocytes (basophils, eosinophils, and neutrophils), resulting in fever, prostration, and bleeding ulcers of the rectum, mouth, and vagina.

agraphia, an abnormal neurological condition characterized by loss of the ability to write, resulting from injury to the language centre in the cerebral cortex. **agraphic,** *adj.*

A:G ratio, the ratio of protein albumin to globulin in the blood serum. On the basis of differential solubility with neutral salt solution the normal values are 3.5 to 5 g/dl for albumin and 2. 5 to 4 g/dl for globulin.

agrypnia. See **insomnia**.

agrypnocoma, a coma in which there is some degree of wakefulness.

agrypnotic, 1. insomniac. **2.** a drug or other substance that prevents sleep.

agyria, 1. an abnormal condition caused by excessive absorption and tissue deposition of silver salts. It is marked by a slate-grey colouration of the skin and mucous membranes. **2.** a cerebral cortex abnormality in which the gyri are poorly developed.

"aha" reaction, (in psychology) a sudden realization or inspiration, experienced especially during creative thinking.

AHF, abbreviation for **antihaemophilic factor**.

AHH, abbreviation for **aryl hydrocarbon hydroxylase**.

Ahumada-del Castillo syndrome, a form of secondary amenorrhoea that may be associated with a pituitary gland tumour.

AI, abbreviation for **artificial intelligence**.

AID, abbreviation for **artificial insemination-donor**.

AIDS, abbreviation for **acquired immune deficiency syndrome**.

AIDS related complex (ARC), a subclinical form of acquired immune deficiency syndrome (AIDS). Signs and symptoms may include weight loss, fever, malaise, lethargy, oral thrush, and immunological abnormalities characteristic of AIDS.

AIH, abbreviation for **artificial insemination-husband**.

ainhum. See **autoamputation**.

air, the colourless, odourless gaseous mixture constituting the earth's atmosphere. It consists of 78% nitrogen, 21% oxygen, almost 1% argon, small amounts of carbon dioxide, hydrogen, and ozone, traces of helium, krypton, neon, and xenon, and varying amounts of water vapour.

airborne contaminants, materials in the atmosphere that can affect the health of persons in the same or nearby environments. Particularly vulnerable are tissues of the upper respiratory tract and lungs.

air cells of the nose. See **nasal sinus**.

air embolism, the abnormal presence of air in the cardiovascular system, resulting in obstruction of the flow of blood through the vessel. Air may be inadvertently introduced by injection, during intravenous therapy or surgery, or traumatically, as by a puncture wound.

air encephalography. See **encephalography**.

air entrainment, the movement of room air into the chamber of a jet nebulizer used to treat respiratory diseases. It increases the rate of nebulization and the amount of liquid administered per unit of time.

airflow pattern, the pattern of movement of respiratory gases through the respiratory tract. The pattern is affected by such factors as gas density and viscosity.

air-fluidized bed, a bed with body support provided by thousands of tiny soda-lime glass beads suspended by pressurized warm air.

air pump, a pump that forces air in or out of a cavity or chamber.

air sickness. See **motion sickness**.

air spaces, the alveolar ducts, alveolar sacs, and alveoli of the respiratory system.

air thermometer, a thermometer using air as its expansible medium.

airway, any tubular passage for the movement of air into and out of the lungs, such as the trachea and bronchi, a respiratory anaesthesia device, or an oropharyngeal tube used for mouth-to-mouth resuscitation. An airway with a diameter greater than 2 mm is defined as a large, or central, airway; one smaller than 2 mm is called a small, or peripheral, airway.

airway clearance, ineffective, an individual's inability to clear secretions or obstructions from the respiratory tract to maintain airway patency. Ineffective airway clearance results in abnormal breath sounds, change in the rate or depth of respiration, tachypnoea, cough, cyanosis, and dyspnoea.

airway conductance, the instantaneous volumetric gas flow rate in the airway per unit of pressure difference between the mouth, nose, or other airway opening and the alveoli. It is also the reciprocal of airway resistance. It is indicated by the symbol G_{aw}.

airway division, one of the 18 segments of the bronchopulmonary system. The segments are usually numbered from 1 to 10 for both the right and left lungs.

airway obstruction, an abnormal condition of the respiratory system characterized by a mechanical impediment to the delivery or to the absorption of oxygen in the lungs, as in bronchospasm, choking, croup, laryngospasm, chronic obstructive lung disease, goitre, tumour, or pneumothorax.

airway resistance, the ratio of pressure difference between the mouth, nose, or other airway opening and the alveoli to the simultaneously measured resulting volumetric gas flow rate. It is indicated by the symbol R_{aw}.

AK, abbreviation for above the knee, a term referring to amputations, amputees, prostheses, and orthoses.

akathisia, an abnormal condition characterized by restlessness and agitation, as seen in tardive dyskinesia. **akathisiac,** *adj.*

akembe, a form of purpura prevalent in Africa and characterized by blisters on the mucous membranes of the mouth, a skin rash, and platelet deficiency.

akinesia, an abnormal state of motor and psychic hypoactivity or muscular paralysis.

akinetic, *adj.*

akinetic apraxia, the inability to perform a spontaneous movement.

akinetic mutism, a state in which a person is unable or refuses to move or to make sounds, resulting from neurological or psychological disturbance.

akinetic seizure, a type of seizure disorder observed in children. It is a brief, generalized seizure in which the child suddenly falls to the ground.

Al, symbol for **aluminum.**

ala, *pl.* **alae, 1.** any winglike structure. **2.** the axilla.

Ala, abbreviation for **alanine.**

ALA, abbreviation for **aminolevulinic acid.**

ala auris, the auricle of the ear.

ala cerebelli, the ala of the central lobule of the cerebellum.

ala cinerea, the triangular area on the floor of the fourth ventricle of the brain from which the autonomic fibres of the vagus nerve arise.

alactasia. See **lactase deficiency.**

ala nasi, the outer flaring cartilaginous wall of each nostril.

alanine (Ala), a nonessential amino acid found in many proteins in the body. It is degraded in the liver to produce pyruvate and glutamate.

alanine aminotransferase (ALT), an enzyme normally present in the serum and tissues of the body, especially the tissues of the liver. This enzyme catalyses the transfer of an amino group from l-alanine to alphaketoglutarate, forming pyruvate and l-glutamate.

Al-Anon, an international organization that offers guidance and counselling for the relatives, friends, and associates of alcoholics.

ala of the ethmoid, a small projection on each side of the crista galli of the ethmoid bone. Each ala fits into a corresponding depression of the frontal bone.

ala of the ilium, the upper flaring portion of the iliac bone.

ala of the sacrum, the flat extension of bone on each side of the sacrum.

alar ligament, one of a pair of ligaments that connects the axis to the occipital bone and limits rotation of the cranium.

alarm reaction, the first stage of the general adaptation syndrome, characterized by the mobilization of the various defence mechanisms of the body or the mind to cope with a stressful situation of a physical or emotional nature.

alastrim, a mild form of smallpox, thought to be caused by a weak strain of *Poxvirus variolae.*

Alateen, an international organization that offers guidance and counselling for the children of alcoholics.

ala vomeris, an extension of bone on each side of the upper border of the vomer.

alba, literally,"white," as in *linea alba.*

Albers-Schönberg disease {Heinrich E. Albers-Schönberg, Hamburg radiologist, b. 1865}, a form of osteopetrosis characterized by marblelike calcification of bones.

Albert's disease, an inflammation of the bursa that lies between the Achilles tendon and the calcaneus. It is most frequently caused by injury. If treatment is delayed, the inflammation may cause erosion of the calcaneus.

albinism, an abnormal congenital condition characterized by partial or total lack of melanin pigment in the body. Total albinos have pale skin that does not tan, white hair, pink eyes, nystagmus, astigmatism, and photophobia.

Albright's syndrome {Fuller Albright, Boston physician, b. 1900}, a disorder characterized by fibrous dysplasia of bone, isolated brown macules on the skin, and endocrine dysfunction. It causes precocious puberty in girls but not in boys.

albumin, a water-soluble, heat-coagulable protein containing carbon, hydrogen, oxygen, nitrogen, and sulfur. Various albumins are found in practically all animal tissues and in many plant tissues.

albumin A, a blood serum constituent that gathers in cancer cells but is deficient in circulation in cancer patients.

albumin (human), a plasma-volume expander prescribed in the treatment of hypoproteinaemia and hypovolaemic shock.

albuminuria. See **proteinuria.**

alcalase, a protein enzyme contained in concentrations of about 60 ppm in certain laundry detergents. It is a cause of enzymatic detergent asthma.

alclometasone dipropionate, a topical corticosteroid prescribed for the relief of symptoms of inflammation and pruritus of corticosteroid-responsive dermatoses.

Alcock's canal {Joseph Alcock, English surgeon, b. 1784}, a canal formed by the obturator internus muscle and the obturator fascia through which the pudendal nerve and vessels pass.

alcohol, 1. (USP) a preparation containing at least 92. 3% and not more than 93.8% by weight of ethyl alcohol, used as a topical antiseptic and solvent. **2.** a clear, colourless, volatile liquid that is miscible with water, chloroform, or ether, obtained by the fermentation of carbohydrates with yeast. **3.** a compound derived from a hydrocarbon by replacing one or more hydrogen atoms with an equal number of hydroxyl (OH) groups. Depending on the number of hydroxyl radicals, alcohols are classified as monohydric, dihydric, trihydric. Some kinds of alcohol are **rubbing alcohol, sugar alcohol,** and **unsaturated alcohol.**

alcoholic cirrhosis. See **cirrhosis.**

alcoholic fermentation, the conversion of carbohydrates to ethyl alcohol.

alcoholic hallucinosis, a form of alcoholic psychosis characterized primarily by auditory hallucinations, abject fear, and delusions of persecution. The condition develops in acute alcoholism as withdrawal symptoms shortly after stopping or reducing the intake of alcohol.

alcoholic hepatitis, acute toxic liver injury associated with excess ethanol consumption. This is characterized by necrosis, polymorphonuclear inflammation, and in many instances Mallory bodies.

alcoholic ketoacidosis, the fall in blood pH (acidosis) sometimes seen in alcoholics and associated with a rise in serum ketone bodies (acetone, beta-hydroxybutyric acid, and acetoacetic acid).

alcoholic-nutritional cerebellar degeneration, a sudden, severe incoordination in the lower extremity, characteristic of poorly nourished alcoholics. The patient walks, if at all, with an ataxic or wide-based gait.

alcoholic paranoia, paranoia associated with chronic alcoholism.

alcoholic psychosis, any of a group of severe mental disorders, such as pathological intoxication, delirium tremens, and acute hallucinosis, characterized by brain damage or dysfunction that results from the excessive use of alcohol.

Alcoholics Anonymous (AA), an international nonprofit organization, founded in 1935, consisting of abstinent alcoholics whose purpose is to help other alcoholics stop drinking and maintain sobriety through group support, shared experiences, and faith in a power greater than themselves.

alcoholic trance, a state of automatism resulting from ethanol intoxication.

alcoholism, the extreme dependence on excessive amounts of alcohol, associated with a cumulative pattern of deviant behaviours. Alcoholism is a chronic illness with frequent medical consequences of central nervous system depression and cirrhosis of the liver. The severity of each of these is increased in the absence of food intake. The severe form of alcohol withdrawal is called delirium tremens.

alcohol poisoning, poisoning caused by the ingestion of any of several alcohols, of which ethyl, isopropyl, and methyl are the most common. Ethyl alcohol (grain alcohol) is found in whiskies, brandy, gin, and other beverages. Isopropyl alcohol is more toxic: Ingestion of 8 ounces may result in respiratory or circulatory failure. Methyl alcohol (wood alcohol) is extremely poisonous: In addition to nausea, vomiting, and abdominal pain, it may cause blindness, and death may follow the consumption of only 2 ounces.

alcohol withdrawal syndrome, the clinical symptoms associated with cessation of alcohol consumption. These may include tremor, hallucinations, autonomic nervous system dysfunction, and seizures.

ALD, abbreviation for **adrenoleukodystrophy**.

aldehyde, any of a large category of organic compounds derived from a corresponding alcohol by the removal of two hydrogen atoms, as in the conversion of ethyl alcohol to acetaldehyde. Each aldehyde is characterized by a carbonyl (-CHO) group in its empiric formula and can be converted into a corresponding acid by the addition of one oxygen atom, as in the conversion of acetaldehyde to acetic acid.

aldolase, an enzyme found in muscle tissue that catalyses the step in anaerobic glycolysis involving the breakdown of fructose 1,6-diphosphate to glyceraldehyde 3-phosphate.

aldose, the chemical form of monosaccharides in which the carbonyl group is an aldehyde.

aldosterone, a steroid hormone produced by the adrenal cortex to regulate sodium and potassium balance in the blood.

aldosteronism, a condition characterized by hypersecretion of aldosterone, occurring as a primary disease of the adrenal cortex or, more often, as a secondary disorder in response to various extra-adrenal pathological processes. Primary aldosteronism, also called **Conn's syndrome,** may be caused by adrenal hyperplasia or by an aldosterone-secreting tumour. Secondary aldosteronism is associated with increased plasma renin activity and may be induced by the nephrotic syndrome, hepatic cirrhosis, idiopathic oedema, congestive heart failure, trauma, burns, or other kinds of stress.

aldosteronoma, *pl.* aldosteronomas, aldosteronomata, an aldosterone-secreting adenoma of the adrenal cortex that is usually small and occurs more frequently in the left than the right adrenal gland, causing hyperaldosteronism with salt retention, expansion of the extracellular fluid volume, and increased blood pressure.

aleukaemic leukaemia, a type of leukaemia in which the total leukocyte count remains within normal limits and few abnormal forms appear in the peripheral blood.

aleukaemic myelosis. See **myeloid metaplasia**.

aleukia, a marked reduction in or the complete absence of white blood cells or blood platelets.

aleukocythemic leukaemia. See **aleukaemic leukaemia**.

Alexander technique, a body-focused mental health therapy introduced by Frederick Alexander. It focuses on individual variations in body musculature, posture, and the breathing process and the correction of defects.

alexia, an abnormal neurological condition characterized by an inability to comprehend written words. **alexic,** *adj.*

alexithymia, an inability to consciously experience and communicate feelings. Stuart

alfa. See **alpha.**

ALG, abbreviation for antilymphocyte globulin.

alga, *pl.* **algae,** any of a large group of nonmotile, or motile, marine plants containing chlorophyll. Many genera and species of algae are found worldwide in fresh water, in salt water, and on land. All belong to the phylum Thallophyta. **algal,** *adj.*

algid malaria, a form of malaria caused by the protozoan Plasmodium falciparum, characterized by coldness of the skin, profound weakness, and severe diarrhoea.

algodystrophy, a painful wasting of the muscles of the hands, often accompanied by tenderness and a loss of bone calcium.

ALGOL, abbreviation for *algorithmic language*, a type of computer language.

algolagnia, a form of sexual perversion characterized by sadism or masochism.

algologist, 1. a person who specializes in the study of or the treatment of pain. **2.** also called phycologist. a person who specializes in the study of algae.

algology, 1. the branch of medicine that is concerned with the study of pain. **2.** also called phycology. the branch of science that is concerned with algae.

algophobia, an anxiety disorder characterized by an abnormal, pervasive fear of experiencing pain or of witnessing pain in others.

algorithm, 1. a step-by-step procedure for the solution of a problem by computer, using specific mathematic or logical operations. **2.** an explicit protocol with well-defined rules to be followed in solving a health care problem.

algor mortis, the reduction in body temperature and accompanying loss of skin elasticity that occur after death.

alienation, the act or state of being estranged or isolated.

alignment, 1. the arrangement of a group of points or objects along a line. **2.** the placing or maintaining of body structures in their proper anatomic positions, such as repairing a fractured bone.

alimentary bolus. See **bolus,** def. **1.**

alimentary canal. See **digestive tract.**

alimentation. nourishment.

aliphatic, pertaining to fat or oil, specifically to those hydrocarbon compounds that open chains of carbon atoms, such as the fatty acids, rather than ring structures.

aliphatic acid, an acid of a nonaromatic hydrocarbon characterized by an open carbon chain.

aliphatic alcohol, an alcohol that contains an open chain or fatty series of hydrocarbons. Examples include ethyl alcohol and isopropyl alcohol.

alkalaemia, a condition of increased pH of the blood.

alkali, a compound with the chemical characteristics of a base. Alkalis combine with fatty acids to form soaps, turn red litmus blue, and enter into reactions that form water-soluble carbonates. **alkaline,** *adj.* **alkalinity,** *n.*

alkali burn, tissue damage caused by exposure to an alkaline compound like lye. The victim should be immediately taken to a medical facility if the tissue damage is more than slight and superficial.

alkaline-ash, residue in the urine having a pH of higher than 7.

alkaline-ash producing foods, foods that may be ingested in order to produce an alkaline pH in the urine, thereby reducing the incidence of acidic urinary calculi, or that may be avoided in order to reduce the incidence of alkaline calculi. Some of the foods that result in alkaline ash are milk, cream, fruit (except prunes, plums, and cranberries), vegetables (except corn and lentils), almonds, chestnuts, coconuts, and olives.

alkaline phosphatase, an enzyme present in bone, the kidneys, the intestine, plasma, and teeth. It may be elevated in the serum in some diseases of the bone and liver and in some other illnesses.

alkaline reserve, an additional amount of sodium bicarbonate the body produces to maintain an arterial blood pH of 7.40 when the carbon dioxide level increases as a result of hypoventilation.

alkalinity, pertaining to the acid-base relationship of any solution that has fewer hydrogen ions or more hydroxyl ions than pure water, which is an arbitrarily neutral standard with a pH of 7.00.

alkalinize, 1. to make a substance alkaline, as through the addition of a base. **2.** to become alkaline.

alkali poisoning, a toxic condition caused by the ingestion of an alkaline agent like liquid ammonia, lye, and some detergent powders. Emergency treatment includes giving copious amounts of water or milk to dilute the alkali. Vomiting is not induced, and mild acids are not administered.

alkaloid, any of a large group of organic compounds produced by plants, including many pharmacologically active substances, such as atropine, caffeine, cocaine, morphine, nicotine, and quinine.

alkalosis, an abnormal condition of body fluids, characterized by a tendency toward a pH level greater than 7.44, as from an excess of alkaline bicarbonate or a deficiency of acid. Respiratory alkalosis may be caused by hyperventilation, resulting in an excess loss of carbon dioxide and a carbonic acid deficit. Metabolic acidosis may result from an excess intake or retention of bicarbonate, loss of gastric acid in vomiting, potassium depletion, or any stimulus that increases the rate of sodium-hydrogen exchange.

alkaptonuria, a rare inherited disorder resulting from the incomplete metabolism of tyrosine, an amino acid, in which abnormal amounts of glycosuric acid are excreted, staining the urine dark. **alkaptonuric,** *adj.*

alkene, an unsaturated aliphatic hydrocarbon containing one double bond in the carbon chain, such as ethylene.

alkyl, a hydrocarbon molecule from which one of the hydrogen atoms has been removed, producing an alkyl radical.

alkylamine, an amine in which an alkyl group replaces one to three of the hydrogen atoms that are attached to the nitrogen atom, such as methylamine.

alkylating agent, any substance that contains an alkyl radical and is therefore capable of replacing a free hydrogen atom in an organic compound. Because this type of chemical reaction results in interference with mitosis and cell division, such agents are particularly useful in the treatment of cancer.

alkylation, a chemical reaction in which a hydrogen atom in an organic compound is replaced by an alkyl radical from an alkylating agent.

ALL, abbreviation for **acute lymphoblastic leukaemia.**

allantoidoangiopagus, conjoined monozygotic twin fetuses of unequal size that are united by the vessels of the umbilical cord. **allantoidoangiopagous,** *adj.*

allantoin, a chemical compound (5-ureidohydantoin), $C_4H_6N_4O_3$, that occurs as a white crystallizable substance found in many plants and in the allantoic and amniotic fluids and fetal urine of primates.

allantois, a tubular extension of the yolk sac endoderm that extends with the allantoic vessels into the body stalk of the embryo. In human embryos, allantoic vessels become the umbilical vessels and the chorionic villi. **allantoic,** *adj.*

allele, 1. one of two or more alternative forms of a gene that occupy corresponding loci on homologous chromosomes. **2.** also called allelomorph. one of two or more contrasting characteristics transmitted by alternative genes.

allelomorph. See **allele.**

Allen correction, multichromatic analysis of reaction to correct for background absorbance.

allergen, a substance that can produce a hypersensitive reaction in the body but is not necessarily intrinsically harmful. Some common allergens are pollen, animal dander, house dust, feathers, and various foods. The body normally protects itself against allergens or antigens by the complex chemical reactions of the humoral immune and the cell-mediated immune systems. **allergenic,** *adj.*

allergenic extract, an extract of the protein of a substance to which a person may be sensitive. The extract, which may be prepared from a wide variety of substances from food to fungi, can be used for diagnosis or for desensitization therapy.

allergic, 1. of or pertaining to allergy. **2.** having an allergy.

allergic alveolitis. See **diffuse hypersensitivity pneumonia.**

allergic asthma, a form of asthma caused by the exposure of the bronchial mucosa to an inhaled airborne antigen. This allergen causes the production of antibodies that bind to mast cells in the bronchial tree. The mast cells then release histamine, which stimulates contraction of bronchial smooth muscle and causes mucosal oedema. Psychological factors may provoke asthma attacks in bronchi already sensitized by allergens.

allergic bronchopulmonary aspergillosis, a form of aspergillosis that occurs in asthmatics when the fungus *Aspergillus fumigatus,* growing within the bronchial lumen, causes a hypersensitivity reaction. The characteristics of the condition are similar to those of asthma, including dyspnoea and wheezing.

allergic conjunctivitis, an abnormal condition characterized by hyperaemia of the conjunctiva caused by an allergy. Common allergens that cause this condition are pollen, grass, topical medications, air pollutants, occupational irritants, and smoke. It is bilateral and usually starts before puberty and lasts about 10 years, commonly recurring in a seasonal pattern.

allergic coryza, acute rhinitis caused by exposure to any allergen to which the person is hypersensitive.

allergic cutaneous angiitis. See **allergic vasculitis.**

allergic interstitial pneumonitis. See **diffuse hypersensitivity pneumonia.**

allergic reaction, a hypersensitive response to an allergen to which an organism has previously been exposed and to which the organism has developed antibodies. Subsequent exposure causes the release of histamine and a variety of symptoms including urticaria, eczema, dyspnoea, bronchospasm, diarrhoea, rhinitis, sinusitis, laryngospasm, and anaphylaxis.

allergic rhinitis, inflammation of the nasal passages, usually associated with watery nasal discharge and itching of the nose and eyes, because of a localized sensitivity reaction to house dust, animal dander, or an antigen, commonly pollen. The condition may be seasonal, as in hay fever, or perennial, as in allergy to dust or animals.

allergic vasculitis, an inflammatory condition of the blood vessels that is induced by an allergen. Allergic cutaneous vasculitis is characterized by itching, malaise, and a slight fever and by the presence of papules, vesicles, urticarial wheals, or small ulcers on the skin.

allergy, a hypersensitive reaction to intrinsically harmless antigens, most of which are environmental. Allergies are classified according to types I, II, III, and IV hypersensitivity. Types I, II, and III involve different immunoglobulin antibodies and their interaction with different antigens. Type IV allergy is associated with contact dermatitis and T cells, which react directly with the antigen and cause local inflammation. Allergies are divided into those that produce immediate or antibody-mediated reactions and those that produce delayed or cell-mediated reactions. Immediate allergic reactions involve types I, II, and III hypersensitivity and antigen-antibody reactions that activate certain enzymes, creating an imbalance between these enzymes and their inhibitors. Some common symptoms of allergy are bronchial congestion, conjunctivitis, oedema, fever, urticaria, and vomiting. Severe allergic reactions, such as anaphylaxis, can cause systemic shock and death. When allergic reactions are life threatening, steroids, may be administered intravenously. For milder diseases, such as serum sickness and hay fever, antihistamines are usually administered.

allergy testing, any one of the various procedures used in identifying the specific allergens that afflict the patients involved. Such tests are helpful in prescribing treatment to prevent allergic reactions or to reduce their severity. The most common kinds of allergy testing include the intradermal, scratch, patch, conjunctival, and use tests.

all fours position, the sixth stage in the Rood system of ontogenetic motor patterns. The lower trunk and lower extremities are brought into a cocontraction pattern while stretching of the trunk and limb girdles develops cocontractions of the trunk flexors and extensors.

allied health personnel. See **paramedical personnel**.

alligator forceps, 1. a forceps with heavy teeth and a double clamp, employed in orthopaedic surgery. **2.** a forceps with long, thin, angular handles and interlocking teeth.

alloaesthesia, a referred pain or other sensation that may be perceived on the same or opposite side of the body but not at the site stimulated.

allodiploid, 1. also allodiploidic. of or pertaining to an individual, organism, strain, or cell that has two genetically distinct sets of chromosomes derived from different ancestral species, as occurs in hybridization. **2.** such an individual, organism, strain, or cell.

allodiploidy, the state or condition of having two genetically distinct sets of chromosomes derived from different ancestral species.

alloeroticism, alloerotism. See **hetero-eroticism**.

allogamy. See **cross fertilization**.

allogenic, 1. (in genetics) denoting an individual or cell type that is from the same species but genetically distinct. **2.** (in transplantation biology) denoting tissues that are from the same species but antigenically distinct; homologous.

allograft, the transfer of tissue between two genetically dissimilar individuals of the same species, such as a tissue transplant between two humans who are not identical twins.

allohexaploid, allohexaploidic. See **allopolyploid**.

allometric growth, the increase in size of different organs or parts of an organism at various rates.

allometron, a quantitative change in the proportional relationship of the parts of an organism as a result of the evolutionary process.

allometry, the measurement and study of the changes in proportions of the various parts of an organism in relation to the growth of the whole or within a series of related organisms. **allometric,** *adj.*

allopathic physician, a physician who treats disease and injury with active interventions, such as medical and surgical treatment, intended to bring about effects opposite from those produced by the disease or injury.

allopathy, a system of medical therapy in which a disease or an abnormal condition is treated by creating an environment that is antagonistic to the disease or condition; for example, an antibiotic toxic to a pathogenic organism is given in an infection, or an iron supplement may be given to increase the synthesis of haemoglobin in iron deficiency anaemia.

allopentaploid, allopentaploidic. See **allopolyploid**.

alloplastic manoeuvre, (in psychology) a process that is part of adaptation, involving an adjustment or change in the external environment.

alloploid, alloploidic. See **allodiploid, allopolyploid**.

alloploidy. See **allodiploidy, allopolyploidy**.

allopolyploid, 1. also allopolyploidic. of or pertaining to an individual, organism, strain, or cell that has more than two genetically distinct sets of chromosomes derived from two or more different ancestral species, as occurs in hybridization. They are referred to as allotriploid, allotetraploid, and so on, depending on the number of multiples of haploid sets of chromosomes they contain. **2.** such an individual, organism, strain, or cell.

allopolyploidy, the state or condition of having more than two genetically distinct sets of chromosomes from two or more ancestral species. See **mosaic**.

allopurinol, a xanthine oxidase inhibitor prescribed in the treatment of gout and other hyperuricaemic conditions.

allorhythmia, any arrhythmia that tends to be repetitive.

all-or-none law, 1. the principle in neurophysiology that if a stimulus is strong enough to trigger a nerve impulse, the entire impulse is discharged. A weak stimulus will not produce a weak reaction. **2.** the principle that the heart muscle, under any stimulus above a threshold level, will respond either with a maximum strength contraction or not at all.

allosteric sites, the sites, other than the active site or sites, of an enzyme that bind regulatory molecules.

allotetraploid, allotetraploidic. See **allopolyploid**.

allotriploid, allotriploidic. See **allopolyploid**.

allowable error, the amount of error that can be tolerated without invalidating the medical usefulness of the analytical result. Allowable error is defined as having a 95% limit of analytical error; only one sample in 20 can have an error greater than this limit.

alloxan, an oxidation product of uric acid that is found in the human intestine in diarrhoea. Because it can destroy the insulin-secreting islet cells of the pancreas, alloxan may cause diabetes.

alloy, a mixture of two or more metals or of substances with metallic properties. Most alloys are formed by mixing molten metals that dissolve in each other.

aloe, the inspissated juice of various species of Aloe plants, formerly used as a cathartic but generally discontinued because it often causes severe intestinal cramps.

alopecia, partial or complete lack of hair resulting from normal ageing, endocrine disorder, drug reaction, anticancer medication, or skin disease. Kinds of **alopecia** include **alopecia areata, alopecia totalis,** and **alopecia universalis**.

alopecia areata, a disease of unknown cause in which there are well-defined bald patches, usually round or oval, on the head and other hairy parts of the body. The condition is usually self-limited and clears completely within 6 to 12 months without treatment.

alopecia totalis, an uncommon condition characterized by the loss of all the hair on the scalp. The cause is unknown, and the baldness is usually permanent. No treatment is known.

alopecia universalis, a total loss of hair on all parts of the body, occasionally an extension of alopecia areata.

alpha, the first letter of the Greek alphabet, often used in chemical nomenclature to distinguish one variation in a chemical compound from others. Also **alfa**.

alpha-adrenergic blocking agent. See **antiadrenergic**.

alpha-adrenergic receptor. See **alpha receptor**.

alpha alcoholism, a mild form of alcoholism in which the dependence is psychological rather than physical.

alpha-aminoisovalerianic acid. See **valine**.

alpha decay, a type of radioactivity which results in the emission of alpha particles. See **alpha particle**.

alpha fetoprotein (AFP), a protein normally synthesized by the liver, yolk sac, and GI tract of a human fetus, but which may be found elevated in the sera of adults having certain malignancies.

alpha-galactosidase, a form of the enzyme that catalyzes the conversion of alpha-D-galactoside to D-galactose.

alpha haemolysis, the development of a greenish zone around a bacterial colony growing on blood-agar medium, characteristic of pneumococci and certain streptococci and caused by the partial decomposition of haemoglobin.

alpha-hydroxypropionic acid. See **lactic acid**.

alpha$_2$-interferon, a protein molecule that has been found effective in controlling the spread of common colds caused by rhinoviruses. It is administered as a nasal spray.

alpha-methyldopa. See **methyldopa**.

alphanumeric, pertaining to a system of characters in which information is coded in combinations of letters and numerals. The characters, which also may include punctuation, are used commonly in computer programming to code signals or data.

alpha particle, a particle emitted from certain radioactive nuclei, consisting of two protons and two neutrons, equivalent to a helium nucleus. Not used in medicine since their extremely short range is not clinically useful and presents a hazard to health if ingested.

alpha receptor, any one of the postulated adrenergic components of receptor tissues that responds to norepinephrine and to various blocking agents. The activation of the alpha receptors causes such physiological responses as increased peripheral vascular resistance, dilatation of the pupils, and contraction of pilomotor muscles.

alpha redistribution phase, a period following intravenous administration of a drug when the blood level begins to fall from its peak.

alpha rhythm. See **alpha wave**.

alpha state, a condition of relaxed, peaceful wakefulness devoid of concentration and sensory stimulation. It is characterized by the alpha rhythm of brain wave activity and is accompanied by feelings of tranquillity and a lack of tension and anxiety.

alpha-tocopherol. See **vitamin E**.

alphavirus, any of a group of very small

togaviruses consisting of a single molecule of single-stranded DNA within a lipoprotein capsule.

alpha wave, one of the four types of brain waves, characterized by a relatively high voltage or amplitude and a frequency of 8 to 13 Hz. Alpha waves are the "relaxed waves" of the brain.

Alport's syndrome, a form of hereditary nephritis with symptoms of glomerulonephritis, haematuria, progressive sensorineural hearing loss, and occasional ocular disorders.

alprazolam, an antianxiety agent is prescribed in the treatment of anxiety disorders or the short-term relief of the symptoms of anxiety.

alprostadil, a proprietary form of prostaglandin E$_1$ used to maintain the patency of ductus arteriosus in certain neonates. It is recommended as a palliative therapy for neonates awaiting surgery to correct congenital heart defects, such as tetralogy of Fallot and tricuspid atresia.

ALS, abbreviation for amyotrophic lateral sclerosis.

alseroxylon, a combination of reserpine and other alkaloids extracted from *Rauwolfia serpentina*. It is used in oral sedatives and antihypertensive medications.

Älstrom syndrome, an inherited disease characterized by multiple end organ resistance to hormones. Clinical features include retinal degeneration leading to childhood blindness, vasopressin-resistant diabetes insipidus, and hypogonadism.

ALT, abbreviation for **alanine aminotransferase**.

altered state of consciousness, any state of awareness that differs from the normal awareness of a conscious person. Altered states of consciousness have been achieved, especially in Eastern cultures, by many individuals using various techniques, such as long fasting, deep breathing, whirling, and chanting.

alternate generation, a type of reproduction in which a sexual generation alternates with one or more asexual generations, as in many plants and lower animals.

alternate tapping, a technique employing gentle taps and used to stimulate balance in anti-gravity positions.

alternating current (AC), an electric current that reverses direction, according to a consistent sinusoidal pattern.

alternating pulse, See **pulsus alternans**.

alternation of generations. See **alternate generation**.

alternation rules, (in psychology) the sociolinguistic rules that establish options available to a person when he or she is speaking to someone else.

alternative inheritance, the acquisition of all genetic traits and conditions from one parent, as in self-pollinating plants and self-fertilizing animals.

alternative pathway of complement activation, a process of antibody formation in which activation of the C3 step occurs without prior activation of C1, C4, and C2.

alternobaric vertigo, a condition of dysequilibrium caused by unequalized pressure differences in the middle ear, as may be experienced by divers during ascent.

alt.h., abbreviation for the Latin prescription term *alternis horis*, meaning "every other hour."

altitude, pertaining to any location on earth with reference to a fixed surface point, which is usually sea level. Several types of health effects are associated with altitude extremes, including a greater intensity of ultraviolet radiation that results from a thinner atmosphere.

altitude sickness, a syndrome associated with the relatively low concentrations of oxygen in the atmosphere at altitudes encountered during mountain climbing or travel in unpressurized aircraft. The acute symptoms may include dizziness, headache, irritability, breathlessness, and euphoria.

altruism, a sense of concern for the welfare of others. It may be expressed at the level of the individual or the larger social system.

alum, a topical astringent, used primarily in lotions and douches.

aluminium (Al), a widely used metallic element and the third most abundant of all the elements. Its atomic number is 13; its atomic weight is 26.97. It is a component of many antacids, antiseptics, astringents, and styptics. Aluminium hydroxychloride is the most commonly used agent in antiperspirants and is also effective as a deodorant.

aluminium acetate solution, an astringent used in ear drops and lotions for inflammatory and exudative skin conditions and wounds.

alveolar adenocarcinoma, a neoplasm in which the tumour cells form alveoli.

alveolar air, the respiratory gases in an alveolus, or air sac, of the lung.

alveolar air equation, a method of calculating the approximate alveolar oxygen tension from the arterial partial pressure of carbon dioxide, fractional inspired oxygen, and the ratio of carbon dioxide production to oxygen consumption.

alveolar-arterial end-capillary gas pressure difference, the gas pressure difference that exists between alveolar gas and pulmonary capillary blood as the latter leaves the alveolus. It is measured in torr units.

alveolar-arterial gas pressure difference, the difference between the measured or calculated mean partial pressure of a gas, such as CO_2, in the alveoli and the simultaneously measured partial pressure of that gas in systemic arterial blood. It is measured in torr units.

alveolar canal, any of the canals of the maxilla through which the posterior superior alveolar blood vessels and the nerves to the upper teeth pass.

alveolar-capillary membrane, a lung tissue structure through which diffusion of oxygen and carbon dioxide molecules occurs during the respiration process.

alveolar cell carcinoma, a malignant pulmonary neoplasm that arises in a bronchiole and spreads along alveolar surfaces. This form of lung cancer is characterized clinically by a severe cough and copious sputum.

alveolar dead space. See **dead space**.

alveolar distending pressure, the pressure difference between the alveolus and the intrapleural space.

alveolar duct, any of the air passages in the lung that branch out from the respiratory bronchioles. From the ducts arise the alveolar sacs.

alveolar fibre, any one of the many white collagenous fibres of the peridontal ligament that extend from the alveolar bone to the intermediate plexus where their terminations mix with those of the cemental fibres.

alveolar fistula. See **dental fistula**.

alveolar gas, the gas mixture within the gas-exchange regions of the lungs, reflecting the combined effects of alveolar ventilation and respiratory gas exchange, or the expired gas that has come from the alveoli and gas exchange regions.

alveolar gas volume, the aggregate volume of gas in the lung regions within which respiratory gas exchange occurs. It is indicated by the symbol V_A.

alveolar macrophages, defence cells within the lungs that act by engulfing and digesting foreign substances that may be inhaled into the alveoli.

alveolar microlithiasis, a disease characterized by the presence of calcium phosphate deposits in the alveolar sacs and ducts. It is familial in about half of cases.

alveolar oedema, an accumulation of fluid within the alveoli.

alveolar pressure (P_A), the pressure in the alveoli of the lungs.

alveolar process, the portion of the maxilla or the mandible that forms the dental arch and serves as a bony investment for the teeth.

alveolar proteinosis, a disorder marked by the accumulation of plasma proteins, lipoproteins, and other blood components in the alveoli of the lungs.

alveolar ridge, the bony ridge of the maxilla or the mandible that contains the alveoli of the teeth.

alveolar soft part sarcoma, a tumour in subcutaneous or fibromuscular tissue, consisting of numerous large round or polygonal cells in a netlike matrix of connective tissue.

alveolar ventilation, the volume of air that ventilates all the perfused alveoli, measured as minute volume in litres. The figure is also the difference between total ventilation and dead space ventilation. The normal average is between 4 and 5 litres per minute.

alveolectomy, the excision of a portion of the alveolar process for aiding the extraction of a tooth or teeth, the modification of the alveolar contour after tooth extraction, or the preparation of the mouth for dentures.

alveoli, small outpouchings of walls of alveolar space through which gas exchange takes place between alveolar air and pulmonary capillary blood.

alveolitis, an allergic pulmonary reaction to the inhalation of antigenic substances characterized by acute episodes of dyspnoea, cough, sweating, fever, weakness, and pain in the joints and muscles. Kinds of alveolitis include bagassosis, farmer's lung, and pigeon breeder's disease.

alveolus, *pl.* **alveoli,** a small saclike structure. Often used interchangeably with acinus. **alveolar,** *adj.*

alymphocytosis, an abnormal reduction in the total number of lymphocytes circulating in the blood.

Alzheimer's disease, presenile dementia, characterized by confusion, memory failure, disorientation, restlessness, agnosia, speech disturbances, inability to carry out purposeful movements, and hallucinations. The disease usually begins in later middle life with slight defects in memory and behaviour and occurs with equal frequency in men and women.

am, abbreviation for an ammonium cation.

Am, symbol for **americium**.

AMA, abbreviation for **American Medical Association**.

amalgam, 1. a mixture or combination. **2.** an alloy of mercury and another metal or metals.

amalgam carrier, (in dentistry) an instrument for carrying plastic amalgam for inserting into a prepared tooth cavity or mould.

amalgam carver, a dental instrument for shaping plastic amalgams used in some tooth cavity fillings.

amalgam condenser, (in dentistry) an instrument used for compacting plastic amalgam in filling teeth.

amalgam core, a rigid base for the retention of a cast crown restoration, used in the replacement of a damaged tooth crown.

amalgam tattoo, a discolouration of the gingiva or buccal membrane caused by particles of silver amalgam filling material that became embedded under the surface.

Amanita, a genus of mushrooms. Some species, such as *Amanita phalloides,* are poisonous, causing hallucinations, GI upset, and pain that may be followed by liver, kidney, and central nervous system damage.

amantadine hydrochloride, an antiviral and dopamine-releasing drug prescribed in the prophylaxis and early treatment of influenza, and for symptomatic treatment of parkinsonian symptoms.

amasesis, the inability to chew food, caused by paralysis of the muscles of mastication, impaired teeth, poorly fitted dentures, or a psychiatric problem.

amastia, absence of the breasts in women caused by a congenital defect, an endocrine disorder resulting in faulty development, lack of development of secondary sex characteristics, or a bilateral mastectomy.

amaurosis, blindness, especially lack of vision resulting from an extraocular cause, such as disease of the optic nerve or brain, diabetes, renal disease, or systemic poisoning produced by excessive use of alcohol or tobacco, rather than from damage to the eye itself. **amaurotic,** *adj.*

amaurosis congenita of Leber. See **Leber's congenital amaurosis**.

amaurosis fugax, transient episodic blindness.

amaurosis partialis fugax, transitory partial blindness, usually caused by vascular insufficiency of the retina or optic nerve as a result of carotid artery disease.

amaurotic familial idiocy. See **Tay-Sachs disease**.

amazia. See **amastia**.

amber mutation, (in molecular genetics) a genetic alteration in which a polypeptide chain terminates prematurely, because an erroneous nucleotide code signals the end of the chain.

ambient, pertaining to the surrounding area or atmosphere.

ambient air standard, the maximum tolerable concentration of any air pollutant, such as lead, nitrogen dioxide, sodium hydroxide, or sulphur dioxide.

ambient pressure, the atmospheric pressure, or pressure in the environment or surrounding area. It is given a reference value of zero (0) cm H_2O.

ambiguous genitalia, external genitalia that are not normal and morphologically typical of either sex, as occurs in pseudohermaphroditism.

ambiopia. See **diplopia**.

ambivalence, 1. a state in which a person experiences conflicting feelings, attitudes, drives, desires, or emotions, such as love and hate, tenderness and cruelty, pleasure and pain. **2.** uncertainty and fluctuation caused by an inability to make a choice between opposites. **3.** a continuous oscillation or fluctuation. **ambivalent,** *adj.*

ambivert, a person who possesses some of the characteristics of both introversion and extraversion.

amblyopia, reduced vision in an eye that appears to be structurally normal when examined with an ophthalmoscope. Kinds of amblyopia are alcoholic amblyopia, suppression amblyopia, tobacco amblyopia, and toxic amblyopia.

ambulance, an emergency vehicle usually used for the transport of patients to hospital in cases of accident, trauma, or sudden, severe illness.

ambulatory, able to walk, hence describing a patient who is not confined to bed, or designating a health service for people who are not hospitalized.

ambulatory automatism, aimless wandering or moving about or performance of mechanical acts without conscious awareness of the behaviour.

ambulatory care, health services provided on an outpatient basis to those who visit a hospital or clinic and depart after treatment on the same day.

ambulatory schizophrenia, a mild form of schizophrenia, characterized by a tendency to respond to questions with vague and irrelevant answers. The person also may seem somewhat eccentric and wander aimlessly.

ambulatory surgery centre, a medical facility designed and equipped to handle relatively minor surgery cases, such as cataracts, herniorrhaphy, and meniscectomy, which do not require overnight hospitalization.

amelanic melanoma a melanoma that lacks melanin.

amelanotic,, of or pertaining to tissue that is unpigmented because it lacks melanin.

amelia, 1. a birth defect, marked by the absence of one or more limbs. The term may be modified to indicate the number of legs or arms missing at birth, such as tetramelia for the absence of all four limbs. **2.** a psychological trait of apathy or indifference associated with certain forms of psychosis.

amelification, the differentiation of ameloblasts, or enamel cells, into the enamel of the teeth.

ameloblast, an epithelial cell from which tooth enamel is formed. **ameloblastic** *adj.*

ameloblastic fibroma, an odontogenic neoplasm in which there is a simultaneous proliferation of mesenchymal and epithelial tissues but no development of dentin or enamel.

ameloblastic haemangioma, a highly vascular tumour of cells covering the dental papilla.

ameloblastic odontoma, an odontogenic tumour characterized by an ameloblastoma within an odontoma.

ameloblastic sarcoma, a malignant odontogenic tumour, characterized by the proliferation of epithelial and mesenchymal tissue without the formation of dentin or enamel.

ameloblastoma, a highly destructive, malignant, rapidly growing tumour of the jaw.

amelodentinal, pertaining to both the enamel

and dentin of the teeth.

amelogenesis, the formation of the enamel of the teeth. **amelogenic,** *adj.*

amelogenesis imperfecta, a hereditary dental defect characterized by a brown colouration of the teeth and resulting from either severe hypocalcification or hypoplasia of the enamel.

amenorrhoea, the absence of menstruation. Amenorrhoea is normal before sexual maturity, during pregnancy, after menopause, and during the intermenstrual phase of the monthly hormonal cycle but is otherwise caused by dysfunction of the hypothalamus, pituitary gland, ovary, or uterus, by the congenital absence or surgical removal of both ovaries or the uterus, or by medication. Primary amenorrhoea is the failure of menstrual cycles to begin. Secondary amenorrhoea is the cessation of menstrual cycles once established. **amenorrhoeic.** *adj.*

amentia, 1. an obsolete term for congenital mental retardation. See learning disability. **2.** also called confusional insanity, a state of mind characterized by apathy and disorientation, bordering on stupor, as in Stearns' alcoholic amentia.

American Academy of Nursing (AAN), the honorary organization of the American Nurses' Association, created to recognize superior achievement in nursing in order to promote advances and excellence in nursing practice and education.

American College of Physicians (ACP), a national professional organization of physicians in the United States.

American College of Surgeons (ACS), a national professional organization of surgeons in the United States.

American Medical Association (AMA), a professional association whose membership is made up of licensed doctors in the United States, including practitioners in all recognized medical specialties as well as general primary care physicians.

American Nurses' Association (ANA), the national professional association of registered nurses in the United States.

americium (Am), an artificially produced radioactive element of the actinide group. Its atomic number is 95; its atomic weight is 243.

Ameslan abbreviation for *American Sign Language,* a method of communication with the deaf that relies primarily on the position, shape, and motion of the hands and fingers for the transmission of concepts and messages.

Ames test, a method for testing substances for possible carcinogenicity by exposing a strain of Salmonella bacteria to a sample of the substance.

amethocaine hydrochloride, a local anaesthetic used in ophthalmology and skin preparations.

ametropia, a condition characterized by an optic defect involving an error of refraction, such as astigmatism, hyperopia, or myopia. **ametropic,** *adj.*

amide-compound local anaesthetic, a local anaesthetic containing an amide ($CONH_2$) group. Some kinds of amide-compound local anaesthetics are bupivacaine and prilocaine.

amidobenzene. See **aniline**.

amikacin sulphate, an aminoglycoside antibiotic prescribed in the treatment of various severe infections that are resistant to other antibiotics.

amiloride hydrochloride, a potassium-sparing diuretic used in the treatment of congestive heart failure or hypertension. It is often given with a thiazide diuretic.

amine, (in chemistry) any organic compound that contains nitrogen.

amine pump, informal. an active transport system in the presynaptic nerve endings that takes up released amine neurotransmitters.

aminoacetic acid. See **glycine**.

amino acid, an organic chemical compound composed of one or more basic amino groups and one or more acidic carboxyl groups. Twenty of the more than 100 amino acids that occur in nature are the building blocks of peptides, polypeptides, and proteins. The eight essential amino acids are isoleucine, leucine, lysine, methionine, phenylalanine, threonine, tryptophan, and valine. Arginine and histidine are essential in infants. Cysteine and tyrosine are quasi-essential because they may be synthesized from methionine and phenylalanine, respectively. The main nonessential amino acids are alanine, asparagine, aspartic acid, glutamine, glutamic acid, glycine, proline, and serine.

aminoaciduria the abnormal presence of amino acids in the urine that usually indicates an inborn metabolic defect, as in cystinuria.

aminobenzene. See **aniline**.

aminobenzoic acid, a metabolic product of the catabolism of the amino acid tryptophan, which is used as a topical sunscreen agent.

aminoglycoside antibiotic. See **antibiotic**.

aminolaevulinic acid (ALA), the aliphatic precursor of haem. It may be detected in the urine of some patients with porphyria, liver disease, and lead poisoning.

aminophylline, a xanthine bronchodilator prescribed in the treatment of bronchial asthma, emphysema, and bronchitis.

aminosalicylic acid. See **paraaminosalicylic acid**.

aminosuccinic acid. See **aspartic acid**.

aminotransferase, an enzyme that catalyses the transfer of an amino group from an alpha-amino acid to an alpha-keto acid, with pyridoxal phosphate and pyridoxamine phosphate acting as coenzymes. Aspartate amino transferase (AST), normally present in serum and various tissues, is released by damaged cells, and, as a result, a high serum level of AST may be diagnostic in myocardial infarction or hepatic disease. Alanine aminotransferase (ALT), a normal constituent of serum and various tissues, may be present in high concentrations in the sera of patients with acute liver disease.

amiodarone hydrochloride, an oral anti-arrhythmic drug prescribed for the treatment of tachycardia associated with Wolff-Parkinson-White syndrome. It is used for other arrhythmias only when other drugs have failed.

amitosis, direct cell division in which there is simple fission of the nucleus and cytoplasm. It does not involve the complex stages of chromatin separation of the chromosomes that occur in mitosis. **amitotic,** *adj.*

amitriptyline, a tricyclic antidepressant used in the treatment of depression and neurogenic pain.

AML, abbreviation for **acute myeloblastic leukaemia**.

ammonia, a colourless aromatic gas consisting of nitrogen and hydrogen, produced by the decomposition of nitrogenous organic matter. Some of its many uses are as an aromatic stimulant, a detergent, and an emulsifier.

ammoniacal fermentation, the production of ammonia and carbon dioxide from urea by the enzyme urease.

ammonium ion, an NH_4^+ ion formed by the reaction of ammonia (NH_3) with a hydrogen ion (H^+).

amnesia, a loss of memory caused by brain damage or by severe emotional trauma. Kinds of amnesia are anterograde amnesia, hysterical amnesia, posttraumatic amnesia, and retrograde amnesia.

amnestic apraxia, the inability to carry out a movement in response to a request because of a lack of ability to remember the request rather than to a loss of motor function.

amniocentesis, an obstetric procedure in which a small amount of amniotic fluid is removed for laboratory analysis. It is usually performed between the sixteenth and twentieth weeks of gestation to aid in the prenatal diagnosis of fetal abnormalities.

amnion, a membrane, continuous with and covering the fetal side of the placenta, that forms the outer surface of the umbilical cord.

amnionitis, an inflammation of the amnion. The condition may develop after early rupture of the fetal membranes.

amnioscopy direct visual examination of the fetus and amniotic fluid with an endoscope that is inserted into the amniotic cavity through the uterine cervix or an incision in the abdominal wall.

amniotic pertaining to the amnion.

amniotic band syndrome, an abnormal condition of fetal development characterized by the development of fibrous bands within the uterus that entangle the fetus, leading to deformities in structure and function.

amniotic fluid, a liquid produced by the fetal membranes and the fetus, also known as 'liquor amnii'. It surrounds the fetus throughout pregnancy, usually totalling about 1000 ml at term. In addition to providing the fetus with physical protection, the amniotic fluid is a medium of active chemical exchange. Amniotic fluid itself is clear, though desquamated fetal cells and lipids give it a cloudy appearance.

amniotic sac, a thin-walled bag that contains the fetus and amniotic fluid during pregnancy, having a capacity of 4 to 5 L at term. The wall of the sac extends from the margin of the placenta. The amnion, chorion, and decidua that make up the wall are each a few cell layers thick. The intact sac and its fluid provide for the equilibration of hydrostatic pressure within the uterus and, during labour, effect the uniform transmission of the force of uterine contractions to the cervix for dilatation.

amniotomy the artificial rupture of the fetal membranes (ARM). It is usually performed to stimulate the onset of labour.

A-mode, amplitude modulated scan in diagnostic ultrasonography. A one-dimensional display where returning echoes are represented by a vertical displacement of the horizontal time base on a TV monitor. The distance between vertical displacements represents the distance betwen reflecting interfaces.

amoeba, a microscopic, single-celled, parasitic organism. Several species may be parasitic in humans, including *Entamoeba coli* and *E. histolytica.* **amoebic,** *adj.*

amoebiasis, an infection of the intestine or liver by species of pathogenic amoebas, particularly *Entamoeba histolytica,* acquired by ingesting food or water contaminated with infected faeces. Mild amoebiasis may be asymptomatic; severe infection may cause profuse diarrhoea, acute abdominal pain, jaundice, anorexia, and weight loss.

amoebic abscess, a collection of pus formed by disintegrated tissue in a cavity, usually in the liver, caused by the protozoan parasite *Entamoeba histolytica.*

amoebic dysentery, an inflammation of the intestine caused by infestation with *Entamoeba histolytica* and characterized by frequent, loose stools flecked with blood and mucus.

amoebicide, a drug or other agent that is destructive to amoebas.

amorph, 1. inactive gene; a mutant allele that has little or no effect on the expression of a trait. **2.** abbreviation for amorphous, such as amorph IZS (amorphous insulin zinc suspension).

amorphic, (in genetics) of or pertaining to a gene that is inactive or nearly inactive so that it has no determinable effect.

amorphous crystals, shapeless, ill-defined crystals, usually phosphates.

amoxapine, an antidepressant similar to the tricyclics. It is prescribed in the treatment of depression.

amoxycillin, a semisynthetic oral penicillin antibiotic similar to ampicillin. It is used in the treatment of infections caused by susceptible gram-negative or gram-positive bacteria.

AMP, abbreviation for adenosine monophosphate.

ampere (A) {André M. Ampère, French physicist, b. 1775}, a unit of measurement of the amount of electric current. An ampere, according to the metre-kilogram-second (MKS) system, is the amount of current passed through a resistance of 1 ohm by an electrical potential of 1 volt.

amperometry, the measurement of current at a single applied potential.

amphetamines, a group of nervous system stimulants, including amphetamine and its chemical congener dextramphetamine, that are subject to abuse because of their ability to produce wakefulness and euphoria. Abuse leads to compulsive behaviour, paranoia, hallucinations, and suicidal tendencies. They have few legitimate medical applications but are used in the treatment of narcolepsy and childhood hyperkinesia.

amphiarthrosis. See **cartilaginous joint**.

amphigenesis. See **amphigony**.

amphigenetic, 1. produced by the union of gametes from both sexes. **2.** bisexual; having both testicular and ovarian tissue.

amphigenous inheritance, the acquisition of genetic traits and conditions from both parents.

amphigonadism true hermaphroditism; having both testicular and ovarian tissue. **amphigonadic,** adj.

amphigony, sexual reproduction. **amphigonic** adj.

amphikaryon, a nucleus containing the diploid number of chromosomes. **amphikaryotic,** adj.

amphimixis, 1. the union of germ cells in reproduction so that both maternal and paternal hereditary characteristics are derived; interbreeding. **2.** (in psychoanalysis) the union and integration of oral, anal, and genital libidinal impulses in the development of heterosexuality.

amphipathic, pertaining to a molecule having two sides with characteristically different properties, such as a detergent, which has both a polar (hydrophilic) end and a nonpolar (hydrophobic) end but is long enough so that each end demonstrates its own solubility characteristics.

amphoric breath sound, an abnormal, resonant, hollow blowing sound heard with a stethoscope. It indicates a cavity opening into the bronchus, or a pneumothorax.

amphoteric, a substance that can have a positive, zero, or negative charge, depending on conditions.

amphotericin B an antifungal medication used topically or systemically in the treatment of fungal infections.

ampicillin a semisynthetic penicillin used in the treatment of infections caused by a broad spectrum of sensitive gram-negative and gram-positive organisms.

amplification, 1. (in molecular genetics) a process in which the amount of plasmid DNA is increased in proportion to the amount of bacterial DNA by treatment with certain substances, including chloramphenicol. **2.** the replication in bulk of an entire gene library. **amplify,** v.

amplitude, width or breadth of range or extent, such as amplitude of accommodation or amplitude of convergence.

amplitude of accommodation (AA), the total accommodative power of the eye, determined by the difference between the refractive power for farthest vision and that for nearest vision.

amplitude of convergence, the difference in the power needed to turn the eyes from their far point to their near point of convergence.

AMPS, Assessment of Motor and Process Skills involving the performance of designated tasks, which is scored by the occupational therapist. AMPS procedure was developed by Dr Anne Fisher.

ampule, a small, sterile glass or plastic container that usually contains a single dose of a solution to be administered parenterally. Also spelled ampoule.

ampulla, a rounded, saclike dilatation of a duct, canal, or any tubular structure, such as the lacrimal duct, semicircular canal, uterine tube, rectum, or vas deferens.

ampulla of Vater. See **hepatopancreatic ampulla**.

ampullary aneurysm. See **saccular aneurysm**.

ampullary tubal pregnancy a kind of tubal pregnancy in which implantation occurs in the ampulla of one of the uterine tubes.

amputation, the surgical removal of a part of the body or a limb or part of a limb, performed to treat recurrent infections or gangrene in peripheral vascular disease, to remove malignant tumours, and in severe trauma. With the patient under general anaesthesia, the part is removed and a shaped flap is cut from muscular and cutaneous tissue to cover the end of the bone, with a section left open for drainage if infection is present. Kinds of amputation include closed amputation, congenital amputation, open amputation, primary amputation, and secondary amputation.

amputation neuroma, a form of traumatic neuroma that may develop near the stump after the amputation of an extremity.

amputee, a person who has had one or more extremities traumatically, congenitally, or surgically removed.

amrinone lactate, an intravenous cardiac inotropic drug prescribed in the short-term management of congestive heart failure in patients who do not respond to therapy with digitalis, diuretics, and vasodilators. It is not available commercially in the United Kingdom.

Amsler grid {Marc Amsler, Swiss ophthalmologist, b. 1891}, a checkerboard grid of intersecting dark horizontal and vertical lines with one dark spot in the middle. To discover a visual field defect, the person simply covers or closes one eye and looks at the spot with the other.

Amsterdam dwarf, a person affected with de Lange's syndrome, in which short stature and severe mental retardation are associated with many other abnormalities.

amu, abbreviation for **atomic mass unit**.

amusia, a form of agnosia characterized by a loss of the ability to recognize melodies.

amyelinic neuroma, a tumour that contains only nonmyelinated nerve fibres.

amyl alcohol, a colourless, oily liquid that is only slightly soluble in water but can be mixed with ethyl alcohol, chloroform, or ether.

amyl alcohol tertiary. See **amylene hydrate**.

amylase, an enzyme that catalyses the hydrolysis of starch into smaller carbohydrate molecules. Alpha-amylase, found in saliva, pancreatic juice, malt, certain bacteria, and moulds, catalyses the hydrolysis of starches to dextrins, maltose, and maltotriose. Beta-amylase, found in grains, vegetables, and malt, is involved in the hydrolysis of starch to maltose.

amylene hydrate, a clear, colourless liquid with a camphorlike odour, miscible with alcohol, chloroform, ether, or glycerin and used as a solvent and a hypnotic.

amylic fermentation, the formation of amyl alcohol from sugar.

amyl nitrite, an inhaled vasodilator prescribed to relieve the vasospasm of angina pectoris. It is also used in the treatment of cyanide poisoning, and as a recreational drug for its ability to relax the anal sphincter during anal intercourse and, reputedly, to heighten orgasm.

amylobarbitone, a barbiturate sedative-hypnotic used for the relief of severe intractable insomnia in patients already taking barbiturates.

amyloidosis, a disease in which a waxy, starchlike, glycoprotein (amyloid) accumulates in tissues and organs, impairing their function. There are two major forms of the condition. **Primary amyloidosis** usually occurs with multiple myeloma. Patients with **secondary amyloidosis** usually suffer from another chronic infectious or inflammatory disease, as tuberculosis, osteomyelitis, rheumatoid arthritis, or Crohn's disease. The cause of both types of amyloidosis is unknown. Almost all organs are affected, most often the heart, lungs, tongue, and intestines in primary amyloidosis, and the kidneys, liver, and spleen in the secondary type.

amylopectinosis. See **Andersen's disease**.

amyotonia, an abnormal condition of skeletal muscle, characterized by a lack of tone, weakness, and wasting, usually the result of motor neuron disease. **amyotonic,** *adj.*

amyotrophic lateral sclerosis (ALS), a degenerative disease of the motor neurons, characterized by atrophy of the muscles of the hands, forearms, and legs spreading to involve most of the body. It results from degeneration of the motor neurons, beginning in middle age.

ana (aa), (in prescriptions) "so much of each," indication of the amount of each ingredient to be compounded. Usually written as an abbreviation.

ANA, abbreviation for **American Nurses' Association**.

anabolic steroid, any one of several compounds structurally related to testosterone. Such compounds promote general growth, oppose the effects of endogenous oestrogens, and have masculinizing effects. All such compounds cause a mixed androgenic-anabolic effect. Anabolic steroids are used clinically in the treatment of aplastic anaemia, red-cell aplasia, and haemolytic anaemia and in anaemias associated with renal failure, myeloid metaplasia, and leukaemia.

anabolism, constructive metabolism characterized by the conversion of simple substances into the more complex compounds of living matter. **anabolic** *adj.*

anacatadidymus, conjoined twins that are fused in the middle but separated above and below.

anaclisis, 1. a condition, normal in childhood but pathological in adulthood, in which a person is emotionally dependent on other people. **2.** a condition in which a person consciously or unconsciously chooses a love object because of a resemblance to the mother, father, or other person who was an important source of comfort and protection in infancy. **anaclitic** *adj.*

anaclitic depression, a syndrome occurring in infants, usually after sudden separation from the mothering person. Symptoms include apprehension, withdrawal, incessant crying, refusal to eat, sleep disturbances, leading to impairment of the infant's physical, social, and intellectual development.

anacrotic pulse, (on a sphygmographic tracing) a pulse characterized by one transient drop in amplitude on the curve of the primary elevation. It is seen in valvular aortic stenosis.

anacusis, a total loss of hearing.

anadicrotic pulse, (on a sphygmographic tracing) a pulse characterized by two transient drops in amplitude on the curve of primary elevation.

anadidymus, conjoined twins that are united at the pelvis and lower extremities but are separated in the upper half.

anadipsia, extreme thirst, often occurring in the manic phase of manic-depressive psychosis. The condition is the result of dehydration caused by the excessive perspiration, continuous urination, and relentless physical activity produced by the intense excitement characteristic of the manic phase.

anaemia, a disorder characterized by a decrease in haemoglobin in the blood to levels below the normal range, decreased red cell production or increased red cell destruction, or blood loss. A separate and distinct morphological classification system describes anaemia by the haemoglobin content of the red cells (normochromic or hypochromic) and by differences in red cell size (macrocytic, normocytic, or microcytic).

anaemia of pregnancy, a condition of pregnancy characterized by a reduction in the concentration of haemoglobin in the blood. It may be physiolological or pathological. In physiological anaemia of pregnancy, the reduction in concentration results from dilution because the plasma volume expands more than the red blood cell volume. In pathological anaemia of pregnancy, the oxygen-carrying capacity of the blood is deficient because of disordered erythrocyte production or excessive loss of erythrocytes through destruction or bleeding.

anaemic anoxia, a condition characterized by a deficiency of oxygen in body tissues, resulting from a decrease in the number of erythrocytes in the blood or in the amount of haemoglobin.

anaerobe, a microorganism that grows and lives in the complete or almost complete absence of oxygen. An example is *Clostridium botulinum.* Some kinds of anaerobes are facultative anaerobe and obligate anaerobe.

anaerobic 1. pertaining to the absence of air or oxygen. **2.** able to grow and function without air or oxygen.

anaerobic catabolism, the breakdown of complex chemical substances into simpler compounds, with the release of energy, in the absence of oxygen.

anaerobic exercise, muscular exertion sufficient to result in metabolic acidosis because of accumulation of lactic acid as a product of muscle metabolism.

anaerobic glycolysis. See **glycolysis**.

anaerobic infection, an infection caused by an anaerobic organism, usually occurring in deep puncture wounds that exclude air or in tissue that has diminished oxygen-reduction potential as a result of trauma, necrosis, or overgrowth of bacteria. Kinds of anaerobic infection are gangrene and tetanus.

anaerobic myositis. See **gas gangrene**.

aneroid not containing a liquid, used especially to describe a device in contrast to one performing a similar function that does contain liquid, such as aneroid sphygmomanometer, which does not contain a column of liquid mercury.

anaeroid barometer, a device consisting of a flexible spring in a sealed, evacuated metal box that is used to measure atmospheric pressure.

anaesthesia, the absence of normal sensation, especially sensitivity to pain, as induced by an anaesthetic substance or by hypnosis or as occurs with traumatic or pathophysiological damage to nerve tissue. Anaesthesia induced for medical or surgical purposes may be topical, local, regional, or general and is described according to the anaesthetic agent used, the method or procedure followed, the area or organ anaethetized, or the age or class of the patient served.

anaesthesia dolorosa, a severe tactile or spontaneous, paradoxical pain in an anaesthetized area.

anaesthetic, a drug or agent that is capable of producing a complete or partial loss of feeling (anaesthesia).

anaesthetic apparatus, an apparatus for administering inhalant anaesthetic agents.

anaesthetics, the branch of medicine that is concerned with the relief of pain and with the administration of medication to relief pain during surgery.

anaesthetic screen, a metal inverted U-shaped frame that attaches to the sides of the operating table, 12 to 18 inches above a patient's upper chest. It is covered with a sheet to prevent contamination of an operative site on the chest or abdomen by airborne infection from the patient or the anaesthetist and to provide a wide sterile field for the surgeon.

anaesthetist, a physician trained in the administration of anaesthetics and in the provision of respiratory and cardiovascular support during anaesthetic procedures.

anal, of or pertaining to the anus.

anal agenesis. See **imperforate anus**.

anal canal, the final portion of the alimentary tract, about 4 cm long, between the rectal ampulla and the anus.

anal character, (in psychoanalysis) a kind of personality exhibiting patterns of behaviour originating in the anal phase of infancy, characterized by extreme orderliness, obstinacy, perfectionism, cleanliness, punctuality, and miserliness, or their extreme opposites.

anal crypt, the depression between rectal columns that encloses networks of veins that, when inflamed and swollen, are called haemorrhoids.

analeptic. See **central nervous system stimulant**.

anal eroticism, (in psychoanalysis) libidinal fixation at or regression to the anal stage of psychosexual development, often reflected in such personality traits as miserliness, stubbornness, and overscrupulousness.

anal fissure, a linear ulceration or laceration of the skin of the anus.

anal fistula, an abnormal opening on the cutaneous surface near the anus, usually resulting from a local crypt abscess and also common in Crohn's disease. A perianal fistula may or may not communicate with the rectum.

analgesia, a lack of pain without loss of consciousness.

analgesia algera. See **anaesthesia dolorosa**.

analgesic 1. relieving pain. **2.** a drug that relieves pain. The opiate (narcotic) analgesics act on the central nervous system and alter the patient's perception; they are more often used for severe pain. The nonnarcotic analgesics may act at the site of the pain or centrally, do not produce tolerance or dependence, and do not alter the patient's perception; they are used for mild to moderate pain.

analgesic cocktail, informal. an individualized mixture of drugs used for pain relief in specific syndromes.

anal membrane. See **cloacal membrane**.

anal membrane atresia. See **imperforate anus**.

analogue, 1. a substance, tissue, or organ that is similar in appearance or function to another but differing in origin or development, such as the eye of a fly and the eye of a human. **2.** a drug or other chemical compound that resembles another in structure or constituents but has different effects. Also spelled analog.

analogue computer, a computer that processes information as a physical quantity, such as voltage, amperage, weight, or length and presents results of calculations that can be continuously varied and measured.

analogue signal, a continuous electric signal representing a specific condition, such as temperature or ECG waveforms.

analogue-to-digital converter, a device for converting analogue information, such as temperature or ECG waveforms, into digital form for processing by a digital computer.

anal reflex, a superficial neurological reflex obtained by stroking the skin or mucosa of the region around the anus, which normally results in a contraction of the external anal sphincter.

anal sadism, (in psychoanalysis) a sadistic form of anal eroticism, manifested by such behaviour as aggressiveness and selfishness.

anal stage, (in psychoanalysis) the pregenital period in psychosexual development, occurring between 1 and 3 years of age, when preoccupation with the function of the bowel and the sensations associated with the anus are the predominant source of pleasurable stimulation.

anal stenosis. See **imperforate anus**.

analysand a person undergoing psychoanalysis.

analysis, the separation of substances into their constituent parts and the determination of the nature, properties, and composition of compounds. In chemistry, qualitative analysis is the determination of the elements present in a substance; quantitative analysis is the determination of how much of each element is present in a substance. Analysis is also an informal term for psychoanalysis. **analytic,** *adj.* analyse, v.

analysis of variance (ANOVA), a series of statistical procedures for determining the differences, attributable to chance alone, among two or more groups of scores.

analyst, 1. a psychoanalyst. **2.** a person who analyses the chemical, physical, or other properties of a substance or product.

analyte, any substance that is measured. The term is usually applied to a component of a biological section.

analytical psychology, 1. the system in which phenomena, such as sensations and feelings, are analysed and classified by introspective rather than by experimental methods. **2.** also called **Jungian psychology,** a system of analysing the psyche according to the concepts developed by Carl Gustav Jung. It differs from the psychoanalysis of Sigmund Freud in stressing a "racial" or collective unconscious and a mystic, religious factor in the development of the personal unconscious and in minimizing the importance of sexual influence on early emotional and psychological development.

anamnesis, 1. remembrance of the past. **2.** the accumulated data concerning a medical or psychiatric patient and the patient's background, including family, previous environment, experiences, and, particularly, recollections, for use in analysing his condition.

anaphase, the third of four stages of nuclear division in mitosis and in each of the two divisions of meiosis. In mitosis and the second meiotic division the centromeres divide, and the two chromatids, which are arranged along the equatorial plane of the spindle, separate and move to the opposite poles of the cell, forming daughter chromosomes. In the first meiotic division the pairs of homologous chromosomes separate from each other and move intact to the opposite poles of the spindle.

anaphia the loss of the ability to perceive tactile stimuli.

anaphylactic hypersensitivity an IgE- or IgG-dependent, immediate-acting humoral hypersensitivity response to an exogenous antigen. Histamine, kinins, and other substances are released from mast cells, causing vasodilatation and muscle contraction. Systemic anaphylaxis, atopic allergies, hayfever, and insect-sting reactions are all anaphylactic hypersensitivity reactions.

anaphylactic shock, a severe and sometimes fatal systemic hypersensitivity reaction to a sensitizing substance, such as a drug, vaccine, certain food, serum, allergen extract, insect venom, or chemical. This condition may occur within seconds from the time of exposure to the sensitizing factor and is commonly marked by respiratory distress and vascular collapse. The more quickly any systemic atopic reaction occurs in the individual after exposure, the more severe the associated shock is likely to be. The involved allergen enters the systemic circulation and triggers an incomplete humoral response that allows the allergen to combine with IgE and cause the release of histamine. Also entering into the reaction are IgG and IgM, which cause the release of complement fractions, further stimulating histamine action.

anaphylactoid purpura. See **Henoch-Schönlein purpura**.

anaphylatoxin a polypeptide derived from complement. It mediates changes in mast cells leading to the release of histamine and other pharmacologically active substances.

anaphylaxis, an exaggerated hypersensitivity reaction to a previously encountered antigen. The response, which is mediated by antibodies of the IgE class of immunoglobulins, causes the release of histamine, kinin, and substances that affect smooth muscle. The reaction may be a localized wheal and flare of generalized itching, hyperaemia, angioneurotic oedema, and in severe cases vascular collapse, bronchospasm, and shock. The severity of symptoms depends on the original sensitizing dose of the antigen, the amount and distribution of antibodies, and the route of entry and size of the dose of antigen producing anaphylaxis. Penicillin injection is the most common cause of anaphylactic shock. Kinds of anaphylaxis are **aggregate anaphylaxis, antiserum anaphylaxis, cutaneous anaphylaxis, cytotoxic anaphylaxis, indirect anaphylaxis,** and **inverse anaphylaxis. anaphylactic, anaphylactoid,** *adj.*

anaplasia, a change in the structure of cells and in their orientation to each other characterized by a loss of differentiation and reversion to a more primitive form. Anaplasia is characteristic of malignancy. **anaplastic,** *adj.*

anaplastic astrocytoma. See **glioblastoma multiforme**.

anarthria, a loss of control of the muscles of speech, resulting in the inability to utter words. The condition is usually caused by damage to a central or peripheral motor nerve.

anasarca, generalized, massive oedema. Anasarca is often observed in oedema associated with renal disease when fluid retention continues for an extended period of time. **anasarcous,** *adj.*

anastomosis *pl.* **anastomoses,** a surgical joining of two ducts or blood vessels to allow flow from one to the other. It may be performed to bypass an aneurysm or a vascular or arterial occlusion. Kinds of anastomoses are end-to-end anastomosis, side-to-side anastomosis.

anastomosis at elbow joint, a convergence of blood vessels at the elbow joint, consisting of various veins and portions of the brachial and deep brachial arteries and their branches.

anatomical crown, the portion of the dentin of a tooth, covered by dental enamel.

anatomical curve, the curvature of the different segments of the vertebral column. In the lateral contour of the back, the cervical curve appears concave, the thoracic curve appears convex, and the lumbar curve appears concave.

anatomical dead space. See **dead space**.

anatomical height of contour, a line that encircles and designates the greatest convexity of a tooth.

anatomical impotence. See **impotence**.

anatomical position, a position of the body in which a person stands erect, facing directly forward, feet pointed forward slightly apart, arms hanging down at the sides with palms facing forward.

anatomical snuffbox, a small, cuplike depression on the back of the hand near the wrist formed by the tendons reaching toward the thumb and index finger as the thumb is abducted, the wrist flexed, and the digits extended.

anatomic zero joint position, the beginning point of a joint range of motion.

anatomy, 1. the study, classification, and description of structures and organs of the body. Kinds of anatomy are **applied anatomy, comparative anatomy, descriptive anatomy, gross anatomy, microscopic anatomy,** and **surface anatomy. 2.** the structure of an organism. **3.** a text on anatomy. **4.** *archaic.* dissection of a body.

ancillary pertaining to something that is subordinate, auxiliary, or supplementary.

anconeus, one of seven superficial muscles of the posterior forearm. A small triangular muscle, it originates on the dorsal surface of the lateral condyle and inserts in the olecranon process of the ulna. It functions to extend the forearm.

ancrod, the venom of the Malayan pit viper, used to remove fibrinogen from the circulation, thus preventing clotting of the blood.

Ancylostoma, a genus of nematode that is an intestinal parasite and causes hookworm disease.

ancylostomiasis hookworm disease, more specifically that caused by *Ancylostoma duodenale, A. braziliense,* or *A. cannium.*

Andersen's disease {Dorothy H. Andersen, American pediatrician, b. 1901}, a rare glycogen storage disease characterized by a genetic deficiency of branching enzyme (amylo-1:4, 1:6 transglucosidase), causing the deposition in tissues of abnormal glycogen with long inner and outer chains.

andreioma, andreoblastoma. See **arrhenoblastoma.**

Andresen removable orthodontic appliance, an activator-type of orthodontic device intended to function as a passive transmitter and stimulator of forces of the perioral muscles by inducing or directing oral forces for the improvement of tooth position and jaw relationship.

androgamone, a gamone secreted by the male gamete.

androgen, any steroid hormone that increases male characteristics. Natural hormones, such as testosterone and its esters and analogues, are primarily used as substitutional therapy during the male climacteric. Androgens may be administered orally or parenterally. **androgenic,** *adj.*

androgynous 1. (of a man or woman) having some characteristics of both sexes. Social role, behaviour, personality, and appearance are reflections of individuality and are not determined by gender. **2.** hermaphroditic. **androgyny,** *n.*

android, pertaining to something that is typically masculine, or manlike, such as an android pelvis.

android pelvis, a type of pelvis in which the structure is characteristic of the male. The bones are thick and heavy, and the inlet is heart-shaped.

androma. See **arrhenoblastoma.**

andropause a change of life for members of the male sex may be expressed in terms of a reordering of life. It is associated with a decline in androgen levels that occurs in men during their late forties or early fifties.

androsterone, a male sex hormone. The greater potency of several other male sex hormones has relegated androsterone largely to historic biochemical interest.

anecdotal, pertaining to medical knowledge based on isolated observations and not yet verified by controlled scientific studies.

anechoic (in ulrasonography) free of echoes or without echoes.

anencephaly, congenital absence of the brain and spinal cord in which the cranium does not close and the vertebral canal remains a groove. Transmitted genetically, anencephaly is not compatible with life.

anergic stupor, a kind of dementia characterized by quietness, listlessness, and nonresistance.

anergy, 1. lack of activity. **2.** an immunodeficient condition characterized by a lack of or diminished reaction to an antigen or group of antigens. This state may be seen in advanced tuberculosis and other serious infections, acquired immune deficiency syndrome, and some malignancies. **anergic,** *adj.*

anetoderma, an idiopathic, patchy atrophy and looseness of the skin for which there is no known effective treatment.

aneuploid, 1. of or pertaining to an individual, organism, strain, or cell that has a chromosome number that is not an exact multiple of the normal, basic haploid number characteristic of the species. **2.** such an individual, organism, strain, or cell. Also **aneuploidic/aneuploidy,** any variation in chromosome number that involves individual chromosomes rather than entire sets. There may be fewer chromosomes, as in Turner's syndrome, or more chromosomes, as in Down's syndrome. Compare **euploidy.**

aneurysm, a localized dilation of the wall of a blood vessel, usually caused by atherosclerosis and hypertension, or less frequently, by trauma, infection, or a congenital weakness in the vessel wall. An arterial aneurysm may be a saccular distension affecting only part of the circumference of the vessel, it may be a fusiform or cylindroid dilatation of a section of the vessel, or it may be a longitudinal dissection between layers of the vascular wall. An aneurysm may rupture, causing haemorrhage, or thrombi may form in the dilated pouch and give rise to emboli that may obstruct smaller vessels. Kinds of aneurysms include **aortic aneurysm, bacterial aneurysm, berry aneurysm, cerebral aneurysm, compound aneurysm, dissecting aneurysm, fusiform aneurysm, mycotic aneurysm, racemose aneurysm, Rasmussen's aneurysm, saccular aneurysm, varicose aneurysm** and **ventricular aneurysm. aneurysmal,** *adj.*

aneurysmal bone cyst, a cystic bone lesion that tends to develop in the metaphyseal region of long bones but may occur in any bone, including the vertebrae. It produces pain and swelling.

aneurysm needle, a needle equipped with a handle, used to ligate aneurysms.

angel dust. See **phencyclidine hydrochloride (PCP).**

anger, an emotional reaction characterized by extreme displeasure, rage, indignation, or hostility. It is considered to be of pathological origin when such a response does not realistically reflect a person's actual circumstances.

angiitis, an inflammatory condition of a vessel, chiefly a blood or lymph vessel. A kind of angiitis is consecutive angiitis.

angina, 1. a spasmodic, cramplike choking feeling. **2.** a term now used primarily to denote the paroxysmal thoracic pain and choking feeling caused by anoxia of the myocardium (angina pectoris). **3.** a descriptive feature of various diseases characterized by a feeling of choking, suffocation, or crushing pressure and pain. Kinds of angina are **intestinal angina, Ludwig's angina, Prinzmetal's angina,** and **streptococcal angina. anginal,** *adj.*

angina decubitus, a condition characterized by periodic attacks of angina pectoris that occur when the person is lying down.

angina dyspeptica, a painful condition caused by gaseous distention of the stomach that mimics angina pectoris.

angina epiglottidea, a painful condition caused by inflammation of the epiglottis.

angina pectoris, a paroxysmal thoracic pain caused most often by myocardial anoxia as a result of atherosclerosis of the coronary arteries. The pain usually radiates down the inner aspect of the left arm and is frequently accompanied by a feeling of suffocation and impending death. Attacks of angina pectoris are often related to exertion, emotional stress, and exposure to intense cold.

angina sine dolore, a painless episode of coronary insufficiency.

angina trachealis. See **croup.**

angioblastic meningioma, a tumour of the blood vessels of the meninges covering the spinal cord or the brain.

angioblastoma, *pl.* **angioblastomas, angioblastomata,** a tumour of blood vessels in the brain. Kinds of angioblastomas are **angioblastic meningioma** and **cerebellar angioblastoma.**

angiocardiogram, a radiograph of the heart and the vessels of the heart.

angiocatheter, a hollow, flexible tube inserted into a blood vessel to withdraw or instil fluids.

angiochondroma, *pl.* **angiochondromas, angiochondromata,** a cartilaginous tumour characterized by an excessive formation of blood vessels.

angioedema. See **angioneurotic oedema.**

angioendothelioma. See **haemangioendothelioma.**

angiofibroma, *pl.* **angiofibromas, angiofibromata,** an angioma containing fibrous tissue.

angiogenesis, the formation of new blood vessels, a common property of malignant tissue.

angiogenin, a protein that mediates the formation of blood vessels. It is used experi-

mentally to stimulate the development of new blood vessels in wound healing, stroke, or coronary heart disease.

angioglioma, *pl.* **angiogliomas, angiogliomatas,** a highly vascular tumour composed of neuroglia.

angiography, radiographic technique to visualise the internal anatomy of the heart and blood vessels after the intravascular introduction of radiopaque contrast medium. **angiographic,** *adj;* **angiograph,** *n.*

angiohaemophilia. See **von Willebrand's disease.**

angiokeratoma, *pl.* **angiokeratomas, angiokeratomata,** a vascular horny neoplasm on the skin, characterized by clumps of dilated blood vessels, clusters of warts, and thickening of the epidermis, especially the scrotum and the dorsal aspect of the fingers and toes.

angiokeratoma circumscriptum, a rare skin disorder characterized by discrete papules and nodules in small patches on the legs or on the trunk.

angiokeratoma corporis diffusum, an uncommon familial disease in which phopholipids are stored in many parts of the body, especially the blood vessels, causing vasomotor, urinary, and cutaneous disorders and, in some cases, muscular abnormalities.

angiolipoma, *pl.* **angiolipomas, angiolipomata,** a benign neoplasm containing blood vessels and tissue.

angioma, *pl.* **angiomas, angiomata,** any benign tumour made up primarily of blood vessels (haemangioma) or lymph vessels (lymphangioma). Most angiomas are congenital; some, like cavernous haemangiomas, disappear spontaneously.

angioma arteriale racemosum, a vascular neoplasm characterized initially by the intertwining of many small, newly formed, dilated blood vessels.

angioma cavernosum. See **cavernous haemangioma.**

angioma cutis, a naevus composed of a network of dilated blood vessels.

angioma lymphaticum. See **lymphangioma.**

angiomatosis, a condition characterized by the presence of numerous vascular tumours. A kind of angiomatosis is the Osler-Weber-Rendu syndrome.

angiomyoma, *pl.* **angiomyomas, angiomyomata,** a benign tumour composed of vascular and muscular tissue elements.

angiomyoneuroma. See **glomangioma.**

angiomyosarcoma, *pl.* **angiomyosarcomas, angiomyosarcomata,** a malignant tumour containing vascular, muscular, and connective tissue elements.

angioneuroma. See **glomangioma.**

angioneurotic anuria, an abnormal condition characterized by an almost complete absence of urination caused by destruction of tissue in the renal cortex.

angioneurotic oedema, an acute, painless,

dermal, subcutaneous or submucosal swelling of short duration involving the face, neck, lips, larynx, hands, feet, genitalia, or viscera. It may result from food or drug allergy, infection, or emotional stress, or it may be hereditary.

angiosarcoma, a rare malignant tumour consisting of endothelial and fibroblastic tissue that proliferates and eventually surrounds vascular channels.

angiospasm, a sudden transient constriction of a blood vessel.

angiotensin I the decapeptide precursor of the vasoactive compound angiotensin II produced by the action of the enzyme renin on angiotensinogen.

angiotensin II a polypeptide occurring in the blood causing vasoconstriction, increased blood pressure, and the release of aldosterone from the adrenal cortex. Angiotensin II is formed from angiotensin I by the angiotensin converting enzyme (ACE).

angiotensin-converting enzyme (ACE), a protein (dipeptidyl carboxypeptidase) that catalyses the conversion of angiotensin I to angiotensin II by removing two terminal amino acids.

angiotensinogen, a serum globulin produced in the liver that is the precursor of angiotensin I.

angiotensin sensitivity test (AST), a test for sensitivity to angiotensin II by infusion of angiotensin-II-amide into the right cubital vein.

angle, 1. the space or the shape formed at the intersection of two lines, planes, or borders may be measured in degrees of a circle. **2.** (in anatomy and physiology) the geometric relationship between the surfaces of the body structures and the positions affected by movement.

angle board, (in radiography) a device used to reproduce angles between the patient's head, the central ray of the x-ray beam, and the x-ray film.

angle-closure glaucoma. See **glaucoma**.

angle former, (in dentistry) one of a series of paired cutting instruments having cutting edges at an angle other than a right angle in relation to the axis of the blade.

angle of incidence, the angle at which an ultrasound beam hits the interface between two different types of tissues, as the facing surfaces of bone and muscle.

angle of Louis, the sternal angle between the manubrium and the body of the sternum.

angle of mandible, the angular relationship between the body and the ramus of the mandible.

angle of Treitz, a sharp curve of flexure at the junction of the duodenum and jejunum.

Angle's classification [Edward H Angle, American orthodontist, b.1855], a classification of the various types of malocclusion.

angstrom (Å), [Anders J. Angström, Swedish physicist, b 1814], a unit of measure of length equal to 0.1 nanometre (1/10,000,000 metre)

angular cheilitis, inflammation at the corner of the mouth.

angular movement, one of the four basic kinds of movement allowed by the various joints of the skeleton in which the angle between two adjoining bones is decreased, as in flexion, or increased, as in extension.

angular vein, one of a pair of veins of the face, formed by the junction of the frontal and the supraorbital veins.

angulated fracture, a fracture in which the fragments of bone are angulated.

angulation, 1. an angular shape or formation. **2.** the discipline of precisely measuring angles, as in the mechanical drafting and surveying. **3.** (in radiography) the direction of the primary beam of radiation in relation to the object being radiographed and the film used to record its image.

anhedonia, the inability to feel pleasure or happiness from experiences that are ordinarily pleasurable, **anhedonic,** *adj.*

anhidrosis, an abnormal condition characterized by inadequate perspiration.

anhidrotic, 1. of or pertaining to anhidrosis. **2.** an agent that reduces or suppresses sweating.

anhydride, a chemical compound derived by the abstraction of water from a substance, especially an acid.

anhydrous, lacking water.

anicteric, pertaining to the absence of jaundice.

anicteric hepatitis, a mild form or hepatitis in which there is not jaundice (icterus), usually seen in infants and young children.

anidean, formless; shapeless; denoting an undifferentiated mass, as an anideus. Also anidian, anidous.

anideus, an anomalous, rudimentary conceptus consisting of a simple rounded mass with little indication of the body parts. A kind of anideus is embryonic anideus.

aniline, an oily, colourless poisonous liquid with a strong odour and burning taste, formerly extracted from the indigo plant and now made synthetically using nitrobenzene and used in the manufacture of aniline dyes.

anilinparasulphonic acid. See **sulphanilic acid**.

anima, 1. the soul or life. **2.** (in Jungian psychology) a person's true, inner, unconscious being or personality, as distinguished from overt personality, or persona. **3.** (in analytical psychology) the female component of the male personality.

animal pole, the active, formative part of the ovum protoplasm that contains the nucleus and bulk of the cytoplasm and where the polar bodies from. In mammals it is also the site where the inner cell mass gives rise to the ectoderm.

animus, 1. the active or rational soul, the animating principle of life. **2.** the male component of the female personality. **3.** (in psychiatry) a deep seated antagonism that is usually controlled but may erupt with virulence under stress.

anion, a negatively charged ion that is attracted to the positive electrode (anode) in electrolysis.

anion gap, the difference between the concentrations of serum cations and anions determined by measuring the concentrations of sodium cations and chloride and bicarbonate anions. It is helpful in the diagnosis and treatment of acidosis.

anise, the fruit of the *Pimpinella anisum* plant. Extract of anise is used in the preparation of carminatives and expectorants.

aniseikonia, an abnormal ocular condition in which each eye perceives the same image as being of a different form and size.

anisocytosis, an abnormal condition of the blood characterized by red blood cells of variable and abnormal size.

anisogamete, a gamete that differs considerably in size and structure from the one with which it unites, as the macrogamete and microgamete of certain sprosoa. **anisogametic,** *adj.*

anisogamy, sexual conjugation of gametes that are of unequal size and structure, as in certain thallophytes and sporozea. **anisogamous,** *adj.*

anisognathic, of or pertaining to an abnormal condition in which the maxillary and the mandibular arches or jaws are of significantly different sizes in the same individual.

anisokaryosis, significant variation in the size of the nucleus of cells of the same general type. **anisokaryotic,** *adj.*

anisomastia, a condition in which one female breast is larger than the other.

anisometropia, a condition characterized by a difference in the refractive powers of the eyes.

anisopia, a condition in which the visual power of one eye is greater than that of the other.

anisopoikilocytosis, an abnormal condition of the blood characterised by red blood cells of variable and abnormal size and shape.

ankle, 1. the joint of the tibia, the talus, and the fibula. **2.** the part of the leg where this joint is located.

ankle bandage, a figure-of-eight bandage looped under the sole of the foot and around the ankle. The heel may be covered or left exposed, although covering is preferable because it prevents "window oedema".

ankle bone. See **talus**.

ankle clonus, an involuntary tendon reflex that causes repeated flexion and extension of the foot, associated with an upper motor neuron lesion.

ankle-foot orthosis (AFO), any of a variety of protective external devices that can be applied to the ankle area to prevent injury in athletic activity, to protect a previous injury and to compensate for chronic joint instability.

ankle reflex. See **Achilles tendon reflex**.

ankyloglossia, an oral defect, characterized by an abnormally short lingual frenum that limits tongue movement and impairs the speech. It may be surgically corrected by a frenotomy.

ankylosing spondylitis, a chronic inflammatory disease of unknown origin, first affecting the spine and adjacent structures, and commonly progressing to eventual fusion (ankylosis) of the involved joints. In extreme cases the patient develops a forward flexion of the spine, called a "poker spine" or "bamboo spine".

ankylosis, 1. fixation of a joint, often in an abnormal position, usually resulting from destruction of articular cartilage and subchondral bone, as occurs in rheumatoid arthritis. **2.** also called arthrodesis, fusion. surgically induced fixation of a joint to relieve pain or provide support.

anlage, (in embryology) the undifferentiated layer of cells from which a particular organ, tissue or structure develops; primordium rudiment.

ANLL, abbreviation for **acute nonlymphoblastic leukaemia**. See **acute myeloblastic leukaemia**.

annihilation, the total transformation of matter into energy.

annular. See **anular**.

annular ligament. See **anular ligament**.

anode, a positively-charged electrode, such as the anode of an x-ray tube.

anode cut-off, loss of density observed on the part of a radiograph, usually when using a large field size, due to absorption of part of the x-ray beam within the anode.

anodic stripping voltammetry, a process of electroanalytical chemistry used to detect trace metals.

anodomia. See **anosmia**.

anodontia, a congenital defect in which some or all of the teeth are missing.

anodyne, a drug that relieves or lessens pain.

anomaly, 1. deviation from what is regarded as normal. **2.** congenital malformation, such as the absence of a limb or the presence of an extra finger. **anomalous,** *adj.*

anomia, a form of aphasia characterized by the inability to name objects, caused by a lesion in the temporal lobe of the brain.

anomie, a state of apathy, alienation, anxiety, personal disorientation, and distress, resulting from the loss of social norms and goals previously valued. Also spelled anomy.

anoopsia, a strabismus in which one or both eyes are deviated upward.

Anopheles, a genus of mosquito, many species of which transmit malaria-causing parasites to humans.

anopia, blindness resulting from a defect in or the absence of one or both eyes.

anoplasty, a restorative operation on the anus.

anorchia, congenital absence of one or both testes.

anorectal, of or pertaining to the anal and rectal portions of the large intestine.

anorectic, 1. of or pertaining to anorexia. **2.** lacking appetite. **3.** a drug causing a loss of appetite.

anorexia, lack or loss of appetite, resulting in the inability to eat. **anorexic, anorectic,** *adj.*

anorexia nervosa, a psychoneurotic disorder characterized by a prolonged refusal to eat, resulting in emaciation, amenorrhoea, emotional disturbance concerning body image, and an abnormal fear of becoming obese.

anorthopia, a visual distortion in which straight lines appear to be curved or angular.

anosigmoidoscopy, a procedure in which an endoscope is used for direct examination of the lining of the anus, rectum, and colon.

anosmia, loss or impairment of the sense of smell, commonly occurring as a temporary condition resulting from a head cold or respiratory infection or when intranasal swelling or other obstruction prevents odours from reaching the olfactory region. It becomes a permanent condition when the olfactory neuroepithelium or any part of the olfactory nerve is destroyed. Kinds of anosmia are **anosmia gustatoria** and **preferantial anosmia. anosmatic, anosmic,** *adj.*

anosmia gustatoria, the inability to smell foods.

anosognosia, an abnormal condition characterized by a real or feigned inability to perceive a defect, especially paralysis, on one side of the body, possibly attributable to a lesion in the right parietal lobe of the brain.

anosphrasia, anosphresia. See **anosmia.**

ANOVA, abbreviation for **analysis of variance.**

anovular menstruation, menstrual bleeding that occurs even though ovulation has not taken place.

anovulation, failure of the ovaries to produce, mature, or release eggs, as a result of ovarian immaturity or postmaturity; or altered ovarian function, as in pregnancy and lactation; of primary ovarian dysfunction, as in ovarian dysgenesis; or of disturbance of the interaction of the hypothalamus, pituitary gland and ovary, caused by stress or disease. **anovulatory** *adj.*

anoxaemia, a deficiency of oxygen in the blood.

anoxia, an abnormal condition characterized by a lack of oxygen. Anoxia may be local or systemic and may be the result of an inadequate supply of oxygen to the respiratory

system or of an inability of the blood to carry oxygen to the tissues or of the tissues to absorb the oxygen from the circulation. Kinds of anoxia include **cerebral anoxia** and **stagnant anoxia. anoxic,** *adj.*

ansa, *pl.* **ansae,** (in anatomy) a looplike structure resembling a curved handle of a vase.

ansa cervicalis, one of three loops of nerves in the cervical plexus, branches of which innervate the infrahyoid muscles.

antacid, 1. of or pertaining to a substance that reduces gastric acidity. **2.** a drug or dietary substance that buffers, neutralizes or absorbs hydrochloric acid in the stomach.

antagonist, 1. one who contends with or is opposed to another. **2.** any agent, such as a drug or muscle, that exerts an opposite action to that of another or competes for the same receptor sites. **3.** (in dentistry) a tooth in the upper jaw that articulates during mastication or occlusion with a tooth in the lower jaw. **antagonistic,** *adj.*, **antagonize,** *v.*

antalgic, avoiding or attempting to counteract pain by the alteration of normal posture or by gait.

antecardium. See **epigastric region.**

antecubital, in front of the elbow; at the bend of the elbow.

anteflexion, bending forwards, as in the body of the uterus on the cervix.

antegonial notch, a depression or concavity commonly present at the junction of the ramus and the mandible, near the attachment of the anterior margin of the masseter.

antenatal, pertaining to the period spanning conception and labour.

antenatal care, care of a pregnant woman during the time in the maternity cycle that begins with conception and ends with the onset of labour.

antenatal diagnosis. See **prenatal diagnosis.**

anterior (A), 1. in front of a structure. **2.** of or pertaining to a surface or part situated toward the front or facing forward.

anterior Achilles bursitis. See **Albert's disease.**

anterior asynclitism. See **asynclitism.**

anterior atlantoaxial ligament, one of five ligaments connecting the atlas to the axis. It is fixed to the inferior boarder of the anterior arch of the atlas and to the ventral surface of the body of the axis.

anterior atlantooccipital membrane, one of two broad, densely woven fibrous sheets that form part of the atlantooccipital joint between the atlas and the occipital bone.

anterior cardiac vein, one of several small vessels that return deoxygenated blood from the ventral portion of the myocardium of the right ventricle to the right atrium.

anterior common ligament. See **anterior longitudinal ligament**

anterior crural nerve. See **femoral nerve**

anterior cutaneous nerve, one of a pair of cutaneous branches of the cervical plexus. It arises from the second and the third cervical nerves, bends around the middle of the sternocleidomastoideus, crosses the muscle obliquely, passes beneath the platysma, and divides into the ascending and descending branches.

anterior determinants of cusp, (in dentistry) the characteristics of the anterior teeth that determine the cusp elevations and the fossa depressions in restoration of the postcanine teeth.

anterior fontanelle, a diamond-shaped area between the frontal and two parietal bones just above the baby's forehead at the junction of the coronal and sagittal sutures. Also known as the bregma.

anterior guide, (in dentistry) the portion of an articulator that is contracted by the incisal guide pin to maintain the selected separation of the upper and lower members of the articulator.

anterior longitudinal ligament, the broad, strong ligament attached to the ventral surfaces of the vertebral bodies. it extends from the occipital bone and the anterior tubercle of the atlas to the sacrum.

anterior mediastinal node, a node in one of the three groups of thoracic visceral nodes of the lyphatic system that drains lymph from the nodes of the thymus, pericardium, and sternum.

anterior mediastinum, a caudal portion of the mediastinum in the middle of the thorax, bounded ventrally by the body of the sternum and parts of the fourth through the seventh ribs and dorsally by the parietal pericardium, extending downward as far as the diaphragm.

anterior nares, the ends of the nostrils that open anteriorly into the nasal cavity and allow the inhalation and exhalation of air. The anterior nares connect with the nasal fossae.

anterior neuropore, the opening of the embryonic neural tube in the anterior portion of the forebrain.

anterior tibial artery, one of the two divisions of the popliteal artery, arising in back of the knee, dividing into six branches, and supplying various muscles of the leg and foot.

anterior tibial node, one of the small lymph glands of the lower limb, lying on the interosseous membrane near the proximal portion of the anterior tibial vessels.

anterior tooth, any one of the incisors or canine teeth.

anterocclusion, (in dentistry) a malocclusion in which the mandibular teeth are anterior to their normal position relative to the teeth in the maxillary arch.

anterograde amnesia, the inability to recall memories of events occurring after the event that precipitated the amnesia.

anterolateral thoracotomy a chest surgery technique in which entry to the chest is made with an incision below the breast but above the costal margins.

anteroposterior, from the front to the back of the body, commonly associated with the direction of the roentgenographic beam.

anteroposterior vaginal repair, a surgical procedure in which the upper and lower walls of the vagina are reconstructed to correct relaxed tissue.

anteversion, 1. the position of an organ in which the organ is tilted forward on its axis, away from the midline, as in uterine anteversion. **2.** (in dentistry) the tipping or the tilting of teeth or other mandibular structures more anteriorly than normal. **3.** the angulation created in the transverse plane between the neck and shaft of the femur.

anthelmintic, 1. of or pertaining to a substance that destroys or prevents the development of parasitic worms, such as filariae, flukes, hookworms, roundworms, schistosomes, tapeworms, threadworms, trichinae, and whipworms. **2.** an anthelmintic drug. An anthelmintic may interfere with parasites' carbohydrate metabolism, inhibit their respiratory enzymes, block their neuromuscular function, or render them susceptible to destruction by the host's macrophages.

anthracosis, a chronic lung disease occurring in coal miners, characterized by the deposit of coal dust in the lungs and the formation of black nodules on the bronchioles and resulting in focal emphysema.

anthracosis linguae. See *parasitic glossitis.*

anthrax, a disease affecting primarily farm animals (cattle, goats, pigs, sheep, and horses), caused by the bacterium *Bacillus anthracis.* Anthrax in animals is usually fatal. Humans most often acquire it when a break in the skin comes into direct contact with infected animals and their hides, or by inhaling the spores of the bacterium.

anthropoid pelvis, a type of pelvis in which the inlet is oval; the anteroposterior diameter is much greater than the transverse, and, because of the posterior inclination of the sacrum, the posterior portion of the space in the true pelvis is much greater than the anterior portion.

anthropometry, the science of measuring the human body as to height, weight, and size of component parts, including measurement of skinfolds, to study and compare the relative proportions under normal and abnormal conditions. **anthropometric,** *adj.*

antiadrenergic, 1. of or pertaining to the blocking of the effects of impulses transmitted by the adrenergic postganglionic fibres of the sympathetic nervous system. **2.** an antiadrenergic agent. Drugs which block the response to adrenergic stimulation by binding to adrenergic receptor sites are classified as alpha-blockers or beta-blockers, depending on which subset of receptors they bind to, and hence which effects of adrenergic stimulation they inhibit. Other antiadrenergic drugs may interfere with the synthesis or release of endogenous adrenaline or noradrenaline.

antianabolic, pertaining to drugs or other agents that inhibit or retard anabolic processes, such as cell division or the creation of new tissue by protein synthesis.

antianaemic, 1. of or pertaining to a substance or procedure that counteracts or prevents a deficiency of erythrocytes. **2.** an agent used to treat or to prevent anaemia.

antianginal drug, any medication that has the effect of dilating the coronary arteries, thereby improving the blood flow to the myocardium to prevent symptoms of angina pectoris.

antiantibody, an immunoglobulin formed as the result of the administration of an antibody that acts as an immunogen. The antiantibody then interacts with the antibody.

antianxiety agent. See **anxiolytic**.

antiarrhythmic, 1. of or pertaining to a procedure or substance that prevents, alleviates, or corrects an abnormal cardiac rhythm. **2.** an agent, usually a drug, used to treat a cardiac arrhythmia. The betaadrenergic blocking agent propranolol may be used in treating arrhythmias. Verapamil and other calcium antagonists control arrhythmias by inhibiting calcium ion influx across the cell membrane of cardiac muscle, thus slowing atrioventricular conduction and prolonging the effective refractory period within the atrioventricular node.

antibacterial, 1. of or pertaining to a substance that kills bacteria or inhibits their growth or replication. **2.** an antibacterial agent. Antibiotics synthesized chemically or derived from various microorganisms exert their bactericidal or bacteriostatic effect by interfering with the production of the bacterial cell wall, by interfering with protein synthesis, nucleic acid synthesis, or cell membrane integrity, or by inhibiting other critical biosynthetic pathways in the bacteria.

antiberiberi factor. See **thiamine**.

antibiotic, 1. of or pertaining to the ability to destroy or interfere with the development of a living organism. **2.** an antimicrobial agent, usually antibacterial, derived from cultures of a microorganism or produced semisynthetically, used to treat infections. The penicillins exert their action by inhibiting mucopeptide synthesis in bacterial cell walls. Aminoglycoside antibiotics interfere with the synthesis of bacterial proteins and are used primarily for the treatment of infections caused by gram-negative organisms. Macrolide antibiotics interfere with protein synthesis of susceptible bacteria without affecting nucleic acid synthesis. The

tetracyclines are primarily bacteriostatic and are thought to exert their effect by inhibiting bacterial protein synthesis. The cephalosporins inhibit bacterial cell wall synthesis. Chloramphenicol, a broad-spectrum antibiotic initially derived from *Streptomyces venezuelae,* inhibits bacterial protein synthesis.

antibiotic anticancer agent, a drug that has both antibiotic and anticancer activity, but which is used clinically for its anticancer effect. Examples include bleomycin, dactinomycin, daunorubicin, and mitomycin.

antibiotic sensitivity tests, a laboratory method for determining the susceptibility of bacterial infections to therapy with antibiotics. After the infecting organism has been recovered from a clinical specimen, it is cultured and tested against several antibiotic drugs. If the growth of the organism is inhibited by the action of the drug, it is reported as sensitive to that antibiotic.

antibody (Ab), an immunoglobulin, essential to the immune system, produced by lymphoid tissue in response to bacteria, viruses, or other antigenic substances. An antibody is specific to an antigen. Each class of antibody is named after its action. Among the many antibodies are agglutinins, bacteriolysins, opsonins, precipitin.

antibody absorption, the process of removing or tying up undesired antibodies in an antiserum reagent by allowing it to react with undesired antigens.

antibody instructive theory, a theory that each antigenic contact in the life of an individual develops a new antibody, as when an immunoglobulin-covered B cell comes in contact with an antigen and subsequently produces plasma cells and memory cells.

antibody specific theory, (in immunology) a theory of antibody formation proposed by F.M. Burnet, stating that preprogrammed, or precommitted, clones of lymphoid cells that are produced in the fetus are capable of interacting with a limited number of antigenic determinants with which the host may come in contact. The theory holds that the body contains an enormous number of diverse clones of cells, each genetically programmed to synthesize a different antibody.

antibromic. See **deodorant**.

anticancer diet, a diet, based on recommendations of the American Cancer Society (ACS), National Cancer Institute (NCI), and National Academy of Sciences, to reduce risk factors associated with eating habits. It includes a fat intake of not more that 30% of total calories and a daily intake of high-fibre foods.

anticholinergic, 1. of or pertaining to a blockade of acetylcholine receptors that results in the inhibition of the transsynaptic transmission of nerve impulses. **2.** an anticholinergic agent that functions by competing with the neurotransmitter acetylcholine for its receptor sites at synaptic junctions. Anticholinergic drugs reduce spasms of smooth muscle in the bladder, bronchi, and intestine; relax the iris sphincter; decrease gastric, bronchial, and salivary secretions; decrease perspiration; and accelerate impulse conduction through the myocardium by blocking vagal impulses.

anticholinergic agent. See **anticholinergic.**

anticholinesterase a drug that inhibits or inactivates the action of acetylcholinesterase. Drugs of this class cause acetylcholine to accumulate at the junctions of various cholinergic nerve fibres and their effector sites or organs, allowing potentially continuous stimulation of cholinergic fibres throughout the central and peripheral nervous systems. They are used as insectides, in the treatment of myasthenia gravis, and in reversing the action of non-depolarizing muscle relaxants.

anticipatory adaptation, the act of adapting to a potentially distressing situation before actually confronting the problem, as when a person tries to relax before learning the results of a medical examination.

anticipatory grief, feelings of grief that develop before, rather than after, the loss of a loved one.

anticipatory guidance, the psychological preparation of a patient to help relieve fear and anxiety of an event expected to be stressful, such as the preparation of a child for surgery by explaining what will happen.

anticoagulant, 1. of or pertaining to a substance that prevents or delays coagulation of the blood. **2.** an anticoagulant drug. Heparin, obtained from the liver and lungs of domestic animals, is a potent anticoagulant that interferes with the formation of thromboplastin, with the conversion of prothrombin to thrombin, and with the formation of fibrin from fibrinogen. Coumarin derivatives, such as warfarin, act as vitamin K antagonists and are active after oral administration.

anticoagulant therapy, treatment by anticoagulant drugs of conditions such as deep vein thrombosis.

anticodon, (in genetics) a sequence of three nucleotides in transfer RNA that pairs complementarily with a specific codon of messenger RNA during protein synthesis to specify a particular amino acid in the polypeptide chain.

anticonvulsant, 1. of or pertaining to a substance or procedure that prevents or reduces the severity of epileptic or other convulsive seizures. **2.** an anticonvulsant drug. Hydantoin derivatives, such as phenytoin, apparently exert their anticonvulsant effect by stabilizing the cell membrane and decreasing intracellular sodium, with the result

that the excitability of the epileptogenic focus is reduced. Carbamazepine, primidone, valproate and phenobarbitone are among the other drugs prescribed to limit or prevent seizures.

antideformity positioning and splinting, the use of splints, braces, or similar devices to prevent or control contractures or other musculoskeletal deformities that may result from disuse, burns, or other injuries.

antidepressant, 1. of or pertaining to a substance or a measure that prevents or relieves depression. **2.** an antidepressant agent. Tricyclic antidepressant agents block re-uptake of amine neuro~trans~mitters, but the exact mechanism of the antidepressant action is unknown. Monoamine oxidase (MAO) inhibitors increase the concentration of adrenaline, noradrenaline, and serotonin in storage sites in the nervous system. Specific serotonin reuptake inhibitors (SSRIs) prevent the reuptake of serotonin by neurons, increasing synaptic concentrations.

antidiarrhoeal, a drug or other agent that relieves the symptoms of diarrhoea. Antidiarrhoeals work by absorbing water from the digestive tract, by altering intestinal motility, by altering electrolyte transport, or by adsorption of toxins or microorganisms.

antidiuretic, 1. of or pertaining to the suppression of urine formation. **2.** an antidiuretic agent. Antidiuretic hormone (vasopressin), produced in hypothalamic nuclei and stored in the posterior lobe of the pituitary gland, suppresses urine formation by stimulating the resorption of water in distal tubules and collecting ducts of the kidneys. **antidiuresis,** *n.*

antidiuretic hormone (ADH), a hormone that decreases the production of urine by increasing the reabsorption of water by the renal tubules. ADH is secreted by cells of the hypothalamus and stored in the posterior lobe of the pituitary gland. It is released in response to a decrease in blood volume or an increased concentration of sodium or other substances in plasma, or by pain, stress, or the action of certain drugs.

antidote, a drug or other substance that opposes the action of a poison. An antidote may coat the stomach and prevent absorption, make the toxin inert, or oppose the action of the poison.

anti-D (RHo) immunoglobulin, a passive immunizing agent used to prevent Rh sensitization postabortion, postmiscarriage, postpartum and after ectopic pregnancy.

antidromic conduction, the conduction of a neural impulse backward from a receptor in the midportion of an axon. It is an unnatural phenomenon and may be produced experimentally.

antiembolism hose, elasticized stockings worn to prevent the formation of emboli and thrombi, especially in patients after surgery or those restricted to bed. Return flow of the venous circulation is promoted, preventing venous stasis and dilatation of the veins, conditions that predispose to varicosities and thromboembolic disorders.

antiemetic, 1. of or pertaining to a substance or procedure that prevents or alleviates nausea and vomiting. **2.** an antiemetic drug or agent. In motion sickness, hyoscine and antihistamines provide relief. In other situations, dopamine antagonists, such as domperidone and haloperidol, specific 5-HT3 antagonists, or corticosteroids, are more effective.

antiepileptic. See **anticonvulsant**.

antifebrile. See **antipyretic**.

antifungal, 1. of or pertaining to a substance that kills fungi or inhibits their growth or reproduction. **2.** an antifungal, antibiotic drug. Amphotericin B and ketoconazole, both effective against a broad spectrum of fungi, probably act by binding to sterols in the fungal cell membrane and changing the membrane's permeability. Griseofulvin, another broad-spectrum antifungal agent, binds to the host's new keratin and renders it resistant to further fungal invasion. Miconazole and clotrimazole inhibit the growth of common dermatophytes, including yeastlike *Candida albicans,* and nystatin is effective against yeast and yeastlike fungi.

antigalactic, pertaining to a drug or other agent that prevents or reduces milk secretion.

anti-GBM disease, an immunologically mediated kidney disorder involving the glomerular basement membrane (GBM), which is damaged in the antigen-antibody reaction. The kidney itself may serve as the antigenic target in the reaction.

antigen, a substance, usually a protein, that causes the formation of an antibody and reacts specifically with that antibody.

antigen-antibody reaction, a process of the immune system in which immunoglobulin-coated B cells recognize an intruder or antigen and stimulate antibody production to protect the body against infection. The T cells of the body assist in the antigen-antibody reaction, but the B cells play the key role. Antigen-antibody reactions activate the complement system of the body, amplifying the humoral immunity response of the B cells and causing lysis of the antigenic cells. Antigen-antibody reactions involve the binding of antigens to antibodies to form antigen-antibody complexes that may render the toxic antigen harmless, agglutinize antigens on the surface of microorganisms, or activate the complement system by exposing the complement-binding sites on the antibody molecule. Antigen-antibody reactions normally produce immunity, but they can also produce allergy,

autoimmunity, and fetomaternal haematological incompatibility. In immediate allergic reactions, antigens provoke the production of specific anti~bodies that may circulate freely in the serum or may become attached to specific cells. Autoimmunity makes it impossible for the immune system to distinguish between self and a foreign substance.

antigen determinant, a small area on the surface of an antigen molecule that fits a combining site of an antibody molecule and binds the antigen in the formation of an antigen-antibody complex. Antigen determinants commonly consist of a sequence of amino acids that decrees the shape of these reactive areas.

antigenicity the quality of causing the production of antibodies. The degree of antigenicity depends on the kind and amount of the particular substance, the condition of the host, and the degree to which the host is sensitive to the antigen and able to produce antibodies.

antigerminal pole. See **vegetal pole**.

antiglobulin, an antibody against human globulin, occurring naturally or prepared in laboratory animals. Specific antiglobulins are used in the detection of specific antibodies, as in blood typing.

antiglobulin test, a test for the presence of antibodies that coat and damage red blood cells as a result of any of several diseases or conditions. The test can detect Rh antibodies in maternal blood and is used to anticipate haemolytic disease of the newborn.

antigravity muscles, the muscle groups involved with stabilization of joints or other body parts by opposing the effects of gravity on the body.

antihaemophilic C factor. See **factor XI**.

antihaemophilic factor (AHF), blood factor VIII, a systemic haemostatic. It is prescribed in the treatment of haemophilia A, a deficiency of factor VIII.

antihaemorrhagic, any drug or agent used to prevent or control bleeding, such as thromboplastin or thrombin, either of which mediates the blood clotting process. Martindale

antihistamine, any substance capable of reducing the physiological and pharmacological effects of histamine, including a wide variety of drugs that block histamine receptors. Many such drugs are readily available as nonprescriptive medicines for the management of allergies. These substances do not stop the release of histamine, and the ways in which they act on the central nervous system (CNS) are not completely understood. The antihistamines are divided into H_1 and H_2 blockers depending on the responses to histamine they prevent. **antihistaminic,** *adj.*

antihypercholesterolaemic, a drug that prevents or controls an increase of cholesterol in the blood. Examples include clofibrate and colestipol.

antihypertensive, 1. of or pertaining to a substance or procedure that reduces high blood pressure. **2.** an antihypertensive agent. Various drugs achieve their antihypertensive effect by preventing the release of the pressor amine noradrenaline from peripheral nerves by blocking its postsynaptic effect; by a direct vasodilator action; by an action within the CNS; or by antagonizing angiotensin-converting enzyme (ACE) and reducing the production of the pressor substance angiotensin II. Thiazides and other diuretic agents reduce blood pressure by decreasing blood volume.

antiinfection vitamin. See **vitamin A**.

antiinflammatory, 1. of or pertaining to a substance or procedure that counteracts or reduces inflammation. **2.** an antiinflammatory drug or agent. The basis of the antiinflammatory effect of salicylates and nonsteroidal antiinflammatory agents, such as indomethacin, appears to involve inhibition of prostaglandin biosynthesis.

antiinitiator, a substance that is a potential co-carcinogen but that may protect cells against cancer development if given before exposure to an initiator.

antileprotic, a drug or other agent that is effective in treating leprosy.

antilipidaemic, 1. of or pertaining to a regimen, diet, or agent that reduces the amount of lipids in the serum. **2.** a drug used to reduce the amount of lipids in the serum.

antilymphocyte globulin (ALG), an antibody preparation used as an immunosuppressive agent in the treatment of rejection reactions in organ transplant recipients.

antimalarial, 1. of or pertaining to a substance that destroys or suppresses the development of malaria plasmodia or to a procedure that exterminates the mosquito vectors of the disease, such as spraying insecticides or draining swamps. **2.** an antimalarial drug that destroys or prevents the development of plasmodia in human hosts.

antimessage, a strand of RNA that cannot act as mRNA because of its negative coding sequence. It must be converted to a positive-strand sequence by a viral transcriptase before it can function as a messenger.

antimetabolite, a substance that resembles a normal human metabolite and interferes with its function in the body, usually by competing for the metabolite's receptors or enzymes.

antimicrobial, 1. of or pertaining to a substance that kills microorganisms or inhibits their growth or replication. **2.** an agent that kills or inhibits the growth or replication of microorganisms.

antimitochondrial antibody, an antibody

that acts specifically against mitochondria. These antibodies are not normally present in the blood of healthy people. A laboratory test for the presence of the antibodies in the blood is a valuable diagnostic aid in liver disease.

antimitotic, pertaining to the inhibition of cell division.

anti-Monson curve. See **reverse curve**.

antimony, a bluish, crystalline metallic element occurring in nature, both free and as salts. Various antimony compounds are used in the treatment of filariasis, leishmaniasis, lymphogranuloma, schistosomiasis, and trypanosomiasis and as an emetic.

antimony poisoning, poisoning caused by the ingestion or inhalation of antimony or antimony compounds, characterized by vomiting, sweating, diarrhoea, and a metallic taste in the mouth. Irritation of the skin or mucous membrane may result from external exposure. Severe poisoning resembles arsenic poisoning.

antimorph, a mutant gene that inhibits or antagonizes the normal influence of its allele in the expression of a trait.

antimuscarinic, inhibiting the stimulation of the postganglionic parasympathetic receptor.

antimutagen, 1. any substance that reduces the rate of spontaneous mutations or counteracts or reverses the action of a mutagen. **2.** any technique that protects cells against the effects of mutagenic agents. **antimutagenic,** *adj.*

antimycotic. See **antifungal**.

antineoplastic, 1. of or pertaining to a substance, procedure, or measure that prevents the proliferation of malignant cells. **2.** a drug that controls or kills cancer cells. Most drugs used in the treatment of cancer are cytotoxic but are generally more damaging to dividing cells than to resting cells. Cycle-specific antineoplastic agents are more effective in killing proliferating cells than in killing resting cells, and phase-specific agents are most active during a specific phase of the cell cycle. Most anticancer drugs prevent the proliferation of cells by inhibiting the synthesis of DNA by various mechanisms.

antineoplastic antibiotic. See **antibiotic anticancer agent**.

antineuritic vitamin. See **thiamine**.

antinuclear antibody (ANA), an autoantibody that reacts with nuclear material. Antinuclear antibodies are found in the blood serum of patients with rheumatoid arthritis, systemic lupus erythematosus, Sjögren's syndrome, polymyositis, and a number of nonrheumatic disorders.

antioestrogen drug, any of a group of drugs which prevent the production of oestrogens. They are most commonly used in the treatment of oestrogen-dependent cancers.

antioxidant, a chemical or other agent that inhibits or retards oxidation of a substance to which it is added. Examples include butylated hydroxyanisole (BHA) and butylated hydroxytoluene (BHT), which are added to foods containing fats or oils to prevent oxygen from combining with the fatty molecules, thereby causing them to become rancid.

antiparallel, (in molecular genetics) the condition in which molecules, such as strands of DNA, are parallel but point in opposite directions.

antiparasitic, 1. of or pertaining to a substance or procedure that kills parasites or inhibits their growth or reproduction. **2.** an antiparasitic drug including **amoebicides, anthelmintics, antimalarials, schistosomicides, trichomonacides,** and **trypanosomicides.**

antiparkinsonian, of or pertaining to a substance or procedure used to treat Parkinson's disease. Drugs for this neurological disorder are of two kinds: those that compensate for the lack of dopamine in the corpus striatum of parkinsonian patients, and anticholinergic agents that counteract the activity of the abundant acetylcholine in the striatum.

antiperistaltic, 1. of or pertaining to a substance that inhibits or diminishes peristalsis. **2.** an antiperistaltic agent. Opiates, such as codeine, morphine and loperamide hydrochloride, are antiperistaltic agents used to provide symptomatic relief in diarrhoea. Anticholinergic (parasympatholytic) drugs reduce spasms of intestinal smooth muscle and are frequently prescribed to decrease excessive GI motility.

antipernicious anaemia factor. See **cyanocobalamin.**

antiprotoplasmatic, pertaining to agents that damage the protoplasm of cells.

antipruritic, 1. of or pertaining to a substance or procedure that tends to relieve or prevent itching. **2.** an antipruritic drug. Topical anaesthetics, corticosteroids, and antihistamines are used as antipruritic agents.

antipsychotic, 1. of or pertaining to a substance or procedure that counteracts or diminishes symptoms of a psychosis. **2.** an antipsychotic drug. Phenothiazine derivatives are the most frequently prescribed antipsychotics for use in the treatment of schizophrenia and other major affective disorders.

antipyretic, 1. of or pertaining to a substance or procedure that reduces fever. **2.** an antipyretic agent. Such drugs act on the thermodetection set point of the hypothalamic heat regulatory centre, causing vasodilatation and sweating. Tepid sponging or a lukewarm bath may decrease an elevated temperature, and hypothermia produced by a cooling blanket is sometimes used for patients with a prolonged, high fever.

antipyretic bath, a bath in which tepid water is used to reduce the temperature of the body.

antirachitic, pertaining to an agent used to treat rickets.

antiscorbutic vitamin. See **ascorbic acid.**

antiseborrhoeic, pertaining to a drug or agent that is applied to the skin to control seborrhoea or seborrhoeic dermatitis.

antisense, (in molecular genetics) a strand of DNA containing the same sequence of nucleotides as messenger RNA (mRNA).

antisepsis, destruction of microorganisms to prevent infection.

antiseptic, 1. tending to inhibit the growth and reproduction of microorganisms. **2.** a substance that tends to inhibit the growth and reproduction of microorganisms.

antiseptic dressing, a dressing treated with an antiseptic, germicide, or bacteriostat, applied to a wound or an incision to prevent or treat infection.

antiseptic gauze, gauze permeated with an antiseptic solution, sometimes packaged in individual, sealed packets.

antiserum, *pl.* **antisera,** serum of an animal or human containing antibodies against a specific disease, used to confer passive immunity to that disease. Antisera do not provoke the production of antibodies. There are two types of antiserum. Antitoxic antiserum neutralizes the toxin produced by specific bacteria, but it does not kill the bacteria. Antimicrobial serum acts to destroy bacteria by making them more susceptible to the leukocytic action.

antiserum anaphylaxis, an exaggerated reaction of hypersensitivity in a normal person caused by the injection of serum from a sensitized individual.

antisialogogue, a drug that reduces saliva secretion.

antisocial personality, a person who exhibits attitudes and overt behaviour contrary to the customs, standards, and moral principles accepted by society.

antisocial personality disorder, a condition characterized by repetitive behavioural patterns that lack moral and ethical standards and bring a person into continuous conflict with society. Symptoms include aggressiveness, callousness, impulsiveness, irresponsibility, hostility, a low frustration level, a marked emotional immaturity, and poor judgment.

antisocial reaction. See **antisocial personality disorder.**

antispasmodic, a drug or other agent that prevents smooth muscle spasms, as in the uterus, digestive system, or urinary tract.

antistreptolysin-O test (ASOT, ASLT) a streptococcal antibody test for finding and measuring serum antibodies to streptolysin-

O, an exotoxin produced by most group A and some group C and G streptococci. The test is often used as an aid in the diagnosis of rheumatic fever.

antithermic. See **antipyretic.**

antithymocyte globulin (ATG) a gamma globulin fraction that has been rendered immune to T lymphocytes.

antithyroid drug, any one of several preparations that can inhibit the synthesis of thyroid hormones and which are commonly used in the treatment of hyperthyroidism. In the body such substances interfere with the incorporation of iodine into the hormones thyroxine and triiodothyronine.

antitoxins, a subgroup of antisera usually prepared from the serum of horses immunized against a particular bacterial toxin, such as botulinum toxin or tetanus toxin. They have been used in the passive immunization of unimmunized individuals exposed to risk of infection, but often provoke allergic reactions and have been mostly replaced by immunoglobulin preparations form pooled human donors.

antitrypsin, a protein, produced in the liver, that blocks the action of trypsin and other proteolytic enzymes.

antitubercular, any of a group of drugs used to treat tuberculosis. At least two drugs, and usually three, are required in combination in tuberculosis therapy.

antitussive, 1. against a cough. **2.** any of a large group of drugs that act on the central and peripheral nervous systems to suppress the cough reflex. Because the cough reflex is necessary for clearing the upper respiratory tract of obstructive secretions, antitussives should not be used with a productive cough.

antivenom, a preparation of venom-neutralizing antibodies prepared from the serum of immunized animals. Antivenoms confer passive immunity and are given as a part of emergency first aid for various snake and insect bites.

antiviral, 1. destructive to viruses. **2.** any of a group of drugs used to treat viral infections.

antivitamin, a substance that inactivates a vitamin.

antixerophthalmic vitamin. See **vitamin A.**

Anton's syndrome, a form of anosognosia in which a person with partial or total blindness denies being visually impaired, despite medical evidence to the contrary.

antral gastritis, an abnormal narrowing of the antrum, or distal portion of the stomach. The narrowing is not a true gastritis, but a radiographic finding that may represent a gastric ulcer or tumour.

antrum cardiacum, a constricted passage from the oesophagus to the stomach, lying just inside the opening formed by the cardiac sphincter.

antrum of Highmore. See **maxillary sinus.**

anular, describing a ring-shaped lesion surrounding a clear, normal, unaffected disc of skin.

anular ligament, a ligament that encircles the head of the radius and holds it in the radial notch of the ulna. Distal to the notch, the anular ligament forms a complete fibrous ring.

anulus, a ring of circular tissue, such as the whitish tympanic anulus around the perimeter of the tympanic membrane.

anuresis. See **anuria.**

anuria, the inability to urinate, the cessation of urine production, or a urinary output of less than 100 to 250 ml per day. Anuria may be caused by kidney failure or dysfunction, a decline in blood pressure below that required to maintain filtration pressure in the kidney, or an obstruction in the urinary passages. Although patients can live up to 2 weeks with anuria, death may occur within 24 hours of the total loss of urinary function. Kinds of anuria include **angioneurotic anuria, calculus anuria, obstructive anuria, postrenal anuria, prerenal anuria,** and **renal anuria. anuric, anuretic,** *adj.*

anus the opening at the terminal end of the anal canal.

anxiety, of a feeling of apprehension, uneasiness, agitation, uncertainty, and fear resulting from the anticipation of some threat or danger, usually of intrapsychic rather than external origin, whose source is generally unknown or unrecognized. Kinds of anxiety include castration anxiety, free-floating anxiety, separation anxiety, and situational anxiety.

anxiety attack, an acute, psychobiological reaction manifested by intense anxiety and panic. Symptoms vary according to the individual and the intensity of the attack but typically include palpitations, shortness of breath, dizziness, faintness, profuse sweating, pallor of the face and extremities, GI discomfort, and a vague feeling of imminent death.

anxiety disorder, a neurotic disorder characterized by persistent anxiety. The symptoms range from mild, chronic tenseness, with feelings of timidity, fatigue, apprehension, and indecisiveness, to more intense states of restlessness and irritability that may lead to aggressive acts or indecisiveness.

anxiety dream, a dream that occurs during rapid-eye-movement (REM) sleep and is accompanied by restlessness and a gradual increase in pulse rate.

anxiety hierarchy, a hierarchic or ranked relationship among various anxiety-producing stimuli.

anxiety management, individuals are encouraged to take control of disruptive phenomena within their lives by employing identified management strategies. These may include enhancing awareness of personal mental/physical responses and the practice of specific techniques e.g. relaxation training.

anxiolytic, a sedative or minor tranquillizer used primarily to treat episodes of anxiety. Kinds of anxiolytics include benzodiazepines, hydroxyzine and meprobamate.

aorta, the main trunk of the systemic arterial circulation, comprising of four parts: the ascending aorta, the arch of the aorta, the thoracic portion of the descending aorta, and the abdominal portion of the descending aorta. It starts at the aortic opening of the left ventricle, where it has a diameter of about 3 cm, rises a short distance toward the neck, bends to the left and dorsally over the root of the left lung, descends within the thorax on the left side of the vertebral column, and passes through the aortic hiatus of the diaphragm into the abdominal cavity.

aortic aneurysm, a localized dilatation of the wall of the aorta caused by atherosclerosis, hypertension, or, less frequently, syphilis. The lesion may be a saccular distention, a fusiform or cylindroid swelling of a length of the vessel, or a longitudinal dissection between the outer and middle layers of the vessel wall.

aortic arch. See **arch of the aorta.**

aortic arch syndrome, any of a group of occlusive conditions of the aortic arch producing a variety of symptoms related to obstruction of the large branch arteries, including the innominate, left common carotid, or left subclavian. Such conditions as atherosclerosis, Takayasu's arteritis, and syphilis may cause aortic arch syndrome.

aortic balloon pump. See **intraaortic balloon pump.**

aortic body, any of specialized nerve cells located in the arch of the aorta where they monitor levels of oxygen and hydrogen ions in the cardiovascular system.

aortic body reflex, a normal chemical reflex initiated by a decrease in oxygen concentration in the blood and, to a lesser degree, by increased carbon dioxide and hydrogen ion concentrations that act on chemoreceptors in the wall of the arch of the aorta and result in nerve impulses that cause the respiratory centre in the medulla to increase respiratory activity.

aortic regurgitation, the flow of blood from the aorta back into the left ventricle.

aortic stenosis, a cardiac anomaly characterized by a narrowing or stricture of the aortic valve because of congenital malformation or of fusion of the cusps, as may result from rheumatic fever. Aortic stenosis obstructs the flow of blood from the left ventricle into the aorta, causing decreased cardiac output and pulmonary vascular congestion.

aortic valve, a valve in the heart between the left ventricle and the aorta. It is composed of three semilunar cusps that close in diastole to prevent blood from flowing back into the left ventricle from the aorta.

aortitis, an inflammatory condition of the aorta, occurring most frequently in tertiary syphilis and occasionally in rheumatic fever. Kinds of aortitis are rheumatic aortitis and syphilitic aortitis.

aortography, a radiographic technique in which the aorta and its branches are injected with any of various contrast media for visualization. **aortogram,** *n.,* **aortographic,** *adj.*

aortopulmonary fenestration, a congenital anomaly characterized by an abnormal fenestration in the ascending aorta and the pulmonary artery cephalad to the semilunar valve, allowing oxygenated and unoxygenated blood to mix.

aosmic. See **anosmia.**

apareunia, an inability to perform sexual intercourse because of a physical or psychological sexual dysfunction.

apathetic hyperthyroidism, a form of thyrotoxicosis that tends to affect mainly older adults, who have stereotyped "senile" physical features and are apathetic and inactive rather than hyperkinetic in behaviour.

apathy, an absence or suppression of emotion, feeling, concern, or passion; an indifference to things found generally to be exciting or moving. **apathetic,** *adj.*

apatite, an inorganic mineral composed of calcium and phosphate that is found in the bones and teeth.

aperient, a mild laxative.

Apert's syndrome {Eugene Apert, French paediatrician, b. 1868}, a rare condition characterized by an abnormal craniofacial appearance in combination with partial or complete syndactyly of the hands and the feet.

aperture an opening or hole in an object or anatomical structure. See specific apertures.

aperture of frontal sinus, an external opening of the frontal sinus into the nasal cavity.

aperture of glottis, an opening between the true vocal cords and the arytenoid cartilages.

aperture of larynx, an opening between the pharynx and larynx.

aperture of sphenoid sinus, a round opening between the sphenoid sinus and nasal cavity, situated just above the superior nasal concha.

apex, *pl.* **apices,** the top, the end, or the tip of a structure, such as the apex of the heart or the apices of the teeth.

apex beat, a pulsation of the left ventricle of the heart, palpable and sometimes visible at the fifth intercostal space.

apex cordis, the pointed lower border of the heart. It is directed downward, forward, to the left, and usually located at the level of the fifth intercostal space.

apexification, (in dentistry) the process of induced tooth root development, or apical closure of the root by the deposit of hard tissue.

apexigraph, (in dentistry) a device used for determining the position of the apex of a tooth root.

apex pulmonis, the rounded upper border of each lung, projecting above the clavicle into the root of the neck.

Apgar score {Virginia Apgar, American anaesthetist, b. 1909}, a scoring system used to assess a baby's condition following birth. It is done at 1 minute, 5 minutes, and every 5 minutes thereafter if there is cause for concern. A score of 0 to 2 is given for each of five factors: respiratory effort, heart rate, muscle tone, colour and response to stimulation, thus the highest score possible is 10, indicating good condition.

aphagia, a condition characterized by the loss of the ability to swallow as a result of organic or psychological causes. A kind of aphagia is aphagia algera.

aphagia algera, a condition characterized by the refusal to eat or swallow because doing so causes pain.

aphakia, (in ophthalmology) a condition in which part or all of the crystalline lens of the eye is absent, usually because it has been surgically removed, as in the treatment of cataracts.   **aphakic, aphacic,** *adj.*

aphasia, an abnormal neurological condition in which language function is defective or absent because of an injury to certain areas of the cerebral cortex. The deficiency may be sensory or receptive, in which language is not understood, or expressive or motor, in which words cannot be formed or expressed.

aphemia, a loss of the ability to speak, applied to emotional disorders as well as neurological causes.

apheresis, a procedure in which blood is temporarily withdrawn, one or more components are selectively removed, and the remainder of the blood is reinfused into the donor. The process is used in treating various disease conditions in the donor and for obtaining blood elements for treating other patients or for research purposes.

aphonia, a condition characterized by loss of the ability to produce normal speech sounds because of overuse of the vocal cords, organic disease, or psychological causes, such as hysteria. Kinds of aphonia include aphonia paralytica and spastic aphonia. **aphonic, aphonous,** *adj.*

aphonia clericorum, a condition characterized by a loss of the voice from overuse.

aphonia paralytica, a condition characterized by a loss of the voice because of paralysis or disease of the laryngeal nerves.

aphonic speech, abnormal speech in which vocalizations are whispered.

aphoria, a condition in which physical weakness is not improved as a result of exercise.

aphrasia, a form of aphasia in which a person may be able to speak or understand single words but is not able to communicate with words that are arranged in meaningful phrases or sentences.

aphronia, (in psychiatry) a condition characterized by an impaired ability to make common-sense decisions.   **aphronic,** *n., adj.*

aphthous fever. See **foot-and-mouth disease.**

aphthous stomatitis, a recurring condition characterized by the eruption of painful ulcers (commonly called canker sores) on the mucous membranes of the mouth.

aphthous ulcer, oral ulceration characterised by painful and recurrent lesions which last for 10 to 14 days. Recurrent aphthae are classified as minor, major and herpetiform.

apical, 1. of or pertaining to the summit or apex. **2.** of or pertaining to the end of a tooth root.

apical curettage, (in dentistry) debridement of the apical surface of a tooth and removal of diseased soft tissues in the surrounding bony crypt.

apical fibre, any one of the many fibres of the periodontal ligament that radiate apically from tooth to bone.

apical lordotic view, a radiograph of the lungs achieved by positioning the patient leaning backward at an angle of approximately 45 degrees.

apical odontoid ligament, a ligament connecting the axis to the occipital bone. It extends from the process of the axis to the anterior margin of the foramen magnum.

apical pulse, the heartbeat as taken with the bell or disk of a stethoscope placed on the apex, or pointed extremity, of the heart.

apicectomy, the surgical removal of the apex or the apical portion of a tooth root, usually in conjunction with apical curettage or root canal therapy.

APKD, abbreviation for **adult polycystic disease**.

aplasia, 1. a developmental failure resulting in the absence of an organ or tissue. **2.** in haematology, a failure of the normal process of cell generation and development.

aplasia cutis congenita, the congenital absence of a localized area of skin. The defect is usually covered by a thin, translucent membrane or scar tissue, or it may be raw and ulcerated.

aplastic, 1. pertaining to the absence or defective development of a tissue or organ. **2.** failure of a tissue to produce normal daughter cells by mitosis.

aplastic anaemia, a deficiency of all of the formed elements of the blood, representing a failure of the cell-generating capacity of the bone marrow. It may be caused by neoplastic disease of the bone marrow or by destruction of the bone marrow by exposure to toxic chemicals, ionizing radiation, or medications.

apneustic breathing, a pattern of respirations

characterized by a prolonged inspiratory phase followed by expiration apnoea.

apneustic centre, an area of nerve tissue in the lower portion of the pons that controls the inspiratory phase of respiration.

apnoea, an absence of spontaneous respiration. Kinds of apnoea include cardiac apnoea, deglutition apnoea, periodic apnoea of the newborn, primary apnoea, reflex apnoea, secondary apnoea, and sleep apnoea. **apnoeic,** *adj.*

apocrine gland {Gk apo from, krinein to separate}, one of the large, deep exocrine glands located in the axillary, anal, genital, and mammary areas of the body. The apocrine glands become functional after puberty, and they secrete sweat.

apodial symmelia. See **sirenomelia.**

apoenzyme, an enzyme without any associated cofactors or with less than the entire amount of cofactors or prosthetic groups.

apogee, the climax of a disease or the period of greatest severity of signs and symptoms, usually followed by a crisis.

apolipoprotein, the protein component of lipoprotein complexes.

aponeurosis, *pl.* **aponeuroses,** a strong sheet of fibrous connective tissue that serves as a tendon to attach muscles to bone or as fascia to bind muscles together.

aponeurosis of the obliquus externus abdominis, the strong membrane that covers the entire ventral surface of the abdomen and lies superficial to the rectus abdominis. Fibres from both sides of the aponeurosis interlace in the midline to form the linea alba.

apophyseal, pertaining to an apophysis.

apophyseal fracture, a fracture that separates an apophysis of a bone from the main osseous tissue at a point of strong tendinous attachment.

apophysis, any small projection, process, or outgrowth, usually on a bone.

apophysitis, a condition characterized by the inflammation of an outgrowth or swelling, expecially a bony outgrowth that is not separated from the bone.

apoplexy, 1. obsolete. a cerebrovascular accident, resulting in paralysis. **2.** a haemorrhage within an organ. **apoplectic,** *adj.*

apoprotein, a polypeptide chain not yet complexed to its specific prosthetic group.

apothecaries' measure, a system of graduated liquid volumes originally based on the minim, formerly equal to one drop of water but now standardized to 0.06 ml; 60 minims equals 1 fluid dram, 8 fluid drams equals 1 fluid ounce, 16 fluid ounces equals 1 pint, 2 pints equals 1 quart, 4 quarts equals 1 gallon.

apothecaries' weight, a system of graduated amounts arranged in order of heaviness and based upon the grain, formerly equal to the weight of a plump grain of wheat but now standardized to 65 mg; 20 grains equals one scruple, 3 scruples equals 1 dram, 8 drams equals 1 ounce, 12 ounces equals 1 pound.

apoxesis. See **apical curettage.**

apparatus, a device or a system composed of different parts that act together to perform some special function, as the attachment apparatus or tissues that support the teeth.

apparent death. See **death.**

apparent focal spot, the area in an x-ray tube from which x-ray photons appear to be emitted. The smaller the apparent focal spot, the less the penumbra of the beam.

appendage, an accessory structure attached to another part or organ.

appendectomy, the surgical removal of the vermiform appendix through an incision in the right lower quadrant of the abdomen. The operation is performed in acute appendicitis to remove an inflamed appendix before it ruptures.

appendiceal, of or pertaining to the vermiform appendix. Also appendicial, appendical.

appendicitis, inflammation of the vermiform appendix, usually acute, which if undiagnosed leads rapidly to perforation and peritonitis. The most common symptom is constant pain in the right lower quadrant of the abdomen around McBurney's point, which the patient describes as having begun as intermittent pain in midabdomen. To decrease the pain, the patient keeps his knees bent to avoid tension of abdominal muscles. Appendicitis is characterized by vomiting, a low-grade fever of 37.2° to 39° C, an elevated white blood count, rebound tenderness, a rigid abdomen, and decreased or absent bowel sounds. Appendicitis is most apt to occur in teenagers and young adults and is more frequent in males.

appendix, *pl.* **appendixes, appendices, 1.** an accessory part of a main structure. **2.** See **vermiform appendix.**

appendix dyspepsia, an abnormal condition characterized by the impairment of the digestive function associated with chronic appendicitis.

appendix epididymidis, a cystic structure sometimes found on the head of the epididymis. It represents a remnant of the mesonephros.

appendix epiploica, *pl.* **appendices epiploicae,** one of the fat pads scattered through the peritoneum along the colon and the upper part of the rectum, especially along the transverse and the sigmoid parts of the colon.

appendix vermiformis. See **vermiform appendix.**

apperception, 1. mental perception or recognition. **2.** (in psychology) a conscious process of understanding or perceiving in terms of a person's previous knowledge, experiences, emotions, and memories. **apperceptive,** *adj.*

appliance, a device or instrument designed for a specific purpose, such as a dental orthodontic device.

application software, a computer program written to perform specific tasks or process particular kinds of information, such as payroll, inventory, or classification systems.

applied anatomy, the study of the structure and morphology of the organs of the body as it relates to the diagnosis and treatment of disease. Kinds of applied anatomy are pathological anatomy, radiological anatomy, and surgical anatomy.

applied chemistry, the application of the study of chemical elements and compounds to industry and the arts.

applied psychology, 1. the interpretation of historical, literary, medical, or other data according to psychological principles. **2.** any branch of psychology that emphasizes practical rather than theoretical approaches and objectives, such as clinical psychology, child psychology, industrial psychology, and educational psychology.

applied science. See **science.**

apposition, the placing of objects in close proximity, as in the layering of tissue cells or juxtapositioning facing surfaces side-by-side.

appositional growth, an increase in size by the addition of new tissue or similar material at the periphery of a particular part or structure, as in the addition of new layers in bone and tooth formation.

approach-approach conflict, a conflict resulting from the simultaneous presence of two or more incompatible impulses, desires, or goals, each of which is desirable.

approach-avoidance conflict, a conflict resulting from the presence of a single goal or desire that is both desirable and undesirable.

appropriate for gestational age infant, a newborn infant whose size, growth, and maturation are normal for gestational age, whether delivered prematurely, at term, or later than term.

approximate, to bring two tissue surfaces close together, as in the repair of a wound or to bring the bones of a joint together, as in physiotherapy.

approximation, (in psychiatry) the movement of one individual toward another in the development of an interpersonal relationship.

approximator, a medical instrument used to draw together the edges of divided tissues, as in closing a wound or in repairing a fractured rib.

apractognosia. See **constructional apraxia.**

apraxia, an impairment in the ability to perform purposeful acts or to manipulate objects. The condition is primarily neurological but occurs in several forms. Ideational apraxia is characterized by impairment caused by a loss of the perception of the use of an object. Motor apraxia is characterized by an inability to use an object or perform a task without any loss of perception of the use of the object or the goal of the task. Amnestic apraxia is characterized by an inability to perform the function because of an inability to remember the command to perform it. Apraxia of speech is an articulatory disorder caused by brain damage and resulting in an inability to programme the position of speech muscles and the sequence of muscle movements necessary to produce understandable speech. **apraxic,** *adj.*

aprosody, a speech defect characterized by the absence of the normal variations in pitch, intonation, and rhythm of word formation.

aprosopia, a congenital anomaly characterized by the absence of part or all of the facial structures. The condition is usually associated with other malformations.

aptitude, a natural ability, tendency, talent, or capability to learn, understand, or acquire a particular skill: mental alertness.

aptitude test, any of a variety of standardized tests for measuring an individual's ability to learn certain skills.

AQ, abbreviation for achievement quotient .

aqua amnii. See **amniotic fluid.**

aqueduct, any canal, channel, or passage through or between body parts, as the aqueduct of Sylvius in the brain.

aqueduct of Sylvius. See **cerebral aqueduct.**

aqueous, 1. watery or waterlike. **2.** a medication prepared with water.

aqueous humour, the clear, watery fluid circulating in the anterior and posterior chambers of the eye.

Ar, symbol for **argon.**

AR, abbreviation for **assisted respiration** .

arabinosylcytosine. See **cytarabine.**

arachidonic acid, an essential fatty acid that is a component of lecithin and a basic material for the biosynthesis of some prostaglandins .

arachnodactyly, a congenital condition of having long, thin, spiderlike fingers and toes, which is seen in Marfan's syndrome.

arachnoid, a delicate, fibrous structure resembling a cobweb or spiderweb, such as the arachnoid membrane. **arachnoidal,** *adj.*

arachnoidea encephali, the arachnoid membrane surrounding the brain.

arachnoidea spinalis, a continuation of the arachnoid membrane of the brain, extending along the spinal cord as far as the cauda equina with sheaths that cover the various spinal nerves as they pass outward to the intervertebral foramina.

arachnoid membrane, a thin, delicate membrane enclosing the brain and the spinal cord, interposed between the pia mater and the dura mater.

arachnoid of the brain. See **arachnoidea encephali.**

arachnoid of the spinal cord. See **arach-**

noidea spinalis.

Aran-Duchenne muscular atrophy [Francois A. Aran, French physician, b. 1817; Guillaume B. A. Duchenne, French neurologist, b. 1806]. a form of amyotrophic lateral sclerosis affecting the hands, arms, shoulders. and legs at the onset before becoming more generalized.

arbitrary inference, a form of cognitive distortion in which a judgement based on insufficient evidence leads to an erroneous conclusion.

arbitrator, an impartial person appointed to resolve a dispute between parties. **arbitration,** *n.*

arborization test. See **ferning test**.

arbovirus, any one of more than 300 arthropod-borne viruses that cause infections characterized by a combination of two or more of the following: fever, rash, encephalitis, and bleeding into the viscera or skin. Dengue, yellow fever, and equine encephalitis are abroviral infections.

ARC, abbreviation for **AIDS-related complex**.

arch, any anatomical structure that is curved or has a bowlike appearance.

arch bar, any one of various types of wires. bars, or splints that conform to the arch of the teeth, used in the treatment of fractures of the jaws and in the stabilization of injured teeth.

archenteric canal. See **neurenteric canal**.

archenteron, *pl.* **archentera,** the primitive digestive cavity formed by the invagination into the gastrula in the embryonic development of many animals. **archenteric,** *adj.*

archetype, 1. an original model or pattern from which a thing or group of things is made or evolves. **2.** (in analytical psychology) an inherited primordial idea or mode of thought derived from the experiences of the human race and present in the unconscious of the individual in the form of drives, moods, and concepts. **archetypal, archetypic, archetypical,** *adj.*

archiblastoma, *pl.* **archiblastomas, archiblastomata,** a tumour composed of cells derived from the layer of tissue surrounding the germinal vesicle.

archigaster. See **archenteron**.

archinephric canal, archinephric duct. See **pronephric duct**.

archinephron. See **pronephros**.

archistome. See **blastopore**.

architectural barriers, architectural features of homes and public buildings that limit access and mobility of disabled persons.

arch length, the length of a dental arch, usually measured through the points of contact between adjoining teeth.

arch length deficiency, the difference in any dental arch between the required length to accommodate all the natural teeth and the actual space available.

arch of the aorta, one of the four portions of the aorta, giving rise to three arterial branches called the innominate, left common carotid, and left subclavian arteries.

arch width, the width of a dental arch, which varies in all diameters between the left and right opposite teeth and is determined by direct measurement between the canines, the first molars, and the second premolars.

arch wire, an orthodontic wire fastened to two or more teeth through fixed attachments, used to cause or guide tooth movement.

arcing spring contraceptive diaphragm, a kind of contraceptive diaphragm in which the flexible metal spring that forms the rim is a combination of a flexible coil spring and a flat band spring made of stainless steel.

arcuate scotoma, an arc-shaped blind area that may develop in the field of vision of a glaucoma patient. It is caused by damage to nerve fibres in the retina.

arcus senilis, an opaque ring, grey to white in colour, that surrounds the periphery of the cornea. The condition is caused by deposits of fat granules in the cornea or hyaline degeneration and occurs primarily in older persons.

ARDS, abbreviation for **acute respiratory distress syndrome**.

area, (in anatomy) a limited anatomical space that contains a specific structure of the body or within which certain physiological functions predominate, such as the aortic area and the association areas of the cerebral cortex.

area under the concentration curve (AUC), a method of measurement of the bioavailability of a drug based on a plot of blood concentrations sampled at frequent intervals. It is directly proportional to the total amount of unaltered drug in the patient's blood.

areflexia, a neurologic condition characterized by the absence of the reflexes.

Arenavirus, a genus of viruses usually transmitted to humans by oral or cutaneous contact with the excreta of wild rodents. Individual arenaviruses are identified with specific geographical areas, such as Bolivian haemorrhagic fever, and Argentine haemorrhagic fever.

areola *pl.* **areolae, 1.** a small space or a cavity within a tissue. **2.** a circular area of a different colour surrounding a central feature, such as the discolouration about a pustule or vesicle. **3.** the part of the iris around the pupil.

areola mammae, the pigmented, circular area surrounding the nipple of each breast.

areolar gland, one of the large sebaceous glands in the areolae encircling the nipples on the breasts of women. The glands secrete a lipoid fluid that lubricates and protects the nipple.

ture-sensitive device that activates an alarm and automatically stops an intravenous infusion when infiltration of the intravenous fluid occurs. The device detects any cooling of the skin at the intravenous site, a common sign of infiltration.

automaticity, a property of specialized excitable tissue that allows self-activation through spontaneous development of an action potential, as in the pacemaker cells of the heart.

automatic mallet condenser. See **mechanical condenser**.

automatic speech, speech composed of or containing words or phrases spoken without voluntary control, often consisting of expletives, profanities, and greetings.

automation, use of a machine designed to follow repeatedly and automatically a predetermined sequence of individual operations.

automatism, 1. (in physiology) involuntary function of an organ system independent of apparent external stimuli, such as the beating of the heart, or dependent on external stimuli but not consciously controlled, such as the dilatation of the pupil of the eye. **2.** (in philosophy) the theory that the body acts as a machine and that the mind, whose processes depend solely on brain activity, is a noncontrolling adjunct of the body. **3.** (in psychology) mechanical, repetitive, and undirected behaviour that is not consciously controlled, as seen in psychomotor epilepsy, hysterical states, and such acts as sleepwalking. Kinds of automatism include ambulatory automatism, command automatism, and immediate posttraumatic automatism.

autonomic, 1. having the ability to function independently without outside influence. **2.** of or pertaining to the autonomic nervous system.

autonomic drug, any of a large group of drugs that mimic or modify the function of the autonomic nervous system.

autonomic dysreflexia, a dysreflexia that is the result of impaired function of the autonomic nervous system caused by simultaneous sympathetic and parasympathetic activity.

autonomic hyperreflexia, a neurological disorder characterized by a discharge of sympathetic nervous system impulses as a result of stimulation of the bladder, large intestine, or other visceral organs.

autonomic nervous system, the part of the nervous system that regulates involuntary vital function, including the activity of the cardiac muscle, the smooth muscle, and the glands. It has two divisions: The sympathetic nervous system accelerates heart rate, constricts blood vessels, and raises blood pressure; the parasympathetic nervous system slows heart rate, increases intestinal peristalsis and gland activity, and relaxes sphincters.

autonomic neuropathy, self-controlling, functionally independent disturbances in the peripheral nervous system.

autonomic reflex, any of a large number of normal reflexes governing and regulating the functions of the viscera. Autonomic reflexes control such activities of the body as blood pressure, heart rate, peristalsis, sweating, and urination.

autonomous bladder. See **flaccid bladder**.

autonomy, the quality of having the ability or tendency to function independently. **autonomous,** adj.

autonomy drive, a behavioural trait characterized by the attempt of an individual to master the environment and to impose the person's purposes on it.

autopentaploid, autopentaploidic. See **autopolyploid**.

autoplastic manoeuvre, (in psychology) a process that is part of adaptation, involving an adjustment within the self.

autoplasty, a plastic surgery procedure in which autografts, or parts of the patient's own tissues, are used to replace or repair body areas damaged by disease or injury.

autopolyploid, 1. also autopolyploidic. of or pertaining to an individual, organism, strain, or cell that has more than two genetically identical or nearly identical sets of chromosomes that are derived from the same ancestral species. **2.** such an individual, organism, strain, or cell.

autopolyploidy, the state or condition of having more than two identical or nearly identical sets of chromosomes.

autopsy, a postmortem examination performed to confirm or determine the cause of death. **autopsic, autopsical,** adj.

autopsy pathology, the study of disease by the examination of the body after death by a pathologist.

autoradiography, method to test the uniformity of radioactive material within a sealed source, where the source self-exposes an x-ray film.

autoserous treatment, therapy of an infectious disease by inoculating the patient with the patient's own serum.

autosite, the larger, more normally formed member of unequal or asymmetrical, conjoined twins on whom the other smaller fetus depends for various physiological functions and for nutrition and growth. **autositic.** adj.

autosomal, 1. pertaining to or characteristic of an autosome. **2.** pertaining to any condition transmitted by an autosome.

autosomal dominant inheritance, a pattern of inheritance in which the transmission of a dominant gene on an autosome causes a characteristic to be expressed. Affected individuals have an affected parent unless the condition is the result of a fresh mutation. Half of the children of a heterozygous affected parent are affected. All of the children of a homozygous affected parent are affected.

autosomal inheritance, a pattern of inheritance in which the transmission of traits depends on the presence or absence of certain genes on the autosomes. The pattern may be dominant or recessive. Kinds of autosomal inheritance are autosomal dominant inheritance and autosomal recessive inheritance.

autosomal recessive inheritance, a pattern of inheritance in which the transmission of a recessive gene on an autosome results in a carrier state if the person is heterozygous for the trait and in the affected state if the person is homozygous for the trait. One fourth of the children of two unaffected heterozygous parents are affected. All of the children of two homozygous affected parents are affected.

autosome, any chromosome that is not a sex chromosome and that appears as a homologous pair in the somatic cell. Humans have 22 pairs of autosomes, which are involved in transmitting all genetic traits and conditions other than those that are sex-linked.

autosplenectomy, a progressive shrinking of the spleen that may occur in sickle cell anaemia. The spleen is replaced by fibrous tissue and becomes nonfunctional.

autosuggestion, an idea, thought, attitude, or belief suggested to oneself, often as a formula or incantation, as a means of controlling one's behaviour.

autotetraploid, autotetraploidic. See **autopolyploid**.

autotopagnosia, the inability to recognize or localize the various parts of the body because of organic brain damage.

autotransfusion, the collection, anticoagulation, filtration, and reinfusion of blood from an active bleeding site. It may be used in cases of major trauma or in major surgery when blood can be collected from a sterile site.

autotriploid, autotriploidic. See **autopolyploid**.

autumn fever. See **leptospirosis**.

auxanology, the scientific study of growth and development. **auxanological,** *adj.*

auxesis, *pl.* **auxeses,** an increase in size or volume because of cell expansion rather than of an increase in the number of cells or tissue elements; hypertrophy. **auxetic,** *adj., n.*

auxilliary enzyme, in a coupled assay system, an enzyme that links the enzyme being measured with an indicator enzyme.

auxiliary storage, a storage device for adding to the main storage of the computer, employing such media as floppy disks, hard disks, cassette tapes, magnetic tapes, or cartridge tapes.

available arch length, the length or space in a dental arch that is available for all the natural teeth of an individual.

avantin. See **isopropyl alcohol**.

avascular, 1. (of a tissue area) not receiving a sufficient supply of blood. **2.** (of a kind of tissue) not having blood vessels.

aversion therapy, a form of behaviour therapy in which punishment or unpleasant or painful stimuli, such as electric shock or drugs that induce nausea, are used in the suppression of undesirable behaviour.

aversive stimulus, a stimulus, such as electric shock, that causes psychological or physical pain.

avidin, a glycoprotein in raw egg white with strong affinity for biotin.

avidity, a measure of the binding strength of antibodies to multiple antigenic determinants on natural antigens.

avitaminosis, a condition resulting from a deficiency of or the lack of absorption or use of one or more essential vitamins in the diet.

AV nicking, a vascular abnormality on the retina of the eye, visible on ophthalmological examination, in which a vein is compressed by an arteriovenous crossing. The vein appears "nicked," because of constriction or spasm.

Avogadro's law {Count Amedeo Avogadro, Italian physicist, b. 1776}, a law in physics stating that equal volumes of all gases at a given temperature and pressure contain the identical number of molecules.

avoidance, (in psychiatry) a conscious or unconscious defence mechanism, physical or psychological, by which an individual tries to avoid or escape from unpleasant stimuli, conflicts, or feelings, such as anxiety, fear, pain, or danger.

avoidance-avoidance conflict, a conflict resulting from the confrontation of two or more alternative goals or desires that are equally aversive and undesirable.

avoidance conditioning, the establishment of certain patterns of behaviour to avoid unpleasant or painful stimuli.

avoidant personality, a personality disorder characterized by hypersensitivity to rejection and a reluctance to start a relationship because of a fear of not being accepted uncritically.

avoirdupois weight, the system of weights in which there are 7000 grains, 256 drams, or 16 ounces to 1 pound. One ounce in this system equals 28.35 g, and 1 pound equals 453.59 g.

avulsed teeth, teeth that have been forcibly displaced from their normal position. Also spelled evulsed teeth.

avulsion, the separation, by tearing, of any part of the body from the whole, such as an umbilical cord torn in the process of delivering the placenta. **avulse,** *v.*

avulsion fracture, a fracture caused by the tearing away of a fragment of bone where a strong ligamentous or tendinous attachment forcibly pulls the fragment away from osseous tissue.

awake anaesthesia, an anaesthetic procedure in which analgesia and anaesthesia are accomplished without loss of consciousness and the concomitant need for life support equipment, personnel, and expertise. Dental procedures and certain kinds of surgery are performed using awake anaesthesia.

awareness context of death, the awareness by a terminally ill patient that he or she is dying and the awareness of the patient's knowledge by the nurse or other health professionals caring for the person.

AWOL, abbreviation for **absent without leave.**

axetil, a contraction for 1-acetoxyethyl.

axial (A), **1.** pertaining to or situated on the axis of a structure or part of the body. **2.** (in dentistry) relating to the long axis of a tooth.

axial current, the central part of the blood current.

axial gradient, **1.** the variation in metabolic rate in different parts of the body. **2.** the development toward the body axis or its parts in relation to the metabolic rate in the various parts.

axial illumination. See **illumination.**

axial neuritis. See **parenchymatous neuritis.**

axial spillway, a groove that crosses a cusp ridge or a marginal ridge and extends onto an axial surface of a tooth.

axilla, *pl.* **axillae,** a pyramid-shaped space forming the underside of the shoulder between the upper part of the arm and the side of the chest.

axillary anaesthesia. See **brachial plexus anaesthesia.**

axillary artery, one of a pair of continuations of the subclavian arteries that starts at the outer border of the first rib and ends at the distal border of the teres major, where it becomes the brachial artery.

axillary nerve, one of the last two branches of the posterior cord of the brachial plexus before the posterior cord becomes the radial nerve.

axillary node, one of the lymph glands of the axilla that help fight infections in the chest, armpit, neck, and arm and drain lymph from those areas. The 20 to 30 axillary nodes are divided into the lateral group, the anterior group, the posterior group, the central group, and the medial group.

axillary vein, one of a pair of veins of the upper limb that begins at the junction of the basilic and the brachial veins near the distal border of the teres major and becomes the subclavian vein at the outer border of the first rib.

axis, *pl.* **axes,** **1.** (in anatomy) a line that passes through the centre of the body, or a part of the body, such as the frontal axis, binauricular axis, and basifacial axis. **2.** the second cervical vertebra about which the atlas rotates, allowing the head to be turned, extended, and flexed.

axis artery, one of a pair of extensions of the subclavian arteries, running into and supplying the upper limb, continuing into the forearm as the palmar interosseous artery.

axis cylinder. See **axon.**

axis traction, the process of pulling the fetal head with obstetric forceps in a direction in line with the path of least resistance, following the curve of Carus through the mother's birth canal.

axoaxonic synapse, a type of synapse in which the axon of one neuron comes in contact with the axon of another neuron.

axodendritic synapse, a type of synapse in which the axon of one neuron comes in contact with the dendrites of another neuron.

axodendrosomatic synapse, a type of synapse in which the axon of one neuron comes in contact with both the dendrites and the cell body of another neuron.

axon, the cylindrical extension of a nerve cell that conducts impulses away from the neuron cell body. Axons may be bare or sheathed in myelin.

axon flare, vasodilatation, reddening, and increased sensitivity of skin surrounding an injured area, caused by an axon reflex.

axonotmesis, an interruption of the axon with subsequent wallerian degeneration of the distal nerve segment.

axoplasmic flow, the continuous pulsing, undulating movement of the cytoplasm between the cell body of a neuron, where protein synthesis occurs, and the axon fibre to supply it with the substances vital for the maintenance of activity and for repair.

axosomatic synapse, a type of synapse in which the axon of one neuron comes in contact with the cell body of another neuron.

azatadine maleate, an antihistamine with antiserotoninergic, anticholinergic, and sedative effects used in the treatment of allergic rhinitis and chronic urticaria.

azathioprine, an immunosuppressant used to prevent organ rejection after transplantation and in the treatment of lupus erythematosus and other systemic inflammatory diseases.

azidothymidine (AZT). See **zidovudine.**

azlocillin, a semisynthetic penicillin antibiotic used for lower respiratory tract, urinary tract, skin, and bone and joint infections and bacterial septicaemia caused by susceptible strains of microorganisms, mainly *Pseudomonas aeruginosa.*

azo dye, a type of nitrogen-containing compound used in commercial colouring materials. Some forms of the chemical are potential carcinogens.

azoospermia, lack of spermatozoa in the semen. It may be caused by testicular dysfunction or by blockage of the tubules of the epididymis, or it may be induced by vasectomy.

azotaemia, the retention in the blood of excessive amounts of nitrogenous compounds. The condition is caused by failure of the kidneys to remove urea from the blood. **azotaemic,** *adj.*

AZT, abbreviation for **azidothymidine.**

azul, azula. See **pinta.**

azygos. See **azygous.**

azygospore, a spore that is produced directly from a gamete that does not undergo conjugation, as in certain algae and fungi.

azygous, occurring as a single entity or part, such as any unpaired anatomical structure; not part of a pair. Also azygos. **azygos,** n.

azygous lobe, a congenital anomaly of the lung caused by a fold of pleural tissue carried by the azygous vein during descent into the thorax during embryonic development. This produces an extra lobe in the right upper lung.

azygous vein, one of the seven veins of the thorax. Beginning opposite the first or second lumbar vertebra, it ends in the superior vena cava.

B

B, symbol for boron.

Ba, symbol for barium.

BA, abbreviation for Bachelor of Arts.

babbling, a stage in speech development characterized by the production of strings of speech sounds in vocal play.

Babcock's operation {William W. Babcock, American surgeon, b. 1872}, the extirpation of a varicosed saphenous vein by inserting an acorn-tipped sound, tying the vein to the sound, and drawing it out.

babesiosis {Victor Babés, Rumanian bacteriologist, b. 1854}, an infection caused by protozoa of the genus *Babesia*. The infective organism is introduced into the host through the bite of ticks of the species *Ixodes dammini*.

Babinski's reflex {Josef F.F. Babinski, French neurologist, b. 1857}, dorsiflexion of the big toe with extension and fanning of the other toes elicited by firmly stroking the lateral aspect of the sole of the foot. The reflex is normal in newborn infants and abnormal in children and adults.

baby, 1. an infant or young child, especially one who is not yet able to walk or talk. **2.** to treat gently or with special care.

Baby Fae, a pseudonym for a human infant who received the first transplant of a baboon heart. The procedure occurred at Loma Linda University Medical Centre in California in October 1984. The recipient, an infant girl, was born with hypoplastic left heart syndrome (HLHS). Death 20 days later was attributed to progressive graft necrosis, complicated by acute renal and pulmonary insufficiency.

baby talk, 1. the speech patterns and sounds of young children learning to talk, characterized by mispronunciation, imperfect syntax, repetition, and phonetic modifications, such as lisping or stuttering. **2.** the intentionally oversimplified manner of speech, imitative of young children learning to talk, used by adults in addressing children or pets. **3.** the speech patterns characteristic of regressive stages of various mental disorders, especially schizophrenia.

bacampicillin hydrochloride, a semi-synthetic penicillin prescribed in the treatment of respiratory tract, urinary tract, skin, and gonococcal infections.

Bachelor of Nursing (BN), an academic degree awarded on satisfactory completion of a 3- or 4-year course of study in a university or college of higher education. The recipient also qualifies as a registered nurse.

Bacillaceae, a family of *Schizomycetes* of the order *Eubacteriales,* consisting of grampositive, rod-shaped cells that can produce cylindrical, ellipsoid, or spherical endospores. Some are parasitic on insects and animals and are pathogenic.

bacillary dysentery. See **shigellosis.**

Bacillus Calmette-Guérin (BCG) {Léon C.A. Calmette, French bacteriologist, b. 1863; Camille Guérin, French bacteriologist, b. 1872}, an attenuated strain of tubercle bacilli, used in many countries as a vaccine against tuberculosis, most often administered intradermally, with a multiple-puncture disc. It appears to prevent the more serious forms of tuberculosis and to give some protection to persons living in areas where tuberculosis is prevalent.

bacilliform, rod-shaped, like a bacillus.

bacilluria, the presence of bacilli in the urine.

Bacillus, a genus of aerobic, gram-positive spore-producing bacteria in the family Bacillaceae, order Eubacteriales, including 33 species, three of which are pathogenic.

Bacillus anthracis, a species of gram-positive, facultative anaerobe that causes anthrax.

bacillus Calmette-Guérin vaccine. See **BCG vaccine.**

back, the posterior portion of the trunk of the body between the neck and the pelvis. The back is divided by a middle furrow that lies over the tips of the spinous processes of the vertebrae. The upper cervical vertebrae cannot be felt in this furrow, but the seventh cervical vertebra is easily distinguished just above the more prominent first thoracic vertebra. The skeletal portion of the back includes the thoracic and the lumbar vertebrae and both scapulas. The root of the spine of the scapula is on a level in the back with the spine of the third thoracic vertebra, and the inferior angle of the scapula is on a level with the spine of the seventh thoracic vertebra.

backache, pain in the lumbar, lumbosacral, or cervical regions of the back, varying in sharpness and intensity. Causes may include muscle strain or other muscular disorders or pressure on the root of a nerve, such as the sciatic nerve, caused in turn by a variety of factors, including a ruptured vertebral disc. Treatment may include heat, ultrasound, devices to provide support for the affected area, bed rest, surgical intervention, and medications to relieve pain and relax spasm of the muscle of the affected area.

back-action condenser, (in dentistry) an instrument for compacting amalgams that has a U-shaped shank to develop the condensing force from a pulling motion rather than the more common pushing motions.

backcross, 1. (in genetics) the cross of a first filial generation hybrid with one of the parents or with a genotype that is identical to the parental strain. **2.** the organism or strain produced by such a cross.

background radiation, naturally occurring radiation emitted by materials in the soil, ground waters, and building material, radioactive substances in the body, especially potassium 40 (^{40}K), and cosmic rays from outer space. Each year the average person is exposed to 300 µSv of cosmic radiation, 400 µSv from rocks and soils, 800 µ inhaled (radon-222), 370 µSv ingested from food and drink and 250 µSv from medical exposures. This gives a total average annual exposure of 2.15 µSv.

back pressure, pressure that builds in a vessel or a cavity as fluid is accumulated.

backscatter radiation. See scattered radiation.

backtracking, a communication technique in which patient and therapist review what has been discussed previously to regain focus.

backup, a duplicate computer, data file, equipment, or procedure for use in the event of failure of storage media or of components.

backward failure, cardiac failure marked by elevated venous pressure and diminished arterial pressure. It develops when the ventricle cannot empty and the blood backs up in the pulmonary veins and the lungs, causing pulmonary oedema.

baclofen, an antispastic agent prescribed for the alleviation of spasticity.

bacteraemia, the presence of bacteria in the blood. **bacteraemic,** *adj.*

bacteraemic shock. See septic shock.

bacteria, *sing.* bacterium, any of the small unicellular microorganisms of the class Schizomycetes. The genera vary morphologically, being spherical (cocci), rod-shaped (bacilli), spiral (spirochetes), or comma-shaped (vibrios).

bacterial aneurysm, a localized dilatation in the wall of a blood vessel caused by the growth of bacteria, often following septicaemia or bacteraemia and usually occurring in peripheral vessels.

bacterial endocarditis, an acute or subacute bacterial infection of the endocardium or the heart valves or both. The condition is characterized by heart murmur, prolonged fever, bacteraemia, splenomegaly, and embolism.

bacterial food poisoning, a toxic condition resulting from the ingestion of food contaminated by certain bacteria. Acute infectious gastroenteritis caused by various species of *Salmonella* is characterized by fever, chills, nausea, vomiting, diarrhoea, and general discomfort beginning 8 to 48 hours after ingestion and continuing for several days. Food poisoning caused by the neurotoxin of *Clostridium botulinum* is characterized by GI symptoms, disturbances of vision, weakness or paralysis of muscles, and, in severe cases, respiratory failure.

bacterial kinase, 1. a kinase of bacterial origin. **2..** a bacterial enzyme that activates plasminogen, the precursor of plasmin.

bacterial meningitis. See meningitis.

bacterial plaque, a film comprised of microorganisms and mucoprotein which forms on all surfaces, teeth, soft tissues and oral appliances, and which can be removed by brushing. It is the major cause of periodontal disease and is responsible for breaking down sugars into acids.

bacterial protein, a protein produced by a bacterium.

bacterial resistance, the ability of certain strains of bacteria to develop a tolerance toward specific antibiotics.

bactericidal, destructive to bacteria.

bactericidin, an antibody that kills bacteria in the presence of complement.

bacteriological sputum examination, a laboratory procedure to determine the presence or absence of bacteria in a specimen of a patient's sputum. Part of the specimen is examined microscopically and part is mixed with culture media and allowed to incubate for more specific examination later.

bacteriologist, a specialist in bacteriology.

bacteriology, the scientific study of bacteria. **bacteriological,** *adj.*

bacteriolysin, an antibody that causes the breakdown of a particular species of bacterial cell.

bacteriolysis, the breakdown of bacteria intracellularly or extracellularly. **bacteriolytic,** *adj.*

bacteriophage, any virus that causes lysis of host bacteria, including the blue-green "algae." Bacteriophages resemble other viruses in that each is composed of either ribonucleic acid or deoxyribonucleic acid. **bacteriophagic,** *adj.*, **bacteriophagy,** *n.*

bacteriophage typing, the process of identifying a species of bacteria according to the type of virus that attacks it.

bacteriostatic, tending to restrain the development or the reproduction of bacteria.

bacteriuria, the presence of bacteria in the urine.

bacteroid, 1. of, pertaining to, or resembling bacteria. **2.** a structure that resembles a bacterium. Also **bacterioid. bacteroidal, bacterioidal,** *adj.*

Bacteroides, a genus of obligate anaerobic bacilli normally found in the colon, mouth, genital tract, and upper respiratory system.

Severe infection may result from the invasion of the bacillus through a break in the mucous membrane.

BAEP, abbreviation for **brainstem auditory-evoked potential**.

bag, a flexible or dilatable sac or pouch designed to contain gas, fluid, or semisolid material such as crushed ice. Several types of bags are used in medical or surgical procedures to dilate the anus, vagina, or other body openings.

bagasse, the crushed fibres or the residue of sugar cane.

bagassosis, a self-limited lung disease caused by an allergic response to bagasse, the fungi-laden, dusty debris left after the syrup has been extracted from sugar cane.

bagging, *informal.* the artificial respiration performed with a ventilator or respirator bag, such as an Ambu bag or Hope resuscitator. The bag is squeezed to deliver air to the patient's lungs as the mask is held over the mouth.

bag of waters. the membranous sac of amniotic fluid surrounding the fetus in the uterus of a pregnant woman. See **amnion.**

Bain Breathing Circuit, a continuous-flow anaesthetic system that does not require a soda-lime absorber.

Bainbridge reflex {Francis A. Bainbridge, English physiologist, b. 1874}, a cardiac reflex consisting of an increased pulse rate, resulting from stimulation of stretch receptors in the wall of the left atrium.

Baker's cyst, a cyst that forms at the back of the knee. It is often associated with rheumatoid arthritis and may appear only when the leg is straightened.

BAL, abbreviation for **British anti-lewisite.** See **dimercaprol.**

balance, 1. an instrument for weighing. **2.** a normal state of physiological equilibrium. **3.** a state of mental or emotional equilibrium. **4.** to bring into equilibrium.

balanced anaesthesia, *informal.* one of a number of variable techniques of general anaesthesia in which no single anaesthetic agent or preset proportion of the combination of agents is used; rather, an individualized mixture of anaesthetics is prescribed according to the needs of a particular patient for a particular operation.

balanced articulation, the simultaneous contacting of the upper and lower teeth as they glide over each other when the mandible is moved from centric relation to various eccentric relations.

balanced diet, a diet containing all of the essential nutrients that cannot be synthesized in adequate quantities by the body, in amounts adequate for growth, energy needs, nitrogen equilibrium, repair of wear, and maintenance of normal health.

balanced occlusion, 1. an occlusion of the teeth that presents a harmonious relation of the occluding surfaces in centric and eccentric positions within the functional range of mandibular positions and tooth size. **2.** the simultaneous contacting of the upper and lower teeth on both sides and in the anterior and posterior occlusal areas of the jaws.

balanced polymorphism, in a population, the recurrence of an equalized mixture of homozygotes and heterozygotes for specific genetic traits, which are maintained from generation to generation by the forces of natural selection.

balanced suspension, a system of splints, ropes, slings, pulleys, and weights for suspending the lower extremities of the body, used as an aid to healing and recuperation from fractures or from surgical operations.

balanced traction, a system of balanced suspension that supplements traction in the treatment of fractures of the lower extremities or after various operations affecting the lower parts of the body.

balanced translocation, the transfer of segments between nonhomologous chromosomes in such a way that there are changes in the configuration and total number of chromosomes, but each cell or gamete contains no more and no less than the normal amount of diploid or haploid genetic material.

balancing factors, events that contribute to the production and outcome of a crisis.

balancing side, (in dentistry) the side of the mouth opposite the working side of a dentition or denture.

balanic, of or pertaining to the glans penis or the glans clitoridis.

balanitis, inflammation of the glans penis.

balanitis xerotica obliterans, a chronic skin disease of the penis, characterized by a white indurated area surrounding the meatus.

balanoplasty, an operation involving plastic surgery of the glans penis.

balanoposthitis, a generalized inflammation of the glans penis and prepuce, characterized by soreness, irritation, and discharge, occurring as a complication of bacterial or fungal infection.

balanopreputial, of or pertaining to the glans penis and the prepuce.

balanorrhagia, balanitis in which pus is discharged copiously from the penis.

balantidiasis, an infection caused by ingestion of cysts of the protozoan *Balantidium coli.* In some cases the organism is a harmless inhabitant of the large intestine, but infection with *B. coli* usually causes diarrhoea.

Balantidium coli, the largest and the only ciliated protozoan species that is pathogenic to humans, causing balantidiasis.

baldness, absence of hair, especially from the scalp.

Balkan frame, an overhead rectangular frame, attached to the bed of an orthopaedic patient, for use in attaching splints, suspending or changing the position of immobilized limbs, and for continuous traction involving weights and pulleys.

Balkan tubulointerstitial nephritis, a chronic kidney disorder marked by renal insufficiency, proteinuria, tubulointerstitial nephritis, and anaemia. The disease is endemic in the Balkans but is not hereditary.

ball, a relatively spherical mass, such as one of the chondrin balls imbedded in hyaline cartilage.

ball-and-socket joint, a synovial joint in which the globular head of an articulating bone is received into a cuplike cavity, such as in hip and shoulder joints.

ballism, an abnormal neuromuscular condition characterized by uncoordinated swinging of the limbs and jerky movements.

ballismus, an abnormal condition characterized by violent flailing motions of the arms and, occasionally, the head, resulting from injury to the subthalamic nucleus. Hemiballismus is a unilateral form of the condition. The term may be used interchangeably with ballism.

ballistic movement, a high-velocity musculoskeletal movement, such as a tennis serve, requiring reciprocal organization of agonistic and antagonistic synergies.

ballistocardiogram, a record of the motion of the body caused by the thrust of the heart during systolic ejection of the blood into the aorta and the pulmonary arteries. The ballistocardiogram is a sensitive tool that is useful in measuring cardiac output and the force of contraction of the heart.

ball of the foot, the part of the foot composed of the heads of the metatarsals and their surrounding fatty fibrous tissue pad.

balloon angioplasty, a method of dilating or reopening an obstructed blood vessel by threading a small catheter, followed by a balloon, into the vessel. The balloon is then inflated to widen the blood vessel.

balloon septostomy. See **Rashkind procedure.**

balloon-tip catheter, a catheter bearing a nonporous inflatable sac around its distal end. After insertion of the catheter the sac can be inflated with air or sterile water, introduced via injection into a special port at the proximal end of the catheter. Kinds of balloon-tip catheters include **Foley catheter, Swan-Ganz catheter.**

ballottable head, a fetal head that has not descended or become fixed in the maternal bony pelvis. The fetal head is given a sharp tap on one side and is felt to bounce to the other side by examining fingers.

ballottement, a technique of palpating an organ or floating structure by bouncing it gently and feeling it rebound.

ball thrombus, a relatively round, coagulated mass of blood, containing platelets, fibrin, and cellular fragments, that may obstruct a blood vessel or an orifice, usually the mitral valve of the heart.

ball-valve action, the intermittent opening and closing of an orifice by a buoyant, ball-shaped mass, which acts as a valve. Some kinds of objects that may act in this manner are kidney stones, gallstones, and blood clots.

balm, 1. a healing or a soothing substance, such as any of various medicinal ointments. **2.** an aromatic plant of the genus *Melissa* that relieves pain.

balsam, any of a variety of aromatic resinous saps, generally from evergreens, usually containing benzoic or cinnamic acid, and used as ingredients in inhalants.

bamboo spine, the characteristically rigid spine of advanced ankylosing spondylitis.

band {ME *bande* strip}, **1.** (in anatomy) a bundle of fibres, as seen in striated muscle, that encircles a structure or binds one part of the body to another. **2.** (in dentistry) a strip of metal that fits around a tooth and serves as an attachment for orthodontic components. **3.** *informal.* the immature form of a segmented granulocyte characterized by a sausage-shaped nucleus.

band adapter, an instrument for aiding in the fitting of an orthodontic band to a tooth.

bandage, 1. a strip or roll of cloth or other material that may be wound around a part of the body in a variety of ways to secure a dressing, maintain pressure over a compress, or immobilize a limb or other part of the body. **2.** to apply a bandage.

bandage shears, a sturdy pair of scissors used to cut through bandages. The blades of most bandage shears are angled to the shaft of the instrument, and the lower blade has a rounded blunt protuberance to facilitate insertion under the bandage without harming the patient's skin.

band cell, any one of the developing granular leukocytes in circulating blood, characterized by a curved or indented nucleus.

banding, (in genetics) any of several techniques of staining chromosomes with fluorescent stains or chemical dyes that produce a series of lateral light and dark areas whose intensity and position are characteristic for each chromosome.

Bandl's ring, the extreme thickening of the retraction ring of normal labour. This occurs if labour is obstructed; it is palpable across the abdomen and is a sign of imminent uterine rupture.

bandpass, a measure of the number of times per second an electron beam can be modulated. It is a factor that influences horizontal resolution on a cathode-ray tube.

band pusher, an instrument used for adapting metal orthodontic bands to the teeth.

band remover, an instrument used for removing orthodontic bands from the teeth.

Bangkok haemorrhagic fever. See **dengue**

fever.

bank blood, anticoagulated, preserved blood collected from donors in units of approximately 470 ml and stored under refrigeration for future use.

bank nurse, a nurse who is available for assignment to duty on an ad hoc basis, usually to assist in times of unusually heavy work loads or to assume the duties of absent nursing personnel.

Banting treatment {William Banting, English coffin-maker, b. 1787}, a therapeutic regimen for obesity, consisting of a low-carbohydrate, high-protein diet.

Banti's syndrome {Guido Banti, Italian pathologist, b. 1852}, a serious, progressive disorder involving several organ systems, characterized by portal hypertension, splenomegaly, anaemia, leukopenia, GI tract bleeding, and cirrhosis of the liver.

bar, a measure of air pressure. It is equal to 1000 millibars, or 10^6 dynes/cm^2, or approximately 1 standard atmosphere (1 atm).

baralyme (BL), a mixture of calcium and barium compounds used to absorb exhaled carbon dioxide in an anaesthesia rebreathing system.

barber's itch. See sycosis barbae.

barbiturate, a derivative of barbituric acid that acts as a sedative, hypnotic, or anticonvulsant. These derivatives have a general depressant action on the central nervous system. They are addictive and have largely been superseded by less toxic drugs.

barbiturism, 1. acute or chronic poisoning by any of the derivatives of barbituric acid. **2.** addiction to a barbiturate.

Bard-Pic syndrome {Louis Bard, French anatomist, b. 1857; Adrian Pic, French physician, b. 1863}, a condition characterized by progressive jaundice, enlarged gallbladder, and cachexia, associated with advanced pancreatic cancer.

Bard's sign {Louis Bard, French anatomist, b. 1857}, the increased oscillations of the eyeball in organic nystagmus when the patient tries to visually follow a target moved from side to side across the line of sight.

bar graph, a graph in which frequencies are represented by bars extending from the ordinate or the abscissa, allowing the distribution of the entire sample to be seen at once.

bariatrics, the field of medicine that focuses on the treatment and the control of obesity and diseases associated with obesity.

baritosis, a benign form of pneumoconiosis caused by an accumulation of barium dust in the lungs. The condition is most likely to affect persons involved in the mining and processing of barite, a barium product used in the manufacture of paints.

barium (Ba), a pale yellow, metallic element classified with the alkaline earths. Its atomic number is 56; its atomic weight is 137.36.

Barium sulphate in suspension is used as a radiopaque contrast medium primarily in radiography of the GI tract.

barium enema, a rectal infusion of barium sulphate, a radiopaque contrast medium, which is retained in the lower intestinal tract, for diagnosing obstruction, tumours or other abnormalities during radiographic examination.

barium meal, the ingestion of barium sulphate, a radiopaque contrast medium, for the radiographic examination of the oesophagus, stomach, and duodenum in the diagnosis of such conditions as dysphagia, peptic ulcer, and fistulas.

barium sulphate, a radiopaque contrast medium used as a diagnostic aid in x-ray examination of the GI tract.

barium swallow. See barium meal.

Barlow's disease. See infantile scurvy.

Barlow's syndrome, an abnormal cardiac condition characterized by an apical systolic murmur, a systolic click, and an electrocardiogram indicating inferior ischaemia.

barognosis, *pl.* **barognoses** the ability to perceive and evaluate weight, especially that held in the hand.

barograph, an instrument that continuously monitors barometric pressure and provides a record on paper of pressure changes.

barometer an instrument for measuring atmospheric pressure, commonly consisting of a slender tube filled with mercury, sealed at one end, and inverted into a reservoir of mercury. At sea level the normal height of mercury in the tube is 760 mm. **barometric,** *adj.*

barometric pressure. See atmospheric pressure.

baroreceptor, one of the pressure-sensitive nerve endings in the walls of the atria of the heart, the vena cava, the aortic arch, and the carotid sinus. Baroreceptors stimulate central reflex mechanisms that allow physiological adjustment and adaptation to changes in blood pressure via vasodilatation or vasoconstriction.

barosinusitis. See aerosinusitis.

barotitis. See aerotitis.

barotitis media. See aerotitis media.

barotrauma, physical injury sustained as a result of exposure to increased environmental pressure, such as may occur among deep-sea divers or caisson workers.

Barr body. See sex chromatin.

barrel chest, a large, rounded thorax, considered normal in some stocky individuals and certain others who live in high-altitude areas and consequently develop increased vital capacities. Barrel chest may also be a sign of pulmonary emphysema.

Barr-Epstein virus. See Epstein-Barr virus.

Barré's pyramidal sign {Jean A. Barré, French neurologist, b. 1880}, the inability of a hemiplegic to maintain a flexed position on the side of the lesion when placed in a prone attitude with the lower limbs flexed 90 degrees at the knees.

Barrett's syndrome {Norman R. Barrett, English surgeon, b. 1903}, a disorder of the lower oesophagus marked by a benign ulcerlike lesion in columnar epithelium, resulting most often from chronic irritation of the oesophagus by gastric reflux of acidic digestive juices.

barrier, 1. a wall or other obstacle that can restrain or block the passage of substances. **2.** something nonphysical that obstructs or separates, as barriers to communication or compliance. **3.** (in radiography) any device that intercepts beams of x-rays.

barrier creams, ointments, lotions, and similar preparations applied to exposed areas of the skin to protect skin cells from exposure to various allergens, irritants, and carcinogens.

barrier nursing, nursing care of a patient in isolation, performed to prevent the spread of infection by creating an aseptic barrier around the patient.

Barthel Index (BI), a disability profile scale developed by D.W. Barthel in 1965 to evaluate a patient's self-care abilities in 10 areas including bowel and bladder control. The patient is scored from 0 to 15 points in various self-care categories, depending on his or her need for help.

bartholinitis, an inflammatory condition of one or both Bartholin's glands, caused by bacterial infection. The condition is characterized by swelling of one or both glands, pain, and the development of an abscess in the infected gland.

Bartholin's cyst {Caspar T. Bartholin, Danish anatomist, b. 1655}, a cyst that arises from one of the vestibular glands or from its ducts, filling with clear fluid that replaces the suppurative exudate characteristic of chronic inflammation.

Bartholin's duct, the major duct of the sublingual gland.

Bartholin's gland, one of two small, mucus-secreting glands located on the posterior and lateral aspect of the vestibule of the vagina.

Bartonella {Alberto Barton, Peruvian bacteriologist, b. 1871}, a genus of small, gram-negative flagellated pleomorphic coccobacilli. Members of the genus are intracellular parasites that infect red blood cells and the epithelial cells of the lymph nodes, liver, and spleen. They are transmitted at night by the bite of a sandfly of the genus *Phlebotomus*.

bartonellosis, an acute infection caused by *Bartonella bacilliformis,* transmitted by the bite of a sandfly. It is characterized by fever, severe anaemia, bone pain, and skin lesions. Untreated, the infection is often fatal.

Barton forceps. See **obstetric forceps.**

Barton's fracture {John R. Barton, American surgeon, b. 1794}, a fracture of the distal articular surface of the radius, which may be accompanied by the dorsal dislocation of the carpus on the radius.

Bartter's syndrome {Frederick C. Bartter, American physiologist, b. 1914}, a rare hereditary disorder, characterized by hyperplasia of the juxtaglomerular apparatus and secondary hyperaldosteronism.

barye, a measure of atmospheric pressure equal to 1 dyne/cm^2, or 1/1000 of a millibar.

basal, of or pertaining to the fundamental or the basic, as basal anaesthesia, which produces the first stage of unconsciousness, and the basal metabolic rate, which indicates the lowest metabolic rate.

basal anaesthesia, 1. a state of unconsciousness just short of complete surgical anaesthesia in depth, in which the patient does not respond to words but still reacts to pinprick or other noxious stimuli. **2.** narcosis produced by injection or infusion of potent sedatives alone, without added narcotics or anaesthetic agents. **3.** any form of anaesthesia in which the patient is completely unconscious, in contrast to awake anaesthesia.

basal body temperature, the temperature of the body taken in the morning, orally or rectally, after at least 8 hours of sleep and before doing anything else, including getting out of bed, smoking a cigarette, moving around, talking, eating, or drinking.

basal-body-temperature method of family planning, a natural method of family planning that relies on the identification of the fertile period of the menstrual cycle by noting the progesterone-mediated rise in basal body temperature of 0.5° to 1° F that occurs with ovulation. The fertile period is considered to continue until the temperature is above the baseline for 5 days; the rise occurs slowly during all 5 days or increases rapidly, reaching a plateau at which it remains for 3 or 4 days. The days after that period are considered "safe" unfertile days.

basal bone, 1. (in prosthodontics) the osseous tissue of the mandible and the maxillae, except for the rami and the processes, which provides support for artificial dentures. **2.** (in orthodontics) the fixed osseous structure that limits the movement of teeth in the creation of a stable occlusion.

basal cell, any one of the cells in the base layer of stratified epithelium.

basal cell acanthoma. See **basal cell papilloma.**

basal cell carcinoma, a malignant, epithelial cell tumour that begins as a papule and enlarges peripherally, developing a central crater that erodes, crusts, and bleeds. The primary cause of the cancer is excessive exposure to the sun or to x-rays.

basal cell papilloma, a benign, epidermal neoplasm characterized by multiple yellow or brown raised oval lesions that usually develop in middle age.

basal gangla, the islands of grey matter within each cerebral hemisphere, the most important being the caudate nucleus, the putamen, and the pallidium.

basal lamina, a thin, noncellular layer of ground substance lying just under epithelial surfaces.

basal layer. See **stratum basale.**

basal membrane, a sheet of tissue that forms the outer layer of the choroid and lies just under the pigmented layer of the retina.

basal metabolic rate (BMR), the amount of energy used in a unit of time by a fasting, resting subject to maintain vital functions. The rate, determined by the amount of oxygen used, is expressed in calories consumed per hour per square metre of body surface area or per kilogram of body weight.

basal metabolism, the amount of energy needed to maintain essential basic body functions, such as respiration, circulation, temperature, peristalsis, and muscle tone, measured when the subject is awake and at complete rest, has not eaten for 14 to 18 hours, and is in a comfortable, warm environment.

basaloid carcinoma, a rare, malignant neoplasm of the anal canal containing areas that resemble basal cell carcinoma of the skin.

basaloma. See **basal cell carcinoma.**

basal seat, (in dentistry) the oral tissues and structures that support a denture.

basal seat area, the portion of the oral structures that is available to support a denture.

basal seat outline, (in dentistry) a profile on the mucous membrane or on a cast of the entire oral area to be covered by a denture.

basal temperature. See **basal body temperature.**

basal tidal volume, the tidal volume of a healthy person at complete rest, with all bodily functions at a minimal level of activity, adjusted for age, weight, and sex.

base, 1. a chemical compound that combines with an acid to form a salt. **2.** a molecule or radical that takes up or accepts protons. **3.** the major ingredient of a compounded material, particularly one that is used as a medication.

base analogue, an analogue of one of the purine or the pyrimidine bases normally found in ribonucleic acid or deoxyribonucleic acid.

Basedow's goitre {Karl A. von Basedow, German physician, b. 1799}, an enlargement of the thyroid gland, characterized by the hypersecretion of thyroid hormone after iodine therapy.

base excess, a measure of metabolic alkalosis or metabolic acidosis.

base-forming food, a food that increases the pH of the urine. Base-forming foods include mainly fruits, vegetables, and dairy products, which are sources of sodium and potassium.

baseline, 1. a known value or quantity with which an unknown is compared when measured or assessed. **2.** (in radiography) any of several basic anatomical planes or locations used for positioning purposes.

baseline behaviour, a specified frequency and form of a particular behaviour during preexperimental or pretherapeutic conditions.

baseline condition, an environmental condition during which a particular behaviour reflects a stable rate of response before the introduction of experimental or therapeutic conditions.

baseline fetal heart rate, the fetal heart rate pattern between uterine contractions.

basement lamina. See **basal lamina.**

basement membrane, the fragile, noncellular layer of tissue that secures the overlying layers of stratified epithelium.

base of the heart, the portion of the heart opposite the apex, directed to the right side of the body. It forms the upper border of the heart, lies just below the second rib, and involves primarily the left atrium, part of the right atrium, and portions of the great vessels.

base of the skull, the floor of the skull, containing the anterior, middle, and posterior cranial fossae and numerous foramina, such as the optic foramen, foramen ovale, foramen lacerum, and foramen magnum.

base pair, a pair of nucleotides in a nucleic acid. One of the pair must be a purine, the other a pyrimidine.

base pairing, (in molecular genetics) the association in nucleic acids of the purine bases adenine and guanine with the pyrimidine bases cytosine, thymine, and uracil.

baseplate, a temporary form that represents the base of a denture, used for making records of maxillomandibular relationships, arranging artificial teeth, or for trial placement in the mouth to ensure a precise fit of a denture.

base ratio, the ratio of molar quantities of the bases in ribonucleic and deoxyribonucleic acids.

bas-fond, the bottom or fundus of any structure, especially the fundus of the urinary bladder.

BASIC, abbreviation for beginner's *a*ll-purpose *s*ymbolic *i*nstruction *c*ode, a computer programing language considered the easiest form of programing language to learn.

basic amino acid, an amino acid that has a positive electric charge in solution. The basic amino acids are arginine, histidine, and lysine.

basic group identity, (in psychiatry) the shared social characteristics, such as world view, language, and value and ideological system, that evolve from membership in an ethnic group.

basic health services, the minimum degree of

health care considered to be necessary to maintain adequate health and protection from disease.

basic human needs, the things required for survival and normal mental and physical health, such as food, water, shelter, and love.

basic salt, a salt that contains an unreplaced hydroxide ion from the base generating it, such as Ca(OH)Cl.

basifacial, pertaining to the lower portion of the face.

basilar, of or pertaining to a base or a basal area.

basilar artery, the single arterial trunk formed by the junction of the two vertebral arteries at the base of the skull, extending from the inferior to the superior border of the pons, dividing into the left and right cerebral arteries.

basilar artery insufficiency syndrome, the composite of clinical indicators associated with insufficient blood flow through the basilar artery, a condition that may be caused by arterial occlusion.

basilar artery occlusion, an obstruction of the basilar artery, resulting in dysfunction involving cranial nerves III through XII, cerebellar dysfunction, hemiplegia or quadriplegia, and loss of proprioception.

basilar membrane, the cellular structure that forms the floor of the cochlear duct and is supported by bony and fibrous projections from the cochlear wall.

basilar plexus, the venous network interlaced between the layers of the dura mater over the basilar portion of the occipital bone.

basilar sulcus, the sulcus that cradles the basilar artery, in the midline of the pons.

basilic vein, one of the four superficial veins of the arm, beginning in the ulnar part of the dorsal venous network and running proximally on the posterior surface of the ulnar side of the forearm. It is joined by the median cubital vein, then ascends to join the brachial vein to form the axillary vein.

basiloma, *pl.* **basilomas, basilomata,** a carcinoma composed of basal cells. A kind of basiloma is **basiloma terebrans**.

basiloma terebrans, a basal cell epithelioma that is invasive.

basioccipital, of or pertaining to the basilar process of the occipital bone.

basion, the midpoint on the anterior margin of the foramen magnum of the occipital bone, opposite the opisthion in the middle of the posterior margin.

basis pedunculi cerebri. See **crus cerebri**.

basket cell, a degenerated leukocyte seen on a blood smear during laboratory examination.

Basle Nomina Anatomica (BNA), an international system of anatomical terminology adopted at Basel, Switzerland.

basophil, a granulocytic white blood cell characterized by a segmented nucleus that contains granules that stain blue when exposed to a basic dye. Basophils represent 1% or less of the total white blood cell count.

basophilic adenoma, a tumour of the pituitary gland composed of cells that can be stained with basic dyes.

basophilic leukaemia, an acute or chronic malignant neoplasm of blood-forming tissues, characterized by large numbers of immature basophilic granulocytes in peripheral circulation and in tissues.

basophilic stipplig, the abnormal presence of punctate, basophilic granules in the red blood cells, observed under the microscope on a gram-stained smear of the blood. Stippling is characteristic of lead poisoning.

basosquamous cell carcinoma, a malignant epidermal tumour composed of basal and squamous cells.

Bassen-Kornzweig syndrome. See **abetalipoproteinaemia**.

BASW, abbreviation for **British Association for Social Work.**

batch processing, a processing mode used with some large computers in which only one user is serviced at a time and groups of similar transactions are accumulated to be processed simultaneously.

bath, (in the hospital) a cleansing procedure performed daily by or for almost all patients to help prevent infection, preserve the unbroken condition of the skin, stimulate circulation, promote oxygen intake, maintain muscle tone and joint mobility, and provide comfort.

bath blanket, a thin, lightweight blanket used to cover a patient during a bath or bed bath.

bathaesthesia, a deep sensibility, such as that associated with organs or structures beneath the surface of the body, such as muscles and joints.

bathmic evolution. See **orthogenic evolution**.

bathycardia, an abnormal but nonpathological condition characterized by an unusually low position of the heart in the chest.

Batten's disease {Frederick E. Batten, English neurologist, b. 1865}, a progressive childhood encephalopathy with disturbed metabolism of polyunsaturated fatty acids.

battered baby. See **child abuse.**

battery, 1. a complex of two or more electrolytic cells connected together to form a single source providing direct current or voltage. **2.** a series or a combination of tests to determine the cause of a particular illness or the degree of proficiency in a particular skill or discipline. **3.** the unlawful use of force on a person. See **assault.**

Battey bacillus, any of a group of atypical mycobacteria, including *Mycobacteria avium* and *M. intracellulare*, that cause a chronic pulmonary disease resembling tuberculosis.

battledore placenta, a condition in which the

umbilical cord is inserted into the margin of the placenta.

Battle's sign {William H. Battle, English surgeon, b. 1855}, a small haemorrhagic spot behind the ear that appears in cases may indicate a fracture of a bone of the lower skull.

batyl alcohol, an alcohol found in fish liver oil that is used to treat bracken poisoning in cattle.

baud {J.M.E. Baudot, French inventor, b. 1845}, binary units per second, used as a measure of the speed with which a computer device transmits information.

Baynton's bandage {Thomas Baynton, English surgeon, b. 1761}, a spiral adhesive wrap applied to the leg over a dressing, used in the treatment of indolent ulcers of the leg.

bayonet angle former, a hoe-shaped paired cutting instrument for accenting angles in a Class 3 tooth cavity.

bayonet condenser, (in dentistry) an instrument for compacting restorative material. It has an offset nib device and a shank with right angle bends for varying the line of force.

BBB, abbreviation for **blood-brain barrier**.

B cell, a type of lymphocyte that originates in the bone marrow. A precursor of the plasma cell on suitable antigenic stimulation, it is one of the two lymphocytes that play a major role in the body's immune response.

BCG, abbreviation for Bacillus Calmette-Guérin.

BCG vaccine, an active immunizing agent prepared from Bacillus Calmette-Guérin. It is prescribed most commonly for immunization against tuberculosis.

BCNU. See **carmustine.**

B complex vitamins, a large group of water soluble substances that includes **vitamin B_1** (thiamine), vitamin doxine), vitamin B_{12} (cyanocobalamin), biotin, choline, carnitine, folic acid, inositol, and **paraaminobenzoic acid.** The B complex vitamins are essential in converting carbohydrates into glucose to provide energy, for metabolism of fats and proteins, for normal functioning of the nervous system, for maintenance of muscle tone in the GI tract, and for the health of skin, hair, eyes, mouth, and liver. They are found in brewer's yeast, liver, whole grain cereals, nuts, eggs, meats, fish, and vegetables and are produced by the intestinal bacteria. Maintaining milk-free diets or taking antibiotics may destroy these bacteria. Symptoms of vitamin B deficiency include nervousness, depression, insomnia, neuritis, anaemia, alopecia, acne or other skin disorders, and hypercholesterolaemia.

b.d. See **b.i.d.**

Be, symbol for **beryllium.**

BE amputation, an amputation of the arm below the elbow.

beaded, 1. of or having a resemblance to a row of beads. **2.** of or pertaining to bacterial colonies that develop along the inoculation line in various stab cultures. **3.** of or pertaining to stained bacteria that develop more deeply stained beadlike granules.

beaker cell. See **goblet cell.**

beam, a bedframe fitting for pulleys and weights, used in the treatment of patients requiring weight traction. See **Balkan frame.**

BEAM, abbreviation for **brain electric activity map**.

beam alignment, (in radiography, radiotherapy) coincidence of radiation and light beam.

beam collimation, (in radiography, radiotherapy) restriction of the size of the radiation beam using adjustable diaphragms.

beam hardening, (in radiation dosimetry) the process of increasing the quality of an x-ray beam by the use of a filter to remove low-energy x-ray photons. See also **beam quality.**

beam quality, (in radiation dosimetry) a measure of the penetrating power of the x-ray beam, usually given in terms of its **half-value layer.**

beam-splitting mirror, (in radiography) image distributor which allows the output image of an image intensifier to be both viewed on a video monitor and recorded onto film simultaneously.

bean, the pod-enclosed flattened seed of numerous leguminous plants. Beans used in pharmacological preparations are alphabetized by specific name.

Beau's lines, white transverse lines across a nail plate associated with interruption in growth of the nail plate.

beat, the force of contraction of the heart muscle, which may be detected and recorded as the pulse.

Becker's muscular dystrophy, a chronic degenerative disease of the muscles, characterized by progressive weakness. It occurs in childhood between 8 and 20 years of age. It is transmitted genetically as an autosomal recessive trait.

Beck I operation, a surgical procedure to provide collateral circulation to the heart. The operation roughens the surface of the epicardium and the parietal lining of the pericardium, applies an irritant to these surfaces, partially closes the coronary sinus at the right atrium, and grafts the parietal pericardium and the mediastinal fat to the myocardium.

Beck II operation, an operation in two stages that provides collateral circulation to the heart. In the first stage a venous graft is placed between the aorta and the coronary sinus. In the second stage, the coronary sinus is partially closed to force oxygenated blood from the aorta to flow into the coronary vessels.

Beck's Depression Inventory (BDI), a system of classifying a total of 18 criteria of depressive illness. It was developed by A.T. in the 1970s as a diagnostic and therapeutic tool.

Beck's triad {Claude S. Beck, American surgeon, b. 1894}, a combination of three symptoms that characterize cardiac compression: high venous pressure, low arterial pressure, and a small, quiet heart.

Beckwith's syndrome {John B. Beckwith, American pathologist, b. 1933}, an hereditary disorder of unknown cause associated with neonatal hypoglycaemia and hyperinsulinism. Clinical manifestations include gigantism, macroglossia, omphalocele or umbilical hernia, visceromegaly, and other abnormalities.

beclomethasone dipropionate, a glucocorticoid prescribed in an inhaler in the treatment of asthma.

becquerel (Bq) {Antoine H. Becquerel, French physicist, b. 1852}, the SI unit of radioactivity, equal to one radioactive decay per second.

bed, (in anatomy) a supporting matrix of tissue, as the nail beds of modified epidermis over which the fingernails and the toenails move as they grow.

bedbug, a blood-sucking arthropod of either the species *Cimex lectularius* or the species *C. hemipterus* that feeds on humans and other animals. The bite causes itching, pain, and redness.

Bedford finger stall, a removable finger splint that holds the injured finger in a brace or cast, along with the adjacent finger.

Bednar's aphthae {Alois Bednar, Austrian paediatrician, b. 1816}, the small, yellowish, slightly elevated ulcerated patches that occur on the posterior portion of the hard palate of infants who place infected objects in their mouths.

bed rest, the restriction of a patient to bed for therapeutic reasons for a prescribed period.

bedside manner, the behaviour of a nurse or doctor as perceived by a patient.

bedwetting. See **enuresis.**

beef tapeworm. See *Taenia saginata.*

beef tapeworm infection, an infection caused by the tapeworm *Taenia saginata,* transmitted to humans when they eat contaminated beef. The infection is rarely found in Western Europe, where beef is carefully inspected and is thoroughly cooked before eating. See **tapeworm infection.**

bee sting, an injury caused by the venom of bees, usually accompanied by pain and swelling. The stinger of the honeybee usually remains implanted and should be removed. Pain may be alleviated by application of an ice pack or a paste of sodium bicarbonate and water. Hypersensitive individuals are encouraged to carry emergency treatment supplies with them when the possibility of bee sting exists.

behaviour, 1. the manner in which a person acts or performs. **2.** any or all of the activities of a person, including physical actions, which are observed directly, and mental activity, which is inferred and interpreted. Kinds of behaviour include **abnormal behaviour, automatic behaviour, invariable behaviour,** and **variable behaviour.**

behavioural isolation, social isolation that occurs because of a person's socially unacceptable behaviour.

behavioural objective, a goal in therapy or research that concerns an act or a specific behaviour or pattern of behaviours.

behavioural reflex. See **conditioned response.**

behavioural science, any of the various interrelated disciplines, such as psychiatry, psychology, sociology, and anthropology, that observes and studies human activity, including psychological and emotional development, interpersonal relationships, values, and mores.

behaviour disorder, any of a group of antisocial behaviour patterns occurring primarily in children and adolescents, such as overaggressiveness, overactivity, destructiveness, cruelty, truancy, lying, disobedience, perverse sexual activity, criminality, alcoholism, and drug addiction.

behaviourism, a school of psychology founded by John B. Watson that studies and interprets behaviour by observing measurable responses to stimuli without reference to consciousness, mental states, or subjective phenomena, such as ideas and emotions.

behaviourist, a follower of the school of behaviourism.

behaviourist psychology. See **behaviourism.**

behaviour modification. See **behaviour therapy.**

behaviour systems model, a conceptual framework describing factors that may affect the stability of a person's behaviour. The model examines systems of behaviour, not the behaviour of an individual at any particular time.

behaviour therapy, a kind of psychotherapy that attempts to modify patterns of behaviour by the application of experimental psychology to the contingencies which maintain unwanted or maladaptive behaviours.

Behçet's disease {Hulusi Behçet, Turkish dermatologist, b. 1889}, a rare and severe illness of unknown cause, mostly affecting young males and characterized by severe uveitis and retinal vasculitis.

Behla's bodies. See **Plimmer's bodies.**

BEI, abbreviation for butanol extractable iodine.

BEIR-III Report, a report, *"The Biological Effects of Low Doses of Ionizing Radiation,"* by the National Academy of Sciences; it estimates the risk of cancer deaths from exposure to radiation at various dose levels.

bejel, a nonvenereal form of syphilis prevalent among children in the Middle East and North Africa, caused by the spirochete *Treponema pallidum II.* The primary lesion is usually on or near the mouth, appearing as a mucous patch, followed by the development of pimplelike sores on the trunk, arms, and legs.

Békésy audiometry {George von Békésy, Hungarian-American physicist, b. 1899}, a method of testing hearing in which the subject presses a signal button while listening to a pure tone that is progressively diminished in intensity and releases the button when the sound no longer is heard. Continuous and interrupted tones are used in the test.

bel {Alexander G. Bell, Canadian inventor, b. 1847}, a unit that expresses intensity of sound. It is the logarithm (to the base 10) of the ratio of the power of any specific sound to the power of a reference sound. The most common reference sound has a power of 10^{-16} watts per cm^2, or the approximate minimum intensity of sound at 1000 cycles per second, that is perceptible to the human ear.

belching. See **eructation.**

belladonna, the dried leaves, roots, and flowering or fruiting tops of *Atropa belladonna,* a common perennial called deadly nightshade, containing the alkaloids hyoscine and hyoscyamine.

bellows murmur, a blowing sound, such as air moving in and out of a bellows.

bellows ventilator, a respiratory care device in which oxygen and other gases are mixed in a bellows that contracts and expands as system pressure is increased or decreased in the chamber surrounding the bellows.

Bell's law {Charles Bell, Scottish surgeon, b. 1774}, an axiom stating that the ventral spinal roots are motor and the dorsal spinal roots are sensory.

Bell's palsy {Charles Bell, Scottish surgeon, b. 1774}, a paralysis of the facial nerve, resulting from trauma to the nerve, compression of the nerve by a tumour, or, possibly, an unknown infection. The person may not be able to open an eye or close the mouth. Plastic surgery may reduce the deformity.

Bell's phenomenon, a sign of peripheral facial paralysis, manifested by the upward and outward rolling of the eyeball when the affected individual tries to close the eyelid.

belly. See **abdomen.**

belly button. See **umbilicus.**

belt restraint, a device used to secure a patient on a stretcher or in a chair.

Bence Jones protein {Henry Bence Jones, English physician, b. 1813}, a protein found almost exclusively in the urine of patients with multiple myeloma.

bench research, *informal.* (in medicine) any research done in a controlled laboratory setting using other than human subjects.

bending fracture, a fracture indirectly caused by the bending of an extremity, such as of the foot or the big toe.

bendrofluazide, a diuretic and antihypertensive prescribed in the treatment of hypertension and oedema.

bends. See **decompression sickness.**

Benedict's qualitative test {Stanley R. Benedict, American biochemist, b. 1884}, a test for sugar in the urine based on the reduction by glucose of cupric ions to a coloured cuprous oxide precipitate when it is placed in an alkaline solution.

benign, (of a tumour) noncancerous and therefore not an immediate threat, even though treatment may be required eventually for health or cosmetic reasons. See **benign neoplasm.**

benign hypertension, a misnomer implying an innocent elevation of blood pressure.

benign intracranial hypertension. See **pseudotumour cerebri.**

benign juvenile melanoma, a benign, pink or fuchsia raised papule with a scaly surface, usually on a cheek and occurring most commonly in children between 9 and 13 years of age.

benign mesenchymoma, a benign neoplasm that has two or more definitely recognizable mesenchymal elements in addition to fibrous tissue.

benign neoplam, a tumour, characteristically localized, that has a fibrous capsule, limited potential for growth, a regular shape, and cells that are well differentiated. A benign neoplasm does not invade surrounding tissue or metastasize to distant sites. It causes harm only by pressure and does not usually recur after surgical excision. Some kinds of benign neoplasms are **adenoma, fibroma, haemangioma,** and **lipoma.**

benign nephrosclerosis, a renal disorder marked by arteriolosclerotic lesions in the kidney. It is associated with hypertension.

benign prostatic hypertrophy, enlargement of the prostate gland, common among men after the age of 50. The condition is not malignant or inflammatory but is usually progressive and may lead to obstruction of the urethra and to interference with the flow of urine, possibly causing frequency of urination, the need to urinate during the night, pain, and urinary tract infections.

benign pseudohypertrophic muscular dystrophy. See **er's muscular dystrophy.**

benign stupor, a state of apathy or lethargy, such as occurs in severe depression.

benign suicide, (in psychology) indirect self-destructive behaviour. It is most likely to occur in older persons who find it impossible to deal with the loss of a loved one and refuse to eat, take medications, or take care of other needs.

benign thrombocytosis. See **thrombocytosis.**

benign tumour, a neoplasm that does not invade other tissues or metastasize in other sites. A benign tumour is usually well encapsulated, and its cells exhibit less anaplase than those of a malignant growth.

Bennet's small corpuscle. See **Drysdale's corpuscle.**

Bennett angle {Norman G. Bennett, English dentist, b. 1870}, (in dentistry) the angle formed by the sagittal plane and the path of the advancing condyle during lateral mandibular movement.

Bennett hand tool test, a test used in occupational therapy and prevocational testing to measure hand function and coordination and speed in performance.

Bennett's fracture {Edward H. Bennett, Irish surgeon, b. 1837}, a fracture that runs obliquely through the base of the first metacarpal bone and into the carpometacarpal joint, detaching the greater part of the articular facet.

bent fracture, an incomplete greenstick fracture.

bentonite {Fort Benton, Montana}, colloidal, hydrated aluminum silicate used as a bulk laxative and as a base for skin care preparations.

bentonite test, a flocculation test for the presence of rheumatoid factor in patient blood samples. After sensitized bentonite particles are added to the serum, the test is considered positive for rheumatoid arthritis if adsorption has occurred with 50% of the particles.

benz, abbreviation for a benzoate carboxylate anion.

benzalkonium chloride, a disinfectant and fungicide prepared in an aqueous solution in various strengths, often used as a preservative in pharmaceutical products.

benzene poisoning, a toxic condition caused by ingestion of benzene, the inhalation of benzene fumes, or exposure to benzene-related products such as toluene or xylene, characterized by nausea, headache, dizziness, and incoordination. In acute cases respiratory failure or ventricular fibrillation may cause death.

benzo(a)pyrene dihydrodiol epoxide (BPDE-I), a carcinogenic derivative of benzo(a)pyrene associated with tobacco smoke.

benzocaine, a local anaesthetic agent derived from aminobenzoic acid, used in many over-the-counter compounds for pruritus and pain.

benzodiazepine, one of a group of psychotropic agents, including the minor tranquillizers chlordiazepoxide, diazepam, lorazepam, and oxazepam, prescribed to alleviate anxiety, and the hypnotics flurazepam, nitrazepam, and temazepam. Diazepam is also prescribed to relieve spasm of the muscles and to increase the seizure threshold. All drugs in this group have anxiolytic, hypnotic, and anticonvulsant and muscle relaxant activity to different degrees.

benzoic acid, a keratolytic agent, usually used with salicylic acid as an ointment in the treatment of athlete's foot and ringworm of the scalp.

benzoyl peroxide, an antibacterial, keratolytic, drying agent prescribed in the treatment of acne.

benztropine mesylate, an anticholinergic and used in the treatment of all forms of parkinsonism.

benzyl alcohol, a clear, colourless, oily liquid, derived from certain balsams, used as a topical anaesthetic and as a bacteriostatic agent in solutions for injection.

benzyl benzoate, a clear, oily liquid with a pleasant, aromatic odour. It is used to destroy lice and scabies, as a solvent, and as an insect repellant.

benzyl carbonol. See **phenylethyl alcohol.**

benzylpenicillin sodium (penicillin G), an antibacterial prescribed in the treatment of many infections, including syphilis, rheumatic fever, and glomerulonephritis.

bereavement, the reaction to the loss of a loved one. It may be accompanied by insomnia, hyperactivity, low mood, and other effects.

Berger rhythm, Berger wave. See **alpha wave.**

Berger's disease, a kidney disorder characterized by recurrent episodes of macroscopic haematuria, proteinuria, and a granular deposition of IgA from the glomerular mesangium. The onset of disease is usually in childhood or early adulthood, and males are affected twice as often as females.

Bergonié-Tribondeau law {Jean A. Bergonié, French radiologist, b. 1857; Louis Frédéric A. Tribondeau, French physician, b. 1872}, (in radiotherapy) a rule stating that the radiosensitivity of tissue depends on the number of undifferentiated cells, their mitotic activity, and the length of time they are actively proliferating.

beriberi, a disease of the peripheral nerves caused by a deficiency of or an inability to assimilate thiamine. It is frequently the result of a diet limited to polished white rice. Symptoms are fatigue, diarrhoea, appetite and weight loss, disturbed nerve function causing paralysis and wasting of limbs, oedema, and heart failure. Kinds of beriberi include **alcoholic beriberi, atrophic beriberi, cardiac beriberi,** and **cerebral beriberi.**

berkelium (Bk), an artificial radioactive transuranic element. Its atomic number is 97; its atomic weight is 247.

berlock dermatitis, an abnormal skin condition, characterized by hyperpigmentation and skin lesions, caused by a unique reaction to psoralen-type photosynthesizers, commonly used in perfumes, colognes, and pomades, such as oil of bergamot. This condition affects mostly women and children and may result from the use of products containing psoralens and from exposure to ultraviolet light. Also spelled **Berloque dermatitis.**

Bernard-Soulier syndrome, a coagulation disorder characterized by an absence of or a deficiency in the ability of the platelets to aggregate because of the relative lack of an essential glycoprotein in the membranes of the platelets. The use of aspirin may provoke haemorrhage in people who have this condition.

Bernoulli's principle {Daniel Bernoulli, Swiss scientist, b. 1700}, (in physics) a principle stating that the sum of the velocity, and the kinetic energy of a fluid flowing through a tube is constant. The greater the velocity, the less the lateral pressure on the wall of the tube. Thus, if an artery is narrowed by an atherosclerotic plaque, the flow of blood through the constriction increases in velocity and decreases in lateral pressure.

Bernstein test. See **acid-perfusion test.**

berry aneurysm, a small, saccular dilatation of the wall of a cerebral artery, occurring most frequently at the junctures of vessels in the circle of Willis.

berylliosis, poisoning that results from the inhalation of dusts or vapours containing beryllium or beryllium compounds. It is characterized by granulomas, pulmonary fibrosis, dry cough, shortness of breath, and chest pain.

beryllium (Be), a steel-grey, lightweight metallic element. Its atomic number is 4; its atomic weight is 9.012. Beryllium occurs naturally as beryl and is used in metallic alloys and in fluorescent powders.

bestiality, 1. a brutal or animal-like character or nature. **2.** conduct or behaviour characterized by beastlike appetites or instincts. **3.** sexual relations between a human being and an animal.

beta, the second letter of the Greek alphabet, employed as a combining form with chemical names to distinguish one of two or more isomers or to indicate the position of substituted atoms in certain compounds.

beta-adrenergic blocking agent. See **antiadrenergic.**

beta-adrenergic receptor. See **beta receptor.**

beta-adrenergic stimulating agent. See **adrenergic drug.**

beta-alaninaemia, an inherited metabolic disorder marked by a deficiency of an enzyme, beta-alanine-alpha-ketoglutarate amino transferase. The clinical signs include seizures, somnolence, and, if uncorrected, death.

beta cells, 1. insulin-producing cells situated in the islets of Langerhans. The insulin-producing function of the beta cells tends to accelerate the movement of glucose, amino acids, and fatty acids out of the blood and into the cellular cytoplasm, countering glucagon function of alpha cells. **2.** the basophilic cells of the anterior lobe of the pituitary gland.

beta decay, a type of radioactive decay which results in the emission of negative or positive **beta particles.**

beta fetoprotein, a protein found in fetal liver and in some adults with liver disease. It is identical with normal liver ferritin.

beta-galactosidase. See **lactase.**

beta haemolysis, the development of a clear zone around a bacterial colony growing on blood agar medium, characteristic of certain pathogenic bacteria.

beta-haemolytic streptococci, the pyogenic streptococci of groups A, B, C, E, F, G, H, K, L, M, and O that cause haemolysis of red blood cells in blood agar in the laboratory. These organisms cause most of the acute streptococcal infections seen in humans.

beta-hydroxyisovaleric aciduria, an inherited metabolic disease caused by a deficiency of an enzyme needed to metabolize the amino acid leucine.

beta-ketobutyric acid. See **acetoacetic acid.**

betamethasone, a glucocorticoid prescribed as a topical ans systemic antiinflammatory agent.

beta-naphthylamine, an aromatic amine used in aniline dyes and a cause of bladder cancer in humans.

beta-oxidation, a catabolic process in which fatty acids are used by the body as a source of energy.

beta particle, an electron or positron emitted from the nucleus of an atom during radioactive decay of the atom. Beta particles have a range of up to 10 metres in air and several cms in soft tissue, depending on their energy.

beta phase, the period immediately following the alpha, or redistribution, phase of drug administration. During the beta phase the blood level of the drug falls more slowly as it is metabolized and excreted from the body.

beta receptor, any one of the adrenergic components of receptor tissues that responds to adrenaline. Activation of beta receptors causes various physiological reactions, as relaxation of the bronchial muscles and an increase in the rate and force of cardiac contraction.

beta rhythm. See **beta wave.**

betatron, a cyclic accelerator that produces high-energy electrons and may be used for external beam radiotherapy.

beta wave, one of the four types of brain waves, characterized by relatively low voltage and a frequency of more than 13 Hz. Beta waves are the "busy waves" of the brain, recorded by electroencephalograph from the frontal and the central areas of the cerebrum when the patient is awake and alert with eyes open.

betaxolol hydrochloride, a drug used topically for the relief of ocular hypertension and chronic open-angle glaucoma.

bethanechol chloride, a cholinergic prescribed in the treatment of faecal and urinary retention and neurogenic.

bevel, 1. any angle, other than a right angle, between two planes or surfaces. **2.** (in dentistry) any angle other than 90 degrees between a tooth cut and a cavity wall in the preparation of a tooth cavity.

bezoar, a hard ball of hair and vegetable fibre that may develop within the intestines of humans but more often is found in the stomachs of ruminants.

B-galactosidase. See **lactase.**

bhang. See **cannabis.**

Bi, symbol for **bismuth.**

bias, 1. an oblique or a diagonal line. **2.** a prejudiced or subjective attitude. **3.** (in statistics) the systematic distortion of a statistic caused by a particular sampling process. **4.** (in electronics) a voltage applied to an electronic device, such as a vacuum tube or a transistor, to control operating limits.

biasing, a method of treating neuromuscular dysfunction by contracting a muscle against resistance, causing the muscle spindles to readjust to the shorter length.

bibliotherapy, a type of group therapy in which books, poems, and newspaper articles are read in the group to help stimulate thinking about events in the real world and to foster relations between group members.

bicarbonate of soda. See **sodium bicarbonate.**

bicarbonate precursor, an injection of sodium lactate used in the treatment of metabolic acidosis. It is metabolized in the body to sodium bicarbonate.

bicarbonate therapy, a procedure to increase a patient's stores of bicarbonate when there are signs of severe acidosis.

bicarbonate transport, the route by which most of the carbon dioxide is carried in the bloodstream. Once dissolved in the blood plasma, the carbon dioxide combines with water to form carbonic acid, which immediately ionizes into hydrogen and bicarbonate ions.

biceps brachii, the long fusiform muscle of the upper arm on the anterior surface of the humerus, arising from two heads above the scapula. The short head arises in a tendon from the corocoid process, the long head arises in the glenoid cavity. Both parts of the muscle converge in a flattened tendon that inserts into the radius of the forearm. It flexes the arm and the forearm and supinates the hand. The long head draws the humerus toward the glenoid fossa, strengthening the shoulder joint.

biceps femoris, one of the posterior femoral muscles. It has two heads at its origin. The long head arises from the tuberosity of the ischium and from the inferior part of the sacrotuberous ligament; the short head arises from the linea aspera and from the lateral intermuscular septum. The fibres passing from both heads join in a tendon that inserts into the lateral side of the fibula, and by a few fibres, into the lateral condyle of the tibia. The tendon of insertion forms the lateral hamstring. The biceps femoris flexes the leg and rotates it laterally and extends the thigh and tends to rotate it laterally.

biceps flexor cubiti. See **biceps brachii.**

biceps reflex, a contraction of a biceps muscle produced when the tendon is tapped with a percussor in testing deep tendon reflexes.

biclour, abbreviation for a bichloride noncarboxylate anion.

biconcave, concave on both sides, especially as applied to a lens. **biconcavity,** *n.*

biconvex, convex on both sides, especially as applied to a lens. **biconvexity,** *n.*

bicornate, having two horns or processes.

bicornate uterus, an abnormal uterus that may be either a single or a double organ with two horns, or branches.

bicuspid, 1. having two cusps or points. **2.** one of the two premolar teeth between the molars and canines of the upper and lower jaw.

bicuspid valve. See **mitral valve.**

b.i.d., (in prescriptions) abbreviation for bis in die, a Latin phrase meaning "twice a day." The times of administration are commonly 9 AM and 7 PM.

bidactyly, an abnormal condition in which the second, third, and fourth digits on the same hand are missing and only the first and fifth are represented. **bidactylous,** *adj.*

bidermoma, *pl.* bidermomas, bidermomata, a teratoid neoplasm composed of cells and tissues originating in two germ layers.

bidet, a fixture resembling a toilet bowl, with a rim to sit on and usually equipped with plumbing implements, for cleaning the genital and rectal areas of the body.

bidirectional printer, a computer-driven printer that prints characters as the printing head moves in either direction.

biduotertian fever, a form of malaria characterized by overlapping paroxysms of chills, fever, and other symptoms, caused by infection with two strains of *Plasmodium*, each having its own cycle of symptoms, such as in quartan and tertian malaria.

bifid, split into two parts.

bifocal {L *bis* + *focus* hearth}, **1.** of or pertaining to the characteristic of having two foci. **2.** (of a lens) having two areas of different focal lengths.

bifurcation, a splitting into two branches, such as the trachea, which branches into the two bronchi at about the level of the fifth thoracic vertebra.

Bigelow's lithotrite {Henry J. Bigelow, American surgeon, b. 1818}, a long-jawed lithotrite, passed through the urethra, for crushing a calculus in the bladder.

bigeminal pulse, an abnormal pulse in which two beats in close succession are followed by a pause during which no pulse is felt.

bigeminy, 1. an association in pairs. **2.** a cardiac arrhythmia characterized by two beats in rapid succession followed by a longer interval. **bigeminal,** *adj.*

bilabe, a narrow forceps used to remove small calculi from the bladder.

bilaminar, pertaining to or having two layers.

bilaminar blastoderm, the stage of embryonic development before mesoderm formation in which only the ectoderm and entoderm primary germ layers have formed.

bilateral, 1. having two sides. **2.** occurring or appearing on two sides. A patient with bilateral hearing loss may have partial or total deafness in both ears. **3.** having two layers.

bilateral long-leg spica cast, an orthopaedic device of plaster of Paris, fibreglass, or other casting material that encases and immobilizes the trunk cranially as far as the nipple line and both legs caudally as far as the toes. A horizontal crossbar to improve immobilization connects the parts of the cast encasing both legs at ankle level.

Bilbao tube, a long, thin, flexible tube that is used to inject barium into the small intestine. The tube is guided with a stiff wire to the end of the duodenum under fluoroscopic control.

bile, a bitter, yellow-green secretion of the liver. Stored in the gallbladder, bile receives its colour from the presence of bile pigments, such as bilirubin. Bile passes from the gallbladder through the common bile duct in response to the presence of a fatty meal in the duodenum. Bile emulsifies these fats, preparing them for further digestion and absorption in the small intestine. **biliary,** *adj.*

bile acid, a steroid acid of the bile, produced during the metabolism of cholesterol. On hydrolysis bile acid yields glycine and cholic acid.

bile duct. See **biliary duct.**

bile pigments, a group of substances that contribute to the colours of bile, which may range from a yellowish-green to brown. A common bile pigment is bilirubin.

bile solubility test, a bacteriological test used in the differential diagnosis of pneumococcal and streptococcal infection.

Bilharzia, See *Schistosoma.*

bilharziasis, See **schistosomiasis.**

biliary, of or pertaining to bile or to the gallbladder and its ducts, which transport bile. These are often called the **biliary tract** or the **biliary system.** Also **bilious.**

biliary atresia, congenital absence or underdevelopment of one or more of the biliary structures, causing jaundice and early liver damage.

biliary calculus, a stone formed in the biliary tract, consisting of bile pigments and calcium salts. Biliary calculi may cause jaundice, right upper quadrant pain, obstruction, and inflammation of the gallbladder.

biliary cirrhosis, an inflammatory condition in which the flow of bile through the ductules of the liver is obstructed.

biliary colic, a type of smooth muscle or visceral pain specifically associated with the passing of stones through the bile ducts.

biliary duct, a duct through which bile passes from the liver to the duodenum.

biliary fistula, an abnormal passage from the gallbladder, a bile duct, or the liver to an internal organ or the surface of the body.

biliary obstruction, blockage of the common or cystic bile duct, usually caused by one or more gallstones. It impedes bile drainage and produces an inflammatory reaction. See **cholecystectomy.**

biliary tract cancer, a relatively rare malignancy in an extrahepatic bile duct, occurring slightly more often in men than in women, characterized by progressive jaundice, pruritus, weight loss, and, in the later stages, severe pain. The tumour is an adenocarcinoma; it may be papillary or flat and ulcerated.

bilingulate, having two tongues or two tonguelike structures.

bilious, 1. of or pertaining to bile. **2.** characterized by an excessive secretion of bile. **3.** characterized by a disorder affecting the bile.

bilirubin, the orange-yellow pigment of bile, formed principally by the breakdown of haemoglobin in red blood cells after termination of their normal life-span. In a healthy person about 250 mg of bilirubin are produced daily, and the majority of that is eventually excreted from the body in the stool. The characteristic yellow pallor of jaundice is caused by the accumulation of bilirubin in the blood and in the tissues of the skin.

bilirubinuria, the presence of bilirubin in urine.

biliuria, the presence of bile in the urine.

biliverdin, a greenish bile pigment formed in the breakdown of haemoglobin and converted to bilirubin.

Billings method, a way of estimating ovulation time by changes in the cervical mucus that occur during the menstrual cycle.

Billroth's operation I {Christian A. Billroth,

Austrian surgeon, b. 1829}, the surgical removal of the pylorus in the treatment of gastric cancer. The proximal end of the duodenum is anastomosed to the stomach.

Billroth's operation II, the surgical removal of the pylorus and duodenum. The cut end of the stomach is anastomosed to the jejunum through the transverse mesocolon.

bilobate, having two lobes.

bilobulate, having two lobules. Also **bilobular.**

bilocular, 1. divided into two cells. 2. containing two cells. Also **biloculate.**

bimanual, of or pertaining to the functioning of both hands.

bimanual palpation, the examination of a woman's pelvic organs conducted by the examiner placing one hand on the abdomen and one or two fingers of the other hand in the vagina.

bimaxillary, of or pertaining to the right and left maxilla.

bimodal distribution, the distribution of quantitative data around two separate modes. It is suggestive of two separate normally distributed populations from which the data are drawn.

bimolecular reaction (E^2), an elimination reaction in which more than one kind of molecule is involved. It may follow first-order, second-order, or more complicated chemical kinetics.

binangle, a surgical instrument that has a shank with two offsetting angles to keep the cutting edge of the instrument within 3 mm of the shaft axis.

binary fission, direct division of a cell or nucleus into two equal parts. It is the common form of asexual reproduction of bacteria, protozoa, and other lower forms of life.

binary number, a number represented in the binary system, and usually represented by 0s and 1s. See **binary system.**

binary system, a number system based on the number two, used in digital computers. Each digit, represented by a zero or one, represents a power of two. Thus the decimal number 47 (actually representing $4 \times 10^2 + 7 \times 10^0$) is expressed in binary notation as 101111 (that is, $1 \times 2^5 + 0 \times 2^4 + 1 \times 2^3 + 1 \times 2^2 + 1 \times 2^1 + 1 \times 2^0$).

binaural stethoscope, a stethoscope having two earpieces.

bind, 1. to bandage or wrap in a band. **2.** to join together with a band or with a ligature. **3.** (in chemistry) to combine or unite molecules by employing reactive groups within the molecules or by using a binding chemical.

binder, a bandage made of a large piece of material to fit and support a specific body part.

binding energy, the amount of energy required to remove a particle from the orbit or nucleus of an atom.

Binet age {Alfred Binet, French psychologist, b. 1857}, the mental age of an individual, especially a child, as determined by the Binet-Simon tests, which are evaluated on the basis of tested intelligence of the "normal" individual at any given age. The Binet age corresponding to "profoundly retarded" is 1 to 2 years; to "severely retarded," 3 to 7 years; and to "mildly retarded," 8 to 12 years.

binocular, 1. pertaining to both eyes, especially regarding vision. **2.** a microscope, telescope, or field glass that can accommodate viewing by both eyes.

binocular fixation, the process of having both eyes directed at the same object at the same time.

binocular ophthalmoscope, an ophthalmoscope having two eyepieces through which stereoscopic examination of the eye may be made.

binocular parallax, the difference in the angles formed by the sight lines to two objects situated at different distances from the eyes. Binocular parallax is a major factor in depth perception.

binocular perception, the visual ability to judge depth or distance by virtue of having two eyes.

binocular vision, the use of both eyes simultaneously so that the images perceived by each eye are combined to appear as a single image.

binomial, containing two names or terms.

binovular, developing from two distinct ova, as in dizygotic twins. Also **diovular.**

binovular twins. See **dizygotic twins.**

bioactive, of or pertaining to a substance that has an effect on or causes a reaction in living tissue.

bioactivity, any response from or reaction in living tissue.

bioassay, the laboratory determination of the concentration of a drug or other substance in a specimen by comparing its effect on an organism or an isolated tissue with that of a standard preparation.

bioavailability, the degree of activity or amount of an administered drug or other substance that becomes available for activity in the target tissue.

biochemical genetics. See **molecular genetics.**

biochemical marker, any hormone, enzyme, antibody, or other substance that is detected in the urine or other body fluids or tissues that may serve as a sign of a disease or other abnormality.

biochemistry, the chemistry of living organisms and life processes.

biochromatic analysis, the spectrophotometric monitoring of a reaction at two wavelengths. It is used to correct for background colour.

bioelectrical impedance analysis (BIA), a

method of measuring the fat composition of the body, compared to other tissues, by its resistance to electricity.

bioelectricity, electric current that is generated by living tissues, such as nerves and muscles.

bioenergetics, a system of exercises based on the concept that natural healing will be enhanced by bringing into harmony the patient's body rhythms and the natural environment.

bioequivalent, 1. (in pharmacology) of or pertaining to a drug or pharmaceutical preparation that has the same effect on the body as another preparation, usually one identical or nearly identical in its chemical formulation. **2.** a bioequivalent drug. **bioequivalence,** *n.*

biofeedback, a process providing a person with visual or auditory information about the autonomical and physiological functions of his or her body, such as blood pressure, muscle tension, and brain wave activity, usually through use of instrumentation.

bioflavonoid, a generic term for any of a group of coloured flavones found in many fruits and essential for the absorption and metabolism of ascorbic acid.

biogenesis, 1. the doctrine that living material can originate only from preexisting life and not from inanimate matter. **2.** the origin of life and living organisms; ontogeny and phylogeny. **biogenetic,** *adj.*

biogenetic law. See **recapitulation theory**.

biogenic, 1. produced by the action of a living organism, such as fermentation. **2.** essential to life and the maintenance of health, such as food, water, and proper rest.

biogenic amine, one of a large group of naturally occurring biologically active compounds most of which act as neurotransmitters. The most dominant, noradrenaline, is involved in such physiological functions as emotional reactions, memory, sleep, and arousal from sleep.

biogenous, 1. biogenetic. **2.** biogenic.

biogeny. See **biogenesis**.

biological, 1. pertaining to living organisms and their products. **2.** any preparation made from living organisms or the products of living organisms and used as a diagnostic, preventive or therapeutic agent. Biologicals include **antitoxins, vaccines,** some **hormones,** and **blood products**.

biological activity, the inherent capacity of a substance, such as a drug or toxin, to alter one or more of the chemical or physiological functions of a cell. The capacity has relationships not only to the physical and chemical nature of the substance but also to its concentration and the duration of cellular exposure to the substance.

biological assay. See **bioassay**.

biological half-life, the time required for the body to eliminate one half of an administered dose of any substance by regular physiological processes.

biological monitoring, 1. a process of measuring the levels of various physiological substances, drugs, or metabolites within a patient during diagnosis or therapy. **2.** the measurement of toxic substances in the environment and the identification of health risks to the population.

biological plausibility, a method of reasoning used to establish a cause and effect relationship between a biological factor and a particular disease.

biological preparation, any preparation made from living organisms or the products of living organisms and used as diagnostic, preventive, or therapeutic agents. Kinds of biological preparations are **antigens, antitoxins, serums,** and **vaccines**.

biological psychiatry, a school of psychiatric thought that stresses the physical, chemical, and neurological causes of and treatments for mental and emotional disorders.

biological vector. See **vector**.

biology, the scientific study of plants and animals. Some branches of biology are **biometry, ecology, molecular biology,** and **palaeontology**.

biomagnetic therapy, a form of magnetotherapy, involving treatment using very small magnets which are placed on certain acupuncture points.

biome, the total group of biological communities existing in and characteristic of a given geographical region, such as a desert, woodland, or marsh.

biomechanics, the study of mechanical laws and their application to living organisms, especially the human body and its locomotor system. **biomechanic, biomechanical,** *adj.*

biomechanical adaptation, a process in the use of orthotic treatment to enable a disabled person to resume normal function of a body part with the aid of a device, such as an ankle-foot brace. The process of adaptation includes the central nervous system input received during therapeutic exercises with the orthotic appliance.

biomedical engineering, a system of techniques in which knowledge of biological processes is applied to solve practical medical problems and to answer questions in biomedical research.

bionics, the science of applying electronic principles and devices, such as computers and solid state miniaturized circuitry, to medical problems, such as artificial pacemakers used to correct abnormal heart rhythms. **bionic,** *adj.*

biophore, a theoretical basic hereditary unit contained in the germ plasm from which all living cells develop and all inherited characteristics are transmitted.

biopotentials, electrical charges produced by various tissues of the body, particularly muscle tissue during contractions.

biopsy, 1. the removal of a small piece of living tissue from an organ or other part of the body for microscopic examination to confirm or establish a diagnosis, estimate prognosis, or follow the course of a disease. **2.** the tissue excised for examination. **3.** *informal.* to excise tissue for examination. Kinds of biopsy include **aspiration biopsy, needle biopsy, punch biopsy,** and **brush biopsy. bioptic,** *adj.*

biopsychic, of or pertaining to psychic factors as they relate to living organisms.

biopsychology. See **psychobiology.**

biopsychosocial, of or pertaining to the complex of biological, psychological, and social aspects of life.

bioptome tip catheter, a catheter with a special tip designed for obtaining endomyocardial biopsy samples. The bioptome tip device is used to monitor heart transplant patients for early signs of tissue rejection.

biorhythm, any cyclical, biological event or phenomenon, such as the sleep cycle, the menstrual cycle, or the respiratory cycle. **biorhythmic,** *adj.*

biostatistics, numerical data on births, deaths, diseases, injuries, and other factors affecting the general health and condition of human populations.

biosynthesis, any one of thousands of chemical reactions continually occurring throughout the body in which molecules form more complex biomolecules. **biosynthetic,** *adj.*

biotaxis, the ability of living cells to develop into certain forms and arrangements. **biotactic,** *adj.*

biotaxy, 1. biotaxis. **2.** the systematic classification of living organisms according to their anatomical characteristics; taxonomy.

biotechnology, 1. the study of the relationships between humans or other living organisms and machinery, such as the ability of aeroplane pilots to perform tasks when traveling at supersonic speeds. **2.** the industrial application of the results of biological research, particularly in fields such as recombinant DNA or gene splicing. See **recombinant DNA.**

biotelemetry, the transmission of physiological data, such as ECG and EEG recordings, heart rate, and body temperature by radio or telephone systems.

biothesiometer, a portable device allowing quantitive measurement of vibratory detection thresholds.

biotic potential, the possible growth rate of a population of organisms under ideal conditions, including absence of predators and maximum nutrients and space for expansion.

biotin, a colourless, crystalline, water-soluble B complex vitamin that acts as a coenzyme in fatty acid production and in the oxidation of fatty acids and carbohydrates.

biotin deficiency syndrome, an abnormal condition caused by a deficiency of biotin, characterized by dermatitis, hyperaesthesia, muscle pain, anorexia, slight anaemia, and changes in electrocardiographic activity of the heart.

biotope, a specific biological habitat or site.

biotransformation, the chemical changes a substance undergoes in the body, such as by the action of enzymes.

Biot's respiration {Camille Biot, French physician, b. 1878}, an abnormal respiratory pattern, characterized by irregular breathing with periods of apnoea.

biovular twins. See **dizygotic twins.**

biparental inheritance. See **amphigenous inheritance.**

biparietal, of or pertaining to the two parietal bones of the head, such as the biparietal diameter.

biparietal diameter, the distance between the protuberances of the two parietal bones of the skull.

bipartite, having two parts.

biped, 1. having two feet. **2.** any animal with only two feet.

bipedal, capable of locomotion on two feet.

bipenniform, (of bodily structure) having the bilateral symmetry of a feather, such as the pattern formed by the fasciculi that converge on both sides of a muscle tendon in the rectus femoris.

biperiden, a synthetic anticholinergic drug used in the treatment of Parkinson's disease and drug-induced extrapyramidal disorders. Biperiden hydrochloride is administered orally, and biperiden lactate is administered intramuscularly or intravenously.

biphasic, having two phases, parts, aspects, or stages.

bipolar, 1. having two poles, such as in certain electrotherapeutic treatments using two poles or in certain bacterial staining that affects only the two poles of the microorganism under study. **2.** (of a nerve cell) having an afferent and an efferent process.

bipolar disorder, a major affective disorder characterized by episodes of mania and depression. One or the other phase may be predominant at any given time, one phase may appear alternately with the other, or elements of both phases may be present simultaneously. Characteristics of the manic phase are excessive emotional displays, excitement, euphoria, hyperactivity accompanied by elation, boisterousness, impaired ability to concentrate, decreased need for sleep, and seemingly unbounded energy, often accompanied by delusions of grandeur. In the depressive phase, marked apathy and underactivity are accompanied by feelings of profound sadness, loneliness, guilt, and lowered self-esteem.

bipolar lead, 1. an electrocardiographic conductor having two electrodes placed on different body regions, with each electrode contributing significantly to the record. **2.** *informal.* a tracing produced by such a lead on an electrocardiograph.

bipotentiality, the characteristic of acting or reacting according to either of two potentials.

bird breeder's lung. See **pigeon breeder's lung**.

bird face retrognathism, an abnormal facial profile with an undeveloped mandible, which may be caused by interference of condylar growth associated with trauma or condylar infection.

bird headed dwarf, a person affected with Seckel's syndrome, a congenital disorder characterized by a proportionate shortness of stature; a proportionately small head with hypoplasia of the jaws, large eyes, and a beaklike protrusion of the nose; learning difficulties; and various other defects.

birth, 1. the event of being born, the coming of a new person out of its mother into the world. **2.** the child-bearing event, the bringing forth by a mother of a baby.

birth canal, *informal.* the passage that extends from the inlet of the true pelvis to the vaginal orifice through which an infant passes during vaginal birth.

birth control. See **contraception**.

birth defect. See **congenital anomaly**.

birthing chair, a chair used in labour and delivery which allows the woman to sit straight up or to recline. The upright position appears to shorten the time in labour, particularly the second or expulsive stage of labour, probably because of gravity and increased participation of the mother. However, use of a birthing chair may increase the amount of blood lost by the mother.

birth injury, trauma suffered by a baby while being born.

birthmark. See **naevus**.

birth plan, a formal written listing of preferences and choices for childbirth, prepared by a woman, usually in conjunction with her partner, midwife or antenatal teacher, before she goes into labour. Some hospitals give women a pre-printed form to fill in as a guide.

birth rate, the proportion of the number of births in a specific area during a given period to the total population of that area, usually expressed as the number of births per 1000 of population.

birth trauma, any physical injury suffered by an infant during the process of delivery.

birth weight, the measured heaviness of a baby when born.

bisacodyl, a stimulant laxative prescribed in the treatment of acute or chronic constipation.

bisect, to divide into two equal lengths or parts.

bisexual, 1. hermaphroditic; having gonads of both sexes. **2.** possessing physical or psychological characteristics of both sexes. **3.** engaging in both heterosexual and homosexual activity. **4.** desiring sexual contact with persons of both sexes.

bisexual libido, (in psychoanalysis) the tendency in a person to seek sexual gratification with people of either sex.

bisferious pulse, an arterial pulse that has two palpable peaks, the second of which is slightly stronger than the first.

Bishop's score, a method of assessing the favourability of the cervix prior to induction of labour. The factors assessed are: dilatation, consistency, position and effacement of the cervix in relation to the ischial spines.

bis in die (b.d., b.i.d.), a Latin phrase, used in prescriptions, meaning "twice a day." It is more commonly used in its abbreviated form.

bismuth (Bi), a reddish, crystalline, trivalent metallic element. Its atomic number is 83; its atomic weight is 209. It is combined with various other elements, such as oxygen, to produce numerous salts used in the manufacture of many pharmaceutical substances.

bismuth gingivitis, a symptom of metallic poisoning caused by bismuth administered in the treatment of systemic disease. It is characterized by a dark bluish line along the gingival margin.

bismuth stomatitis, an abnormal oral condition caused by systemic use of bismuth compounds over prolonged periods, characterized by a blue-black line on the inner aspect of the gingival sulcus or pigmentation of the buccal mucosa, a sore tongue, metallic taste, and a burning sensation in the mouth.

bit, abbreviation for binary digit, a single digit of a binary number.

bite, 1. the act of cutting, tearing, holding, or gripping with the teeth. **2.** the lingual portion of an artificial tooth between its shoulder and incisal edge. **3.** an occlusal record or relationship.

biteblock, (in radiotherapy) a block placed in the patient's mouth during treatment to reproduce the position of, and immobilize, the tongue and mandible.

bite block. See **occlusal rim**.

biteguage, a prosthetic dental device that helps attain proper occlusion of the teeth rooted in the maxilla and the mandible.

biteguard, a resin appliance that covers the occlusal and incisal surfaces of the teeth. It is designed to stabilize the teeth and provide a platform for the excursive glides of the mandible.

biteguard splint, a device for covering the occlusal and incisal surfaces of the teeth and for protecting them from traumatic occlusal forces during immobilization and stabilization processes.

bitelock, a dental device for retaining the

occlusion rims in the same relation outside the mouth as inside the mouth.

bitemporal, of or pertaining to both temples or both temporal bones.

biteplane, a removable dental appliance for covering the occlusal surfaces of the teeth and to prevent their articulation.

biteplate, a device used in dentistry as a diagnostic or a therapeutic aid for prosthodontics or for orthodontics.

bite reflex, a swift, involuntary biting action that may be triggered by stimulation of the oral cavity.

bite wing film, a type of dental x-ray film that has a central tab or wing on which the teeth close to maintain film position during radiographic examination.

bite wing radiograph, a kind of dental x-ray that reveals approximately the coronal portions of maxillary and mandibular teeth and portions of the interdental septa on the same film.

Bithynia, a genus of snails, species of which act as intermediate hosts to *Opisthorchis.*

biting in childhood, a natural behaviour trait and reflex action in infants, acquired at about 5 to 6 months of age in response to the introduction of solid foods in the diet and the beginning of the teething process. The activity represents a significant modality in the psychosocial development of the child, because it is the first aggressive action the infant learns, and through it the infant learns to control the environment.

Bitot's spots {Pierre Bitot, French surgeon, b. 1822}, white or grey triangular deposits on the bulbar conjunctiva adjacent to the lateral margin of the cornea, a clinical sign of vitamin A deficiency.

bitrochanteric lipodystrophy, an abnormal and excessive deposition of fat on the buttocks and the outer aspect of the upper thighs, occurring most commonly in women.

bitterling test, a Japanese test for pregnancy in which a female bitterling fish is immersed in 1 L of fresh water containing 10 ml of the urine of the woman being tested. If the woman is pregnant, the long oviduct of the bitterling grows from its belly.

biuret test, a method for detecting urea and other soluble proteins in serum.

bivalent, 1. also **divalent.** (in genetics) a pair of synapsed homologous chromosomes that are attached to each other by chiasmata during the early first meiotic prophase of gametogenesis. **2.** See **valence,** def. **1.** **bivalence,** *n.*

bivalent chromosome, a pair of synapsed homologous chromosomes during the early stages of gametogenesis.

bivalve cast, an orthopaedic cast used for immobilizing a section of the body for the healing of one or more broken bones or for correction or the maintenance of correction

of an orthopaedic deformity. The cast is cut in half to monitor and detect pressure under the cast.

bizarre leiomyoma. See **epithelioid leiomyoma**.

BK, abbreviation for *below the knee,* a term referring to amputations, amputees, prostheses, and orthoses.

Bk, symbol for **berkelium**.

black damp. See **damp**.

Black Death, *informal.* bubonic plague, especially the fourteenth century epidemic in Europe that killed over 25,000,000 people.

black eye, an eyelid contusion. It is usually treated for the first 24 hours with ice packs to reduce swelling, then treated with hot compresses to aid in resorption of blood from the haematoma.

black fever. See **kala-azar**.

black hairy tongue. See **parasitic glossitis**.

blackhead. See **comedo**.

black light. See **Wood's light**.

black lung disease. See **anthracosis, pneumoconiosis**.

blackout, *informal.* a temporary loss of vision or consciousness resulting from cerebral ischaemia.

black plague. See **bubonic plague**.

black tongue. See **parasitic glossitis**.

blackwater fever, a serious complication of chronic falciparum malaria, characterized by jaundice, haemoglobinuria, acute renal failure, and the passage of bloody dark red or black urine because of massive intravascular haemolysis.

black widow spider, a poisonous arachnid found in many parts of the world. The venom injected with its bite causes perspiration, abdominal cramps, nausea, headaches, and dizziness of various levels of intensity.

black widow spider antivenom, a passive immunizing agent prescribed in the treatment of black widow spider bite.

bladder, 1. a membranous sac serving as a receptacle for secretions. **2.** the urinary bladder.

bladder cancer, the most common malignancy of the urinary tract. It is characterized by a tumour or by multiple growths that tend to recur in a more aggressive form. The risk for developing bladder cancer is increased with cigarette smoking and exposure to carcinogens, such as aniline dyes, and with the use of beta-naphthylamine, mixtures of aromatic hydrocarbons, or benzidine and its salts, used in chemical, paint, plastics, rubber, textile, petroleum, and wood industries and in medical laboratories. Other predisposing factors are chronic urinary tract infections, calculous disease, and schistosomiasis; in Egypt, where *Schistosoma haematobium* infestations are extremely common, the bladder is the most frequent site of cancer. Early symptoms of a bladder cancer include haematuria, frequent

blue asphyxia. See **asphyxia livida**.

blue baby, an infant born with cyanosis caused by a congenital heart lesion, such as transposition of the great vessels, by tetralogy of Fallot, or by incomplete expansion of the lungs (congenital atelectasis).

blue bloater. See **chronic bronchitis**.

blue naevus, a sharply circumscribed, usually benign, steel blue skin nodule. It is found on the face or upper extremities, grows very slowly, and persists throughout life. Any sudden change in the size of such a lesion demands surgical attention and biopsy. The dark colour is caused by large, densely packed melanocytes deep in the dermis of the naevus.

blue spot, 1. one of a number of small greyish blue spots that may appear near the armpits or around the groins of individuals infested with lice, such as in pediculosis corporis and pediculosis pubis. **2.** one of a number of dark blue or mulberry hued round or oval spots that may appear as a congenital condition in the sacral regions of certain children and usually disappear spontaneously as the affected individual matures.

blunt dissection, a dissection performed by separating tissues along natural lines of cleavage, without cutting.

blunthook, 1. a sturdy hook-shaped bar used in obstetrics for traction between the abdomen and the thigh in cases of difficult breech deliveries. **2.** a hook-shaped device with a blunt end used in embryotomy.

blunting, a decrease in the intensity of emotional expression from the level one would normally expect as a reaction to a specific situation.

blurred film fault, a defect in a photograph or radiograph that appears as an indistinct or blurred image.

blush, a brief, diffuse erythema of the face and neck, commonly the result of dilation of superficial small blood vessels in response to heat or sudden emotion.

B lymphocyte. See **B cell**.

BMA, abbreviation for **British Medical Association**.

B-mode, brightness modulation, an imaging technique used in ultrasound scanning in which bright dots on an oscilloscope screen represent echos and the intensity of the brightness indicates the strength of the echo.

BMI, abbreviation for **body mass index**.

BMR, abbreviation for **basal metabolic rate**.

BN, abbreviation for **Bachelor of Nursing**.

Boas' test {Ismar I. Boas, German physician, b. 1858}, **1.** a test for hydrochloric acid in the contents of the stomach. **2.** a test for lactic acid in a sample of gastric juice that depends on the oxidation of the lactic acid to aldehyde and formic acid by the action of sulphuric acid and manganese. **3.** a test for gastric motility in which a fasting patient drinks 400 ml of water that has been tinted green by the addition of chlorophyll solution.

Bodansky unit {Aaron Bodansky, American biochemist, b. 1887}, the quantity of phosphatase in 100 ml of serum needed to liberate 1 mg of phosphorous as phosphate ion from sodium betaglycerophosphate in 1 hour at 37° C. It is used to express the measure of certain enzymes, such as acid phosphatase in the body.

body, 1. the whole structure of an individual with all the organs. **2.** a cadaver or a corpse. **3.** the largest or the main part of any organ, such as the body of the tibia or the body of the vastus lateralis.

body cavity, any of the spaces in the chest and abdomen that contain body organs.

body fluid, a fluid contained in the three fluid compartments of the body: the blood plasma of the circulating blood, the interstitial fluid between the cells, and the cell fluid within the cells. Blood plasma and interstitial fluid make up the extracellular fluid; the cell fluid is the intracellular fluid. The chemical constituents of the fluids vary greatly; for example, sodium is present in large amounts in both compartments of the extracellular fluid but is nearly absent in the intracellular fluid; protein is present in the blood plasma and cell fluid but not in the interstitial fluid.

body image, a person's subjective concept of his or her physical appearance. The mental representation, which may be realistic or unrealistic, is constructed from self-observation, the reactions of others, and a complex interaction of attitudes, emotions, memories, fantasies, and experiences, both conscious and unconscious.

body image disturbance, a disruption in the way a person perceives his or her body image. Defining characteristics include verbal or nonverbal responses to a real or perceived change in structure or function, a missing body part, personalization of the missing part by giving it a name, refusal by the person to look at a part of the body, negative feelings about the body, trauma to a nonfunctioning part, a change in general social involvement or life-style, and a fear of rejection by others.

body jacket, an orthopaedic cast that encases the trunk of the body but does not extend over the cervical area. It is used to help immobilize the trunk for the healing of spinal injuries and scoliosis and for postoperative positioning and immobilization after spinal surgery.

body language, a set of nonverbal signals, including body movements, postures, gestures, spatial positions, facial expressions, and bodily adornment, that give expression to various physical, mental, and emotional states.

body mass index (BMI), a measure achieved by the formula Weight/Height^2 = BMI. May be used to indicate ranges of so-called healthy and unhealthy weights in clinical settings where professional intervention may be necessary, e.g. anorexia nervosa may be defined in terms of a BMI that ranges from 13.5 or below to 20. Obesity may be defined in terms of a BMI that ranges from 20 to 40, It should not be used as a single reference point for diagnosis, and should be combined with other measures of nutritional state and psychological health.

body mechanics, the field of physiology that studies muscular actions and the function of muscles in maintaining the posture of the body.

body movement, motion of all or part of the body, especially at a joint or joints. Some kinds of body movements are abduction, adduction, extension, flexion, and rotation.

body odour, a fetid smell associated with stale perspiration. Freshly secreted perspiration is odourless, but after exposure to the atmosphere and bacterial activity at the surface of the skin, chemical changes occur to produce the odour.

body of Retzius {Magnus G. Retzius, Swedish anatomist, b. 1842}, any one of the masses of protoplasm containing pigment granules at the lower end of a hair cell of the organ of Corti in the internal ear.

body plethysmograph, a device for studying alveolar pressures, lung volumes, and airway resistance. The patient sits or reclines in an airtight compartment and breathes normally. The pressure changes in the alveoli are reciprocated in the compartment and are recorded automatically.

body position, attitude or posture of the body. Some kinds of body position are anatomical position, decubitus, Fowler's position, prone, supine, and Trendelenburg position.

body resorption, the release of calcium into the blood from destruction of bone tissue cells.

body righting reflex, any one of the neuromuscular responses to restore the body to its normal upright position when it has been displaced.

body scheme, a Piagetian term for a cognitive structure that develops in infants in the sensorimotor period during the first 2 years of life as they learn to differentiate between themselves and the world around them.

body-scheme disorder. See **autotopagnosia**.

body stalk, the elongated part of the embryo that is connected to the chorion.

body surface area. See **surface area**.

body systems model, (in nursing education) a conceptual framework in which illness is studied in relation to the functional systems of the body. In this model, nursing care is directed toward manipulating the patient's environment in such a way that the signs and symptoms of the health problem are alleviated.

body temperature, the level of heat produced and sustained by the body processes. Variations and changes in body temperature are major indicators of disease and other abnormalities. Heat is generated within the body through metabolism of food and lost from the body surface through radiation, convection, and evaporation of perspiration. Heat production and loss are regulated and controlled in the hypothalamus and brainstem. Diseases of the hypothalamus or interference with the other regulatory centres may produce abnormally low body temperatures. Normal adult body temperature, as measured orally, is 37° C. Oral temperatures ranging from 36° C to 37.5° C are consistent with good health, depending on the physical activity of the person, the ambient temperature, and the particular normal body temperature for that person. Axillary temperature is usually 0.5° C lower than the oral temperature. Rectal temperatures may be 0.2° to 0.5° C higher than oral readings. Body temperature appears to vary 0.5° to 1° C throughout the day, with lows recorded early in the morning and peaks between 6 PM and 10 PM.

body temperature, altered, failure to maintain body temperature within normal range. Risk factors include extremes of age or weight; exposure to cool-to-cold or warm-to-hot environments; dehydration; inactivity or vigorous activity; medications causing vasoconstriction or vasodilation; altered metabolic rate; sedation; inappropriate clothing for environmental temperature; and illness or trauma affecting temperature regulations.

body type, the general physical appearance of an individual human body.

Boeck's sarcoid. See **sarcoidosis**.

Boerhaave's syndrome {Hermann Boerhaave, Dutch physician, b. 1668}, a condition marked by spontaneous rupture of the oesophagus, leading to mediastinitis and pleural effusion. Emergency care is needed, with surgery and drainage, to save the life of the patient.

Bohr effect {Christian Bohr, Danish physiologist, b. 1855}, the effect of CO_2 and H^+ on the affinity of haemoglobin for molecular O_2. Increasing P_{CO} and H^+ decrease oxyhaemoglobin saturation, whereas decreasing concentrations have the opposite effect.

boil, a skin abscess. See **furuncle**.

boiling point {ME *boilen* to make bubbles; L *pungere* to prick}, the temperature at which a substance passes from the liquid to the gaseous state at a particular atmospheric pressure.

bole, any of a variety of soft, friable clays of various colours, although usually red from iron oxide.

Bolivian haemorrhagic fever, an infectious

disease caused by an arenavirus, generally transmitted from infected rodents to humans through contamination of food by rodent urine, though direct transmission between people has also been observed. The patient experiences chills, fever, headache, muscle ache, anorexia, nausea, and vomiting.

bolus, 1. a round mass, specifically a masticated lump of food ready to be swallowed. **2.** a large round preparation of medicinal material for oral ingestion, usually soft and not prepackaged. **3.** a dose of a medication or a contrast material, radioactive isotope, or other pharmaceutical preparation injected all at once intravenously. **4.** in radiotherapy, tissue equivalent material used to achieve a plane surface and more uniform dose distribution.

bolus tube feeding, delivery of nutrients by tube into stomach. Volume of feed required over a 24 hour period is determined and divided up into suitable smaller volumes. These are introduced by syringe at regular intervals.

Bombay phenotype, a rare genetic trait involving the phenotypical expression of the ABO blood groups. Cells of such individuals are phenotypically of blood type O, even though they are genotype AB, and the serum contains anti-A, anti-B, and anti-H antigens. The trait is named after the city in which it was first reported.

bonding, the attachment process that occurs between an infant and the parents, especially the mother, and is significant in the formation of affectionate ties that later influence both the physical and psychological development of the child. Especially important in initiating bonding is eye to eye contact, fondling of the infant, soothing talk, and other affectionate behaviour that begins to create positive emotional ties. Mothers are more concerned with physically touching and holding the infant, whereas fathers are more intent on forming a sense of absorption, preoccupation, and visual interest in the child—what has been called paternal engrossment. Although bonding is considered primarily an emotional response, it is possible that there may be some biochemical and hormonal interaction in the mother stimulating the response, but studies are still inconclusive.

bond specificity, the nature of enzyme action that causes the disruption of only certain bonds between atoms.

bone, 1. the dense, hard, and slightly elastic connective tissue, comprising the 206 bones of the human skeleton. It is composed of compact osseous tissue surrounding spongy cancelous tissue permeated by many blood vessels and nerves and enclosed in membranous periosteum. Long bones contain yellow marrow in longitudinal cavities and red marrow in their articular ends. Red marrow also fills the cavities of the flat and the short bones, the bodies of the vertebrae, the cranial diploe, the sternum, and the ribs. Blood cells are produced in active red marrow. Osteocytes form bone tissue in concentric rings around an intricate haversian system of interconnecting canals that accommodates blood vessels, lymphatic vessels, and nerve fibres. **2.** any single element of the skeleton, such as a rib, the sternum, or the femur.

bone cancer, a skeletal malignancy occurring as a primary sarcomatous tumour in an area of rapid growth or, more frequently, as a metastasis from cancer elsewhere in the body. Primary bone tumours are comparatively rare. In adults bone cancer is strongly linked to exposure to ionizing radiation. Paget's disease, hyperparathyroidism, chronic osteomyelitis, old bone infarcts, and fracture callosities increase the risk of bone tumours, but most osseous malignancies are metastatic lesions found most often in the spine or pelvis and less often in sites away from the trunk. Bone cancers progress rapidly but are often difficult to detect; pain that increases at night may be the only symptom. The most common osseous malignancies are osteosarcomas, followed by chrondrosarcomas, fibrosarcomas, and Ewing's sarcoma.

bone cutting forceps, a kind of forceps with long handles, single or double joints, and heavy blades.

bone graft, the transplantation of a piece of bone from one part of the body to another to repair a skeletal defect. In some cases animal bone may be transplanted to a human.

bone marrow, specialized, soft tissue filling the spaces in cancelous bone of the epiphyses. Fatty, **yellow marrow** is found in the compact bone of most adult epiphyses. **Red marrow** is found in many bones of infants and children and in the spongy bone of the proximal epiphyses of the humerus and femur and in the sternum, ribs, and vertebral bodies of adults. It is composed of myeloid tissue and is essential in the manufacture and maturation of red blood cells.

bone marrow puncture, aspiration of marrow from bone cavity (usually sternum or iliac crest), with a marrow puncture needle, for diagnosis of blood disorders.

bone marrow transplant, the transplantation of bone marrow from healthy donors to stimulate production of formed blood cells. The bone marrow is removed from the donor by aspiration and infused intravenously into the recipient.

bone resorption, apical progression of the level of the alveolar crest, associated with inflammatory or dystrophic periodontal disease and resulting in decreased bone support for the teeth.

Bonnevie-Ullrich syndrome. See **Turner's syndrome**.

Bonwill's triangle {William G. A. Bonwill, American dentist, b. 1833}, an equilateral triangle with 4 inch (10 cm) sides formed by lines from the contact points of the lower central incisors (or the median line of the residual ridge of the mandible) to the condyle on either side and from one condyle to the other.

booster injection, a vaccine or toxoid, usually given in a smaller amount than for primary immunization, given to an immune individual maintain the immune response at an appropriate level.

Boothby-Lovelace-Bulbulian (BLB) mask, an apparatus for the administration of oxygen, consisting of a mask fitted with an inspiratory-expiratory valve and a rebreathing bag.

boracic acid. See boric acid.

borate, any salt of boric acid. Borate salts and boric acid, although formerly used as mild antiseptic irrigation solutions, especially for ophthalmic conditions, are highly poisonous when taken internally or absorbed through a cut, abrasion, or other wound in the skin, and are seldom used nowadays.

borborygmus, *pl.* **borborygmi** an audible abdominal sound produced by hyperactive intestinal peristalsis. Borborygmi are rumbling, gurgling, and tinkling noises heard in auscultation.

borderline, 1. personality disorder characterized by emotional lability and splitting. **2.** schizotypal personality disorder. **3.** mild schizophrenia.

Bordetella {Jules J.B.V. Bordet, Belgian bacteriologist, b. 1870}, a genus of gram-negative coccobacilli, some species of which are pathogens of the respiratory tract of humans, including *Bordetella bronchiseptica, B. parapertussis,* and *B. pertussis.*

boric acid, a white, odourless powder or crystalline substance used as a buffer and formerly employed as a topical antiseptic and eye wash.

Bornholm disease. See epidemic pleurodynia.

boron (B), a nonmetallic element, similar to aluminum. Its atomic number is 5; its atomic weight is 10.8. Elemental boron occurs in the form of dark crystals and as a greenish yellow amorphous mass. Certain concentrations of this element are toxic to plant and animal life, but plants need traces of boron for normal growth. It is the characteristic element of boric acid, used chiefly as a dusting powder and ointment for minor skin disorders.

Borrelia {Amédé Borrel, French bacteriologist, b. 1867}, a genus of coarse, unevenly coiled, helical spirochetes, several species of which cause tickborne and louseborne infections. Many animals serve as reservoirs and hosts for *Borrelia.*

boss, a swelling, eminence, or protruberance on an organ, such as a tumour or overgrowth on a bone surface.

Boston exanthem, an epidemic disease characterized by scattered, pale red maculopapules on the face, chest, and back, occasionally accompanied by small ulcerations on the tonsils and soft palate. It is caused by echovirus 16 and requires no treatment.

bottle feeding, feeding an infant or young child from a bottle with a rubber teat on the end, sometimes called artificial feeding because it is done as a substitute for or supplement to breastfeeding.

bottle mouth syndrome, dental caries occurring in children between 18 months and 3 years of age as a result of being given bottles of sweetened juice or other sugary drinks to suck on too often or for too long at a time.

botulism, an often fatal form of food poisoning caused by an endotoxin produced by the bacillus *Clostridium botulinum.* The toxin is ingested in food contaminated by *C. botulinum,* although it is not necessary for the live bacillus to be present if the toxin has been produced. In rare instances, the toxin may be introduced into the human body through a wound contaminated by the organism. Botulism develops without gastric distress and may not occur for up to 1 week after the contaminated food has been ingested. Botulism is characterized by a period of lassitude and fatigue followed by visual disturbances. Muscles may become weak, and the victim often develops dysphagia.

bouba. See yaws.

Bouchard's node {Charles J. Bouchard, French physician, b. 1837}, an abnormal cartilaginous or bony enlargement of a proximal interphalangeal joint of a finger, usually occurring in degenerative diseases of the joints.

bougie, a thin, cylindrical instrument made of rubber, waxed silk, or other flexible material for insertion into canals of the body in order to dilate, examine, or measure them.

boulimia. See bulimia.

boundary, (in psychology) an aspect of group relations in which limits on interpersonal interaction are clearly defined.

boundary lubrication, a coating of a thin layer of molecules on each weight-bearing surface of a joint to facilitate a sliding action by the opposing bone surfaces.

boundary maintenance mechanisms, (in psychology) behaviour and practices that exclude members of some groups from the customs and values of another group.

bound carbon dioxide, carbon dioxide that is transported in the bloodstream as part of a sodium bicarbonate molecule, as distinguished from dissolved carbon dioxide, or bicarbonate ion.

bounding pulse, a pulse that, on palpation, feels full and springlike because of an increased thrust of cardiac contraction or an increased volume of circulating blood within the elastic structures of the vascular system.

bouquet fever. See **dengue fever.**

Bourneville's disease. See **tuberous sclerosis.**

boutonneuse fever, an infectious disease caused by *Rickettsia conorii*, transmitted to humans through the bite of a tick. The onset of the disease is characterized by a lesion called a tache noire, or black spot, at the site of the infection, fever lasting from a few days to 2 weeks, and a papular erythematous rash that spreads over the body to include the skin of the palms and soles.

boutonniere deformity, an abnormality of a finger marked by the fixed flexion of the proximal interphalangeal joint and the hyperextension of the distal interphalangeal joint.

bovine spongiform encephalopathy (BSE), a fatal encephalopathy affecting cattle, thought to be related to scrapie in sheep and Creutzfeldt-Jacob disease in humans.

Bowditch's law. See **all-or-none law.**

bowel. See **intestine.**

bowel training, a method of establishing regular evacuation by reflex conditioning, used in the treatment of faecal incontinence, impaction, chronic diarrhoea, and autonomic hyperreflexia. In patients with autonomic hyperreflexia, distention of the rectum and bladder causes paroxysmal hypertension, restlessness, chills, diaphoresis, headache, elevated temperature, and bradycardia.

Bowen's disease, Bowen's precancerous dermatosis. See **intraepidermal carcinoma.**

bowleg. See **genu varum.**

Bowman's capsule {Sir William Bowman, English surgeon, b. 1816}, the cup-shaped end of a renal tubule containing a glomerulus.

bowtie filter, (in radiology) a special bowtie-shaped filter that may be used in computed tomography procedures to compensate for the shape of the patient's head or body.

boxer's fracture, a fracture of one or more metacarpal bones, usually the fourth or the fifth, caused by punching a hard object. Such a fracture is often distal, angulated, and impacted.

boxing, (in dentistry) the forming of vertical walls, most commonly made of wax, to produce the desired shape and size of the base of a cast.

Boyle's law {Robert Boyle, English scientist, b. 1627}, (in physics) a law stating that the product of the volume and pressure of a gas compressed at a constant temperature remains constant.

BP, abbreviation for **blood pressure.**

BPDE-I, abbreviation for **benzo(a)pyrene dihydrodiol epoxide.**

Br, symbol for **bromine.**

brace, an orthotic device, sometimes jointed, to support and hold any part of the body in the correct position to allow function, such as a leg brace that permits walking and standing.

brachial, of or pertaining to the arm.

brachial artery, the principal artery of the upper arm that is the continuation of the axillary artery. It has three branches and terminates at the radial and the ulnar arteries.

brachialis, a muscle of the upper arm, covering the anterior part of the elbow joint and the distal half of the humerus. It functions to flex the forearm.

brachial plexus, a network of nerves in the neck, passing under the clavicle and into the axilla, originating in the fifth, sixth, seventh, and eighth cervical and first two thoracic spinal nerves and innervating the muscles and skin of the chest, shoulders, and arms.

brachial plexus anaesthesia, an anaesthetic block of the region innervated by the anterior divisions of the last four cervical and first two thoracic nerves. The plexus extends from the transverse processes to the apex of the axilla, where the terminal nerves are formed.

brachial plexus paralysis. See **Erb's palsy.**

brachial pulse, the pulse of the brachial artery, palpated in the antecubital space.

brachiocephalic, of or relating to the arm and head.

brachiocephalic arteritis. See **Takayasu's arteritis.**

brachiocephalic artery, brachiocephalic trunk. See **innominate artery.**

brachiocephalic vein. See **innominate vein.**

brachiocubital, pertaining to the arm and forearm.

brachioradialis, the most superficial muscle on the radial side of the forearm. It functions to flex the forearm.

brachioradialis reflex, a deep tendon reflex, elicited by striking the lateral surface of the forearm proximal to the distal head of the radius, characterized by normal slight elbow flexion and forearm supination.

brachycephaly, a congenital malformation of the skull in which premature closure of the coronal suture results in excessive lateral growth of the head, giving it a short, broad appearance with a cephalic index of between 81 and 85. **brachycephalic, brachycephalous,** *adj.*

brachydactyly, a condition of abnormally short fingers or toes.

brachytherapy, the use of radioactive sources placed at a short distance from the lesion to be irradiated in order to give a high radiation dose to the lesion with minimum dose to surrounding normal tissues. See **interstitial therapy, intracavitary therapy.**

Bradford frame {Edward H. Bradford, American surgeon, b. 1848}, a rectangular orthopaedic frame made of pipes to which heavy movable straps of canvas are attached, running from side to side to support a patient in a prone or supine position. The straps can be removed to permit the patient to urinate or defaecate while remaining immobile.

Bradford solid frame, a rectangular orthopaedic device of metal covered with canvas to aid in immobilization, especially of children in traction. The main purpose of the device is to assist in maintaining proper immobilization, positioning, and alignment by controlling movement.

Bradford split frame, a rectangular orthopaedic device of metal covered with two separate pieces of canvas fastened at both ends of the frame. Used especially in paediatrics to aid in the immobilization of children in traction, it is divided in the middle by a large opening designed to accommodate the excretory functions of an incontinent patient in a hip spica cast. The division also allows for the upper and lower extremities of the patient to be elevated separately and for the maintenance of a clean and dry cast. For an incontinent child, a plastic funnel leading into the bedpan is positioned below the opening in the frame.

bradycardia, an abnormal circulatory condition in which the myocardium contracts steadily but at a rate of less than 60 contractions a minute. The heart normally slows during sleep, and in some physically fit people the pulse may be quite slow. Cardiac output is decreased, causing faintness, dizziness, chest pain, and eventually syncope and circulatory collapse.

bradycardia-tachycardia syndrome, a heart disorder characterized by a heart rate that alternates between abnormally slow and abnormally rapid rhythms.

bradykinesia, an abnormal condition characterized by slowness of all voluntary movement and speech, such as caused by parkinsonism, other extrapyramidal disorders, and certain tranquillizers.

bradykinin, a peptide of nonprotein origin containing nine amino acid residues. It is produced from α_2-globulin by kallikrein, and it is a potent vasodilator.

bradypnoea, an abnormally slow rate of breathing.

Bragg curve {Sir William H. Bragg, English physicist, b. 1862}, in radiation dosimetry, a graphical representation of the ionization pattern of a charged particle, such as an electron. Ionization density increases as the particle travels along its track, reaching a maximum at the end of its track.

Braille {Louis Braille, French teacher of blind, b. 1809}, a system of printing for the blind consisting of raised dots or points that can be read by touch.

brain, the portion of the central nervous system contained within the cranium. It consists of the cerebrum, cerebellum, pons, medulla, and midbrain.

brain concussion, a violent jarring, or shaking, or other blunt, nonpenetrating injury to the brain caused by a sudden change in momentum of the head. After a mild concussion there may be a transient loss of consciousness followed, on awakening, by a headache. Severe concussion may cause prolonged unconsciousness and disruption of certain vital functions of the brainstem, such as respiration and vasomotor stability.

brain death, an irreversible form of unconsciousness characterized by a complete loss of brain function while the heart continues to beat. The usual clinical criteria for brain death include the absence of reflex activity, movements, and respiration. The pupils are dilated and fixed. A diagnosis of brain death requires that the electric activity of the brain be evaluated and shown to be absent on two electroencephalograms performed 12 to 24 hours apart.

brain electric activity map (BEAM), a topographical map of the brain areas that show electric potentials evoked by a flash of light. Potentials recorded at 4-millisecond intervals are converted into a many-coloured map of the brain, showing them to be positive or negative.

brain fever, *informal.* any inflammation of the brain or meninges.

brain oedema. See **cerebral oedema**.

brain scan, radiographic investigation of the brain using either computed tomography, magnetic resonance or radionuclide imaging.

brainstem, the portion of the brain comprising the medulla oblongata, the pons, and the mesencephalon. It performs motor, sensory, and reflex functions and contains the corticospinal and the reticulospinal tracts. The 12 pairs of cranial nerves from the brain arise mostly from the brainstem.

brainstem auditory evoked potential (BAEP), the most reliable evoked potential for predicting nerve damage during surgery in the auditory nerve region. A clicking sound is made, and the EEG waves from the auditory area of the patient's brain are observed. Cessation or absence of electricl activity may indicate damage or destruction.

brain tumour, a neoplasm of the intracranial portion of the central nervous system that is usually invasive but does not spread beyond the cerebrospinal axis. Intracranial tumours in children are usually the result of a developmental defect. In adults 20% to 40% of malignancies in the brain are metastatic lesions from cancers in the breast, lung, GI tract, kidney, or a malignant melanoma. The origin of primary brain tumours is not

lead. Calcium is the fifth most abundant element in the human body and occurs mainly in the bone. The body requires calcium ions for the transmission of nerve impulses, muscle contraction, blood coagulation, cardiac functions, and other processes. It is a component of extracellular fluid and of soft tissue cells. Abnormally high levels of ionized calcium in the extracellular fluid can produce muscle weakness, lethargy, and coma. A relatively small decrease from the normal level of this element can produce tetanic seizures.

calcium antagonist. See **calcium channel blocker**.

calcium channel blocker, a drug that inhibits the flow of calcium ions across the membranes of smooth muscle cells. By reducing the calcium flow, smooth muscle tone is relaxed and the risk of muscle spasms is diminished. Calcium channel blockers are used primarily in the treatment of hypertension and angina pectoris.

calcium chloride, the chloride salt of calcium used to replenish calcium in the blood. It is given intravenously in the treatment of hypocalcaemia, as an antidote for magnesium poisoning, and to increase the tone of cardiac muscle during resuscitation.

calcium pump, a theoretical, energy-requiring mechanism for transmitting calcium ions across a cell membrane from a region of low calcium ion concentration to one of higher concentration.

calculus, *pl.* **calculi,** an abnormal stone formed in body tissues by an accumulation of mineral salts. Kinds of calculi include biliary calculus and urinary calculus.

calculus anuria, the cessation of urine production caused by renal calculi.

Caldwell-Moloy pelvic classification {William E. Caldwell, American obstetrician, b. 1880; Howard C. Moloy, American gynaecologist, b. 1903}, a system for classifying the structure of the bony pelvis of the female. The types in this system are android, anthropoid, gynaecoid, and platypelloid.

calefacient, 1. making or tending to make anything warm or hot. **2.** an agent that imparts a sense of warmth when applied, such as a hot-water bottle or a hot compress.

calendar method of family planning. See **natural family planning method**.

calf, *pl.* **calves,** the fleshy mass at the back of the leg below the knee, composed chiefly of the gastrocnemius muscle.

calf bone. See **fibula**.

calibre, the diameter of a tube or a canal, as any of the blood vessels.

californium (Cf), an artificial element in the actinide group. Its atomic number is 98; its atomic weight is 251. Californium 252 is a radioisotope which emits alpha particles and neutrons. The neutrons may be used in brachytherapy applications.

calipers, an instrument with two hinged, adjustable, curved legs, used to measure the thickness or the diameter of a convex body or solid.

caliper splint, a splint for the leg consisting of two metal rods running from the back of a band around the thigh or from a cushioned ring around the lower portion of the pelvis. The rods are attached to a metal plate under the shoe below the arch of the foot.

Calliphoridae, a family of medium-sized to large flies that belong to the order Diptera, serve as pathogenic vectors, and may cause intestinal or nasopharyngeal myiasis in humans.

callomania, an abnormal psychological condition characterized by delusions of personal beauty.

callosal fissure, a groove following the convex aspect of the corpus callosum.

callosity. See **callus**.

callosomarginal fissure, a long, irregular groove on the medial surface of a cerebral hemisphere. It divides the cingulate gyrus from the medial frontal gyrus and from the paracentral lobule.

callus, 1. a common, usually painless thickening of the epidermis at locations of external pressure or friction. **2.** bony deposit formed between and around the broken ends of a fractured bone during healing. **callous,** *adj.*

calmodulin, a calcium-binding protein that mediates a variety of biochemical and physiological processes, including the contraction of muscles and the release of noradrenaline.

calor, heat, as that generated by inflammation of tissues or that from the normal metabolic processes of the body.

caloric, of or pertaining to heat or calories.

calorie, 1. the amount of heat required to raise 1 g of water 1°C at atmospheric pressure. **2.** a quantity of heat equal to 1000 small calories. **3.** a unit, equal to the large calorie, used to denote the heat expenditure of an organism and the fuel or energy value of food. **caloric,** *adj.*

calorific, pertaining to the production of heat.

calorigenic, of or pertaining to a substance or process that produces heat or energy or that increases the consumption of oxygen.

calorimeter, a device used for measuring quantities of heat generated by friction, by chemical reaction, or by the human body. **calorimetric,** *adj.*

calorimetry, the measurement of the amounts of heat radiated and the amounts of heat absorbed. **calorimetric,** *adj.*

calvaria, the skull cap or superior portion of the skull, which varies greatly in shape from individual to individual. In some persons the calvaria is relatively oval, in others it is more circular.

calvities, the condition of baldness. **calvous,** *adj.*

calyx, *pl.* **calyces, calyxes, 1.** a cup-shaped organ. **2.** a renal calyx. **3.** the wall of an ovarian follicle after expulsion of the ovum at ovulation. Also spelled calix.

cambium layer, 1. the loose, inner cellular layer of the periosteum that develops during ossification. **2.** a cellular layer of formative tissue that lies between the wood and the bark in plants.

camera, (in anatomy) any cavity or chamber, as those of the eye or the heart.

cAMP, abbreviation for cyclic adenosine monophosphate.

camphor, a colourless or white crystalline substance with a penetrating odour and pungent taste, occurring naturally in certain plants, especially *Cinnamomum camphora.*

camphor poisoning, a severe toxic condition resulting from the accidental ingestion of camphorated oils. Symptoms may include headache, hallucinations, nausea, vomiting, diarrhoea, convulsions, and kidney failure.

camptodactyly, the permanent flexion of one or more fingers. **campodactylic,** *adj.*

camptomelia, a congenital anomaly characterized by bending of one or more limbs, causing permanent bowing or curving of the affected area. **camptomelic,** *adj.*

Campylobacter, a genus of bacteria found in the family Spirillaceae. The type species is C. fetus, which consists of several subspecies that cause human infections, as well as abortion and infertility in cattle.

camsylate, a contraction for camphorsulphonate.

Camurati-Engelmann disease, an inherited disorder of bone development marked by an onset of symptoms of muscular pain, weakness, and wasting, mainly in the legs, during childhood. The symptoms vary individually from mild to disabling. In some cases there may be compression of nerve tissue. The symptoms usually subside during early adulthood.

canal, 1. (in anatomy) a narrow tube or channel. Some kinds of canals are adductor canal, Alcock's canal, and alveolar canal. **2.** (in dentistry) one of the accessory root canals and collateral pulp canals in the teeth.

canaliculus, *pl.* **canaliculi,** a very small tube or channel, like the tiny haversian canaliculi throughout bone tissue.

canalization, the formation of canals or of passages through any tissue.

canal of Schlemm {Friedrich Schlemm, German anatomist, b. 1795}, a tiny vein at the angle of the anterior chamber of the eye that connects with the pectinate villi, draining the aqueous humour and funneling it into the bloodstream.

canavanine, an amino acid antagonist present in alfalfa sprouts in concentrations of about 15,000 ppm, or 1.5% by weight. Canavanine can displace arginine in cellular proteins.

cancellous, (of tissue) latticelike, porous, spongy. Cancellous tissue is normally present in the interior of many bones, where the spaces are usually filled with marrow.

cancer, 1. a neoplasm characterized by the uncontrolled growth of anaplastic cells that tend to invade surrounding tissue and to metastasize to distant body sites. **2.** any of a large group of malignant neoplastic diseases characterized by the presence of malignant cells. Each cancer is distinguished by the nature, site, or clinical course of the lesion. The basic origin of cancer is undetermined, but many potential causes are recognized such as, cigarette smoking, exposure to carcinogenic chemicals, ionizing radiation, and ultraviolet rays. Many viruses induce malignant tumours in animals, and viral particles are detected in some human tumours. The high incidence of various kinds of cancer in certain families suggests that genetic susceptibility is an important factor. An excess rate of malignant tumors in organ transplant recipients after immunosuppressive therapy indicates that the immune system plays a major role in controlling the proliferation of anaplastic cells. The age-adjusted death rate for oral cancer is almost 10 times higher in Hong Kong than in Denmark, and that for prostate cancer is more than 10 times greater in Sweden than in Japan, but leukaemia mortality is similar throughout the world. In the United Kingdom, cancer is second only to cardiovascular disease as a cause of mortality. Surgery remains the major form of treatment, but irradiation is widely used as preoperative, postoperative, or primary therapy; chemotherapy, with single or multiple antineoplastic agents, is often highly effective.

cancer bodies. See **Russell's bodies.**

cancericidal, of or pertaining to a substance or procedure capable of destroying cancer cells.

cancer in situ. See **carcinoma in situ.**

cancer of the small intestine, a neoplastic disease of the duodenum, jejunum, or ileum. Its characteristics vary, depending on the kind of tumour and the site, but may include abdominal pain, vomiting, weight loss, diarrhoea, intermittent bowel obstruction, GI bleeding, or a mass deep in the right abdomen. Adenocarcinomas, the most common tumours, occur more frequently in the duodenum or upper jejunum and form polypoid or constricting napkin-ring growths. Lymphomas, found most often in the lower small intestine, are associated with a malabsorption syndrome. Surgery, including a wide resection of mesenteric lymph nodes, is indicated for adenocarcinomas. Irradiation is not effective in ablation of these tumours but is recommended postoperatively for lymphomas to treat metastatic lesions.

cancer staging, a system for describing the

extent of a malignant tumour and its metastases, used to plan appropriate treatment and predict prognosis. Staging involves a careful physical examination, diagnostic procedures, and, ultimately, surgical exploration. The standardized system developed by the American Joint Committee for Cancer Staging and End Results Reporting uses the letter T to represent the tumour, N for the regional lymph node involvement, M for distant metastases, and numeric subscripts in each category to indicate the degree of dissemination. According to this system $T_1N_0M_0$ designates a small, localized tumour; $T_2N_1M_0$ is a larger primary tumor that has extended to regional nodes; and $T_4N_3M_3$ is a very large lesion involving regional nodes and distant sites. The Ann Arbor System classifies Hodgkin's disease as Stages I to IV according to the number and location of involved lymph nodes in relation to the diaphragm and the involvement of extralymphatic organs or tissues, based on numerous diagnostic procedures and by a staging laparotomy. Other systems may be used for staging breast carcinoma, colorectal cancer, and cutaneous melanoma.

cancer-ulcer, a carcinomatous ulceration.

cancriform, of or pertaining to a lesion resembling a cancer.

cancroid, 1. of or pertaining to a lesion resembling a cancer. **2.** a moderately malignant skin cancer.

cancrumoris, acute necrotising gingivitis frequently affecting young children in association with systemic diseases such as malnutrition, measles and malaria. It may spread to the cheeks causing necrosis and destroying the tissues of the cheek so that teeth are exposed through the affected area.

candela, See **candle.**

Candida, a genus of yeastlike fungi including the common pathogen, *Candida albicans.*

Candida albicans, a common, budding, yeastlike, microscopic fungal organism normally present in the mucous membranes of the mouth, intestinal tract, and vagina and on the skin of healthy people. Under certain circumstances, it may cause superficial infections of the mouth or vagina and, less commonly, serious invasive systemic infection and toxic reaction.

Candida vaginitis. See **candidiasis.**

candidiasis, any infection caused by a species of *Candida*, usually *Candida albicans*, characterized by pruritus, a white exudate, peeling, and easy bleeding. Nappy rash, intertrigo, vaginitis, and thrush are common topical manifestations of candidiasis.

Candiru fever, an arbovirus infection transmitted to humans by the bite of a sandfly, characterized by an acute fever, headache, and muscle aches.

candle, (in optics) the basic unit of measurement for luminous intensity, equal to 1/60 of the luminous intensity of a square centimetre of a black body heated to 1773.5°C or the solidification temperature of platinum, adopted in 1948 as the international standard of luminous intensity.

cane, a sturdy wooden or metal shaft, or walking stick, used to give support and mobility to an ambulatory but partially disabled person.

canine fossa, (in dentistry) either of the wide depressions on the external surface of each maxilla, superolateral to the canine tooth socket.

canine tooth, any one of the four teeth, two in each jaw, situated immediately lateral to the incisor teeth in the human dental arches. The canine teeth are larger and stronger than the incisors, and they project beyond the level of the other teeth in both arches. Their roots sink deeply into the bones, causing marked prominences on the alveolar arch. The canines erupt as deciduous teeth about 16 to 20 months after birth. The eruption of the permanent canines occurs during the eleventh or the twelfth year of life.

canker, an ulcer or sore, especially in the mouth.

canker sore, an ulcerous lesion of the mouth, characteristic of aphthous stomatitis.

cannabis, a psychoactive drug derived from the flowering tops of hemp plants. It has no currently acceptable clinical use in the United Kingdom but has been employed in the treatment of glaucoma and as an antiemetic in some cancer patients to counter the nausea and vomiting associated with chemotherapy. Cannabis is a Class A, Schedule I drug under the Misuse of Drugs Act 1971 and Misuse of Drugs regulations 1985. The common hemp from which cannabis is obtained is an herbaceous annual of which *Cannabis sativa* is the sole species. All parts of the plant contain psychoactive substances or cannabinoids, the highest concentrations of which are in the resin of the flowering tops of the plant.

cannabism, a condition associated with excessive or extended use of cannabis drugs. It is characterized by anxiety, disorientation, hallucinations, memory defects, and paranoia.

cannon wave, a powerful "a" wave in the jugular pulse, characteristic of a complete heart block and of premature ventricular beats of the heart. Cannon waves are caused by the contraction of the right atrium of the heart immediately after contraction of the right ventricle has closed the tricuspid valve.

cannula, *pl.* **cannulas, cannulae,** a flexible tube containing a stiff, pointed trocar that may be inserted into the body, guided by the trocar. As the trocar is removed, a body fluid may be passed through the cannula to the outside. **cannular, cannulate,** *adj.*

cannulation, the insertion of a cannula into a

body duct or cavity, as into the trachea, bladder, or a blood vessel. **cannulate, cannulize,** v.

cantharis, *pl.* **cantharides,** the dried insects Cantharis vesicatoria containing cantharidin, formerly used as a topical vesicant, and with a reputation as an aphrodisiac ('Spanish fly').

canthus, *pl.* **canthi,** the angle at the medial and the lateral margins of the eyelids. **canthic,** *adj.*

cap, abbreviation for Latin capiat, "let him or her take," used in prescriptions.

CAP, (in molecular genetics) abbreviation for catabolic activator protein. CAP participates in initiating the transcription of RNA in organisms without a true nucleus, as bacteria.

capacitance vessels, 1. the blood vessels that hold the major portion of the intravascular blood volume. **2.** the veins that are downstream from the arterioles, capillaries, and venules.

capacitation, the process in which the spermatozoon, after it reaches the ampulla of the uterine tube, undergoes a series of changes that lead to its ability to fertilize an ovum.

capacitor discharge unit, an x-ray unit incorporating a high tension capacitor usually used in techniques requiring small values of milliAmpere-seconds.

capacity factor, the ratio of the elution volume of a substance to the void volume in the column.

capillaritis, an abnormal condition characterized by a progressive pigmentary disorder of the skin without inflammation but with dilatation.

capillarity. See **capillary action.**

capillary, one of the tiny blood vessels (about 0.008 mm in diameter) joining arterioles and venules. Through their walls, which consist of a single layer of endothelial cells, blood and tissue cells exchange various substances.

capillary action, the action involving molecular adhesion by which the surface of a liquid in a tube is either elevated or depressed, depending on the cohesiveness of the liquid molecules.

capillary angioma. See **cherry angioma.**

capillary bed, a capillary network.

capillary flames. See **telangiectatic naevus.**

capillary fracture, any thin hairlike fracture.

capillary haemangioma, a blood-filled birthmark or a benign tumour consisting of closely packed, small blood vessels. Commonly found in infants, it first grows, then spontaneously disappears in early childhood without treatment.

capillary pulse. See **Quincke's pulse.**

capillary refilling, the process of blood returning to a portion of the capillary system after being interrupted briefly. A capillary refill of more than 3 seconds is considered a sign of sluggish digital circulation, and a time of 5 seconds is regarded as abnormal.

capillary resistance test, see **tourniquet test.**

capillary tufting, an abnormal condition in which pulmonary capillaries project as tufts, or small masses, into the alveoli.

capillovenous, of or pertaining to the venous capillaries.

capillus, *pl.* **capilli,** one of the hairs of the body, especially one of the hairs of the scalp.

capitate, having the shape of a head.

capitate bone, one of the largest carpal bones, located at the centre of the wrist and having a rounded head that fits the concavity of the scaphoid and the lunate bones.

capitulum, *pl.* **capitula,** a small, rounded prominence on a bone where it articulates with another bone.

capitulum humeri, a rounded eminence at the distal end of the humerus. It articulates with the radius.

capnograph an instrument used in anaesthesia, respiratory physiology, and respiratory therapy to produce a tracing, or capnogram, which shows the proportion of carbon dioxide in expired air.

capnometry, the measurement of carbon dioxide in a volume of gas, usually by methods of infrared absorption or mass spectrometry.

capotement, a splashing sound made by fluid movements in a dilated stomach.

capreomycin, an antibiotic prescribed in the treatment of tuberculosis caused by capreomycin-susceptible strains of Mycobacterium tuberculosis when the primary agents are ineffective or cannot be used.

capric acid, a white, crystalline substance with a rancid odour, occurring as a glyceride in natural oils.

caproic acid, a fatty acid that occurs in milk fat and some plant oils. It is used in the production of artificial flavours.

capsid, the layer of protein enveloping a virion.

capsomere, one of the building blocks of a viral capsid. It consists of groups of identical protein molecules and is visible in an electron microscope.

capsula. See **capsule.**

capsular pattern, a series of limitations of joint movement when the joint capsule is a limiting structure. It occurs only in synovial joints that are controlled by muscles.

capsular swelling test. See **quellung reaction.**

capsule, 1. a small, soluble container, usually made of gelatin, used for enclosing a dose of medication for swallowing. **2.** a membranous shell surrounding certain microorganisms, such as the pneumococcus bacterium. **3.** a well-defined anatomical structure that encloses an organ or part, such as the capsule of the adrenal gland.

capsulectomy, the surgical excision of a capsule, usually the capsule of a joint or the capsule of the lens of the eye.

capsule of Tenon. See **fascia bulbi**.

capsule of the kidney, the fatty enclosure of the kidney, consisting of adipose tissue continuous at the hilus with the fat of the renal sinus.

capsuloma, *pl.* **capsulomas, capsulomata,** a neoplasm of the renal capsule or the subcapsular area.

capsulotomy, an incision into the capsule of the eye, such as in an operation to remove a cataract.

captopril, an angiotensin-converting enzyme inhibitor prescribed for the treatment of severe hypertension.

caput, *pl.* **capita, 1.** the head. **2.** the enlarged or prominent extremity of an organ or part.

caput costae, the head of a rib; it articulates with a vertebral body.

caput epididymidis, the head of the epididymis.

caput femoris, the head of the femur; it fits into the acetabulum.

caput fibulae, the head of the fibula; it articulates with the lateral condyle of the tibia.

caput humeri, the head of the humerus; it fits into the glenoid cavity of the scapula.

caput mallei, the head of the malleus.

caput mandibulae, the articular process of the ramus of the mandible.

caput ossis metacarpalis, the metacarpal head; it articulates with the proximal phalanx of the same digit.

caput phalangis, the articular head at the distal end of the proximal and middle phalanges.

caput radii, the head of the radius; it articulates with the capitulum of the humerus.

caput stapedis, the head of the stapes.

caput succedaneum, a localized pitting oedema in the scalp of a fetus that may overlie sutures of the skull. It is usually formed during labour as a result of the circular pressure of the cervix on the fetal head.

carapace, a horny shield or shell covering the dorsal surface of an animal, such as a turtle.

carate. See **pinta**.

carb, abbreviation for a **carbonate noncarboxylate anion**.

carbam, abbreviation for a **carbamate carboxylate anion**.

carbamate, any of a group of anticholinesterase enzymes that cause reversible inhibition of cholinesterase. They are used in certain medications and insecticides. Some carbamates are toxic and may cause convulsions and death through ingestion or skin contact.

carbamate kinase, a liver enzyme that catalyses the transfer of a phosphate group from adenosine triphosphate, associated with ammonia and carbon dioxide, to form adenosine diphosphate and carbamoylphosphate.

carbamazepine, an anticonvulsant and analgesic prescribed in the treatment of seizure disorders, trigeminal neuralgia, and diabetes insipidus.

carbamino compound, a chemical complex formed by the binding of carbon dioxide molecules to plasma proteins. .

carbamino-haemoglobin, a chemical complex formed by carbon dioxide and haemoglobin after the release of oxygen by the haemoglobin to a tissue cell. The action is similar to that of the formation of a carbamino compound. It accounts for nearly 25% of the carbon dioxide released in the lung.

carbenicillin disodium, a semisynthetic penicillin antibiotic prescribed in the treatment of infections caused by *Pseudomas aeruginosa* and *Proteus spp*.

carbidopa, a peripheral decarboxylase inhibitor prescribed in combination with levodopa in the treatment of idiopathic Parkinson's disease, to prevent the breakdown of levodopa outside the brain.

carbocyclic. See **closed-chain**.

carbohydrate, any of a group of organic compounds, the most important being sugar, starch, cellulose, and gum. They are classified according to molecular structure as mono-, di-, tri-, poly-, and heterosaccharides. Carbohydrates constitute the main source of energy for all body functions and are necessary for the metabolism of other nutrients. They are synthesized by all green plants and in the body are either absorbed immediately or stored in the form of glycogen. They can also be manufactured in the body from some amino acids and the glycerol component of fats.

carbohydrate loading, a dietary practice of some endurance atheletes, such as marathon runners, intended to increase glycogen stores in the muscle tissue. A period of carbohydrate abstinence designed to deplete stored glycogen is followed by a diet high in complex carbohydrates. The practice is controversial and not universally practised.

carbohydrate metabolism, the sum of the anabolic and catabolic processes of the body involved in the synthesis and breakdown of carbohydrates, principally galactose, fructose, and glucose. Energy-rich phosphate bonds are produced in many metabolic reactions requiring carbohydrates.

carbolated camphor, a mixture of 1.5 parts camphor with 1 part each of alcohol and phenol, used as an antiseptic dressing for wounds.

carbolic acid, a poisonous, colourless to pale pink crystalline compound obtained from coal tar distillation and converted to a clear liquid with a strong odour and burning taste by the addition of water.

carbolic acid poisoning. See **phenol poisoning**.

carbon (C), a nonmetallic, chiefly tetravalent element. Its atomic number is 6; its atomic weight is 12.011. Carbon occurs in pure form in diamond and graphite and is a component of all living tissue. Most of the study of organic chemistry focuses on the vast number of carbon compounds. Carbon is essential to the chemistry of the body, participating in many metabolic processes and acting as a component of carbohydrates, amino acids, triglycerides, deoxyribonucleic and ribonucleic acids, and many other compounds. Carbon dioxide produced in glycolysis is important in the acid-base balance of the body and in controlling respiration.

carbon 11, a radioisotope of carbon with a half-life of 20 minutes. It is produced by a cyclotron and emits positrons.

carbon 14, a beta-emitter with a half-life of 5760 years. It occurs naturally, arising from cosmic rays, and is used as a tracer in studying various aspects of metabolism and in dating relics that contain natural carbonaceous materials.

carbon arc lamp, an electric lamp producing a strong white light of adjustable intensity from an arc of current between carbon electrodes.

carbonate, a $CO_3^=$ anion. Carbonates are in equilibrium with bicarbonates in water and frequently occur in compounds as insoluble salts, such as calcium carbonate.

carbon cycle, the steps by which carbon in the form of carbon dioxide is extracted from and returned to the atmosphere by living organisms. The process starts with the photosynthetic production of carbohydrates by plants, progresses through the consumption of carbohydrates by animals and human beings, and ends with the exhalation of carbon dioxide and also with the release of carbon dioxide during the decomposition of plants and animals.

carbon damp. See **damp**.

carbon dioxide (CO_2), a colourless, odourless gas produced by the oxidation of carbon. Carbon dioxide, as a product of cell respiration, is carried by the blood to the lungs and is exhaled. The acid-base balance of body fluids and tissues is affected by the level of carbon dioxide and its carbonate compounds. Solid carbon dioxide (dry ice) is used in the treatment of some skin conditions.

carbon dioxide narcosis, a condition of severe hypercapnia, with symptoms of confusion, tremors, convulsions, and coma, that may occur if blood levels of carbon dioxide are increased to 70 mg Hg or higher.

carbon dioxide pressure. See **carbon dioxide tension**.

carbon dioxide retention, any increased partial pressure and body stores of carbon dioxide resulting from impaired carbon dioxide elimination. Respiratory acidosis may result from carbon dioxide retention.

carbon dioxide response, the ventilatory reaction to increased concentrations of carbon dioxide gas. Responses normally increase in a linear curve up to a concentration of 8% or 10%. It flattens slightly near the peak and falls off at concentrations of about 20%. At concentrations around 25%, the person is conscious but is unable to perform simple tasks.

carbon dioxide stores, the volume of carbon dioxide contained in the body as a gas and also in the form of carbonic acid, carbonate, bicarbonate, and carbamino-haemoglobin. During a steady state of respiration and circulation, the quantity of carbon dioxide stores remains constant.

carbon dioxide tension, the partial pressure of carbon dioxide gas, expressed as Pco_2, which is proportional to its percentage in the blood or lungs. A high rate of ventilation causes a lower alveolar Pco_2; a lower rate of breathing leads to higher amounts of alveolar and blood carbon dioxide.

carbon dioxide therapy, the therapeutic inhalation of a low concentration of carbon dioxide gas. Such therapy may be used to dilate the blood vessels, stimulate the cardiovascular brain centres, and overcome hyperventilation. It is used in the treatment of hiccupping (singultation).

carbon dioxide titration curve, a line plotted on a graph showing the blood pH and total carbon dioxide concentration changes that result from the addition or removal of carbon dioxide.

carbon fibre, a material consisting of graphite fibres in a plastic matrix used in radiological devices for radiolucency combined with strength.

carbonic anhydrase, an enzyme that assists in the hydration of carbon dioxide to carbonic acid in the red blood cell so it can be transported from the tissue cell to the lungs.

carbonic anhydrase inhibitor, a substance that decreases the rate of carbonic acid and H^+ production in the kidney, thereby increasing the excretion of solutes and the rate of urinary output.

carbon monoxide, a colourless, odourless, poisonous gas produced by the combustion of carbon or organic fuels in a limited oxygen supply. Carbon monoxide combines irreversibly with haemoglobin, preventing the formation of oxyhaemoglobin and reducing the oxygen supply to the tissues.

carbon monoxide poisoning, a toxic condition in which carbon monoxide gas has been inhaled and absorbed by erythrocytes in the circulation, displacing oxygen from the red blood cells and decreasing the capacity of the blood to carry oxygen to the cells of the body. Headache, dyspnoea, drowsiness, confusion, cherry-pink skin, unconsciousness, and apnoea occur in sequence as the level of carbon monoxide in the blood increases. Treatment includes removal of the victim from the toxic environment, resuscitation, and administration of oxygen.

carbon tetrachloride, a colourless, volatile, toxic liquid used as a solvent and in fire extinguishers. Ingestion of the liquid or inhalation of the fumes usually results in headaches, nausea, depression, abdominal pain, and convulsions. In poisoning by inhalation, ventilatory assistance and oxygen may be necessary.

carboxyfluoroquinolone, any of a group of oral quinolone antibiotics that is generally effective against Enterobacteriaceae and shows varying activity against *Pseudomonas* and other species. The drugs differ in their oral absorption.

carboxyhaemoglobin, a compound produced by the exposure of haemoglobin to carbon monoxide.

carboxyl, a monovalent radical COOH characteristic of organic acids. The hydrogen of the radical can be replaced by metals to form salts.

carbuncle, a large staphylococcal infection containing purulent matter in deep, interconnecting, subcutaneous pockets. Eventually pus discharges to the skin surface through openings. Common sites for carbuncles are the back of the neck and the buttocks.

carbunculosis, an abnormal condition characterized by a cluster of deep painful abscesses that drain through multiple openings onto the skin surface, usually around hair follicles. Carbunculosis is a form of folliculitis, most commonly caused by the coagulase-positive *Staphylococcus aureus*. The lesions caused by this condition may result in fever and malaise.

carcinectomy, the excision of a cancer.

carcinoembryonic antigen (CEA), an antigen present in very small quantities in adult tissue. A greater than normal amount is suggestive of cancer.

carcinogen, a substance or agent that causes the development or increases the incidence of cancer.

carcinogenesis, the process of initiating and promoting cancer.

carcinogenic, of or pertaining to the ability to cause the development of a cancer.

carcinoid, a small yellow tumour derived from argentaffin cells in the GI mucosa that secrete serotonin, other catecholamines, and similar compounds.

carcinoid syndrome, the systemic effects of serotonin-secreting carcinoid tumours manifested by flushing, diarrhoea, cramps, skin lesions resembling pellagra, laboured

breathing, palpitations, and valvular heart disease, especially of the pulmonary valve. Treatment includes surgical excision of the tumour.

carcinolysis, the destruction of cancer cells, as by the action of an antineoplastic drug. **carcinolytic,** *adj.*

carcinoma, *pl.* **carcinomas, carcinomata,** a malignant epithelial neoplasm that tends to invade surrounding tissue and to metastasize to distant regions of the body. It develops most frequently in the skin, large intestine, lungs, stomach, prostate gland, cervix, or breast. The tumour is characteristically firm, irregular, and nodular, with a well-defined border in some places. It usually cannot be clearly dissected and excised without removing normal surrounding tissue. Macroscopically, it is whitish with diffuse, dark haemorrhagic patches, and it has yellow areas of necrosis in the centre. **carcinomatous,** *adj.*

carcinoma basocellulare. See **basal cell carcinoma.**

carcinoma cutaneum. See **basal cell carcinoma, squamous carcinoma.**

carcinoma en cuirasse, a rare neoplasm accompanying advanced breast cancer and characterized by progressive extensive fibrosis and rigidity of the skin of the chest, neck, back, and, occasionally, abdomen.

carcinoma fibrosum. See **scirrhous carcinoma.**

carcinoma gigantocellulare. See **giant cell carcinoma.**

carcinoma in situ, a premalignant neoplasm that has not invaded the basement membrane but shows cytological characteristics of invasive cancer. Such neoplastic changes in stratified squamous or glandular epithelium are frequently seen on the uterine cervix and also occur in the anus, bronchi, buccal mucosa, esophagus, eye, lip, penis, uterine endometrium, vagina, and lesions of senile keratosis.

carcinoma lenticulare, a form of carcinoma tuberosum or scirrhous skin cancer characterized by the development of many small, relatively flat nodules that often coalesce to form larger areas resembling a fungous infection.

carcinoma medullare, carcinoma molle. See **medullary carcinoma.**

carcinoma mucocellulare. See **Krukenberg's tumour.**

carcinoma scroti, an epithelial cell carcinoma of the scrotum.

carcinoma simplex, an undifferentiated epithelial tumor in which the stroma and neoplastic epithelial cells do not have a definite microscopic pattern.

carcinoma spongiosum, a carcinoma that is soft and spongy with small and large cavities in it.

carcinoma telangiectaticum, a neoplasm of

the capillaries of the skin causing dilatation of the vessels and red spots on the skin that blanch with pressure.

carcinomatoid, resembling a carcinoma.

carcinomatosis, an abnormal condition characterized by the extensive spread of carcinoma throughout the body.

carcinomatous, pertaining to carcinoma. Also **carcinous.**

carcinoma tuberosum. See **tuberous carcinoma.**

carcinoma villosum. See **villous carcinoma.**

carcinomectomy. See **carcinectomy.**

carcinophilia, the property in which there is an affinity for carcinomatous tissue. **carcinophilic,** adj.

carcinosarcoma, pl. **carcinosarcomas, carsinosarcomata,** a malignant neoplasm composed of carcinomatous and sarcomatous cells. Tumours of this type may occur in the oesophagus, thyroid gland, and uterus.

carcinosis, pl. **carcinoses,** a condition characterized by the development of many carcinomas throughout the body. Kinds of carcinoses are carcinosis pleurae, miliary carcinosis, pulmonary carcinosis.

carcinosis pleurae, a secondary malignancy of the pleura in which nodules develop throughout the membranes.

carcinostatic, of or pertaining to the tendency to slow or halt the growth of a carcinoma.

carcinous, carcinomatous.

cardia, 1. the opening between the oesophagus and the cardiac portion of the stomach. **2.** the portion of the stomach surrounding the oesophagogastric connection, characterized by the absence of acid cells. **3.** an obsolete term formerly and vaguely used to describe the heart and the region around the heart. **cardiac,** adj.

cardiac, 1. of or pertaining to the heart. **2.** pertaining to a person with heart disease. **3.** of or pertaining to the proximal part of stomach.

cardiac aneurysm. See **ventricular aneurysm.**

cardiac apnoea, abnormal, temporary absence of respiration, as in Cheynes-Stokes respiration.

cardiac arrest, a sudden cessation of cardiac output and effective circulation, usually precipitated by ventricular fibrillation and, in some instances, by ventricular asystole. When cardiac arrest occurs, delivery of oxygen and removal of carbon dioxide stop, tissue cell metabolism becomes anaerobic, and metabolic and repiratory acidosis ensue.

cardiac arrhythmia, an abnormal rate or rhythm of atrial or ventricular myocardial contraction. The condition may be caused by a defect in the ability of the sinoatrial node to maintain its pacemaker function, or by a failure of the bundle of His, the bundle branches, or the Purkinje network to conduct the contractile impulse. Kinds of arrhythmia include bradycardia, extrasystole, heart block, premature atrial contraction, premature ventricular contraction, tachycardia.

cardiac asthma, an attack of asthma associated with heart disease, such as ventricular failure, and characterized by predominant pulmonary congestion with some bronchoconstriction.

cardiac catheter, a long, fine catheter designed to be passed into the heart through a blood vessel.

cardiac catheterization, a diagnostic procedure in which a catheter is introduced into a large vein or artery, usually of an arm or a leg, and threaded through the circulatory system to the heart.

cardiac compression. See **cardiac tamponade.**

cardiac conduction defect, any impairment of the electrical pathways and the specialized muscular fibres that conduct action impulses to contract the atria and the ventricles.

cardiac cycle, the cycle of events during which an electrical impulse is conducted through special fibres over the muscle of the myocardium, from the sinoatrial (SA) node to the atrioventricular (AV) node, to the bundle of His and the bundle branches, and to the Purkinje fibres, causing contraction of the atria followed by contraction of the ventricles. Contraction occurs with depolarization of the muscle fibres; recovery requires repolarization. Deoxygenated blood enters the right atrium of the heart from the superior vena cava and is pumped through the tricuspid valve into the right ventricle. With ventricular contraction, the blood is pumped through the pulmonary valve into the pulmonary artery and the lungs for oxygenation. Oxygen-rich blood is returned to the heart through the branches of the pulmonary veins to the left atrium and is then passed through the mitral valve into the left ventricle. With ventricular contraction, the blood is pumped through the aortic semilunar valve into the aorta for peripheral circulation. On electrocardiogram the cycle is shown as a series of waves, called P, Q, R, S, and T waves, that includes the QRS complex and two segments that connect the waves, the PR segment and the ST segment.

cardiac decompensation, a condition of heart failure in which the heart is unable to fulfill its normal function of ensuring adequate cellular perfusion to all parts of the body without assistance. Causes may include myocardial infarction, increased work load, infection, toxins, or defective heart valves.

cardiac failure. See **heart failure.**

cardiac impulse, the movement of the thorax, caused by the beating of the heart. It is readily palpable and easily recorded.

cardiac index, a measure of the cardiac output of a patient per square metre of body surface area. It is obtained by dividing the cardiac output in litres per minute by the body surface area.

cardiac insufficiency, the inability of the heart to perform its normal functions properly.

cardiac massage, repeated, rhythmic compression of the heart applied directly, during surgery, or through the intact chest wall in an effort to maintain circulation after cardiac arrest or ventricular fibrillation.

cardiac monitor, a device for the continuous observation of cardiac function.

cardiac monitoring, a continuous check on the functioning of the heart with an electronic instrument that provides an electrocardiographic reading on an oscilloscope.

cardiac murmur, an abnormal sound heard during auscultatory examination of the heart, caused by the flow of blood into a chamber or through a valve or by a valve opening or closing. A murmur is classified by the time of its occurrence during the cardiac cycle, the duration, and the intensity of the sound on a scale of I to V.

cardiac muscle, a special striated muscle of the myocardium, containing dark intercalated disks at the junctions of abutting fibers. Cardiac muscle is an exception among involuntary muscles, which are characteristically smooth. Its contractile fibrillae resemble those of skeletal muscle but are only one third as large in diameter, are richer in sarcoplasm, and contain centrally located instead of peripheral nuclei.

cardiac output, the volume of blood expelled by the ventricles of the heart, equal to the amount of blood ejected at each beat (the stroke output), multiplied by the number of beats in the period of time used in the computation. A normal heart in a resting adult ejects from 2.5 to 4 L of blood per minute. A decreased output at rest is usually indicative of a late stage in abnormal cardiac performance; its failure to increase during exercise occurs much earlier in a malfunctioning heart.

cardiac output, decreased, a state in which the amount of blood pumped by an individual's heart is sufficiently reduced that it is inadequate to meet the needs of the body's tissues. Defining characteristics include variations in blood pressure, arrhythmias, fatigue, jugular vein distention, colour changes of the skin and mucous membranes, oliguria, decreased peripheral pulses, cold and clammy skin, rales, dyspnoea, orthopnoea, and restlessness.

cardiac pacemaker. See **pacemaker**.

cardiac plexus, one of several nerve complexes situated close to the arch of the aorta. The cardiac plexuses contain sympathetic and parasympathetic nerve fibres that leave the plexuses, accompany the right and the left coronary arteries, and enter the heart to terminate in the sinoatrial and atrioventricular nodes and in the atrial myocardium.

cardiac radionuclide imaging, examination of the heart, using a radiopharmaceutical. For example, following the intravenous administration of thallium 201 chloride for myocardial perfusion studies using a gamma camera.

cardiac reserve, the potential capacity of the heart to function well beyond its basal level, responding to the demands of various physiological and psychological changes.

cardiac resuscitation. See **cardiopulmonary resuscitation**.

cardiac sphincter, a ring of muscle fibres at the juncture of the oesophagus and stomach.

cardiac standstill, the complete cessation of ventricular contractions and ejection of blood by the heart.

cardiac stimulant, a pharmacological agent that increases the action of the heart. Cardiac glycosides, such as digitoxin, digoxin, and lanatoside, increase the force of myocardial contractions and decrease the heart rate and conduction velocity, allowing more time for the ventricles to relax and become filled with blood. They are used in the treatment of congestive heart failure, atrial flutter and fibrillation, paroxysmal atrial tachycardia, and cardiogenic shock. Adrenaline, a potent vasopressor and cardiac stimulant, is sometimes used to restore heart rhythm in cardiac arrest. Isoprenaline hydrochloride may be used in treating heart block. Dopamine is employed in the short-term treatment of cardiac decompensation resulting from depressed contractility.

cardiac tamponade, compression of the heart produced by the accumulation in the pericardial sac of fluid or of blood resulting from the rupture of a blood vessel of the myocardium, as by a penetrating wound.

cardiac valve. See **heart valve**.

cardinal frontal plane, the plane that divides the body into front and back portions.

cardinal horizontal plane. See **transverse plane**.

cardinal ligament, a sheet of subserous fascia extending across the female pelvic floor as a continuation of the broad ligament. It is embedded in the adipose tissue on each side of the vagina and is formed by the fasciae of the vagina and the cervix converging at the lateral borders of these organs.

cardinal position of gaze, (in ophthalmology) one of six positions to which the normal eye may be turned. Each position requires the function of a specific ocular muscle and a cranial nerve.

cardinal sagittal plane. See **median plane**.

cardinal symptom. See **symptom.**

cardiocirculatory, of or pertaining to the heart and the circulation.

cardiogenic shock, an abnormal condition often characterized by low cardiac output in association with acute myocardial infarction and congestive heart failure. Cardiogenic shock is fatal in about 80% of cases, and immediate therapy is necessary to save affected individuals. Depending on the signs, therapy may include the administration of fluids, diuretics, or vasoactive drugs and the application of various devices such as pacing catheters.

cardiogram, an electronically recorded tracing of cardiac activity.

cardiography, the technique of graphically recording the movements of the heart by means of a cardiograph.

cardiologist, a doctor or surgeon specializing in the diagnosis and treatment of disorders of the heart.

cardiology, the study of the anatomy, normal functions, and disorders of the heart.

cardiolysis, an operation that separates the heart and the pericardium from the sternal periosteum in a procedure to correct adhesive mediastinopericarditis.

cardiomegaly, hypertrophy of the heart caused frequently by pulmonary hypertension and also occurring in arteriovenous fistula, congenital aortic stenosis, ventricular septal defect, patent ductus arteriosus, and Paget's disease.

cardiomyopathy, any disease that affects the myocardium, as alcoholic cardiomyopathy.

cardiomyopexy, a surgical procedure in which the blood supply from the nearby pectoral muscles of the chest is diverted directly to the coronary arteries of the heart.

cardioplasty, a surgical procedure to correct a defect in the cardiac sphincter of the oesophagus that frequently leads to cardiospasm.

cardioplegia, 1. paralysis of the heart. **2.** the arrest of myocardial contractions by injection of chemicals, hypothermia, or electrical stimuli for the purpose of performing surgery on the heart.

cardiopulmonary, of or pertaining to the heart and the lungs.

cardiopulmonary arrest. See **cardiac arrest.**

cardiopulmonary bypass, a procedure used in heart surgery in which the blood is diverted from the heart and lungs by means of a pump oxygenator and returned directly to the aorta.

cardiopulmonary resuscitation (CPR), a basic emergency procedure for life support, consisting of artificial respiration and manual external cardiac massage. It is used in cases of cardiac arrest to establish effective circulation and ventilation in order to prevent irreversible cerebral damage resulting from anoxia. External cardiac massage compresses the heart between the lower sternum and the thoracic vertebral column. During compressions, blood is forced into systemic and pulmonary circulation, and venous blood refills the heart when the compression is released. Mouth-to-mouth breathing or a mechanical form of ventilation is used concomitantly with CPR to oxygenate the blood being pumped through the circulatory system.

cardiorrhaphy, an operation in which the heart muscle is sutured.

cardioscope, an obsolete device for inspecting and manipulating the internal structures of the heart.

cardiospasm, a form of achalasia characterized by a failure of the cardia at the distal end of the oesophagus to relax, causing dysphagia and regurgitation, and sometimes requiring surgical division of the muscle.

cardiotachometer, an instrument that continuously monitors and records the heartbeat.

cardiotomy, 1. an operation in which the heart is incised. **2.** an operation in which the cardiac end of the stomach or cardiac orifice is incised.

cardiotonic, 1. of or pertaining to a substance that tends to increase the efficiency of contractions of the heart muscle. **2.** a pharmacological agent that increases the force of heart contractions.

cardiotoxic, having a toxic or injurious effect on the heart.

cardiovascular, of or pertaining to the heart and blood vessels.

cardiovascular assessment, an evaluation of the condition, function, and abnormalities of the heart and circulatory system.

cardiovascular disease, any one of numerous abnormal conditions characterized by dysfunction of the heart and blood vessels. Some common kinds of cardiovascular disease are atherosclerosis, cor pulmonale, rheumatic heart disease, syphilitic heart disease, and systemic hypertension.

cardiovascular system, the network of structures, including the heart and the blood vessels, that pump and convey the blood throughout the body. The system includes thousands of miles of vessels, capillaries, and venules and is vital to maintaining homeostasis. Numerous control mechanisms of the system assure that the blood is delivered to the structures where it is most needed and at the proper rate. The system delivers nutrients and other essential materials to the fluids surrounding the cells and removes waste products, which are conveyed to excretory organs, such as the kidneys and the intestine. The cardiovascular system functions in close association with the respiratory system, transporting oxygen inhaled into the lungs and conveying carbon dioxide to the lungs for expiration.

cardioversion, the restoration of the heart's normal sinus rhythm by delivery of a synchronized electric shock through two metal paddles placed on the patient's chest. Cardioversion is used in the treatment of atrial fibrillation and in ventricular, nodal, and atrial arrhythmias.

carditis, an inflammatory condition of the muscles of the heart, usually resulting from infection. In most cases more than one layer of muscles is involved. Chest pain, cardiac arrhythmia, circulatory failure, and damage to the structures of the heart may occur. Kinds of carditis are **endocarditis, myocarditis,** and **pericarditis.**

care plan. See **nursing care plan.**

caries, an abnormal condition of a tooth or a bone characterized by decay, disintegration, and destruction of the structure. Kinds of caries include dental caries, radiation caries, and spinal caries.

carina, *pl.* **carinae,** any structure shaped like a ridge or keel, such as the carina of the trachea, that projects from the lowest tracheal cartilage.

cariocas, a form of lateral movement in a gait cycle in which the side-stepping leg is brought successively behind and then in front of the stance leg.

cariogenic, tending to produce caries.

carisoprodol, a skeletal muscle relaxant prescribed for the relief of muscle spasm.

carmalum See **carmine dye.**

carminative, 1. of or pertaining to a substance that relieves flatulence and abdominal distention. **2.** a carminative agent that relieves gaseous distention and painful spasms, especially after meals.

carmine dye, a red colouring substance, produced by the addition of alum to an extract of cochineal, used for staining specimens in histology.

carmustine, a lipid-soluble nitrosourea, 1,3-bis(2-chloroethyl)-1-nitrosourea, used as a cytotoxic agent in the treatment of brain tumours, multiple myeloma, Hodgkin's disease, and non-Hodgkin's lymphomas.

carneous, having the quality of flesh.

carneous mole, see **missed abortion.**

carnitine, a substance found in skeletal and cardiac muscle and certain other tissues that functions as a carrier of fatty acids across the membranes of the mitochondria. It is used therapeutically in treating heart diseases.

carnivore, an animal belonging to the order *Carnivora,* classified as a flesheater, with appropriate teeth and a characteristically simple stomach and a short intestine for such a diet. **carnivorous,** *adj.*

carotene, a red or orange hydrocarbon found in carrots, sweet potatoes, milk fat, egg yolk, and leafy vegetables, such as beet greens, spinach, and broccoli. Carotene is a provitamin and in the body is converted into vitamin A.

Also spelled **carotin, carrotene, carrotine.**

carotenaemia, the presence of high levels of carotene in the blood resulting in an abnormal yellow appearance of the plasma and skin.

carotenoid, any of a group of red, yellow, or orange highly unsaturated pigments that are found in some animal tissue and in foods, such as carrots, sweet potatoes, and leafy green vegetables. Many of these substances are necessary for the formation of vitamin A in the body. Also spelled **carotinoid.**

carotenosis. See **carotenaemia.**

carotid, of or pertaining to the carotid artery.

carotid body, a small structure containing neural tissue at the bifurcation of the carotid arteries. It monitors the oxygen content of the blood and assists in regulating respiration.

carotid-body reflex, a normal chemical reflex initiated by a decrease in oxygen concentration in the blood and, to a lesser degree, by increased carbon dioxide and hydrogen ion concentrations that act on chemoreceptors at the bifurcation of the common carotid arteries and result in nerve impulses that cause the respiratory centre in the medulla to increase respiratory activity.

carotid-body tumour, a benign, round, firm growth that develops at the bifurcation of the common carotid artery. The tumour ometimes may cause dizziness, nausea, and vomiting, especially if it impedes the flow of blood because pressure is increased in the vascular system.

carotid plexus, any one of three nerve plexuses associated with the carotid arteries.

carotid pulse, the pulse of the carotid artery, palpated by gently pressing a finger in the groove between the larynx and the sternocleidomastoid muscle in the neck.

carotid sinus, a dilatation of the arterial wall at the bifurcation of the common carotid artery. It contains sensory nerve endings from the vagus nerve that respond to changes in blood pressure.

carotid sinus reflex, the decrease in the heart rate as a reflex reaction from pressure on or within the carotid artery at the level of its bifurcation.

carotid sinus syndrome, a temporary loss of consciousness that sometimes accompanies convulsive seizures because of the intensity of the carotid sinus reflex when pressure builds in one or both carotid sinuses.

carotodynia, a tenderness along the length of the common carotid artery.

carpal, of or pertaining to the carpus, or wrist.

carpal tunnel, a conduit for the median nerve and the flexor tendons, formed by the carpal bones and the flexor retinaculum.

carpal tunnel syndrome, a common painful disorder of the wrist and hand, induced by compression on the median nerve between the inelastic carpal ligament and other structures within the carpal tunnel. The median nerve innervates the palm and the radial side of the hand; compression of the nerve causes weakness, pain with opposition of the thumb, and burning, tingling, or aching, sometimes radiating to the forearm and to the shoulder joint.

carpometacarpal (CMC) joint, any of the joints formed by the distal row of carpal bones and the bases of the metacarpals. The joints are essential for prehensile patterns.

carpopedal spasm, a spasm of the hand, or thumbs, or foot, or toes that sometimes accompanies tetany.

carpus, the wrist, made up of eight bones arranged in two rows. The proximal row consists of the scaphoid, lunate, triangular, and pisiform. The distal row consists of the trapezium, trapezoid, capitate, and hamate.

carrier, 1. a person or animal who harbours and spreads an organism causing disease in others but who does not become ill. **2.** one whose chromosomes carry a recessive gene.

Carrión's disease. See **bartonellosis**.

Carroll Quantitative Test of Upper Extremity Function, a six-part test of the ability of the patient to grasp and lift objects of different shapes and sizes.

carrying angle, the angle at which the humerus and radius articulate.

carry-over, contamination of a specimen by the previous one.

car sickness. See **motion sickness**.

cartilage, a nonvascular supporting connective tissue composed of various cells and fibers, found chiefly in the joints, the thorax, and various rigid tubes, such as the larynx, trachea, nose, and ear. Temporary cartilage, such as that comprising most of the fetal skeleton at an early stage, is later replaced by bone. Permanent cartilage remains unossified, except in certain diseases and, sometimes, in advanced age. Kinds of permanent cartilage are hyaline cartilage, white fibrocartilage, and yellow cartilage. **cartilaginous,** *adj.*

cartilage graft, the transplantation of cartilage. It is used to correct congenital ear and nose defects in children and to treat severe injuries in adults.

cartilage-hair hypoplasia, a genetic disorder, inherited as an autosomal recessive trait, characterized by dwarfism caused by hypoplasia of the cartilage, multiple skeletal abnormalities, and excessively sparse, short, fine, brittle hair that is usually light coloured.

cartilaginous joint, a slightly movable joint in which cartilage unites bony surfaces. Two types of articulation involving cartilaginous joints are synchondrosis and symphysis.

CARTOS, abbreviation for *computer-aided reconstruction* by tracing of serial sections, a technique in which serial, hand-drawn copies of electron micrographs are pro-grammed on a computer for display on a television screen. The image can be manipulated for study of all dimensions of the structure.

caruncle, a small, fleshy projection, as one of the lacrimal caruncles at the inner canthus of the eye or the hymenal caruncles that are the hymenal remnants.

carunculae hymenales, remnants of a ruptured hymen that appear as irregular projections of normal skin around the introitus to the vagina.

cascade, any process that develops in stages, with each stage dependent on the preceding one, often producing a cumulative effect.

cascade humidifier, a bubbling respiratory care device in which gases travel down a tower and pass through a grid into a chamber of heated water.

cascara, a stimulant laxative prepared from the bark of the *Rhamnus purshianus* tree, used to treat constipation.

caseation, a form of tissue necrosis in which there is loss of cellular outline and the appearance is that of crumbly cheese. It is typical of tuberculosis. **caseate,** *v.*

caseation necrosis, necrosis that transforms tissue into a dry cheeselike mass.

case-control study, a retrospective type of scientific investigation in which a group of patients with a particular disease or disorder, such as myocardial infarction, is compared with a control group of persons who have not developed that medical problem.

case fatality rate, the number of registered deaths caused by any specific disease, expressed as a percentage of the total number of reported cases of a specific disease.

case management, the assignment of a health care provider to assist a patient in assessing health and social service systems and to assure that all required services are obtained.

case nursing, a health care system in which one nurse is assigned to a single patient for delivery of total nursing care.

caseous, cheeselike; describing the mixture of fat and protein that appears in some body tissues undergoing necrosis.

caseous fermentation, the coagulation of soluble casein through the action of rennin.

cassette. See **x-ray cassette**.

cast, 1. a stiff, solid dressing formed with plaster of paris or other material around a limb or other body part to immobilize it during healing. **2.** a mould of a part or all of a patient's teeth and internal jaw area for fitting prostheses or dentures. **3.** a tiny structure formed by deposits of mineral or other substances on the walls of renal tubules, bronchioles, or other organs. Casts often appear in samples of urine or blood collected for laboratory examination. **4.** the deviation of an eye from the normal parallel lines of vision, such as in strabismus.

cast core, a metal casting, employing a post in

the root canal for retaining an artificial tooth crown.

casting, (in dentistry) the process by which crowns, inlays, and other metallic restorations are produced.

castor oil, an oil derived from *Ricinus communis*, used as a stimulant laxative. It is used for the treatment of constipation.

castration, the surgical excision of one or both testicles or ovaries, performed most frequently to reduce the production and secretion of certain hormones that may stimulate the proliferation of malignant cells in women with breast cancer or in men with cancer of the prostate.

castration anxiety, 1. the fantasized fear of injury or loss of the genital organs, possibly as a reaction to a repressed feeling of punishment for forbidden sexual desires. **2.** a general threat to the masculinity or femininity of a person or an unrealistic fear of bodily injury or loss of power.

castration complex. See **castration anxiety.**

casuistics, the recording and the study of the cases of any disease.

CAT, abbreviation for computerized axial tomography.

catabasis, *pl.* **catabases,** the phase in which a disease declines. **catabatic,** *adj.*

catabiosis, the normal ageing of cells. **catabiotic,** *adj.*

catabolic activator protein. See **CAP.**

catabolism, a complex, metabolic process in which energy is liberated for use in work, energy storage, or heat production by the destruction of complex substances by living cells to form simple compounds. **catabolic,** *adj.*

catacrotism, an anomaly of the pulse, characterized by one or more small additional waves in the descending limb of the pulse tracing. **catacrotic,** *adj.*

catagen. See **hair.**

catalase, a heme enzyme, found in almost all biological cells, that catalyses the decomposition of hydrogen peroxide to water and oxygen.

catalepsy, an abnormal state characterized by a trancelike level of consciousness and postural rigidity. It occurs in hypnosis and in certain organic and psychological disorders, such as schizophrenia, epilepsy, and hysteria.

catalysis, an increase in the rate of any chemical reaction, caused by a chemical material that is neither part of the process itself nor consumed or affected by the reaction. **catalytic,** *adj.*

catalyst, a substance that influences the rate of a chemical reaction without being permanently altered by the process. Most catalysts, including enzymes in living organisms, accelerate chemical reactions; negative catalysts retard such reactions.

catamnesis, the medical history of a patient from the onset of an illness.

cataphylaxis, 1. the migration of leukocytes and antibodies to the site of an infection. **2.** the deterioration of the natural defence system of the body. **cataphylactic,** *adj.*

cataplexy, a condition characterized by sudden muscular weakness and hypotonia, caused by emotions, as anger, fear or surprise, often associated with narcolepsy. **cataplectic,** *adj.*

cataract, an abnormal progressive condition of the lens of the eye, characterized by loss of transparency. A grey-white opacity can be seen within the lens, behind the pupil. Most cataracts are caused by degenerative changes, occurring most often after 50 years of age. The tendency to develop cataracts is inherited. **Congenital cataracts** are usually hereditary but may be caused by viral infection during the first trimester of gestation. If cataracts are untreated, sight is eventually lost. At first vision is blurred; then, bright lights glare diffusely, and distortion and double vision may develop. Uncomplicated cataracts of old age (**senile cataracts**) are usually treated with excision of the lens and prescription of special contact lenses or glasses.

catarrh, *obsolete.* inflammation of the mucous membranes with discharge, especially inflammation of the air passages of the nose and the trachea. **catarrhal, catarrhous,** *adj.*

catarrhal dysentery, See **sprue.**

catastrophic reaction, 1. the uncoordinated response to a drastic shock or a sudden threatening condition, such as often occurs in the victims of car crashes and disasters. **2.** response to sudden insight into one's own mental disorder, e.g. dementia.

catatonia, a state or condition characterized by conspicuous motor disturbance, manifested usually as immobility with extreme muscular rigidity or, less commonly, as excessive, impulsive activity. **catatonic,** *adj.*

catatonic excitement, a state of extreme agitation that may occur when a patient is unable to maintain catatonic immobility.

catatonic schizophrenia, a form of schizophrenia characterized by alternating periods of extreme withdrawal and extreme excitement. During the withdrawal stage stupor, muscular rigidity, mutism, blocking, negativism, and catalepsy (cerea flexibilitas) may be seen; during the period of excitement, purposeless and impulsive activity may range from mild agitation to violence.

catatonic stupor, a form of catatonia marked by a lack of response; it may be related to a patient's fear of losing the ability to control his or her impulses.

cat-bite fever. See **cat-scratch fever.**

CAT-CAM, abbreviation for **contoured adducted controlled alignment method.**

catchment area, the specific geographic area for which a particular institution, such as a hospital, health centre or school, is responsible.

catch-up growth, an acceleration of the growth rate following a period of growth retardation caused by a secondary deficiency, such as acute malnutrition or severe illness. The phenomenon, which is routinely seen in premature infants, involves rapid increase in weight, length, and head circumference and continues until the normal individual growth pattern is resumed.

cat-cry syndrome, a rare, congenital disorder recognized at birth by a kittenlike cry caused by a laryngeal anomaly. The condition is associated with a defect in chromosome 5. Other characteristics include low birth weight, microcephaly, "moon face," wide-set eyes, strabismus, and low-set misshaped ears. Infants are hypotonic; heart defects and mental and physical retardation are common.

catecholamine, any one of a group of sympathomimetic compounds composed of a catechol molecule and the aliphatic portion of an amine. Some catecholamines are produced naturally by the body and function as key neurologic chemicals. Catecholamines are also synthesized as drugs used in the treatment of various disorders, such as anaphylaxis, asthma, cardiac failure, and hypertension. Some important endogenous catecholamines are dopamine, adrenaline, and noradrenaline.

catechol-o-methyl transferase (COMT), an enzyme that deactivates the catecholamines adrenaline and noradrenaline.

cat-eye syndrome, a rare, congenital autosomal anomaly, marked by the presence of an extra, small chromosome 22 and pupils that resemble the vertical pupils of a cat.

categoric data, (in research) any data that are classified by name rather than by number, such as race, religion, ethnicity, or marital status.

catgut, a nonabsorbable suture material, prepared from the intestines of sheep, used to close surgical wounds.

catharsis, 1. a cleansing or purging. **cathartic,** *n.* **2.** the therapeutic release of pent-up feelings and emotions by open discussion of ideas and thoughts. **3.** the process of bringing repressed ideas and feelings into the consciousness by the technique of free association, often in conjunction with hypnosis and the use of hypnotic drugs.

cathartic. See **laxative.**

catheter, a hollow, flexible tube that can be inserted into a vessel or cavity of the body to withdraw or to instill fluids. Kinds of catheters include urinary catheter, Foley catheter, and intrauterine catheter.

catheter hub, a threaded plastic connection at the end of an intravenous catheter.

catheterization, the introduction of a catheter into a body cavity or organ to inject or

remove a fluid. The most common procedure is the insertion of a catheter into the bladder through the urethra for the relief of urinary retention and for emptying the bladder completely before surgery. Sterile, aseptic techniques are necessary to prevent infection. For indwelling catheters, attention is given to maintaining continuous free drainage and to the increased possibility of infection. Kinds of catheterization are **cardiac catheterization,** and **hepatic vein catheterization. catheterize,** *v.*

cathexis, the conscious or unconscious attachment of emotional feeling and importance to a specific idea, person, or object. Translatgion of a German word, 'Besetzung', used by Freud. **cathectic,** *adj.*

cathode, the electrode at which reduction occurs.

cathode ray, a stream of electrons emitted by the negative electrode of a gaseous discharge device when the cathode is bombarded by positive ions, such as in a cathode ray tube or an oscilloscope. The ray is usually focused by electromagnets that control its direction and position on a screen coated with a phosphor to create a visible pattern.

cathode ray oscilloscope, an instrument that produces a visual representation of electric variations by means of the fluorescent screen of a cathode ray tube. Oscilloscopes are used to display patients' brain waves and heart beats for monitoring and diagnostic purposes.

cathode ray tube (CRT), a vacuum tube that focuses a beam of electrons onto a spot on a screen coated with a phosphor, creating a visible image of information on the face of the tube.

cation, a positively charged ion that in solution is attracted to the negative electrode.

cation-exchange resin, any one of various insoluble organic polymers with high molecular weights that exchange their cations for other ions in solution.

catoptric, of or pertaining to a reflected image or reflected light, such as from a mirror.

CAT scan. See **computed tomography.**

cat scratch fever, a disease that results from the scratch or bite of a healthy cat. Inflammation and pustules are found on the scratched skin, and lymph nodes in the neck, head, groin, or axilla swell 2 weeks later.

cat's eye amaurosis, a monocular blindness, with a bright reflection from the pupil caused by a white mass in the vitreous humor resulting from inflammation or a malignant lesion.

caudad, toward the tail or end of the body, away from the head.

cauda equina, the lower end of the spinal cord at the first lumbar vertebra and the bundle of lumbar, sacral, and coccygeal nerve roots that descend through the spinal canal of the sacrum and coccyx.

caudal, signifying a position toward the distal end of the spine.

caudal anaesthesia, the injection of a local anaesthetic agent into the caudal portion of the spinal canal through the sacrum. It is performed in labour and in such procedures as culdoscopy and anorectal and genitourinary surgery.

caudate, having a tail.

caudate process, a small elevation of tissue that extends obliquely from the lower extremity of the caudate lobe of the liver to the visceral surface of the right lobe.

caul, the intact amniotic sac covering the baby's head at birth. The sac usually ruptures or is ruptured during the course of labour or delivery; when it remains intact, it must be torn or cut to allow the baby to breathe.

cauliflower ear, a thickened, deformed ear caused by repeated trauma, such as that suffered by boxers.

caumaesthesia, an abnormal condition in which a patient has a low temperature but experiences a sense of intense heat. **caumaesthetic,** *adj.*

causalgia, a severe sensation of burning pain, often in an extremity, sometimes with local erythema of the skin. It is the result of injury to a peripheral sensory nerve.

causal hypothesis, (in research) a hypothesis that predicts a cause-and-effect relationship among the variables to be studied.

causal hypothesis testing study, (in nursing research) an experimental design used in testing a hypothesis that predicts a cause-and-effect relationship within the data to be studied.

causality, (in research) a relationship between one phenomenon or event (A) and another (B) in which A precedes and causes B and the direction of influence and the nature of the effect are predictable and reproducible and may be empirically observed.

cause, any process, substance, or organism that produces an effect or condition.

caustic, 1. any substance that is destructive to living tissue, such as silver nitrate, nitric acid, or sulphuric acid. **2.** exerting a burning or corrosive effect.

caustic poisoning, the accidental ingestion of strong acids or alkalis, resulting in burns and tissue damage to the mouth, esophagus, and stomach. The victim experiences immediate pain, swelling, and oedema. The pulse may be weak and rapid. Respirations become shallow, and oedema may close the airway. Administration of "neutralizing" substances is not recommended because of the risk of a heat-producing chemical reaction.

cautery, 1. a device or agent that scars and burns the skin, such as in the coagulation of tissue by heat or caustic substances. **2.** a destructive effect produced by a cauterizing agent.

cautery knife, a surgical knife that cuts tissue and cauterizes it to prevent bleeding. The knife is connected to an electric source that generates the heat necessary for cauterization.

cavalry bone. See **rider's bone.**

Cavell, Edith, (1865-1915), an English nurse who trained at the London Hospital. In 1907 she became the head of a nurses' training school in Brussels, with the task of raising nursing standards to match those of Britain. After the Germans occupied Belgium in World War I, she nursed or sheltered more than 200 fleeing soldiers and helped them reach Holland. She was arrested by the Germans, tried, and shot on October 12, 1915. Her execution brought her widespread fame.

cavernoma. See **cavernous haemangioma.**

cavernous, containing cavities or hollow spaces.

cavernous angioma. See **cavernous haemangioma.**

cavernous body of the clitoris, cavernous body of the penis. See **corpus cavernosum.**

cavernous haemangioma, a benign, congenital tumour consisting of large, blood-filled, cystic spaces. The scalp, face, and neck are the most common sites.

cavernous lymphangioma. See **lymphangioma cavernosum.**

cavernous rale, an abnormal hollow, metallic sound heard during auscultation of the thorax. It is caused by contraction and expansion of a pulmonary cavity during respiration and indicates a pathological condition.

cavernous sinus, one of a pair of irregularly shaped, bilateral venous channels between the sphenoid bone of the skull and the dura mater. It is one of the five anterior inferior venous sinuses that drain the blood from the dura mater into the internal jugular vein.

cavernous sinus syndrome, an abnormal condition characterized by oedema of the conjunctiva, the upper eyelid, and the root of the nose and by paralysis of the third, the fourth, and the sixth nerves. It is caused by a thrombosis of the cavernous sinus.

cavernous sinus thrombosis, a syndrome, usually secondary to infections near the eye or nose, characterized by orbital oedema, venous congestion of the eye, and palsy of the nerves supplying the extraocular muscles.

cavitary, 1. denoting the presence of one or more cavities. **2.** any entozoon having a body cavity or an alimentary canal.

cavitate, the act of rapidly forming and collapsing vapour pockets or bubbles in a flowing fluid with low pressure areas, often causing damage to surrounding structures.

cavitation, 1. the formation of cavities within the body, such as those formed in the lung by tuberculosis. **2.** any cavity within the body, such as the pleural cavities.

cavity, 1. a hollow space within a larger structure, such as the peritoneal cavity or the oral cavity. **2.** nontechnical. a space in a tooth formed by dental caries.

cavity classification, the taxonomy of carious lesions according to the tooth surfaces on which they occur, such as labial, buccal, or occlusal; and type of surface, such as pitted or smooth.

cavosurface angle, (in dentistry) the angle formed by the junction of the wall of a prepared cavity with the external surface of the tooth.

cavosurface bevel, the incline of the cavosurface angle of a prepared tooth cavity wall relative to the enamel wall.

cavum, *pl.* **cava, 1.** any hollow or cavity. **2.** the inferior or superior vena cava.

Cb, symbol for **columbium.**

CBF, abbreviation for **cerebral blood flow.**

CCK, abbreviation for **cholecystokinin.**

CCU, abbreviation for **coronary care unit.**

Cd, symbol for **cadmium.**

CD, abbreviation for **controlled drug.**

CDE, the major symbols used in one system for the nomenclature of the Rh system, in which D is the same as Rh_0, the major determining factor of Rh positivity.

Ce, symbol for **cerium.**

CEA, abbreviation for **carcinoembryonic antigen.**

ceasmic, pertaining to or characterized by a persistent embryonic fissure or abnormal cleavage of parts.

ceasmic teratism, a congenital anomaly, caused by developmental arrest, in which parts of the body that should be fused remain in their fissured embryonic state, such as in cleft palate.

cefaclor, a cephalosporin antibiotic used in the treatment of bacterial infections.

cefadroxil monohydrate, a cephalosporin antibiotic used in the treatment of bacterial infections.

cefotaxime sodium, an injectable cephalosporin antibiotic used in the treatment of bacterial infections.

cefoxitin sodium, an injectable cephalosporin antibiotic used in the treatment of bacterial infections.

ceftazidime, an injectable cephalosporin antibiotic used in the treatment of severe bacterial infections.

ceftizoxime sodium, an injectable cephalosporin antibiotic used in the treatment of severe bacterial infections.

ceftriaxone sodium, an injectable cephalosporin antibiotic used in the treatment of severe bacterial infections.

cefuroxime axefil, cefuroxime sodium, cephalosporin antibiotics used in the treatment of bacterial infections.

cell, the fundamental unit of all living tissue. Eukaryotic cells consist of a nucleus, cytoplasm, and organelles surrounded by a cytoplasmic membrane. Within the nucleus are the nucleolus and chromatin granules that develop into chromosomes. Organelles within the cytoplasm include the endoplasmic reticulum, ribosomes, the Golgi complex, mitochondria, lysosomes, and the centrosome. Prokaryotic cells are similar but lack a nucleus. The specialized nature of body tissue reflects the specialized structure and function of its constituent cells.

cella, *pl.* **cellae** an enclosed space.

cell biology, the science that deals with the structures, living processes, and functions of cells, especially human cells.

cell body, the part of a cell that contains the nucleus and surrounding cytoplasm exclusive of any projections or processes, such as the axon and dendrites of a neuron or the tail of a spermatozoon. It is concerned more with the metabolism of the cell than with a specific function.

cell cycle, the sequence of events that occurs during the growth and division of tissue cells.

cell death, 1. terminal failure of a cell to maintain the essential life functions. **2.** the point in the process of dying at which vital functions have ceased at the cellular level.

cell division, the continuous process by which a cell divides in four stages; prophase, metaphase, anaphase, and telophase. Preliminary to prophase, the centrosome of the cell divides into two parts, which become oriented at opposite poles of the nucleus. During the prophase, previously dispersed chromatin condenses into chromomeres strung along a threadlike chromonema composed of deoxyribonucleic acid. During metaphase, the chromosomes become oriented in the equatorial plane with a clear area directed toward the two centrosomes. Each centromere divides during late metaphase and early anaphase. In telophase, the chromosomes form a compact mass, lose their individuality, and disperse into the chromatin of the intermitotic nucleus.

cell line, a colony of animal cells developed as a subculture from a primary culture.

cell-mediated immune response, a delayed type IV hypersensitivity reaction, mediated primarily by sensitized T cell lymphocytes as opposed to antibodies.

cell-mediated immunity. See **cellular immunity.**

cell membrane, the outer covering of a cell, often having projecting microvilli and containing the cellular cytoplasm. The cell membrane controls the exchange of materials between the cell and its environment.

cell theory, the proposition that cells are the basic units of all living substance and that cellular function is the essential process of life.

cellular hypersensitivity reaction. See **cell-mediated immune response.**

cellular immunity, the mechanism of acquired immunity characterized by the dominant role of small T cell lymphocytes, such as in resistance to infectious diseases, in delayed hypersensitivity reactions, resistance to cancer, autoimmune diseases, graft rejection, and certain allergies.

cellular infiltration, the migration and grouping of cells within tissues throughout the body.

cellulitis, an infection of the skin characterized most commonly by local heat, redness, pain, and swelling, and occasionally by fever, malaise, chills, and headache. Abscess and tissue destruction usually follow if antibiotics are not taken.

cellulose, a colourless, insoluble, nondigestible, transparent solid carbohydrate that is the primary constituent of the skeletal substances of the cell walls of plants.

cell wall, the structure that covers and protects the cell membrane in some kinds of cells, such as certain bacteria and all plant cells.

celosomia, a congenital malformation characterized by a fissure or absence of the sternum and ribs and protrusion of the viscera.

celosomus, a fetus with celosomia.

Celsius (C) {Anders Celsius, Swedish scientist, b. 1701}, denoting a temperature scale in which 0° is the freezing point of water and 100° is the boiling point of water at sea level.

cement, 1. a sticky or mucilaginous substance that helps neighboring tissue cells stick together. **2.** any of a variety of dental materials used to fill cavities or to hold bridgework or other dental prostheses in place. **3.** a material used in the fixation of a prosthetic joint in adjacent bones, such as methyl methacrylate.

cemental fibre, any one of the many fibres of the periodontal membrane that extend from the cementum to the intermediate plexus.

cement lining, (in dentistry) a layer of insulated dental cement, sometimes medicated, pressed into the bottom of a prepared cavity to protect the pulp, to reduce the bulk of metallic restoration, or eliminate undercuts in a tapered preparation.

cementifying fibroma, 1. an intrabony lesion that is not associated with the teeth, composed of fibrous connective tissue enclosing foci of calcified material resembling cementum. **2.** a rare odontogenic tumour composed of varying amounts of fibrous connective tissue resembling cementum. **3.** a central lesion of the jaws.

cementoblastoma, *pl.* **cementoblastomas, cementoblastomata,** an odontogenic fibrous tumour consisting of cells developing into cementoblasts but containing only a small amount of calcified tissue.

cementoma, *pl.* **cementomas, cementomata,** an accumulation of cementum existing free at the apex of a tooth, probably caused by trauma rather than neoplastic growth.

cementopathia, periodontitis resulting from disease or defect of the cementum.

cementum, the bonelike connective tissue that covers the roots of the teeth and helps to support them.

cen, abbreviation for **centromere**.

cenogenesis, the development of physical characteristics that are absent in earlier forms of a species, as an adaptive response to environmental conditions. Also spelled **coenogenesis, caenogenesis, kenogenesis.**

censor, 1. a person who monitors or evaluates books, newspapers, plays, works of art, speech, or other means of expression in order to suppress certain kinds of information. **2.** (in psychoanalysis) a psychic suppression that allows unconscious thoughts to rise to consciousness only if they are heavily disguised.

centesis, a perforation or a puncture, such as a paracentesis, abdominocentesis, or thoracocentesis.

centigrade, See **Celsius**.

centimetre (cm), the metric unit of measurement equal to one hundredth of a metre, or 0.3937 inches.

centimetre-gram-second system (cgs, CGS), the internationally accepted scientific system of expressing length, mass, and time in basic units of centimetres, grams, and seconds. The CGS system has been replaced by the Système International d'Unités (SI) or the International System of Units, based on the metre, kilogram, and second.

centipoise {Jean L. M. Poiseuille, French physiologist, b. 1799}, a measure of the viscosity of a liquid, equal to one hundredth of a poise.

central, pertaining to or situated at a centre.

central amaurosis, blindness caused by a disease of the central nervous system.

central canal of spinal cord, the conduit that runs the entire length of the spinal cord and contains most of the 140 ml of cerebrospinal fluid in the body of the average individual. The central canal of the spinal cord lies in the centre of the cord between the ventral and the dorsal grey commissures and extends cranialward into the medulla oblongata, where it opens into the fourth ventricle of the brain.

central chemoreceptor, any of the sensory nerve cells or chemical receptors that are located in the medulla of the brain.

central chondrosarcoma, a malignant cartilaginous tumour that forms inside a bone.

central control hypothesis, a concept that the subcortical nervous system is regulated by internal control mechanisms in the form of templates inherited phylogenetically from animal ancestors.

central fissure. See **central sulcus**.

central implantation. See **superficial implantation**.

central lobe, one of the lobes constituting

each of the cerebral hemispheres, lying hidden in the depths of the lateral sulcus. The central lobe can be seen only if the lips of the sulcus are parted or cut away.

central nervous system (CNS), one of the two main divisions of the nervous system of the body, consisting of the brain and the spinal cord. The central nervous system processes information to and from the peripheral nervous system and is the main network of coordination and control for the entire body. The spinal cord extends various types of nerve fibres from the brain and acts as a switching and relay terminal for the peripheral nervous system. The 12 pairs of cranial nerves emerge directly from the brain. Sensory nerves and motor nerves of the peripheral system leave the spinal cord separately between the vertebrae but unite to form 31 pairs of spinal nerves containing sensory fibres and motor fibres. More than 10 billion neurons constitute but one tenth of the brain cells, the other cells consisting of neuroglia. Flowing through various cavities of the central nervous system, such as the ventricles of the brain, the subarachnoid spaces of the brain and spinal cord, and the central canal of the spinal cord is the cerebro~spinal fluid. The brain and the spinal cord are composed of grey matter and white matter. The grey matter contains primarily nerve cells and associated processes; the white matter consists of bundles of predominantly myelinated nerve fibres.

central nervous system depressant, any drug that decreases the function of the central nervous system, such as alcohol, barbiturates, and hypnotics. Central nervous system depressants elevate the seizure threshold; this property makes some of them useful as anticonvulsants. Others are used recreationally and can produce physical dependence in a relatively short period of time. Sudden withdrawal of central nervous system depressants that have been used in high doses for prolonged periods can result in rebound excitation and seizures, and can even be fatal.

central nervous system stimulant, a substance that quickens the activity of the central nervous system by increasing the rate of neuronal discharge or by blocking an inhibitory neurotransmitter. Many natural and synthetic compounds stimulate the central nervous system, but only a few are used therapeutically. Many, such as caffeine and the amphetamines are used recreationally.

central nervous system syndrome (CNS syndrome), a constellation of neurological and emotional signs and symptoms that results from a massive whole-body dosage of radiation.

central nervous system tumour, a neoplasm of the brain or spinal cord that characteristically does not spread beyond the cerebrospinal axis, although it may be highly invasive locally and have widespread effects on body functions. Many brain tumours are metastatic lesions from primary cancer in the breast, lung, GI tract, kidney, or a site of melanoma.

central neuritis. See **parenchymatous neuritis.**

central neurogenic hyperventilation (CNHV), a pattern of breathing marked by rapid and regular respirations at a rate of about 25 per minute. Increasing regularity, rather than rate, is an important diagnostic sign because it indicates an increasing depth of coma.

central processing unit (cpu, CPU), a component of a computer that controls the encoding and execution of instructions.

central ray (CR), the portion of the x-ray beam that is directed towards the centre of the film or of the object being radiographed.

central scotoma, an area of blindness or site of depressed vision involving the macula of the retina.

central sleep apnoea, a form of sleep apnoea resulting from a decreased respiratory centre output. It may involve primary brainstem medullary depression.

central stimulant. See **central nervous system stimulant.**

central sulcus, a cleft separating the frontal from the parietal lobes of the brain.

central tendon, a broad connective tissue sheet that forms the diaphragm. It is composed of interlacing fibres that arise from the lumbar vertebrae, the costal margin, and the xiphoid process of the sternum.

central venous catheter, a catheter that is threaded through the internal jugular, antecubital, or subclavian vein, usually with the tip resting in the superior vena cava or the right atrium.

central venous oxygen saturation (CVS_{O_2}), the oxygen saturation in the vena cava. The CVS_{O_2} is measured through a central venous catheter and is useful in measuring cardiac output.

central venous pressure (CVP), the blood pressure in the large veins of the body, as distinguished from peripheral venous pressure in an extremity. It is measured with a water manometer that may be attached to the head of a patient's bed and to a central venous catheter inserted into the vena cava.

central venous pressure (CVP) monitor, a device for measuring and recording the venous blood pressure by means of an indwelling catheter and a pressure manometer.

central venous return, the blood from the venous system that flows into the right atrium through the vena cava.

central vision, vision that results from images falling on the macula of the retina.

centre, 1. the middle point of the body or

geometric entity, equidistant from points on the periphery. **2.** a group of neurons with a common function, such as the accelerating centre in the brain that controls the heartbeat.

centrencephalic, of, pertaining to, or involving the centre of the encephalon.

centre of gravity, the midpoint or centre of the weight of a body or object. In the standing adult human the centre of gravity is in the midpelvic cavity, between the symphysis pubis and the umbilicus.

centric jaw relationship (CJR), the relationship of the mandible to the maxilla when the condyles are in the most retruded unrestrained position in the glenoid fossa, from which lateral excursions of the jaw can be made.

centrifugal, 1. denoting a force that is directed outward, away from a central point or axis, such as the force that keeps the moon in its orbit around the earth. **2.** a direction away from the head.

centrifugal analyser, equipment that uses centrifugal force to mix the sample aliquot with reagent and a spinning rotor to pass the reaction mixture through a detector.

centrifugal current, an electric current in the body with the positive pole near the nerve centre and the negative pole at the periphery.

centrifuge, a device for separating components of different densities contained in liquid by spinning them at high speeds. Centrifugal force causes the heavier components to move to one part of the container, leaving the lighter substances in another. **centrifugal,** *adj.,* **centrifuge,** *v.*

centrilobular, pertaining to, or situated at the centre of a lobule.

centriole, an intracellular organelle, usually as a component of the centrosome. Often occurring in pairs, centrioles are associated with cell division. They appear to aid in the formation of the spindle that develops during mitosis.

centripetal, 1. denoting an afferent direction, such as that of a sensory nerve impulse travelling toward the brain. **2.** denoting the direction of a force pulling an object toward an axis of rotation or constraining an object to a specific curved path.

centripetal current, an electric current passing through the body from a peripheral positive electrode to a negative pole near the nerve centre.

centromere, the specialized, constricted region of the chromosome that joins the two chromatids to each other and attaches to the spindle fibre in mitosis and meiosis. During cell division the centromeres split longitudinally, half going to each of the new daughter chromosomes.

centrosome, a self-propagating cytoplasmic organelle, which consists of the centrosphere and the centrioles. It is located near the nucleus and functions as the dynamic centre of the cell, especially during mitosis.

centrosphere, the differentiated, condensed area of cytoplasm surrounding the centrioles in the centrosome of the cell.

centrum, *pl.* **centra,** any kind of center, especially one related to a structure of the body, as the centrum semi-ovale of a cerebral hemisphere.

cephal-. See **cephalo**.

cephalad, toward the head, away from the end, or tail.

cephalalgia, headache, often combined with another word to indicate a specific type of headache, such as histamine cephalalgia.

cephalexin, a cephalosporin antibiotic used by mouth in the treatment of bacterial infections.

cephalgia. See **cephalalgia, headache**.

cephalhaematoma, a swelling on the head, due to an effusion of blood between the periosteum and bone. This occurs during labour. It may take weeks to subside, but no treatment is necessary.

-cephalia, a combining form meaning '(condition of the) head': *hemicephalia, megacephalia, notancephalia.*

cephalic, of or pertaining to the head.

-cephalic, a combining form meaning 'relating to the head': *holocephalic, megalocephalic, postcephalic.*

cephalic presentation, a classification of fetal position in which the head of the fetus is at the uterine cervix.

cephalic vein, one of the four superficial veins of the upper limb. It receives deoxygenated blood from the dorsal and the palmar surfaces of the forearm.

cephalo-, cephal-, a combining form meaning 'pertaining to the head': *cephalocaudal, cephalocentesis, cephalogenesis.*

cephalocaudal, pertaining to the long axis of the body, or the relationship between the head and the base of the spine.

cephalomelus, a deformed individual with a structure resembling an arm or a leg protruding from the head.

cephalometry, scientific measurement of the head, such as that performed in dentistry to determine appropriate orthodontic procedures for correcting malocclusions and other abnormal conditions. **cephalometric,** *adj.*

cephalopagus. See **craniopagus**.

cephalopelvic, pertaining to a relationship between the fetal head and the maternal pelvis.

cephalopelvic disproportion (CPD), an obstetric condition in which the fetal head is too large or a mother's birth canal too small to permit normal labour or birth.

cephalosporin, a semisynthetic derivative of an antibiotic originally derived from the microorganism *Cephalosporium acre-*

monium. Cephalosporins are similar in structure to penicillins except for a beta-lactam-dihydrothiazine ring in place of the beta-lactam-thiazolidin in penicillin.

cephalothoracoiliopagus. See **synadelphus**.

cephalothoracopagus, a conjoined twin fetus attached at the head, neck, and thorax.

-cephaly, -cephalia, a combining form meaning '(specified) condition of the head': *macrencephaly, platycephaly, trochocephaly.*

cephazolin sodium, a cephalosporin antibiotic used in the treatment of bacterial infections.

cephradine, a cephalosporin antibiotic used in the treatment of certain bacterial infections.

cer-, a combining form meaning 'wax': *ceraceous, cerate, cerumen.*

ceramics, (in dentistry) the technology of making dental restorations from fused porcelain and other glasses.

cerato-, kerato-, a combining form meaning 'pertaining to the cornea or to horny tissue': *ceratocricoid, ceratohyal, ceratopharyngeus.*

cercaria, *pl.* **cercariae** a wormlike form of trematode. It develops in a freshwater snail and is released into the water. Cercariae enter the body of the next host by ingestion, by direct invasion through the skin, or through a cut or other break in the skin. They encyst and complete their development in various organs of the body. Each species tends to migrate to one organ, such as *Fasciola hepatica,* which becomes a liver fluke.

cerclage, 1. an orthopaedic procedure in which the ends of an oblique bone fracture or the chips of a broken patella are bound together with a wire loop or a metal band to hold the bone fragments in position until healed. **2.** a procedure in which a taut silicone band is applied around the sclera to restore contact between the retina and the choroid when the retina is detached. **3.** an obstetric procedure in which a nonabsorbable suture is used for holding the cervix closed to prevent spontaneous abortion in a woman who has an incompetent cervix.

cerea flexibilitas, a cataleptic state, frequently observed in catatonic schizophrenia, in which the limbs retain for an indefinite period of time the positions in which they are placed.

cerebellar, of or pertaining to the cerebellum.

cerebellar angioblastoma, a tumour in the cerebellum composed of a mass of blood vessels. It may be cystic and is frequently associated with von Hippel-Lindau disease.

cerebellar artery occlusion, an obstruction of one of the arteries supplying the cerebellum.

cerebellar atrophy, any of several diseases characterized by deterioration and wasting

of tissues of the cerebellum.

cerebellar cortex, the superficial grey matter of the cerebellum covering the white substance in the medullary core and consisting of two layers, an external molecular layer and an internal granule cell layer. The layers are separated by an incomplete stratum of Purkinje cells.

cerebellar cortical degeneration. See **alcoholic nutritional cerebellar degeneration**.

cerebellar speech, abnormal speech seen in diseases of the cerebellum. It is characterized by slow, jerky, and slurred articulation that may be intermittent and explosive or monotonous and unvaried in pitch.

cerebellopontine, leading from the cerebellum to the pons varolii.

cerebellospinal, leading from the cerebellum to the spinal cord.

cerebellum, *pl.* **cerebellums, cerebella,** the part of the brain located in the posterior cranial fossa behind the brainstem. It consists of two lateral cerebellar hemispheres, or lobes, and a middle section called the vermis. Three pairs of peduncles link it with the brain stem. Its functions are concerned with coordinating voluntary muscular activity.

cerebr-, a combining form meaning 'pertaining to the cerebrum': *cerebralgia, cerebrocardiac, cerebropathy.*

cerebral, of or pertaining to the cerebrum.

-cerebral, a combining form referring to the brain: *craniocerebral, medicerebral, postcerebral.*

cerebral aneurysm, an abnormal localized dilatation of a cerebral artery, most commonly the result of congenital weakness of the muscle layer of the vessel wall. Cerebral aneurysms may also be caused by infection, such as subacute bacterial endocarditis or syphilis, by neoplasms, arteriosclerosis, and trauma. Cerebral aneurysms may occur in infancy or old age and may be fusiform dilatations of the entire circumference of an artery or saccular outcroppings of the side of a vessel, which may be as small as a pinhead or as large as an orange but are usually the size of a pea.

cerebral angiography, a radiographic technique for visualizing the vascular system of the brain by injecting a radiopaque contrast medium into a selected artery. **cerebral angiogram,** *n.*

cerebral anoxia, a condition in which oxygen is deficient in brain tissue. This state can exist for no more than 4 to 6 minutes before the onset of irreversible brain damage.

cerebral aqueduct, the narrow conduit, between the third and the fourth ventricles in the midbrain, that conveys the cerebrospinal fluid.

cerebral cortex, a thin layer of grey matter on the surface of the cerebral hemisphere, folded into gyri with about two thirds of its area buried in fissures. It integrates higher mental functions, general movement, visceral functions, perception, and behavioural reactions. It has been classified many different ways, with reference according to supposed phylogenetic and ontogenetic differences, structure, cell, and fibre layers, and function areas. Research has described more than 200 areas on the basis of differences in myelinated fibre patterns and has defined 47 separate function areas with different cell designs.

cerebral dominance, the specialization of each of the two cerebral hemispheres in the integration and control of different functions. In 90% of the population, the left cerebral hemisphere specializes in or dominates the ability to speak and write and the ability to understand spoken and written words. In the other 10% of the population, either the right hemisphere or both hemispheres dominate the speech and writing abilities. The right cerebral hemisphere perceives tactual stimuli and visual spatial relationships better than the left cerebral hemisphere.

cerebral embolism, a cerebrovascular accident caused by an embolus that blocks the flow of blood through the vessels of the cerebrum, resulting in tissue ischaemia distal to the occlusion.

cerebral evoked potential. See **evoked potential (EP).**

cerebral gigantism, an abnormal condition characterized by excessive weight and size at birth, accelerated growth during the first 4 or 5 years after birth without any increase in the level of growth hormone, and then reversion to normal growth.

cerebral haemorrhage, a haemorrhage from a blood vessel in the brain. Three criteria used to classify cerebral haemorrhages are location (subarachnoid, extradural, subdural), the kind of vessel involved (arterial, venous, capillary), and origin (traumatic, degenerative). Each kind of cerebral haemorrhage has its own clinical characteristics. Most cerebral haemorrhages occur in the region of the basal ganglia and are caused by the rupture of a sclerotic artery as a result of hypertension. Other causes of rupture include congenital aneurysm, cerebrovascular infarction, and head trauma.

cerebral hemiplegia, paralysis of one side of the body caused by a lesion in the brain.

cerebral hemisphere, one of the halves of the cerebrum. The two cerebral hemispheres are divided by a deep longitudinal fissure and are connected medially at the bottom of the fissure by the corpus callosum. Prominent grooves subdivide each hemisphere into four major lobes. The hemispheres consist of external grey substance, internal white substance, and internal grey substance and are covered by cerebral cortexes at the surface.

cerebral localization, **1.** the determination of various areas in the cerebral cortex associated with specific functions, such as the 47 areas of Brodmann. **2.** the diagnosis of a cerebral condition, such as a brain lesion, by determining the area of the brain affected, a determination made by analysis of the signs manifested by the patient and of electroencephalograms.

cerebral nerve. See **cranial nerves.**

cerebral oedema, an accumulation of fluid in the brain tissues. Causes can include an infection, tumour, and trauma. Brain tissues are compressed. Early symptoms are involuntary muscle contractions, dilated pupils, and a gradual loss of consciousness. Cerebral oedema can be fatal.

cerebral palsy, a motor function disorder caused by a permanent, nonprogressive brain defect or lesion present at birth or shortly thereafter. The neurological deficit may result in spastic hemiplegia, monoplegia, diplegia, or quadriplegia, athetosis or ataxia, seizures, paraesthesia, varying degrees of mental retardation, and impaired speech, vision, and hearing. The disorder is usually associated with premature or abnormal birth and intrapartum asphyxia, causing damage to the nervous system. Walking is usually delayed, and, when attempted, the child manifests a typical scissors gait. The arms may be affected only slightly, but the fingers are often spastic. Deep-tendon reflexes are exaggerated, and there may be slurred speech, delay in acquiring sphincter control, and athetotic movements of the face and hands. Treatment is individualized and may include the use of braces, surgical correction of deformities, speech therapy, and various muscle relaxants and anticonvulsants.

cerebral perfusion pressure (CPP), a measure of the amount of blood flow to the brain. It is calculated by subtracting the intracranial pressure from the mean systemic arterial blood pressure.

cerebral tabes. See **general paresis.**

cerebral thrombosis, a clotting of blood in any cerebral vessel, such as the middle cerebral artery or the ascending parietal artery.

cerebral vascular. See **cerebrovascular.**

cerebriform carcinoma. See **medullary carcinoma.**

cerebrocerebellar atrophy, a deterioration of the cerebellum caused by certain abiotrophic diseases.

cerebroid, resembling the substance of the brain.

cerebroma, *pl.* **cerebromas, cerebromata,** any unusual mass of brain tissue.

cerebromedullary tube. See **neural tube.**

cerebroretinal angiomatosis, a hereditary disease characterized by congenital, tumourlike vascular nodules in the retina and cerebellum.

cerebroside, any of a group of glycolipids found in the brain and other tissue of the nervous system, especially the myelin sheath.

cerebrospinal, pertaining to or involving the brain and the spinal cord.

cerebrospinal fluid (CSF), the fluid that flows through and protects the four ventricles of the brain, the subarachnoid space, and the spinal canal. It is composed mainly of secretions of the choroid plexi in the lateral ventricles and in the third and the fourth ventricles of the brain. Openings in the roof of the fourth ventricle allow the fluid to flow into the subarachnoid spaces around the brain and the spinal cord. Samples of the fluid may be removed by lumbar puncture between the third and the fourth lumbar vertebrae.

cerebrospinal nerves, the 12 pairs of cranial nerves and 31 pairs of spinal nerves that originate in the brain and spinal cord.

cerebrotendinous xanthomatosis. See **van Bogaert's disease.**

cerebrovascular, of or pertaining to the vascular system and blood supply of the brain. Also **cerebral vascular.**

cerebrovascular accident (CVA), an abnormal condition of the blood vessels of the brain characterized by occlusion by an embolus or cerebrovascular haemorrhage, resulting in ischaemia of the brain tissues normally perfused by the damaged vessels.

cerebrum, *pl.* **cerebrums, cerebra,** the largest and uppermost section of the brain, divided by a central sulcus into the left and the right cerebral hemispheres, and connected by the corpus callosum. The internal structures of the hemispheres merge with those of the diencephalon and further communicate with the brain stem through the cerebral peduncles. The cerebrum performs sensory functions, motor functions, and less easily defined integration functions associated with various mental activities. Some of the processes that are controlled or affected by the cerebrum are memory, speech, writing, and emotional response. **cerebral,** *adj.*

cerium (Ce), a ductile, grey rare-earth element. Its atomic number is 58; its atomic weight is 140.13. A compound of cerium, cerium oxalate, is used as a sedative, an antiemetic, and an antitussive.

ceroid, a golden, waxy pigment appearing in the cirrhotic livers of some individuals, in the GI tract, in the nervous system, and in the muscles.

ceroma, *pl.* **ceromas, ceromata,** a neoplasm that has undergone waxy degeneration.

certification, a process in which an individual, an institution, or an educational programme is evaluated and recognized as meeting certain predetermined standards. Certification is usually made by a nongovernmental agency.

certify, 1. to guarantee formally that certain requirements have been met based on expert knowledge of significant, pertinent facts. **2.** to attest, by a legal process, that someone is insane. **3.** to attest to the fact of someone's death in writing, usually on a form as required by local authority. **4.** to declare that a person has satisified certain requirements for membership or acceptance into a professional or other group.   **certification,** *n.,* **certifiable,** *adj.*

cerulean, sky-blue in colour.

ceruloplasmin, a glycoprotein in plasma that transports 96% of the plasma copper.

cerulytic, pertaining to a drug or other agent that dissolves cerumen.

cerumen, a yellowish or brownish waxy secretion produced by vestigial apocrine sweat glands in the external ear canal.

ceruminolytic. See **cerulytic.**

ceruminosis, excessive buildup of cerumen or earwax in the external auditory canal. It can cause discomfort, symptoms of hearing loss, and irritation leading to the development of infection.

ceruminous gland, one of a number of tiny structures in the external ear canal, believed to be modified sweat glands. They secrete a waxy cerumen instead of watery sweat.

cervic-, a combining form meaning 'pertaining to the neck': *cervicectomy, cervicitis, cervicobrachial.*

cervical, 1. of or pertaining to the neck or the region of the neck. **2.** of or pertaining to the constricted area of a necklike structure, such as the neck of a tooth or the cervix of the uterus.

cervical adenitis, an abnormal condition characterized by enlarged, tender lymph nodes of the neck.

cervical amputation, the removal of the neck of the uterus.

cervical canal, the canal within the uterine cervix, which protrudes into the vagina. The uterine end of the canal is closed at the internal os and, in the nullipara, at the distal end by the external os. The canal is a passageway through which the menstrual flow escapes and, vastly dilated and effaced by labour, through which the infant must come to be delivered vaginally. Sperm must travel upward through the canal to reach the uterus and uterine tubes.

cervical cancer, a neoplasm of the uterine cervix that can be detected in the early, curable stage by the Papanicolaou (Pap) test. Factors associated with the development of cervical cancer are coitus at an early age, many sexual partners, genital herpesvirus infections, multiparity, and poor obstetric and gynaecological care. Early cervical neoplasia is usually asymptomatic, but there may be a watery vaginal discharge or occasional spotting of blood; advanced lesions may cause a dark, foul-smelling vaginal discharge, leakage from bladder or rectal fistulas, anorexia, weight loss, and back and leg pains. About 90% of cervical tumours are squamous cell carcinomas, fewer than 10% are adenocarcinomas, and others are mixtures of these kinds, or, in rare cases, sarcomas. Tumours on the surface of the cervix may be huge, polypoid masses whereas endophytic lesions tend to be small and hard; ulcerative lesions may cause extensive erosion. Cervical cancer invades the tissues of adjacent organs and may metastasize through lymphatic channels to distant sites, including the lungs, bone, liver, brain, and paraaortic nodes.

cervical cap, a contraceptive device consisting of a small rubber cup fitted over the uterine cervix to prevent spermatozoa from entering the cervical canal

cervical cauterization, treatment, whereby abnormal cells of the superficial tissues of the cervix are destroyed by cautery.

cervical conization, the excision of a cone-shaped section of tissue from the endocervix.

cervical disc syndrome, an abnormal condition characterized by compression or irritation of the cervical nerve roots in or near the intervertebral foramina before the roots divide into the anterior and the posterior rami. Cervical disc syndrome may be caused by ruptured intervertebral discs, degenerative cervical disc disease, or cervical injuries. The form caused by ruptured cervical intervertebral discs or by degenerative disease may produce varying degrees of malalignment, causing nerve root compression. Most cervical disc syndromes are caused by injuries that involve hyperextension, which results in compression of the anatomic structures. Flexion injuries in the cervical area do not result in nerve compression. Pain, the most common symptom, usually emanates from the cervical area but may radiate down the arm to the fingers and increase with cervical motion. Other signs and symptoms associated with cervical disc syndrome may be paraesthesia, headache, blurred vision, decreased skeletal function, and weakened hand grip. Examination may reveal varying degrees of muscular atrophy, sensory abnormalities, muscular weakness, and decreased reflexes.

cervical endometritis, an inflammation of the inner lining of the cervix uteri.

cervical erosion, a condition in which the squamous epithelium of the cervix is abraded as a result of irritation caused by infection or trauma, such as childbirth, and is replaced by columnar epithelium.

cervical fistula, an abnormal passage from the cervix to the vagina or bladder that may be caused by a malignant lesion, radiotherapy, surgical trauma, or injury during childbirth.

cervical mucus method of family planning. See **ovulation method of family planning.**

cervical os. See **external cervical os, internal cervical os.**

cervical plexus, the network of nerves formed by the ventral primary divisions of the first four cervical nerves. The plexus is located opposite the cranial aspect of the first four cervical vertebrae. It communicates with certain cranial nerves and numerous muscular and cutaneous branches.

cervical plexus anaesthesia, nerve block at any point below the mastoid process from C_2 to the second cervical vertebra transverse process of the sixth cervical vertebra. This method is used for operations on the area between the jaw and clavicle.

cervical polyp, an outgrowth of columnar epithelial tissue of the endocervical canal, usually attached to the wall of the canal by a slender pedicle. Often there are no symptoms, but multiple or abraded polyps may cause bleeding, especially with contact during coitus. Polyps are most common in women over 40 years of age. The cause is not known.

cervical smear, a small amount of the secretions and superficial cells of the cervix, secured with a sterile applicator or special small wooden or plastic spatula from the external os of the uterine cervix. For a Pap smear, it is obtained from the squamocolumnar junction of the uterine cervix and from the vaginal vault and endocervical canal. The specimen is spread on a specially labelled glass slide and sent for cytological examination by a special laboratory.

cervical spondylosis, a form of degenerative joint and disc disease affecting the cervical vertebrae and resulting in compression of the associated nerve roots. Symptoms include pain or loss of feeling in the affected arm and shoulder, and stiffness of the cervical spine.

cervical stenosis, a narrowing of the canal between the body of the uterus and the cervical os.

cervical tenaculum. See **tenaculum.**

cervical triangle, one of two triangular areas formed in the neck by the oblique course of the sternocleidomastoideus. The anterior triangle is bounded by the midline of the throat anteriorly, the sternocleidomastoideus laterally, and the body of the mandible superiorly. The posterior triangle is bounded by the clavicle inferiorly and by the borders of the sternocleidomastoideus and the trapezius superiorly.

cervical vertebra, one of the first seven segments of the vertebral column. They differ from the thoracic and the lumbar vertebrae by the presence of a foramen in each transverse process. The first cervical vertebra has no body, supports the head, and contains a smooth, oval facet for articulation with the dens of the second cervical vertebra. The seventh cervical vertebra has a very long, prominent spinous process that is nearly horizontal in direction and is often used as a palpable reference for locating the other cervical spines.

cervicitis, acute or chronic inflammation of the uterine cervix. **Acute cervicitis** is infection of the cervix marked by redness, oedema, and bleeding on contact. Symptoms do not always occur but may include any or all of the following: discharge from the vagina, pelvic pressure or pain, scant bleeding with intercourse, and itching or burning of the external genitalia. Chronic cervicitis is a persistent inflammation of the cervix usually occurring among women in their reproductive years.

cervico-, a combining form meaning 'neck': *cervicodynia, cervicolabial, cervicotomy.*

cervicodynia, pain in the neck.

cervicofacial actinomycosis. See **actinomycosis.**

cervicolabial, pertaining to or situated in the labial area of the neck of an incisor or a canine tooth.

cervicouterine, pertaining to or situated at the cervix of the uterus.

cervicovaginitis, an inflammation of the cervix and vagina.

cervicovesical, of or pertaining to the cervix of the uterus and the bladder.

cervix, the part of the uterus that protrudes into the cavity of the vagina. The cervix is divided into the supravaginal portion and the vaginal portion. The supravaginal portion is separated ventrally from the bladder by the parametrium. The vaginal portion of the cervix projects into the cavity of the vagina and contains the cervical canal.

ceryl alcohol, a fatty alcohol present in many waxes.

cestode. See **tapeworm.**

cestode infection, cestodiasis. See **tapeworm infection.**

cestoid, 1. resembling a tapeworm. **2.** a tapeworm of the Cestoda subclass.

cetyl alcohol, a fatty alcohol, derived from spermaceti, used as an emulsifier and stiffening agent in creams and ointments.

cetylpyridinium chloride, an antiinfective used as a preservative in pharmaceutical preparations, as a topical cleanse, and in oral hygiene products.

cevitamic acid. See **ascorbic acid.**

Cf, symbol for **californium.**

CF test, abbreviation for **complement-fixation test.**

cGMP, abbreviation for **cyclic guanosine monophosphate.**

cgs, CGS, abbreviation for **centimetre-gram-second system.**

Ch¹, symbol for **Christchurch chromosome.**

Chaddock reflex {Charles G. Chaddock, American neurologist, b. 1861}, an abnormal reflex, induced by firmly stroking the ulnar surface of the forearm, characterized by flexion of the wrist and extension of the fingers in fanlike position.

Chaddock's sign {Charles G. Chaddock}, a variation of Babinski's reflex, elicited by firmly stroking the side of the foot just distal to the lateral malleolus, characterized by extension of the great toe and fanning of the other toes.

chafe an irritation of the skin by friction, such as when rough material rubs against an unprotected area of the body.

chafing, superficial irritation of the skin by friction.

chain, 1. a length of several units linked together in a linear pattern, such as a polypeptide chain of amino acids or a chain of atoms forming a chemical molecule. **2.** a group of individual bacteria linked together, such as streptococci formed by a chain of cocci. **3.** the serial relationship of certain structures essential to function, such as the chain of ossicles in the middle ear.

chain ligature, an interlocking ligature that ties off a pedicle at several places by passing a long thread through the pedicle at different points.

chain reaction, 1. (in chemistry) a reaction that produces a compound needed for the reaction to continue. **2.** (in physics) a reaction that perpetuates itself by the proliferating fission of nuclei and the release of atomic particles that cause more nuclear fissions.

chain reflex, a series of reflexes, each stimulated by the preceding one.

chain-stitch suture, a continuous surgical stitch in which each loop of the suture is secured by the next loop.

chalasia, abnormal relaxation or incompetence of the cardiac sphincter of the stomach, resulting in reflux of the gastric contents into the oesophagus with subsequent regurgitation.

chalazion, a small, localized swelling of the eyelid resulting from obstruction and retained secretions of the meibomian glands.

chalice cell. See **goblet cell.**

chalicosis, a type of fibrosis that results from the inhalation of calcium dusts. Respiratory impairment is generally caused by the presence of free silica in the calcium dust.

chalkitis, an abnormal condition characterized by inflammation of the eyes, caused by rubbing the eyes with the hands after touching or handling brass.

challenge, a method of testing the sensitivity of an individual to a hormone, allergen, or other substance by administering a sample. To challenge the person's sensitivity to a particular antigen, a small amount may be injected to determine whether the immune system will react by producing appropriate antibodies.

chalone, any one of numerous polypeptide inhibitors that is elaborated by a tissue and functions like a hormone on specific target organs.

chamaeprosopy. a facial appearance characterized by a low brow and a broad face with a facial index of 90 or less. **chamaeprosopic,** *adj.*

chamber, 1. a hollow but not necessarily empty space or cavity in an organ, as in the anterior and posterior chambers of the eye or the atrial and ventricular chambers of the heart. **2.** a room or closed space used for research or therapeutic purposes, such as a decompression chamber or hyperbaric oxygen chamber.

Chamberlain's line {W. E. Chamberlain, American radiologist, b. 1891}, a line that extends from the posterior of the hard palate to the dorsum of the foramen magnum.

Chamberlen forceps {Peter Chamberlen, English stetrician, b. 1560}, one of the earliest kinds of obstetric forceps, introduced in the seventeenth century.

chancre, 1. a skin lesion, usually of primary syphilis, that begins at the site of infection as a papule and develops into a red, bloodless, painless ulcer with a scooped-out appearance. The chancre teems with *Treponema pallidum* spirochetes and is highly contagious. **2.** a papular lesion or ulcerated area of the skin that marks the point of infection of a nonsyphilitic disease, such as tuberculosis.

chancroid, a highly contagious, sexually transmitted disease caused by infection with a bacillus, *Haemophilus ducreyi*. It characteristically begins as a papule, usually on the skin of the external genitalia; it then grows and ulcerates, other papules form, and, if untreated, the bacillus spreads, causing buboes in the groin.

change agent, a role in which communication skills, education, and other resources are applied to help a client adjust to changes caused by illness or disability.

change of life, informal. the female climacteric; menopause.

channel, a passageway or groove that conveys fluid, such as the central channels that connect the arterioles with the venules.

channel ulcer, a rare type of peptic ulcer found in the pyloric canal between the stomach and the duodenum.

chaotic atrial tachycardia, a form of atrial tachycardia marked by an abnormal electrocardiogram tracing in which the P wave, representing contraction of the atria, is irregular in time and variable in shape.

chapped, pertaining to skin that is roughened, cracked, or reddened by exposure to cold or excessive surface evaporation. Stinging and burning sensations often accompany the disorder. Prevention is by protection against exposure to cold and wind.

character, 1. the integrated composite of traits and behavioural tendencies that enable a person to react in a relatively consistent way to the customs and mores of society. **2.** any letter, number, symbol, or punctuation mark, usually composed of eight bits or one byte, that can be transmitted as output by a computer.

character analysis, a systematic investigation of the personality of an individual with special attention to psychological defences and motivations, usually undertaken to improve behaviour.

character disorder, a chronic, habitual, maladaptive, and socially unacceptable pattern of behaviour and emotional response.

characteristic curve, (in radiography) a graphical representation of the relationship between the density (amount of blackening) on a radiograph, and the radiation exposure. The exposure is usually plotted on a logarithmic scale in order to compress a wide range of exposures.

characteristic radiation, the emission of electromagnetic radiation as a result of the interaction of high-speed electrons with matter. An electron ejects an inner-shell electron of a target atom, and subsequent electron transitions result in the emission of characteristic radiation. The type of radiation depends on the difference in binding energies of the shells involved.

character neurosis. See **character disorder**.

charcoal. See **activated charcoal**.

Charcot-Bouchard aneurysm {Jean M. Charcot, French neurologist, b. 1825; Charles J. Bouchard, French physician, b. 1837}, a small, round aneurysm of a small artery of the cerebral cortex or basal ganglia, which some authorities believe is the cause of massive cerebral haemorrhage.

Charcot-Leyden crystal {Jean M. Charcot; Ernst V. von Leyden, German physician, b. 1832}, any one of the crystalline structures shaped like narrow, double pyramids found in the sputum of individuals suffering from bronchial asthma. They are also found in the faeces of patients with dysentery.

Charcot-Marie-Tooth atrophy {Jean M. Charcot; Pierre Marie, French neurologist, b. 1853; Howard H. Tooth, English neurologist, b. 1856}, a progressive hereditary disorder characterized by degeneration of the peroneal muscles of the fibula, resulting in clubfoot, foot drop, and ataxia.

Charcot's fever {Jean M. Charcot}, a syndrome characterized by a recurrent fever, jaundice, and abdominal pain in the right upper quadrant occurring with inflammation of the bile ducts.

Charcot's joint, See **neuropathic joint disease**.

charlatan, a totally unqualified individual posing as an expert, especially an individual pretending to be a physician. **charlatanical,**

adj.

Charles' law. See **Gay-Lussac's law.**

charley horse, a painful condition of the quadricep or hamstring muscles characterized by soreness and stiffness. It is the result of a strain, tear, or bruise of the muscle.

chart, 1. informal. a patient record. **2.** to note data in a patient record, usually at prescribed intervals.

charta, *pl.* **chartae,** a piece of paper, especially one treated with medicine, as for external application, or with a chemical for a special purpose, such as litmus paper.

chauffeur's fracture, any fracture of the radial styloid, produced by a twisting or a snapping type injury.

Chaussier's areola {Francois Chaussier, French anatomist, b. 1746}, an areola of indurated tissue surrounding a malignant pustule.

CHC, abbreviation for **Community Health Council.**

check ligament. See **alar ligament.**

check-up, a thorough study or examination of the health of an individual.

Chediak-Higashi syndrome {Moises Chediak, twentieth century French physician; Ototaka Higashi, twentieth century Japanese physician}, a congenital, autosomal disorder, characterized by partial albinism, photo-phobia, massive leukocytic inclusions, psychomotor abnormalities, recurrent infections, and early death.

cheek, a fleshy prominence, especially the fleshy protuberances on both sides of the face between the eye and the jaw and the ear and the nose and mouth.

cheekbone. See **zygomatic bone.**

cheilitis an abnormal condition of the lips characterized by inflammation and cracking of the skin.

cheilocarcinoma, *pl.* **cheilocarcinomas, cheilocarcinomata,** a malignant epithelial tumour of the lip.

cheiloplasty, surgical correction of a defect of the lip.

cheilorraphy, a surgical procedure that sutures the lip, such as in the repair of a congenitally cleft lip or a lacerated lip.

cheilosis, a disorder of the lips and mouth characterized by scales and fissures, resulting from a deficiency of riboflavin in the diet.

cheiralgia, a pain in the hand, especially the pain associated with arthritis. **cheiralgic,** *adj.*

cheiromegaly, an abnormal condition characterized by excessively large hands. **cheiromegalic,** *adj.*

cheiroplasty, an operation involving plastic surgery of the hand. **cheiroplastic,** *adj.*

chelate, 1. (of a metal ion and two or more polar groups of a single molecule) to form a bond, thus creating a ringlike complex. **2.** (in medicine) a compound composed of a central metal ion and an organic molecule with multiple bonds, arranged in ring formations, used especially in chemotherapeutic treatments for metal poisoning. **3.** of or pertaining to chelation.

chelating agent, a substance that promotes chelation. Chelating agents are used in the treatment of metal poisoning.

chelation, a chemical reaction in which there is a combination with a metal to form a ring-shaped molecular complex in which the metal is firmly bound and sequestered.

cheloid. See **keloid.**

cheloidosis. See **keloidosis.**

chemabrasion, a method of treating scars, chromatosis, or other skin disorders by applying chemicals that remove the surface layers of skin cells.

chemical, 1. a substance composed of chemical elements or a substance produced by or used in chemical processes. **2.** pertaining to chemistry.

chemical action, any process in which natural elements and compounds react with each other to produce a chemical change or a different compound; for example, hydrogen and oxygen combine to produce water.

chemical agent, any chemical power, active principle, or substance that can produce an effect in the body by interacting with various body substances, such as aspirin, which produces an analgesic effect.

chemical antidote, any substance that reacts chemically with a poison to form a compound that is harmless.

chemical burn, tissue damage caused by exposure to a strong acid or alkali, such as phenol, creosol, mustard gas, or phosphorus. Emergency treatment includes washing the surface with copious amounts of water to remove the chemical and, if the damage is more than slight and superficial, immediate transport to a hospital accident and emergency department.

chemical cauterization the corroding or burning of living tissue by a caustic chemical substance, such as potassium hydroxide.

chemical diabetes. See **impaired glucose tolerance.**

chemical energy. See **energy.**

chemical gastritis, inflammation of the stomach caused by the ingestion of a chemical compound.

chemical indicator, a commercially prepared device that monitors all or part of the physical conditions of the sterilization cycle. It usually consists of a sensitive ink dye that changes colour under certain conditions.

chemical mediator, a neurotransmitter chemical, such as acetylcholine.

chemical name, the exact designation of the chemical structure of a drug as determined by the rules of accepted systems of chemical nomenclature. For example, N,N-bis-(2-chloroethyl)-N'-(3-hydroxypropyl) phosphordiamidic acid cyclic acid monohydrate is the chemical name of cyclophosphamide, a drug used in cancer chemotherapy.

chemical plaque control, use of antiseptics to control bacterial plaque. Antiplaque agents are delivered in mouthwashes, toothpastes and gels.

chemical shift, the slight departure in the nuclear magnetic resonance spectrum of an element, such as hydrogen, when it is a constituent in a complex biomolecule, from the spectrum for a sample containing that element in pure form.

chemical warfare, the wageing of war with poisonous chemicals and gases.

cheminosis, any disease caused by a chemical substance.

chemistry, the science dealing with the elements, their compounds, and the chemical structure and interactions of matter. Kinds of chemistry include inorganic chemistry and organic chemistry.

chemistry, normal values, the amounts of various substances in the normal human body, determined by testing a large sample of people presumed to be healthy. Normal values are expressed in ranges of numbers and can vary from laboratory to laboratory.

chemodifferentiation, a stage in embryonic development that precedes and controls specialization and differentiation of the cells into rudimentary organs.

chemonucleolysis, a method of dissolving the nucleus pulposus of an intervertebral disc by the injection of a chemolytic agent, such as the enzyme chymopapain.

chemoprophylaxis, the use of antimicrobial drugs to prevent the acquisition of pathogens in an endemic area or to prevent their spread from one body area to another.

chemoreceptor, a sensory nerve cell activated by chemical stimuli, such as a chemoreceptor in the carotid that is sensitive to the P_{CO_2} in the blood, signalling the respiratory centre in the brain to increase or decrease respiration.

chemoreflex, any reflex initiated by the stimulation of chemical receptors, such as the carotid and aortic bodies, which respond to changes in carbon dioxide, hydrogen ion, and oxygen concentrations in the blood.

chemosis, an abnormal oedematous swelling of the mucous membrane covering the eyeball and lining the eyelids that is usually the result of local trauma or infection.

chemostat, a device that assures a steady rate of cell division in bacterial populations by maintaining a constant environment.

chemosurgery, the destruction of malignant, infected, or gangrenous tissue by the application of chemicals. The technique is used successfully to remove skin cancers.

chemotaxis, a response involving movement that is positive (toward) or negative (away from) to a chemical stimulus.

chemotherapeutic agent, a chemical agent used to treat diseases. The term usually refers to a medication used to treat cancer by killing cancer cells.

chemotherapy, the treatment of infections and other diseases with chemical agents. In modern usage, chemotherapy usually refers to the use of chemicals to destroy cancer cells on a selective basis. The cytotoxic agents used in cancer treatments generally function in the same manner as ionizing radiation; they do not kill the cancer cells directly but instead impair their ability to replicate. Chemotherapeutic agents are often used in combination with radiation treatments for their synergistic effect.

chenodeoxycholic acid, a secondary bile acid. It is used to dissolve cholesterol gallstones, as an alternative to surgery.

cherry angioma, a small, bright red, clearly circumscribed vascular tumour on the skin. It occurs most often on the trunk but may be found anywhere on the body. The lesion is very common.

cherry red spot, an abnormal red circular area of the choroid, seen through the fovea centralis of the eye and surrounded by a contrasting white oedema. It is associated with cases of infantile cerebral sphingolipidosis and sometimes appears in the late infantile form of amaurotic familial idiocy.

cherubism, an abnormal hereditary condition characterized by progressive bilateral swelling at the angle of the mandible, especially in children.

chest. See **thorax**.

chest cavity. See **body cavity**.

chest drain, a catheter inserted through the thorax into the chest cavity for removing air or fluid.

chest lead 1. an electrocardiographic conductor in which the exploring electrode is placed on the chest or precordium. The indifferent electrode is placed on the patient's back for a CB (chest back) lead, on the front of the chest for a CF (chest front) lead, on the left arm for a CL (chest left) lead, and on the right arm for a CR (chest right) lead. **2.** informal. the tracing produced by such a lead on an electrocardiograph.

chest pain, a physical complaint that requires immediate diagnosis and evaluation. Chest pain may be symptomatic of cardiac disease, such as angina pectoris, myocardial infarction, or pericarditis, or of disease of the lungs, such as pleurisy, pneumonia, or pulmonary embolism or infarction. The source of chest pain may also be musculoskeletal, GI, or psychogenic. Over 90% of severe chest pain is caused by coronary disease, spinal root compression, or psychological disturbance. Specific cardiovascular conditions associated with chest pain are myocardial infarction, angina pectoris, pericarditis, and a dissecting aneurysm of the thoracic aorta. Musculoskeletal conditions include rib fractures, swelling of the rib cartilage, and muscle strain. GI conditions associated with chest pain include oesophagitis, peptic ulcers, hiatus hernia, and pancreatitis.

chest physiotherapy. See **cupping and vibrating, percussion**.

chest wall percussion. See **percussion**.

chewing reflex, a pathological sign in brain-damaged adults, characterized by repetitive chewing motions when the mouth is stimulated.

Cheyne-Stokes respiration (CSR) {John Cheyne, Scottish physician, b. 1777; William Stokes, Irish physician, b. 1804}, an abnormal pattern of respiration, characterized by alternating periods of apnoea and deep, rapid breathing. The respiratory cycle begins with slow, shallow breaths that gradually increase to abnormal depth and rapidity. Respiration gradually subsides as breathing slows and becomes shallower, climaxing in a 10- to 20-second period without respiration before the cycle is repeated.

CHF, abbreviation for **congestive heart failure**.

ch'i, a Chinese concept of a fundamental life energy that flows in orderly ways along meridians, or channels, in the body.

Chiari-Frommel syndrome {Johann B. Chiari, German physician, b. 1817; Richard Frommel, German gynaecologist, b. 1854}, a hormonal disorder that occurs after a pregnancy in which weaning does not spontaneously end lactation.

Chiari's syndrome. See **Budd-Chiari syndrome**.

chiasm, 1. the crossing of two lines or tracts, as the crossing of the optic nerves at the optic chiasm. **2.** (in genetics) the crossing of two chromatids in the prophase of meiosis. **chiasmal, chiasmic,** *adj.*

chiasma, *pl.* **chiasmata** {Gk, lines that cross}, (in genetics), the visible point of connection between homologous chromosomes during the first meiotic division in gametogenesis. The X-shaped configurations form during the late prophase stage and provide the means by which exchange of genetic material occurs. **chiasmatic, chiasmic.** *adj.*

chiasmatypy. See **crossing over**.

chiasmic. See **chiasm, chiasma**.

chickenpox, an acute, highly contagious viral disease caused by a herpesvirus, varicella zoster virus (VZV). It occurs primarily in young children and is characterized by crops of pruritic vesicular eruptions on the skin. The disease is transmitted by direct contact with skin lesions or, more commonly, by droplets spread from the respiratory tract of infected persons, usually in the prodromal period or the early stages of the rash. The vesicular fluid and the scabs are infectious

until entirely dry. Indirect transmission through uninfected persons or objects is rare. The diagnosis is usually made by physical examination and by the characteristic appearance of the disease. The virus may be identified by culture of the vesicle fluid.

chief cell, 1. any one of the columnar epithelial cells or the cuboidal epithelial cells that line the gastric glands and secrete pepsinogen and intrinsic factor, which is needed for the absorption of vitamin B_{12} and the normal development of red blood cells. Anaemia is caused by the absence of intrinsic factor. **2.** any one of the epithelioid cells with pale-staining cytoplasm and a large nucleus containing a prominent nucleolus. **3.** any one of the polyhedral epithelial cells, within the parathyroid glands.

chief complaint, a subjective statement made by a patient describing the patient's most significant or serious symptoms or signs of illness or dysfunction.

chigger, the larva of *Trombicula* mites found in tall grass and weeds. It sticks to the skin and causes irritation and severe itching.

chigoe, a flea found in tropical and subtropical America and Africa. The pregnant female flea burrows into the skin of the feet, causing an inflammatory condition that may lead to spontaneous amputation of a toe.

chikungunya encephalitis, an arbovirus infection characterized by a high fever that begins abruptly, muscle aches, a rash, and pain in the joints. It is transmitted by the bite of a mosquito and occurs mainly in Africa, Asia, and on some Pacific islands.

chilblain, redness and swelling of the skin because of excessive exposure to cold. Burning, itching, blistering, and ulceration, similar to a thermal burn, may occur. Treatment includes protection against cold and injury, and gentle warming.

child, 1. a person of either sex between the time of birth and adolescence. **2.** an unborn or recently born human being; fetus, neonate, infant. **3.** an offspring or descendant; a son or daughter or a member of a particular tribe or clan. **4.** one who is like a child or immature.

child abuse, the physical, sexual, or emotional maltreatment of a child. It may be overt or covert and often results in permanent physical or psychiatric injury, mental impairment, or sometimes death. Child abuse is the result of multiple and complex factors involving both the parents and the child, compounded by various stressful environmental circumstances, such as poor socioeconomic conditions, inadequate physical and emotional support within the family, and any major life change or crisis, especially those crises arising from marital strife. Parents at high risk for abuse are characterized as having unsatisfied needs, difficulty in forming adequate interpersonal relationships, unrealistic expectations of the child, and a lack of nuturing experience, often involving neglect or abuse in their own childhoods. Obvious physical marks on a child's body, as burns, welts, or bruises, and signs of emotional distress, including symptoms of failure to thrive, are common indications of some degree of neglect or abuse. Often, radiographs to detect healed or new fractures of the extremities or diagnostic tests to identify sexual molestation are necessary.

childbirth. See **birth.**

child development, the various stages of physical, social, and psychological growth that occur from birth through adulthood.

childhood, 1. the period in human development that extends from birth until the onset of puberty. **2.** the state or quality of being a child.

childhood aphasia, an inability to process language because of a brain dysfunction in childhood.

childhood-onset pervasive developmental disorders, disturbances in thought, affect, social relatedness, and behaviour that emerge between the ages of 30 months and 12 years.

childhood polycystic disease. See **polycystic kidney disease.**

child psychiatry, the branch of psychiatry that specializes in the diagnosis, aetiology and treatment of the psychopathological syndromes and symptoms of children. Such conditions are associated with early pathology, tactile hypersensitivity and homoeostatic disorders, and include poor infant-parent attachment, infantile autism, anaclitic depression, avoidance reaction, persistent stranger and separation anxiety, early signs of aggression, hyperactivity, cyclic vomiting and disturbances in sleeping, eating and elimination.

childhood schizophrenia, a form of schizophrenia, occurring before the onset of puberty, resulting from organic brain damage or from environmental conditions. It is characterized by autistic withdrawal into fantasy, obsessional attachments, failure to communicate verbally, repetitive gestures, emotional unresponsiveness, and a severely impaired sense of identity. Two kinds of childhood schizophrenia are **early infantile autism** and **symbiotic infantile psychotic syndrome.**

childhood triad, three types of behaviour - arson, bedwetting, and cruelty to animals - that may predict emerging sociopathy when they occur consistently and in combination.

child neglect, the failure by parents or guardians to provide for the basic needs of a child by physical or emotional deprivation that interferes with normal growth and development or that places the child in jeopardy.

child psychology, the study of the mental, emotional, and behavioural development of infants and children.

child welfare, any service sponsored by the social services or special organizations that provide for the physical, social, or psychological care of children in need.

chill, 1. the sensation of cold caused by exposure to a cold environment. **2.** an attack of shivering with pallor and a feeling of coldness, often occurring at the beginning of an infection and accompanied by a rapid rise in temperature.

Chilomastix, a genus of flagellate protozoa, as *Chilomastix mesnili,* a nonpathogenic intestinal parasite of humans.

chimera, an organism carrying cell populations derived from two or more different zygotes of the same or of different species. It may be a natural phenomenon, such as in a bone marrow graft.

chimerism, a state in bone marrow transplantation in which bone marrow and host cells exist compatibly without signs of graft-versus-host rejection disease.

chin, the raised triangular portion of the mandible below the lip. It is formed by the mental protuberance.

chip, 1. a relatively small piece of a bone or tooth. **2.** to break off or cut away a small piece.

chip fracture, any small fragmental fracture, usually one involving a bony process near a joint.

chiralgia, a pain in the hand, particularly one that does not result from a nerve injury or disease.

chirality. See **handedness.**

chiroplasty a surgical procedure to restore an injured or congenitally deformed hand to normal use.

chiropodist, see **podiatrist.**

chiropody see **podiatry.**

chiropractic, a system of therapy based on the theory that the state of a person's health is determined in general by the condition of his or her nervous system. In most cases treatment provided by chiropractors involves the mechanical manipulation of the spinal column. Some practitioners employ radiology for diagnosis and use physiotherapy and diet in addition to spinal manipulation. Chiropractic does not employ drugs or surgery.

chirospasm. See **writer's cramp.**

chisel fracture, any fracture in which there is an oblique detachment of a bone fragment from the head of the radius.

chi square, (in statistics) a statistical test for an association between observed data and expected data represented by frequencies. The test yields a statement of the probability of the obtained distribution having occurred by chance alone.

Chlamydia, **1.** a microorganism of the genus

Chlamydia. **2.** a genus of microorganisms that live as intracellular parasites, have a number of properties in common with gram-negative bacteria, and are currently classified as specialized bacteria. *Chlamydia trachomatis*, an organism that lives in the conjunctiva of the eye and the epithelium of the urethra and cervix, is responsible for inclusion conjunctivitis, lymphogranuloma venereum, and trachoma. *Chlamydia psittaci* is an organism that infects birds and causes a type of pneumonia in humans.

chloasma, tan or brown pigmentation, particularly of the forehead, cheeks, and nose, commonly associated with pregnancy or the use of oral contraceptives.

chloracne, a skin condition characterized by small, black follicular plugs and papules on exposed surfaces, especially on the arms, face, and neck of workers in contact with chlorinated compounds, such as cutting oils, paints, varnishes, and lacquers.

chloral camphor, a mixture of equal parts of camphor and chloral hydrate, used externally as a sedative.

chloral hydrate, a sedative and hypnotic used for the relief of insomnia.

chlorambucil, an alkylating agent used in the treatment of a variety of malignant diseases, including chronic lymphocytic leukaemia and Hodgkin's disease.

chloramphenicol, an antibacterial and antirickettsial used in the treatment of serious bacterial infections.

chlordane poisoning. See **chlorinated organic insecticide poisoning.**

chlordiazepoxide, a minor tranquillizer prescribed in the treatment of anxiety and alcohol withdrawal symptoms.

chlorhexidine, an antimicrobial agent used as a surgical scrub, hand rinse, and topical antiseptic.

chlorhydria, an excessive level of hydrochloric acid in the stomach.

chloride, a compound in which the negative element is chlorine. Chlorides are salts of hydrochloric acid; the most common is sodium chloride (table salt).

chloride shift, an exchange of chloride ions in red blood cells in peripheral tissues in response to P_{CO_2} of blood. The shift reverses in the lungs.

chloriduria, an excessive level of chlorides in the urine.

chlorinated organic insecticide poisoning, poisoning resulting from the inhalation, ingestion, or absorption of DDT and other insecticides containing chlorophenothane, as heptachlor, dieldrin, and chlordane. It is characterized by vomiting, weakness, malaise, convulsions, tremors, ventricular fibrillation, respiratory failure, and pulmonary oedema.

chlorine (Cl), a yellowish-green, gaseous element of the halogen group. Its atomic number is 17; its atomic weight is 35.453. It has a strong, distinctive odour, is irritating to the respiratory tract, and is poisonous if ingested or inhaled. It occurs in nature chiefly as a component of sodium chloride in sea water and in salt deposits. It is used as a bleach and as a disinfectant to purify water for drinking or for use in swimming pools.

chlormezanone, an anxiolytic and muscle relaxant used to treat anxiety and muscle spasm.

chloroform, a nonflammable, volatile liquid that was the first inhalation anaesthetic to be discovered. Chloroform is a dangerous anaesthetic drug: A difference of only 10% in drug-plasma levels can result in hypotension, myocardial and respiratory depression, cardiogenic shock, ventricular fibrillation, coma, and death.

chloroformism, 1. the habit of inhaling chloroform for its narcotic effect. **2.** the anaesthetic effect of chloroform.

chloroleukaemia, a kind of myelogenous leukaemia in which specific tumour masses are not seen at autopsy but body fluids and organs are green.

chlorolymphosarcoma, *pl.* **chlorolymphosarcomas, chlorolymphosarcomata,** a greenish neoplasm of myeloid tissue occurring in patients with myelogenous leukaemia. The mononuclear cells in the peripheral blood are believed to be lymphocytes rather than myeloblasts, such as found with chloroma.

chloroma, *pl.* **chloromas, chloromata,** a malignant, greenish neoplasm of myeloid tissue occurring anywhere in the body in patients with myelogenous leukaemia.

chloromyeloma. See **chloroma.**

chlorophyll, a plant pigment capable of absorbing light and converting it to energy for the oxidation and reduction involved in the photosynthesis of carbohydrates.

chlorophyll test. See **Boas' test.**

chloroquine, an antimalarial prescribed in the prophylaxis and treatment of malaria. It is also used in the treatment of rheumatoid arthritis and some forms of lupus erythematosus.

chlorothiazide, an antihypertensive and diuretic used in the treatment of hypertension and oedema.

chlorpheniramine maleate, an antihistamine prescribed in the treatment of a variety of allergic reactions, including rhinitis, skin rash, and pruritus.

chlorpromazine, a phenothiazine tranquilizer and antiemetic prescribed in the treatment of psychotic disorders, severe nausea and vomiting, and intractable hiccups.

chlorpropamide, an oral sulphonyurea hypoglycaemic prescribed in the treatment of mild, stable non-insulin-dependent diabetes mellitus.

chlortetracycline hydrochloride, an antibiotic prescribed in the treatment of a variety of bacterial infections.

chlorthalidone, a diuretic and antihypertensive prescribed in the treatment of high blood pressure and oedema.

choana, *pl.* **choanae, 1.** a funnel-shaped channel. **2.** See **posterior nares.**

choanal atresia, a congenital anomaly in which a bony or membranous occlusion blocks the passageway between the nose and pharynx.

choke, to interrupt respiration by compression or obstruction of larynx or trachea.

choke damp. See **damp.**

chokes, a respiratory condition, occurring in decompression sickness, characterized by shortness of breath, substernal pain, and a nonproductive cough caused by bubbles of gas in the blood vessels of the lungs.

choking, the condition in which a respiratory passage is blocked by constriction of the neck, an obstruction in the trachea, or swelling of the larynx. It is characterized by sudden coughing and a red face that rapidly becomes cyanotic. The person cannot breathe and clutches his or her throat.

cholangeostomy, a surgical operation to form an opening in a bile duct.

cholangiocarcinoma, a cancer of the biliary epithelium in the liver. It tends to occur mainly in patients who have had ulcerative colitis or an infestation of liver flukes.

cholangiography, a radiographic technique for visualizing the biliary tract by the introduction of a radiopaque contrast medium, either intravenously, or percutaneously, or endoscopically for example. **cholangiogram,** *n.*

cholangiohepatoma, *pl.* **cholangiohepatomas, cholangiohepatomata,** a neoplasm in which there is an abnormal mixture of liver cord cells and bile ducts.

cholangiolitis, an abnormal condition characterized by inflammation of the fine tubules of the bile duct system, which may cause cholangiolitic cirrhosis. **cholangiolitic,** *adj.*

cholangioma, *pl.* **cholangiomas, cholangiomata,** a neoplasm of the bile ducts.

cholangiopancreatography, a radiographic technique to visualize the biliary tract and pancreatic duct by endoscopic retrograde introduction of a radiopaque contrast medium. **cholangiopancreatogram.**

cholangitis, inflammation of the bile ducts, caused either by bacterial invasion or by obstruction of the ducts by calculi or a tumour. The condition is characterized by severe right upper quadrant pain, jaundice (if an obstruction is present), and intermittent fever.

cholecalciferol. See **vitamin D₃.**

cholecystectomy, the surgical removal of the gallbladder, performed to treat cholelithiasis and cholecystitis. The gallbladder is excised and the cystic duct ligated; the common duct is searched, and any stones found are removed. A T-tube is left in place to ensure adequate bile drainage; a Penrose drain may be left in a separate stab wound to prevent the formation of an abcess.

cholecystitis, acute or chronic inflammation of the gallbladder. Acute cholecystitis is usually caused by a gallstone that cannot pass through the cystic duct. Pain is felt in the right upper quadrant of the abdomen, accompanied by nausea, vomiting, eructation, and flatulence. Chronic cholecystitis, the more common type, has an insidious onset. Pain, often felt at night, may follow a fatty meal. Complications include biliary calculi, pancreatitis, and carcinoma of the gallbladder.

cholecystography, a radiographic technique for visualizing the gallbladder and common bile duct by introduction of a radioapaque contrast medium orally. **cholecystogram,** *n.*

cholecystokinin, a hormone, produced by the mucosa of the upper intestine, that stimulates contraction of the gallbladder and the secretion of pancreatic enzymes.

choledocholithiasis. See **biliary calculus.**

choledocholithotomy, a surgical operation to make an incision in the common bile duct to remove a stone.

cholelithiasis, the presence of gallstones in the gallbladder. The condition affects about 20% of the population over 40 years of age and is more prevalent in women and in persons with cirrhosis of the liver. Patients complain of abdominal discomfort, eructation, and intolerance to certain foods.

cholelithic dyspepsia, an abnormal condition characterized by sudden attacks of indigestion associated with the dysfunction of the gallbladder.

cholelithotomy, a surgical operation to remove gallstones through an incision in the gallbladder.

cholera, an acute bacterial infection of the small intestine, characterized by severe diarrhoea and vomiting, muscular cramps, dehydration, and depletion of electrolytes. The symptoms are caused by toxic substances produced by the infecting organism, Vibrio cholerae. The profuse, watery diarrhoea, as much as a litre an hour, depletes the body of fluids and minerals.

choleragen, an exotoxin, produced by the *cholera vibrio*, that stimulates the secretion of electrolyte and water into the small intestine in Asiatic cholera.

cholera vaccine, an active immunizing agent used for immunization against cholera.

choleretic, 1. stimulating the production of bile either by cholepoiesis or by hydrocholeresis. **2.** a choleretic agent.

choleric, having a hot temper or an irascible nature.

cholestasis, interruption in the flow of bile through any part of the biliary system, from liver to duodenum. It is essential to discover whether the cause is within the liver (intrahepatic) or outside it (extrahepatic). Symptoms of both types include jaundice, pale and fatty stools, dark urine, and intense itching over the skin.   **cholestatic,** *adj.*

cholestatic hepatitis, inflammation of the liver caused by hepatitis infection that produces interruption of the flow of bile in the intrahepatic ducts.

cholesteatoma, a cystic mass composed of epithelial cells and cholesterol that is found in the middle ear and occurs as a congenital defect or as a serious complication of chronic otitis media.

cholesterase, an enzyme in the blood and other tissues that forms cholesterol and fatty acids by hydrolysing cholesterol esters.

cholesteraemia. See **cholesterolaemia**.

cholesterol, a fat-soluble crystalline steroid alcohol found in animal fats and oils, and egg yolk, and widely distributed in the body, especially in the bile, blood, brain tissue, liver, kidneys, adrenal glands, and myelin sheaths of nerve fibres. It facilitates the absorption and transport of fatty acids and acts as the precursor for the synthesis of vitamin D at the surface of the skin, as well as for the synthesis of the various steroid hormones. Increased levels of serum cholesterol may be associated with the pathogenesis of atherosclerosis.

cholesterolaemia, 1. the presence of excessive amounts of cholesterol in the blood. **2.** the abnormal condition of having excessive amounts of cholesterol in the blood.

cholesteroleresis, the increased elimination of cholesterol in the bile.

cholesterol metabolism, the anabolic and catabolic processes in the synthesis and degradation of cholesterol in the body. Ingested cholesterol is quickly absorbed. It is also synthesized in the liver and by most other tissues of the body.

cholesterolopoiesis, the elaboration of cholesterol by the liver.

cholesterolosis, an abnormal condition in which there are deposits of cholesterol within large macrophages in the submucosa of the gallbladder.

cholesteryl ester storage disease, an inherited disorder in which there is an accumulation of neutral lipids, such as cholesterol esters and glycerides, in body tissues. A form of the disorder affecting infants, with symptoms in the first weeks after birth, is Wolman's disease.

cholestyramine, an ion exchange resin, bile acid binder, and hypolipidaemic agent prescribed for primary hyperlipidaemia and for pruritus resulting from partial biliary obstruction.

choline, one of the B complex vitamins, essential for the metabolism of fats in the body. It is a primary component of acetylcholine, the neurotransmitter, and functions with inositol as a basic constituent of lecithin. The richest sources of choline are liver, kidneys, brains, wheat germ, brewer's yeast, and egg yolk.

choline esters, a group of cholinergic drugs that mimic acetylcholine at body sites where acetylcholine is the neurotransmitter.

cholinergic, 1. of or pertaining to nerve fibres that elaborate acetylcholine at the myoneural junctions. **2.** the tendency to transmit or to be stimulated by or to stimulate the elaboration of acetylcholine.

cholinergic blocking agent, any agent that blocks the action of acetylcholine and substances similar to acetylcholine. Such agents, in effect, block the action of cholinergic nerves that transmit impulses by the release of acetylcholine at their synapses.

cholinergic crisis, a pronounced muscular weakness and respiratory paralysis caused by excessive acetylcholine, often apparent in patients suffering from myasthenia gravis as a result of overmedication with anticholinesterase drugs.

cholinergic nerve, a nerve that releases the neurotransmitter acetylcholine at its synapse. The cholinergic nerves include all the preganglionic sympathetic and the preganglionic parasympathetic nerves, the postganglionic parasympathetic nerves, the somatic motor nerves to skeletal muscles, and some nerves to sweat glands and to certain blood vessels.

cholinergic stimulant. See **cholinergic**.

cholinergic urticaria an abnormal and usually transient vascular reaction of the skin, often associated with sweating in susceptible individuals subjected to stress, strong exertion, or hot weather.

cholinesterase, an enzyme that acts as a catalyst in the hydrolysis of acetylcholine to choline and acetate. It is important in terminating the physiological action of acetylcholine.

chondral, of or pertaining to cartilage.

chondrectomy, the surgical excision of a cartilage.

chondriocont, a threadlike or rod-shaped mitochondrion.

chondriome, the total mitochondria content of a cell, taken as a unit.

chondriomite, a single granular mitochondrion or a group of such organelles appearing in a chain formation.

chondriosome. See **mitochondrion**.

chondritis, any inflammatory condition affecting the joints.

chondroadenoma. See **adenochondroma**.

chondroangioma, *pl.* **chondroangiomas, chondroangiomata,** a benign, mesenchymal tumour containing vascular and cartilaginous elements.

chondroblast, any one of the cells that develops from the mesenchyma and forms cartilage.

chondroblastoma, *pl.* **chondroblastomas, chondroblastomata,** a benign tumour, derived from precursors of cartilage cells, that develops most frequently in epiphyses of the femur and humerus.

chondrocalcinosis, an arthritic disease in which calcium deposits are found in the peripheral joints. It resembles gout and is often found in patients over 50 years of age who have osteoarthritis or diabetes mellitus.

chondrocarcinoma, *pl.* **chondrocarcinoma, chondrocarcinomata,** a malignant epithelial tumour in which there is cartilaginous metaplasia.

chondroclast, a giant multinucleated cell associated with the resorption of cartilage. **chondroclastic,** *adj.*

chondrocostal, of or pertaining to the ribs and the costal cartilages.

chondrocyte, any one of the polymorphic cells that form the cartilage of the body. **chondrocytic,** *adj.*

chondrodysplasia, an inherited disease characterized by abnormal growth at the ends of bones, particularly the long bones of the arms and legs.

chondrodysplasia punctata, an inherited form of dwarfism characterized by ichthyotic skin lesions, radiographic epiphyseal stippling, and a pug nose. There are two types of the anomaly, a benign Conradi-Hunermann form and a lethal rhizomelic form.

chondrodystrophia calcificans congenita, an inherited defect characterized by many small opacities in the epiphyses of the long bones. Dwarfism, contractures, cataracts, mental retardation, and short stubby fingers develop as the infant grows into childhood.

chondrodystrophy, a group of disorders in which there is abnormal conversion of cartilage to bone, particularly in the epiphyses of the long bones.

chondroectodermal dysplasia, an inherited form of dwarfism marked by distal limb shortening, postaxial polydactyly, and cardiovascular abnormalities.

chondroendothelioma, *pl.* **chondroendotheliomas,** chondroendotheliomata a benign mesenchymal tumour containing cartilaginous and endothelial components.

chondrofibroma, *pl.* **chondrofibromas, chondrofibromata,** a fibrous tumour containing cartilaginous components.

chondrogenesis, the development of cartilage. **chondrogenetic,** *adj.*

chondroid, resembling cartilage.

chondrolipoma, *pl.* **chondrolipomas, chondrolipomata,** a benign mesenchymal tumour containing fatty and cartilaginous components.

chondroma, *pl.* **chondromas, chondromata,** a benign, fairly common tumour of cartilage cells that grows slowly within cartilage (enchondroma) or on the surface (ecchondroma). Kinds of chondromas are joint chondroma and synovial chondroma. **chondromatous,** *adj.*

chondromalacia, a softening of cartilage. Chondromalacia fetalis is a lethal congenital form of the condition in which the stillborn infant is born with soft and pliable limbs. Chondromalacia patellae occurs in young adults after knee injury and is characterized by swelling and pain and by degenerative changes, which are revealed on examination by x-ray.

chondroma sarcomatosum. See **chondrosarcoma.**

chondromatosis, a condition characterized by the presence of many cartilaginous tumours. A kind of chondromatosis is synovial chondromatosis.

chondromere, a cartilaginous, embryonic vertebra and its costal component.

chondromyoma, *pl.* **chondromyomas, chondromyomata,** a benign mesenchymal tumour containing myomatous and cartilaginous tissue.

chondromyxofibroma, a benign tumour that develops from cartilage-forming connective tissue. The lesion, typically a firm, greyish-white, somewhat rubbery mass, tends to occur in the knee and small bones of the foot.

chondromyxoid, composed of cartilaginous and myxoid elements.

chondromyxoid fibroma. See **chondromyxofibroma.**

chondrophyte, an abnormal mass of cartilage. **chondrophytic,** *adj.*

chondroplast. See **chondroblast.**

chondroplasty, the surgical repair of cartilage.

chondrosarcoma, *pl.* **chondrosarcomas, chondrosarcomata,** a malignant neoplasm of cartilaginous cells or their precursors that occurs most frequently on long bones, the pelvic girdle, and the scapula. Kinds of chondrosarcomas are central chondrosarcoma and mesenchymal chondrosarcoma. **chondrosarcomatous,** *adj.*

chondrosarcomatosis, a condition characterized by multiple, malignant cartilaginous tumours.

chondrosis, 1. the development of the cartilage of the body. **2.** a cartilaginous tumour.

chondrotomy, a surgical procedure for dividing a cartilage.

CHOP, an anticancer drug combination of cyclophosphamide, doxorubicin, vincristine, and prednisolone.

chopping, a therapeutic exercise to improve the strength and coordination of upper trunk nerves and muscles by lifting the arms overhead and bringing them down in a chopping or slashing movement.

chordae tendineae, *sing.* **chorda tendinea**, the strands of tendon that anchor the cusps of the mitral and the tricuspid valves to the papillary muscles of the ventricles of the heart, preventing prolaspe of the valves into the atria during ventricular contraction.

chordal canal. See **notochordal canal**.

chorda spinalis. See **spinal cord**.

chorda umbilicalis. See **umbilical cord**.

chordee, a congenital defect of the genitourinary tract resulting in a ventral curvature of the penis, caused by a fibrous band of tissue instead of normal skin along the corpus spongiosum.

chordencephalon, the portion of the central nervous system that develops in the early weeks of pregnancy from the neural tube and includes the mesencephalon, the rhombencephalon, and the spinal cord. **chordencephalic,** *adj.*

chorditis, 1. inflammation of a spermatic cord. **2.** inflammation of the vocal cords or of the vocal folds.

chordoid, resembling the notocord or notochordal tissue.

chordoma, *pl.* **chordomas, chordomata**, a rare, congenital tumour of the brain developing from the fetal notochord.

chordotomy, an operation in which the anterolateral tracts of the spinal cord are surgically divided to relieve pain.

chorea, a condition characterized by involuntary, purposeless, rapid motions, as flexing and extending the fingers, raising and lowering the shoulders, or grimacing.

chorea gravidarum, a form of chorea occurring during a first pregnancy subsequent to an episode of Sydenham's chorea in childhood.

chorea minor. See **Sydenham's chorea**.

choreiform, resembling the rapid jerky movements associated with chorea.

choreoathetoid cerebral palsy, a form of cerebral palsy characterized by both choreiform (jerky, ticlike twitching) and athetoid (slow, writhing) movements.

chorioadenoma, *pl.* **chorioadenomas, chorioadenomata**, an epithelial cell tumour of the outermost fetal membrane that is intermediate in the malignant development of a hydatid mole to invasive choriocarcinoma.

chorioadenoma destruens, an invasive hydatidiform mole in which the chorionic villi of the mole penetrate into the myometrium and parametrium of the uterus and metastasize to distant parts of the body.

chorioallantoic graft, the grafting of tissue onto the chorioallantoic membrane of the egg of a hen to improve the environment for embryonic growth.

chorioamnionic, of or pertaining to the chorion and the amnion.

chorioamnionitis, an inflammatory reaction in the amniotic membranes caused by organisms in the amniotic fluid.

choriocarcinoma, *pl.* **choriocarcinomas, choriocarcinomata**, an epithelial malignancy of fetal origin that develops from the chorionic portion of the products of conception, usually from a hydatidiform mole. The primary tumour usually appears in the uterus as a soft, dark red, crumbling mass.

choriocele, a hernia or protrusion of the tissue of the choroid layer of the eye.

chorioepithelioma. See **choriocarcinoma**.

choriogenesis, the development of the chorion after the trophoblast anchors to the uterine tissue and extends primary villi into the intervillous space. **choriogenetic,** *adj.*

choriomeningitis. See **lymphocytic choriomeningitis**.

chorion, (in biology) the outermost membrane derived from the trophoblast. It develops villi about 2 weeks after fertilization and is vascularized by allantoic vessels 1 week later. It gives rise to the placenta and persists until birth as the outer of the two layers of membrane containing the amniotic fluid and the fetus.

chorionic carcinoma, chorionic epithelioma. See **choriocarcinoma**.

chorionic gonadotropin (CG), a chemical component of the urine of pregnant women. This glycoprotein hormone is secreted by the placental trophoblastic cells. It is composed of two subunits, alpha and beta human chorionic gonadotropin. The alpha subunit is nearly identical to similar subunits of the follicle-stimulating, luteinizing, and thyroid-stimulating hormones. The specific hormonal effects of chorionic gonadotropin are activated by the beta portion. They include stimulation of the corpus luteum to secrete oestrogen and progesterone and to decrease lymphocyte activation.

chorionic villi tiny vascular fibrils on the surface of the chorion that infiltrate the maternal blood sinuses of the endometrium and help form the placenta.

chorioretinitis, an inflammatory condition of the choroid and retina of the eye, usually as a result of parasitic or bacterial infection. It is characterized by blurred vision, photophobia, and distorted images.

chorioretinopathy, a noninflammatory process caused by disease that involves the choroid and the retina.

choroid, a thin, highly vascular membrane covering the posterior five sixths of the eye between the retina and sclera.

choroidal malignant melanoma, a tumour of the choroid coat that grows into the vitreous humour, causing detachment and degeneration of the overlying retina.

choroiditis, an inflammatory condition of the choroid membrane of the eye.

choroidocyclitis, an abnormal condition characterized by inflammation of the choroid and the ciliary processes.

choroidoretinitis. See **chorioretinopathy**.

choroid plexectomy, a surgical procedure for the reduction of cerebrospinal fluid production in the ventricles of the brain in hydrocephalus, usually in the newborn.

choroid plexus, any one of the tangled masses of tiny blood vessels contained within the ventricles of the brain.

Christchurch chromosome (Ch¹) {Christchurch, city on South Island of New Zealand}, an abnormally small acrocentric chromosome of the G group, involving any members of chromosome pairs 21 or 22, in which the short arms are missing or partially deleted.

Christmas disease. See **haemophilia B.**

Christmas factor. See **factor IX.**

chromaffin, having an affinity for strong staining with chromium salts, especially strong staining of the cells of the adrenal, the coccygeal, and the carotid glands, certain cells of the adrenal medulla, and the cells of the paraganglions. Also **chromaphil.**

chromaffin body. See **paraganglion.**

chromaffin cell, any one of the special cells comprising the paraganglia and connected to the ganglia of the coeliac, the renal, the suprarenal, the aortic, and the hypogastric plexuses. The chromaffin cells of the adrenal medulla secrete two catecholamines, adrenaline and noradrenaline, which affect smooth muscle, cardiac muscle, and glands in the same way as sympathetic stimulation, increasing and prolonging sympathetic effects.

chromaffinoma. See **phaeochromocytoma.**

chromaphil. See **chromaffin.**

chromatic, 1. of or pertaining to colour. **2.** stainable by a dye. **3.** of or pertaining to chromatin. Also **chromatinic.**

chromatic dispersion, the splitting of light into its various component wavelengths or frequencies, such as with a prism.

chromatid, one of the two identical threadlike filaments of a chromosome.

chromatid deletion, the breakage of a chromatid. The breakage may be caused by a single-hit chromatid produced by radiation. The fragments are isochromatids.

chromatin, the material within the cell nucleus from which the chromosomes are formed. It consists of fine, threadlike strands of deoxyribonucleic acid attached to a protein base, usually histone. During cell division, portions of the chromatin condense and coil to form the chromosomes. A kind of chromatin is sex chromatin. **chromatinic,** *adj.*

chromatin-negative, pertaining to or descriptive of the nuclei of cells that lack sex chromatin, specifically characteristic of the normal male, but also occurring in certain chromosomal abnormalities.

chromatin nucleolus. See **karyosome.**

chromatin-positive, pertaining to or descriptive of the nuclei of cells that contain sex chromatin, specifically characteristic of the normal female, but occurring also in certain chromosomal abnormalities.

chromatism, 1. an abnormal condition characterized by hallucinations in which the affected individual sees coloured lights. **2.** abnormal pigmentation.

chromatogram, 1. the record produced by the separation of gaseous substances or dissolved chemical substances moving through a column of absorbent material that filters out the various absorbates in different layers. **2.** any graphic record produced by any chromatographic method.

chromatography, any one of several processes for separating and analysing various gaseous or dissolved chemical materials according to differences in their absorbency with respect to a specific substance and according to their different pigments. Some kinds of chromatography are column chromatography, displacement chromatography, gas chromatography, ion-exchange chromatography, and paper chromatography. **chromatographic,** *adj.*

chromatopsia, 1. an abnormal condition characterized by a visual defect that makes colourless objects appear tinged with colour. **2.** a form of colour blindness characterized by the imperfect perception of various colours. It may be caused by a deficiency in one or more of the retinal cones or from defective nerve circuits that convey colour-associated impulses to the cerebral cortex. The most common defect in colour sense is the inability to distinguish red from green.

chromatosis, a condition of abnormal skin pigmentation in any part of the body.

chromaesthesia, 1. the colour sense that depends on the mixture of wavelengths in the light that enters the eye and the response of the different types of retinal cones associated with colour vision. **2.** an abnormal condition characterized by the confusion of other senses, such as taste and smell, with imagined sensations of colour.

chromhidrosis a rare, functional disorder in which apocrine sweat glands secrete coloured sweat.

chromic myopia, a kind of colour blindness characterized by the ability to distinguish colours only of those objects that are close to the eye.

chromium (Cr), a hard, brittle, metallic element. Its atomic number is 24; its atomic weight is 51.9. Traces of chromium occur in plants and animals, and there is evidence this element may be important in human nutrition, especially in carbohydrate metabolism. Chromium 51 isotope is used in blood studies.

chromobacteriosis, an extremely rare, usually fatal systemic infection caused by a bacillus *Chromobacterium violaceum,* found in fresh water in tropical and subtropical regions, which enters the body through a break in the skin.

chromoblastomycosis, an infectious skin disease caused by any of a variety of fungi and characterized by the appearance of pruritic, warty nodules that develop in a cut or other break in the skin.

chromocentre. See **karyosome.**

chromogen, a substance that absorbs light, producing colour.

chromomere, any of the series of beadlike structures that lie along the chromonema of a chromosome during the early stages of cell division.

chromomycosis. See **chromoblastomycosis.**

chromonema, *pl.* **chromonemata,** the coiled filament along which the chromomeres lie that forms the central part of the chromatid of the chromosome during cell division.

chromophilic, denoting a cell, tissue, or microorganism that is easily stained, particularly certain leukocytes.

chromophobe adenoma. See **chromophobic adenoma.**

chromophobia, 1. the resistance of certain cells and tissues to stains. **2.** a morbid aversion to colours. **chromophobe,** *n.*

chromophobic, denoting a cell, tissue, or microorganism that is not easily stained, particularly certain cells of the anterior lobe of the pituitary gland.

chromophobic adenoma, a tumour of the pituitary gland composed of cells that do not stain with acid or basic dyes.

chromoplasm. See **chromatin.**

chromosomal aberration, any change in the structure or number of any of the chromosomes for a given species, which can result in anomalies of varying severity. In humans, a number of disorders are directly associated with chromosomal defects, including Down's syndrome, Turner's syndrome, and Kleinfelter's syndrome.

chromosomal nomenclature, a standard nomenclature that serves to identify the complement of chromosomes in an individual according to the number of chromosomes, sex, and the deletion or addition of a specific chromosome or part of a chromosome. Complement in a normal female is recorded as 46,XX, and for a normal male, 46,XY. Chromosomal aberrations are designated by indicating the total chromosomal number, sex complement, and the group or specific chromosome in which the addition or deletion occurs. The short arm of a chromosome is designated "p," the long arm is "q," and a translocation is "t".

chromosome, any one of the threadlike structures in the nucleus of a cell that function in the transmission of genetic information. Each consists of a double strand of the nucleoprotein deoxyribonucleic acid (DNA), which is coiled in a helix formation and attached to a protein base, usually a histone. The genes, which contain the genetic material that controls the inheritance of traits, are arranged in a linear pattern along the entire length of each DNA strand. Each species has a characteristic number of chromosomes in the somatic cell, which in humans is 46 and includes 22 homologous pairs of autosomes and one pair of sex chromosomes, with one member of each pair being derived from each parent. Kinds of chromosomes include **accessory chromosome, Christchurch chromosome, daughter chromosome, gametic chromosome, giant chromosome, homologous chromosomes, Philadelphia chromosome, sex chromosome, somatic chromosome, W chromosome,** and **Z chromosome. chromosomal,** *adj.*

chromosome banding. See **banding.**

chromosome coil, the spiral formed by the coiling of two or more chromonemata of the chromatid within the chromosome.

chromosome complement, the normal number of chromosomes found in the somatic cell of any given species. In humans it is 46, consisting of 22 pairs of homologous autosomes and one pair of sex chromosomes.

chromosome 5p syndrome. See **cat-cry syndrome.**

chromosome mapping. See **mapping.**

chromosome puff, a band of accumulated chromatic material located at a specific site on a giant chromosome. It is indicative of gene activity, specifically DNA and RNA synthesis, for the particular locus.

chromosome walking, the process by which overlapping molecular clones that span large chromosomal intervals are isolated.

chromotrope, 1. a component of tissue that stains metachromatically with metachromatic dyes. **2.** any one of several dyes differentiated by numeric suffixes. **chromotropic,** *adj.*

chronaxie, (in electroneuromyography) a measure of the shortest duration of an electric stimulus needed to excite nerve or muscle tissue.

chronic, (of a disease or disorder) developing slowly and persisting for a long period of time, often for the remainder of the lifetime of the individual.

chronic airway obstruction, a type of respiratory disorder in which the patient, when at rest, appears to breathe at a normal rate and does not show signs of respiratory distress. However, there may be prolongation of the expiratory phase with pursed-lip breathing.

chronic alcoholic delirium. See **Korsakoff's psychosis.**

chronic alcoholism, a pathological condition resulting from the habitual use of alcohol in excessive amounts. Symptoms include anorexia, diarrhoea, weight loss, neurological and psychiatric disturbances (most notably depression), and fatty deterioration of the liver, sometimes leading to cirrhosis.

chronic appendicitis, 1. a type of appendicitis characterized by thickening or scarring of the vermiform appendix, caused by previous inflammation. **2.** an obsolete term for chronic pain in the appendiceal area without any evidence of inflammation.

chronic brain syndrome (CBS), an abnormal condition that is caused by impairment of the cerebral tissue function, characterized by loss of memory and disorientation. It may occur in dementia paralytica, cerebral arteriosclerosis, brain trauma, and Huntington's chorea.

chronic bronchitis, a very common debilitating respiratory disease, characterized by greatly increased production of mucus by the glands of the trachea and bronchi and resulting in a cough with expectoration for at least 3 months of the year for more than 2 consecutive years.

chronic care, a pattern of medical and nursing care that focuses on long-term care of people with chronic diseases or conditions, either at home or in hospital.

chronic carrier, an individual who acts as host to pathogenic organisms for an extended period of time without displaying any signs of disease.

chronic cervicitis. See **cervicitis**.

chronic cholecystitis. See **cholecystitis**.

chronic chorea. See **Huntington's chorea**.

chronic cystic mastitis. See **fibrocystic disease**.

chronic disease, a disease that persists over a long period of time as compared with the course of an acute disease. The symptoms of chronic disease are usually less severe than those of the acute phase of the same disease.

chronic gastritis. See **gastritis**.

chronic glaucoma. See **glaucoma**.

chronic glomerulonephritis, a noninfectious disease of the glomerulus of the kidney characterized by proteinuria, haematuria, oedema, and decreased production of urine.

chronic hypoxia, a usually slow, insidious reduction in oxygen flow to the tissue cells resulting from gradually destructive or fibrotic lung diseases, congenital or acquired heart disorders, or chronic blood loss. There is usually an absence of acute symptoms, but the person develops persistent mental and physical fatigue, shows sluggish mental responses, and complains of a loss of ability to perform physical tasks.

chronic idiopathic thrombocytopenic purpura. See **idiopathic thrombocytopenic purpura**.

chronic illness, any illness that persists over a long period of time and affects physical, emotional, intellectual, social, or spiritual functioning.

chronic intestinal ischaemia. See **intestinal angina**.

chronic interstitial nephritis. See **interstitial nephritis**.

chronicity, pertaining to a state of being chronic.

chronic lingual papillitis, an inflammatory disorder of the tongue, sometimes extending to the buccal mucosa and palate, characterized by irregularly scattered red patches, thinning of the lingual papillae, severe burning pain, and shedding of epidermal tissue.

chronic lymphoblastic leukaemia (CLL), a neoplasm of blood-forming tissues, characterized by a proliferation of small, long-lived lymphocytes, chiefly B cells, in bone marrow, blood liver, and lymphoid organs. No treatment is curative, but remissions may be induced by chemotherapy with chlorambucil and glucocorticoids or by thymic, splenic, or total body irradiation.

chronic mastitis. See **mastitis**.

chronic mucocutaneous candidiasis, an abnormal condition and rare form of candidiasis, characterized by lesions of the skin, viral infections, and recurrent respiratory tract infections. This disease usually occurs during the first year of life but can develop as late as the 20s. It affects both men and women and is associated with an inherited defect of the cell-mediated immune system and apparently allows autoantibodies to develop against target organs. The humoral immune system functions normally in this disease. The onset of infections associated with the disease may precede endocrinopathy.

chronic myeloblastic leukaemia (CML), a malignant neoplasm of blood-forming tissues, characterized by a proliferation of granular leukocytes and, often, of megakaryocytes. The disease is marked by malaise, fatigue, heat intolerance, bleeding gums, purpura, skin lesions, weight loss, hyperuricaemia, abdominal discomfort, and massive splenomegaly.

chronic nephropathy, a kidney disorder characterized by generalized or local damage to the tubulointerstitial areas of the kidney. The condition frequently results from more than a single cause, such as diabetes and a bacterial infection. Symptoms include polyuria, renal acidosis, oedema, proteinuria, and blood in the urine.

chronic obstructive pulmonary disease (COPD), a progressive and irreversible condition characterized by diminished inspiratory and expiratory capacity of the lungs. The person complains of dyspnoea with physical exertion, of difficulty in inhaling or exhaling deeply, and sometimes of a chronic cough.

chronic (open-angle) glaucoma. See **glaucoma**.

chronic pain, pain that continues or recurs

over a prolonged period, caused by various diseases or abnormal conditions, as rheumatoid arthritis. Chronic pain is often less intense than the acute pain. The person with chronic pain does not display increased pulse and rapid respiration because these autonomic reactions to pain cannot be sustained for long periods.

chronic pyelonephritis. See **pyelonephritis.**

chronic tuberculous mastitis, a rare infection of the breast resulting from extension of tuberculosis of underlying ribs.

chronic undifferentiated schizophrenia, a condition marked by the symptoms of more than one of the classic types of schizophrenia—simple, paranoid, catatonic, or hebephrenic.

chronograph, a device that records small intervals of time, such as a stopwatch. **chronographic,** *adj.*

chronological, 1. arranged in time sequence. **2.** of or pertaining to chronology.

chronological age, the age of an individual expressed as a period of time that has elapsed since birth, as the age of an infant, which is expressed in hours, days, or months, and the age of children and adults, expressed in years.

chronopsychophysiology, the science of physiological cyclic processes in the body.

chronotropism, the act or process of affecting the regularity of a periodic function, especially interference with the rate of heartbeat. **chronotropic,** *adj.*

chrysiasis, an abnormal condition characterized by the deposition of gold in the tissues of the body.

Chua K'a, a holistic counselling system of muscle tension release that emphasizes clarification and cleansing of the mind and emotions.

Churg-Strauss syndrome, an allergic disorder marked by granulomatosis, usually of the lungs, and often involving the circulatory system.

Chvostek's sign {Franz Chvostek, Austrian surgeon, b. 1835}, an abnormal spasm of the facial muscles elicited by light taps on the facial nerve in patients who are hypocalcaemic. It is a sign of tetany.

Chvostek-Weiss sign. See **Chvostek's sign.**

chyle, the cloudy liquid products of digestion taken up by the small intestine. Consisting mainly of emulsified fats, chyle passes through fingerlike projections in the small intestine. **chylous,** *adj.*

chyliform ascites. See **chylous ascites.**

chyloid, resembling the chyle that fills the lacteals of the small intestine during the digestion of fatty foods.

chylomicron, minute droplets of the lipoproteins measuring less than 0.5 mm in diameter. Chylomicrons consist of about 90% triglycerides with small amounts of cholesterol, phospholipids, and protein. They are synthesized in the GI tract and carry dietary glycerides from the intestinal mucosa into the plasma.

chylothorax, a condition marked by the effusion of chyle from the thoracic duct into the pleural space.

chylous ascites, an abnormal condition characterized by an accumulation of chyle in the peritoneal cavity.

chyluria, a condition characterized by the milky appearance of the urine because of the presence of chyle.

chylus. See **chyle.**

chyme, the viscous, semifluid contents of the stomach present during digestion of a meal.

chymopapain, a proteolytic enzyme isolated from the fruit of Carica papaya and related to papain.

chymosin. See **rennin.**

chymotrypsin, 1. a proteolytic enzyme, produced by the pancreas, that catalyses the hydrolysis of casein and gelatin. **2.** a yellow crystalline powder prepared from an extract of ox pancreas, used in treating digestive disorders.

chymotrypsinogen, a substance, produced in the pancreas, that is the zymogen precursor to the enzyme chymotrypsin. It is converted to chymotrypsin by trypsin.

Ci, abbreviation for **curie.**

cibophobia, an abnormal or morbid aversion to food or to eating.

cicatricial entropion. See **cicatrix, entropion.**

cicatricial stenosis, the narrowing of a duct or tube because of the formation of scar tissue.

cicatrix, *pl.* **cicatrices,** scar tissue that is avascular, pale, contracted, and firm after the earlier phase of skin healing characterized by redness and softness. **cicatricial,** *adj.* **cicatrize,** *v.*

cicutism, poisoning caused by water hemlock, resulting in cyanosis, dilated pupils, convulsions, and coma.

cigarette smoking, the inhalation of the gases and hydrocarbon vapours generated by slowly burning tobacco in cigarettes. The practice is partly due to the effect on the nervous system of the nicotine contained in the smoke. In addition to nicotine, nearly 1000 other chemicals have been identified in cigarette smoke.

ciguatera poisoning, a nonbacterial food poisoning that results from eating fish contaminated with the ciguatera toxin. Characteristics of ciguatera poisoning are vomiting, diarrhoea, tingling or numbness of extremities and the skin around the mouth, itching, muscle weakness, and pain.

cilia, *sing.* **cilium, 1.** the eyelids or eyelashes. **2.** small, hairlike processes on the outer surfaces of some cells, aiding metabolism by producing motion, eddies, or current in a fluid. **ciliary,** *adj.*

ciliary body, the thickened part of the vascular tunic of the eye that joins the iris with the anterior portion of the choroid.

ciliary canal, the spaces of the iridocorneal angle.

ciliary gland, one of the numerous tiny, modified sweat glands arranged in several rows near the free margins of the eyelids.

ciliary margin, the peripheral border of the iris, continuous with the ciliary body.

ciliary movement, the waving motion of the hairlike processes projecting from the epithelium of the respiratory tract and from certain microorganisms.

ciliary mucus transport, the movement of particles from the upper respiratory tract by means other than exhalation, particularly through the wave motion of cilia lining the tract and the mucous layer.

ciliary muscle, a semitransparent, circular band of smooth muscle fibres attached to the choroid of the eye, the chief agent in adjusting the eye to view near objects.

ciliary process, any one of about 80 tiny fleshy projections on the posterior surface of the iris, forming a frill around the margin of the crystalline lens of the eye.

ciliary reflex. See **accommodation reflex.**

ciliary ring, a small grooved band of tissue, about 4 mm wide, that forms the posterior part of the ciliary body of the eye.

ciliary zone, an outer circular area on the anterior surface of the iris, separated from the inner circular area by the angular line. The ciliary zone contains the stroma of the iris.

Ciliata, a class of protozoa of the subphylum Ciliophora, characterized by cilia throughout the life cycle.

ciliate, of or having cilia, as certain epithelial cells of the body or protozoa of the class Ciliata.

ciliated epithelium, any epithelial tissue that projects cilia from its surface, such as portions of the epithelium in the respiratory tract.

ciliospinal reflex, a normal brainstem reflex initiated by scratching or pinching the skin of the back of the neck, resulting in dilatation of the pupil.

cimetidine, a histamine H_2-receptor antagonist used to inhibit the production and secretion of acid in the stomach in the treatment of duodenal ulcer and other conditions where reduction in gastric acid is useful.

Cimex lectularius. See **bedbug.**

cinchona, the dried bark of the stem or root of species of Cinchona, containing the alkaloids quinine and quinidine.

cinchonism, a condition resulting from excessive ingestion of cinchona bark or its alkaloid derivatives. Cinchonism is characterized by deafness, headache, ringing in the ears, and signs of cerebral congestion.

cineangiocardiography, see **cineradiography.**

cineangiogram. See **cineradiography.**

cinefluorography. See **cineradiography.**

cinematics. See **kinematics.**

cineradiography, recording the image on the output phosphor of an image intensifier on a rapid sequence camera using celluloid roll film. May be used in cardiac catheterization or certain GI studies.

cingulate, 1. having a zone or a girdle, usually with transverse markings. **2.** of or pertaining to a cingulum.

cingulate sulcus. See **callosomarginal fissure.**

cingulectomy, the surgical excision of a portion of the cingulate gyrus in the frontal lobe of the brain and the immediately surrounding tissue.

cingulotomy, a procedure in brain surgery to alleviate intractable pain by producing lesions in the tissue of the cingulate gyrus of the frontal lobe.

cinnamon, the aromatic inner bark of several species of Cinnamomum, a tree native to the East Indies and China. Saigon cinnamon is commonly used as a carminative, an aromatic stimulant, or a spice. **cinnamic,** *adj.*

CIPM, abbreviation for **Comité International des Poids et Mesures.**

circadian dysrhythmia, the biological and psychological stress effects of jet lag, or rapid travel through several time zones. In addition to a shift in normal time eating and sleeping patterns, medication schedules and other therapies may be disrupted.

circadian rhythm, a pattern based on a 24-hour cycle, especially the repetition of certain physiological phenomena, as sleeping and eating.

circinate, having a ring-shaped outline or formation; annular.

circle, (in anatomy) a circular or nearly circular structure of the body, as the circle of Willis and circle of Zinn. **circular,** *adj.*

circle of Carus. See **curve of Carus.**

circle of Willis {Thomas Willis, English physician, b. 1621}, a vascular network at the base of the brain, formed by the interconnection of the internal carotid, anterior cerebral, posterior cerebral, anterior communicating, and posterior communicating arteries.

circuit, a course or pathway, particularly one through which an electric current passes. Current passes through a closed or continuous circuit and stops if the circuit is open, interrupted, or broken.

circuit training, a method of physical exercise in which activities are arranged in sets so that the participant moves quickly from one activity to another with a minimum of rest between sets.

circular bandage, a bandage wrapped around an injured part, usually a limb.

circular fibre, any one of the many fibres in the free gingiva that encircle the teeth.

circular fold, one of the numerous annular projections in the small intestine. They vary in size and frequency and are formed by mucous and submucous tissue.

circulation, movement of an object or substance through a circular course so that it returns to its starting point, such as the circulation of blood through the circuitous network of arteries and veins.

circulation time, normal, the time required for blood to flow from one part of the body to another. It involves injecting a traceable dye or radioisotope into a vein and timing its reappearance in an artery at the point of injection.

circulatory failure, failure of the cardiovascular system to supply the cells of the body with a volume of blood adequate to meet the metabolic demands of the cells.

circulatory fluid. See **blood, lymph**.

circulatory system, the network of channels through which the nutrient fluids of the body circulate.

circulus arteriosus minor, the small artery encircling the outer circumference of the iris.

circumanal, of or pertaining to the area surrounding the anus.

circumcision, a surgical procedure in which the prepuce of the penis or, rarely, the prepuce of the clitoris is excised. Ritual circumcision is required by the religions of approximately one sixth of the population of the world.

circumcorneal, pertaining to the area of the eye surrounding the cornea.

circumduction, 1. the circular movement of a limb or of the eye. **2.** the motion of the head of a bone within an articulating cavity, as the hip joint. Circumduction is a combination of abduction, adduction, extension, and flexion.

circumferential fibrocartilage, a structure made of fibrocartilage, in which fibrocartilaginous rims surround the margins of various articular cavities, as the glenoid labra of the hip and the shoulder.

circumferential implantation. See **superficial implantation**.

circumlocution, the use of pantomime or nonverbal communication or word substitution by a patient to avoid revealing that a word has been forgotten.

circumoral, of or pertaining to the area of the face around the mouth.

circumscribed scleroderma. See **morphea**.

circum-speech, (in psychiatry) behavioural characteristics associated with conversation. They include body language, maintenance of personal space between individuals, handsweeps, head nods, and task-oriented activities such as walking or knitting while carrying on a conversation.

circumstantiality, (in psychiatry) a speech pattern in which a patient has difficulty in separating relevant from irrelevant information while describing an event. Circumstantiality may be a sign of chronic brain dysfunction.

circumvallate papilla. See **papilla**.

circus movement, 1. an unusual and involuntary rolling or somersaulting, because of injured neurological mechanisms that control body posture, such as the cerebral pedicles or the vestibular apparatus. **2.** an unusual circular gait caused by injury to the brain or to basal nerve centres. **3.** a mechanism associated with the excitatory wave of the atrium of the heart that travels a circular path characterized by a gap between the refractory and the excitatory tissue.

cirrhosis, a chronic degenerative disease of the liver in which the lobes are covered with fibrous tissue, the parenchyma degenerates, and the lobules are infiltrated with fat. Gluconeogenesis, detoxification of drugs and alcohol, bilirubin metabolism, vitamin absorption, GI function, hormonal metabolism, and other functions of the liver deteriorate. Cirrhosis is most commonly the result of chronic alcohol abuse but can be the result of nutritional deprivation or hepatitis or other infection. The symptoms of cirrhosis are the same regardless of the cause: nausea, flatulence, anorexia, weight loss, ascites, light-coloured stools, weakness, abdominal pain, varicosities, and spider angiomas. Kinds of cirrhosis are biliary cirrhosis, fatty cirrhosis, and posthepatic cirrhosis.

cirsoid aneurysm. See **racemose aneurysm**.

cis configuration, 1. the presence of the dominant alleles of two or more pairs of genes on one chromosome and the recessive alleles on the homologous chromosome. **2.** the presence of the mutant genes of a pair of pseudoalleles on one chromosome and the wild-type genes on the homologous chromosome. **3.** (in chemistry) a form of isomerism in which two substituent groups are on the same side of a double bond.

cisplatin, a cytotoxic platinum complex used in the treatment of a wide variety of cancers, including metastatic testicular and ovarian tumours.

cisterna, *pl.* **cisternae,** a cavity that serves as a reservoir for lymph or other body fluids. Kinds of cisternae include cisterna chyli and cisterna subarachnoidea.

cisterna chyli, a dilatation at the beginning of the thoracic duct. It receives the two lumbar lymphatic trunks and the intestinal lymphatic trunk.

cisternal puncture, the insertion of a needle into the cerebellomedullary cistern to withdraw cerebrospinal fluid for examination. The puncture is made between the atlas and the occipital bone.

cisterna subarachnoidea, any one of many small subarachnoid spaces that serve as reservoirs for cerebrospinal fluid.

cistron, a fragment or portion of DNA that codes for a specific polypeptide. It is the smallest unit functioning as a transmitter of genetic information. **cistronic,** *adj.*

cisvestism, the practice of wearing attire appropriate to the sex of the individual involved but not suitable to the age, occupation, or status of the wearer.

cit, abbreviation for a **citrate carboxylate anion.**

citrate, 1. any salt or ester of citric acid. **2.** the act of treating with a citrate or citric acid. **citration,** *n.*

citric acid, a white, crystalline, organic acid soluble in water and alcohol. It is extracted from citrus fruits or obtained by fermentation of sugars and is used as a flavouring agent in foods, carbonated beverages, and certain pharmaceutical products.

citrin, a crystalline flavonoid concentrate that is used as a source of bioflavonoid.

citrovorum factor. See **folinic acid**.

citrulline, an amino acid that is produced from ornithine during the urea cycle and is subsequently transformed to arginine by the transfer of a nitrogen atom from aspartate.

citrullinaemia, a disorder of amino acid metabolism caused by a deficiency of an enzyme, argininosuccinic acid synthetase. The clinical features include vomiting, convulsions, and coma.

C/kg, a unit of radiation exposure in the SI system. It represents coulombs per kilogram of air, as in the relationship, 1 roentgen (R) $= 2.58 \times 10^{-4}$ °C/kg of air.

Cl, symbol for chlorine.

clairvoyance, the alleged power or ability to perceive or be aware of objects or events without the use of the physical senses.

clairvoyant, 1. pertaining to or characterized by clairvoyance. **2.** one who allegedly possesses the powers of clairvoyance.

clam poisoning. See **shellfish poisoning**.

clamp, an instrument with serrated tips and locking handles, used for gripping, holding, joining, supporting, or compressing an organ or vessel.

clamp forceps. See **pedicle clamp**.

clang association, the mental connection between dissociated ideas made because of similarity in the sounds of the words used to describe the ideas. Also spelled klang association.

clapping, (in massage) the procedure of making percussive movements on the body of a patient by lowering the cupped palms alternately in a series of rapid, stimulating blows.

clarification (in psychology) an intervention technique designed to guide the patient in focusing on and recognizing gaps and inconsistencies in his or her statements.

clarify, (in chemistry) to clear a turbid liquid by allowing any suspended matter to settle, by adding a substance that precipitates any suspended matter, or by heating. **clarification,** *n.*

Clark's rule {Cecil Clark, 20th century English chemist}, a method of calculating the approximate paediatric dosage of a drug for a child using this formula: weight in pounds/150 × adult dose.

clasmocytic lymphoma. See **histiocytic malignant lymphoma**.

clasp, 1. (in dentistry) a sleevelike fitting that is fastened over a tooth to hold a partial denture in place. **2.** (in surgery) any device for holding tissues together, especially bones.

clasp-knife reflex, an abnormal sign in which a spastic limb resists passive motion and then suddenly gives way, similar to the blade of a jackknife.

clasp torsion, the twisting of a dental retentive clasp arm on its long axis.

classical caesarean section, a method for surgically delivering a baby through a vertical midline incision of the upper segment of the uterus.

classical conditioning, a form of learning in which a previously neutral stimulus comes to elicit a given response through associative training.

classical typhus. See **epidemic typhus**.

classic apraxia. See **ideomotor apraxia**.

classification, a process in data collection and analysis in which data are grouped according to previously determined characteristics. **classify,** *v.*

classification schemes, systems of organizing data or information, usually involving categories of items with similar characteristics. An example is the International Classification of Diseases (ICD) compiled by the World Health Organization (WHO).

claudication, a weakness of the legs accompanied by cramplike pains in the calves caused by poor circulation of the blood to the leg muscles.

claustrophobia, a morbid fear of being in or becoming trapped in enclosed or narrow places.

claustrum, *pl.* **claustra, 1.** a barrier, as a membrane that partially closes an aperture. **2.** a thin sheet of grey matter, composed chiefly of spindle cells, situated lateral to the external capsule of the brain and separating the internal capsule from white matter of the insula.

clavicle, a long, curved, horizontal bone just above the first rib, forming the ventral portion of the shoulder girdle. It articulates medially with the sternum and laterally with the acromion of the scapula and accommodates the attachment of numerous muscles.

clavicular notch, one of a pair of oval depressions at the superior end of the sternum.

clavus. See **corn.**

clawfoot. See **pes cavus.**

clawhand, an abnormal condition of the hand characterized by extreme flexion of the middle and distal phalanges and hyperextension of the metacarpophalangeal joints.

claw-type traction frame, an orthopaedic apparatus that holds various pieces of traction equipment, such as the pulleys, the ropes, and the weights by which traction is applied to various parts of the body or by which various parts of the body are suspended.

clean-catch specimen, a urine specimen that is as free from bacterial contamination as possible without the use of a catheter.

cleansing enema, an enema, usually composed of soapsuds, administered to remove all formed faecal material from the colon.

clearance, the removal of a substance from the blood via the kidneys. Kidney function can be tested by measuring the amount of a specific substance excreted in the urine in a given length of time.

clear cell, 1. a type of cell found in the parathyroid gland that does not take on a colour with the ordinary tissue stains used for microscopic examination. **2.** the principal cell of most renal cell carcinomas and, occasionally, of ovarian and parathyroid tumours. **3.** a specific type of epidermal cell, probably of neural origin, that has a dark-staining nucleus but clear cytoplasm with haematoxylin and eosin stain.

clear cell carcinoma, 1. a malignant tumour of the tubular epithelium of the kidney that contain abundant clear cytoplasm. **2.** an uncommon ovarian neoplasm characterized by cells with clear cytoplasm.

clear cell carcinoma of the kidney. See **renal cell carcinoma.**

clearing agent, a chemical, such as ammonium thiosulfate (a constituent of fixer), used in the processing of exposed x-ray film to remove unexposed and undeveloped silver halide from the emulsion.

clearing test, a range of motion test that moves the joint to its limits, stretching the capsule and other soft tissues in an attempt to reproduce symptoms. If no symptoms are produced, the joint is cleared as a cause of a musculoskeletal disorder.

clear-liquid diet, a diet that supplies fluids and provides minimal residue. The diet is nutritionally inadequate and is usually prescribed for a limited amount of time, as 1 day, postoperatively.

cleavage, 1. the series of repeated mitotic cell divisions occurring in the ovum immediately after fertilization to form a mass of cells that transforms the single-celled zygote into a multicellular embryo capable of growth and differentiation. At this initial stage, as the zygote remains uniform in size, the cleavage cells, or blastomeres, become smaller with each division. **2.** the act or process of cleaving or splitting, primarily the splitting of a complex molecule into two or more simpler molecules. Kinds of cleavage include determinate cleavage, equal cleavage, indeterminate cleavage, partial cleavage, total cleavage, and unequal cleavage.

cleavage cavity. See **blastocoele.**

cleavage cell. See **blastomere.**

cleavage fracture, any fracture that splits cartilage with the avulsion of a small piece of bone from the distal portion of the lateral condyle of the humerus.

cleavage line, any one of a number of linear striations in the skin that delineate the general structural pattern and tension of the subcutaneous fibrous tissue. They correspond closely to the crease lines on the surface of the skin and are present in all areas of the body but are visible only in certain sites, such as the palms of the hands and soles of the feet.

cleavage nucleus. See **segmentation nucleus.**

cleavage plane, 1. the area in a fertilized ovum where cleavage takes place; the axis along which any cell division occurs. **2.** any plane within the body where organs or structures can be separated with minimal damage to surrounding tissue.

cleft, 1. divided. **2.** a fissure, especially one that originates in the embryo, as the branchial cleft or the facial cleft.

cleft foot, an abnormal condition in which the division between third and fourth toes extends into the metatarsum of the foot.

cleft lip, a congenital anomaly consisting of one or more clefts in the upper lip resulting from the failure in the embryo of the maxillary and median nasal processes to close.

cleft-lip repair, the surgical correction of a unilateral or bilateral congenital interruption of the upper lip, usually resulting from the embryological failure of the median nasal and maxillary processes to unite.

cleft palate, a congenital defect characterized by a fissure in the midline of the palate, resulting from the failure of the two sides to fuse during embryonic development. The fissure may be complete, extending through both the hard and soft palates into the nasal cavities, or it may show any degree of incomplete or partial cleft.

cleft-palate repair, the surgical correction of a congenital fissure in the midline of the partition separating the oral and nasal cavities. Palatine clefts range from a simple separation in the uvula to an extensive fissure involving the soft and hard palate and extending forward unilaterally or bilaterally through the alveolar ridge. A cleft lip often accompanies a cleft palate.

cleft uvula, an abnormal congenital condition in which the uvula is split into halves because of the failure of the posterior palatine folds to unite.

cleidocranial dysostosis, a rare, abnormal hereditary condition characterized by defective ossification of the cranial bones and by the complete or partial absence of the clavicles. The defective ossification of the cranial bones delays the closing of the cranial sutures and results in large fontanelles.

cleidocranial dystrophia. See **cleidocranial dysostosis.**

clemastine, an antihistamine used in the treatment of symptoms of allergic rhinitis and other conditions.

cleptomania. See **kleptomania.**

click, (in cardiology) an extra heart sound that occurs during systole.

client, 1. a person who is recipient of a professional service. **2.** a recipient of health care regardless of the state of health. **3.** a recipient of health care who is not ill or hospitalized. **4.** a patient.

client-centred therapy, a nondirective method of group or individual psychotherapy in which the role of the therapist is to listen to and then reflect or restate without judgment or interpretation the words of the client.

client interview. See **patient interview.**

climacteric. See **menopause.**

climacteric melancholia. See **involutional melancholia.**

climate, a composite of the prevailing weather conditions that characterizes any particular geographic region. **climatic,** *adj.*

climax, a peak of intensity, such as a sexual orgasm or the high point of a fever.

climbing fibre, a type of nerve fibre that carries impulses to the Purkinje cells of the cerebellar cortex.

clindamycin hydrochloride, an antibiotic used in the treatment of certain serious bacterial infections, and topically in the treatment of acne.

clinic, 1. a department in a hospital where persons not requiring hospitalization may receive medical care. **2.** a group practice of doctors. **3.** a meeting place for doctors and medical students where instruction can be given at the bedside of a patient or in a similar setting. **4.** a seminar or other scientific medical meeting. **5.** a detailed published report of the diagnosis and treatment of a health care problem.

clinical, 1. of or pertaining to a clinic. **2.** of or pertaining to direct, bedside medical care. **3.** of or pertaining to materials or equipment used in the care of a sick person.

clinical crown, 1. the portion of a tooth that is covered by enamel and visible in the mouth. **2.** the portion of a tooth that is occlusal to the deepest part of the gingival crevice.

clinical-crown/clinical-root ratio, the proportion between the length of the portion of the teeth lying coronal to the epithelial attachment and the length of the portion of the root lying apical to the epithelial attachment. The ratio is useful in the diagnosis and prognosis of periodontal disease.

clinical cytogenetics, the branch of genetics that studies the relationship between chromosomal abnormalities and pathological conditions.

clinical diagnosis, a diagnosis made on the basis of knowledge obtained by medical history and physical examination alone, without benefit of laboratory tests or x-ray films.

clinical disease, a stage in the history of a pathological condition that begins with anatomical or physiological changes sufficient to produce recognizable signs and symptoms of a disease.

clinical genetics, a branch of genetics that studies inherited disorders and investigates the possible genetic factors that may influence the occurrence of any pathological condition.

clinical horizon, the imaginary line above which detectable signs and symptoms of a disease first begin to appear.

clinical humidity therapy, respiratory therapy in which water is added to the therapeutic gases to make them more comfortable to breathe.

clinical laboratory, a laboratory in which tests directly related to the care of patients are performed.

clinical nurse specialist (CNS), a registered nurse who has acquired advanced knowledge and clinical skills in a specific area of nursing and health care.

clinical-pathology conference, a teaching conference in which a case is presented to a clinician who then demonstrates the process of reasoning that leads to his diagnosis. A pathologist then presents an anatomical diagnosis, based on the study of tissue removed at surgery or obtained in autopsy.

clinical pathology, the laboratory study of disease by a pathologist using techniques appropriate to the specimen being studied.

clinical psychology, the branch of psychology concerned with the application of psychological theory and research to the assessment and treatment of dysfunctional behaviours and cognitions, learning difficulties, and group relations.

clinical research centre, an organization, often associated with a medical school or a teaching hospital, that studies, analyses, correlates, and describes medical cases. Such centres usually have extensive laboratory facilities and specialized staff.

clinical trials, organized studies to provide large bodies of clinical data for statistically valid evaluation of treatment.

Clinitron bed, a special bed containing an air-fluidization mattress that conforms to the body shape of the patient.

clinocephaly, a congenital anomaly of the head in which the upper surface of the skull is saddle-shaped or concave. **clinocephalic, clinocephalous,** *adj.*

clinodactyly, a congenital anomaly characterized by abnormal lateral or medial bending of one or more fingers or toes. **clinodactylic, clinodactylous,** *adj.*

clinometer, an instrument used to measure angular convergence of the eyes or the degree of paralysis of extraocular muscles.

clioquinoh, an antiamoebic and topical antiinfective used in the treatment of eczema, athlete's foot and other fungal infections.

clip, a surgical device used for grasping the skin to align the edges of a wound and to stop bleeding, especially of the smaller blood vessels.

clipped speech. See **scamping speech.**

clitoris, the vaginal erectile structure homologous to the corpora cavernosa of the penis. It consists of two corpora cavernosa within a dense layer of fibrous membrane, joined along their inner surfaces by an incomplete fibrous septum.

CLL, abbreviation for **chronic lymphocytic leukaemia.**

cloaca, *pl.* **cloacae, 1.** (in embryology) the end of the hindgut before the developmental division into the rectum, the bladder, and the primitive genital structures. **2.** (in pathology) an opening into the sheath of tissue around a necrotic bone.

cloacal membrane, a thin sheath that separates the internal and external portions of the cloaca in the developing embryo.

cloacal septum. See **urorectal septum.**

clobetasol propionate, a very potent topical corticosteroid prescribed for the short term treatment of inflammation and pruritis associated with certain types of severe dematitis.

clofibrate, a hypolipidaemic used in the treatment of high blood levels of cholesterol, triglycerides, or both.

clomiphene citrate, a nonsteroidal antioestrogen that acts to stimulate ovulation. It is prescribed principally in the treatment of anovulatory infertility in women.

clomiphene stimulation test, a test used to evaluate gonadal function in males who show signs of abnormal pubertal development. Clomiphene, a nonsteroidal analogue of oestrogen, stimulates the hypothalamic-pituitary system to raise FSH and LH levels of the blood.

clonal selection theory. See **antibody specific theory.**

clonazepam, an anticonvulsant used in the prevention of seizures in all forms of epilepsy, and the management of status epilepticus and myoclonus.

clone, a group of genetically identical cells or organisms derived from a single common cell or organism through mitosis.

clonidine hydrochloride, a centrally acting alpha-adrenergic agonist used for the reduction of high blood pressure, and for prophy-

laxis of migraine and postmenapausal flushing.

clonorchiasis, an infestation of liver flukes.

Clonorchis sinensis, the Chinese or Oriental liver fluke, a form of tapeworm that is acquired by humans who eat raw or imperfectly cooked fish that is the intermediate host of the parasite.

clonus, an abnormal pattern of neuromuscular activity, characterized by rapidly alternating involuntary contraction and relaxation of skeletal muscle.

C-loop, a surgically formed loop of bowel with a C-shape.

clor, abbreviation for a **chloride noncarboxylate anion.**

clorazepate dipotassium, a benzodiazopine minor tranquillizer used in the treatment of anxiety.

closed amputation, a kind of amputation in which one or two broad flaps of muscular and cutaneous tissue are retained to form a cover over the end of the bone. It is performed only when no infection is present.

closed-angle glaucoma. See **glaucoma.**

closed bite, 1. an abnormal overbite. **2.** a decrease in the occlusal vertical dimension produced by various factors, such as tooth abrasion and insufficient eruption of supportive posterior teeth.

closed-chain, (in organic chemistry) of or pertaining to a compound in which the carbon atoms are bonded together to form a closed ring.

closed-circuit breathing, any breathing system in which a contained gas mixture is rebreathed, either directly or after recirculation through a water or carbon dioxide absorbing unit. An example is a spirometer.

closed-circuit helium dilution, a technique for measuring residual lung volume and functional residual capacity by having a patient breathe through a spirometer containing a known concentration of helium.

closed drainage. See **drainage.**

closed group, a group in which all members are admitted at the same time and vacancies that occur in the membership are unfilled.

closed system, a system that does not interact with its environment.

closed-system helium dilution method, a technique for measuring functional residual capacity and residual volume.

closed-wound suction, any one of several techniques for draining potentially harmful fluids, such as blood, pus, serosanguineous fluid, and tissue secretions from surgical wounds. The technique is used as an aid to many operations, such as mastectomies, augmentations, plastic and reconstructive procedures, and urological and urogenital procedures. Closed-wound suction devices usually consist of disposable transparent containers attached to suction tubes and portable suction pumps. Closed-wound suction also allows irrigation of the wound with special flow controls to permit a periodic change in the flow direction of solutions.

closing capacity (CC), (in respiratory therapy) the sum of the closing volume and the residual volume of gas in the lungs.

closing volume (CV), the volume of gas remaining in the lungs when the small airways begin to close during a controlled maximum exhalation.

clostridial,, of or pertaining to anaerobic spore-forming bacteria of the genus *Clostridium*.

clostridial myonecrosis. See **myonecrosis.**

Clostridium, a genus of spore-forming, anaerobic bacteria of the *Bacillaceae* family involved in gas gangrene, botulism, food poisoning, cellulitis, wound infections, and tetanus.

closure, 1. the surgical closing of a wound by suture. **2.** a visual phenomenon in which the mind "sees" an entire figure when only a portion is actually visible.

closylate, a contraction for p-chlorobenzenesulfonate.

clot. See **blood clot.**

clot retraction, when blood clots, the clot retracts, normally 42-62% after 1 hour at 37 °C, but less if platelets or fibrinogen are deficient.

clotrimazole, an antifungal used topically in the treatment of a variety of superficial fungal infections and for candidal vulvovaginitis.

clotting. See **blood clotting.**

clotting factor assays, method of identifying exactly which clotting factor(s) is defective in cases of haemorrhagic disorder.

clotting time, the time required for blood to form a clot, tested by collecting 4 ml of blood in a glass tube and examining it for clot formation.

cloud baby, a newborn who appears well and healthy but is a carrier of infectious bacterial or viral organisms. The infant may contaminate the surrounding environment with airborne droplets from the respiratory tract forming clouds of the organisms.

clove, the dried flower bud of *Eugenia caryophyllata*. It contains the lactone caryophyllin and a volatile oil used as a dental analgesic, a germicide, and a salve.

cloverleaf nail, a surgical nail shaped in cross section like a cloverleaf, used especially in the repair of fractures of the femur.

cloverleaf skull deformity, a congenital defect characterized by a trilobed skull resulting from the premature closure of multiple cranial sutures during embryonic development.

clubbing, an abnormal enlargement of the distal phalanges, usually associated with cyanotic heart disease or advanced chronic pulmonary disease but sometimes occurring with biliary cirrhosis, colitis, chronic dysentery, and thyrotoxicosis. Clubbing occurs in all the digits but is most easily seen in the fingers.

clubfoot, a congenital deformity of the foot, sometimes resulting from intrauterine constriction and characterized by unilateral or bilateral deviation of the metatarsal bones of the forefoot. Ninety-five percent of clubfoot deformities are equinovarus, characterized by medial deviation and plantar flexion of the forefoot, but a few are calcaneovalgus, or calcaneovarus, characterized by lateral deviation and dorsiflexion either outward from or inward toward the midline of the body.

club hair, a hair in the resting, or final, stage of the growth cycle.

clubhand, a congenital disorder in which the hand develops abnormally as a widened stump at the end of the wrist with stunted fingers.

cluster analysis, (in statistics) a complex technique of data analysis of numeric scale scores that produces clusters of variables related to one another. The technique is performed with a computer.

cluster breathing, a breathing pattern in which a closely grouped series of respirations is followed by apnoea. The activity is associated with a lesion in the lower pontine region of the brainstem.

cluster headache. See **histamine headache.**

cluttering, a speech defect characterized by a rapid, confused, nervous delivery with uneven rhythmic patterns and the omission or transposition of various letters or syllables.

Cm, symbol for **curium.**

CMF, a cytotoxic drug combination of cyclophosphamide, methotrexate, and fluorouracil, used in the management of breast cancer.

CML, abbreviation for **chronic myelocytic leukaemia.**

CMRNG, abbreviation for **chromosomally mediated resistant** *Neisseria gonorrhoea*.

CMV, abbreviation for **cytomegalovirus.**

CNS, abbreviation for **central nervous system.**

CNS sympathomimetic, a drug, such as cocaine or amphetamine, whose effects mimic those of sympathetic nervous system stimulation.

CNS syndrome. See **central nervous system syndrome.**

Co, symbol for **cobalt.**

CO, 1. symbol for carbon monoxide. **2.** abbreviation for cardiac output.

CO$_2$, symbol for **carbon dioxide.**

coagulase, an enzyme produced by bacteria, particularly the *Staphylococcus aureus*, that promotes the formation of thrombi.

coagulation, 1. the process of transforming a liquid into a solid, especially of the blood. **2.** (in colloid chemistry) the transforming of the liquid dispersion medium into a gelatinous mass. **3.** the hardening of tissue by some physical means, as by electrocoagulation or photocoagulation.

coagulation current, an electric current delivered by a needle ball or other variously shaped points that coagulates tissue.

coagulation factor, one of 13 factors in the blood, the interactions of which are responsible for the process of blood clotting. The factors, using standardized numeric nomenclature, are factor I, fibrinogen; factor II, prothrombin; factor III, tissue thromboplastin; factor IV, calcium ions; factors V and VI, proaccelerin or labile factors; factor VII, proconvertin or stable factor; factor VIII, antihaemophilic globulin; factor IX, plasma thromboplastin component (PTC); factor X, factor; factor XI, plasma thromboplastin antecedent (PTA); factor XII, Hageman factor or glass factor; factor XIII, fibrin stabilizing factor or Laki-Lorand factor.

coagulation necrosis. See **necrosis**.

coagulation time. See **clotting time**.

coagulopathy, a pathological condition affecting the ability of the blood to coagulate.

coal tar, a topical antipruritic and keratoplastic used in the treatment of chronic skin diseases, such as eczema and psoriasis.

Coanda effect, a phenomenon of fluid movement similar to the Bernoulli effect in which passage of a stream of gas next to a wall results in a pocket of turbulence that makes the gas stream adhere to the wall. The principle is used in fluidic ventilators.

coaption, fitting together, such as the two edges of a wound.

coarct, the act of narrowing or constricting, especially the lumen of a blood vessel.

coarctation, a stricture or contraction of the walls of a vessel as the aorta.

coarctation of the aorta, a congenital cardiac anomaly characterized by a localized narrowing of the aorta, which results in increased pressure proximal to the defect and decreased pressure distal to it. Symptoms of the condition are directly related to the pressure changes created by the constriction. Clinical manifestations include dizziness, headaches, fainting, epistaxis, reduced or absent femoral pulses, and muscle cramps in the legs from tissue anoxia during increased exercise.

coarse, (in physiology) involving a wide range of movements, such as those associated with tremors and other involuntary movements of the skeletal muscle.

coarse fremitus, a rough, loud, tremulous vibration of the chest wall noted on palpation of the chest during a physical examination as the person inhales and exhales.

coat, 1. a membrane that covers the outside of an organ or part. **2.** one of the layers of a wall of an organ or part, especially a canal or a vessel.

cobalamin, a generic term for a chemical portion of the vitamin B_{12} group.

cobalt (Co), a metallic element that occurs in the minerals cobaltite, smaltite, and linnaeite. Its atomic number is 27; its atomic weight is 58.9. Cobalt is a component of vitamin B_{12}, is found in most common foods, and is readily absorbed by the GI tract. Certain amounts of cobalt stimulate the production of erythropoietin.

cobalt 60 (^{60}Co), a radioactive isotope of the silver-white metallic element cobalt with a mass number of 60 and a half-life of 5.2 years. ^{60}Co emits gamma rays of 1.17 MeV and 1.33 MeV and is used in brachytherapy and external beam radiotherapy.

COBOL, abbreviation for common business oriented language, a high-level compiler computer language for programming.

coca, a species of South American shrubs, native to Bolivia and Peru and cultivated in Indonesia. It is a natural source of cocaine.

cocaine hydrochloride, a local anaesthetic and CNS stimulant. It was originally derived from coca leaves but can also be prepared synthetically. In solution the drug is an effective topical anaesthetic commonly used in the examination and treatment of the eye, ear, nose, and throat. The vasoconstrictive action of the drug slows bleeding and limits absorption. Prolonged or frequent use may damage the mucous membranes. Cocaine is a Class A, Schedule A drug under the Misuse of Drugs Act 1971 and the Misuse of Drugs Regulations 1985, because of its high abuse potential. Cocaine base (crack, freebase) is also abused, has no medical use and is subject to the same legal controls as the hydrochloride.

cocarcinogen, an agent that, by itself, does not transform a normal cell into a cancerous state but in concert with another can effect the transformation.

coccidioidomycosis, an infectious fungal disease caused by the inhalation of spores of the bacterium *Coccidioides immitis*, which is carried on windborne dust particles. The disease is endemic in hot, dry regions of North and South America. Primary infection is characterized by symptoms resembling those of the common cold or influenza. Secondary infection, occurring after a period of remission, is marked by low-grade fever, anorexia and weight loss, cyanosis, dyspnoea, haemoptysis, focal skin lesions resembling erythema nodosum, and arthritic pain in the bones and joints.

coccidiosis, a parasitic disease of tropical and subtropical regions caused by the ingestion of oocysts of the protozoa Isospora belli or I. hominis. Symptoms include fever, malaise, abdominal discomfort, and watery diarrhoea.

coccus, *pl.* **cocci,** a bacterium that is round,

spheric, or oval, as gonococcus, pneumococcus, staphylococcus, streptococcus. **coccal,** *adj.*

coccygeal vertebra, one of the four segments of the vertebral column that fuse to form the adult coccyx. They are considered rudimentary vertebrae and have no pedicles, laminae, or spinous processes.

coccygeus, one of two muscles in the pelvic diaphragm. Stretching across the pelvic cavity like a hammock, it is a triangular sheet of muscle and tendinous fibers, dorsal to the levator ani, arising from the spine of the ischium and from the sacrospinous ligament. It acts to draw the coccyx ventrally, helping to support the pelvic floor.

coccygodynia, a pain in the coccygeal area of the body.

coccyx, *pl.* **coccygs,** the beaklike bone joined to the sacrum by a disk of fibrocartilage at the base of the vertebral column. It is formed by the union of three to five rudimentary vertebrae. **coccygeal,** *adj.*

cochineal, a red dye prepared from the dried female insects of the species *Coccus cacti* containing young larvae.

cochlea, a conic bony structure of the inner ear, perforated by apertures for passage of fibers of the acoustic nerve. Part of the osseous labyrinth, it is a spiral tunnel about 30 mm long with two full and three quarter-turns, resembling a tiny snail shell. **cochlear,** *adj.*

cochlear canal, a bony spiral tunnel within the cochlea of the internal ear. It contains one opening that communicates with the tympanic cavity, a second that connects with the vestibule, and a third that leads to a tiny canal opening on the inferior surface of the temporal bone.

cochlear duct. See cochlear canal.

cochlear toxicity, toxic effects of drugs that may result in hearing disorders, such as tinnitus.

cockroach, the common name of members of the *Blattidae* family of insects that infest homes, workplaces, and other areas inhabited by humans. Cockroaches transmit a number of disease agents, including bacteria, protozoa, and eggs of parasitic worms.

cocontraction, the simultaneous contraction of agonist and antagonist muscles around a joint to hold a position.

code, 1. (in law) a published body of statutes, as a civil code. **2.** a collection of standards and rules of behaviour, as a dress code. **3.** a symbolic means of representing information for communication or transfer, as a genetic code. **4.** a system of notation that allows information to be transmitted rapidly, such as Morse code, or in secrecy, such as a cryptographic code.

codeine phosphate, an opiate used to treat mild to moderate pain, diarrhoea, and as an antitussive.

code of ethics, a statement encompassing the set of rules by which practitioners of a profession are expected to conform.

coding, the process of organizing information into categories, which are assigned codes for the purposes of sorting, storing, and retrieving the data.

cod-liver oil, a pale-yellow, fatty oil extracted from the fresh livers of the codfish and other related species. It is a rich source of vitamins A and D.

Codman's tumour. See chondroblastoma.

codominant, of or pertaining to the alleles or to the trait resulting from the full expression of both alleles of a pair in a heterozygote, as the AB or MNS blood group antigens. **codominance,** *n.*

codon, a unit of three adjacent nucleotides in a DNA or messenger RNA molecule that designates a specific amino acid in the polypeptide chain during protein synthesis.

coefficient, a mathematical relationship between factors that can be used to measure or evaluate a characteristic under specified conditions.

Coelenterates, a phylum of marine animals that includes jellyfish, sea anemones, hydroids, and corals.

coelenteron, *pl.* **coelentera,** the digestive cavity of those animals having only two germ layers, such as the hydra and jellyfish.

coeliac artery, a thick visceral branch of the abdominal aorta, arising caudal to the diaphragm, usually dividing into the left gastric, the common hepatic, and the splenic arteries.

coeliac disease, an inborn error of metabolism characterized by the inability to hydrolyse peptides contained in gluten. The disease affects adults and young children, who suffer from abdominal distention, vomiting, diarrhoea, muscle wasting, and extreme lethargy. Most patients respond well to a high-protein, high-calorie, gluten-free diet.

coeliac plexus. See solar plexus.

coeliac rickets, arrested growth and osseous deformities resulting from malabsorption of fat and calcium.

coeliocolpotomy, an incision into the abdomen through the vagina.

coelioma, *pl.* **coeliomas, coeliomata,** an abdominal neoplasm, especially a mesothelial tumour of the peritoneum.

coelioscope. See laparoscope.

coeliothelioma, *pl.* **coeliotheliomas, coeliotheliomata,** a mesothelioma of the abdomen.

coelom, the body cavity of the developing embryo. A kind of coelom is extraembryonic coelom. Also spelled **coelome, celom. coelomic, celomic,** *adj.*

coelosomy, a congenital anomaly characterized by the protrusion of the viscera from the body cavity.

coenesthesia, the general sense of existing,

derived as the aggregate of all the various stimuli and reactions throughout the body at any specific moment to produce a feeling of health or illness.

coenzyme, a nonprotein substance that combines with an apoenzyme to form a complete enzyme or holoenzyme. Coenzymes include some of the vitamins.

coffee, the dried and roasted ripe seeds of Coffea arabica, *C. liberica,* and *C. robusta* trees that grow in tropical areas. Coffee contains the alkaloid caffeine.

coffee-ground vomitus, dark brown vomitus the colour and consistency of coffee grounds, composed of gastric juices and old blood and indicative of slow upper GI bleeding.

cognition, the mental process characterized by knowing, thinking, learning, and judging. **cognitive,** *adj.*

cognitive, pertaining to the mental processes of comprehension, judgment, memory, and reasoning, as contrasted with emotional and volitional processes.

cognitive-behavioural psychotherapy, a form of therapy based on recent developments in cognitive psychology, which hypothesizes that changes in cognitive structure can lead to changes in behaviour. Therapy aims to identify behaviours which the client wishes to change along with the cognitive processes which apparently maintain these behaviours. The client is helped to learn the skills necessary to undertake cognitive restructuring in order to bring about the desired changes in behaviour in relation to his or her own short and long term goals.

cognitive development, the developmental process by which an infant becomes an intelligent person, acquiring, with growth, knowledge and the ability to think, learn, reason, and abstract.

cognitive dissonance, a state of tension resulting from a discrepancy in a person's emotional and intellectual frame of reference for interpreting and coping with his or her environment.

cognitive function, an intellectual process by which one becomes aware of, perceives, or comprehends ideas.

cognitive learning, 1. learning that is concerned with acquisition of problem-solving abilities and with intelligence and conscious thought. 2. a theory that defines learning as behavioural change based on the acquisition of information about the environment.

cognitive psychology, the study of the development of thought, language, and intelligence in infants and children.

cognitive restoration, an intervention technique designed to restore cognitive functioning.

cognitive restructuring, a change in attitudes, values, or beliefs that limit a person's self-expression; it occurs as a result of insight or behavioural achievement.

cognitive structuring, the process of reviewing with a patient the changes that have occurred in the patient's thinking to show a sense of change and a sense of playing an active role in bringing about that change.

cognitive therapy, any of the various methods of treating mental and emotional disorders that help a person change attitudes, perceptions, and patterns of thinking.

cogwheel rigidity, an abnormal rigor in muscle tissue, characterized by jerky movements when the muscle is passively stretched.

cohabit, to live together in a sexual relationship when not married.

cohere, to stick together, as similar molecules of a common substance.

coherence, 1. the property of sticking together, as the molecules within a common substance. 2. (in psychology) the logical pattern of expression and thought evident in the speech of a normal, stable individual. **coherent,** *adj.*

coherent perception of reality, an agreement between family members' perceptions of their emotional reality and the views of outside observers.

cohesiveness, 1. (in psychiatry) a force that attracts members to a group and causes them to remain in the group. 2. (in dentistry) a property of annealed pure gold that allows it to be used as a filling material.

cohesive termini, (in molecular genetics) the complementary single-stranded ends projecting from a double-stranded DNA segment that can be joined to introduced fragments.

cohort, (in statistics) a collection or sampling of individuals who share a common characteristic, such as members of the same age or the same sex.

cohort study, (in research) a study concerning a specific subpopulation, such as the children born between December and May in 1975 and the children born in the same months in 1955.

coil. See **intrauterine contraceptive device.**

coiled tubular gland, one of the many multicellular glands that contain a coiled, tube-shaped secretory portion, such as the sweat glands.

coinnervation. See **cocontraction.**

coitus, the sexual union of two people of opposite sex in which the penis is introduced into the vagina, typically resulting in mutual excitation and usually orgasm. **coital,** *adj.*

coitus interruptus. See **withdrawal method.**

colation, the act of filtering or straining, as urine is often strained for medical examination.

colchicine, a gout suppressant used in the treatment of acute gout and prophylaxis during initial therapy with other drugs.

cold, 1. the absence of heat. 2. a contagious

viral infection of the upper respiratory tract, usually caused by a strain of rhinovirus. It is characterized by rhinitis, tearing, low-grade fever, and malaise and is treated symptomatically with rest, mild analgesia, decongestants, and an increased intake of fluids.

cold abscess, a site of infection that does not show common signs of heat, redness, and swelling.

cold agglutinin, a nonspecific antibody, found on the surface of red blood cells in certain diseases, that may cause clumping of the cells at temperatures below 4° C and may cause haemolysis.

cold-blooded, unable to regulate body heat, as fishes, reptiles, and amphibians that have internal temperatures that are close to the temperatures of the environments in which they live.

cold cautery. See **cryocautery**.

cold environment, a human environment arbitrarily designated as one in which the temperature is below 10 °C. The human body generally begins to experience some functional impairment when unprotected in temperatures below 15 °C. The body's haemostatic mechanism reacts with vasoconstriction, reducing heat loss to the environment. When vasoconstriction no longer eases the thermal strain between the skin and the environment, muscular hypertonus and shivering become mechanisms for maintaining body temperature.

cold haemoglobinuria. See **haemoglobinuria**.

cold injury, any of several abnormal and often serious physical conditions caused by exposure to cold temperatures.

cold-pressor test, a test for the tendency to develop essential hypertension. One hand of the individual is immersed in ice water for about 60 seconds. An excessive rise in the blood pressure or an unusual delay in the return of normal blood pressure when the hand is removed from the water is believed to indicate that the individual is at risk for hypertension.

cold-sensitive mutation, a genetic alteration resulting in a gene that functions at a high temperature and not at a low temperature.

cold sore. See **herpes simplex**.

colectomy, surgical excision of part or all of the colon, performed to treat cancer of the colon or severe chronic ulcerative colitis.

colestipol hydrochloride, a hypolipidaemic that acts by sequestering bile acids in the intestine, thus reducing plasma levels of cholesterol. It is prescribed in the treatment of hyperlipidaemia.

colic, 1. sharp visceral pain resulting from torsion, obstruction, or smooth muscle spasm of a hollow or tubular organ, such as a ureter or the intestines. Kinds of colic include biliary colic, infantile colic, and renal colic. **2.** of or pertaining to the colon. **colicky,** *adj.*

colicinogen an episome in some strains of *Escherichia coli* that induces secretion of a colicin, a protein lethal to other strains of the bacterium.

coliform, 1. of or pertaining to the colon-aerogenes group, or the *Escherichia coli* species of microorganisms, constituting most of the intestinal flora in humans and other animals. **2.** having the characteristic of a sieve or cribriform structure, such as some of the porous bones of the skull.

colistin sulphate, a polymyxin antibiotic prescribed topically in the treatment of infections of the eye, systemically for serious gram-negative infections, and by mouth as a component of gut sterilization regimens. It is not absorbed from the GI tract.

colitis, an inflammatory condition of the large intestine, either one of the episodic, functional, irritable bowel syndromes or one of the more serious chronic, progressive, inflammatory bowel diseases. Irritable bowel syndrome is characterized by bouts of colicky pain and diarrhoea or constipation, often resulting from emotional stress. **colitic,** *adj.*

collaborative power structure, an arrangement whereby adult family members of a functional family make major decisions and are in agreement about power distribution.

collagen, a protein consisting of bundles of tiny reticular fibrils, which combine to form the white glistening inelastic fibres of the tendons, the ligaments, and the fascia. **collagenous,** *adj.*

collagen disease, any of the various abnormal conditions characterized by extensive disruption of the connective tissue, as inflammation and fibrinoid degeneration. Some collagen diseases are polyarteritis nodosa, rheumatoid coronary arteritis, and ankylosing spondylitis.

collagenoblast, a cell that differentiates from a fibroblast and functions in the formation of collagen. It can also transform into cartilage and bone tissue by metaplasia.

collagenous fibre, any one of the tough, white fibres that constitute much of the intercellular substance and the connective tissue of the body.

collagen vascular disease, any of a group of acquired disorders that have in common diffuse immunological and inflammatory changes in small blood vessels and connective tissue. Common features of most of these entities include arthritis, skin lesions, iritis and episcleritis, pericarditis, pleuritis, subcutaneous nodules, myocarditis, vasculitis, and nephritis.

collapse, 1. *nontechnical.* a state of extreme depression or a condition of complete exhaustion because of physical or psychosomatic problems. **2.** an abnormal condition characterized by shock. **3.** the abnormal sagging of an organ or the obliteration of its cavity.

collar, any structure that encircles another, usually around its neck, such as the periosteal bone collars that form around the diaphyses of young bones.

collarbone. See **clavicle.**

collateral, 1. secondary or accessory. **2.** (in anatomy) a small branch, such as any one of the arterioles or venules in the body.

collateral fissure, a fissure separating the subcalcarine and the subcollateral gyri of the cerebral hemisphere.

collateral pulp canal, (in dentistry) a branch of the pulp canal that emerges from the root at a place other than the apex.

collateral ventilation, the ventilation of pulmonary air spaces through indirect pathways, such as pores in alveolar septa.

collecting tubule, any one of the many relatively large straight tubules of the kidney that funnel urine into the renal pelvis. The collecting tubules play an important role in maintaining the fluid balance of the body by allowing water to osmose through their membranes into the interstitial fluid in the renal medulla.

collective bargaining, the use of collective action by employees in negotiating working conditions and economic issues with their employer.

collective unconscious, (in analytical psychology) that portion of the unconscious common to all human beings.

college, 1. an organization of individuals with common professional training and interests, such as the Royal College of Nurses. **2.** an institution of higher learning.

College of Radiographers, the professional body for radiographers in the United Kingdom.

Colles' fascia {Abraham Colles, Irish surgeon, b. 1773; L, band}, the deep layer of the subcutaneous fascia of the perineum, constituting a distinctive structure in the urogenital region of the body. It is a strong, smooth sheet of tissue containing elastic fibres.

Colles' fracture {Abraham Colles}, a fracture of the radius at the epiphysis within 1 inch of the joint of the wrist, easily recognized by the dorsal and lateral position of the hand that it causes.

colligative, (in physical chemistry) of or pertaining to those properties of matter that depend on the concentration of particles, such as molecules and ions, rather than the chemical properties of any substance.

collimator, (in radiography, radiotherapy) a device for limiting the size and shape of the radiation beams.

colliquation, the degeneration of a tissue of the body to a liquid state, usually associated with necrotic tissue.

colliquative, characterized by the profuse discharge of fluid, as in suppurating wounds and structures of the body that are infected.

collision tumour, a tumour formed as two separate growths, developing close to each other, join.

collodion, a clear or a slightly opaque, highly inflammable liquid composed of pyroxylin, ether, and alcohol. It dries to a strong, transparent film.

collodion baby, an infant whose skin at birth is covered with a scaly, parchmentlike membrane.

colloid, a state or division of matter in which large molecules or aggregates of molecules that do not precipitate, and that measure between 1 and 100 nm, are dispersed in another medium.

colloidal sulphur, a form of very finely divided sulphur that is used topically in the treatment of acne and other skin disorders.

colloid carcinoma, a former term for mucinous carcinoma.

colloid chemistry, the science dealing with the composition and nature of chemical colloids.

colloid goitre, a greatly enlarged, soft thyroid gland in which the follicles are distended with colloid.

colloid osmotic pressure, an abnormal condition of the kidney caused by the pressure of concentrations of large particles, such as protein molecules, that will not pass through a membrane.

collyrium, an ophthalmic liquid containing medications to be instilled into the eye.

coloboma, *pl.* **colobomas, colobomata,** a congenital or pathological defect in the ocular tissue of the body, usually affecting the iris, ciliary body, or choroid by forming a cleft that extends inferiorly. **colobomatous,** *adj.*

coloenteritis. See **enterocolitis.**

colon, the portion of the large intestine extending from the caecum to the rectum. It has four segments: ascending colon, transverse colon, descending colon, and sigmoid colon. **colonic,** *adj.*

colonic. See **colon.**

colonic fistula, an abnormal passage from the colon to the surface of the body or an internal organ or structure.

colonic irrigation, a procedure for washing the inner wall of the colon by filling it with water, then draining it. It is not considered an enema, but rather a technique for removing any material that may be present high in the colon.

colonization, the presence and multiplication of microorganisms without tissue invasion or damage.

colonoscopy, the examination of the mucosal lining of the colon using a colonoscope, an elongated endoscope.

colon stasis. See **atonia constipation.**

colony, 1. (in bacteriology) a mass of micro-organisms in a culture that originates from a single cell. Some kinds of colonies, according to different configurations, are smooth colonies, rough colonies, and dwarf colonies. **2.** (in cell biology) a mass of cells in a culture or in certain experimental tissues, such as a spleen colony.

colony counter, a device used for counting colonies of bacteria growing in a culture and usually consisting of an illuminated, transparent plate that is divided into sections of known area.

coloproctitis, an inflammation of both the colon and rectum.

coloptosis, the prolapse or downward displacement of the colon.

colorectal cancer, a malignant neoplastic disease of the large intestine, characterized by melaena, a change in bowel habits, and the passing of blood. The high incidence of colorectal cancer in the western world, as contrasted with the low incidence in Japan and rural Africa, suggests that a diet high in refined carbohydrates and beef and low in roughage may be a causative factor. Most lesions of the large bowel are adenocarcinomas; one half arise in the rectum, one fifth in the sigmoid colon, approximately one sixth in the caecum and ascending colon, and the rest in other sites.

colorimetry, 1. measurement of the intensity of colour in a fluid or substance. **2.** measurement of colour in the blood by use of a colorimeter to determine haemoglobin concentration. **colorimetric,** *adj.*

colosigmoidoscopy, the direct examination of the sigmoid portion of the colon with a sigmoidoscope.

colostomate, a person who has undergone a colostomy.

colostomy, surgical creation of an artificial anus on the abdominal wall by incising the colon and bringing it out to the surface, performed for cancer of the colon and benign obstructive tumours, and severe abdominal wounds. A colostomy may be single-barrelled, with one opening, or double-barrelled, with distal and proximal loops open onto the abdomen. A type of colostomy is loop colostomy.

colostomy irrigation, a procedure used by those with a colostomy to clear the bowel of faecal matter and to help establish an evacuation schedule.

colostrum, the fluid secreted by the breast during pregnancy and the 3 to 4 days postpartum before lactation begins, consisting of immunologically active substances and white blood cells, water, protein, fat, and carbohydrate in a thin, yellow, serous fluid.

colotomy, a surgical incision into the colon, usually performed through the abdominal wall.

colour blindness, an abnormal condition characterized by an inability to distinguish clearly colours of the spectrum. In most cases it is not a blindness but a weakness in perceiving them distinctly. There are two forms of colour blindness. **Daltonism** is the most common form and is characterized by an inability to distinguish reds from greens. It is an inherited, sex-linked disorder. **Total colour blindness,** or **achromatic vision,** is characterized by an inability to perceive any colour at all. Only white, grey, and black are seen. It may be the result of a defect in or the absence of the cones in the retina.

colour dysnomia, an inability to name colours despite an ability to match and distinguish them. It may be caused by expressive aphasia.

colour index, the ratio between the concentration of haemoglobin and the number of red blood cells in any given sample of blood. The colour index is computed by dividing the concentration of haemoglobin by the approximate number of red blood cells.

Colour Index, a publication of dyers, colorists, and textile chemists that specifies all the standard industrial pigments and stains according to five-digit numbers. For example, methylene blue is assigned number 52015.

colour vision, a recognition of colour as the result of changes in the pigments of the cones in the retina that react to varying intensities of red, green, and blue light.

colpalgia, a pain in the vagina.

colpectomy, the surgical excision of the vagina.

colpitis, a vaginal inflammation.

colpocystitis, an inflammation of the vagina and urinary bladder.

colpocystocele the prolapse of the urinary bladder into the vagina, usually through the anterior vaginal wall.

colpohysterectomy, vaginal hysterectomy.

colporrhaphy, a surgical procedure in which the vagina is sutured, as for the purpose of narrowing the vagina.

colposcope, a lighted instrument with lenses for direct examination of the surfaces of the vagina and cervix.

colposcopy, an examination of the vagina and cervix with a colposcope.

colpotomy, any surgical incision into the wall of the vagina.

columbium, former name for niobium.

column chromatography, the process of separating and analysing a group of substances according to the differences in their absorption affinities for a given absorbent as evidenced by pigments deposited during filtration through the same absorbent contained in a glass cylinder or tube. The substances are dissolved in a liquid that is passed through the absorbent. The absorbates move down the column at different rates and leave behind a band of pigments that is subsequently washed with a pure solvent to "develop" discrete pigmented bands that constitute a chromatograph.

coma, a state of profound unconsciousness, characterized by the absence of spontaneous eye movements, response to painful stimuli, and vocalization. The person cannot be aroused. Coma may be the result of trauma, brain tumour, haematoma, toxic condition, acute infectious disease with encephalitis, vascular disease, poisoning, diabetic acidosis, or intoxication.

comatose, pertaining to a state of coma, or abnormally deep sleep, caused by illness or injury.

combat fatigue, any of a variety of disorders resulting from exhaustion, the stress of combat, or the cumulative emotions and psychological strain of warfare or similar situations. It is characterized by anxiety, depression, memory and sleep disorders, and various related symptoms. See also **posttraumatic stress disorder**.

combat psychiatry, a system of psychiatric care developed from the treatment of soldiers in combat during World War II. Its goals were to return soldiers to duty within a brief time period and to prevent the development of deep-seated psychiatric illnesses. The techniques later became the basis for crisis intervention in the treatment of civilian patients.

combination chemotherapy, the use of two or more anticancer drugs at the same time.

combined anaesthesia. See **balanced anaesthesia**.

combined carbon dioxide, the portion of the total carbon dioxide that is contained in blood carbonate and can be calculated as the difference between the total and dissolved carbon dioxide.

combined cycling ventilator, a mechanical ventilator that has more than one cycling mechanism, such as equipment that may have time cycling or pressure cycling as a backup to a volume cycling control device.

combined modality treatment, the use of chemotherapy in combination with surgery or radiation or both in the treatment of cancer.

combined oxygen, the oxygen that is physically bound to haemoglobin as oxyhaemoglobin (HbO_2) One gram-molecular weight of oxygen can combine with 16,700 g of haemoglobin, and each gram of haemoglobin can take up and carry 1.34 ml of oxygen.

combined patterns, pertaining to a method of evaluating the neuromuscular functions of a patient through tests that reveal the degree of coordination between movement patterns of the trunk and the extremities.

combined system disease, a disorder of the nervous system caused by a deficiency of vitamin B_{12} that results in pernicious anaemia and degeneration of the spinal cord and peripheral nerves, marked by increased difficulty in walking, a feeling of vibration in the legs, and a loss of sense of position. Also known as subacute combined degeneration of the spinal cord.

combining form, a component of a word, often derived from Latin or Greek. It may be a root, a prefix, or a suffix, or all three. For example, in the words *arthralgia, encephalitis, hepatomegaly,* and *oliguria,* the combining forms are *arthr-, -algia, en-, -cephal, -itis, hepato-, -megaly, olig-,* and *-uria.*

combining sites, 1. concave features on antibody molecules that serve as locations for binding antigens. Because of possible variations, each kind of antibody can provide combining sites for a specific antigen. **2.** locations on protein molecules where drugs or other substances may become bound by electrochemical attraction.

combustion, the process of burning or oxidation, which may be accompanied by light and heat. Oxygen itself does not burn, but oxygen supports combustion. The rate of combustion is influenced by both oxygen concentration and its partial pressure.

comedo, *pl.* **comedones,** blackhead, the basic lesion of acne vulgaris, caused by an accumulation of keratin and sebum within the opening of a hair follicle. It is dark because of the effect of oxygen on sebum, not because of the presence of dirt.

comedocarcinoma, *pl.* **comedocarcinomas, comedocarcinomata,** a malignant intraductal neoplasm of the breast, in which the central cells degenerate and may be easily expressed from the cut surface of the tumour.

comedogenicity, the ability of certain drugs or agents, such as anabolic steroids, to produce acne comedones.

comfort measure, any action taken to promote comfort of the patient, such as a change in position, or the prewarming of a stethoscope or a bedpan.

Comité International des Poids et Mesures (CIPM), a group of scientists that meets periodically to define the international (SI) units of physical quantities, as the volume of a litre, the length of a metre, or the precise amount of time in a minute.

command, an order given to the computer to execute a specific instruction, as a code that evokes a particular programme or performs a particular function.

command automatism, a condition characterized by an abnormal mechanical responsiveness to commands, usually followed without critical judgment, such as may be seen in hypnosis and certain psychotic states.

command hallucination, a psychotic condition in which the patient hears and obeys voices that command him or her to perform certain acts.

commensal, (of two different organisms) living together in an arrangement that is not harmful to either and may be beneficial to both.

comminuted, crushed or broken into a number of pieces.

comminuted fracture, a fracture in which there are several breaks in the bone, creating numerous fragments.

commissure, 1. a band of nerve fibre or other tissue that crosses from one side of the body to the other, usually connecting two structures or masses of tissue. **2.** a site of union of two anatomic parts, as the corner of the eye, lips, or labia.

commissurotomy, the surgical division of a fibrous band or ring connecting corresponding parts of a body structure.

commitment, 1. the placement or confinement of an individual in a specialized hospital or other institutional facility. **2.** the legal procedure of admitting a mentally ill person to an institution for psychiatric treatment. **3.** a pledge or contract to fulfill some obligation or agreement, used especially in some forms of psychotherapy or marriage guidance counselling.

committed effective dose equivalent, (in radiobiology) ionizing radiation dose received by a given tissue, organ or the whole body, due to intake of radionuclides.

Committee on the Safety of Medicines, a UK government body which monitors the safety of drug products, its duties include operation of the yellow card scheme. See yellow card scheme.

common bile duct, the duct formed by the juncture of the cystic duct and hepatic duct.

common carotid artery, one of the major arteries supplying blood to the head and neck. Each divides into an external common carotid and an internal common carotid. Branches supply the face, scalp, neck, throat, brain, and other tissues.

common carotid plexus, a network of nerves on the common carotid artery, supplying sympathetic fibres to the head and the neck, with branches that accompany the cranial blood vessels.

common cold. See **cold**.

Common Foundation Programme, the first part of the pre-registration nursing programme in the UK when students of all specialities learn together, studying the core components, in theory and practice.

common hepatic artery, the visceral branch of the celiac trunk of the abdominal aorta, passing to the pyloris and dividing into five branches.

common iliac artery, a division of the abdominal aorta, starting to the left of the fourth lumbar vertebra and dividing into external and internal iliac arteries.

common iliac node, a node in one of the seven groups of parietal lymph nodes serving the abdomen and the pelvis.

common iliac vein, one of the two veins that are the sources of the inferior vena cava, formed by the union of the internal and the external iliac veins.

communicability period, the usual time span during which contact with an infected person is most likely to result in spread of the infection.

communicable, contagious; transmissible by direct or indirect means, as a communicable disease.

communicable disease, any disease transmitted from one person or animal to another directly, by contact with excreta or other discharges from the body; or indirectly, via substances or inanimate objects, such as contaminated drinking glasses, toys, or water; or via vectors, as flies, mosquitoes, ticks, or other insects. Many communicable diseases, by law, must be reported to the local health authority.

communicating hydrocephalus. See **hydrocephalus**.

communication, any process in which a message containing information is transferred, especially from one person to another, via any of a number of media.

communication channels, (in communication theory) any gesture, action, sound, written word, or visual image used in transmitting messages.

communication, impaired verbal, a state in which an individual experiences a decreased or absent ability to use or understand language in human interaction. Defining characteristics include an inability to speak the dominant language of the culture, slurring, stuttering, difficulty in forming words or sentences, difficulty in expressing thoughts verbally, inappropriate verbalization, dyspnoea, disorientation, and the absence of speech.

communication theme, (in psychiatry) a recurrent concept or idea that ties together components of communication. Kinds of communication themes include **content theme,** in which a single concept links varied topics of discussion; **mood theme,** in which the underlying idea is the emotion communicated by the individual; and **interaction theme,** in which a particular idea best describes the dynamics between communicating participants.

communication theory, a theory that describes a model of a system of communication consisting of a source of information (the sender), a transmitter, a communication channel, a source of noise (interference), a receiver, and a purpose for the message.

community, a group of people who reside in a designated geographical area and who share common interests or bonds.

community-acquired infection, an infection acquired from the environment, including infections acquired indirectly from the use of medications. Community-acquired infections are distinguished from nosocomial, or hospital-acquired, diseases by the types of organisms that affect patients who are recovering from a disease or injury.

community care, the care of patients and clients in their own homes, or in community-based health centres, rather than in hospital wards or clinics. Health professionals involved in community care include general practitioners, district nurses, health visitors, practice nurses and community midwives.

community pharmacist, a general practice pharmacist working outside the hospital service.

Community Health Council (CHC), originated in the first reorganization of the NHS in 1974, the function of the CHC is monitor health services in its geographical area and provide advice to health authorities. Members are appointed to CHCs by various interested organizations ranging from local and health authorities to trades unions. Although CHCs can act on behalf of health service users, the extent to which they can represent users' interests and views is debatable.

community medicine, a branch of medicine that is concerned with the health of the members of a community, municipality, or region.

community mental health, a treatment philosophy based on the social model of psychiatric care that advocates a comprehensive range of mental health services to be made readily available to all members of the community.

community mental health centre, a community-based centre that provides comprehensive mental health services, including ambulatory and inpatient care.

community psychiatric nurse (CPN), a Registered Nurse (Mental) who specializes in working with clients in the community. Such a nurse will often have a personal caseload of clients and a nurse-therapist aspect to his or her role.

community psychiatric nursing, the care given by specially trained mental health nurses, to clients in their own homes, and outside institutions.

community psychiatry, the branch of psychiatry concerned with the development of an adequate and coordinated program of mental health care for residents of specified catchment areas.

community reintegration, the return and acceptance of a disabled person as a participating member of the community.

compact bone, hard, dense bone that is usually found at the surface of skeletal structures, as distinguished from spongy cancellous bone.

comparative anatomy, the study of the morphology and function of all living animals from the simplest to the most highly specialized animals.

comparative embryology, the study of the similarities and differences among various organisms during the embryological period of development.

comparative method, the analytical method to which the test method is compared in the comparison-of-methods experiment.

comparative physiology, the study of the similarities and differences of the vital processes found in various species of living organisms to determine fundamental physiological relationships.

comparative psychology, 1. the study of human behaviour as it relates to or differs from animal behaviour. **2.** the study of the psychological and behavioural differences among various peoples.

compartment model, a mathematical representation of the body or an area of the body created to study physiological or pharmacological kinetics. A compartment model can simulate all of the biological processes involved in the kinetic behaviour of a drug after it has been introduced into the body, leading to a better understanding of the drug's pharmacodynamic effects.

compartment syndrome, a pathological condition caused by the progressive development of arterial compression and reduced blood supply.

compatibility, 1. the quality or state of existing together in harmony; congruity. **2.** the orderly, efficient integration of the elements of one system with those of another. **3.** the formation of a stable chemical or biochemical system, specifically in medication, so that two or more drugs can be administered at the same time without producing undesired side effects or without cancelling or changing the therapeutic effects of the others. **4.** (in immunology) the degree to which the body's defence system will tolerate the presence of foreign material, such as transfused blood, grafted tissue, or transplanted organs, without an immune reaction. Usually, complete compatibility exists between identical twins. **5.** (in blood grouping or crossmatching) the lack of reaction between blood groups so that there is no agglutination when the red blood cells of one sample are mixed with the serum of another sample; no reaction from transfused blood. **compatible,** *adj.*

compendium, *pl.* **compendia,** a collected body of information on the standards of strength, purity, and quality of drugs. The official compendia in the United Kingdom are the *British Pharmacopoeia,* and the *British National Formulary.*

compensated flow meter, a gas therapy device with a scale that is calibrated against a constant pressure of 50 psi instead of the atmosphere.

compensated gluteal gait, one of the more common abnormal gaits associated with a weakness of the gluteus medius. It is a variation of the Trendelenburg gait and involves the dropping of the pelvis on the unaffected side of the body during the walking cycle between the moment of heelstrike on the affected side and the moment of heelstrike on the unaffected side.

compensated heart failure, an abnormal cardiac condition in which heart failure is compensated for by such mechanisms as increased sympathetic adrenergic stimulation of the heart, fluid retention with increased venous return, increased end-diastolic ventricular volume and fibre length, and hypertrophy.

compensating current, an electric current that neutralizes the intensity of a muscle current.

compensating curve, the curvature of alignment of the occlusal surfaces of the teeth, developed to compensate for the paths of the condyles as the mandible moves from centric to eccentric positions.

compensating filter, (in radiology) a device, such as a wedge fashioned from aluminium or plastic that is positioned over a body area to compensate for differences in radiopacity.

compensation, 1. the process of counterbalancing any defect in bodily structure or function. **2.** (in cardiology) the process of maintaining an adequate blood flow through such normal cardiac and circulatory mechanisms as tachycardia, fluid retention with increased venous return, and hypertrophy. Failure of the heart to compensate and to provide the required cardiac output indicates a diseased heart muscle. **3.** (in psychiatry) a complex defence mechanism that allows one to avoid the unpleasant or painful emotional stimuli that result from a feeling of inferiority or inadequacy. A kind of compensation is **dosage compensation**.

compensation neurosis, an unconscious process by which one prolongs the symptoms resulting from an injury or disease in order to receive secondary gains, especially money.

compensator. A device used in radiotherapy to correct for irregularities in body surfaces by providing a differential attenuation of the beam before it reaches the patient.

compensatory hypertrophy, an increase in the size or the function of an organ or part to counterbalance a structural or functional defect.

compensatory pause, a longer than normal period between heartbeats. This increased refractory period may be associated with premature ventricular contractions. Because the stimulus is out of phase, it interferes with the usual sequence of excitability and refractoriness, resulting in a lag before the next contraction.

competence, 1. (in embryology) the total capacity of an embryonic cell to react to determinative stimuli in various ways of differentiation. **2.** the ability of bacteria to take up donor DNA molecules.

competitive antagonist. See **antimetabolite**.

competitive-binding assay, an analytical procedure based on the reversible binding of a ligand to a binding protein.

competitive displacement, the tendency of one drug to displace another at a protein-binding site when both drugs are taken at the same time. The bound drug becomes less pharmacologically active than the free drug.

competitive identification, the unconscious modelling of one's personality on that of another as a means of outdoing or bettering the other person.

competitive inhibitor, an inhibitor of an enzyme reaction that competes with the substrate by binding at the active site.

complaint, 1. (in law) a pleading by a plaintiff made under oath to initiate a suit. It is a statement of the formal charge and the cause for action against the defendant. **2.** *informal.* any ailment, problem, or symptom identified by the client, patient, member of the person's family, or other knowledgeable person.

complement, one of 11 complex, enzymatic serum proteins. In an antigen-antibody reaction, complement causes lysis.

complement abnormality, an unusual condition characterized by deficiencies or by dysfunctions of any of the nine functional components of the enzymatic proteins of blood serum. The components are labelled C1 through C9. Theoretically, any of the nine complement components may be lacking. The most common abnormalities are C2 and C3 deficiencies and C5 familial dysfunction. Patients with complement deficiencies or with complement dysfunctions may be more susceptible to infections and to collagen vascular diseases. Some patients with lupus erythematosus or dermatomyositis have displayed complement abnormalities. Studies indicate that primary complement deficiencies may be inherited. Secondary complementary deficiencies may stem from immunological reactions, such as drug-induced serum disease, which depletes complement.

complemental inheritance, the acquisition or expression of a trait or condition from the presence of two independent pairs of nonallelic genes. Both of the genes must be present for the characteristic to appear in the phenotype.

complementarity, pertaining to a relationship in which differences are maximal.

complementary feed, an artificial feed given as a supplement to an infant that is mainly breast fed.

complementary gene, either member of two or more nonallelic gene pairs that interact to produce an effect not expressed in the absence of any of the pairs.

complementary transactions, (in psychiatry) transactions that may continue indefinitely as the parties involved keep relating from the same ego state.

complement cascade, a biochemical process involving the C1 to C9 complement components in which one complement interacts with another in a specific sequence called a complement pathway. The reaction sequence is C1, 4, 2, 3, 5, 6, 7, 8, 9 (the first complements being out of numerical sequence for historical reasons). The cascade effect leads to an accumulation of fluid in a cell and finally lysis of the membrane, causing the cell to rupture.

complement fixation, an immunological reaction in which an antigen combines with an antibody and its complement, causing the complement factor to become inactive or "fixed".

complement-fixation test (C-F test), any serological test in which complement fixation is detected, indicating the presence of a particular antigen. Specific C-F tests are used to aid in the diagnosis of amoebiasis, Rocky Mountain spotted fever, trypanosomiasis, and typhus.

complete abortion, termination of pregnancy in which the conceptus is expelled or removed in its entirety.

complete fistula, an abnormal passage from an internal organ or structure to the surface of the body or to another internal organ or structure.

complete fracture, a bone break that completely disrupts the continuity of osseous tissue across the entire width of the bone involved.

complete health history, a health history that includes a history of the present illness, a health history, social history, occupational history, sexual history, and a family health history.

complete rachischisis, a rare congenital fissure of the entire vertebral column and spinal cord, resulting from the failure of the embryonic neural tube to close.

complete response (CR), the total disappearance of a tumour.

complex, 1. a group of items, as chemical molecules, that are related in structure or function as are the iron and protein portions of haemoglobin or the cobalt and protein portions of vitamin B_{12}. **2.** a combination of signs and symptoms of disease that forms a syndrome. **3.** (in psychology) a group of associated ideas with strong emotional overtones affecting a person's attitudes.

complex carbohydrate, a carbohydrate, such as starch, that is composed of a large number of glucose molecules, so called to distinguish it from simple sugars.

complex cavity, a cavity that involves more than one surface of a tooth.

complex fracture, a closed fracture in which the soft tissue surrounding the bone is severely damaged.

complex odontoma. See **composite odontoma.**

complex protein, a protein that contains a simple protein and at least one molecule of another substance, as a glycoprotein, nucleoprotein, or haemoglobin.

complex spatial relations, the perceptual relationship of one figure or part of a figure to another.

complex sugars, sugar molecules that can be hydrolysed or digested to yield two molecules of the same or different simple sugars, as sucrose, lactose, and maltose.

compliance, 1. fulfillment by the patient of the care-giver's prescribed course of treatment. **2.** (in respiratory physiology) a measure of distensibility of the lung volume produced by a unit pressure change.

compliance factor, a measure of the amount of trapped tidal volume in a mechanical ventilating system associated with expansion of the flexible tubing when pressure is applied.

complication, a disease or injury that develops during the treatment of an earlier disorder. The complication frequently alters the prognosis.

component, a significant part of a larger unit.

component therapy, a kind of transfusion in which specific blood components are administered instead of whole blood. Packed red cells or platelet-rich plasma suspensions may be transfused in larger quantities than would be possible if whole blood were used.

composite core, a buildup of composite resin, designed and installed to retain an artificial tooth crown.

composite odontoma, an odontogenic tumour composed of abnormally arranged calcified enamel and dentine.

compos mentis, the quality of having a sound mind.

compound, 1. (in chemistry) a substance composed of two or more different elements, chemically combined in definite proportions, that cannot be separated by physical means. **2.** any substance composed of two or more different ingredients. **3.** to make a substance by combining ingredients, such as a pharmaceutical. **4.** denoting an injury characterized by multiple factors, such as a compound fracture.

compound aneurysm, a localized dilatation of an arterial wall in which some of the layers are distended and others are ruptured or dissected.

compound fracture, a fracture in which the broken end or ends of the bone have torn through the skin.

compound melanocytoma. See benign juvenile melanoma.

compound tubuloalveolar gland, one of the
many multicellular glands with more than
one secretory duct that contains both tube-
shaped and sac-shaped portions, as the salivary glands.

compress, a soft pad, usually made of cloth,
used to apply heat, cold, or medications to
the surface of a body area. A compress also
may be applied over a wound to help control
bleeding.

compressed air hazards. See decompression sickness.

compressibility factor, a measure of the
amount of tidal volume that may be trapped
in a mechanical ventilator system in relation
to the water pressure applied. It is expressed
in millilitres of gas per centimetre of water
pressure.

compressible volume, a part of the tidal volume of gas produced by a mechanical ventilator that does not reach the patient because
of compression of the gas and expansion of
the flexible tubing in the equipment.

compression, the act of pressing, squeezing,
or otherwise applying pressure to an organ,
tissue, or body area. Kinds of pathological
compression include compression fracture,
in which bone surfaces are forced
against each other, causing a break, and
compression paralysis, marked by paralysis
of a body area caused by pressure on a
nerve.

compression fracture, a bone break, especially in a short bone, that disrupts osseous
tissue and collapses the affected bone.

compression neuropathy, any of several disorders involving damage to sensory nerve
roots or peripheral nerves, caused by mechanical pressure or localized trauma and
characterized by paraesthesia, weakness, or
paralysis.

compressive atelectasis, a loss of the ability
of the lung to move air in and out of the
atelectatic region because of intrathoracic
pressures that compress the alveoli. The condition may result from a pulmonary embolism.

compressor naris, the transverse part of the
nasalis muscle that serves to depress the cartilage of the nose and to draw the ala toward
the septum.

compromise, an action that may involve a
change in a person's behaviour, as in substituting goals or delaying satisfaction of needs
in one area to reduce stress in another.

compromise body image, a new body image
acquired by a patient as part of his or her
adjustment to a physical dysfunction. A
compromise body image incorporates and
modifies unacceptable features of the condition through psychological defence mechanisms.

compromised host, a person who is less-
than-normally able to resist infection, because of immunosuppressive therapy, immunological defect, severe anaemia, or concurrent disease or condition, including
metastatic malignancy, cachexia, or severe
malnutrition.

Compton scatter {Arthur H. Compton,
American physicist, b. 1892}, the principal
interaction process of photons with tissue
in the 40 keV to 4 MeV energy range.
At the lower energies, most of the photon
energy is scattered, whereas at higher
energies, most of the photon energy is
absorbed.

compulsion, an irresistible, repetitive, irrational impulse to perform an act that is usually contrary to one's ordinary judgments or
standards yet results in overt anxiety if it is
not completed.

compulsive idea, a recurring, irrational idea
that persists in the mind, usually resulting in
an irresistible urge to perform some inappropriate act.

compulsive personality, a type of character
structure in which there is a pattern of
chronic and obsessive adherence to rigid
standards of conduct. The compulsive person is likely to follow repetitive patterns of
behaviour, such as snapping the fingers,
crossing the legs, or refusing to walk on
cracks in the sidewalk.

compulsive personality disorder, a condition in which an irrational preoccupation
with order, rules, ritual, and detail interferes
with everyday functioning and normal behaviour.

compulsive polydipsia, a compelling urge to
drink excessive amounts of liquid. Extreme
cases can result in death from water intoxication and electrolyte imbalance.

compulsive ritual, a series of acts a person
feels must be carried out even though he or
she recognizes the behaviour to be useless
and inappropriate.

compuphobia, an irrational fear of working
with computers.

computed radiography, a technique which
uses a charged plate and dedicated reader to
provide a digitized radiographic image for
processing in a laser imager.

computed tomography (CT), an x-ray technique that produces an image representing a
detailed cross section of tissue structure. The
procedure employs a narrowly collimated
beam of x-rays that rotates in a continuous
360-degree motion around the patient to
image the body in cross-sectional slices. An
array of detectors, positioned at several angles, records those x-rays that pass through
the body. The image is created by computer.
Formerly called computerized axial
tomography.

computer, an electronic device for processing and storing large amounts of informa-

tion very quickly.

computer-assisted learning (CAL), a teaching process employing a computer in the presentation of instructional materials, often in such a way as to require the student to interact with it.

computerized axial tomography (CAT). See **computed tomography**.

conation, the mental process characterized by desire, impulse, volition, and striving.

concanavalin A, a haemagglutinin, isolated from the meal of the jack bean, that reacts with polyglucosans in the blood of mammals causing agglutination.

concatenates, long molecules formed by continuous repeating of the same molecular subunit.

concave-convex joint relationship, the relative shape of each component of a joint's articulating surfaces. One surface is usually concave and the other convex.

concavity, a deep depression or inward curving surface of an organ or body structure.

concealed accessory pathway, (in cardiology) an extramuscular tract between the atria and ventricles that conducts only in a retrograde direction.

concealed bigeminy, (in cardiology) a bigeminal cardiac arrhythmia that may not be revealed on an electrocardiogram except through the appearance of odd numbers of P waves between manifest extrasystoles.

concealed junctional extrasystole, a junctional impulse that arises in and discharges the atrioventricular junction but fails to reach either atria or ventricles.

conceive, to become pregnant.

concentrate, 1. to decrease the bulk of a liquid and increase its strength per unit of volume by the removal of inactive ingredients through evaporation or other means. **2.** a substance, particularly a liquid, that has been strengthened and reduced in volume through such means.

concentration gradient, a gradient that exists across a membrane separating a high concentration of a particular ion from a low concentration of the same ion.

concentric, describing two or more circles that have a common centre.

concentric contraction, a common form of muscle contraction that occurs in rhythmic activities when the muscle fibres shorten as tension develops.

concentric fibroma, a fibrous tumour surrounding the uterine cavity.

concept, a construct or abstract idea or thought that originates and is held within the mind. **conceptual,** *adj.*

conception, 1. the beginning of pregnancy, usually taken to be the instant that a spermatozoon enters an ovum and forms a viable zygote. **2.** the act or process of fertilization. **3.** the act or process of creating an idea or notion. **4.** the idea or notion created; a general impression resulting from the interpretation of a symbol or set of symbols.

conceptive, 1. able to become pregnant. **2.** pertaining to or characteristic of the mental process of forming ideas or impressions.

conceptual disorder, a disturbance in thought processes, in cognitive activities, or in the ability to formulate concepts.

conceptual framework, a group of concepts that are broadly defined and systematically organized to provide a focus, a rationale, and a tool for the integration and interpretation of information.

conceptus, the product of conception; the fertilized ovum and its enclosing membranes at all stages of intrauterine development, from the time of implantation to birth.

concha, a body structure that is shell shaped, as the cavity in the external ear that surrounds the external auditory canal meatus.

concoction, a remedy prepared from a mixture of two or more drugs or substances that have been heated.

concomitant, designating one or more of two or more things, occurring simultaneously, that may or may not be interrelated or produced as a result of the others; accompanying.

concomitant symptom, any symptom that accompanies a primary symptom.

concordance, (in genetics) the expression of one or more specific traits in both members of a pair of twins.　**concordant,** *adj.*

concreteness, pertaining to the content of a communication that is not vague, but which includes specific feelings, behaviours, and experiences or situations.

concrete operation, a thought process based on concrete rather than abstract points of reference.

concrete thinking, a stage in the development of the cognitive thought processes in the child. During this phase, thought becomes increasingly logical and coherent so that the child is able to classify, sort, order, and organize facts while still being incapable of generalizing or dealing in abstractions.

concretion. See **calculus**.

concurrent disinfection, the daily handling and disposal of contaminated material or equipment.

concurrent nursing audit. See **nursing audit**.

concurrent sterilization, a method of preparing an infant-feeding formula in which all ingredients and equipment are sterilized before mixing the formula.

concurrent validity, validity of a test or a measurement tool that is established by concurrently applying a previously validated tool or test to the same phenomena, or data base, and comparing the results.

concussion, 1. a violent jarring or shaking, as caused by a blow or an explosion. **2.** informal. brain concussion.

condensation, 1. a reduction to a denser form, such as from water vapour to a liquid. **2.** (in psychology) a process often present in dreams in which two or more concepts are fused so that a single symbol represents the multiple components.

condensation nuclei, neutral particles, such as dust, in the atmosphere that are able to absorb or adsorb water and grow in size. At relatively high humidities, they form fogs or hazes. Condensation nuclei consisting of sulphuric or nitric acid vapours or nitrogen oxides may be a source of respiratory irritants.

condenser, (in dentistry) an instrument for compacting restorative material into a prepared tooth cavity. It has a working end, or nib, with a flat or serrated face.

condition, 1. a state of being, specifically in reference to physical and mental health or well-being. **2.** anything that is essential for or that restricts or modifies the appearance or occurrence of something else. **3.** to train the body or mind, usually through specific exercises and repeated exposure to a particular state or thing. **4.** (in psychology) to subject a person or animal to conditioning or associative learning so that a specific stimulus will always elicit a particular response.

conditioned avoidance response, a learned reaction that is performed either consciously or unconsciously to avoid an unpleasant or painful stimulus or to prevent such stimuli from occurring.

conditioned escape response, a learned reaction that is performed either consciously or unconsciously to stop or to escape from an aversive stimulus.

conditioned orientation response (COR), the desired response in an audiometry technique used in hearing tests for children under the age of 2 years. A toy mounted on a loudspeaker moves or lights up after presentation of a test tone. If later test sounds are audible to the child, he or she will look toward the toy after hearing a tone.

conditioned reflex, a reflex developed gradually by training in association with a specific, repeated external stimulus.

conditioned response, an automatic reaction to a stimulus that does not normally elicit such response but which has been learned through training. Such responses are produced by repeated association of some physiological function or behavioural pattern with an unrelated stimulus or event.

conditioning, a form of learning based on the development of a response or set of responses to a stimulus or series of stimuli. Kinds of conditioning are classical conditioning and operant conditioning.

condom {Doctor Condon, 18th century English physician}, a soft, flexible sheath that covers the penis and prevents semen from entering the vagina in sexual intercourse, used to avoid the transmission of an infection and to prevent conception.

conduct disorder, (in psychiatry) behaviour in an adolescent that is unacceptable in the social environment and could be considered criminal in an adult.

conduction, 1. (in physics) a process in which heat is transferred from one substance to another because of a difference in temperature; a process in which energy is transmitted through a conductor. **2.** (in physiology) the process by which a nerve impulse is transmitted.

conduction anaesthesia, a loss of sensation, especially pain, in a region of the body, produced by injecting a local anaesthetic along the course of a nerve or nerves to inhibit the conduction of impulses to and from the area supplied by that nerve or nerves.

conduction aphasia, a dissociative speech phenomenon in which there is no difficulty in comprehending words seen or heard and in which there is no dysarthria, yet the patient has problems in self-expression. The patient may substitute words similar in sound or meaning for the correct ones but is unable to repeat from dictation, to spell, and to read aloud.

conduction system, specialized tissue that carries electrical impulses, such as bundle branches and Purkinje fibres.

conduction velocity, the speed with which an electrical impulse can be transmitted through excitable tissue, as in the movement of a contraction impulse through His-Purkinje fibres of the heart.

conductive hearing loss, a form of hearing loss in which sound is inadequately conducted through the external or middle ear to the sensorineural apparatus of the inner ear. Sensitivity to sound is diminished, but clarity is not changed.

conductive tissue. See **nerve.**

conductor, 1. any substance through which electrons flow easily. **2.** (in psychiatry) a family therapist who uses his or her own personality to give direction to a family in therapy.

conduit, 1. an artificial channel or passage that connects two organs or different parts of the same organ. **2.** a tube or other device for conveying water or other fluids from one region to another.

condylar fracture, any fracture of the round end of a hinge joint, usually occurring at the distal end of the humerus or at the distal end of the femur, frequently detaching a small bone fragment that includes the condyle.

condylar guide, a mechanical device on a dental articulator, designed to guide articular movement similar to that produced by the paths of the condyles in the temporomandibular joints.

condyle, a rounded projection at the end of a

bone that anchors muscle ligaments and articulates with adjacent bones.

condyloid joint, a synovial joint in which a condyle is received into an elliptic cavity, as the wrist joint. A condyloid joint permits no axial rotation but allows flexion, extension, adduction, abduction, and circumduction.

condyloma, *pl.* **condylomata,** a wartlike growth on the anus, vulva, or glans penis.

condyloma acuminatum, *pl.* condylomata acuminata, a soft, wartlike or papillomatous growth common on warm and moist skin and the mucous membrane of the genitalia.

condyloma latum, *pl.* **condylomata lata,** a flat, moist, papular growth that appears in secondary syphilis in the coronal sulcus of the perineum or on the glans penis.

cone, 1. a photoreceptor cell in the retina of the eye that enables a person to visualize colours. There are three kinds of retinal cones, one for each of the colours, blue, green, and red; other colours are seen by stimulation of more than one type of cone. **2.** a cone-shaped device attached to x-ray equipment to collimate the beam. **conic, conical,** *adj.*

cone biopsy, surgical removal of a cone-shaped segment of the cervix, including both epithelial and endocervical tissue.

cone of light, 1. a triangular reflection observed during an ear examination when the light of an otoscope is focused on the image of the malleus. **2.** the group of light rays entering the pupil of the eye and forming an image on the retina.

confabulation, the fabrication of experiences or situations, often recounted in a detailed and plausible way to fill in and cover up gaps in the memory.

confession, making known to another person a real or imagined transgression.

confidentiality, the nondisclosure of certain information except to another authorized person.

configuration, the hardware, software, and peripherals assembled to work as a computer unit in a specific situation.

configurationism. See **Gestalt psychology.**

confinement, 1. a state of being held or restrained within a specific place in order to hinder or minimize activity. **2.** the final phase of pregnancy during which labour and childbirth occur; parturition.

confinement deprivation, an emotional disorder that may result when an individual is separated from familiar surroundings or denied contact with familiar persons or objects.

conflict, 1. a mental struggle, either conscious or unconscious, resulting from the simultaneous presence of opposing or incompatible thoughts, ideas, goals, or emotional forces, such as impulses, desires, or drives. **2.** a painful state of consciousness caused by the arousal of such opposing forces and the inability to resolve them. **3.** (in psychoanalysis) the unconscious emotional struggle between the demands of the id and those of the ego and superego or between the demands of the ego and the restrictions imposed by society. Kinds of conflict include **approach-approach conflict, approach-avoidance conflict, avoidance-avoidance conflict, extrapsychic conflict,** and **intrapsychic conflict.**

confluence of the sinuses, the wide junction of the superior sagittal, the straight, and the occipital sinuses with the two large transverse sinuses of the dura mater.

confrontation test, a method of assessing the visual field of a patient by moving an object into the periphery of each of the visual quadrants. The test is conducted while one eye is covered and the vision of the other is fixed on a point straight ahead. The patient reports when the moving object is first detected.

confusion, a mental state characterized by disorientation regarding time, place, or person, causing bewilderment, perplexity, lack of orderly thought, and inability to choose or act decisively. **confusional,** *adj.*

confusional insanity. See **amentia.**

confusional state, a mild form of delirium that may be experienced by an elderly person or a patient with preexisting brain disease. The confusional state may be triggered by a sudden or unexpected change in the person's environment.

congener, one of two or more things that are similar or closely related in structure, function, or origin. Examples of congeners are muscles that function identically and chemical compounds similar in composition and effect. **congenerous,** *adj.*

congenital, present at birth, as a congenital anomaly or defect.

congenital absence of sacrum and lumbar vertebrae, an abnormal condition present at birth and characterized by varying degrees of deformity, ranging from the absence of the lower segment of the coccyx to the absence of the entire sacrum and all lumbar vertebrae.

congenital adrenal hyperplasia, a group of disorders that have in common an enzyme defect resulting in low levels of cortisol and increased secretion of ACTH. The disorder leads to pseudohermaphroditism in female infants and macrogenitosomia in male infants.

congenital amputation, the absence of a fetal limb or part at birth, previously attributed to amputation by constricting bands in utero but now regarded as a developmental defect.

congenital anomaly, any abnormality present at birth, particularly a structural one, which may be inherited genetically, acquired during gestation, or inflicted during parturition.

congenital cardiac anomaly, any structural

or functional abnormality or defect of the heart or great vessels existing from birth. Congenital heart disease is a major cause of neonatal distress and is the most common cause of death in the newborn other than problems related to prematurity. Kinds of congenital cardiac anomalies include **atrial septal defect, coarctation of the aorta, tetralogy of Fallot, transposition of the great vessels, tricuspid atresia,** and **ventricular septal defect.**

congenital cloaca. See **persistent cloaca.**

congenital cytomegalovirus (CMV) disease. See **cytomegalic inclusion disease.**

congenital dermal sinus, a channel present at birth, extending from the surface of the body and passing between the bodies of two adjacent lumbar vertebrae to the spinal canal.

congenital dislocation of the hip, a congenital orthopaedic defect in which the head of the femur does not articulate with the acetabulum, because of an abnormal shallowness of the acetabulum.

congenital facial diplegia. See **Möbius' syndrome.**

congenital glaucoma, a rare form of glaucoma affecting infants and young children, resulting from a congenital closure of the iridocorneal angle by a membrane that obstructs the flow of aqueous humour and increases the intraorbital pressure. The condition is progressive, usually bilateral, and may damage the optic nerve.

congenital goitre, an enlargement of the thyroid gland at birth. It may be caused by a deficiency of enzymes required for the production of thyroxine.

congenital heart disease. See **congenital cardiac anomaly.**

congenital hypoplastic anaemia. See **Diamond-Blackfan syndrome.**

congenital megacolon. See **Hirschsprung's disease.**

congenital nonspherocytic haemolytic anaemia, a large group of blood disorders made up of a number of similar inherited diseases, each with a deficiency of one of the enzymes of red-cell glycolysis. Most are associated with varying degrees of haemolysis.

congenital oculofacial paralysis. See **Möbius' syndrome.**

congenital polycystic disease. See **polycystic kidney disease.**

congenital pulmonary arteriovenous fistula, a direct connection between the arterial and venous systems of the lung pres~ent at birth that results in a right-to-left shunt and permits unoxygenated blood to enter systemic circulation. The fistula may be single or multiple and may occur in any part of the lung.

congenital scoliosis, an abnormal condition present at birth, characterized by a lateral curvature of the spine, resulting from specific congenital rib and vertebral anomalies. The aetiological and pathological characteristics of congenital scoliosis are divided into six categories. Category I is associated with partial unilateral failure of the formation of a vertebra. Category II is associated with complete unilateral failure of the formation of a vertebra. Category III is associated with bilateral failure of segmentation with the absence of disc space. Category IV is associated with the unilateral failure of segmentation with the unsegmented bar. Category V is associated with the fusion of ribs. Category VI is associated with any condition not covered in the other categories. Category IV scoliosis seems to progress more rapidly and cause the greatest degree of deformity.

congenital short neck syndrome, a rare congenital malformation of the cervical spine in which the cervical vertebrae are fused, usually in pairs, into one mass of bone, resulting in decreased neck motion and decreased cervical length, sometimes with neurological involvement. When the deformity involves nerve-root compression, symptoms of peripheral nerve involvement, as pain or a burning sensation, may be evident, accompanied by paralysis, hyperaesthesia, or paraesthesia.

congenital subluxation of the hip. See **congenital dislocation of the hip.**

congestion, abnormal accumulation of fluid in an organ or body area. The fluid is often blood, but it may be bile or mucus.

congestive atelectasis, severe pulmonary congestion characterized by diffuse injury to alveolar-capillary membranes, resulting in haemorrhagic oedema, stiffness of the lungs, difficult ventilation, and respiratory failure.

congestive heart failure (CHF), an abnormal condition characterized by circulatory congestion caused by cardiac disorders, especially myocardial infarction of the ventricles. This condition usually develops chronically in association with the retention of sodium and water by the kidneys. Acute congestive heart failure may develop after myocardial infarction of the left ventricle and cause a significant shift of blood from the systemic to the pulmonary circulation before the typical retention of sodium and water occurs.

conglomerate silicosis, a severe form of silicosis marked by conglomerate masses of mineral dust in the lungs, causing acute shortness of breath, coughing, and production of sputum. The patient usually develops cor pulmonale.

Congolese red fever. See **murine typhus.**

congruent communication, a communication pattern in which the person sends the same message on both verbal and nonverbal levels.

conic papilla. See **papilla.**

conization, the removal of a cone-shaped sample of tissue, as in a cone biopsy.

conjoined manipulation, the use of both hands in obstetric and gynaecological procedures, with one positioned in the vagina and the other on the abdomen.

conjoined tendon. See **inguinal falx**.

conjoined twins, two fetuses developed from the same ovum who are physically united at birth. Conjoined twins result when separation of the blastomeres in early embryonic development does not occur until a late cleavage phase and is incomplete, causing the fused condition.

conjoint family therapy, a form of psychotherapy in which a single nuclear family is seen, and the issues and problems raised by family members are addressed by the therapist.

conjugate, (in pelvimetry) the measurement of the female pelvis to determine whether the presenting part of a fetus can enter the birth canal.

conjugated oestrogen, a mixture of sodium salts of oestrogen sulphates, chiefly those of oestrone, equilin, and 17-alpha-dihydroequilin, blended to approximate the average composition of oestrogenic substances in the urine of pregnant mares. Conjugated oestrogens may be prescribed to relieve postmenopausal vasomotor symptoms, for the treatment of atrophic vaginitis, female hypogonadism, primary ovarian failure, and palliation in advanced prostatic carcinoma and metastatic breast cancer.

conjugated protein, a compound that contains a protein molecule united to a nonprotein substance.

conjugation, (in genetics) a form of sexual reproduction in unicellular organisms in which the gametes temporarily fuse so that genetic material can transfer from the donor male to the recipient female, where it is incorporated, recombined, and then passed on to the progeny through replication.

conjugon, an episome that induces bacterial conjugation.

conjunctiva, the mucous membrane lining the inner surfaces of the eyelids and anterior part of the sclera. The palpebral conjunctiva lines the inner surface of the eyelids and is thick, opaque, and highly vascular. The **bulbar conjunctiva** is loosely connected, thin, and transparent, covering the sclera of the anterior third of the eye.

conjunctival burns, chemical burns of the conjunctiva. Emergency treatment involves bathing the eye with copious amounts of water until the chemical has been neutralized. The injured eye should be examined and treated by an ophthalmologist to prevent complications.

conjunctival oedema. See **chemosis**.

conjunctival fornix. See **inferior conjunctival fornix, superior conjunctival fornix**.

conjunctival reflex, a protective mechanism for the eye in which the eyelids close whenever the conjunctiva is touched.

conjunctival test, a procedure used to identify offending allergens by instilling the eye with a dilute solution of the allergenic extract.

conjunctivitis, inflammation of the conjunctiva, caused by bacterial or viral infection, allergy, or environmental factors. Red eyes, a thick discharge, sticky eyelids in the morning, and inflammation without pain are characteristic.

connecting fibrocartilage, a disc of fibrocartilage found between many joints, especially those with limited mobility, such as the spinal vertebrae. Each disc is composed of concentric rings of fibrous tissue separated by cartilaginous laminae.

connective tissue, tissue that supports and binds other body tissue and parts. It derives from the mesoderm of the embryo and is dense, containing large numbers of cells and large amounts of intercellular matenal. The intercellular material is composed of fibres in a matrix or ground substance that may be liquid, gelatinous. or solid, such as in bone and cartilage. Kinds of connective tissue are bone, cartilage, and fibrous connective tissue.

connective tissue disease. See **collagen vascular disease**.

Conor's disease. See **Marseilles fever**.

Conradi's disease. See **chondrodystrophia calcificans congenita**.

consanguinity, a hereditary or "blood" relationship between persons by having a common parent or ancestor.

conscience, 1. the moral, self-critical sense of what is right and wrong. **2.** (in psychoanalysis) the part of the superego system that monitors thoughts, feelings, and actions and measures them against internalized values and standards.

conscious, 1. (in neurology) capable of responding to sensory stimuli; awake, alert; aware of one's external environment. **2.** (in psychiatry) that part of the psyche or mental functioning in which thoughts, ideas, emotions, and other mental content are in complete awareness.

consciousness, a clear state of awareness of self and the environment in which attention is focused on immediate matters.

conscious proprioception, the conscious awareness of body position and movement of bodily segments. It is regulated by the lemniscal system through pathways that begin in joint receptors and end in the parietal lobe of the cerebral cortex; it enables the cortex to refine voluntary movements.

conscious sedation. See **awake anaesthesia**

consecutive angiitis, an inflammatory condition of blood or lymph vessels resulting from a similar process in surrounding tissues.

consensual, pertaining to a reflex action in which stimulation of one part of the body results in a response in another part.

consensual light reflex, a normally present crossed reflex in which light directed at one eye causes the opposite pupil to contract.

consensually validated symbols, symbols that are accepted by enough people that they have an agreed-upon meaning.

consensual reaction to light, the constriction of the pupil of one eye when the other eye is illuminated. Stimulation of either optic nerve causes constriction of both pupils.

consensual validation, a mutual agreement by two or more people about a particular meaning that is to be attributed to verbal or nonverbal behaviour.

consensus sequence, (in molecular genetics) a sequence in a strand of RNA nucleotides that is used as a site for the insertion of a splice of an RNA sequence from another source into the segment.

consenting adult, an adult who willingly agrees to participate in an activity with one or more other adults. The term is usually applied to sexual activity.

consequences, stimulus events following a behaviour that strengthen or weaken that behaviour. They may be either reinforcers or punishers.

conservation of energy, (in physics) a law stating that in any closed system the total amount of energy is constant.

conservation of matter, (in physics) a law stating that matter can neither be created nor destroyed and that the amount of matter in the universe is finite.

conservation principles of nursing, a conceptual framework for nursing that is directed toward maintaining the wholeness or integrity of the patient when the normal ability to cope is disturbed or exceeded by stress. Nursing intervention is determined by the patient's need to conserve energy and to maintain structural, personal, and social integrity. The nurse acts as a "conservationist ".

consolidation, 1. the combining of separate parts into a single whole. **2.** a state of solidification. **3.** (in medicine) the process of becoming solid, as when the lungs become firm and inelastic in pneumonia.

consolidation of individuality and emotional constancy, (in psychiatry) the fourth and final subphase in Mahler's system of the separation individuation phase of preoedipal development. It begins towards the end of the second year.

constancy, an absence of variation in quality of distinctive features despite location, rotation, size, or colour of an object.

constant positive airway pressure. See con-

tinuous positive airway pressure (CPAP).

constant positive pressure ventilation. See **continnous positive pressure ventilation (CPPV).**

constant pressure generator, a generator that provides or generates a constant gas pressure throughout the inspiratory cycle of breathing. The pressure may range from a low value such as 12 cm H_2O, to a high value of as much as 3500 cm H_2O, as required.

constant region, an area of an immunoglobulin molecule in which the amino acid sequence is relatively constant.

constant touch, a technique to diagnose the sensibility of an injured body part by pressing the eraser end of a pencil or another object in various areas to determine the ability of the person to detect the pressure.

constipation, difficulty in passing stools or an incomplete or infrequent passage of hard stools. Among the organic causes are intestinal obstruction, diverticulitis, and tumours. Functional impairment of the colon may occur in elderly or bedridden patients who fail to respond to the urge to defecate. **constipated,** *adj.*

constipation, colonic, a pattern of elimination characterized by hard, dry stools resulting from a delay in passage of food residue. Defining characteristics include decreased frequency, hard dry stool, straining at stool, painful defaecation, abdominal distention, a palpable mass, rectal pressure, headache, appetite impairment, and abdominal pain.

constipation, perceived, a state in which an individual makes a self-diagnosis of constipation and ensures a daily bowel movement through use of laxatives, enemas, and suppositories. The defining characteristic is an expectation of a daily bowel movement, which may be expected at the same time every day, with the resulting overuse of laxatives, enemas, and suppositories.

constipation, rectal, a pattern of elimination that is characterized by stool retention, normal stool consistency. and delayed elimination, resulting from biopsychosocial disruptions. There is also abdominal discomfort, rectal fullness, and a change in flatus.

constitutional delay, a period in the development of a child during which growth may be interrupted. In some cases constitutional delay may be associated with an illness or stressful event.

constitutional psychology, the study of the relationship of individual psychological makeup to body morphology and organic functioning.

constitutive resistance, the bacterial resistance to antibiotics that is contained in the DNA molecules of the organism. The trait can be passed on to daughter cells through cell division.

constriction, an abnormal closing or reduction in the size of an opening or passage of the body, as in vasoconstriction of a blood vessel.

constriction ring, a band of contracted uterine muscle that forms a stricture around part of the fetus during labour, usually after premature rupture of the membranes and sometimes impeding labour.

constrictive pericarditis, a fibrous thickening of the pericardium caused by gradual scarring or fibrosis of the membrane that resists the normal dilation of the heart chambers during the blood-filling phases of the cardiac cycle.

constrictor, a muscle that causes a narrowing of an opening, as the ciliary body fibres that control the size of the pupil.

constructional apraxia, a form of apraxia characterized by the inability to copy drawings or to manipulate objects to form patterns or designs. It is caused by a right hemisphere lesion.

constructive aggression, an act of self-assertiveness in response to a threatening action for purposes of self-protection and preservation.

constructive interference, (in ultrasonography) an increase in amplitude of sound waves that results when multiple waves of equal frequency are transmitted precisely in phase.

construct validity, validity of a test or a measurement tool that is established by demonstrating its ability to identify the variables that it proposes to identify.

consultation, a process in which the help of a specialist is sought to identify ways to handle problems in patient management or in the planning and implementation of health care programmes.

consumption, an obsolete term for tuberculosis.

consumption coagulopathy. See **disseminated intravascular coagulation (DIC)**

contact, 1. the touching or bringing together of two surfaces, as those of upper and lower teeth. **2.** the bringing together either directly or indirectly, as through the handling of food or clothing, of two individuals so as to allow the transmission of an infectious organism from one to the other. **3.** a person who has been exposed to an infectious disease.

contact dermatitis, a skin rash resulting from exposure to a primary irritant or to a sensitizing antigen. In the nonallergic type, a primary irritant, such as an alkaline detergent or an acid, causes a lesion similar to a thermal burn. In the allergic type, sensitizing antigens, on first exposure, result in an immunological change in certain lymphocytes. Poison ivy and nickel dermatitis are common examples of delayed hypersensitivity reaction.

contact factor. See **factor XII.**

contact lens, a small, curved, glass or plastic lens shaped to fit the person's eye and to correct refraction. Contact lenses float on the precorneal tear film.

contact shield, a protective device constructed of metal or other material that is positioned directly over the eyes or gonads of a patient to be exposed to an x-ray beam.

contagious, communicable, such as a disease that may be transmitted by direct or indirect contact. **contagion,** *n.*

contagious disease. See **communicable disease.**

contamination, a condition of being soiled, stained, touched, or otherwise exposed to harmful agents, making an object potentially unsafe for use as intended or without barrier techniques.

content validity, validity of a test or a measurement as a result of the use of previously tested items or concepts within the tool.

context, (in communications theory) the setting, meaning, and language of a message.

continence, the ability to control bladder or bowel function.

continent ileostomy, an ileostomy that drains into a surgically created pouch or reservoir in the abdomen. Involuntary discharge of intestinal contents is prevented by a valve created from the ileum.

contingency contracting, a formal agreement between a psychotherapist and a patient undergoing behaviour therapy regarding the consequences of certain actions by both parties.

contingency management, any of a group of techniques used in behaviour therapy that attempts to modify a behavioural response by controlling the consequences of that response. Kinds of contingency management include contingency contracting shaping, and token economy.

continuing education, (in nursing) formal, organized, educational programmes designed to promote and update the knowledge, skills, and professional attitudes of nurses. Continuing education is not to be confused with academic, degree-granting programmes, such as advanced education or postgraduate education.

continuity theory, a concept that an individual's personality does not change as the person ages, with the result that his or her behaviour becomes more predictable.

continuous anaesthesia, a method for maintaining regional nerve block in anaesthesia for surgical operations or labour in which an anaesthetic solution drips either at intervals or at a low rate of flow. The procedure is named according to the area infiltrated: continuous spinal, caudal, epidural, peridural, or lumbar.

continuous fever, a fever that persists steadily for a prolonged period of time.

continuous negative chest wall pressure, a negative pressure (below ambient pressure) that is applied to the chest wall during the entire respiratory cycle, thus providing increased transpulmonary pressure.

continuous positive airway pressure (CPAP), (in respiratory therapy) ventilation assisted by a flow of air delivered at a constant pressure throughout the respiratory cycle. It is performed for patients who can initiate their own respirations but who are not able to maintain adequate arterial oxygen levels without assistance. CPAP may be given through a ventilator and endotracheal tube, through a nasal cannula, or into a hood over the patient's head.

continuous positive pressure ventilation (CPPV), a positive pressure above ambient pressure maintained at the upper airway throughout the breathing cycle. The term is usually applied to positive end expiratory pressure (PEEP) and mechanical ventilation.

continuous reinforcement, a schedule of reinforcement in which omission of a response is followed by the reinforcer.

continuous tremor, fine, rhythmic, purposeless movements that persist during rest but sometimes disappear briefly during voluntary movements.

continuous tube feeding, delivery of nutrients by tube into the stomach, duodenum or jejunum. Feeding is controlled by enteral feeding pump and is continued over the 24 hour period providing the volume of feed required.

continuum, *pl.* **continua,** 1. a continuous series or whole. 2. (in mathematics) a system of real numbers.

contoured adducted trochanteric controlled alignment method (CATCAM), a design for an artificial lower limb for persons who have undergone above the knee amputations.

contra bevel, 1. (in dentistry) the angle between a cutting blade and the base of the periodontal pocket when the blade is held so that it separates the sulcular epithelium from the external epithelium of the gingiva. 2. (in dentistry) an external bevel of a tooth preparation extending onto a buccal or lingual cusp from an intracoronal restoration.

contraception, a process or technique for the prevention of pregnancy by means of a medication, device, or method that blocks or alters one or more of the processes of reproduction in such a way that sexual union can occur without impregnation. Kinds of contraception include **cervical cap, condom, contraceptive diaphragm, intrauterine device, natural family-planning method, oral contraceptive, spermatocide,** and **sterilization.**

contraceptive, any device or technique that prevents conception.

contraceptive diaphragm, a contraceptive device consisting of a hemisphere of thin rubber bonded to a flexible ring, inserted in the vagina together with spermaticidal jelly or cream so that spermatozoa cannot enter the uterus, thus preventing conception.

contraceptive diaphragm fitting, a procedure, performed in the doctor's surgery or family planning clinic, in which a contraceptive diaphragm is selected according to the clinical assessment of certain anatomical factors specific to the woman being fitted.

contraceptive effectiveness, the effectiveness of a method of contraception in preventing pregnancy. It is sometimes represented as a percentage but more accurately as the number of pregnancies per 100 woman-years. A contraceptive method that results in a pregnancy rate of less than 10 pregnancies per 100 woman-years is considered highly effective.

contraceptive method, any act, device, or medication for avoiding conception or a viable pregnancy.

contract, 1. an agreement or a promise that meets certain legal requirements, including competence of both or all parties to the contract, proper lawful subject matter, mutuality of agreement, mutuality of obligation, and consideration (the giving of something of value in payment for the obligation undertaken). 2. to make such an agreement or promise. **contractual,** *adj.*

contractile ring dysphagia, an abnormal condition characterized by difficulty in swallowing because of an overreactive interior oesophageal sphincteric mechanism that induces painful sticking sensations under the lower sternum.

contractility, (in cardiology) the force of a heart contraction when preload and afterload are constant.

contraction, 1. a reduction in size, especially of muscle fibres. 2. an abnormal shrinkage. 3. (in labour) a rhythmic tightening of the musculature of the upper uterine segment that begins mildly and becomes very strong late in labour, occurring as frequently as every 2 minutes, and lasting over 1 minute. 4. abnormal smallness of the birth canal or part of it, a cause of dystocia. **Inlet contraction** exists if the anteroposterior diameter is 10 cm or less or if the transverse diameter is 11.5 cm or less. **Midpelvic contraction** exists if the sum of the measurements in centimetres of the interspinous diameter (normally 10.5 cm) and the posterior sagittal diameter (normally 5 cm) is 13.5 cm or less. **Outlet contraction** exists if the intertuberous diameter is 8 cm or less.

contractore, an abnormal, usually permanent condition of a joint, characterized by flexion and fixation and caused by atrophy and shortening of muscle fibres or by loss of the normal elasticity of the skin, such as from the formation of extensive scar tissue over a joint.

contraindication, a factor that prohibits the

administration of a drug or the performance of a procedure in the care of a specific patient.

contralateral, affecting or originating in the opposite side of a point of reference, such as a point on a body.

contrast, a measure of the differences between two adjacent areas in an image. Contrast may be based on differences in optical density or differences in radiation transmission, or other parameters.

contrast enema. See **barium enema.**

contrast examination, the use of radiopaque materials, such as iodine and barium, to make internal organs visible on x-ray film.

contrast medium, radiopaque or radiolucent material introduced into the body to enable radiographic visualization of internal structures.

contrecoup injury. See **coup.**

control, to exercise restraint or maintain influence over a situation, as in self-control, the conscious limitation or suppression of impulses.

control cable, a stainless steel wire, usually contained in a flexible stainless steel housing, used to move a prosthesis, such as an artificial arm.

control gene, (in molecular genetics) a gene, such as the operator gene or regulator gene, that controls the transcription of the amino-acid sequence in the structural gene by either inducing or repressing protein synthesis.

control group. See **group.**

controlled area, an area in which the instantaneous dose rate of ionizing radiation exceeds, or is likely to exceed 7.5 uSvh^{-1}, or where any person entering the area might receive a dose which exceeds three tenths of any relevant dose limit.

controlled association, 1. a direct connection of relevant ideas as the result of a specific stimulus. 2. a process of bringing repressed ideas into the consciousness in response to words spoken by a psychoanalyst.

controlled drug, a drug whose possession, supply, prescription, storage and destruction are subject to special statutory controls.

controlled hypotension. See **deliberate hypotension.**

controlled oxygen therapy, the administration of oxygen to a patient on a dose-response basis in which oxygen is regarded as a drug and only the smallest amount of gas is used to obtain a desired therapeutic effect.

controlled ventilation, the use of an intermittent positive pressure breathing unit or other respirator that has an automatic cycling device that replaces spontaneous respiration.

control of haemorrhage, the limitation of the flow of blood from a break in the wall of a blood vessel, as by direct pressure, use of a tourniquet, or application of pressure on pressure points proximal to the wound. Direct pressure with a thick compress is applied in such a way that the edges of the wound are brought together. A tourniquet is applied proximal to the site of bleeding only in the most drastic emergency, for the limb may then have to be sacrificed because of tissue anoxia stemming from the use of the tourniquet. Pressure is applied to a pressure point by using firm manual pressure over the main artery supplying the wound. Points used to obtain the pulse may be used as pressure points to stop haemorrhage.

control process, a system of establishing standards, objectives, and methods, and measuring actual performance, comparing results, reinforcing strengths, and taking necessary corrective action.

control unit, a part of the central processing unit that controls the sequence of operations within a computer.

contusion, an injury that does not break the skin, caused by a blow to the body and characterized by swelling, discoloration, and pain. The immediate application of cold may limit the development of a contusion.

convalescence, the period of recovery after an illness, injury, or surgery.

convection, (in physics) the transfer of heat through a gas or liquid by the circulation of heated particles.

convergence, the movement of two objects toward a common point, such as the turning of the eyes inward to see an object close to the face.

convergent evolution, the development of similar structures or functions within widely differing phylogenetic species in response to similar environmental conditions.

convergent strabismus. See **esotropia.**

conversion, 1. changing from one form to another, transmutation. 2. (in obstetrics) the correction of a fetal position during labour. 3. (in psychiatry) an unconscious defence mechanism by which emotional conflicts ordinarily resulting in anxiety are repressed and transformed into symbolic physical symptoms having no organic basis.

conversion disorder, a kind of hysterical neurosis in which emotional conflicts are repressed and converted into sensory, motor, or visceral symptoms having no underlying organic cause, such as blindness, anaesthesia, hypaesthesia, hyperaesthesia, paraesthesia, involuntary muscular movements, paralysis, aphonia, mutism, hallucinations, catalepsy, choking sensations, and respiratory difficulties.

convulsion. See **seizure.**

Cooley's anaemia. See **thalassaemia.**

Coolidge tube, a basic type of hot-cathode x-ray tube that, with modern refinements, has been used by radiologists since it was invented in 1913.

cooling, reducing body temperature by the application of a hypothermia blanket, cold moist dressings, ice packs, or tepid sponging.

cooling rate, the rate at which temperature decreases with time (°C/minute) immediately after the completion of hyperthermia treatment.

Coombs' positive haemolytic anaemia {Robin R. A. Coombs, Bntish immunologist, b. 1921}, a form of anaemia resulting from premature destruction of circulating red blood cells.

Coombs' test, a test for detecting antibodies in the blood. Indirect Ct detects antibody in maternal blood; direct Ct detects antibodies in umbilical cord blood.

cooperative play, any organized play among a group of children in which activities are planned for the purpose of achieving some goal.

coordinated reflex, a sequence of muscular actions occurring in a purposeful, orderly progression, such as the act of swallowing.

COPD, abbreviation for **chronic obstructive pulmonary disease.**

coping, a process by which a person deals with stress, solves problems, and makes decisions. The process has two components, cognitive and noncognitive. The cognitive component includes the thought and learning necessary to identify the source of stress. The noncognitive components are automatic and focus on relieving the discomfort.

coping ability, the degree to which an individual is able to adapt to any stress encountered in the activities of daily life, whether of a physical or psychological nature, through the use of both conscious and unconscious mechanisms.

coping, defensive, a falsely positive self-evaluation based on a self-protective pattern that defends against underlying perceived threats to positive self-regard.

coping mechanism, any effort directed toward stress management, including task oriented and ego-defence mechanisms; the factors that enable an individual to regain emotional equilibrium after a stressful experience.

coping resources, the characteristics of a person, group, or environment that are helpful in assisting individuals to adapt to stress.

coping style, the cognitive, affective, or behavioural responses of a person to problematic or traumatic life events.

COPP, an anticancer drug combination of cyclophosphamide, procarbazine, and prednisone.

copper (Cu), a malleable, reddish-brown, metallic element. Its atomlc number is 29; its atomic weight is 63.54. Copper is a component of several important enzymes in the body and is essential to good health. Copper deficiency in the body is rare because only 2 to 5 mg daily, easily obtained from a variety of foods, is sufficient for a proper bal-

ance. Copper accumulates In individuals with Wilson's disease, primary biliary cirrhosis, and, occasionally, chronic extrahepatic biliary tract obstruction.

coprogogue. See **cathartic.**

coprolalia, the excessive use of obscene language.

coproporphyria, a rare, hereditary, metabolic disorder in which large quantities of nitrogenous substances, called porphyrins, are excreted in the urine. Attacks, with varying GI and neurological symptoms, may be precipitated by certain drugs.

coproporphyrin, any of the nitrogenous organic substances normally excreted in the faeces that are products of the breakdown of bilirubin from haemoglobin decomposition.

copulation. See **coitus.**

cor, 1. the heart. 2. relating to the heart.

coracobrachialis, a muscle with its origin on the scapula and its insertion on the inner side of the humerus. It functions by adducting the shoulder.

coracoid process, the thick, curved extension of the superior border of the scapula, to which the pectoralis minor is attached.

cord, any long, rounded, flexible structure. The body contains many different cords, such as the spermatic, vocal, spinal, nerve, umbilical, and hepatic cords. **cordal,** adj.

corditis, an abnormal inflammation of the spermatic cord, accompanied by pain in the testis, often caused by an infection orginating in the urethra or by tumour, hydrocele, or varicocele.

core, 1. a kind of main computer memory. 2. (in dentistry) a section of a mould, usually of plaster, made over assembled parts of a dental restoration to record and maintain their relationships so that the parts can be reassembled in their original position.

core gender identiy. See **gender identity.**

Cori's disease {Carl F. Cori, b. 1896: Gerty T. Cori, b. 1896: American biochemists}, a rare type of glycogen storage disease, in which a missing enzyme results in abnormally large deposits of glycogen in the liver, skeletal muscles, and heart. Signs are an enlarged liver, hypoglycaemia, acidosis, and, occasionally, stunted growth.

corium, the layer of skin, just below the epidermis, consisting of papillary and reticular layers and containing blood and lymphatic vessels, nerves and nerve endings, glands, and hair follicles.

corkscrew oesophagus, a neurogenic disorder in which normal peristaltic contractions of the oesophagus are replaced by spastic movements occurring spontaneously or with swallowing or gastric acid reflux.

corn, a horny mass of condensed epithelial cells overlying a bony prominence. Corns result from chronic function and pressure.

cornea, the convex, transparent, anterior part of the eye, comprising one sixth of the outermost tunic of the eye bulb. It is a fibrous structure with five layers: the anterior corneal epithelium, continuous with that of the conjunctiva: the anterior limiting layer (Bowman's membrane): the substantia propria: the posterior limiting layer (Descemet's membrane): and the endothelium of the anterior chamber (keratoderma). It is dense, uniform in thickness, and nonvascular.

corneal abrasion, the rubbing off of the outer layers of the cornea.

corneal grafting, transplantation of corneal tissue from one human eye to another, performed to improve vision in corneal scarring or distortion or to remove a perforating ulcer. Under local anaesthesia the affected area is excised: an identical section of clear cornea is cut from the donor eye and sutured in place, using an operating microscope. Postoperatively, the eye is covered with a protective metal shield, and the patient is cautioned to avoid coughing, sneezing, sudden movement, or lifting.

corneal loupe, (in ophthalmology) a loupe designed especially for examining the cornea.

corneal reflex, a protective mechanism for the eye in which the eyelids close when the cornea is touched.

cornification, thickening of the skin by a build up of dead, keratinized epithelial cells.

corn pad, a device that helps relieve the pressure and the pain of a corn by transferring the pressure to surrounding, unaffected areas.

cornual pregnancy, an ectopic pregnancy in one of the straight or curved extensions of the body of the uterus. The cornu of the uterus usually ruptures between 12 and 16 weeks of the pregnancy unless the condition is treated surgically to remove the products of conception.

corona, 1. a crown. **2.** a crownlike projection or encircling structure, such as a process extending from a bone. **coronal, coronoid,** *adj.*

coronal plane. See **frontal plane.**

coronal suture, the serrated transverse suture between the frontal bone and the parietal bone on each side of the skull.

corona radiata, *pl.* **coronae radiatae, 1.** a network of fibres that weaves through the internal capsule of the cerebral cortex and intermingles with the fibres of the corpus callosum. **2.** an aggregate of cells that surrounds the zona pellucida of the ovum.

coronary, 1. (in anatomy) of or pertaining to encircling structures, such as the coronary arteries; of or petaining to the heart. **2.** nontechnical. myocardial infarction or occlusion.

coronary arteriovenous fistula, an unusual congenital abnormality characterized by a direct communication between a coronary artery, usually the right, and the right atrium or ventricle, the coronary sinus, or the vena cava. A large shunt may result in growth failure, limited exercise tolerance, dyspnoea, and anginal pain.

coronary artery, one of a pair of arteries that branch from the aorta, including the left and the right coronary arteries. Since these vessels and their branches supply the heart, any dysfunction or disease that affects them can cause serious, sometimes fatal complications. The branches of the coronary arteries are affected by many different disorders, such as embolic, neoplastic, inflammatory, and noninflammatory diseases.

coronary artery disease, any one of the abnormal conditions that may affect the arteries of the heart and produce various pathological effects, especially the reduced flow of oxygen and nutrients to the myocardium. Any of the coronary artery diseases, such as coronary atherosclerosis, coronary arteritis, or fibromuscular hyperplasia of the coronary arteries, may produce the common characteristic symptom of angina pectoris, which, however, may also be associated with cardiomyopathy, in which the coronary arteries are normal. The most common kind of coronary artery disease is coronary atherosclerosis, now the leading cause of death in the Western world. Coronary atherosclerosis occurs most frequently in populations with regular diets high in calories, total fat, saturated fat, cholesterol, and refined carbohydrates. The risk is also greater among cigarette smokers than nonsmokers and appears to be proportional to the number of cigarettes smoked per day. Atherosclerosis develops with the formation of fatty fibrous plaques that narrow the lumen of the coronary arteries and may lead to thrombosis and myocardial infarction. Treatment of the patient with coronary artery disease concentrates on reducing myocardial oxygen demand or on increasing oxygen supply. Therapy commonly includes the administration of nitrates, such as nitroglycerin, isosorbide dinitrate, or propranolol, a beta-adrenergic blocker.

coronary artery fistula, a congenital anomaly characterized by an abnormal communication between a coronary artery and the right side of the heart or the pulmonary artery.

coronary autoregulation, the process of coronary artery vasodilatation in response to myocardial ischaemia.

coronary bypass, open-heart surgery in which a prosthesis or a section of a blood vessel is grafted onto one of the coronary arteries and connected to the ascending aorta, bypassing a narrowing or blockage in a coronary artery. The operation is performed in coronary artery disease to improve the blood supply to the heart muscle, to reduce the workload of the heart, and to relieve anginal pain.

coronary care nursing, the specialist nursing care provided in hospital in a coronary care unit.

coronary care unit (CCU), a specially equipped hospital area designed for the treatment of patients with sudden, life-threatening cardiac conditions, as acute coronary thrombosis. Such units contain resuscitation and monitoring equipment and are staffed by personnel especially trained and skilled in recognizing and immediately responding to cardiac emergencies with cardiopulmonary resuscitation techniques, the administration of antiarrhythmic drugs, and other appropriate therapeutic measures.

coronary collateralization, the spontaneous development of new blood vessels in or around areas of restricted blood flow to the heart.

coronary occlusion, an obstruction of any one of the coronary arteries, usually caused by progressive atherosclerosis and sometimes complicated by thrombosis. Coronary occlusions are usually caused by an obstruction of a coronary artery that develops gradually from the accumulation of fatty, fibrous plaques that narrow the arterial lumen, reduce the blood flow, and lead to myocardial infarction. In certain heart diseases arterial spasms may narrow the lumen of a coronary artery, blocking blood flow. Occlusion of the circumflex branch of the left coronary artery causes a lateral wall infarction. Occlusion of the anterior descending branch of the left coronary artery causes an infarction of the anterior heart wall. Occlusion of the right coronary artery or one of its branches causes a posterior wall infarction. Many patients who suffer coronary occlusions recover because of fast treatment and collateral circulation provided by extensive arterial anastomoses of the heart.

coronary sinus, the wide venous channel, about 2.25 cm long, situated in the coronary sulcus and covered by muscular fibers from the left atrium. It drains five coronary veins through a single semilunar valve.

coronary thrombosis, a development of a thrombus that blocks a coronary artery, often causing myocardial infarction and death. Coronary thromboses commonly develop in segments of arteries with atherosclerotic lesions.

coronary vein, one of the veins of the heart that drains blood from the capillary beds of the myocardium through the coronary sinus into the right atrium.

coronavirus, a member of a family of viruses that includes several types capable of causing acute respiratory illnesses.

coroner, a public official who investigates the causes and circumstances of a death oc-

curring in certain circumstances, especially a death that may have resulted from unnatural causes.

coronoid fossa, a small depression in the distal, dorsal surface of the humerus that receives the coronoid process of the ulna when the forearm is flexed.

coronoid process of mandible, a prominence on the anterior surface of the ramus of the mandible to which each temporal muscle attaches.

coronoid process of ulna, a wide, flaring projection of the proximal end of the ulna. The proximal surface of the process forms the lower part of the trochlear notch.

corpse, the body of a dead human.

cor pulmonale, an abnormal cardiac condition characterized by hypertrophy of the right ventricle of the heart as a result of hypenension of the pulmonary circulation. Pulmonary hypertension associated with this condition is caused by some disorder of the pulmonary parenchyma or of the pulmonary vascular system between the origin of the left pulmonary artery and the entry of the pulmonary veins into the left atrium. Approximately 85% of patients with cor pulmonale have chronic obstructive pulmonary disease: 25% of patients with emphysema eventually develop cor pulmonale. Pulmonary capillary destruction and pulmonary vasoconstriction decrease the cross-sectional area of the pulmonary vascular bed, increasing pulmonary vascular resistance and causing pulmonary hypertension. The right ventricle dilates and hypertrophies to compensate for the extra work required in forcing blood through the lungs. Some of the early signs of cor pulmonale include chronic cough, exertional dyspnoea, fatigue, wheezing, and weakness.

corpus. See **body.**

corpus cavernosum, a type of spongy erectile tissue within the penis or clitoris. The tissue becomes engorged with blood during sexual excitement.

corpuscle, 1. any cell of the body. **2.** a red or white blood cell. **corpuscular,** *adj.*

corpuscular radiation, the radiation associated with subatomic particles, such as electrons, protons, neutrons, or alpha particles, that travel in streams at various velocities.

corpus luteum, *pl.* **corpora lutea,** an anatomical structure on the surface of the ovary, consisting of a spheroid of yellowish tissue 1 to 2 cm in diameter that grows within the ruptured ovarian follicle after ovulation. It acts as a short-lived endocrine organ that secretes progesterone, which serves to maintain the decidual layer of the endometrium in the richly vascular state necessary for implantation and pregnancy. If conception occurs, the corpus luteum grows and secretes increasing amounts of progesterone.

corpus spongiosum, one of the cylinders of

spongy tissue that, with the corpora cavernosa, form the penis.

corpus vitreum. See **vitreous humour.**

corrected pressure, a method of applying Boyle's law of gas pressures to adjust simultaneously for changes in both pressure and humidity.

corrective emotional experience, a process by which a patient gives up old patterns of behaviour and learns or relearns new patterns by reexperiencing early unresolved feelings and needs.

corrective exercise. See **therapeutic exercise.**

correlation, (in statistics) a relationship between variables that may be negative (inverse), positive or curvilinear.

correlative differentiation, (in embryology) specialization or diversification of cells or tissues caused by an inductor or other external factor.

Corrigan's pulse {Dominic J. Corrigan, Irish physician, b. 1802}, a bounding pulse in which a great surge is felt followed by a sudden and complete absence of force or fullness in the artery. It occurs in excited emotional states, in various abnormal cardiac conditions and as a result of systemic arteriosclerosis.

corrosion of surgical instruments, the rusting of surgical instruments or the gradual wearing away of their polished surfaces because of oxidation and the action of contaminants. It usually occurs because of inadequate cleaning and drying of surgical instruments after use, the use of sterilizing solutions that eat into the surface, overexposure to such solutions, or a faulty autoclave.

corrosive, 1. eating away a substance or tissue, especially by chemical action. **2.** an agent or substance that eats away a substance or tissue.   **corrode,** *v*, **corrosion** *n*.

corrosive gastritis, an acute inflammatory condition of the stomach caused by the ingestion of an acid, alkali, or other corrosive chemical in which the lining of the stomach is eaten away by the corrosive substance.

corrugator supercilii, one of the three muscles of the eyelid. It functions to draw the eyebrow downward and inward, as if to frown.

cortex, *pl.* **cortices,** the outer layer of a body organ or other structure, as distinguished from the internal substance.

cortical apraxia. See **motor apraxia.**

cortical audiometry. See **audiometry.**

cortical blindness, blindness that results from a lesion in the visual centre of the cerebral cortex of the brain.

cortical bone, bone that is 70% to 90% mineralized.

cortical fracture, any fracture that involves the cortex of the bone.

cortical substance of cerebellum. See **cerebellar cortex.**

corticosteroid, any one of the natural or the synthetic hormones associated with the adrenal cortex, which influences or controls key processes of the body, such as carbohydrate and protein metabolism, electrolyte and water balance, and the functions of the cardiovascular system, the skeletal muscle, the kidneys, and other organs. The corticosteroids synthesized by the adrenal glands include the glucocorticoids and the mineralocorticoids. The principal glucocorticoids are cortisol and corticosterone. The only physiologically important mineralocorticoid in humans is aldosterone.

corticotropin. See **adrenocorticotropic hormone.**

corticotropin-releasing factor (CRF), a polypeptide secreted by the hypothalamus into the bloodstream. It triggers the release of ACTH from the pituitary gland.

cortisol, see **hydrocortisone.**

cortisone, a glucocorticoid secreted by the adrenal cortex and also made synthetically. It is used, as cortisone acetate, as an antiinflammatory agent.

Corti's organ. See **organ of Corti.**

Cornebacterium, a common genus of rod-shaped, curved bacilli having many species. The most common pathogenic species are *Corynebacterium acnes,* commonly found in acne lesions, and *C. diphtheriae,* the cause of diphtheria.

coryza, See **rhinitis.**

coryza spasmodica. See **hay fever.**

cosmetic surgery, reconstruction of cutaneous or underlying tissues, usually about the face and neck, performed to correct a structural defect or to remove a scar, birthmark, or some normal evidence of ageing. Kinds of cosmetic surgery include rhinoplasty, rhytidoplasty.

cosmic radiation, high-energy particles with great penetrating power originating in outer space and reaching the earth as normal background radiation. The rays consist partly of high-energy atomic nuclei.

costal, 1. of or pertaining to a rib. **2.** situated near a rib or on a side close to a rib.

costal cartilage. See **cartilage.**

cost analysis, an analysis of the disbursements of a given activity, agency, department, or programme.

cost-benefit ratio, a ratio that represents the relationship of the cost of an activity to the benefit of its outcome or product.

cost capping, informal. a limit on the amount of money that an agency, department, or institution may spend.

cost control, the process of monitoring and regulating of the expenditure of funds by an agency or institution.

cost effectiveness, the extent to which an activity is thought to be as valuable as it is expensive, such as the provision of antenatal care being cost effective in preventing the costly incidence of perinatal morbidity.

Costen's syndrome. See **temporomandibular joint pain-dysfunction syndrome**.

costochondral, of or pertaining to a rib and its cartilage.

costophrenic (CP) angle, the angle at the bottom of the lung where the diaphragm and chest wall meet.

costotransverse articulation, any one of 20 gliding joints between the ribs and associated vertebrae, except for the eleventh and twelfth ribs.

costovertebral, of or relating to a rib and the vertebral column.

costovertebral angle (CVA), one of two angles that outline a space over the kidneys. The angle is formed by the lateral and downward curve of the lowest rib and the vertical column of the spine itself.

cosyntropin, a synthetic form of ACTH that is used in the diagnosis and treatment of adrenal hypofunction disorders, such as Addison's disease.

cot death. See **sudden infant death syndrome**.

co-trimoxazole, a mixture of suphamethoxazole with trimethorim in the proportions 5 to **1.** The two components are synergistic in their antibacterial action and the combination is active against a wide range of bacteria, some protozoa and Pneumocystis carinii. Although still widely used in bacterial infections, especially those of the urinary, respiratory and GI tracts, it is being superseded by less toxic compounds. Its main indication is in the treatment of *Pneumocystis carinii* pneumonia.

Cotton's fracture, a trimalleolar fracture involving medial, lateral, and posterior malleoli.

cotyledon, one of the visible segments on the maternal surface of the placenta. A typical placenta may have 15 to 28 cotyledons, each consisting of fetal vessels, chorionic villi, and intervillous space.

cotyloid cavity. See **acetabulum**.

cough, a sudden, audible expulsion of air from the lungs. Coughing is preceded by inspiration, the glottis is partially closed, and the accessory muscles of expiration contract to expel the air forcibly from the respiratory passages. Coughing is an essential protective response that serves to clear the lungs, bronchi, or trachea of irritants and secretions or to prevent aspiration of foreign material into the lungs. It is a common symptom of diseases of the chest and larynx. Antitussive medications are sometimes prescribed in the treatment of a cough in the absence of mucus or congestion.

cough fracture, any fracture of a rib, usually the fifth or the seventh rib, caused by violent coughing.

coulomb {Charles A. de Coulomb, French physicist, b. 1736}, the Sl unit of electricity equal to the quantity of charge transferred in 1 second across a conductor in which there is a constant current of 1 ampere, or 1 ampere second.

Coulomb's law, (in physics) a law stating that the force of attraction or repulsion between two electrically charged bodies is directly proportional to the strength of the electric charges and inversely proportional to the square of the distance between them.

coulometry, a type of electroanalytical chemistry in which a reagent generated at the surface of an electrode reacts with a substance to be measured. The substance, usually a metal ion, is measured in terms of the coulombs required for the reaction.

Coulter counter {W. H. Coulter, 20th century American engineer}, a trademark for an electric device that rapidly identifies, sorts, and counts the various kinds of cells present in a small specimen of blood.

coumarin, an anticoagulant, prescribed for prophylaxis and treatment of thrombosis and embolism.

Council for Professions Supplementary to Medicine (CPSM), council formed under the Professions Supplementary to Medicine Act 1960, to promote high standards of professional education and conduct in the professions of podiatry, dietetics, medical laboratory science, occupational therapy, orthoptics, physiotherapy and radiotherapy.

counselling, the act of providing advice and guidance to a patient or the patient's family. It helps the patient recognize and manage stress and facilitates interpersonal relationships.

count, a computation of the number of objects or elements present per unit of measurement. Kinds of counts include Addis count, bacteria count, blood count, and platelet count.

counterclaim, (in law) a claim made by a defendant establishing a cause for action in his favour against the plaintiff.

counterconditioning, a process used in behavioural therapy in which a learned response is replaced by an alternative response that is less disruptive.

countercurrent, a change in the direction of the flow of a fluid, such as occurs in the ascending branch of a kidney tubule where osmolality undergoes a reversal after a gradual change in sodium chloride concentrations. counterinjunction, (in transactional analysis) an overt message from the Parent ego state of the mother or father that may be difficult to follow if the message conflicts with earlier parental instructions.

counterphobic behaviour, an expression of reaction to a phobia by a patient who actively seeks exposure to the type of situation that precipitates phobic symptoms.

counterpulsation, 1. the action of a circulatory-assist pumping device synchronized counter to the normal action of the heart. **2.** the process of increasing the intraaortic pressure in diastole by inflation of an intraaortic balloon and deflation of the balloon immediately preceding the next systole.

countershock, (in cardiology) a high-intensity, short-duration electric shock applied to the area of the heart, resulting in total cardiac depolarization.

countersociety, a society that runs counter to or against the established society in which it exists. An example is a street gang that may have its own role models, goals, and system of values.

countertraction, a force that counteracts the pull of traction, especially in orthopaedics, such as the force of body weight resulting from the pull of gravity.

countertransference, the conscious or unconscious emotional response of a psychotherapist or psychoanalyst to a patient.

countertransport, the simultaneous transport of two different substances across the same membrane, each in the opposite direction.

coup, any blow or stroke or the effects of such a blow to the body, usually used with a French word identifying a type of stroke: **1.** coup de sabre, a wound resembling a sword cut. **2.** coup de soleil. See sunstroke. **3.** coup sur coup, adminstration of a drug in small amounts over a short period of time rather than in a single larger dose. **4.** contre coup, an injury most often associated with a blow to the skull in which the force of the impact is transmitted through the skull bones to the opposite side of the head where the bruise, fracture, or other sign of injury appears.

couples therapy, psychotherapy in which couples, who may be married or unmarried but living together, undergo therapy together.

coupling, 1. the act of coming together, joining, or pairing. **2.** (in genetics) the situation in linked inheritance in which the nonalleles of two or more mutant genes are located on the same chromosome and are close enough so that they are likely to be inherited together.

coupling interval, the interval between the dominant heartbeat and a coupled extrasystole.

Courvoisier's law {Ludwig Courvoisier, Swiss surgeon, b. 1843}, a statement that the gallbladder is smaller than usual if a gallstone blocks the common bile duct but is dilated if the common bile duct is blocked as a result of a cause other than a gallstone, such as pancreatic cancer.

couvade, a custom in some non-Western cultures whereby the husband goes through mock labour while his wife is giving birth.

Couvelaire uterus {Alexandre Couvelaire, French obstetrician, b. 1873}, the deep purple colour of the uterus following a severe concealed placental abruption, because the blood has been forced back into the myometrium.

Cowling's rule, a method of calculating the approximate paediatric dosage of a drug for a child using this formula: (age at next birthday/24) x adult dose.

Cowper's gland {William Cowper, English surgeon, b. 1666}, either of two round, peasized glands embedded in the urethral sphincter of the male.

cowpox, a mild infectious disease characterized by a pustular rash, caused by the vaccinia virus transmitted to humans from infected cattle. Cowpox infection usually confers immunity to smallpox, because of the similarity of the variola and vaccinia viruses.

coxa, *pl.* **coxae,** the hip joint: the head of the femur and the acetabulum of the innominate bone.

coxa adducta, coxa flexa. See **coxa vara**.

coxal articulation, the ball-and-socket joint of the hip, formed by the articulation of the head of the femur into the cup-shaped cavity of the acetabulum.

coxa magna, an abnormal widening of the head and neck of the femur.

coxa plana. See **Perthes' disease**.

coxa valga, a hip deformity in which the angle formed by the axis of the head and neck of the femur and the axis of its shaft is signifcantly increased.

coxa vara, a hip deformity in which the angle formed by the axis of the head and neck of the femur and the axis of its shaft is decreased.

coxa vara luxans, a fissure or crack in the neck of the femur with dislocation of the head, caused by coxa vara.

coxsackievirus, ally of 30 serologically different enteroviruses associated with a variety of symptoms and primarily affecting children during warm weather. Among the diseases associated with coxsackievirus infections are herpangina, hand, foot, and mouth disease, epidemic pleurodynia, myocarditis, pericarditis, aseptic meningitis, and several exanthemae.

CPAP, abbreviation for **continuous positive airway pressure**.

CPK isoenzyme fraction, one of several blood-borne enzymes that are released after myocardial necrosis. The isoenzyme of CPK (creatine phosphokinase) is a diagnostic clue to heart damage.

CPN, abbreviation for **community psychiatric nurse**.

CPPB, abbreviation for **continuous positive pressure breathing**.

CPPV, abbreviation for **continuous positive pressure ventilation**.

CPR, abbreviation for **cardiopulmonary resuscitation**.

CPSM, abbreviation for **Council for Professions Supplementary to Medicine**.

cpu, CPU, abbreviation for **central processing unit of a computer**.

Cr, symbol for **chromium**.

CR, abbreviation for **controlled respiration**.

crab louse, a species of body louse, *Phthirus pubis*, that infests the hairs of the genital area and is often transmitted between people by venereal contact.

crack, informal, cocaine base. See **cocaine hydrochloride**.

cracked tooth syndrome, a crack in the tooth structure giving rise to acute pain which is worse on biting. Diagnosis of cracked tooth syndrome can be difficult to detect clinically.

crackle, a fine, bubbling sound heard on auscultation of the lung. It is produced by air entering distal airways and alveoli that contain serous secretions.

cradle cap, a common seborrhoeic dermatitis of infants consisting of thick, yellow, greasy scales on the scalp. Treatment includes oil or ointment to soften the scales, and frequent shampoos.

cramp, 1. a spasmodic and often painful contraction of one or more muscles. **2.** a pain resembling a muscular cramp. Kinds of cramps include **writer's cramp**.

cranial   arachnoid.   See   **arachnoidea encephali**.

cranial arteritis, See **temporal arteritis**.

cranial nerves, the 12 pairs of nerves emerging from the cranial cavity through various openings in the skull. Beginning with the most anterior, they are designated by Roman numerals and named (I) olfactory, (II) optic, (III) oculomotor, (IV) trochlear, (V) trigeminal, (VI) abducens, (VII) facial, (VIII) acoustic, (IX) glossopharyngeal, (X) vagal, (XI) accessory, (XII) hypoglossal. The cranial nerves are attached to the base of the brain and carry impulses for such functions as smell, vision, ocular movement, pupil contraction, muscular sensibility, general sensibility, mastication, facial expression, glandular secretion, taste, cutaneous sensibility, hearing, equilibrium, swallowing, phonation, tongue movement, head movement, and shoulder movement.

cranial osteopathy, osteopathic treatment of the head in which osteopathic techniques are used to deal with the bones and very narrow joints of the skull. It is concerned with the cranial mechanism and balance; disturbance of this physiological balance might be caused by an accident or experience at birth such as a forceps delivery or protracted labour.

craniocervical, pertaining to the junction of the skull and neck, particularly the area of the foramen magnum.

craniodidymus, a two-headed fetus in which the two bodies are fused.

craniofacial dysostosis, an abnormal hereditary condition characterized by acrocephaly, exophthalmos, hypertelorism, strabismus, parrot-beaked nose, and hypoplastic maxilla with relative mandibular prognathism.

craniohypophyseal xanthoma, a condition in which cholesterol deposits are formed around the hypophyses of the bones, as in Hand-Schuller-Christian disease.

craniometaphyseal dysplasia, an inherited bone disorder characterized by paranasal overgrowth, thickening of the skull and jaw, and entrapment of cranial nerves. The patient may experience nasorespiratory infections, associated with bone overgrowth at the sinuses, and malocclusion of the jaws.

craniopagus, conjoined twins that are united at the heads. Fusion can occur at the frontal, occipital, or parietal regions.

craniopharyngeal, of or pertaining to the cranium and the pharynx.

craniopharyngioma, *pl.* **cranoiopharyngiomas, craniopharyngiomata,** a congenital pituitary tumour, appearing most often in children and adolescents, that arises in cells derived from Rathke's pouch or the hypophyseal stalk. The tumour may interfere with pituitary function, damage the optic chiasm, disrupt hypothalamic control of the autonomic nervous system, and result in hydrocephalus.

craniosacral osteopathy. See **cranial osteopathy**.

craniostenosis, a congenital deformity of the skull resulting from premature closure of the sutures between the cranial bones.

craniostosis, premature ossification of the sutures of the skull, often associated with other skeletal defects. The sutures close before or soon after birth. If no surgical correction is made, the growth of the skull is inhibited, the head is deformed, and the eyes and brain are often damaged.

craniotabes, benign, congenital thinness of the top and back of the skull of a newborn, common because the rate of brain growth exceeds the rate of calcification of the skull during the last month of gestation.

craniotomy, any surgical opening into the skull, performed to relieve intracranial pressure, to control bleeding, or to remove a tumour.

craniotubular, pertaining to a bossing, or overgrowth, of bone that results in an abnormal contour and increased bone density.

cranium, the bony skull that holds the brain. It is composed of eight bones: frontal, occipital, sphenoid, and ethmoid bones, and paired temporal and parietal bones.   **cranial,** *adj.*

cravat bandage, a triangular bandage, folded lengthwise. It may be used as a circular, figure-of-eight, or spiral bandage to control bleeding or to tie splints in place.

crawling reflex. See **symmetric tonic neck reflex.**

C-reactive protein (CRP), a protein not normally detected in the serum but present in many acute inflammatory conditions and with necrosis. CRP appears in the serum within 24 to 48 hours of the onset of inflammation. After a myocardial infarction, it is present in 24 hours. CRP disappears when an inflammatory process is suppressed by salicylates and steroids, or both.

cream, 1. the portion of milk rich in butterfat. **2.** any fluid mixture of thick consistency, such as used to apply medication to the surface of the body.

crease, an indentation or margin formed by a doubling back of tissue, such as the folds or creases on the palm of the hand and sole of the foot.

creatine, an important nitrogenous compound produced by metabolic processes in the body. Combined with phosphorus, it forms high energy phosphate.

creatine kinase, an enzyme in muscle, brain, and other tissues that catalyses the transfer of a phosphate group from adenosine triphosphate to creatine, producing adenosine diphosphate and phosphocreatine.

creatinine, a substance formed from the metabolism of creatine, commonly found in blood, urine, and muscle tissue.

creatinine height index (CHI), a measurement of a 24-hour urinary excretion of creatinine, which is generally related to the patient's muscle mass and an indicator of malnutrition, particularly in young males.

creatinism, a condition caused by a congenital absence of the thyroid gland or its secretions.

creative therapies, the therapeutic use of creative techniques in Occupational Therapy. Techniques employed may include art, drama, ceramics, music, writing. The selection and application of these activities is dependent upon the specific, identified needs of the patient/client following a comprehensive assessment.

credentials, a predetermined set of standards, such as certification, establishing that a person or institution has achieved professional recognition in a specific field of health care.

Crede's method {Karl S. Crede, German physician, b. 1819}, a technique for promoting the expulsion of urine by manual compression of the bladder through pressure on the lower abdominal wall.

Crede's prophylaxis {Karl S. Crede}, the instillation of a 1% silver-nitrate solution into the conjunctiva of newborn infants to prevent ophthalmia neonatorum.

creep, a rheological effect of metals and other solid materials that may become elongated or deformed as a result of a load being applied for a long period of time.

creeping eruption, a skin lesion characterized by irregular, wandering red lines made by the burrowing larvae of hookworms and certain roundworms.

cremaster, a thin, muscular layer spreading out over the spermatic cord in a series of loops. It is a continuation of the obliquus internus. It functions to draw the testis up toward the superficial inguinal ring in response to cold or to stimulation of the nerve.

cremasteric reflex, a superficial neural reflex elicited by stroking the skin of the upper inner aspect of the thigh in a male. This normally results in a brisk retraction of the testis on the side of the stimulus.

crenation, the formation of notches or leaf-like, scalloped edges on an object. Red blood cells exposed to a hypertonic saline solution acquire a notched, shrivelled surface because of the osmotic effect of the solution. They are then called crenated red blood cells. **crenate, crenated,***adj.*

creosol, an oily liquid that is one of the active constituents (phenol) of creosote. It should not be confused with cresol.

creosote, a flammable, oily liquid with a smoky odour that is used primarily as a wood preservative. It can be a cause of a wide variety of health problems, ranging from cancer and corneal damage to convulsions.

crepitus, 1. flatulence or the noisy discharge of fetid gas from the intestine through the anus. **2.** a sound like a crackling noise associated with gas gangrene, the rubbing of bone fragments, or the rales of a consolidated area of the lung in pneumonia.

cresc-, a combining form meaning 'to grow': crescograph.

crescendo angina, a form of anginal discomfort associated with ischaemic electrocardiographic changes, marked by increased frequency, provocation, intensity, or character.

cresol, a mixture of three isomers in a liquid with a phenolic odour. It is derived from coal tar and used in synthetic resins and disinfectants. Symptoms of chronic poisoning include skin eruptions, digestive disorders, uraemia, jaundice, nervous disorders, vertigo, and mental changes.

CREST syndrome, abbreviation for **calcinosis, Raynaud's phenomenon, oesophageal dysfunction, sclerodactyly,** and **telangiectasis,** which may occur for varying periods of time in patients with scleroderma.

cretin dwarf, a person in whom short stature is caused by infantile hypothyroidism and severe deficiency of thyroid hormone.

cretinism, a condition characterized by severe congenital hypothyroidism and often associated with other endocrine abnormalities. Typical signs of cretinism include dwarfism, mental deficiency, puffy facial features, dry skin, large tongue, umbilical hernia, and muscular incoordination. The disorder occurs usually in areas where the diet is deficient in iodine and where goitre is endemic. **cretinoid, cretinous,** *adj.,* **cretin,** *n.*

Creutzfeldt-Jakob disease, [Hans G. Creutzfeldt, German neurologist, b. 1885; Alfons M. Jakob, German neurologist, b. 1884}, a rare, fatal encephalopathy caused by a slow virus. The disease occurs in middle age, and symptoms are progressive dementia, dysarthria, muscle wasting, and various involuntary movements, such as myoclonus and athetosis. Deterioration is obvious week to week. Death ensues, usually within a year.

CRF, abbreviation for **corticotropin-releasing factor**.

cribriform carcinoma. See **adenocystic carcinoma**.

crico-, a combining form meaning 'ring'. *cricoderma, cricoid cricoidectomy.*

cricoid, 1. having a ring shape. **2.** a ringshaped cartilage connected to the thyroid cartilage by the cricothyroid ligament at the level of the sixth cervical vertebra.

cricoid pressure, a technique to reduce the risk of the aspiration of stomach contents during induction of general anaesthesia. The cricoid cartilage is pushed against the oesophagus to prevent passive regurgitation.

cricopharyngeal, of or pertaining to the cricoid cartilage and the pharynx.

cricopharyngeal incoordination, a defect in the normal swallowing reflex. The cricopharyngeus muscle ordinarily serves as a sphincter to keep the top of the oesophagus closed except when the person is swallowing, vomiting, or belching. The trachea remains open for breathing, but air normally does not enter the oesophagus during respiration. When the series of neuromuscular actions is not properly coordinated, the patient may choke, swallow air, regurgitate fluid into the nose, or experience discomfort in swallowing food.

cricothyrotomy, an emergency incision into the larynx, performed to open the airway in a person who is choking. A small vertical midline cut is made just below the Adam's apple and above the cricoid cartilage. The incision is opened further with a transverse cut through the cricothyroid membrane, and the wound is held open with a tube that is open at both ends to allow air to move in and out.

cri-du-chat syndrome. See **cat-cry syndrome**.

Crigler-Najjar syndrome [John F. Crigler, Jr. American paediatrician, b. 1919; Victor A. Najjar. American paediatrician, b. 1914}, a congenital, familial, autosomal anomaly, in which glucuronyl transferase, an enzyme, is deficient or absent. The condition is characterized by nonhaemolytic jaundice, an ac-

cumulation of unconjugated bilirubin in the blood, and severe disorders of the central nervous system.

crime, any act that violates a law and may include criminal intent.

Criminal Injuries Compensation Board, a scheme whereby victims of violent crime can receive compensation for their injuries, even if the criminal justice system is not used to dealing with the perpetrator of the violence.

criminal psychology, the study of the mental processes, motivational patterns, and behaviour of criminals.

crin-, a combining form meaning to separate': crinin, crinogenic.

-crinat, a combining form designating an ethacrynic acid-derived diuretic.

-crine, a combining form designating an acridine derivative.

-crinia, a combining form meaning '(condition of) endocrine secretion': haemocrinia, hypercrinia. neurocrinia.

-crisia, 1. a combining form meaning a 'diagnosis': acrisia, urocrisia. **2.** a combining form meaning a '(specified) condition of endocrine secretion': hypercrisia, hyperendocrisia, hypocrisia.

crisis, 1. a turning point for better or worse in the course of a disease, usually indicated by a marked change in the intensity of signs and symptoms. **2.** a turning point in events affecting the emotional state of a person, such as death or divorce.

crisis intervention, (in psychiatry) therapeutic intervention to help resolve a particular and immediate problem. No attempt is made at in-depth analysis.

crisis-intervention unit, a group of health professionals specially trained for rendering emergency psychiatric care to a person or group of persons during a period of crisis, especially instances involving suicide attempts or drug abuse.

crisis resolution, (in psychiatry) the development of effective adaptive and coping devices to resolve a crisis.

crisis theory, a conceptual framework for defining and explaining the phenomena that occur when a person faces a problem that appears to be insoluble.

crisscross inheritance, the acquisition of genetic characteristics or conditions from the parent of the opposite sex.

crista supraventricularis, the muscular ridge on the interior dorsal wall of the right ventricle of the heart.

criterion, *pl.* **criteria,** a standard or rule by which something may be judged, such as a health condition, or a diagnosis established. Usually plural, criteria refers to a set of rules or principles against which something may be measured, such as health care practices.

critical care, See **intensive care**.

critical organs, tissues that are the most sensitive to irradiation, such as the gonads, lymphoid organs, and intestine. The skin, cornea, oral cavity, oesophagus, vagina, cervix, and optic lens are the next most sensitive organs to irradiation.

critical period of development, a specific time during which the environment has its greatest impact on an individual's development.

critical point, the temperature and pressure at which, in a sealed system, the densities of the liquid and gas forms of a substance will be equal and the two are not visibly separated.

critical pressure, the pressure exerted by a vapour in a closed system at the critical temperature.

critical temperature, the highest temperature at which a substance can exist as a liquid outside a sealed system.

Crohn's disease {Burrill B. Crohn, American physician, b. 1884}, a chronic inflammatory bowel disease of unknown origin, usually affecting the ileum, the colon, or both structures. Diseased segments may be separated by normal bowel segments. Crohn's disease is characterized by frequent attacks of diarrhoea, severe abdominal pain, nausea, fever, chills, weakness, anorexia, and weight loss.

-cromil, a combining form designating a cromoglicic acid-type antiallergic agent.

cromoglicic acid. See **cromolyn sodium.**

cromolyn sodium, an antiasthmatic that acts by decreasing allergic bronchospasm resulting from an inhaled allergen. It is prophylactically prescribed in the treatment of bronchial asthma. The drug has no effect after an attack has begun.

Cronkhite-Canada syndrome {Leonard W. Cronkhite, American physician, b. 1919; Wilma J. Canada, American radiologist}, an abnormal familial condition characterized by GI polyposis accompanied by ectodermal defects, such as nail atrophy, alopecia and excessive skin pigmentation. In some individuals it is also accompanied by protein-losing enteropathy, malabsorption, and deficiency of blood calcium, potassium, and magnesium.

cross, (in genetics) any method of crossbreeding or any individual, organism, or strain produced from crossbreeding. Kinds of crosses include **dihybrid cross, monohybrid cross, polyhybrid cross,** and **trihybrid cross.**

cross-bite tooth, any of the posterior teeth that allow the modified buccal cusps of the upper teeth to be positioned in the central fossae of the lower teeth.

crossbreeding, the production of offspring by the mating of plants and animals from different varieties, strains, or species hybridization.

crossed extension reflex, one of the spinal-mediated reflexes normally present in the first 2 months of life. It is demonstrated by the flexion, adduction, and extension of one leg when the foot of the other leg is stimulated.

crossed grid, (in radiography) an assembly of two parallel or focused grids at right angles to each other.

crossed reflex, any neural reflex in which stimulation of one side of the body results in a response on the other side, such as the consensual light reflex.

cross-eye. See **esophoria.**

cross fertilization, 1. (in zoology) the union of gametes from different species or varieties to form hybrids. **2.** (in botany) the fertilization of the flower of one plant by the pollen from a different plant, as opposed to self-fertilization.

cross-hatch grid. See **crossed grid.**

crossing over, the exchange of sections of chromatids between homologous pairs of chromosomes during the prophase stage of the first meiotic division.

crossmatching of blood, a procedure used by blood banks to determine compatibility of a donor's blood with that of a recipient after the specimens have been matched for major blood type. Serum from the donor's blood is mixed with red cells from the recipient's blood, and cells from the donor are mixed with serum from the recipient. If agglutination occurs, an antigenic substance is present and the bloods are not compatible.

crossover, the result of the recombination of genes on homologous pairs of chromosomes during meiosis.

cross resistance, the resistance to a particular antibiotic that also results in resistance against a different antibiotic to which the bacteria may not have been exposed.

cross-sectional, (in statistics) pertaining to the comparative data of two groups of persons at one point in time.

cross-sectional anatomy, the study of the relationship of the structures of the body by the examination of cross sections of the tissue or organ.

cross sensitivity, a sensitivity to one substance that predisposes an individual to sensitivity to other substances that are related in chemical structure.

cross-sequential, (in statistics) pertaining to data that compare several cohorts at different points in time.

cross tolerance, a tolerance to other drugs that develops after exposure to only one agent. An example is the cross tolerance that develops between alcohol and barbiturates.

crotamiton, a scabicide prescribed in treating scabies and other pruritic skin diseases.

croup, an acute viral infection of the upper and lower respiratory tract that occurs pnmarily in infants and young children 3 months to 3 years of age after an upper respiratory tract infection. It is characterized by hoarseness, fever, a distinctive harsh, brassy cough, persistent stridor during inspiration, amd varying degrees of respiratory distress resulting from obstruction of the larynx. The most common causative agents are the parainfluenza viruses, especially type 1, followed by the respiratory syncytial viruses (RSV) and influenza A and B viruses. **croupous, croupy,** *adj.*

Croupette, a trademark for a device that provides cool humidification with the administration of oxygen or of compressed air, used especially in the treatment of paediatric patients. It consists of a nebulizer with attached tubing that connects with a canopy to enclose the patient and contain the humidifying mist.

crown, 1. the upper part of an organ or structure, such as the top of the head. **2.** the portion of a human tooth that is covered by enamel.

crowning, (in obstetrics) the phase at the end of labour in which the fetal head is seen at the introitus of the vagina. The labia are stretched in a crown around the head.

crown/root ratio, the relation of the clinical crown to the clinical root of a tooth.

CRP, abbreviation for **C-reactive protein**.

CRT, abbreviation for **cathode-ray tube**.

cruciate ligament of the atlas, a crosslike ligament attaching the atlas to the base of the occipital bone above and the posterior surface of the body of the axis below.

crude birth rate, the number of births per 1000 people in a population durng 1 year.

crura anthelicis, the two ridges on the external ear marking the superior termination of the anthelix and bounding the triangular fossa.

crural, pertaining to the leg, particularly the upper leg or thigh.

crureus. See **vastus intermedius**.

crus, *pl.* **crura, 1.** the leg, from knee to foot. **2.** a structure resembling a leg, such as crura anthelicis.

crus cerebri, the ventral part of the cerebral peduncle, composed of the descending fibre tracts passing from the cerebral cortex to form the longitudinal fascicles of the pons.

crush syndrome, 1. a severe, life-threatening condition caused by extensive crushing trauma, characterized by destruction of muscle and bone tissue, haemorrhage, and fluid loss resulting in hypovolaemic shock, haematuria, renal failure, and coma. **2.** a severe complication of heroin-induced coma characterized by oedema, vascular occlusion, and lymphatic obstruction.

crust, a solidified, hard outer layer formed by the drying of a bodily exudate, common in such dermatological conditions as eczema, impetigo, seborrhoea, and favus, and during the healing of burns and lesions; a scab.

crutch, a wooden or metal staff, the most common kind of which reaches from the ground almost to the axilla, to aid a person in walking. A padded, curved surface at the top fits under the arm; a grip in the form of a crossbar is held in the hand at the level of the palms to support the body. Kinds of crutches include **axillary crutches, forearm crutches**.

Crutchfield tongs {W. Gayle Crutchfield, American surgeon, b. 1900}, an instrument inserted into the skull to hyperextend the head and neck of patients with fractured cervical vertebrae. The tongs are inserted into small burr holes drilled in each parietal region of the skull; the surrounding skin is sutured and covered with a collodion dressing. A weight is suspended from a rope extending from the centre of the tongs, over a pulley attached to the bed head.

crutch gait, a gait achieved by a person on crutches by alternately bearing weight on one or both legs and on the crutches. In a three-point gait, weight is borne on the noninvolved leg, then on both crutches, then on the noninvolved leg. Four-point gait gives stability but requires bearing weight on both legs. Each leg is used alternately with each crutch. Two-point gait characteristically uses each crutch with the opposing leg. The swing-to and swing-through gaits are often used by paraplegic patients with weightsupporting braces on the legs. Weight is borne on the supported legs, the crutches are placed one stride in front of the person who then swings to that point or through the crutches to a spot in front of them.

crutch palsy, the temporary or permanent loss of sensation or muscle control resulting from pressure on the radial nerve by a crutch.

cry, 1. a sudden, loud, voluntary, or automatic vocalization in response to pain, fear, or a startle reflex. **2.** weeping, because of pain or as an emotional response to depression or grief. **3.** See **cat-cry syndrome**.

crying vital capacity, a measurement of the tidal volume while an infant is crying; may be valuable in monitoring infants with lung diseases that cause changes in functional residual capacity.

cryoanaesthesia, the freezing of a part to achieve adequate deadening of neural sensitivity to pain during brief minor surgical procedures.

cryocautery, the application of any substance, such as solid carbon dioxide, that destroys tissue by freezing.

cryogen, a chemical that induces freezing, used to destroy diseased tissue without injury to adjacent structures. Cell death is caused by dehydration. Kinds of cryogens include carbon dioxide, freon, liquid nitrogen, and nitrous oxide,   **cryogenic,** *adj.*

cryoglobulin, an abnormal plasma protein that precipitates and coalesces at low temperatures and dissolves and disperses at body temperature.

cryoglobulinaemia, an abnormal condition in which cryoglobulins are present in the blood.

cryonics, the techniques in which cold is applied for a variety of therapeutic goals, including brief local anaesthesia, destruction of superficial skin lesions. and preservation of cells, tissue, organs, or the entire body. **cryonic,** *adj.*

cryoprecipitate, 1. any precipitate formed upon cooling a solution. **2.** a preparation rich in factor VIII collected from fresh human plasma that has been frozen and thawed.

cryostat, a device used in surgical pathology that consists of a special microtome used for freezing and slicing sections of tissue for study by a surgical pathologist.

cryosurgery, use of subfreezing temperature to destroy tissue, such as in the destruction of the ganglion of nerve cells in the thalamus in the treatment of Parkinson's disease. The coolant is circulated through a metal probe, chilling it to as low as -160ºC, depending on the chemical used. The moist tissues adhere to the cold metal of the probe and freeze.

cryotherapy, a treatment using cold as a destructive medium for some common skin disorders. Solid carbon dioxide or liquid nitrogen is applied briefly with a sterile cotton-tipped applicator.

crypt, a blind pit or tube on a free surface. Some kinds of crypts are anal **crypt, dental crypt,** and **synovial crypt.**

cryptitis, an inflammation of a crypt, usually a perianal crypt, often accompanied by pain, pruritus, and spasm of the sphincter.

cryptocephalus, a malformed fetus that has a small, underdeveloped head. **cryptocephalic, cryptocephalons,** *adj.* **cryptocephaly,** *n.*

cryptococcosis, an infectious disease caused by a fungus. *Cryptococcus neoformans* which spreads through the lungs to the brain and central nervous system, skin, skeletal system, and urinary tract. Initial symptoms may include coughing or other respiratory effects because the lungs are a primary site of infection. After the fungus spreads to the meninges, neurological symptoms may develop, including headache, blurred vision, and difficulty in speaking.

Cryptococcus, a genus of yeastlike fungi that reproduces by budding rather than by producing spores. Certain pathogenic species exist of which *C. neoformans* is the most important.

Cryptococcus neoformans, a species of yeastlike fungus that causes cryptococcosis, a potentially fatal infection that can affect the lungs, skin, and brain.

cryptodidymus, conjoined twins in which one fetus is small, underdeveloped and concealed within the body of the other more fully formed autosite.

crypt of iris, any one of the small pits in the iris along its free margin encircled by the circulus arteriosus minor.

cryptomenorrhoea, an abnormal condition in which the products of menstruation are retained within the vagina because of an imperforate hymen, or, less often, within the uterus because of an occlusion of the cervical canal. **cryptomenorrhoeal,** *adj.*

cryptophthalmos, a developmental anomaly characterized by complete fusion of the eyelids, usually with defective formation or lack of the eyes.

cryptorchidism, failure of one or both of the testicles to descend into the scrotum.

cry reflex, a normal infantile reaction to pain, hunger, or need for attention. The reflex may be absent in an infant born prematurely or one in poor health.

crystal, a solid inorganic substance, the atoms or molecules of which are arranged in a regular, repeating three-dimensional pattern, which determines the shape of a crystal. **crystalline,** *adj.*

crystalline lens, a transparent structure of the eye, enclosed in a capsule, situated between the iris and the vitreous humour, and slightly overlapped at its margin by the ciliary processes. The capsule of the lens is a transparent, elastic membrane that touches the free border of the iris anteriorly and is secured by the suspensory ligament of the lens. The posterior surface is more convex than the anterior. It is composed of a soft, cortical material, a firm nucleus, and concentric laminae.

crystalloid, a substance in a solution that can be diffused through a semipermeable membrane.

crystalluria, the presence of crystals in the urine. The condition may be a source of urinary tract irritation.

Cs, symbol for **caesium.**

CSF, abbreviation for **cerebrospinal fluid.**

CSM, abbreviation for **Committee on the Safety of Medicines**

CSR, abbreviation for **Cheyne-Stokes respiration.**

CSP, abbreviation for **Chartered Soceity of Physiotherapy.**

CT, abbreviation for **computerized tomography.**

C3 nephritic factor, a C3 complement protein molecule that may be deposited in glomerular capillary walls and mesangial tissues, precipitating or contributing to local immune inflammatory injury and kidney damage.

Cu, symbol for **copper.**

cubital, pertaining to the elbow or the forearm.

cuboid bone, the cuboidal tarsal bone on the lateral side of the foot. It articulates with the calcaneus, lateral cuneiform, and fourth and fifth metatarsal bones.

cue, a stimulus that determines or may prompt

the nature of a person's response.

cuff, an inflatable elastic tube that is placed about the upper arm and expanded with air to restrict arterial circulation during blood pressure examination.

cuffed endotracheal tube, an endotracheal tube with a balloon at one end that may be inflated to tighten the fit of the tube in the lumen of the airway. The balloon forms a cuff that prevents gastric contents from passing into the lungs and gas from leaking back from the lungs.

cuirass, 1. a negative-pressure full body respirator. An electric driven pump is adjusted to match the timing of the patient's spontaneous breathing. **2.** a tightly fitted chest bandage.

cul-de-sac, *pl.* **culs-de-sac, cul-de-sacs,** a blind pouch or caecum, such as the conjunctival cul-de-sac and the dural cul-de-sac.

cul-de-sac of Douglas. See **pouch of Douglas.**

culdocentesis, the use of needle puncture or incision through the vagina to remove intraperitoneal fluid, including purulent material.

culdotomy, an incision or needle puncture of the pouch of Douglas by way of the vagina.

Culex, a genus of humpbacked mosquitoes. It includes species that transmit viral encephalitis and filariasis.

Cullen's sign {Thomas S. Cullen. American gynaecologist, b. 1868}, the appearance of faint, irregularly formed haemorrhagic patches on the skin around the umbilicus. It may appear 1 to 2 days after the onset of anorexia and the severe, poorly localized abdominal pains that are characteristic of acute pancreatitis.

cult, a specific complex of beliefs, rites, and ceremonies maintained by a group in association with some particular person or object.

cultural assimilation, a process by which members of an ethnic minority group lose cultural characteristics that distinguish them from the dominant cultural group.

cultural healer, a member of an ethnic or cultural group who uses traditional methods of healing rather than modern scientific methods to provide health care for other members of the group.

cultural relativism, a concept that health and normality emerge within a social context, and that the content and form of mental health will vary greatly from one culture to another.

culturally relativistic perspective, an ability to understand the behaviour of transcultural patients (those who move from one culture to another) within the context of their own culture.

culture, 1. (in microbiology) a laboratory test involving the cultivation of microorganisms or cells in a special growth medium. **2.** (in psychology) a set of learned values, beliefs, customs, and behaviour that is shared by a group of interacting individuals.

culture-bound, pertaining to a health condition that is specific to a particular culture, such as a belief in the effects of certain kinds of prayer or the "evil eye."

culture medium. See **medium**.

culture procedure, (in bacteriology) any of several techniques for growing colonies of microorganisms to identify a pathogen and to determine which antibiotics are effective in combatting the infection caused by the organism.

culture shock, the psychological effect of a drastic change in the cultural environment of an individual. The person may exhibit feelings of helplessness, discomfort, and disorientation in attempting to adapt to a different cultural group with dissimilar practices, values, and beliefs.

cumulative, increasing by incremental steps with an eventual total that may exceed the expected result.

cumulative action, 1. the increased activity of a therapeutic measure or agent when administered repeatedly. **2.** the increased activity demonstrated by a drug when repeated doses accumulate in the body and exert a greater biological effect than the initial dose.

cumulative dose, the total dose that accumulates from repeated exposure to radiation or a radiopharmaceutical product.

cumulative gene, See **polygene**.

cuneate, (of tissue) wedge-shaped, used especially in describing cells of the nervous system.

cuneiform, (of bone and cartilage) wedge-shaped.

cuneiform bone. See **triangular bone**.

cunnilingus, the oral stimulation of the female genitalia.

cup arthroplasty of the hip joint, the surgical replacement of the head of the femur by a metal or plastic mould to relieve pain and increase motion in arthritis or to correct a deformity. The damaged or diseased bone is removed under general anaesthesia, and the acetabulum and the head of the femur are reshaped. A metal Vitallium cup is inserted between the two and becomes the articulating surface of the femur. Postoperatively, the patient's leg is suspended in traction to hold it in a position of abduction and internal rotation to keep the cup in place. Continued abduction is necessary for 6 weeks. Possible complications include infection, thrombophlebitis, pulmonary embolism, and fat embolism. The patient receives extensive physiotherapy, crutches are necessary to avoid bearing of full weight for 6 months, and an exercise programme must be followed for several years.

cupping, a counterirritant technique of applying a suction device to the skin to draw blood to the surface of the body.

cupric, of or pertaining to copper in its divalent form, as cupric sulphate.

cupulolithiasis, a severe, long-lasting vertigo brought on by movement of the head to certain positions. There are many possible causes, among them otitis media, ear surgery, or injury to the inner ear. In addition to extreme dizziness, signs are nausea, vomiting, and ataxia.

curare, a substance derived from tropical plants of the genus Stryknos. It is a potent muscle relaxant that acts by preventing transmission of neural impulses across the myoneural junctions. Large dosage can cause complete paralysis, but action is usually reversible with anticholinergics.

curariform, 1. chemically similar to curare. **2.** having the effect of curare.

curative treatment. See **treatment.**

cure, 1. restoration to health of a person afflicted with a disease or other disorder. **2.** the favourable outcome of the treatment of a disease or other disorder. **3.** a course of therapy, a medication, a therapeutic measure, or another remedy used in treatment of a medical problem, such as faith healing, fasting, or rest cure.

curette, 1. a surgical instrument shaped like a spoon or scoop for scraping and removing material or tissue from an organ, cavity, or surface. **2.** to remove tissue or debris with such a device. A kind of curette is a Hartmann's curette.

curettage, scraping of material from the wall of a cavity or other surface, performed to remove tumours or other abnormal tissue or to obtain tissue for microscopic examination. Curettage also refers to clearing unwanted material from fistulas and areas of chronic infection.

curie (c, Ci) {Marie S. Curie. Polish-born chemist, b. 1867: Pierre Curie. French scientist. b. 1859}, a unit of radioactivity used before adoption of the becquerel (Bq) as the SI unit. It is equal to 3.70 x 1010 Bq.

curium (Cm) {Marie S. Curie: Pierre Curie}, a radioactive metallic element. Its atomic number is 96: its atomic weight is 247.

Curling's ulcer {Thomas B. Curling, English surgeon, b. 1811}, a duodenal ulcer that develops in people who have severe burns on the surface of the body.

current, 1. a flowing or streaming movement. **2.** a flow of electrons along a conductor in a closed circuit: an electric current. **3.** certain physiological electric activity and characteristics of blood circulation. Physiological currents include abnerval current, action current, axial current, centrifugal current, centripetal current, compensating current, demarcation current, and electrotonic current.

current of injury. See **demarcation current.**

curriculum vitae (CV), *pl.* **curricula vitae,** a summary of educational and professional experiences, including activities and honours, to be used in seeking employment, for biographical citations on professional meeting programmes, or for related purposes.

Curschmann spiral {Heinrich Curschmann, German physician, b. 1846}, one of the coiled fibrils of mucus occasionally found in the sputum of persons with bronchial asthma.

curvature myopia, a type of nearsightedness caused by retractive errors associated with an excessive curvature of the cornea.

curve, (in statistics) a straight or curved line used as a graphic method of demonstrating the distribution of data collected in a study or survey.

curve of Carus {Karl G. Carus, German physician, b. 17891}, the normal axis of the pelvic outlet.

curve of occlusion, 1. a curved occlusal surface that simultaneously contacts the major portion of the incisal and occlusal prominences of the existing teeth. **2.** the curve of dentition on whieh lie the occlusal surfaces of the teeth.

curve of Spee {Ferdinand Graf von Spee, German embryologist, b. 18551}, **1.** the anatomical curvature of the occlusal alignment of the teeth, beginning at the tip of the lower canine, following the buccal cusps of the natural premolars and molars, and continuing to the anterior border of the ramus. **2.** the curve of the occlusal surfaces of the arches in vertical dimension, produced by a downward dipping of the mandibular premolars. with a corresponding adjustment of the upper premolars.

curvilinear trend, (in statistics) a trend in which a graphic representation of the data yields a curved line.

cushingoid {Harvey W. Cushing, American surgeon, b. 1869}, having the habitus and facies characteristic of Cushing's disease: fat pads on the upper back and face, striae on the limbs and trunk, and excess hair on the face.

Cushing's disease {Harvey W. Cushing}, a metabolic disorder characterized by the abnormally increased secretion of adrenocortical steroids caused by increased amounts of adrenocorticotropic hormone (ACTH) secreted by the pituitary, such as by a pituitary adenoma. Excess adrenocortical hormones result in accumulations of fat on the chest, upper back, and face and in oedema, hyperglycaemia, increased gluconeogenesis, muscle weakness, purplish striae on the skin, decreased immunity to infection, osteoporosis with susceptibility to fracture of bones, acne, and facial hirsutism.

Cushing's syndrome {Harvey W. Cushing}, a metabolic disorder resulting from the chronic and excessive production of cortisol by the adrenal cortex or by the administration of glucocorticoids in large doses for several weeks or longer. When occurring spontaneously, the syndrome represents a failure in the body's ability to regulate the secretion of cortisol or adrenocorticotropic hormone (ACTH). (Normally cortisol is produced only in response to ACTH, and ACTH is not secreted in the presence of high levels of cortisol.) The most common cause of the syndrome is a pituitary tumour that causes an increased secretion of ACTH. The patient with Cushing's syndrome has a decreased glucose tolerance, central obesity, round "moon" face, supraclavicular fat pads, a pendulous, striae-covered pad of fat on the chest and abdomen, oligomenorrhoea or decreased testosterone levels, muscular atrophy, oedema, hypokalaemia, and some degree of emotional change. The skin may be abnormally pigmented and fragile; minor infections may become systemic and longlasting.

cusp, 1. a sharp projection or a rounded eminence that rises from the chewing surface of a tooth, such as the two pyramidal cusps that arise from the premolars. **2.** any one of the small flaps on the valves of the heart, as the ventral, dorsal, and medial cusps attached to the right atrioventricular valve.

cuspid valve. See **atrioventricular valve.**

cuspless tooth, a tooth without cuspal prominences on its masticatory surface.

cut, (in molecular genetics) a fissure or split in a double strand of DNA in contrast to a nick in a single strand.

cutaneous, of or pertaining to the skin.

cutaneous absorption, the taking up of substances through the skin.

cutaneous anaphylaxis, a localized, exaggerated reaction of hypersensitivity in the form of a wheal and flare caused by an antigen injected into the skin of a sensitized individual, generally used as a test of sensitivity to various allergens.

cutaneous emphysema. See **subcutaneous emphysema.**

cutaneous horn, a hard, skin-coloured projection of the epidermis, usually on the head or face. The lesion may be precancerous and is usually excised.

cutaneous larva migrans, a skin condition caused by a hookworm, Ancylostoma braziliense, a parasite of cats and dogs. Its ova are deposited in the ground with the faeces of infected animals, develop into larvae, and invade the skin of people, particularly bare feet, but any skin may be involved. Secondary infections often occur if the skin has been broken by scratching.

cutaneous lupus erythematosus. See **discoid lupus erythematosus.**

cutaneous membrane. See **skin.**

cutaneous papilloma, a small brown or flesh-coloured outgrowth of skin, occurring most frequently on the neck of an older person.

cutdown, an incision into a vein with insertion of a polyethylene catheter for intravenous infusion. It is performed when an infusion cannot be started by venipuncture and in hyperalimentation therapy, when highly concentrated solutions are given via catheter into the superior vena cava.

cuticle, 1. epidermis. **2.** the sheath of a hair follicle. **3.** the thin edge of cornified epithelium at the base of a nail.

cutis. See **skin.**

cutis laxa, abnormally loose, relaxed skin resulting from an absence of elastic fibres in the body, usually a hereditary condition.

cutis marmorata. See **livedo.**

cuvette, a small transparent tube or container with specific optical properties that is used in laboratory research and analyses, such as photometric evaluations, colourimetric determinations, and turbidity studies.

CVA, abbreviation for **cerebrovascular accident.**

CVP, abbreviation for **central venous pressure.**

cyanide poisoning, poisoning resulting from the ingestion or inhalation of cyanide from such substances as bitter almond oil, prussic acid, hydrocyanic acid, or potassium or sodium cyanide. Characterized by tachycardia, drowsiness, convulsion, and headache, cyanide poisoning may result in death within 1 to 15 minutes.

cyanocobalamin, a red, crystalline. water-soluble substance with activity similar to that of vitamin B_{12}. It is involved in the metabolism of protein, fats, and carbohydrates, normal blood formation, and neural function. Deficiency is usually caused by the absence of intrinsic factor, which is necessary for the absorption of cyanocobalamin from the GI tract and which results in pernicious anaemia and brain damage. Symptoms of deficiency include nervousness, neuritis, numbness and tingling in the hands and feet, poor muscular coordination, unpleasant body odour, and menstrual disturbances.

cyanogenetic glycosides, chemical compounds contained in foods that release hydrogen cyanide when chewed or digested. This disrupts the structure of the substances, causing cyanide to be released. Although human poisoning from cyanogenetic glycosides is rare, cases have been reported of cyanide poisoning from certain varieties of lima beans, cassava, and bitter almonds.

cyanomethaemoglobin, a haemoglobin derivative formed during nitrite therapy for cyanide poisoning.

cyanosis, bluish discolouration of the skin and mucous membranes caused by an excess of deoxygenated haemoglobin in the blood or a structural defect in the haemoglobin molecule, such as in methaemoglobin. **cyanotic,** *adj.*

cyanotic congenital defect, a congenital heart defect that allows the mixing of unsaturated (venous) blood with saturated (arterial) blood to produce cyanosis.

cyclacillin, a penicillin antibiotic prescribed in the treatment of certain bacterial infections.

cyclamate, an artificial, non nutritive sweetener formerly used in the form of calcium or sodium salt.

cyclandelate, a vasodilator prescribed in the treatment of muscular ischaemia and peripheral vascular obstruction or spasm.

cyclencephaly, a developmental anomaly characterized by the fusion of the two cerebral hemispheres. **cyclencephalic, cyclencephalous,** *adj.* **cyclencephalus,** *n.*

cyclic adenosine monophosphate (cAMP), a cyclic nucleotide formed from adenosine triphosphate by the action of adenyl cyclase. This cyclic compound, known as the ''second messenger,'' participates in the action of catecholamines, vasopressin, adrenocorticotropic hormone, and many other hormones.

cyclic guanosine monophosphate (cGMP), a substance that mediates the action of certain hormones in a manner similar to that of cyclic adenosine monophosphate (cAMP).

cyclic tube feeding, delivery of nutrients by tube into the stomach, duodenum or jejunum. Feeding is controlled by an enteral feeding pump to provide the volume of feed required in 24 hours, allowing for several breaks to be incorporated during that period of time.

cyclitis, inflammation of the ciliary body causing redness of the sclera adjacent to the cornea of the eye.

cyclizine hydrochloride, cyclizine lactate, antihistamines used in the treatment or prevention of motion sickness, labyrinth disorders, and nausea and vomiting.

cyclobenzaprine hydrochloride, a muscle relaxant used in the short-term treatment of muscle spasm.

cyclocephalic, cyclocephalous, cyclocephaly. See **cyclopia**.

cyclomethycaine sulphate, a local anaesthetic agent for use on nontraumatized mucous membranes before clinical examination or instrumentation.

cyclophosphamide, an alkylating agent used in the treatment of a variety of neoplasms and as an immunosuppressant in organ transplants.

cyclopia, a developmental anomaly characterized by fusion of the orbits into a single cavity containing one eye.

cycloplegia, paralysis of the ciliary muscles, as induced by certain ophthalmic drugs to allow examination of the eye.

cycloplegic, 1. of or pertaining to a drug or treatment that causes paralysis of the ciliary muscles of the eye. **2.** one of a group of anticholinergic drugs used to paralyse the ciliary muscles of the eye for ophthalmological examination or surgery. Any of the cycloplegics may cause adverse effects in persons sensitive to anticholinergics.

cyclopropane, a highly flammable and explosive potent anaesthetic gas. It is now used for anaesthesia only when characteristics of other anaesthetic agents contraindicate their use in a specific patient.

cycloserine, an antitubercular used in the treatment of tuberculosis resistant to first-line treatment.

cyclosporin, any of a group of biologically active metabolites of *Tolypocladium inflarum Gams* and certain other fungi. The major forms are cyclosporin A and cyclosporin C, which are cyclic oligopeptides with immunosuppressive, antifungal, and antipyretic effects. As immunosuppressants, cyclosporins affect primarily the T cell lymphocytes.

cyclosporine, an alternative term for cyclosporin A.

cyclothymic disorder, a mild form of bipolar disorder.

cyclothymic personality, a personality characterized by extreme swings in mood from elation to depression.

cyclotomy, a surgical procedure for the correction of a defect in the ciliary muscle of the eye.

cyclotron, a device used to accelerate charged particles or ions. It may be used to produce a high-energy beam of protons or neutrons for external beam radiotherapy, or to manufacture radioisotopes.

cylindrical grasp, the normal position of the hand and fingers when holding cylindrical objects, such as a glass tumbler. The fingers close around the object, which is stabilized against the palm of the hand. It occurs as a reflex action in infants and later is developed into a voluntary gross grasp.

cylindroma, *pl.* **cylindromas, cylindromata, 1.** See adenocystic carcinoma. **2.** a benign neoplasm of the skin, usually of the scalp or face, developing from a hair follicle or sweat gland.

cylindromatous carcinoma. See **adenocystic carcinoma**.

cylindromatous spiradenoma. See **cylindroma**.

cypionate, a contraction for cyclopentanepropionate.

cyproheptadine hydrochloride, an antihistamine with antiserotonergic properties used in the treatment of a variety of hypersensitivity reactions, including rhinitis, skin rash, and pruritus, and in the prophylaxis of resistant cases of migraine.

Cyprus fever. See **brucellosis**.

Cys, abbreviation for **cysteine**.

cyst, a closed sac in or under the skin lined with epithelium and containing fluid or semisolid material, as a sebaceous cyst.

cystadenocarcinoma, a pancreatic tumour that evolves from a mucous cystadenoma. Clinical features include epigastric pain and a palpable abdominal mass.

cystadenoma, *pl.* **cystadenomas, cystadenomata, 1.** an adenoma associated with a cystoma. **2.** an adenoma containing multiple cystic structures.

cystathioninaemia, an inherited metabolic disorder caused by a deficiency of the enzyme cystathionase. It results in an excess of the amino acid methionine. Some patients may be asymptomatic, whereas others show signs of mental retardation.

cystectomy, a surgical procedure in which all or a part of the bladder is removed, as may be required in treating cancer of the bladder.

cysteine (Cys), a nonessential amino acid found in many proteins in the body, including keratin. It is a metabolic precursor of cystine and an important source of sulphur for various body functions.

cystic acne. See **acne conglobata**.

cystic carcinoma, a malignant neoplasm containing cysts or cystlike spaces. Tumours of this kind occur in the breast and ovary.

cystic duct, the duct through which bile from the gallbladder passes into the common bile duct.

cysticercosis, an infection and infestation by the larval stage of the pork tapeworm Taenia solium or the beef tapeworm T. saginata. The eggs are ingested and hatch in the intestine; the larvae invade the subcutaneous tissue, brain, eye, muscle, heart, liver, lung, and peritoneum. The invasive, early phase of the infection is characterized by fever, malaise, muscle pain, and eosinophilia. Epilepsy and personality change may appear if the brain is affected.

cysticercus, a larval form of tapeworm. It consists of a single scolex enclosed in a bladderlike cyst.

cystic fibroma, a fibrous tumour in which cystic degeneration has occurred.

cystic fibrosis, an inherited disorder of the exocrine glands, causing those glands to produce abnormally thick secretions of mucus, elevation of sweat electrolytes, increased organic and enzymatic constituents of saliva, and overactivity of the autonomic nervous system. The glands most affected are those in the pancreas, the respiratory system, and the sweat glands. Cystic fibrosis is usually recognized in infancy or early childhood. When present in infancy, the earliest manifestation is meconium ileus, an obstruction of the small bowel by viscid stool. Other early signs are a chronic cough, frequent, foul smelling stools, and persistent upper respiratory infections. The most reliable diagnostic tool is the sweat test, which shows elevations of both sodium and chloride.

cystic goitre, an enlargement of the thyroid gland containing cysts resulting from mucoid or colloid degeneration.

cystic lymphangioma, a cystic growth formed by lymph vessels: usually congenital, it most frequently occurs in the neck, axilla, or groin of children.

cystic mole. See **hydatid mole**.

cystic myxoma, a tumour of the connective tissue that has undergone cystic degeneration.

cystic neuroma, a neoplasm of nerve tissue that has degenerated and become cystic.

cystic tumour, a tumour with cavities or sacs containing a semisolid or a liquid material.

cystine, a nonessential amino acid found in many proteins in the body, including keratin and insulin. Cystine is a product of the oxidation of two cysteine molecules.

cystinosis, a congenital disease characterized by glucosuria, proteinuria, cystine deposits in the liver, spleen, bone marrow, and cornea, rickets, excessive amounts of phosphates in the urine, and retardation of growth.

cystinuria, 1. abnormal presence in the urine of the amino acid cystine. **2.** an inherited defect of the renal tubules, characterized by excessive urinary excretion of cystine and several other amino acids. In high concentration, cystine tends to precipitate in the urinary tract and form kidney or bladder stones.

cystitis, an inflammatory condition of the urinary bladder and ureters, characterized by pain, urgency and freguency of urination, and haematuria. It may be caused by a bacterial infection, calculus or tumour.

cystocele, protrusion of the urinary bladder through the wall of the vagina, in hernia.

cystography, a radiographic visualization of the urinary bladder, usually a part of intravenous urography.   **cystogram,** *n.*

cystolith. See **vesicle calculus**.

cystoma, *pl.* **cystomas, cystomata,** any tumour or growth containing cysts, especially one in or near the ovary.

cystometry, the study of bladder function by use of a cystometer, an instrument that measures capacity in relation to changing pressure. The urological procedure, cystometrography, measures the amount of pressure exerted on the bladder at varying degrees of capacity. The results of the measurements are traced graphically on a cystometogram.

cystosarcoma phyllodes, a benign breast tumour that grows rapidly and tends to recur if not adequately excised.

cystoscope, an instrument for examining and treating lesions of the urinary bladder, ureter, and kidney. It consists of an outer sheath with a lighting system. a viewing obturator, and a passage for catheters and operative devices.

cystoscopy, the direct visualization of the urinary tract by means of a cystoscope inserted in the urethra. For the examination the bladder is distended with air or water and the patient is in a fasting state. **cystoscopic,** *adj.*

cystourethrogram. See **intravenous urography.**

cytarabine, a cytotoxic antimetabolite used in the treatment of acute and chronic myelocytic leukaemia, acute lymphocytic leukaemia, and erythroleukaemia.

cytoarchitectonic, pertaining to the cellular arrangement within a tissue or structure.

cytoarchitecture, the typical pattern of cellular arrangement within a particular tissue or organ, as in the cerebral cortex. **cytoarchitectural,** *adj.*

cytobiotaxis. See **cytoclesis.**

cytoblast, obsolete. the nucleus of a cell.

cytocentrum. See **centrosome.**

cytocerastic. See **cytokerastic.**

cytochemism, the chemical activity within the living cell, specifically the various reactions to and affinity for chemical substances.

cytochemistry, the study of the various chemicals within a living cell and their actions and functions.

cytocide, any substance that is destructive to cells. **cytocidal,** *adj.*

cytoclesis, the influence exerted by one cell on the action of other cells; the vital principle of all living tissue.

cytoctony, the destruction of cells, specifically the killing of cells in culture by viruses.

cytode, the simplest type of cell, consisting of a protoplasmic mass without a nucleus, such as a bacterium.

cytodieresis, *pl.* cytodiereses, cell division, especially the phenomena involving the division of the cytoplasm. **cytodieretic,** *adj.*

cytodifferentiation, 1. a process by which embryonic cells acquire biochemical and morphological properties essential for specialization and diversification. **2.** the total and gradual transformation from an undifferentiated to a fully differentiated state.

cytogene, a particle within the cytoplasm of a cell that is self-replicating, derived from the genes in the nucleus, and capable of transmitting hereditary information.

cytogenesis, the origin, development, and differentiation of cells. **cytogenetic, cytogenic,** *adj.*

cytogeneticist, one who specializes in cytogenetics.

cytogenetics, the branch of genetics that studies the cellular constituents concerned with heredity, primarily the structure, function, and origin of the chromosomes. One kind of cytogenetics is clinical cytogenetics. **cytogenetic,** *adj.*

cytogenic gland, a glandular organ that secretes living cells, specifically the testes and ovary.

cytogenic reproduction, the formation of a new organism from a unicellular germ cell, either sexually through the fusion of gametes to form a zygote or asexually by means of spores.

cytogenics. See **cytogenetics.**

cytogeny, 1. cytogenetics. **2.** the origin and development of the cell. **cytogenic, cytogenous,** *adj.*

cytogony, cytogenic reproduction.

cytohistogenesis, the structural development and formation of cells. **cytohistogenetic,** *adj.*

cytohyaloplasm. See **hyaloplasm.**

cytoid, like or resembling a cell.

cytoid body, a small white spot on the retina of each eye that is seen by using an ophthalmoscope in examining the eyes of a patient affected with systemic lupus erythematosus.

cytokerastic, pertaining to or characteristic of cellular development from a lower to a higher form or from a simple to more complex arrangement. Also **cytocerastic.**

cytokinesis, the division of the cytoplasm, exclusive of nuclear division, that occurs during the final stages of mitosis and meiosis to form daughter cells: the total of all the changes that occur in the cytoplasm during mitosis, meiosis, and fertilization. **cytokinetic,** *adj.*

cytokine, any of a group of peptides and glycopeptides released by cells of the immune system to influence other cells in the system. Many of these have now been synthesised such as interleukin II and interferons, and used for their immunodulatory and cytotoxic actions.

cytological map, the graphic representation of the location of genes on a chromosome, based on correlating genetic recombination test-crossing results with the structural analysis of chromosomes that have undergone such changes as deletions or translocations as detected by banding techniques. cytological sputum examination, a microscopic examination of a specimen of bronchial secretions, including a search for cells that may be cancerous or otherwise abnormal.

cytologist, one who specializes in the study of cells, specifically one who uses cytological techniques in the differential diagnosis of neoplasms.

cytology, the study of cells, including their formation, origin, structure, function, biochemical activities, and pathology. Kinds of cytology are aspiration biopsy cytology and exfoliative cytology. **cytologic, cytological,** *adj.*

cytolymph. See **hyaloplasm.**

cytolysin, an antibody that dissolves antigenic cells. Kinds of cytolysin are bacteriolysin and haemolysin.

cytolysis, *pl.* cytolyses, the destruction or breakdown of the living cell, primarily by the disintegration of the outer membrane. A kind of cytolysis is immune cytolysis. **cytolytic,** *adj.*

cytomegalic inclusion disease (CID), a viral infection caused by the cytomegalovirus (CMV), a virus related to the herpesviruses, characterized by malaise, fever, lymphadenopathy, pneumonia, hepatosplenomegaly, and superinfection with various bacteria and fungi as a result of the depression of immune response characteristic of herpesviruses. It is primarily a congenitally acquired disease of newborn infants, transmitted in utero from the mother to the fetus. Results may range from spontaneous abortion or fatal neonatal illness to birth of a normal infant.

cytomegalovirus (CMV), a member of a group of large species specific herpes-type viruses with a wide variety of disease effects.

cytomegalovirus disease. See cytomegalic inclusion disease.

cytometer, a device for counting and measuring the number of cells within a given amount of fluid, as blood, urine, or cerebrospinal fluid.

cytometry, the counting and measuring of cells, specifically blood cells. **cytometric,** *adj.*

cytomitome, the fibrillary network within the cytoplasm of a cell, as contrasted with that in the nucleoplasm.

cytomorphology, the study of the various forms of cells and the structures contained within them. **cytomorphologic, cytomorphological,** *adj.* **cytomorphologist,** *n.*

cytomorphosis, *pl.* cytomorphoses, the various changes that occur within a cell during the course of its life cycle.

cyton, the cell body of a neuron or that portion containing the nucleus and its surrounding cytoplasm from which the axon and dendrites are formed.

cytophoresis, 1. a therapeutic technique that uses the principle of centrifugation to remove red or white blood cells or platelets from patients with certain blood disorders. **2.** a laboratory procedure for separating specific components, such as white blood cells or platelets, from donor blood by centrifugation.

cytophotometer, an instrument for measuring light density through stained portions of cytoplasm, used for locating and identifying chemical substances within cells.

cytophotometry, the identification of chemical substances within cells, using a cytophotometer.

cytophysiology, the study of the biochemical processes involved in the functioning of an individual cell, as contrasted with the functioning of organs or tissues. **cytophysiologic, cytophysiological,** *adj.,* **cytophysiologist,** *n.*

cytoplasm, all of the substance of a cell other than the nucleus.

cytoplasmic bridge. See **intercellular bridge.**

cytoplasmic inheritance, the acquisition of traits or conditions controlled by self-replicating substances within the cytoplasm, as mitochondria or chloroplasts, rather than by the genes. The phenomenon occurs in plants and lower animals but has not yet been demonstrated in humans.

cytosine, a major pyrimidine base found in nucleotides and a fundamental constituent of DNA and RNA. In free or uncombined form it occurs in trace amounts in most cells.

cytosine arabinoside. See cytarabine.

cytoskeleton, the cytoplasmic elements, including the tonofibrils, keratin, and other microfibrils, that function as a supportive system within a cell, especially an epithelial cell.

cytosome, a multilayered membrane-bound lamellar body found in type II pneumocytes. It is a precursor of pulmonary surfactant.

cytotoxic, pertaining to a pharmacological compound or other agent that destroys or damages tissue cells.

cytotoxic anaphylaxis, an exaggerated hypersensitivity reaction to an injection of antibodies specific for antigenic substances that occur normally on surfaces of body cells.

cytotoxic drug, any pharmacological compound that inhibits the proliferation of cells within the body. Such compounds as the alkylating agents and the antimetabolites are designed to destroy abnormal cells selectively; they are commonly used in chemotherapy.

cytotoxic hypersensitivity, an IgG or an IgM complement-dependent, immediate-acting hypersensitive humoral response to foreign cells or to alterations of surface antigens on the cells.

cytotoxin, a substance that has a toxic effect on certain cells. An antibody may act as a cytotoxin. **cytotoxic,** *adj.*

cytotrophoblast, the inner layer of cells of the trophoblast of the early mammalian embryo that gives rise to the outer surface and villi of the chorion. **cytotrophoblastic,** *adj.*

CY-VA-DIC, an anticancer drug combination of cyclophosphamide, vincristine, doxorubicin, and dacarbazine.

D

D, 1. symbol for dead space gas. **2.** symbol for **diffusing capacity**. **3.** abbreviation for **dioptre**. **4.** abbreviation for *dexter*, meaning "right."

DA, abbreviation for **developmental age**.

dacarbazine, a cytotoxic alkylating agent used primarily in the treatment of malignant melanoma and Hodgkin's disease.

D/A converter. See **digital-to-analogue converter**.

Dacron cuff, a sheath of Dacron surrounding an atrial or venous catheter to prevent ascending infections and accidental displacement of the catheter.

dacryoadenitis, an inflammation of the lacrimal gland.

dacryocyst, a lacrimal sac at the medial angle of the eye, a normal anatomical feature.

dacryocystectomy, partial or total excision of the lacrimal sac.

dacryocystitis, an infection of the lacrimal sac caused by obstruction of the nasolacrimal duct, characterized by tearing and discharge from the eye.

dacryocystorhinostomy, a surgical procedure for restoring drainage into the nose from the lacrimal sac when the nasolacrimal duct is obstructed.

dacryostenosis, an abnormal stricture of the nasolacrimal duct, occurring either as a congenital condition or as a result of infection or trauma. Dacryocystorhinostomy may be required to correct this condition.

dactinomycin, a cytotoxic antibiotic used in the treatment of a variety of malignant diseases, including Wilms' tumour and rhabdomyosarcoma in children. *Also:* **actinomycin D**.

dactyl, a digit (finger or toe).   **dactylic,** *adj.*

dactylitis, a painful inflammation of the fingers or toes, usually associated with sickle cell anaemia or certain infectious diseases, particularly syphilis or tuberculosis.

daily adjusted progressive resistance exercise (DAPRE), a programme of isotonic exercises that allows for individual differences in the rate at which a patient regains strength in an injured or diseased body part.

Dakin's solution {Henry D. Dakin, American biochemist, b. 1880}, an antiseptic solution containing boric acid and sodium hypochlorite.

daltonism {John Dalton, English chemist, b. 1766}, *informal.* a form of red-green colour blindness. It is genetically transmitted as a sex-linked autosomal recessive trait.

Dalton's law of partial pressures John

Dalton, (in physics) a law stating that the sum of the pressure exerted by a mixture of gases is equal to the total of the partial pressures that could be exerted by the gases if they were separated.

damp, a potentially lethal atmosphere in caves and mines. **Black damp** or **choke damp** is caused by absorption of the available oxygen by coal seams. **Fire damp** is composed of methane and other explosive hydrocarbon gases. **White damp** is another name for carbon monoxide.

damping, (in cardiology) pertaining to a diminishing of the amplitude of a series of waves or oscillations and eventual arrest of any fluctuations.

danazol, a drug with androgenic, anti-oestrogenic and antiprogesteronic activities, that acts to suppress the output of gonadotropins from the pituitary. It is used in the treatment of endometriosis.

dance reflex, a normal response in the neonate to simulate walking by a reciprocal flexion and extension of the legs when held in an erect position with the soles touching a hard surface.

dance therapy, (in psychology) the use of rhythmic body movements or dance to release expression of feelings.

dander, dry scales shed from the skin or hair of animals or feathers of birds that may cause an allergic reaction in some individuals.

dandruff, an excessive amount of scaly material composed of dead, keratinized epithelium shed from the scalp that may be a mild form of seborrhoeic dermatitis. Treatment with a keratolytic shampoo is usually recommended.

Dandy-Walker cyst {Walter E. Dandy, American neurosurgeon, b. 1886; Arthur E. Walker, American surgeon, b. 1907}, a cystic malformation of the fourth ventricle of the brain, resulting from hydrocephalus.

danthron, a stimulant laxative prescribed in the treatment of constipation, usually in combination with the surface active agent poloxamer '188' in co-danthromer.

dantrolene sodium, a skeletal muscle relaxant prescribed in the treatment of severe muscle spasticity and malignant hyperthermia.

DAPRE, abbreviation for **daily adjusted progressive resistance exercise**.

dapsone (DADPS), a sulfone derivative used in the treatment of leprosy and dermatitis herpetiformis.

Darier's disease. See **keratosis follicularis.**

dark adaptation, a normal increase in sensitivity of the retinal rod cells of the eye to detect any light that may be available for vision in a dimly lit environment. The process is accompanied by an adjustment of the pupils to allow more light to enter the eyes.

darkfield microscopy, examination with a darkfield microscope, in which the specimen is illuminated by a peripheral light source. Organisms in specimens that have been prepared for use with a darkfield microscope appear to glow against a dark background.

darkroom, a room designed to exclude white light but providing safe lighting to enable the handling of unprocessed, light-sensitive photographic and x-ray film.

darwinian reflex. See **grasp reflex.**

darwinian theory {Charles R. Darwin, English naturalist, b. 1809}, the theory postulated by Charles Darwin that organic evolution results from the process of natural selection of those variants of plants and animals best suited to survive in their environmental surroundings. **darwinian,** *adj.*, *n. Also:* **darwinism.**

DASE, abbreviation for **Denver Articulation Screening Examination.**

data, *sing.* **datum, 1.** pieces of information, especially those that are part of a collection of information to be used in an analysis of a problem, such as the diagnosis of a health problem. **2.** information stored and processed by a computer.

data analysis, (in research) the phase of a study that includes classifying, coding, and tabulating information needed to perform statistic or qualitative analyses according to the research design and appropriate to the data.

data base, a large store or bank of information, especially in a form that can be processed by computer.

data base management systems (DBMS), a set of computer programmes written to aid a user in the storage and retrieval of large amounts of related information.

data collection, (in research) the phase of a study that includes the gathering of information and identification of sampling units as directed by the research design.

data clustering, the grouping of related information from the patient's health history, physical examination, and laboratory results as part of the process of making a diagnosis.

data retrieval, the recovery of information from an organized filing system, such as a computer data base, index card file, or colour-coded record folders.

data processing, the techniques and practices involved in the manipulation of information by a computer.

datum. See **data.**

daughter chromosome, either of the paired chromatids that during the anaphase stage of mitosis separate and migrate to opposite ends of the cell before division. Each contains the complete genetic information of the original chromosome.

daughter element, an element that results from the radioactive decay of a parent element. An example is technetium 99, which is the daughter element created by the decay of an atom of molybdenum 99.

daughter product. See **decay product.**

daunorubicin hydrochloride, a cytotoxic anthracycline antibiotic prescribed in the treatment of cancer, particularly leukaemia.

Davidson regimen {Edward C. Davidson, American physician}, b. 1894 , a method of treating chronic constipation in children, of developing regular bowel habits, and of identifying those with functional bowel disease or obstructive disorders. The child is then given mineral oil in increasing doses, until four or five loose bowel movements occur daily. Some children, especially those under 2 years of age, require supplemental, fat-soluble vitamins to maintain proper nutrition. The child is placed on a potty-chair at a specific time each day for 5 to 15 minutes; as regular habits develop, the mineral oil is gradually withdrawn over a period of several weeks.

day blindness. See **hemeralopia.**

daydream, a usually non-pathological reverie that occurs while a patient is awake. The content is usually the fulfilment of wishes that are not disguised, and fulfilment is imagined as direct. .

day health care services, the provision of hospitals, nursing homes, or other facilities for health-related services to adult patients who are ambulatory or can be transported and who regularly use such services for a certain number of daytime hours but do not require continuous in-patient care.

day hospital, a psychiatric facility that offers a therapeutic programme during daytime hours for formerly institutionalised patients.

daylight processing, automatic method of removing an x-ray film from a cassette and feeding it into an automatic film processor without requiring a darkroom.

day patient. See **in-patient.**

day sight. See **nyctalopia.**

dB, abbreviation for **decibel.**

DC, abbreviation for **direct current.**

D & C, abbreviation for **dilatation and curettage.**

DDT (dichlorodiphenyltrichloroethane), a non-degradable, water-insoluble, chlorinated hydrocarbon once used worldwide as a major insecticide, especially in agriculture. In recent years, knowledge of its adverse impact on the environment has led to restrictions in its use.

DDT poisoning. See **chlorinated organic insecticide poisoning.**

dead-end host, any animal from which a parasite cannot escape to continue its life cycle. Humans are dead-end hosts for trichinosis, because the larvae encyst in muscle and human flesh is unlikely to be a source of food for other animals susceptible to this parasite.

dead space, 1. a cavity that remains after the incomplete closure of a surgical or traumatic wound, leaving an area in which blood can collect and delay healing. **2.** the amount of lung in contact with ventilating gases but not in contact with pulmonary blood flow. **Alveolar dead space** refers to alveoli that are ventilated by the pulmonary circulation but are not perfused. The condition may exist when pulmonary circulation is obstructed, such as by a thromboembolus. **Anatomical dead space** is an area in the trachea, bronchi, and air passages containing air that does not reach the alveoli during respiration. As a general rule, the volume of air in the anatomical dead space in millilitres is approximately equal to the weight in pounds of the involved individual. Certain lung disorders, such as emphysema, increase the amount of anatomical dead space. **Physiological dead space** is an area in the respiratory system that includes the anatomical dead space together with the space in the alveoli occupied by air that does not contribute to the oxygen-carbon dioxide exchange.

dead space effect, any of several potential adverse effects of dead space resulting from mechanical ventilation, particularly when there is alveolar dead space. In hospitalized patients, this can be responsible for producing hypoxaemia and hypercarbia. A pulmonary embolism can also produce a dead space effect; blood flow in the pulmonary arteries is reduced without impeding ventilation.

deaf, 1. unable to hear; hard of hearing. **2.** people who are unable to hear or who suffer hearing impairment.   **deafness,** *n.*

deaf-mute, a person who is unable to hear or speak because of disability of the brain or the organs of hearing and speech.

deafness, a condition characterized by a partial or complete loss of hearing. In assessing deafness, the patient's ears are examined for drainage, crusts, accumulation of cerumen, or structural abnormality. It is determined if the deafness is conductive or sensory, temporary or permanent, and congenital or acquired in childhood, adolescence, or adulthood. The effect of ageing, when applicable, is evaluated, and a psychosocial assessment is conducted to ascertain if the individual is well adjusted to deafness or reacts to the handicap with fear, anxiety, frustration, depression, anger or hostility. In all cases, the degree of loss and the kind of impairment causing the loss are determined.

deaminase, an enzyme that catalyses the hy-

drolysis of the NH_2 bond in amino compounds. The enzymes are usually named according to the substrate, such as adenosine deaminase, or guanosine deaminase.

deamination, the removal, usually by hydrolysis, of the NH_2 radical from an amino compound.

death, 1. apparent death, the cessation of life as indicated by the absence of heartbeat or respiration. **2. legal death,** the total absence of activity in the brain and central nervous system, the cardiovascular system, and the respiratory system as observed and declared by a doctor.

death instinct, instinctive behaviour that tends to be self-destructive.

death rate, the number of deaths occurring within a specified population during a particular time period, usually expressed in terms of deaths per 1000 persons per year.

death rattle, a sound produced by air moving through mucus that has accumulated in the throat of a dying person after loss of the cough reflex.

death trance, a state in which a person appears to be dead.

debilitating, pertaining to a disease or injury that enfeebles, weakens, or otherwise disables a person.

debility, feebleness, weakness, or loss of strength.

debride, to remove dirt, foreign objects, damaged tissue and cellular debris from a wound or a burn, so as to prevent infection and promote healing. In treating a wound, debridement is the first step in cleansing it. **debridement,** *n.*

debris, the dead, diseased, or damaged tissue and any foreign material that is to be removed from a wound or other area being treated.

decalcification, loss of calcium salts from the teeth and bones caused by malnutrition, malabsorption, or other dietary or physiological factors. It may result from a diet that lacks adequate calcium. Malabsorption may be caused by a lack of vitamin D necessary for the absorption of calcium from the intestine, by an excess of dietary fats that can combine with calcium, by the presence of oxalic acid that can combine with calcium, or by a relative lack of acid in the digestive tract. Other factors include the parathyroid hormone control of the calcium level in the bloodstream, the ratio of calcium to phosphorus in the blood, and the relative activity of osteoblast cells that form calcium deposits in the bones and teeth and osteoclast cells that absorb calcium from bones and teeth.

decanoic acid. See **capric acid.**

decay product, a stable or radioactive nuclide formed directly from the radioactive disintegration of a radionuclide or as a result of successive transformation in a radioactive series.

deceleration, a decrease in the speed or velocity of an object or reaction.

decerebrate posture, the position of a patient, who is usually comatose, in which the arms are extended and internally rotated and the legs are extended with the feet in forced plantar flexion. The posture is usually observed in patients afflicted by compression of the brainstem at a low level.

decibel (dB) {Alexander G. Bell}, a unit of measure of the intensity of sound. A decibel is one-tenth of 1 bel; an increase of 1 bel is perceived as an approximate doubling of loudness, based on a sound-pressure reference level of 0.0002 dyn/cc.

decidua, the epithelial tissue of the endometrium lining the uterus. It envelops the conceptus during gestation and is shed in the puerperium. It is also shed periodically during menstruation.

decidua basalis, the decidua of the endometrium in the uterus that lies beneath the implanted ovum.

decidua capsularis, the decidua of the endometrium of the uterus covering the implanted ovum.

decidua menstrualis, the endometrium shed during menstruation.

decidua parietalis. See **decidua vera**.

decidua vera, the decidua of the endometrium lining the uterus except for those areas beneath and above the implanted and developing ovum, called, respectively, decidua basalis and decidua capsularis.

decidual endometritis, an inflammation or infection of any portion of the decidua during pregnancy.

deciduoma, a tumour of the endometrial tissue of the uterus. A deciduoma tends to develop after a pregnancy, regardless of the outcome of the pregnancy. It may be benign or malignant.

deciduous dentition. See **deciduous tooth**.

deciduous tooth, any one of the set of 20 teeth that appear normally during infancy, consisting of four incisors, two canines, and four molars in each jaw. Deciduous teeth start developing at about the sixth week of fetal life. In most individuals, the first deciduous tooth erupts through the gum about 6 months after birth. Thereafter, one or more deciduous teeth erupt about every month until all 20 have appeared. The deciduous teeth are usually shed between the ages of 6 and 13.

decoction, a liquid extract of water-soluble substances, usually extracted with the aid of boiling water. Herbal remedies are usually decoctions.

decode, to interpret coded information into a form usable by people.

decoded message, (in communication theory) a message as translated by a receiver.

decoic acid. See **capric acid**.

decompensation, the failure of a system, as cardiac decompensation in heart failure.

decomposition, the dissolution of a substance into simpler chemical forms.

decompression, 1. a technique used to readapt an individual to normal atmospheric pressure after exposure to higher pressures, as in diving. **2.** the removal of pressure caused by gas or fluid in a body cavity, as the stomach or intestinal tract.

decompression sickness, a painful, sometimes fatal syndrome caused by the formation of nitrogen bubbles in the tissues of divers, caisson workers, and aviators who move too rapidly from environments of higher to those of lower atmospheric pressures. Gaseous nitrogen then accumulates in the joint spaces and peripheral circulation, impairing tissue oxygenation. Disorientation, severe pain and syncope follow. Treatment is by rapid return of the patient to an environment of higher pressure, followed by gradual decompression.

decongestant, 1. of or pertaining to a substance or procedure that eliminates or reduces congestion or swelling. **2.** a decongestant drug. Antihistaminic agents and adrenergic drugs that cause bronchodilatation or vasoconstriction in the nasal mucosa are used as decongestants.

decontamination, the process of making a person, object or environment free of microorganisms, radioactivity or other contaminants.

decorticate posture, the position of a comatose patient in which the upper extremities are rigidly flexed at the elbows and at the wrists. The decorticate posture indicates a lesion in a mesencephalic region of the brain.

decorticate rigidity. See **decorticate posture**.

decortication, (in medicine) the removal of the cortical tissue of an organ or structure, such as kidney, brain or lung. **decorticate,** *v., adj.*

decrement, a decrease or stage of decline, as of a uterine contraction.

decremental conduction, (in cardiology) conduction that slows progressively as the effectiveness of the propagating impulse gradually decreases.

decubitus, a recumbent or horizontal position, such as lateral decubitus which is lying on one side.

decubitus projection, (in radiography) a position for producing a radiograph of the chest or abdomen of a patient who is lying down, with the central ray parallel to the horizon. Variations of the position include left and right AP oblique, dorsal decubitus, ventral decubitus, and left and right lateral decubitus.

decussate, to cross in the form of an "X," as certain nerve fibres from the retina cross at the optic chiasm. **decussation,** *n.*

deduction, a system of reasoning that leads from a known principle to an unknown, or from the general to the specific. Deductive reasoning is used to test diagnostic hypotheses.

deep brachial artery, a branch of each of the brachial arteries, arising at the distal border of the teres major and supplying the humerus and the muscles of the upper arm.

deep breathing and coughing exercises, the exercises taught to a person to improve breathing or maintain respiratory function, especially after prolonged inactivity or after general anaesthesia. Incisional pain after surgery in the chest or abdomen often inhibits normal respiratory excursion.

deep coma. See **coma**.

deep fascia, the most extensive of three kinds of fascia, comprising an intricate series of connective sheets and bands that hold the muscles and other structures in place throughout the body, wrapping the muscles in grey, felt-like membranes.

deep heat, the application of heat in the treatment of deep body tissues, particularly muscles and tendons.

deep palmar arch, the termination of the radial artery, joining the deep palmar branch of the ulnar artery in the palm of the hand.

deep sensation, the awareness or perception of pain, pressure or tension in the deep layers of skin, muscles, tendons or joints.

deep structure, (in neurolinguistics) the deeper experience and meaning to which surface structures in a communication may refer.

deep temporal artery, one of the branches of the maxillary artery on each side of the head. It branches into the anterior portion and posterior portion to supply the temporalis.

deep tendon reflex (DTR), a brisk contraction of a muscle in response to a sudden stretch induced by a sharp tap on the tendon of insertion of the muscle. Absence of the reflex may have been caused by damage to the muscle, the peripheral nerve, nerve roots, or the spinal cord at that level. Kinds of DTRs include **Achilles tendon reflex, biceps reflex, brachioradialis reflex, patellar reflex,** and **triceps reflex**.

deep vein, one of the many systemic veins that accompany the arteries, usually enclosed in a sheath that wraps both the vein and the associated artery. The larger arteries are usually accompanied by only one deep vein. The deep veins accompanying the smaller arteries occur usually in pairs, one vein on each side of the artery.

deep vein thrombosis, a disorder involving a thrombus in one of the deep veins of the body. Symptoms include tenderness, pain, swelling, warmth and discolouration of the skin. A deep vein thrombus is potentially life threatening, and treatment is directed towards prevention of movement of the thrombus toward the lungs.

deep x-ray therapy. See **external radiation therapy**

deerfly fever. See **tularemia**.

defaecation, the elimination of faeces from the digestive tract through the rectum.

defaecation reflex. See **rectal reflex**.

defaecography, a radiographic technique to demonstrate defaecation by the introduction of radiopaque contrast medium rectally.

defence mechanism, an unconscious, intrapsychic reaction that offers protection to the self. Kinds of defence mechanisms include **compensation, conversion, dissociation, displacement** and **sublimation**.

defensin, a peptide with natural antibiotic activity found within human neutrophils. Three types of defensins have been identified, each consisting of a chain of about 30 amino acids.

defensive radical therapy, (in psychology) a therapeutic technique intended as a survival tactic. The therapist begins at the patient's present state and uses encouragement to help the patient avoid self-defeating behaviour.

deferent duct. See **vas deferens**.

defervescence, the diminishing or disappearance of a fever. **defervescent,** *adj.*

defibrillate, to stop fibrillation of the atria or the ventricles of the heart, usually by delivering an electric shock to the myocardium through the chest wall by the use of a defibrillator.

defibrillation, the termination of ventricular fibrillation, by delivering a direct electric countershock to the patient's precordium.

defibrillator, a device that delivers an electric shock at a preset voltage to the myocardium through the chest wall. It is used for restoring the normal cardiac rhythm and rate when the heart has stopped beating or is fibrillating.

deficiency disease, a condition resulting from the lack of one or more essential nutrients in the diet, metabolic dysfunction, or over-indulgence in a limited number of foods.

deficit, any deficiency or difference from what is normal, such as an oxygen deficit, a cause of hypoxia.

definitive, 1. final; clearly established without doubt or question. **2.** (in embryology) fully formed in the final differentiation of a tissue, structure, or organ. **3.** (in parasitology) of or pertaining to the host in which the parasite undergoes the sexual phase of its reproductive cycle.

definitive host, any animal in which the reproductive stages of a parasite develop. The female *Anopheles* mosquito is the definitive host for malaria. Humans are definitive hosts for pinworms, schistosomes, and tapeworms.

definitive prosthesis, a permanent prosthetic

device that replaces a temporary-fit appliance, such as a pylon.

definitive treatment, any therapy generally accepted as a specific cure of a disease.

defloration, the rupture of the vaginal hymen. Defloration may occur during sexual intercourse, during a gynaecological examination, or by surgery if necessary to remove an obstruction to menstrual flow.

deformity, a condition of being distorted, disfigured, flawed, malformed, or misshapen, which may affect the body in general or any part of it and may be the result of disease, injury or birth defect.

degeneration, the gradual deterioration of normal cells and body functions.

degenerative chorea. See **Huntington's chorea**.

degenerative disease, any disease in which there is deterioration of structure or function of tissue. Some kinds of degenerative disease are arteriosclerosis, cancer and osteoarthritis.

degenerative joint disease. See **osteoarthritis**.

degloving, 1. the exposure of the bony mandibular anterior or posterior regions by oral surgery. **2.** traumatic skin stripping.

deglutition, swallowing.

deglutition apnoea, the normal absence of respiration during swallowing.

degradation, the reduction of a chemical compound to a compound less complex, usually by splitting off one or more groups or subgroups of atoms, as deamination.

dehiscence, the separation of a surgical incision or rupture of a wound closure.

dehydrate, 1. to remove or lose water from a substance. **2.** to lose excessive water from the body. **dehydration,** *n*.

dehydrated alcohol, a clear, colourless, highly hygroscopic liquid with a burning taste, containing at least 99.5% ethyl alcohol by volume.

dehydration, 1. excessive loss of water from the body tissues. Dehydration is accompanied by a disturbance in the balance of essential electrolytes, particularly sodium, potassium and chloride. Signs of dehydration include poor skin turgor, flushed dry skin, coated tongue, oliguria, irritability and confusion. **2.** rendering a substance free from water.

dehydration fever, a fever that frequently occurs in newborns, thought to be caused by dehydration.

dehydration of gingivae, the drying of gingival tissue, often the result of mouth breathing, which lowers the resistance of the gingival tissue to infection.

deinstitutionalization, the practice of discharging certain long-term mentally ill patients from psychiatric hospitals.

Deiters' nucleus {Otto F. C. Deiters, German anatomist, b. 1834}, one of the vestibular nuclei located in the brainstem.

déjà vu, the sensation or illusion that one is encountering a set of circumstances or a place that was previously experienced. The phenomenon results from some unconscious emotional connection with the present experience.

Dejerine-Sottas disease {Joseph J. Dejerine, French neurologist, b. 1849; Jules Sottas, French neurologist, b. 1866}, a rare, congenital spinocerebellar disorder characterized by the development of palpable thickenings along peripheral nerves, degeneration of the peripheral nervous system, pain, paraesthesia, ataxia, diminished sensation and deep tendon reflexes.

del, (in cytogenetics) abbreviation for deletion.

de Lange's syndrome. See **Amsterdam dwarf**.

delayed dentition. See **retarded dentition**.

delayed echolalia, a phenomenon, commonly seen in schizophrenia, involving the meaningless, automatic repetition of overheard words and phrases. It occurs hours, days or even weeks after the original stimulus.

delayed hypersensitivity reaction. See **cell-mediated immune response**.

delayed language, a failure of language use to develop at the expected age, usually because of a hearing defect, brain injury or emotional disturbance.

delayed sensation, a feeling or impression that is not experienced immediately after a stimulus.

delayed treatment seeker, (in psychology) a person who delays seeking treatment for a problematic life event until months or years after the event, usually following a precipitating event such as an anniversary reaction. Stuart

Delecato-Doman theory, a therapeutic concept that full neurological organization of a disabled or mentally retarded child requires that the child pass through developmental patterns covering progressively higher anatomical levels of the nervous system.

deletion (del), (in cytogenetics) the loss of a piece of a chromosome because it has broken away from the genetic material.

deletion syndrome, any of a group of congenital autosomal anomalies that result from the loss of chromosomal genetic material, because of breakage of a chromatid during cell division, as the cat-cry syndrome, which results from the absence of the short arm of chromosome 5.

deliberate biological programming, the Hayflick theory of ageing based on studies showing that human cells contain biological clocks that predetermine death after undergoing mitosis a finite number of times.

deliberate hypotension, an anaesthetic process in which a short-acting hypotensive agent, such as sodium nitroprusside or trimethaphan camsylate, is given to reduce blood pressure and thus bleeding during surgery.

delinquency, 1. negligence or failure to fulfil a duty or obligation. **2.** an offence, fault, misdemeanour or misdeed; a tendency to commit such acts.

delinquent, 1. characterized by neglect of duty or violation of law. **2.** one whose behaviour is characterized by persistent antisocial, illegal, violent or criminal acts; a juvenile delinquent.

délire de toucher, an abnormal desire or irresistable urge to touch or handle objects.

delirious mania, an extreme form of the manic state in which activity is so frenzied, confused and incoherent that it is difficult to discern any link between affect and behaviour.

delirium, 1. a state of frenzied excitement or wild enthusiasm. **2.** an acute organic mental disorder characterized by confusion, disorientation, restlessness, clouding of consciousness, incoherence, fear, anxiety, excitement, and often illusions, hallucinations, usually of visual origin, and at times delusions. The condition is caused by disturbances in cerebral functions that may result from a wide range of metabolic disorders, including nutritional deficiencies and endocrine imbalances; postpartum or postoperative stress; ingestion of toxic substances, as various gases, metals, or drugs, including alcohol; and other causes of physical and mental shock or exhaustion. Kinds of delirium include **acute delirium, delirium tremens, exhaustion delirium, senile delirium,** and **traumatic delirium. delirious,** *adj.*

delirium tremens (DTs), an acute and sometimes fatal psychotic reaction caused by excessive intake of alcoholic beverages over a long period of time. The reaction may follow a prolonged alcoholic binge without an adequate intake of food, occur during a period of abstinence, be precipitated by a head injury or infection, or result from the partial or total withdrawal of alcohol after prolonged drinking. Initial symptoms include loss of appetite, insomnia and general restlessness, followed by agitation, excitement, disorientation, mental confusion, vivid and often frightening hallucinations, acute fear and anxiety, illusions and delusions, coarse tremors of the hands, feet, legs and tongue, fever, increased heart rate, extreme perspiration, GI distress and precordial pain.

delivery, (in obstetrics) the birth of a child; parturition.

DeLorme technique, a method of physical exercise with weights in which sets of repetitions are repeated with rests between sessions. The technique involves the use of heavier weights and fewer repetitions in successive sets.

delta-9-tetrahydrocannabinol (THC), a pharmacologically active ingredient of cannabis that has been used experimentally in treating some cases of nausea and vomiting associated with cancer chemotherapy.

delta optical density analysis, a technique used to diagnose anaemia in a fetus by measuring the proportion of bilirubin decomposition products in the amniotic fluid. The method involves spectrographic examination of a fluid sample. The data are sometimes expressed in terms of δOD_{450}, representing the wavelength in nm at which maximum absorption of light by bilirubin occurs.

delta wave, 1. the slowest of the four types of brain waves, characterized by a frequency of 4 Hz and a relatively high voltage. Delta waves are "deep-sleep waves" associated with a dreamless state. **2.** (in cardiology) a slurring of the QRS portion of an ECG tracing caused by preexcitation.

deltoid, 1. triangular. **2.** of or pertaining to the deltoid muscle that covers the shoulder.

deltoid muscle, a large, thick triangular muscle that covers the shoulder joint and abducts, flexes, extends, and rotates the arm.

delusion, a persistent, aberrant belief or perception held inviolable by a person even though it is illogical, unique and probably wrong. Kinds of delusion include **delusion of being controlled, delusion of grandeur, delusion of persecution, nihilistic delusion** and **somatic delusion.**

delusion of being controlled, the false belief that one's feelings, beliefs, thoughts and acts are governed by some external force, as seen in various forms of schizophrenia.

delusion of grandeur, the gross exaggeration of one's importance, wealth, power or talents, as seen in disorders such as megalomania, general paresis and paranoid schizophrenia.

delusion of persecution, a morbid belief that one is being mistreated and harassed by unidentified enemies, as seen in paranoia and paranoid schizophrenia.

delusion of poverty, (in psychology) a false belief by a person that he or she is impoverished.

delusion of reference. See **idea of reference.**

delusion stupor, the state of lethargy and unresponsiveness observed in catatonic schizophrenia.

demarcation current, an electric current that flows from an uninjured to an injured end of a muscle.

deme, a small, closely related, interbreeding population of organisms or individuals, usually occupying a circumscribed area.

demecarium bromide, an ophthalmic anticholinesterase agent used in the treatment of open-angle glaucoma.

demeclocycline hydrochloride, a tetracycline antibiotic used in the treatment of a variety of infections, and also in the management of inappropriate antidiuretic hormone secretion.

dementia, a progressive, organic mental disorder characterized by chronic personality disintegration, confusion, disorientation, stupor, deterioration of intellectual capacity and function, and impairment of control of memory, judgment and impulses. Dementia may be caused by drug intoxication, hyperthyroidism, pernicious anaemia, paresis, subdural haematoma, benign brain tumour, hydrocephalus, insulin shock and tumour of islet cells of the pancreas. Kinds of dementia include **Alzheimer's disease, dementia paralytica, Pick's disease, secondary dementia, senile dementia** and **toxic dementia**.

dementia paralytica. See **general paresis**.

dementia praecox, an obsolete term for schizophrenia, especially developing in adolescence or early adulthood.

demigauntlet bandage, a glove-like bandage covering only the hand and leaving the fingers free.

demineralization, a decrease in the amount of minerals or inorganic salts in tissues, as occurs in certain diseases.

demispan, a measurement of skeletal size used with elderly people, where actual height is difficult to measure. Demispan is measured with a metal tape anchored between the subject's middle and ring finger and extended along the outstretched arm to the sternal notch.

demography, the study of human populations, particularly the size, distribution and characteristics of members of population groups. Demography is applied in studies of health problems involving ethnic groups, populations of a specific geographical region, or religious groups with special dietary restrictions.

demonstrative, a type of circum-speech that accompanies and illustrates speech. Pasquali **De Morgan's spots**. See **cherry angioma**.

demulcent, 1. any of several oily substances used for soothing and reducing irritation of surfaces that have been abraded or irritated. **2.** soothing, as a counterirritant or balm.

demyelination , the process of destruction or removal of the myelin sheath from a nerve or nerve fibre.

denaturation, 1. the alteration of the basic nature or structure of a substance. **2.** the process of making a potential food or beverage substance unfit for human consumption, although it may still be used for other purposes, such as a solvent.

denatured alcohol, ethyl alcohol made unfit for ingestion by the addition of acetone or methanol, used as a solvent and in chemical processes.

dendrite, a branching process that extends from the cell body of a neuron. Each neuron usually possesses several dendrites.

dendritic, 1. tree-like, with branches that spread towards or into neighbouring tissues, such as dendritic keratitis. **2.** of or pertaining to a dendrite.

dendritic keratitis, a serious herpes virus infection of the eye, characterized by an ulceration of the surface of the cornea resembling a tree with knobs at the ends of the branches. Untreated dendritic keratitis may result in permanent scarring of the cornea with impaired vision or blindness.

dendrodendritic synapse, a type of synapse in which a dendrite of one neuron comes in contact with a dendrite of another neuron.

dengue fever, an acute arbovirus infection transmitted to humans by the Aedes mosquito and occurring in tropical and subtropical regions. Manifestations of dengue usually occur in two phases, separated by a day of remission. In the first attack, the patient experiences fever, extreme weakness, headache, sore throat, muscle pains, and oedema of the hands and feet. The second attack is marked by a return of fever and a bright-red scarlatinaform rash.

dengue haemorrhagic fever shock syndrome (DHFS), a grave form of dengue fever characterized by shock with collapse or prostration; cold, clammy extremities; a weak, thready pulse; respiratory distress; and all of the symptoms of dengue fever. Haemorrhage, bruises, small reddish spots indicating bleeding from skin capillaries, and bloody vomit, urine and faeces may occur and precede circulatory collapse.

denial, 1. refusal or restriction of something requested, claimed or needed, often resulting in physical or emotional deficiency. **2.** an unconscious defence mechanism in which emotional conflict and anxiety are avoided by refusing to acknowledge those thoughts, feelings, desires, impulses or external facts that are consciously intolerable.

denial, ineffective, a conscious or unconscious attempt to disavow the knowledge or meaning of an event to reduce anxiety or fear to the detriment of health. The individual delays or refuses medical attention and does not perceive personal relevance of symptoms or danger. Defining characteristics include self-treatment to relieve symptoms, minimizing of symptoms, displacement of the source of symptoms to other organs, and displacement of fear of impact of the condition.

Denis Browne splint {Sir Denis J. W. Browne, English surgeon, b. 1892}, a splint for the correction of talipes equinovarus (clubfoot), composed of a curved bar attached to the soles of a pair of high-top shoes.

denitrogenation, the elimination of nitrogen from the lungs and body tissues during a period of breathing pure oxygen.

dens, *pl.* **dentes, 1.** a tooth or tooth-like structure or process. The term is sometimes modified to identify a particular tooth, such as dens caninus. **2.** the cone-shaped odontoid process of the axis, or second cervical vertebra.

dens deciduus. See **deciduous tooth**.

dense fibrous tissue, a fibrous connective tissue consisting of compact, strong, inelastic bundles of parallel collagenous fibres that have a glistening white colour.

dens in dente, a tooth-like structure present within the pulp chamber.

densitometer, a device that uses a photoelectric cell to detect differences in the density of light transmitted through a liquid or other material, such as radiographic film.

density, the amount of mass of a substance in a given volume. The greater the mass in a given volume, the greater the density. See also: optical density.

density gradient, the variation of the concentration of a solute in a confined solution.

dens serotinus. See **wisdom tooth**.

dental, of or pertaining to a tooth or teeth.

dental abscess, an abscess that forms in bone or soft tissues of the jaw, as a result of an infection that may follow dental caries or injury to a tooth. Symptoms include pain that may be continuous and exacerbated by hot or cold foods or the pressure of closing the jaws firmly.

dental alveolus, a tooth socket in the mandible or maxilla.

dental amalgam, an alloy of silver, tin and mercury with small amounts of copper and sometimes zinc, used for filling tooth cavities.

dental anaesthesia, any of several anaesthetic procedures used in dental surgery.

dental anomaly, an aberration in which one or more teeth deviate from the normal in form, function or position.

dental appliance, any device used by a dentist for a specific purpose, such as an orthodontic appliance used to correct malocclusion.

dental arch, the curving shape formed by the arrangement of a normal set of teeth.

dental calculus, a salivary deposit of calcium phosphate and calcium carbonate with organic matter on the teeth or a dental prosthesis.

dental canal. See **alveolar canal**.

dental caries, an abnormal destructive condition in a tooth, caused by the complex interaction of food, especially starches and sugars, with bacteria that form dental plaque. This material adheres to the surfaces of the teeth and provides the medium for the growth of bacteria and the production of organic acids that cause breaks in the enamel sheath of the tooth. Enzymes produced by the bacteria then attack the protein compo-

nent of the tooth. This process, if untreated, ultimately leads to the formation of deep cavities and bacterial infection of the pulp chamber and nerves. Kinds of dental caries include **active caries, arrested caries, primary caries** and **secondary caries**.

dental crypt, the space occupied by a developing tooth.

dental engine, an apparatus consisting of a hand instrument to which various rotating tools or drills can be fitted. It is driven by an electric motor.

dental erosion, the chemical or mechanical-chemical destruction of a tooth substance that causes variously shaped concavities at the cementoenamel junctions of teeth. The surfaces of these depressions, unlike those of carious cavities, are hard and smooth.

dental extraction forceps, a type of forceps used for grasping teeth in extractions.

dental film, a type of x-ray film made for either intraoral or panoramic exposure. Intraoral films are small, double-emulsion films without screens but with a lead foil backing to reduce patient dose. Panoramic films are large single-emulsion screen films.

dental fistula, an abnormal passage from the apical periodontal area of a tooth to the surface of oral mucous membrane.

dental floss, a waxed or unwaxed thread used to remove bacterial plaque from the interproximal surfaces of the teeth and around bridges.

dental granuloma, a disorder characterized by a mass of granulation tissue which is surrounded by a fibrous capsule attached to the apex of a pulp-involved tooth.

dental hygienist, a person with special training to provide dental services under the supervision of a dentist. Services supplied by a dental hygienist include dental prophylaxis, application of medications, and provision of dental education at the chairside and in the community.

dental implant, a plastic or metal device that is implanted in the jaw bones to provide permanent support for fixed bridges or dentures when there is insufficient bony ridge to support a denture.

dental plaque. See **bacterial plaque**.

dental pulp, a small mass of connective tissue, blood vessels, and nerves located in a chamber within the dentine and enamel layers of a tooth.

dental restoration. See **restoration**.

dental review committee, a group of dentists and administrative personnel that reviews questionable dental claims and practices and suggests dental care policies.

dental stone. See **artificial stone**.

dental surgery assistant, a person who assists a dentist in the performance of generalized tasks, including chairside assistance, clerical work, and some radiography and dental laboratory work.

dental technician, a person who makes dental prostheses and orthodontic appliances as prescribed by a dentist. Kinds of dental prostheses made by dental technicians include full dentures, partial dentures, crowns, bridgework, and other dental restorations.

dental therapist, a member of the dental team who is professionally trained and qualified to carry out dental treatment prescribed by the dentist and permitted to work in the Community and Hospital Dental Services. Permitted treatment includes simple fillings, the extraction of deciduous teeth, the application of preventive solutions and gels, and oral health education.

dentate fracture, any fracture that causes serrated bone ends that fit together like the teeth of gears.

dentate nucleus, a deep cerebellar nucleus that receives fibres from the lateral zone of the cerebellar cortex and appears to act as a trigger for the motor cortex, governing intentional movements as well as properties of ongoing movements.

denticle, a calcified body in the pulp chamber of a tooth.

dentifrice, a pharmaceutical compound used with a toothbrush for cleaning and polishing the teeth. It typically contains a mild abrasive, a detergent, a flavouring agent and a binder.

dentigerous cyst, an odontogenic cyst arising from the enamel organ of an unerupted tooth.

dentine, the chief material of teeth, surrounding the pulp and situated inside of the enamel and cementum. Harder and denser than bone, it consists of solid organic substratum which is calcified.

dentine eburnation, a change in carious teeth in which softened and decalcified dentine develops a hard, brown, polished appearance.

dentine globule, a small spheric body in peripheral dentine, created by early calcification.

dentinoenamel, pertaining to both dentine and enamel of the teeth.

dentinoenamel junction, the interface of enamel and dentine of a tooth crown, generally conforming to the shape of the crown.

dentinogenesis, the formation of dentine of the teeth.   **dentinogenic,** *adj.*

dentinogenesis imperfecta, hereditary dysplasia of dentine of deciduous and permanent teeth in which brown, opalescent dentine overgrows and obliterates the pulp cavity. The teeth have short roots and wear rapidly.

dentist, a person who practises dentistry and is qualified and licensed to do so. In the UK, undergraduate training involves 5 years at an approved dental school, and a further period of vocational training is mandatory for general dental practice.

dentistry, the practice of prevention and treatment of diseases and disorders of the teeth and of surrounding structures of the oral cavity. Responsibilities include the repair, restoration and replacement of missing teeth, the correction of malocclusions, and the detection of oral and systemic disease and malignancy. There are a number of specialised branches of dentistry which require postgraduate specialist training; these include endodontics, oral medicine and pathology, oral and maxillofacial surgery, orthodontics, paedodontics, periodontics, prosthodontics and forensic dentistry.

dentition, 1. the development and eruption of the teeth. **2.** the arrangement, number, and kind of teeth as they appear in the dental arch of the mouth. **3.** the character of the teeth of an individual or species as determined by their form and arrangement. Kinds of dentition include **artificial dentition, deciduous dentition, delayed dentition, mixed dentition, natural dentition, permanent dentition, precocious dentition, predeciduous dentition, primary dentition** and **secondary dentition.**

dentoalveolar abscess, the formation and accumulation of pus in a tooth socket or the jawbone around the base of a tooth.

dentoalveolar cyst. See **periodontal cyst.**

dentoenamel junction. See **dentinoenamel junction.**

dentofacial, of or pertaining to an oral or gnathic structure.

dentofacial anomaly, an abnormality in which an oral or gnathic structure deviates from the normal in form, function or position.

dentogenesis imperfecta, 1. a genetic disturbance of the dentine, characterized by early calcification of the pulp chambers, marked attrition and an opalescent hue to the teeth. **2.** a localized form of mesodermal dysplasia affecting the dentine of the teeth. It may be hereditary and associated with osteogenesis imperfecta. **3.** a genetic condition that produces defective dentine but normal tooth enamel.

dentogingival fibre, any one of the many fibres that spread like a fan, emerge from the supra-alveolar portion of the cementum and terminate in the free gingiva.

dentogingival junction, the junction between the gingival attachment, a non-keratinized epithelium and the surface of the teeth.

dentoperiosteal fibre, any one of the many fibres that emerge from the supra-alveolar part of the cementum of a tooth and extend into the mucoperiosteum of the attached gingiva.

dentulous dental arch, a dental arch that contains natural teeth.

denture, an artificial tooth or a set of artificial teeth not permanently fixed or implanted.

denture base, 1. the portion of a denture that fits the oral mucosa of the basal seat and supports artificial teeth. **2.** the part of a denture that covers the soft tissue of the mouth, commonly made of resin or a combination of resins and metal.

denture flask, a sectional metal case in which plaster of paris or artificial stone is moulded to process dentures or other resin restorations.

denture hyperplasia, an area of hyperplastic tissue which develops as a result of local irritation caused by a denture; denture granuloma.

denture packing, the laboratory procedure of filling and compressing a denture-base material into a mould in a flask.

denture stomatitis, a mild form of chronic atrophic candidosis usually affecting the mucosa in contact with the upper denture. It is rarely sore and often associated with poor dental hygiene, wearing dentures at night or xerostomia.

Denver Articulation Screening Examination (DASE), a test for evaluating the clarity of pronunciation in children between 2½ and 6 years of age. Each child's performance may be compared with a standardized norm for the age.

Denver classification, the system of identifying and classifying human chromosomes according to the criteria established at the Denver (1960), London (1963) and Chicago (1966) conferences of cytogeneticists. It is based on chromosome size and position of the centromere as determined during mitotic metaphase, and is divided into seven major groups, designated A to G, which are arranged according to decreasing length.

Denver Developmental Screening Test (DDST), a test for evaluating the development in children from 1 month to 6 years of age. The developmental level of motor, social and language skills is expressed as a ratio in which the child's age is the denominator, and the age at which the norm possesses skills equal to those of the child being tested is the numerator.

deodorant, 1. destroying or masking odours. **2.** a substance that destroys or masks odours. Underarm deodorants contain an antiperspirant, such as aluminum chloride, aluminum hydroxyl, aluminum sulphate or aluminum zirconyl hydroxychloride. These aluminum salts form an obstructive hydroxide gel in sweat ducts. Some underarm deodorants contain antibacterial agents or fragrances.

deodorized alcohol, a liquid, free of organic impurities, containing 92. 5% absolute alcohol.

deontologism, a doctrine of ethics that states that moral duty or obligation is binding.

deossification, the loss of mineral matter from bones.

deoxyribonucleic acid (DNA), a large nucleic acid molecule, found principally in the chromosomes of the nucleus of a cell, that is the carrier of genetic information. The genetic information is coded in the sequence of the nitrogenous, molecular subunits of the molecule.

dependence, 1. the state of being dependent. **2.** the total psychophysical state of one addicted to drugs or alcohol who must receive an increasing amount of the substance to prevent the onset of abstinence symptoms.

dependency needs, the sum of the physical and emotional requirements of an infant for survival, including parenting, love, affection, shelter, protection, food and warmth. Reliance on others to satisfy these needs normally decreases with age and maturity.

dependent, of or pertaining to a condition of being reliant on someone or something else for help, support, favour and other need, as a child is dependent on a parent, a narcotics addict is dependent on a drug, or one variable is dependent on another variable. **depend,** *v.*

dependent differentiation. See **correlative differentiation.**

dependent intervention, a therapeutic action based on the written or verbal orders of another health professional.

dependent personality, behaviour characterized by excessive or compulsive needs for attention, acceptance and approval from other people to maintain security and self-esteem.

dependent personality disorder, a mental state characterized by a lack of self-confidence and an inability to function independently.

dependent variable, (in research) a factor that is measured to learn the effect of one or more independent variables.

depersonalization, a feeling of strangeness or unreality concerning oneself or the environment, often resulting from anxiety.

depersonalization disorder, an emotional disturbance characterized by depersonalization feelings in which a dream-like atmosphere pervades the consciousness. The body may not feel like one's own, and important events may be watched with equanimity.

depilation, the removal or extraction of hair from the body, either temporarily by mechanical or chemical means or permanently, by electrolysis, which destroys the hair follicle. **depilate,** *v.*

depilatory, 1. of or pertaining to a substance or procedure that removes hair. **2.** a depilatory agent.

depolarization, the reduction of a membrane potential to a less negative value.

depot, 1. any area of the body in which drugs or other substances are stored and from which they can be distributed. **2.** (of a drug) injected or implanted to be slowly absorbed into the circulation.

depot injection, an injectable formulation of a drug that results in a gradual release of the medication over a period of several days.

depressant, 1. (of a drug) tending to decrease the function or activity of a system of the body. **2.** such a drug; for example, cardiac depressant, respiratory depressant.

depressed fracture, any fracture of the skull in which fragments are depressed below the normal surface of the skull.

depression, 1. a depressed area, hollow or fossa; downward or inward displacement. **2.** a decrease of vital functional activity. **3.** a mood disturbance characterized by feelings of sadness, despair and discouragement resulting from and normally proportionate to some personal loss or tragedy. **4.** an abnormal emotional state characterized by exaggerated feelings of sadness, melancholy, dejection, worthlessness, emptiness and hopelessness, that are inappropriate and out of proportion to reality. Kinds of depression include **agitated depression, anaclitic depression, endogenous depression, involutional melancholia, reactive depression,** and **retarded depression.**   **depressive,** *adj.*

depressor, any agent that reduces activity when applied to nerves and muscles.

depressor septi, one of the three muscles of the nose. It lies between the mucous membrane and the muscular structure of the lip and serves to draw the ala down, constricting the nostril.

deprivation, the loss of something considered valuable or necessary by taking it away or denying access to it. In experimental psychology, animal or human subjects may be deprived of something desired or expected for study of their reactions.

depth dose. See **percentage depth dose.**

depth electroencephalography. See **electroencephalography.**

depth perception, the ability to judge depth or the relative distance of objects in space and to orientate one's position in relation to them. Binocular vision is essential to this ability.

depth psychology, any approach to psychology that emphasizes the study of personality and behaviour in relation to unconscious motivation.

de Quervain's fracture {Fritz de Quervain, Swiss surgeon, b. 1868}, fracture of the navicular bone of the hand, with dislocation of the lunate bone.

de Quervain's thyroiditis {Fritz de Quervain}, an inflammatory condition of the thyroid, characterized by swelling and tenderness of the gland, fever, dysphagia, fatigue, and severe pain in the neck, ears and jaw. The disorder often occurs after a viral infection of the upper respiratory tract, and tends to remit spontaneously and to recur several times.

der, (in cytogenetics) abbreviation for derivative chromosome.

derailment, a schizophrenic pattern of speech in which incomprehensible, disconnected and unrelated ideas replace logical and orderly thought.

derby hat fracture. See **dishpan fracture.**

dereflection, a technique of logotherapeutic psychology directed towards taking a person's mind off a certain goal through a positive redirection to another goal, with emphasis on assets and abilities rather than the problems at hand.

dereistic thought, a type of mental activity in which fantasy is not modified by logic, experience or reality.

derivative, anything that is derived or obtained from another substance or object; for example, organs and tissues are derivatives of the primordial germ cells.

derived protein, a metabolic product of protein hydrolysis, such as proteose, peptone or peptide.

derived quantity, any secondary quantity derived from a combination of base quantities, such as mass, length and time.

dermabrasion, a treatment for the removal of scars on the skin by the use of revolving wire brushes or sandpaper. An aerosol spray is used to freeze the skin for this procedure.

Dermacentor, a genus of ticks. It includes species that transmit Rocky Mountain spotted fever, tularaemia, brucellosis and other infectious diseases.

dermatitis, an inflammatory condition of the skin, characterized by erythema and pain or pruritus. Various cutaneous eruptions occur and may be unique to a particular allergen, disease or infection. Some kinds of dermatitis are **actinic dermatitis, contact dermatitis, rhus dermatitis** and **seborrhoeic dermatitis.**

dermatitis exfoliativa neonatorum. See **Ritter's disease.**

dermatitis herpetiformis, a chronic, severely pruritic skin disease with symmetrically located groups of red, papulovesicular, vesicular, bullous or urticarial lesions that leave hyperpigmented spots.

dermatitis medicamentosa. See **drug rash.**

dermatitis venenata. See **contact dermatitis.**

dermatocyst, a cystic tumour of cutaneous tissues.

dermatofibroma, *pl.* **dermatofibromas, dermatofibromata,** a cutaneous nodule that is painless, round, firm, grey or red, and elevated. It is most commonly found on the extremities.

dermatoglyphics, the study of the skin ridge patterns on fingers, toes, palms of hands and soles of feet. The patterns are used as a basis of identification, but they also have diagnostic value because of associations between certain patterns and chromosomal anomalies.

dermatographia, an abnormal skin condition characterized by wheals that develop from tracing on the skin with the fingernail or a blunted instrument.

dermatologist, a doctor specializing in disorders of the skin.

dermatology, the study of the skin, including the anatomy, physiology, and pathology of the skin and the diagnosis and treatment of skin disorders.

dermatome, 1. (in embryology) the mesodermal layer in the early developing embryo that gives rise to the dermal layers of the skin. **2.** (in surgery) an instrument used to cut thin slices of skin for grafting. **3.** an area on the surface of a body innervated by afferent fibres from one spinal root.

dermatomycosis, a superficial, fungal infection of the skin, characteristically found on parts that are moist and protected by clothing, such as the groin or feet. It is caused by a dermatophyte. **dermatomycotic,** *adj.*

dermatomyositis, a disease of the connective tissues, characterized by pruritic or eczematous inflammation of the skin and tenderness and weakness of the muscles. Muscle tissue is destroyed, and loss is often so severe that the person may become unable to walk or perform simple tasks.

Dermatophagoides farinae, a ubiquitous species of household dust mite responsible for allergic reactions in sensitive individuals.

dermatophyte, any of several fungi that cause parasitic skin disease in humans.

dermatophytid, an allergic skin reaction characterized by small vesicles and associated with dermatomycosis.

dermatophytosis, a superficial fungus infection of the skin, caused by *Microsporum, Epidermophyton* or *Trichophyton* species of dermatophyte. On the trunk and upper extremities this is commonly called "ringworm" infection and is characterized by round or oval, scaly patches with slightly raised borders and clearing centers. On the feet, small vesicles, cracking, itching, scaling and often secondary bacterial infections occur, and are commonly known as "athlete's foot".

dermatoplasty, a surgical procedure in which skin tissue is transplanted to a body surface damaged by disease or injury.

dermatopolyneuritis. See **acrodynia**.

dermatosclerosis, a skin disease characterized by fibrous infiltration of the fatty subcutaneous tissue, leading to patches of thick, leather-like skin.

dermatosis, any disorder of the skin, especially if not associated with inflammation.

dermatosis papulosa nigra, a common abnormal skin condition in blacks consisting of multiple, tiny, benign, skin-coloured or hyperpigmented papules on the cheeks.

dermis. See **corium**.

dermographism. See **dermatographia**.

dermoid, 1. of or pertaining to the skin. **2.** *informal.* a dermoid cyst.

dermoid cyst, a tumour, derived from embryonal tissues. It consists of a fibrous wall lined with epithelium and a cavity containing fatty material, and frequently hair, teeth, bits of bone and cartilage. Kinds of dermoid cysts are **implantation dermoid cyst, inclusion dermoid cyst, thyroid dermoid cyst** and **tubal dermoid cyst.**

DES, abbreviation for **diethylstilboestrol**.

descending aorta, the main portion of the aorta, consisting of the thoracic aorta and the abdominal aorta, that continues from the aortic arch into the trunk of the body and supplies many parts, such as the oesophagus, lymph glands, ribs and stomach.

descending colon, the segment of the colon that extends from the end of the transverse colon at the splenic flexure on the left side of the abdomen down to the beginning of the sigmoid colon in the pelvis.

descending current. See **centrifugal current**.

descending oblique muscle. See **obliquus externus abdominis**.

descending urography. See **intravenous pyelography**.

descensus, the process of falling or descending; prolapse.

descriptive anatomy, the study of the morphology and structure of the body by systems, such as vascular system and nervous system.

descriptive embryology, the study of the changes that occur in cells, tissues and organs during the progressive stages of prenatal development.

descriptive epidemiology, the first stage of epidemiological investigation. It focuses on describing disease distribution by characteristics relating to time, place and person.

descriptive psychiatry, the study of external, readily observable behaviour.

desensitization. See **systemic desensitization.**

desensitize, 1. (in immunology) to render an individual insensitive to any of the various antigens. **2.** (in psychiatry) to relieve an emotionally disturbed person of the stress of phobias and neuroses by encouraging discussion of the anxieties and the stressful experiences that cause the emotional problems involved. **3.** (in dentistry) to remove or reduce the painful response of vital, exposed dentine to irritating substances and temperature changes.

desert fever. See **coccidioidomycosis.**

desert rheumatism. See **coccidioidomycosis.**

desferrioxamine mesylate, a chelating agent prescribed in the treatment of acute iron intoxication and chronic iron overload.

desiccant, any agent or procedure that promotes drying or causes a substance to dry up.

desiccate, 1. to dry thoroughly. **2.** to preserve by drying, especially food.

designer drugs, synthetic organic compounds that are designed as analogues of illicit drugs, with the same effects on the user. Because designer drugs are generally not listed as controlled substances, prosecution of manufacturers, distributors or users is often difficult.

desipramine hydrochloride, a tricyclic antidepressant prescribed in the treatment of depression.

desmocyte. See fibroblast.

desmoid tumour, a neoplasm in skeletal muscle and fascia. The tumour is usually a firm, circumscribed, rubbery mass which is often regarded as overproliferation of scar tissue.

desmopressin, an antidiuretic analogue of vasopressin prescribed in the treatment of diabetes insipidus.

desmosis, any disease of connective tissue.

desmosome, a small, circular, dense area within the intercellular bridge that forms the site of adhesion between certain epithelial cells, especially the stratified epithelium of the epidermis.

desoxymethasone, a potent corticosteroid used typically as an anti-inflammatory agent.

desoxyribonucleic acid. See **deoxyribonucleic acid**.

desquamation, a normal process in which the cornified layer of the epidermis is sloughed in fine scales.

desquamative gingivitis, gingival inflammation.

desquamative interstitial pneumonia, a respiratory disease characterized by an accumulation of cellular matter in the alveoli and bronchial tubes. It leads to a fibrotic condition with symptoms of coughing, chest pain, weight loss and dyspnoea.

destructive aggression, an act of hostility unnecessary for self-protection or preservation, directed towards an external object or person.

destructive interference, (in ultrasonography) a phenomenon that results when propagated waves are out of phase so that maximum molecular compression for one wave occurs at the same point as the maximum rarefaction for the second wave.

detached retina. See **retinal detachment**.

detection bias, a potential artefact in epidemiological data resulting from the use of a particular diagnostic technique or equipment.

detergent, 1. a cleansing agent. **2.** cleansing. **3.** (in respiratory therapy) a wetting agent that is administered to mediate the removal of respiratory tract secretions from airway walls.

deterioration, pertaining to a condition that is gradually worsening.

determinant evolution, the theory that evolution progresses according to a predetermined course.

determinants of occlusion, (in dentistry) the classifiable factors that influence proper closure of the teeth. The common fixed factors are the intercondylar distance, anatomy, mandibular centricity and relationship of the jaws. The common changeable factors are tooth shapes, tooth positions, and vertical dimensions of occlusion, cusp height and fossa depth.

determinate cleavage, mitotic division of the fertilized ovum into blastomeres that are each destined to form a specific part of the embryo. Damage to or destruction of any of these cells results in a malformed organism.

deterministic effect, (in radiobiology) biologic effect of ionising radiation which occurs above a certain threshold dose, depending on the organ or tissue exposed, and where the severity of the effect increases with dose. For example, erythema of the skin, radiation-induced cataract.

detoxification, the removal of a poison or its effects from a patient.

detoxification service, a hospital service providing treatment to diminish or remove from a patient's body the toxic effects of chemical substances, such as alcohol, drugs or poisonous substances to which a person may have been exposed.

detrusor urinae muscle, a complex of longitudinal fibres that form the external layer of the muscular coat of the bladder.

deuterium, a radioactive isotope of the hydrogen atom, used as a tracer.

deuteroplasm. See **deutoplasm**.

deutoplasm, the inactive elements of the protoplasm, primarily the stored nutritive material contained in the yolk.

development, 1. the gradual process of change and differentiation from a simple to a more advanced level of complexity. Kinds of development include **arrested development, mosaic development, psychomotor development, psychosexual development, psychosocial development** and **regulative development. 2.** (in biology) the series of events that occur within an organism from the time of fertilization of the ovum to the adult stage. **developmental,** *adj.*

developmental age (DA), an expression of a child's developmental progress stated in age and determined by standardized measurements, such as body size and dimensions, by social and psychological functioning, by observations of motor skills, and through mental and aptitude tests.

developmental agraphia, a deficiency in a child's ability to learn to form letters and write.

developmental anatomy, the study of differentiation and growth of an organism from one cell to birth.

developmental anomaly, any congenital defect that results from the interference with the normal growth and differentiation of the fetus. Such defects can arise at any stage of embryonic development, vary greatly in type and severity, and are caused by a wide variety of determining factors, including genetic mutations, chromosomal aberrations, teratogenic agents and environmental factors.

developmental arrest. See **arrested development**.

developmental crisis, severe, usually transient, stress that occurs when a person is unable to complete the tasks of a psychosocial stage of development, and is therefore unable to move on to the next stage.

developmental disorder, a form of mental retardation that develops in some children after they have progressed normally for the first 3 or 4 years of life.

developmental dysfunction, any abnormal or impaired process of development or its result.

developmental dyspraxia, a disorder of sensory integration characterized by an impaired ability to plan skilled non-habitual movements.

developmental groove, a fine recessed line in the enamel of a tooth that marks the union of the lobes of the crown in its development.

developmental guidance, (in dentistry) the comprehensive dentofacial orthopaedic control over the growth of jaws and eruption of teeth. The control may be needed throughout the entire growth and maturation of the face, beginning at the earliest detection of a developing malformation.

developmental handling, the moving of a child through part or all of the developmental sequence to enhance expression of normal movement patterns, such as righting and equilibrium reactions.

developmental horizon, any one of 25 stages in the development of the human embryo, from the one-cell stage at conception to the morphologically and physiologically complex organism at the end of the seventh week of gestation.

developmental milestones, significant behaviours which are used to mark the progress of development.

developmental model, 1. a conceptual framework devised to be used as a guide in making a diagnosis, in understanding a developmental process, and in forming a prognosis for continued development. **2.** (in nursing) a conceptual framework describing four stages, or processes, of patient therapy. In the first stage, called orientation, the patient begins a relationship with the nurse or other therapist and begins to clarify the problem with the help of the therapist. In the second stage, called identification, the patient develops a sense of closeness and attachment to the therapist. In the third stage, called exploitation, the patient makes full use of the nursing services offered, begins to assume some control of interactions and becomes more independent. During the last stage, called resolution, the therapeutic relationship is terminated; the patient is independent and no longer needs the nurse or therapist.

developmental physiology, the study of the physiological processes as they relate to embryonic development.

developmental quotient (DQ), the numeric expression of a child's developmental level as measured by dividing the developmental age by the chronological age and multiplying by 100.

developmental task, a physical or cognitive skill that a person must accomplish during a particular age period to continue developing, such as walking, which precedes the development of a sense of autonomy in the toddler period.

developmental theory of ageing, a concept based on the premise that traits and characteristics developed early in life tend to continue into the later years.

deviance, behaviour that is contrary to the accepted standards of a community or culture.

deviant behaviour, actions that exceed the usual limits of accepted behaviour and involve failure to comply with the social norm of the group.

deviate, 1. a person or an act that varies from that which is considered standard, such as a social or sexual deviate, or that which is within a statistical norm. **2.** to vary from that which is considered standard or within a statistical norm. **deviant,** *adj.*, **deviation,** *n.*

deviated septum, a shifted medial partition of the nasal cavity, a condition affecting many adults. The nasal septum more commonly shifts to the left during normal growth, but severe deflection of the septum may significantly obstruct the nasal passages and result in infection, sinusitis, shortness of breath, headache or recurring nosebleeds.

deviation from normal, a quality, characteristic, symptom, or clinical finding that is different from what is commonly regarded as normal, such as an elevated temperature, multiple gestation or an extra digit.

device, an item other than a drug that has application in the healing arts. The term is sometimes restricted to items used directly by, on, or in the patient and not surgical instruments or other equipment used for diagnosis and treatment. Devices include orthopaedic appliances, intra-uterine devices, crutches, artificial heart valves, pacemakers and prostheses.

devil's grip. See **epidemic pleurodynia**.

devitalized, pertaining to tissues with a reduced oxygen supply and blood flow.

devitalized tooth. See **pulpless tooth**.

dewar, (in magnetic resonance imaging) a double chamber used to maintain the temperature of superconducting magnet coils at near absolute zero.

dew point, the temperature at which air becomes saturated with water vapour and the water vapour condenses to liquid. In aerosol therapy, water may condense on containers, tubing and other surfaces when the dew point is reached.

dexamethasone, a glucocorticoid prescribed in the treatment of a variety of inflammatory conditions and also used as an antiemetic.

dexamphetamine sulphate, a central nervous system stimulant prescribed in the treatment of narcolepsy and in the treatment of hyperkinetic disorders in children. It has also been prescribed as an anorectic drug in treating exogenous obesity. The drug is addictive and classified as Class B, Schedule 2, under the Misuse of Drugs Act 1971 and the Misuse of Drugs Regulations 1985.

dextrality. See **right-handedness**.

dextran fermentation, the conversion of dextrose to dextran by the action of *Leuconostoc mesenteroides* dextran (LMD) bacteria.

dextrans, a group of slowly metabolized polysaccharides, used in solution as plasma volume expanders in cases of hypovolaemia due to shock arising from burns, septicaemia or other cause.

dextrocardia, pertaining to the location of the heart in the right hemithorax, either as a result of displacement by disease or a congenital defect.

dextromethorphan hydrobromide, an antitussive related to morphine but lacking narcotic effects. It is prescribed for the suppression of non-productive cough.

dextrose. See **glucose**.

dextrose and sodium chloride injection, a fluid, nutrient and electrolyte replenisher. It is available for parenteral use in a variety of concentrations.

DHFS, abbreviation for **dengue haemorrhagic fever shock syndrome**.

dhobie itch, a form of contact dermatitis associated with the use of laundry marking fluids.

diabetes, 1. a clinical condition characterized by the excessive excretion of urine. **2.** diabetes mellitus.

diabetes insipidus, a metabolic disorder, characterized by extreme polyuria and polydipsia, caused by deficient production or secretion of the antidiuretic hormone (ADH) or an inability of the kidney tubules to respond to ADH. Rarely, the symptoms are self-induced by an excessive water intake. The condition may be acquired, familial, idiopathic or nephrogenic. The patient is usually well and comfortable except for the annoyance of frequent urination and a constant need to drink.

diabetes mellitus (DM), a complex disorder of carbohydrate, fat and protein metabolism that is primarily a result of a relative or complete lack of insulin secretion by the beta cells of the pancreas or of defects of the insulin receptors. The disease is often familial but may be acquired, such as in Cushing's syndrome, as a result of the administration of excessive glucocorticoid. The various forms of diabetes have been organized into a series of categories developed by the National Diabetes Data Group of the National Institutes of Health. Type I diabetes in this classification scheme includes patients dependent on insulin to prevent ketosis. The category is also known as the insulin-dependent diabetes mellitus (IDDM) subclass. This group was previously called juvenile-onset diabetes, brittle diabetes, or ketosis-prone diabetes. Patients with Type II, or non-insulin-dependent diabetes mellitus (NIDDM), are those previously designated as having maturity-onset diabetes, adult-onset diabetes, ketosis-resistant diabetes, or stable diabetes. Type II patients are further subdivided into obese NIDDM and non-obese NIDDM groups. Those with gestational diabetes (GDM), usually identified as Type III, are in a separate subclass composed of women who developed glucose intolerance in association with pregnancy. Type IV, also identified as Other Types of Diabetes, includes patients whose diabetes is associated with a pancreatic disease, hormonal changes, adverse effects of drugs, or genetic or other anomalies. A fifth subclass, the impaired glucose tolerance (IGT) group, includes persons whose plasma glucose levels are abnormal although not sufficiently beyond the normal range to be diagnosed as diabetic. The onset of diabetes mellitus is sudden in children and usually insidious in non-insulin-dependent diabetes mellitus (type II). Characteristically, the course is progressive and includes polyuria, polydipsia, weight loss, polyphagia, hyperglycaemia and glycosuria. The eyes, kidneys, nervous system, skin and circulatory system may be affected, infections are common, and atherosclerosis often develops. Kinds of diabetes mellitus are **gestational diabetes, insulin-dependent diabetes,** and **non-insulin-dependent diabetes**.

diabetes, other types. See other types of diabetes.

diabetic, 1. of or pertaining to diabetes. **2.** affected with diabetes. **3.** a person who has diabetes mellitus.

diabetic amaurosis, blindness associated with diabetes, caused by a proliferative, haemorrhagic form of retinopathy that is characterized by capillary microaneurysms and hard or waxy exudates. Cataracts are also common.

diabetic coma, a life-threatening condition occurring in diabetic patients, caused by inadequate treatment, failure to take prescribed insulin, or, most frequently, infection, surgery, trauma or other stress that increases the body's need for insulin. Without insulin to metabolize glucose, fats are burned for energy, resulting in ketosis and acidosis. Warning signs of diabetic coma include a dull headache, fatigue, inordinate thirst, epigastric pain, nausea, vomiting, parched lips, a flushed face and sunken eyes. The temperature usually rises and then falls; the systolic blood pressure drops, and circulatory collapse may occur.

diabetic diet, a diet prescribed in the treatment of diabetes mellitus, usually containing limited amounts of sugar or readily available carbohydrates and increased amounts of proteins, complex carbohydrates and unsaturated fats. Dietary regulation depends on an individual's needs.

diabetic foot and leg care, the special attention given to prevent the circulatory disorders and infections that frequently occur in the lower extremities of diabetic patients. The patient's legs and feet are examined daily for signs of dry, scaly, red, itching, or cracked skin, blisters, corns, calluses, abrasions, infection, blueness and swelling around varicosities, and thickened, discoloured nails. The feet are bathed daily in tepid water with mild soap, and are dried gently but thoroughly with a soft towel. A lanolin-based lotion is then applied.

diabetic ketoacidosis, an acute, life-threatening complication of uncontrolled diabetes mellitus in which urinary loss of water, potassium, ammonium and sodium results in hypovolaemia, electrolyte imbalance, extremely high blood-glucose levels and the breakdown of free fatty acids causing acidosis, often with coma. The person appears flushed, has hot, dry skin, is restless, uncomfortable, agitated, diaphoretic, and breath has a fruity odour. Coma, confusion, and nausea are often noted. Untreated, the condition invariably proceeds to coma and death.

diabetic retinopathy, a disorder of retinal blood vessels characterized by capillary microaneurysms, haemorrhage, exudates, and the formation of new vessels and connective tissue. The disorder occurs most frequently in patients with long-standing, poorly controlled diabetes. Repeated haemorrhage may result in permanent opacity of the vitreous humour, and blindness may eventually set in.

diabetic treatment, therapy of diabetes mellitus by means of a low carbohydrate diet, insulin injections or oral hypoglycaemic agents, such as chlorpropamide, acetohexamide, tolbuta-mide and tolazamide.

diabetic xanthoma, an eruption of yellow papules or plaques on the skin in uncontrolled diabetes mellitus. The lesion disappears as the metabolic functions are stabilized and the disease is brought under control.

diabetogenic state, a health condition manifested by signs and symptoms of diabetes.

diacet, abbreviation for a **carboxylate diacetate anion.**

diacetic acid. See **acetoacetic acid.**

diacondylar fracture, any fracture that runs across the line of a condyle.

diagnose, to determine the type and cause of a health condition based on the signs and symptoms of the patient, data obtained from laboratory analysis of fluid, tissue specimens and other tests, and family and occupational background information.

diagnosis, *pl.* **diagnoses, 1.** identification of a disease or condition by a scientific evaluation of physical signs, symptoms, history, laboratory tests and procedures. Kinds of diagnoses are clinical diagnosis, differential diagnosis, laboratory diagnosis, nursing diagnosis, and physical diagnosis. **2.** the art of naming a disease or condition. **diagnostic,** *adj.,* **diagnose,** *v.*

diagnostic, pertaining to a diagnosis.

Diagnostic and Statistical Manual of Mental Disorders (DSM), a manual, published by the American Psychiatric Association, listing the official diagnostic classifications of mental disorders. The *DSM* recommends the use of a multiaxial evaluation system as a holistic diagnostic approach. It consists of five axes, each of which refers to a different class of information, including both mental and physical data. Axes I and II include all of the mental disorders, classified broadly as clinical syndromes and personality disorders; axis III contains physical disorders and conditions; and axes IV and V provide a coded outline of supplemental information which may be useful for planning individual treatment and predicting its outcome. Each of the classifications of the mental disorders contains a code that provides a reference to the WHO *International Classification of Diseases (ICD).*

diagnostic anaesthesia, a procedure in which analgesia is induced to a depth adequate to comfortably permit performance of moderately painful diagnostic procedures of short duration. Awake anaesthesia is often used for this purpose.

diagnostician, a person skilled and trained in making diagnoses.

diagnostic imaging, medical imaging including radiography, ultrasonography, computerised tomography, magnetic resonance imaging and radionuclide imaging.

diagnostic position of gaze. See **cardinal position of gaze**.

diagnostic process, the act of determining a patient's health status and evaluating the factors influencing that status.

diagnostic radiography. See **radiography**

diagnostic radiology. See **diagnostic imaging**.

diagnostic services, services related to the diagnosis made by a doctor but which may be performed also by nurses or other health professionals.

diagonal conjugate, a radiographic measurement of the distance from the inferior border of the symphysis pubis to the sacral promontory. The measurement averages around 12. 5 to 13.0 cm.

diakinesis, the final stage in the first meiotic prophase in gametogenesis, in which the chromosomes achieve maximum contraction and are ready to separate.

dialect, a variation of a language different from other forms of the same language in pronunciation, syntax and word meanings.

dialogue, a complex form of computer-assisted instruction in which the student is actively engaged in "true conversation" with a computer.

dialysate, a solution used in dialysis.

dialysis, 1. the process of separating colloids and crystalline substances in solution by the difference in their rate of diffusion through a semipermeable membrane. **2.** a medical procedure for the removal of certain elements from the blood or lymph by virtue of the difference in their rates of diffusion through an external semipermeable membrane or, in the case of peritoneal dialysis, through the peritoneum.

dialysis dementia, a neurological disorder that occurs in some patients undergoing dialysis. The precise cause is unknown, but the effect is believed to be related to chemicals in the dialysing fluid, drugs administered to the dialysis patient, or both.

dialysis disequilibrium syndrome, a disorder caused by a rapid change in extracellular fluid composition during dialysis. The syndrome may be marked by cerebral or neurological disturbances, cardiac arrhythmias and pulmonary oedema.

dialysis fluid, the solution that flows on the opposite side of a semipermeable membrane to blood.

dialyser, 1. a machine used in dialysis. **2.** a semipermeable membrane or porous diaphragm in a dialysis machine.

Diamond-Blackfan syndrome, a rare congenital disorder evident in the first 3 months of life, characterized by severe anaemia, very low reticulocyte count, but normal numbers of platelets and white cells.

diamond stone, (in dentistry) any of the rotary devices that contain diamond chips as an abrasive.

diamorphine, a semisynthetic opiate alkaloid, known informally as heroin. It is used for its potent analgesic properties, and is also widely abused for its psychotropic effects.

diapedesis, the passage of red or white blood corpuscles through the walls of the vessels that contain them without damage to the vessels.

diaphanography, a type of transillumination used to examine the breast, using selected wavelengths of light and special imaging equipment.

diaphanoscopy, examination of an internal structure with a diaphanoscope, an instrument that transilluminates body tissues. It is sometimes used in the diagnosis of breast tumours.

diaphoresis, the secretion of sweat, especially the profuse secretion associated with an elevated body temperature, physical exertion, exposure to heat and mental or emotional stress.

diaphoretic. See **sudorific**.

diaphragm, 1. (in anatomy) a dome-shaped musculofibrous partition that separates the thoracic and abdominal cavities. The convex cranial surface of the diaphragm forms the floor of the thoracic cavity, and the concave surface forms the roof of the abdominal cavity. This partition is pierced by various openings through which pass the aorta, oesophagus and vena cava. **2.** (in optics) an opening that controls the amount of light passing through an optical network. **3.** a thin, membranous partition, as that employed in dialysis. **4.** (in radiography, radiotherapy) a mechanical device used to collimate the beam of radiation to the required size, usually incorporating a light beam to indicate the area of field covered by the radiation beam. **diaphragmatic,** *adj.*

diaphragmatic hernia, the protrusion of part of the stomach through an opening in the diaphragm, most commonly an abnormally enlarged oesophageal hiatus. In some cases, the intestines may also herniate into the chest. The enlargement of the normal opening for the oesophagus may be caused by trauma, congenital weakness, increased abdominal pressure or relaxation of ligaments of skeletal muscles, and permits part of the stomach to slide into the thorax. A sliding hiatus hernia, one of the most common pathological conditions of the upper GI tract, may occur at any age but is most frequent in elderly and middle-aged individuals. A kind of diaphragmatic hernia is **hiatus hernia**.

diaphragmatic node, a node in one of three groups of thoracic parietal lymph nodes, situated on the thoracic side of the diaphragm and consisting of the anterior set, the middle set, and the posterior set.

diaphragm stethoscope, an instrument for

auscultation of bodily sounds. Originally designed by René Laënnec, it consists of a vibrating disk, or diaphragm, which transmits sound waves through tubing to two earpieces.

diaphyseal aclasis, a relatively rare abnormal condition that affects the skeletal system. Characterized by multiple exostoses or bony protrusions, it is hereditary. The characteristic exostoses are radiographically and microscopically similar to osteochondromas.

diaphyseal dysplasia. See **Camurati-Engelmann disease**.

diaphysis, the shaft of a long bone, consisting of a tube of compact bone enclosing the medullary cavity.

diapositive. See **reversal film**.

diarrhoea, 1. the frequent passage of loose, watery stools, generally the result of increased motility in the colon. The stool may also contain mucus, pus, blood or excessive amounts of fat. Conditions in which diarrhoea is an important symptom are dysenteric diseases, malabsorption syndrome, lactose intolerance, irritable bowel syndrome, GI tumours and inflammatory bowel disease. Untreated, diarrhoea may lead to rapid dehydration and electrolyte imbalance. and should be treated symptomatically until proper diagnosis can be made. **2.** in terms of diagnosis, the defining characteristics of diarrhoea include abdominal pain, cramping, increased frequency of elimination, increased frequency of bowel sounds, loose or liquid stools, urgency of defaecation and a change in the colour of the faeces. **diarrhoeal, diarroheic,** *adj.*

diarthrosis. See **synovial joint**.

diastasis, the forcible separation of two parts that are normally joined together, such as the separation of parts of a bone at an epiphysis or the separation of two bones that lack a synovial joint.

diastasis recti abdominis, the separation of the two rectus muscles along the median line of the abdominal wall. In an adult woman, the abnormality is often caused by repeated pregnancies.

diastatic fermentation, the conversion of starch to glucose by the enzyme ptyalin.

diastole, 1. the period of time between contractions of the atria or the ventricles, during which blood enters the relaxed chambers from the systemic circulation and the lungs. Ventricular diastole begins with the onset of the second heart sound and ends with the first heart sound. **2.** phase 4 of the action potential (from the end of phase 3 to the beginning of phase 0).

diastolic, pertaining to diastole, or the blood pressure at the instant of maximum cardiac relaxation.

diastolic augmentation, an increase in arterial diastolic pressure caused by the counterpulsation of a circulatory assistance device, such as an intra-aortic balloon pump.

diastolic blood pressure, the minimum level of blood pressure measured between contractions of the heart. Diastolic pressures for an individual may vary with age, sex, body weight, emotional state and other factors.

diastolic filling pressure, the blood pressure in the ventricle during diastole.

diastrophic, pertaining to a bent or curved condition of bones or distortion of other structures.

diastrophic dwarf, a person in whom short stature is caused by osteochondrodysplasia and is associated with various deformities of the bones and joints, including scoliosis, clubfoot, micromelia, hand defects, multiple joint contractures and subluxations, ear deformities and cleft palate.

diathermy, the production of heat in body tissues for therapeutic purposes by high-frequency currents that are insufficiently intense to destroy tissues or impair their vitality. Diathermy is used in treating chronic arthritis, bursitis, fractures, gynaecological disorders, sinusitis and other conditions.

diathesis, an inherited physical constitution predisposing to certain diseases or conditions, many of which are believed to be associated with the Y chromosome as males appear to be more susceptible than females.

diazepam, a benzodiazepine sedative and tranquilliser used in the treatment of anxiety, muscle tension, and as an anticonvulsant.

diazoxide, a vasodilator used as an antihypertensive. It is prescribed for the emergency reduction of blood pressure in severe hypertension when drastic reduction of the diastolic blood pressure is required. It is also used in some cases of hypoglycaemia for its ability to raise blood pressure.

dic, (in cytogenetics) abbreviation for dicentric.

DIC, abbreviation for **disseminated intravascular coagulation**.

dicephaly, a developmental anomaly in which the fetus has two heads. **dicephalous, dicephalic,** *adj.*, **dicephalus,** *n.*

dichlorodiphenyltrichloroethane.See **DDT**.

dichorial twins, dichorionic twins. See **dizygotic twins**.

dichroic stain, dichroic fog (in radiography) pink/yellow stain on radiographic film due to non-neutralization of the developing agent by the fixer.

dichotomy, a division or separation into two equal parts.

dichotomy planning, the preparation for ongoing and future needs for health care resources of patients as they move along the health/illness continuum.

Dick test {George F. Dick, b. 1881; Gladys R. H. Dick, b. 1881; American physicians}, a skin test for determining sensitivity to an erythrotoxin produced by the group A streptococci that cause scarlet fever.

dicrotic notch, the interval between the two peaks of a dicrotic pulse.

dicrotic pulse, a pulse with two separate peaks, the second usually weaker than the first.

dicyclomine hydrochloride, an anticholinergic used to treat disorders of the GI tract characterized by smooth muscle spasm.

didymitis, an inflammation in a testicle.

didymus, a testis.

dieldrin, a highly toxic pesticide that is also poisonous to humans and animals if ingested, inhaled or absorbed through the skin. It causes dysfunction of the central nervous system and is a possible carcinogen.

diencephalon, the division of the brain between the telencephalon and the mesencephalon. It consists of the hypothalamus, thalamus, metathalamus and epithalamus, and includes most of the third ventricle.

dienoestrol, an oestrogen used as a vaginal cream in the treatment of atrophic vaginitis and kraurosis vulvae.

diet, 1. food and drink considered in relation to their nutritional qualities, composition, and effects on health. **2.** nutrients prescribed, regulated or restricted as to kind and amount for therapeutic or other purposes. **3.** the customary allowance of food and drink regularly provided or consumed. **dietetic,** *adj.*

dietary assessment, assessment of the nutrient intake of an individual or a group of individuals. Methods of assessment include weighed food intakes, dietary recall and food diaries.

dietary fibre, a generic term for non-digestible chemical substances found in plant cell walls and surrounding cellular material, each with a different effect on the various GI functions, such as colon transit time, water absorption and lipid metabolism. The main dietary fibre components are cellulose, lignin, hemicellulose, pectin and gums.

dietetic food diarrhoea. See osmotic diarrhoea.

dietetics, the science of applying nutritional principles to the planning and preparation of foods and regulation of the diet in relation to both health and disease.

diethylcarbamazine citrate, an anthelmintic prescribed in the treatment of ascariasis, filariasis, onchocerciasis and tropical eosinophilia.

diethyl ether. See ether.

diethylpropion hydrochloride, an appetite suppressant prescribed in the treatment of obesity.

diethylstilboestrol (DES), a synthetic hormone with oestrogenic properties.

dietitian, a person who meets all the requirements of active membership in the British Dietetic Association, after completing special educational training in the nutritional care of groups and individuals. A registered dietitian is one who has successfully completed his or her degree and has obtained a State Registration.

Dietl's crisis {Joseph Dietl, Polish physician, b. 1804}, a sudden, excruciating pain in the kidney, caused by distention of the renal pelvis, by the rapid ingestion of very large amounts of liquid, or by a kinking of a ureter that produces temporary occlusion of the flow of urine from the kidney.

differential absorption, the strong absorption of x-rays in high atomic number materials, such as bone, compared to the low absorption of x-rays in low atomic number materials, such as air and soft tissues, due to the photoelectric effect. This difference in absorption results in an x-ray image.

differential diagnosis, the distinction between two or more diseases with similar symptoms by systematically comparing their signs and symptoms.

differential growth, a comparison of the various increases in size or the different rates of growth of dissimilar organisms, tissues or structures.

differential white blood cell count, an examination and enumeration of the distribution of leukocytes in a stained blood smear. The different kinds of white cells are counted and reported as percentages of the total examined.

differentiation, 1. (in embryology) a process in development in which unspecialized cells or tissues are systemically modified and altered to achieve specific and characteristic physical forms, physiological functions, and chemical properties. Kinds of differentiation are **correlative, functional, invisible** and **self-differentiation**. **2.** progressive diversification leading to complexity. **3.** the acquisition of functions and forms different from those of the original. **4.** distinction of one thing or disease from another, as in differential diagnosis. **5.** (in psychology) a mental autonomy or separation of intellect and emotions so that one is not dominated by reactive anxiety of a family or group emotional system. **6.** the first subphase of the separation-individuation phase in Mahler's system of preoedipal development. **differentiate,** *v.*

diffraction, the bending and scattering of wavelengths of light or other radiation, such as the radiation that passes around obstacles in its path. X-ray diffraction is used in the study of the internal structure of cells. The x-rays are diffracted by cell parts into patterns that are indicative of chemical and physical structure.

diffuse, becoming widely spread, such as through a membrane or fluid.

diffuse fibrosing alveolitis. See interstitial pneumonia.

diffuse goitre, an enlargement of all parts of the thyroid gland.

diffuse hypersensitivity pneumonia, an immunologically mediated inflammatory reaction in the lungs, induced by exposure to an allergen or by an adverse reaction to a drug. The disorder is characterized by cough, fever, dyspnoea, malaise, pulmonary oedema, and infiltration of the alveoli with eosinophils and large mononuclear cells.

diffuse idiopathic skeletal hyperostosis, a form of degenerative joint disease in which the ligaments along the spinal column become calcified and lose their flexibility.

diffuse lipoma, diffuse lipomatosis. See **multiple lipomatosis**.

diffuse myocardial fibrosis, a type of heart disease characterized by a generalized distribution of fibrous tissue that replaces normal heart muscle cells.

diffusing capacity, the rate of gas transfer through a unit area of a permeable membrane per unit of gas pressure difference across it. It is affected by specific chemical reactions that may occur in the blood.

diffusing capacity of lungs (D_L), the number of millilitres of a gas that diffuse from the lung across the alveolar-capillary (A-C) membrane into the bloodstream each minute, for each 1 mm Hg difference in the pressure gradient across the membrane.

diffusion, the process in which solid, particulate matter in a fluid moves from an area of higher concentration to an area of lower concentration, resulting in an even distribution of the particles in the fluid.

diffusion constant, a mathematical constant relating to the ability of a substance to spread widely.

diffusion defect, any impairment of alveolar-capillary diffusion caused by pathological changes in any of the structures of the alveolar-capillary membrane and resulting in fewer molecules of oxygen crossing the membrane.

diffusion deposition, the impaction of an aerosol particle on the surface of an alveolar membrane or other airway structure, causing it to settle out of a vapour or gas.

diffusion of gases, a natural process, essential in respiration, in which molecules of a gas pass from an area of high concentration to one of a lower concentration.

diflunisal, a non-steroidal anti-inflammatory agent prescribed for mild to moderate pain and inflammation in osteoarthritis and other musculoskeletal disorders.

digastricus, one of four suprahyoid muscles having two parts, an anterior belly and a posterior belly. The anterior belly acts to open the jaw and draw the hyoid bone forward. The posterior belly acts to draw back and raise the hyoid bone.

DiGeorge's syndrome {Angelo M. DiGeorge, American physician, b. 1821}, a congenital disorder characterized by severe immunodeficiency and structural abnormalities, including hypertelorism, notched, low-set ears, small mouth, downward slanting eyes, cardiovascular defects and absence of the thymus and parathyroid glands.

digest, 1. to soften by heat and moisture. **2.** to break into smaller parts and simpler compounds by mastication, hydrolysis and the action of intestinal secretions and enzymes. **3.** any material that results from digestion or hydrolysis.

digestant, a substance, such as pepsin, that is added to the diet as an aid to the digestion of food.

digestion, the conversion of food into absorbable substances in the GI tract. Digestion is accomplished through the mechanical and chemical breakdown of food into progressively smaller molecules, with the help of glands located both inside and outside the gut. **digestive,** adj.

digestive fever, a slight rise in body temperature that normally accompanies the digestive process.

digestive gland, any one of the many structures that secretes reactive agents involved in the breaking down of food into the constituent absorbable substances needed for metabolism. Some kinds of digestive glands are the salivary glands, gastric glands, intestinal glands, liver and pancreas.

digestive system, the organs, structures and accessory glands of the digestive tube of the body through which food passes from the mouth to the oesophagus, stomach and intestines. The accessory glands secrete digestive enzymes, used by the digestive system to break down food substances in preparation for absorption into the bloodstream before carrying the waste to the intestines for excretion.

digestive tract, a musculomembranous tube, about 9 m long, extending from the mouth to the anus and lined with mucous membrane. Its various portions are the mouth, pharynx, oesophagus, stomach, small intestine and large intestine. The tube, which is part of the digestive system of the body, includes numerous accessory organs.

digital, 1. of or pertaining to a digit, that is, a finger or toe. **2.** resembling a finger or toe. **3.** the characterization or measurement of a signal in terms of a series of numbers rather than in terms of some continuously varying value.

digital angiography, a technique of producing enhanced x-ray images of the heart with computerized fluoroscopy equipment.

digital computer, a computer that processes information in numeric form.

digital fluoroscopy, a method of conducting fluoroscopic examinations with an image intensifier-television system combined with a high-speed digital video image processor.

digital radiography (DR), a method of x-ray image formation that uses a computer to store and manipulate data.

digital subtraction angiography (DSA), a method by which x-ray images of blood vessels filled with contrast material are digitized and then subtracted from images stored before the administration of contrast. Thus, the background is eliminated and only the vessels appear.

digital-to-analogue converter, a device for converting digital information into analogue form for representation as a continuous method of interpreting data, as from an ohm-meter or thermometer.

digitalis, plant material with cardiotonic action, formerly used in the treatment of congestive heart failure and certain cardiac arrhythmias, now superseded by the purified active principals.

digitalis glycoside. See **glycoside**.

digitalis therapy, the administration of a digitalis preparation to a person with a heart disorder to increase the force of myocardial contractions, produce a slower, more regular apical rate and slow the transmission of impulses through the conduction system. Digitalis may be used in treating various cardiac disorders, including atrial fibrillation, atrial septal defect, coarctation of the aorta, congenital heart block, congestive heart failure, endocardial fibroelastosis, great vessel transposition, malformation of the tricuspid valve, myocarditis, paroxysmal atrial tachycardia and patent ductus arteriosus.

digitalization, the administration of digitalis in doses sufficient to achieve maximum pharmacological effects without also producing toxic symptoms.

digitalized, the state of having a therapeutic total body level of a cardiac glycoside.

digitalizing dose, the amount of a cardiac glycoside needed to digitalize a patient.

digitate, having fingers or finger-like projections.

digitate wart, a finger-like, horny projection that arises from a pea-shaped base and occurs on the scalp or near the hairline. Like other warts, it is a benign viral infection of the skin and the adjacent mucous membrane.

digitoxin, a cardiac glycoside obtained from leaves of *Digitalis purpurea*. It is used in the treatment of congestive heart failure and certain cardiac arrhythmias.

digoxin, a cardiac glycoside obtained from leaves of *Digitalis lanata*. It is useed in the treatment of congestive heart failure and certain cardiac arrhythmias.

digoxin immune fab, ovine, a parenteral antidote used to treat life-threatening digoxin or digitoxin toxicity.

diGuglielmo's disease, diGuglielmo's syndrome. See **erythroleukaemia**.

dihybrid, (in genetics) pertaining to or describing a person, organism or strain that is heterozygous for two specific traits.

dihybrid cross, (in genetics) the mating of two individuals, organisms or strains which have different gene pairs that determine two specific traits, or in which two particular characteristics or gene loci are being followed.

dihydric alcohol, an alcohol containing two hydroxyl groups.

dihydroergotamine mesylate, an alpha-adrenergic blocking agent used to treat migraine and cluster headache.

dihydrotachysterol, a rapid-acting form of vitamin D. It is prescribed in the treatment of hypocalcaemia resulting from hypoparathyroidism and pseudohypoparathyroidism.

dilatation, 1. normal physiological increase in the diameter of a body opening, blood vessel or tube, such as the widening of the pupil of the eye in response to decreased light or the widening of the opening of the uterine cervix during labour. **2.** the diameter of the opening of the cervix in labour as measured on vaginal examination, expressed in centimetres.

dilatation and curettage (D & C), dilatation of the uterine cervix and scraping of the endometrium of the uterus, performed to diagnose disease of the uterus, correct heavy or prolonged vaginal bleeding, or empty uterine contents of the products of conception. It is also done to remove tumours, rule out carcinoma of the uterus, remove retained placental fragments postpartum or after an incomplete abortion, and find the cause of infertility.

dilatator naris, the alar portion of the nasalis muscle that dilates the nostril.

dilatator pupillae, a muscle that contracts the iris of the eye and dilates the pupil.

dilate. See **dilatation**.

dilator, a device for expanding a body opening or cavity.

diltiazem, a calcium antagonist used for the treatment of angina pectoris and hypertension.

diluent, a substance, generally a fluid, that makes a solution or mixture thinner, less viscous or more liquid.

dilute, pertaining to a solution in which there is a relatively small amount of solute in proportion to solvent.

diluting agent, (in respiratory therapy) a substance that can modify the viscosity of secretions so that they can be removed easily. Examples include water and hypotonic saline, which can be aerosolized or nebulized.

dimenhydrinate, an antihistamine prescribed in the treatment of nausea and motion sickness.

dimer, a compound formed by the union of two radicals or two molecules of a simpler compound, as a polymer formed from two or more molecules of a monomer.

dimercaprol, a heavy-metal chelating agent. It is used in the treatment of Wilson's disease and for acute arsenic, mercury or gold poisoning resulting from an overdosage with therapeutic mercurial diuretics or gold salts, or from the accidental or deliberate ingestion of mercury, gold or arsenic. Formerly called **British anti-lewisite (BAL)**.

dimethindene maleate, an antihistamine used in the treatment of a variety of allergic reactions, including rhinitis, skin reactions and itching.

dimethoxymethylamphetamine (DOM), a psychedelic agent with no recognised medical use.

dimethyl carbinol. See **isopropyl alcohol.**

dimethyl sulphoxide (DMSO), an anti-inflammatory agent prescribed in the treatment of interstitial cystitis, which is being investigated as a topical anti-inflammatory agent in sports injuries.

Dimitri's disease. See **Sturge-Weber syndrome.**

dinitrochlorobenzene (DNCB), a substance applied topically as a test for delayed hypersensitivity reactions.

dioctyl   sodium   sulphosuccinate.   See **docusate sodium.**

diode, an electronic device which allows current to pass in one direction only.

dioecious, an animal or plant that is sexually distinct, having either male or female reproductive organs.

diolamine, a contraction for diethanolamine.

Dionysian, the personal attitude of one who is uninhibited, mystic, sensual, emotional and irrational, and who may seek to escape from the boundaries imposed by the limits of one's senses.

dioptre, a metric measure of the refractive power of a lens. It is equal to the reciprocal of the focal length of the lens in meters. For example, a lens with a focal length of 0.5 m has a dioptre measure of 2.0 (1/2.0) and when prescribed as a corrective lens for the eye should make printed matter most clearly focused when held 0.5 m from the eyes.

dioptric power, the refractive power of an optic lens as measured in dioptres.

diovular. See **binovular.**

diovulatory, routinely releasing two ova during each ovarian cycle.

dioxin, a contaminant of the herbicide 2,4,5-trichlorophenoxyacetic   acid   (2,4,5-T), widely used throughout the world for weed control. Exposure to dioxin is associated with chloracne and porphyria cutanea tarda (PCT).

DIP, abbreviation for **desquamative interstitial pneumonia.**

diphenadione, an anticoagulant agent used as a rodenticide.

diphenhydramine hydrochloride, an antihistamine prescribed in the treatment of a variety of allergic reactions, including rhinitis, skin rash and pruritus, and in the treatment of motion sickness.

diphenoxylate hydrochloride, an opiate used in the treatment of diarrhoea and intestinal cramping.

diphenylhydantoin. See **phenytoin.**

2,3-diphosphoglyceric acid (DPG), a substance in the erythrocyte that affects the affinity of haemoglobin for oxygen. It is a chief end- product of glucose metabolism.

diphtheria, an acute, contagious disease caused by the bacterium *Corynebacterium diphtheriae*, characterized by the production of a systemic toxin and a false membrane lining of the mucous membrane of the throat. The toxin is particularly damaging to the tissues of the heart and central nervous system, and the dense pseudomembrane in the throat may interfere with eating, drinking and breathing. Untreated, the disease is often fatal, causing heart and kidney failure.

diphtheroid, 1. of or pertaining to diphtheria. **2.** resembling the bacillus *Corynebacterium diphtheriae*.

diphyllobothriasis. See **fish tapeworm infection.**

Diphyllobothrium, a genus of large, parasitic, intestinal flatworms having a scolex with two slitlike grooves.

dipivefrin, an ophthalmic adrenergic drug used in the treatment of open-angle glaucoma.

diplegia, bilateral paralysis of both sides of any part of the body or of like parts on the opposite sides of the body. A kind of diplegia is **facial diplegia.**   **diplegic,** *adj.*

diplococcus, *pl.* **diplococci,** a coccus that occurs in pairs.

diploë, the loose tissue filled with red bone marrow between the two tables of the cranial bones.

diploid, of, or pertaining to an individual, organism, strain or cell that has two complete sets of homologous chromosomes. In humans the normal diploid number is 46. **diploidic,** *adj.*

diploidy, the state or condition of having two complete sets of homologous chromosomes.

diplokaryon, a nucleus that contains twice the diploid number of chromosomes.

Diploma in Medical Ultrasound (DMU), post-qualifying diploma awarded by the College of Radiographers.

Diploma in Nursing, an educational programme following an academic curriculum combined with practical experience in hospital and community settings. It leads to the award of a diploma and registration as a nurse. Post-registration diploma courses are also available.

Diploma in Radionuclide Imaging (DRI), post-qualifying diploma awarded by the College of Radiographers in radionuclide imaging.

Diploma of the College of Radiographers

(DCR), professional qualification of competence to practise radiography awarded by the College of Radiographers in the UK, prior to the development and availability of pre-registration degree courses. The qualification may be awarded in either diagnostic radiography (DCR(R)) or therapeutic radiography (DCR(T)).

diplonema, the loop-like formation of chromosomes in the diplotene stage of the first meiotic prophase of gametogenesis.

diplopagus, conjoined twins that are more or less equally developed, although one or several internal organs may be shared.

diplopia, double vision caused by defective function of the extraocular muscles or a disorder of the nerves that innervate the muscles.

diplornavirus, a double-stranded RNA virus that is the cause of Colorado tick fever. It is related to the reoviruses that are associated with various respiratory infections.

diplosomatia, a congenital anomaly in which fully formed twins are joined at one or more areas of their bodies.

diplotene, the fourth stage in the first meiotic prophase in gametogenesis in which the tetrads exhibit chiasmata between the chromatids of the paired homologous chromosomes and genetic crossing-over occurs.

dipodia, a developmental anomaly characterized by the duplication of one or both feet.

dipolar ion. See **zwitterion.**

dipole, a molecule with areas of opposing electric charges, as hydrogen chloride with a predominance of electrons about the chloride portion and a positive charge on the hydrogen side.

diprop, abbreviation for a carboxylate dipropionate anion.

diprosopus, a malformed fetus that has a double face showing varying degrees of development.

dipsomania, an uncontrollable, often periodic craving for and indulgence in alcoholic beverages; alcoholism.

dipstick, a chemically treated strip of paper used in the analysis of urine or other fluids.

Dip.T.D, abbreviation for the Diploma in Teaching Physiotherapy.

dipus, conjoined twins that have only two feet.

dipygus, a malformed fetus that has a double pelvis, one of which is usually not fully developed.

dipyridamole, an antiplatelet drug used as an adjunct to oral anticoagulation in patients with prosthetic heart valves.

direct-access memory, access to computerized data independently of previously obtained data. The data transfer is directly between the computer memory and peripheral devices.

direct antagonist, one of a pair or a group of muscles that pull in opposite directions and whose combined action keeps the part from moving.

direct calorimetry, the measurement of the amount of heat directly generated by any oxidation reaction, especially one involving a living organism.

direct causal association, a cause-and-effect relationship between a causative factor and a disease with no other factors intervening in the process.

direct contact, mutual touching of two individuals or organisms. Many communicable diseases may be spread by the direct contact between an infected and a healthy person.

direct current, an electric current that flows in one direction only and is substantially constant in value.

direct exposure film, a type of x-ray film designed to be used without intensifying screens, and therefore requiring relatively high radiation exposure but giving very fine image detail.

direct fracture, any fracture occurring at a specific point of injury that is a direct result of that injury.

direct generation. See **asexual generation.**

direct gold, any form of pure gold that may be compacted directly into a prepared tooth cavity to form a restoration.

direct illumination. See **illumination.**

directive therapy, a psychotherapeutic approach in which the psychotherapist directs the course of therapy by intervening to ask questions and offer interpretations.

direct lead, 1. an electrocardiographic conductor in which the exploring electrode is placed directly on the surface of the exposed heart. **2.** *informal.* a tracing produced by such a lead on an electrocardiograph.

direct patient care, (in nursing) care of a patient provided in person by a member of the staff.

direct percussion. See **percussion.**

direct-question interview, an enquiry that usually requires simple one- or two-word responses.

direct reaction to light, the constriction of a pupil receiving increased illumination, as by a flashlight during an ophthalmological examination.

direct relationship. See **positive relationship.**

direct retainer, a clasp, attachment or assembly fastened to an abutment tooth, for the purpose of maintaining a removable restoration in its planned position in relation to oral structures.

direct self-destructive behaviour, any form of suicidal activity, such as suicide threats, attempts or gestures, as well as the act of suicide itself. The intent of the behaviour is death, and the person is aware of this as the desired outcome.

dirofilariasis, a rare human infestation of the dog heartworm, Dirofilaria immitis, which may be transmitted through the bite of any of several species of mosquitoes.

disability, the loss, absence or impairment of physical or mental fitness that is observable and measurable.

disaccharidase deficiency. See **lactase deficiency.**

disaster-action plan, a formal plan of action, usually prepared in written form, for coordinating the response of a hospital staff in the event of a disaster within the hospital or the surrounding community.

disc. See **disk.**

discharge, 1. also evacuate, excrete, secrete. to release a substance or object. **2.** to release a patient from a hospital. **3.** to release an electric charge, which may be manifested by a spark or surge of electricity, from a storage battery, capacitor or other source. **4.** to release a burst of energy from or through a neuron. **5.** a release of emotions, often accompanied by a wide range of voluntary and involuntary reflexes, weeping, rage or other emotional displays, called affective discharge in psychology. **6.** a substance or object discharged.

discharge abstract, items of information compiled from medical records of patients discharged from a hospital, organized and recorded in a uniform format to provide data for statistical studies, reports or research.

discharge coordinator, an individual who arranges with community agencies and institutions for the continuing care of patients after their discharge from a hospital.

discharge planning, a schedule of events often planned by a multidisciplinary team leading to the return of a patient from hospital confinement to a normal life at home.

discharge summary, a clinical report prepared by a doctor or other health professional at the conclusion of treatment, outlining the patient's chief complaint, diagnostic findings, therapy administered and the patient's response to it.

disciform keratitis, an inflammatory condition of the eye that often follows an attack of dendritic keratitis and is believed to be an immunological response to an ocular herpes simplex infection. The condition is characterized by disc-like opacities in the cornea, usually with inflammation of the iris.

disclosing solution, a topically applied dye, used in aqueous solution to stain and reveal plaque and other deposits on teeth.

discoblastula, a blastula formed from the partial cleavage that occurs in a fertilized ovum containing a large amount of yolk.

discocyte, a mature, normal erythrocyte exhibiting one of its many steady-state configurations. It is a biconcave disk without a nucleus.

discography, a radiographic technique for visualizing the intranuclear disc morphology by injecting a radiopaque contrast medium into the centre of the disc. **discogram,** *n.*

discoid lupus erythematosus (DLE), a chronic, recurrent disease, primarily of the skin, characterized by red macules that are covered with scales and extend into follicles. The lesions are typically distributed in a butterfly pattern covering the cheeks and bridge of the nose but may also occur on other parts of the body. The cause of the disease is not established, but there is evidence that it may be an autoimmune disorder. Some cases seem to be induced by certain drugs.

discoid meniscus, an abnormal condition characterized by a discoid rather than semilunar shape of the cartilaginous meniscus of the knee. Common complaints are a "clicking" occurring in the knee joint or the knee joint giving way. These characteristics are often associated with an injury to the knee, but occur also without any history of trauma.

disconfirmation, a dysfunctional communication that negates, discounts or ignores information received from another person.

discordance, (in genetics) the expression of one or more specific traits in only one member of a pair of twins.   **discordant,** *adj.*

discriminator, (in nuclear medicine) an electronic device used in scintillation counters and gamma cameras, which can be set to accept pulses from a photomultiplier tube within certain limits. It is used to eliminate unwanted radiation in the detection and measurement of radioactivity.

discus. See **disk.**

discus articularis, a small oval plate between the condyle of the mandible and the mandibular fossa.

discus interpubicus. See **interpubic disk.**

disease, 1. a condition of abnormal vital function involving any structure, part or system of an organism. **2.** a specific illness or disorder characterized by a recognizable set of signs and symptoms, attributable to heredity, infection, diet or environment.

disease prevention, activities designed to protect patients or other members of the public from actual or potential health threats and their harmful consequences.

disengagement, 1. an obstetrical manipulation in which the presenting part of the baby is dislodged from the maternal pelvis as part of an operative delivery. **2.** the release or detachment of oneself from other persons or responsibilities. **3.** (in transactional family therapy) a role assumed by a therapist in observing and restructuring intervention without becoming actively and directly involved in the problem.

disengagement theory, the psychosocial concept that ageing individuals and society normally withdraw from active engagement with each other.

dishpan fracture, a fracture that depresses the skull.

disinfectant, a chemical that can be applied to objects to destroy micro-organisms.

disinfection, the process of killing pathogenic organisms.

disintegrative psychosis, a mental disorder of childhood that usually has an onset after the age of 3 years and following normal development of speech, social behaviour and other traits. After a vague illness, the child undergoes mental deterioration, eventually reaching a stage of severe mental retardation.

disjunction, (in genetics) the separation of the paired homologous chromosomes during the anaphase stage of the first meiotic division, or of the chromatids during anaphase of mitosis and the second meiotic division.

disk, 1. also spelt (chiefly in ophthalmology) disc. A flat, circular platelike structure, as an articular disk or an optic disc. **2.** *informal.* an intervertebral disk. **3.** a flexible plastic, oxide-coated disk, contained in a special square jacket, for use in a computer disk drive. Also diskette.

disk drive, a computer device containing a disk that spins at high speeds, equipped with a head that allows electric impulses to be written onto and read from the electromagnetic surface.

dislocation, the displacement of any part of the body from its normal position, particularly a bone from its normal articulation with a joint. **dislocate,** *v.*

dismiss, (in law) to discharge or dispose of an action, suit or motion trial. dismissal, n.

disopyramide phosphate, a cardiac depressant prescribed in the treatment of premature ventricular contractions and ventricular tachycardia.

disorganized schizophrenia, a form of schizophrenia characterized by an earlier age of onset, usually at puberty, and a more severe disintegration of the personality than occurs in other forms of the disease. Symptoms include inappropriate laughter and silliness; peculiar mannerisms, like grimaces; talking and gesturing to oneself; regressive, bizarre and often obscene behaviour.

disorientate, to cause to lose awareness or perception of space, time, personal identity or relationships.

disorientation, a state of mental confusion characterized by inadequate or incorrect perceptions of place, time or identity.

disparate twins, twins who are distinctly different from each other in weight and other features.

dispersing agent, a chemical additive used in pharmacology to effect an even distribution of the ingredients throughout a product, such as in dermatological emulsions containing both oil and water.

dispersion, the scattering or dissipation of finely divided material, as when particles of a substance are scattered throughout the volume of a fluid.

dispersion medium. See medium.

displaced fracture, a traumatic bone break in which two ends of a fractured bone are separated from each other. The ends of broken bones in displaced fractures often pierce surrounding skin, as in an open fracture, or may be contained within the skin, as in a closed fracture.

displacement, 1. the state of being displaced or the act of displacing. **2.** (in chemistry) a reaction in which an atom, molecule or radical is removed from combination and replaced by another. **3.** (in physics) the displacing in space of one mass by another, such as the weight or volume of a fluid being displaced by a floating or submerged body. **4.** (in psychiatry) an unconscious defence mechanism for avoiding emotional conflict and anxiety by transferring emotions, ideas or wishes from one object to a substitute that is less anxiety-producing.

dissect, to cut apart tissues for visual or microscopic study using a scalpel, a probe, or scissors. **dissection,** *n.*

dissecting aneurysm, a localized dilatation of an artery, most commonly the aorta, characterized by a longitudinal dissection between the outer and middle layers of the vascular wall. Blood entering a tear in the intimal lining of the vessel causes a separation of weakened elastic and fibromuscular elements in the medial layer, and leads to the formation of cystic spaces filled with ground substance. Rupture of a dissecting aneurysm may be fatal in less than 1 hour.

disseminated intravascular coagulation (DIC), a grave coagulopathy resulting from the overstimulation of the body's clotting and anticlotting processes in response to disease or injury, such as septicaemia, poisonous snake bites, severe trauma or haemorrhage. The primary disorder initiates generalized intravascular clotting, which in turn overstimulates fibrinolytic mechanisms; as a result, the initial hypercoagulability is succeeded by a deficiency in clotting factors with hypocoagulability and haemorrhage.

disseminated lupus erythematosus. See systemic lupus erythematosus.

disseminated multiple sclerosis. See multiple sclerosis.

dissimilar twins. See dizygotic twins.

dissociation, 1. the act of separating into parts or sections. **2.** an unconscious defence mechanism by which an idea, thought, emotion or other mental process is separated from the consciousness and thereby loses emotional significance. **dissociative,** *adj.*

dissociative anaesthesia, an anaesthetic procedure characterized by analgesia and amnenesia without loss of respiratory function or pharyngeal and laryngeal reflexes. This form of anaesthesia may be used to provide analgesia during brief, superficial operative procedures or diagnostic processes.

dissociative disorder, a type of hysterical neurosis in which emotional conflicts are so repressed that a separation or split in the personality occurs, resulting in an altered state of consciousness or a confusion in identity. Symptoms include amnesia, somnambulism, fugue, dream state or multiple personality.

dissolved gas, gas in a simple physical solution, as distinguished from gas that has reacted chemically with a solvent or other solutes and is chemically combined.

distal, 1. away from or being furthest from a point of origin. **2.** away from or being furthest from the midline or a central point, such as a distal phalanx.

distal latency, (in electroneuromyography) the time interval between the stimulation of a compound muscle and the observed response.

distal muscular dystrophy, a rare form of muscular dystrophy, usually affecting adults, characterized by moderate weakness and wasting that begins in the arms and legs and then extends gradually to the proximal and facial muscles.

distal phalanx, any one of the small distal bones in the third row of phalanges of the hand or the foot. Each distal phalanx of the toes is smaller and more flattened than that of a finger.

distal radioulnar articulation, the pivot-like articulation of the head of the ulna and the ulnar notch on the lower end of the radius, involving two ligaments.

distal renal tubular acidosis (distal RTA), an abnormal condition characterized by excessive acid accumulation and bicarbonate excretion. It is caused by the inability of the distal tubules of the kidney to secrete hydrogen ions, thus decreasing the excretion of titratable acids and ammonium and increasing the urinary loss of potassium and bicarbonate. Primary distal RTA occurs mostly in females, adolescents, older children and young adults. It may occur sporadically or as the result of hereditary defects. Secondary distal RTA is associated with numerous disorders, such as cirrhosis of the liver, malnutrition, starvation and various genetic problems.

distal sparing, a condition in which the spinal cord remains intact below a lesion. The reflex arc remains but is not modified by supraspinal influences. As a result, there may be spastic movements distal to the level of the lesion.

distance regulation, behaviour that is related to the control of personal space. Most humans establish a quantum of space between themselves and others that offers security from either psychological or physical threat, while not creating a feeling of isolation.

distance vision, the ability to see objects clearly, usually from more than 20 feet or 6 m away.

distension, the state of being distended or swollen.

distortion, (in psychology) the process of shifting experience in one's perceptions. The distortions of patients tend to influence their views of the world and themselves.

distraction, 1. procedures that prevent or lessen the perception of pain by focusing attention on sensations unrelated to pain. **2.** a method of straightening a spinal column by the forces of axial tension pulling on the joint surfaces, such as applied by a Milwaukee brace.

distress of the human spirit. See spiritual distress.

distributed processing, a combination of local and remote computers in a network connected to a central computer, to distribute the processing and thereby reduce the load on the central computer.

distributive analysis and synthesis, the system of psychotherapy used by the psychobiological school of psychiatry.

distributive care, a pattern of healthcare that is concerned with environment, heredity, living conditions, lifestyle and early detection of pathological effects.

district nurse. an individual educated in hospital and community nursing, who practices primarily in the client's home.

disulfiram, an inhibitor of alcohol metabolism used in the treatment of chronic alcoholism. It causes severe intestinal cramping, diaphoresis and nausea if alcohol is ingested.

disuse phenomena, the physical and the psychological changes, usually degenerative, that result from the lack of use of a part of the body or a body system. Disuse phenomena are associated with confinement and immobility, especially in orthopaedics. The physical changes often induced by continued bed rest constitute problems affecting many key areas and systems of the body, such as the skin, musculoskeletal system, GI tract, cardiovascular system and respiratory system. Unused muscles lose size and strength, often wasting away until they are unable to perform their vital functions of support and contraction. Another disuse phenomenon is contracture, which may result from constant flexion or extension of a body part by the patient on prolonged bed rest. The immobilized patient may experience bone demineralization because of a restricted diet and decreased motility.

diuresis, increased formation and secretion of urine. Diuresis occurs in conditions such as diabetes mellitus and diabetes insipidus.

diuretic, 1. (of a drug or other substance)

tending to promote the formation and excretion of urine. **2.** a drug that promotes the formation and excretion of urine. Diuretic drugs can be classified by chemical structure and pharmacological activity into the following groups: aldosterone antagonists, carbonic anhydrase inhibitors, loop diuretics, mercurials, osmotics, potassium-sparing diuretics and thiazides. A diuretic medication may contain drugs from one or more of these groups.

diurnal, taking place daily, such as sleeping and eating.

diurnal mood variation, a change in mood that is related to the time of day. Examples are commonly found in differences between "night" people" and "morning" people.

diurnal variation, the range of output or excretion rate of a substance in a specimen being collected for laboratory analysis over a 24-hour period.

divalent. See **bivalent.**

divergence, a separation or movement of objects away from each other, as in the simultaneous turning of the eyes outward due to an extraocular muscle defect.

diverticular disease. See **diverticulitis, diverticulosis.**

diverticulitis, inflammation of one or more diverticula. The penetration of faecal matter through the thin-walled diverticula causes inflammation and abscess formation in the tissues surrounding the colon. With repeated inflammation, the lumen of the colon narrows and may become obstructed. During periods of inflammation, the patient will experience crampy pain, particularly over the sigmoid colon, fever, and leukocytosis. Barium enemas and proctoscopy are performed to rule out carcinoma of the colon which exhibits some of the same symptoms. Conservative treatment includes bed rest, intravenous fluids, antibiotics and nil-by-mouth. In acute cases, bowel resection of the affected part greatly reduces mortality and morbidity.

diverticulosis, the presence of pouch-like herniations through the muscular layer of the colon, particularly the sigmoid colon.

diverticulum, *pl.* **diverticula,** a pouch-like herniation through the muscular wall of a tubular organ. A diverticulum may be present in the stomach, the small intestine or, most commonly, the colon. **diverticular,** *adj.*

diving, the act of work or recreation in an underwater environment. The main health effects are related to the increased pressure to which the person is subjected, as the ambient pressure generally increases by 1 atm (14.7 pounds per square inch) for each 33 feet of descent below the water surface.

diving goitre, a large, movable thyroid gland located at times above the sternal notch and at other times below the notch.

diving reflex, an automatic change in the cardiovascular system that occurs when the face and nose are immersed in water. The heart rate decreases and the blood pressure remains stable or increases slightly, while blood flow to all parts of the body except the brain is reduced.

division, 1. an administrative subunit in a hospital, such as a division of medical nursing or a division of surgical nursing. **2.** the separation of something into two or more parts or sections. A kind of division is cell division.

dizygotic, of or pertaining to twins from two fertilized ova.

dizygotic twins, two offspring born of the same pregnancy and developed from two ova that were released from the ovary simultaneously and fertilized at the same time. They may be of the same or opposite sex, differ both physically and in genetic constitution, and have two separate and distinct placentas and membranes, both amnion and chorion.

dizziness, a sensation of faintness or an inability to maintain normal balance in a standing or seated position, sometimes associated with giddiness, mental confusion, nausea and weakness. A patient who experiences dizziness should be carefully lowered to a safe position because of the danger of injury from falling.

DLE, abbreviation for **discoid lupus erythematosus.**

DM, abbreviation for **diabetes mellitus.**

DMSO, abbreviation for **dimethyl sulphoxide.**

DMU, abbreviation for **Diploma in Medical Ultrasound.**

DN, abbreviation for **District Nurse, Diploma of Nursing.**

DNA, abbreviation for **deoxyribonucleic acid.**

DNA chimera, (in molecular genetics) a recombinant molecule of DNA composed of segments from more than one source.

DNA ligase, an enzyme that can repair breaks in a strand of DNA by synthesizing a bond between adjoining nucleotides. Under some circumstances the enzyme can join together loose ends of DNA strands, and in some cases it can repair breaks in RNA.

DNA polymerase, (in molecular genetics) an enzyme that catalyses the assembly of deoxyribonucleoside triphosphates into DNA, with single-stranded DNA serving as the template.

DNCB, abbreviation for **dinitrochlorobenzene.**

DNE, abbreviation for **Diploma of Nursing Education.**

Dobie's globule {William M. Dobie, English physician, b. 1828}, a very small stainable body in the transparent disk of a striated muscle fibre.

dobutamine hydrochloride, a beta-adrenergic stimulating agent prescribed to increase cardiac output in shocked patients, after myocardial infarction, and as an adjunct in cardiac surgery.

Dock, Lavinia Lloyd (1858 1956), an American public health nurse. She advocated an international public health movement and the improvement of education for nurses. With M. Adelaide Nutting, she wrote History of Nursing, a classic in nursing literature.

doctrine of double effect, a concept that an evil or lesser good is morally acceptable if done to achieve a greater good, provided that certain conditions are fulfilled.

doctoral programme in nursing, an educational programme of study that offers preparation for a doctoral degree in the field of nursing designed to prepare nurses for advanced practice and research. Upon successful completion the degree Ph.D is awarded.

documentation, 1. a detailed recording of information. **2.** written material associated with a computer or a programme. Kinds of documentation include user documentation, an instruction manual that provides enough information for the individual to use the system; system documentation, a complete description of the hardware and software that make up a system; and programme documentation, a general and specific description of what a programme does and how it does it.

docusate sodium, a stool softener prescribed in the treatment of constipation.

δOD, abbreviation for delta optic density.

Doederlein's bacillus Albert S. Doederlein, German physician, b. 1860, a gram-positive bacterium present in normal vaginal secretions.

Doehle bodies {Karl G. P. Doehle, German pathologist, b. 1855}, blue inclusions in the cytoplasm of some leukocytes in May-Hegglin anomaly and in blood smears from patients with acute infections.

Döhle-Heller disease. See syphilitic aortitis.

dolichocephaly. See scaphocephaly.

doll's-eye reflex, a normal response in newborns to keep the eyes stationary as the head is moved to the right or left. The reflex disappears as ocular fixation develops.

dolor, any condition of physical pain, mental anguish or suffering from heat. It is one of the four signs of inflammation. The others are calor (heat), rubor (redness) and tumour (swelling).

DOM, abbreviation for **dimethoxymethylamphetamine.**

dome fracture, any fracture of the acetabulum, specifically involving a weight-bearing surface.

dominance, (in genetics) a basic principle stating that not all genes determining a given trait operate with equal vigour. If two genes at a given locus produce a different effect, the gene that is manifest is dominant. **dominant,** *adj.*

dominant gene, one that produces a phenotypic effect regardless of whether its allele is the same or different.

dominant group, a social group that controls the value system and rewards in a particular society.

dominant trait, an inherited characteristic, such as eye colour, likely to appear in an offspring although it may occur in only one parent.

Donath-Landsteiner syndrome {Julius Donath, Austrian physician, b. 1870; Karl Landsteiner, Austrian-American pathologist, b. 1868}, a rare blood disorder, marked by haemolysis minutes or hours after exposure to cold. Systemic symptoms include passage of dark urine, severe pain in the back and legs, headache, vomiting, diarrhoea and moderate reticulocytosis.

donor, 1. a human or other organism that gives living tissue to be used in another body, for example, blood for transfusion or a kidney for transplantation. **2.** a substance or compound that gives part of itself to another substance.

Donovan bodies {Charles Donovan, Irish physician, b. 1863}, encapsulated gram-negative rods of the species *Calymmatobacterium granulomatis*, present in the cytoplasm of mononuclear phagocytes obtained from the lesions of granuloma inguinale.

dopa, an amino acid derived from tyrosine that occurs naturally in plants and animals. It is a precursor of dopamine, epinephrine and norepinephrine.

dopamine hydrochloride, a sympathomimetic catecholamine prescribed in the treatment of shock, hypotension and low cardiac output.

dopaminergic, having the effect of dopamine.

dope, *slang.* morphine, heroin or other opiate, or marijuana or other substance illicitly bought or sold, and often self-administered for sedative, hypnotic, euphoric or other mood-altering purpose.

Doppler effect Christian J. Doppler, Austrian scientist, b. 1803, the apparent change in frequency of sound, light or radio waves emitted by a source as it moves away from or towards an observer. The frequency increases as the source moves toward the observer and decreases as it moves away.

Doppler scanning {Christian J. Doppler}, (in ultrasonography) a technique used in ultrasound imaging to monitor the behaviour of a moving structure, such as flowing blood or a beating heart.

dorsal, pertaining to the back or posterior. **dorsum,** *n.*

dorsal carpal ligament. See retinaculum extensorum manus.

dorsal cutaneous nerve, a nerve that is close to the surface of the foot and ankle, where it may be both visible and palpable.

dorsal decubitus position. See **supine.**

dorsal digital vein, one of the communicating veins along the sides of fingers.

dorsal inertia posture, a tendency of a debilitated or weak person to slip downwards in bed when the head of the bed is raised.

dorsal interventricular artery, the arterial branch of the right coronary artery, branching to supply both ventricles.

dorsalis pedis artery, the continuation of the anterior tibial artery, starting at the ankle joint, dividing into five branches and supplying various muscles of the foot and toes.

dorsalis pedis pulse, the pulse of the dorsalis pedis artery, palpable between the first and second metatarsal bones on the top of the foot.

dorsal lip, the marginal fold of the blastopore during gastrulation in the early stages of embryonic development of many animals.

dorsal rigid posture, a position in which a patient lying in bed holds one or both legs drawn up to the chest. It often involves only the right leg and is intended to relieve abdominal pain.

dorsal scapular nerve, one of a pair of supraclavicular branches from the roots of the brachial plexus. It supplies the rhomboideus major and rhomboideus minor, and sends a branch to the levator.

dorsiflect, to bend or flex backwards, as in the upward bending of the fingers, wrist, foot or toes.

dorsiflexion, flexion towards the back, as accomplished by a muscle.

dorsiflexor, a muscle causing backward flexion of a part of the body, such as the hand or foot.

dorsiflexor gait, an abnormal gait caused by the weakness of the dorsiflexors of the ankle. It is characterized by footdrop during the entire gait cycle, and excessive knee and hip flexion to allow clearance of the involved extremity during the swing phase.

dorsodynia, a pain in the back, particularly in the muscles of the upper back area.

dorsosacral position. See **lithotomy position.**

dorsum sellae, the posterior boundary of the sella turcica of the sphenoid bone. It bears the posterior clinoid process and is an anatomical marker for the location of the pituitary gland at the base of the skull.

dosage, the regimen specifying the size, frequency and number of doses of a therapeutic agent to be administered to a patient.

dosage compensation, (in genetics) the mechanism that counterbalances the number of X-linked gene doses in the sex chromosomes so that they are equal in both the male, which has one X chromosome, and the female, which has two. In mammals this is accomplished by genetic activation of only one of the X chromosomes in the somatic cells of females.

dose, the amount of a drug or other substance to be administered at one time or over a specified period.

dose-area product, measurement of the total amount of radiation used in any single exposure.

dose-area product meter, (in radiography) electronic device which gives an instantaneous readout of the total amount of radiation used in a single exposure, by incorporating a large area ionisation chamber through which the x-ray beam passes.

dose equivalent (DE), a quantity used in radiation-safety work that equates on a unified scale the amount of radiation dose and the physical damages that it might produce. The unit of dose equivalent is the sievert (Sv).

dose fractionation. See **fractionation, def. 5.**

dose limit, annual maximum permitted dose from exposure to ionising radiation resulting from the sum of the effective dose equivalent and the committed effective dose equivalent, to the whole body, or to individual organs and tissues.

dose rate, (in radiobiology) the quantity of absorbed dose delivered per unit time.

dose ratemeter, (in radiotherapy) an instrument for measuring the dose rate of radiation.

dose response, a range of drug effects seen between the minimum dose at which an effect is first observed, and a toxic dose level, where adverse effects result.

dose-response relationship, (in radiobiology) a mathematical relationship between the dose of radiation and the body's reaction to it. In a linear dose-response relationship, the response is proportional to the dose.

dose threshold, (in radiobiology) the minimum amount of absorbed radiation that produces a detectable degree of a given effect.

dosimeter, an instrument to detect and measure accumulated radiation exposure.

double-approach conflict. See **approach-approach conflict.**

double-avoidant conflict. See **avoidance-avoidance conflict.**

double bind, a "no win" situation resulting from two conflicting messages from a person who is crucial to one's survival, such as a verbal message that differs from a nonverbal message.

double-blind study, an experiment designed to test the effect of a treatment or substance using groups of experimental and control subjects in which neither the subjects nor the investigators know which treatment or substance is being administered to which group. In a test of a new drug, the substance may be identified to the investigators only by a code. A double-blind study may be augmented by a cross-over experiment, in which experimental subjects unknowingly become control subjects and vice versa at some point in the study.

double contrast radiography, technique in which two contrast media are used, one radiopaque, the other radiolucent, such as air or CO_2. May be used in barium meals, barium enemas and knee and elbow arthography.

double-emulsion film, x-ray film coated with light-sensitive emulsion on both sides.

double fracture, a fracture consisting of breaks or cracks in two places in a bone, resulting in more than two bone segments.

double gel diffusion. See **immunodiffusion.**

double innervation, innervation of effector organs by fibres of the sympathetic and parasympathetic divisions of the autonomic nervous system. The pelvic viscera, bronchioles, heart, eyes and digestive system are all doubly innervated.

double monster, a fetus that has developed from a single ovum but has two heads, trunks and multiple limbs.

double-needle entry, a technique for injecting a contrast medium or other agent with two needles, one with a larger bore. In discography, a 20-gauge needle is used to perform a spinal puncture, after which a longer, 26-gauge needle is passed through the guide needle to the injection target area.

double quartan fever, a form of malaria in which paroxysms of fever occur in a repeating pattern of 2 consecutive days followed by 1 day of remission. The pattern is usually the result of concurrent infections by two species of the genus Plasmodium, one causing paroxysms every 72 hours and the other every 48 hours.

double tachycardia, the simultaneous but independent firing of two rapid heart contraction impulses, one controlling the atria and one the ventricles.

double vision. See **diplopia.**

double-void, a urinalysis procedure in which the first specimen is discarded and a second, obtained 30 to 45 minutes later, is tested. This method gives a more accurate measure of the amount of glucose in the urine at that particular time.

douche, 1. a procedure in which a litre or more of a solution of a medication or cleansing agent in warm water is introduced into the vagina under low pressure. The woman often performs the procedure herself, sitting on a toilet seat or semi-sitting in a bathtub. **2.** to perform a douche.

Downey cells {Hal Downey, American physician, b. 1877}, lymphocytes identified in one system of classification of the blood cells of patients with infectious mononucleosis. The cells are designated as Downey I, II, or III lymphocytes.

Down's syndrome {John L. Down, English physician, b. 1828}, a chromosome abnormality associated with increasing maternal age. There is either an extra chromosome attached to the 21st pair (trisomy 21), or a translocation usually between chromosomes 14 and 21. The syndrome is always associated with learning disabilities and certain characteristics, including slanting eyes with prominent epicanthic folds, low-set ears, a large protruding tongue, a single palmar crease and Brushfields' spots in the iris.

doxapram hydrochloride, a respiratory stimulant prescribed to improve respiratory function after anaesthesia and during ventilatory failure.

doxepin hydrochloride, a tricyclic antidepressant prescribed in the treatment of depression.

doxorubicin hydrochloride, a cytotoxic anthracycline antibiotic prescribed in the treatment of a variety of malignant diseases.

doxycycline, a tetracycline antibiotic used in the treatment of a variety of bacterial infections.

doxylamine succinate, an antihistamine used in the treatment of acute allergic symptoms produced by the release of histamine.

dp/dt, (in cardiology) the rate of pressure change per unit of time.

DPG, abbreviation for **2,3-diphosphoglyceric acid.**

DQ, abbreviation for **developmental quotient.**

dracunculiasis, a parasitic infection caused by infestation by the nematode *Dracunculus medinensis.* It is characterized by ulcerative skin lesions on the legs and feet that are produced by gravid female worms. People are infected by drinking contaminated water or eating contaminated shellfish.

Dracunculus medinensis, a parasitic nematode of the Mediterranean area that causes dracunculiasis. An American species is *Dracunculus insignis.*

drain, a tube or other opening used to remove air or a fluid from a body cavity or wound. The drain may be a closed system, designed to provide complete protection against contamination, or an open system.

drainage, the removal of fluids from a body cavity, wound or other source of discharge, by one or more methods. **Closed drainage** is a system of tubing and other apparatus attached to the body to remove fluid in an airtight circuit that prevents environmental contaminants from entering the wound or cavity. **Open drainage** is drainage in which discharge passes through an open-ended tube into a receptacle. **Suction drainage** utilizes a pump or other mechanical device to assist in extracting a fluid. **Tidal drainage** is drainage in which a body area is washed out by alternately flooding and then emptied it with the aid of gravity; this is a technique that may be used in treating a urinary bladder disorder.

drainage tube, a heavy-gauge catheter used for the evacuation of air or a fluid from a cavity or wound in the body.

Draize test, a controversial method of testing the toxicity of pharmaceutical and other products to be used by humans, by placing a small amount of the substance in the eyes of rabbits. The eye-irritancy potential of a substance is considered a measure of the possible effect the product could have on similar human tissues.

dram, a unit of mass equivalent to an apothecaries' measure of 60 grains or $^1/_8$ ounce and to $^1/_{16}$ ounce or 27.34 grains avoirdupois.

dramatic play, an imitative activity in which a child fantasizes and acts out various domestic and social roles and situations, as rocking a doll, pretending to be a doctor or nurse, or teaching school.

drape, a sheet of fabric or paper, usually the size of a small bed sheet, for covering all or part of a person's body during a physical examination or treatment. **drape,** *v.*

drawer sign, a diagnostic sign of a ruptured or torn knee ligament. It is tested by having the patient flex the knee at a right angle while the examiner grasps the lower leg just below the knee and moves the leg first towards and then away from himself. The test is positive for knee injury if the head of the tibia can be moved more than a half-inch from the joint.

drawsheet, a sheet that is smaller than a bottom or top sheet of a bed and is usually placed to keep the mattress and bottom linens dry or used to turn or move a patient in bed.

dream, 1. a sequence of ideas, thoughts, emotions, or images that pass through the mind during the rapid-eye-movement stage of sleep. **2.** the sleeping state in which this process occurs. **3.** a visionary creation of the imagination experienced during wakefulness. **4.** (in psychoanalysis) the expression of thoughts, emotions, memories or impulses repressed from the consciousness. **5.** (in analytical psychology) the wishes, emotions and impulses that reflect the personal unconscious and the archetypes that originate in the collective unconscious.

dream analysis, a process of gaining access to the unconscious mind by means of examining the content of dreams, usually through the method of free association.

dream association, a relationship of thoughts or emotions discovered or experienced when a dream is remembered or analysed.

dream state, a condition of altered consciousness in which a person does not recognize the environment and reacts in a manner opposed to his or her usual behaviour, as by flight or an act of violence.

drepanocytic anaemia, sickle cell anaemia.

dress code, the standards set by an institution for the dress of the members of the institution.

dressing, a clean or sterile covering applied directly to wounded or diseased tissue for absorption of secretions, protection from trauma, administration of medications, to keep the wound clean, or to stop bleeding. Kinds of dressings include **absorbent dressing, antiseptic dressing, occlusive dressing, pressure dressing,** and **wet dressing.**

dressing forceps, a kind of forceps that has narrow blades and blunt or notched teeth, designed for dressing wounds, removing drainage tubes or extracting fragments of necrotic tissue.

Dressler's syndrome, an autoimmune disorder that may occur several days after an acute coronary infarction, characterized by fever, pericarditis, pleurisy, pleural effusions and joint pain. It results from the body's immunological response to a damaged myocardium and pericardium.

DRI, abbreviation for **Diploma in Radionuclide Imaging.**

dried factor IX fraction, a haemostatic containing factors II, VII, IX and X. It is used in the treatment of haemophilia B. It is a vitamin K-dependent protein product sythesized in the liver.

drift, 1. antigenic drift, a change that occurs in a strain of virus so that variations appear periodically with alterations in antigenic qualities. **2.** genetic drift, random variations in gene frequency of a population from one generation to the next.

drifting tooth, any one of the teeth that migrate from normal position in the associated dental arch.

Drinker respirator {Philip Drinker, American engineer, b. 1893}, an airtight respirator consisting of a metal tank that encloses the entire body, except for the head. Used for long-term therapy, it alternates positive and negative air pressure within the tank, providing artificial respiration.

drip, 1. the process of a liquid or moisture forming and falling in drops. Kinds of drip are nasal drip and postnasal drip. **2.** the slow but continuous infusion of a liquid into the body, such as into the stomach or a vein. **3.** to infuse a liquid continuously into the body.

drip feed, a method of feeding a liquid formula diet through a tube inserted through the nostrils to the stomach.

drip set, (in intravenous therapy) an apparatus for delivering specific volumes of intravenous solutions within predetermined periods of time and at a specific flow rate. It consists of plastic tubing and a combinaion drip chamber with or without a filter.

drive, 1. a basic, compelling urge. **Primary drive** refers to one that is innate and in close contact with physiological processes. A secondary drive is one that evolves during the process of growth, inciting and directing behaviour. **2.** an electromechanical device that holds a secondary-storage medium and allows for the transfer of data to and from the computer, such as a disk drive or tape drive.

drop, a small spherical mass of liquid. A drop may vary in size with differences in temperature, viscosity and other factors. For therapeutic purposes, a drop is regarded as having a volume of .06 to 0.1 ml, or 1 to 1.5 minims.

drop arm test, a diagnostic test for a tear in the supraspinatus tendon. It is positive if the patient is unable slowly and smoothly to lower the affected arm from a position of 90 degrees of abduction.

drop attack, a form of transient ischaemic attack (TIA) in which a brief interruption of cerebral blood flow results in a person falling to the floor without losing consciousness. The episode may affect the person's sense of balance or leg muscle tone.

droperidol, an antipsychotic, sedative drug of the butyrophenone group, commonly used with a narcotic analgesic (fentanyl) in neuroleptan algesia.

drop foot. See **footdrop.**

droplet infection, an infection acquired by the inhalation of pathogenic micro-organisms suspended in particles of liquid exhaled, sneezed or coughed by another infected person or animal.

dropper, a glass or plastic tube narrowed at one end so it will dispense a liquid medication one drop at a time.

dropsy. See **hydrops.**

Drosophila, a genus of fly, including *Drosophila melanogaster,* the Mediterranean fruit fly, useful in genetic experiments because of the large chromosomes found in its salivary glands and its sensitivity to environmental effects, such as exposure to radiation.

drowning, asphyxiation because of submersion in a liquid.

drox, abbreviation for a non-carboxylate hydroxide anion.

drug, 1. any substance taken by mouth, injected into a muscle, skin, a blood vessel or a cavity of the body, or applied topically to treat or prevent a disease or condition. **2.** *informal.* an abused substance.

drug absorption, the process whereby a drug moves from the muscle, digestive tract or other site of entry into the body through the circulatory system to the target organ or tissue.

drug abuse, the use of a drug for a nontherapeutic, recreational effect. Some of the most commonly abused drugs are alcohol, amphetamines, barbiturates, cocaine, methaqualone and opium alkaloids.

drug addiction, a condition characterized by an overwhelming desire to continue taking a drug to which one has become habituated through repeated consumption because it produces a particular effect, usually an alteration of mental activity, attitude or outlook. Addiction is usually accompanied by a compulsion to obtain the drug, a tendency to increase the dose, a psychological or physical dependence, and is followed by detrimental consequences for the individual and society.

drug administration, the giving by a nurse or other authorized person of a drug to a patient.

drug allergy, hypersensitivity to a pharmacological agent, manifested by reactions ranging from a mild rash to anaphylactic shock, depending on the individual, the allergen and the dose.

drug clearance, the elimination of a drug from the body. The rate of clearance helps to determine the size and frequency of doses required with a particular medication.

drug compliance, pertaining to the reliability of the patient to use a prescribed medication exactly as ordered by the physician. Noncompliance occurs when a patient neglects to take the prescribed dosages at the recommended times or discontinues the drug without consulting the physician.

drug dependence, a psychological craving for or a physiological reliance on a chemical agent, resulting from habituation, abuse or addiction.

drug dispensing, the preparation, packaging, labelling, associated record keeping and transfer of a prescription drug to a patient or an intermediary, such as a nurse, who is responsible for the administration of a drug.

drug distribution, the pattern of absorption of drug molecules by various tissues after the chemical enters the circulatory system. Because of differences in pH, cell membrane functions and other individual tissue factors, most drugs are not distributed equally to all parts of the body.

drug-drug interaction, a modification of the effect of a drug when administered with another drug. The effect may be an increase or a decrease in the action of either substance, or it may be an adverse effect that is not normally associated with either drug.

drug eruption. See **drug rash.**

drug fever, a fever caused by the pharmacological action of a medication, its thermoregulatory action, a local complication of parenteral administration or, most commonly, an immunological reaction mediated by drug-induced antibodies. The onset of fever occurs usually between 7 and 10 days after the medication is begun; a return to normal is seen within 2 days of discontinuation of the drug.

drug-food interaction, the effect produced when some drugs and certain foods or beverages are taken at the same time, as in the case of monoamine oxidase inhibitors that can react dangerously with foods containing the amino acid tyramine.

drug-induced parkinsonism, a syndrome with the clinical features of Parkinson's disease, but caused by the dopamine-blocking actions of neuroleptic drugs.

drug metabolism, the transformation of a drug by the body tissues into a metabolite, which sometimes is the actual therapeutic agent.

drug monograph, a statement that specifies the kinds and amounts of ingredients a drug or class of drugs may contain, directions for the use of the drug, the conditions in which the drug may be used and contraindications to its use.

drug potency, a measure of the effect of one drug as compared to another medication of the same type. The drug that produces the maximum effect in the smallest dose has the greater potency.

drug rash, a skin eruption, usually an allergic reaction, that is caused by a particular drug. When a drug rash occurs as a sensitivity reaction, the skin rash does not occur the first time the drug is taken, but the effect is observed with subsequent uses of the same drug.

drug receptor, any part of a cell, usually an enzyme or large protein molecule, with which a drug molecule interacts to trigger its desired response or effect.

drug rehabilitation centre, an agency that provides long-term care for a gradual return to the community of a person with a chemical or drug dependency.

drug-seeking behaviour, a pattern of seeking narcotic pain medication or tranquilizers with forged prescriptions, false identification, repeatedly asking for replacement of "lost" drugs or prescriptions, complaining of severe pain without an organic basis, and being abusive or threatening when denied drugs.

drug sequestration, the process by which certain drugs are stored in the body tissues. Examples include tetracycline, which may be stored in bone tissue, and chloroquine, which is stored in the liver.

drug tolerance, a condition of cellular adaptation to a pharmacologically active substance so that increasingly larger doses are required to produce the same physiological or psychological effect.

drug trial, the process of determining an adequate and effective therapeutic dose of a specific drug for a particular patient. The trial culminates with (1) an acceptable clinical result, (2) intolerable adverse effects, (3) a poor response after an appropriate blood level is reached, or (4) the drug is administered for a specific time.

drusen, small, white hyaline deposits that develop beneath the retinal pigment epithelium, sometimes appearing as nodules within the optic nerve head. They tend to occur most frequently in persons over the age of 60.

Drug Tariff, a document produced by the UK Department of Health giving details of which items attract remuneration in fulfilment of NHS prescriptions.

DRV, dietary reference value, the Department of Health's estimation of the requirements of energy and nutrients for the population. Requirements for individuals are considered to follow a normal distribution. See **EAR.**

dry catarrh, a dry cough, accompanied by almost no expectoration that occurs in severe coughing spells. It is associated with asthma and emphysema in older people.

dry dressing, a plain dressing containing no medication, applied directly to an incision or a wound to prevent contamination or trauma, or to absorb secretions.

dry eye syndrome, a dryness of the cornea and conjunctiva caused by a deficiency in tear production. The condition results in a sensation of a foreign body in the eye, burning eyes, keratitis and erosion of the epithelial layers of the cornea and conjunctiva.

dry gangrene. See **gangrene,**

dry gas (D), (in respiratory therapy) a gas that contains no water vapour.

dry ice, solid carbon dioxide, with a temperature of about -140° F. It is used in cryotherapy of various skin disorders.

dry rale, an abnormal chest sound produced by air passing through a constricted bronchial tube.

Drysdale's corpuscle {Thomas M. Drysdale, American gynaecologist, b. 1831}, one of a number of transparent cells in the fluid of some ovarian cysts.

dry skin, epidermis lacking moisture or sebum, often characterized by a pattern of fine lines, scaling and itching. Causes include too frequent bathing, low humidity, decreased production of sebum in ageing skin and ichthyosis.

dry socket, an inflamed condition of a tooth socket (alveolus) after extraction. Normally, a blood clot forms over the alveolar bone at the base of the tooth socket after an extraction. If the clot fails to form properly or becomes dislodged, the bone tissue is exposed to the environment and can become infected. Also localised alveolar osteitis.

DSM, abbreviation for *Diagnostic and Statistical Manual of Mental Disorders.* DSM-III-R identifies the revised version of the third edition of the manual.

DSR, abbreviation for **dynamic spatial reconstructor.**

dTc, abbreviation for **d-tubocurarine.**

DTR, abbreviation for **deep tendon reflex.**

DTs, abbreviation for **delirium tremens.**

dual-focus tube, an x-ray tube used for diagnostic imaging. The large focal spot is used when a high tube loading is required at the expense of image sharpness. A small focal spot is used to produce fine, detailed images.

duality of CNS control, a theory that the normal central nervous system is regulated by a check-and-balance feedback programme. The theory is based on studies of posture-movement, mobility-stability, flexion-extension synergies and similar action-reaction examples.

Duane-Hunt law, (in radiation dosimetry) a principle that x-ray energy is inversely proportional to the photon wavelength. As the photon wavelength increases, photon energy decreases, and vice versa. The minimum x-ray wavelength is associated with the maximum x-ray energy.

DUB, a genetically determined human blood factor that is associated with immunity to certain diseases.

Dubin-Johnson syndrome {Isadore N. Dubin, American pathologist, b. 1913; Frank B. Johnson, American pathologist, b. 1919}, a rare, chronic, hereditary hyperbilirubinemia, characterized by non-haemolytic jaundice, abnormal liver pigmentation and abnormal function of the gallbladder.

DuBois formula, a logarithmic method of calculating the number of square meters of body surface area (BSA) of an individual from the height in centimetres, the weight in kilograms, and a constant, 0.007184.

Dubowitz assessment, a system of estimating the gestational age of a newborn child according to such factors as posture, ankle dorsiflexion, and arm and leg recoil.

Dubowitz score, a method of assessing gestation age in a low birthweight baby.

Duchenne-Erb paralysis. See **Erb's palsy.**

Duchenne's disease, a series of three different neurological conditions: spinal muscular atrophy, bulbar paralysis and tabes dorsalis.

Duchenne-Aran disease, muscular atrophy caused by degeneration of the anterior horn cells of the spinal cord and affecting primarily the upper extremities. There is chronic muscle wasting and weakness that first appears in the hands and advances progressively to the arms and shoulders, eventually affecting the legs and other body areas.

Duchenne's muscular dystrophy Guillame B. A. Duchenne, an abnormal congenital condition characterized by progressive symmetrical wasting of the leg and pelvic muscles. It is an X-linked recessive disease that appears insidiously between 3 and 5 years of age and spreads from the leg and pelvic muscles to the involuntary muscles. Associated muscle weakness produces a waddling gait and pronounced lordosis. Muscles rapidly deteriorate, and calf muscles become firm and enlarged from fatty deposits. Affected children develop contractures, have

difficulty climbing stairs, often stumble and fall, and display wing scapulae when they raise their arms.

duck walk. See **metatarsus valgus.**

duct, a narrow tubular structure, especially one through which material is secreted or excreted.

duct carcinoma, a neoplasm developed from the epithelium of ducts, especially in the breast or pancreas.

duct ectasia, an abnormal dilation of a duct by lipids and cellular debris.

ductility, the property of a material that has a large elastic range and tends to deform before failing from stress.

duction, the movement of an individual eyeball from the primary to secondary or tertiary positions of gaze.

ductless gland, a gland lacking an excretory duct, such as an endocrine gland, which secretes hormones into blood or lymph.

duct of Rivinus {Augustus Q. Rivinus. German anatomist, b. 1652}, one of the minor sublingual ducts.

duct of Wirsung. See **pancreatic duct.**

ductus, *pl.* **ductus,** a duct.

ductus arteriosus, a vascular channel in the fetus that joins the pulmonary artery directly to the descending aorta.

ductus deferens. See **vas deferens.**

ductus epididymidis, a tube into which the efferent ductules of the testes empty.

ductus venosus, the vascular channel in the fetus passing through the liver and joining the umbilical vein with the inferior vena cava.

Dukes' classification, a system of identifying stages of colorectal tumours, from A to D, according to the degree of tissue invasion and metastasis. A Dukes' A tumour is one that is confined to the mucosa and submucosa. A B tumour is one that has invaded the musculature but has not involved the lymphatic system. C tumours have invaded the musculature with metastatic involvement of the regional lymph nodes. D tumours are those that have metastasized to distant organ tissues.

dumdum fever. See **kala-azar.**

dump, 1. to preserve the contents of one computer memory by transferring it into another memory. **2.** to print out the contents of a computer memory or other computer-storage medium. **3.** the printout resulting from such an operation.

dumping syndrome, the combination of profuse sweating, nausea, dizziness and weakness experienced by patients who have had a subtotal gastrectomy. Symptoms are felt soon after eating, when the contents of the stomach empty too rapidly into the duodenum.

Dunlop skeletal traction, an orthopaedic mechanism that helps immobilize the upper limb in the treatment of contracture or supracondylar fracture of the elbow. The mechanism employs a system of traction weights, pulleys and ropes. The system is attached to the bone involved with a pin or wire.

Dunlop skin traction, an orthopaedic mechanism that helps immobilize the upper limb in the treatment of contracture and supracondylar fracture of the elbow. The mechanism employs a system of traction weights, pulleys and ropes, and may be applied as adhesive skin traction or non-adhesive skin traction.

duodenal, of or pertaining to the duodenum.

duodenal bulb, the first part of the superior portion of the duodenum, which has a bulblike appearance on x-ray views of the small intestine.

duodenal ulcer, an ulcer in the duodenum, the most common type of peptic ulcer.

duodenography, a radiographic examination to visualize the duodenum, using a barium meal technique.   **duodenogram,** *n*.

duodenojejunal flexure. See **angle of Treitz.**

duodenoscope, an endoscopic instrument, usually fibreoptic, for the visual examination of the duodenum.

duodenoscopy, the visual examination of the duodenum by means of an endoscope.

duodenum, *pl.* **duodena, duodenums,** the shortest, widest and most fixed portion of the small intestine, taking an almost circular course from the pyloric valve of the stomach so that its termination is close to its starting point. It is about 25 cm long and is divided into superior, descending, horizontal and ascending portions.

dup, (in cytogenetics) abbreviation for **duplication.**

duplex inheritance. See **amphigenous inheritance.**

duplex transmission, the passage of a neural impulse in both directions along a nerve fibre.

duplicating film, a single-emulsion film used to copy an ultraviolet x-ray image by exposing it through ultraviolet light.

Dupuytren's contracture {Baron Guillame Dupuytren, French surgeon, b. 1777}, a progressive, painless thickening and tightening of subcutaneous tissue of the palm, causing the fourth and fifth fingers to bend into the palm and resist extension. Tendons and nerves are not involved. An incision is made into the palm, and the thickened tissue is excised carefully to avoid injury to adjacent ligaments.

Dupuytren's fracture. See **Galeazzi's fracture.**

dural sac, the blind pouch formed by the lower end of the dura mater, at the level of the second sacral segment.

dura mater, the outermost and most fibrous of the three membranes surrounding the brain and spinal cord. The dura mater encephali covers the brain, and the dura mater spinalis covers the cord.

duress, (in law) an action compelling another person to do what otherwise would not be done voluntarily. A consent form signed under duress is not valid.

Durozier murmur, a systolic murmur heard over the femoral or another large artery when the artery is compressed. The phenomenon is associated with high arterial pulse pressure or aortic insufficiency.

dust {AS}, any fine, particulate, dry matter. Kinds of dust are inorganic dust and organic dust.

dust fever. See **brucellosis.**

Dutton's relapsing fever {Joseph E. Dutton, English pathologist, b. 1877}, an infection caused by a spirochaete, Borrelia duttonii, which is transmitted by a soft tick, Ornithodoros moubata, found in human dwellings in tropical Africa. The spirochaete enters the lesion through a tick bite, producing a high fever, chills, rapid heartbeat, headache, joint and muscle pain, vomiting and neurological disorders.

duty, (in law) an obligation owed by one party to another. Duty may be established by statute or other legal process, or it may be undertaken voluntarily.

Duverney's fracture {Joseph G. Duverney, French anatomist, b. 1648}, fracture of the ilium just below the anterior superior spine.

dv/dt, (in cardiology) the rate of change of voltage with respect to time.

DVT, abbreviation for **deep vein thrombosis.**

dwarf, 1. an abnormally short, undersized person, especially one whose bodily parts are not proportional. Kinds of dwarfs include **achondroplastic dwarf, Amsterdam dwarf, asexual dwarf, ateliotic dwarf, bird-headed dwarf, Brissaud's dwarf, cretin dwarf, diastrophic dwarf, phocomelic dwarf, pituitary dwarf, primordial dwarf, rachitic dwarf, renal dwarf, Russell dwarf, sexual dwarf, Silver dwarf** and **thanatophoric dwarf. 2.** to prevent or retard normal growth.

dwarfism, the abnormal underdevelopment of the body, characterized predominantly by extreme shortness of stature. Dwarfism has multiple causes, including genetic defects, endocrine dysfunction involving either the pituitary or thyroid glands, chronic diseases, such as rickets, renal failure and intestinal malabsorption defects, and psychosocial stress.

Dwyer instrumentation, one of the two most common surgical methods for correcting the spinal curvature associated with scoliosis. The Dwyer cable method uses a mechanical device that is inserted to assist in maintaining the corrected curvature while the fusion heals.

Dy, symbol for **dysprosium.**

dyad, (in genetics) one of the paired homologous chromosomes consisting of two chromatids, which result from the division of a tetrad in the first meiotic division of gametogenesis. **dyadic,** *adj.*

dyadic interpersonal communication, a process in which two people interact face to face as senders and receivers, such as in a conversation.

dydrogesterone, a synthetic oral progestogen used in the treatment of abnormal uterine bleeding, menopausal vasomotor symptoms, pickwickian syndrome and other conditions amenable to hormonal manipulation.

dye, 1. to apply colouring matter to a substance. **2.** a chemical compound capable of imparting colour to a substance to which it is applied. Medically, dyes are used as stains for tissues, test reagents, therapeutic agents, and to colour pharmaceutical preparations.

dynamic, 1. tending to change or encourage change, such as a dynamic nurse-patient relationship. **2.** (in respiratory therapy) a condition of changing volume.

dynamic cardiac work, the energy transfer that occurs during the process of ventricular ejection of blood.

dynamic compliance, pertaining to the distensibility of the lung, as measured by plethysmography during the breathing cycle.

dynamic equilibrium, the ability of a patient to adjust to displacements of the body's centre of gravity by changing the body's base of support.

dynamic ileus, an intestinal obstruction with associated recurrent and continuous muscle spasma.

dynamic imaging, (in ultrasonography) the imaging of an object in motion at a frame rate that does not cause significant blurring of any one image and at a repetition rate sufficient to adequately represent the movement pattern.

dynamic nurse-patient relationship, a conceptual framework in which the interpersonal aspects of the nurse-patient relationship are analysed. The relationship is affected by the behaviour of the patient, the reaction of the nurse, and the actions of the nurse that are intended to aid the patient.

dynamic psychiatry, the study of motivational, emotional and biological factors as determinants of human behaviour.

dynamic range, 1. (in radiography) the range of voltage or input signals that result in a digital output. **2.** (in audiology) the range of decibels from the faintest sound a person can hear to the level of sound that causes pain.

dynamic response, the accuracy with which a physiological monitoring system, such as an electrocardiograph, will simulate the actual event being recorded.

dynamic spatial reconstructor (DSR), a kind of x-ray machine used in research, permitting moving three-dimensional images of human organs to be examined visually and from any direction.

dynamometer, a device for measuring the degree of force expended in the contraction of a group of muscles, such as a squeeze dynamometer which measures the gross grip strength of the hand muscles.

dysadrenia, abnormal adrenal function characterized by decreased production of hormones, as in hypoadrenalism or hypoadrenocorticism, or by increased secretion of the products of the gland, as in hyperadrenalism or hyperadrenocorticism.

dysaesthesia, a common effect of spinal cord injury characterized by sensations of numbness, tingling, burning or pain felt below the level of the lesion.

dysarthria, difficult, poorly articulated speech, resulting from interference in the control over the muscles of speech, usually because of damage to a central or peripheral motor nerve.

dysautonomia, a dysfunction of the autonomic nervous system that can be a clinical feature of diabetes, parkinsonism, Adie's syndrome, Shy-Drager syndrome or Riley-Day syndrome. A fairly common effect is orthostatic hypotension with syncope and drop attacks.

dysbarism, a reaction to a sudden change in ambient pressure, such as rapid exposure to the lower atmospheric pressures of high altitudes. It is marked by symptoms similar to those of decompression sickness.

dysbetalipoproteinaemia. See **broad beta disease.**

dyscholia, any abnormal condition of the bile, either regarding the quantity secreted or the condition of the constituents.

dyschondroplasia. See **enchondromatosis.**

dyscrasia, an abnormal blood or bone marrow condition, such as leukaemia, aplastic anaemia or Rh incompatibility.

dyscrasic fracture, any fracture caused by the weakening of a specific bone as a result of a debilitating disease.

dysdiadochokinesia, an inability to perform rapidly alternating movements, such as rhythmically tapping the fingers on the knee. The cause is a cerebellar lesion and is related to dysmetria.

dysentery, an inflammation of the intestine, especially of the colon, that may be caused by chemical irritants, bacteria, protozoa or parasites. It is characterized by frequent and bloody stools, abdominal pain and tenesmus.

dysfunctional, (of a body organ or system) unable to function normally. **dysfunction,** *n.*

dysfunctional communication, a communication that results from inaccurate perceptions, faulty internal filters (personal interpretations of information) and social isolation.

dysfunctional stereotype, a stereotype in which the dysfunctional aspects of a culture are emphasized.

dysfunctional thought record, (in psychology) a therapeutic technique in which a patient records his thoughts whenever a strong emotion is experienced. The record is later reviewed by the therapist and patient to explore the causes of the automatic thoughts.

dysfunctional uterine bleeding, abnormal uterine bleeding that is not caused by a tumour, inflammation or pregnancy. It may be characterized by painless, irregular, heavy bleeding, intermenstrual spotting or periods of amenorrhoea. The condition is associated with anovulation and unopposed oestrogen stimulation.

dysgammaglobulinaemia, an inherited immune deficiency disease characterized by blood disorders and a tendency to experience repeated infections. The cause is a deficiency of immunoglobulins needed to produce antibodies.

dysgenesis, 1. defective or abnormal formation of an organ or part, primarily during embryonic development. **2.** impairment or loss of the ability to procreate. A kind of dysgenesis is gonadal dysgenesis. **dysgenic,** adj.

dysgenics, the study of those factors or situations that are genetically detrimental to the future of a race or species.

dysgenitalism, any condition involving the abnormal development of the genital organs.

dysgerminoma, pl. dysgerminomas, dysgerminomata, a rare malignant tumour of the ovary, believed to arise from the undifferentiated germ cells of the embryonic gonad.

dysgnathic anomaly, (in dentistry) an abnormality that extends beyond the teeth, affecting the maxilla, the mandible, or both.

dysgraphia, an impairment of the ability to write, caused by a pathological disorder. **dysgraphic,** adj.

dyshidrosis, a condition in which abnormal sweating occurs. Kinds of dyshidrosis are **hyperhidrosis** and **miliaria.**

dyskeratosis, an abnormal or premature keratinization of epithelial cells.

dyskinesia, an impairment of the ability to execute voluntary movements. Dyskinesia can be an adverse effect of prolonged use of phenothiazine medications in elderly patients or those with brain injuries. **dyskinetic,** adj.

dyskinetic syndrome, a form of cerebral palsy involving a basal ganglia disorder. Clinical features include athetoid movements of the extremities and sometimes the trunk. The movements tend to increase with emotional tension and to diminish during sleep.

dyslexia, an impairment of the ability to read, as a result of a variety of pathological conditions, some of which are associated with the central nervous system. Dyslexic persons often reverse letters and words, cannot adequately distinguish the letter sequences in written words, and have difficulty determining left from right. **dyslexic,** adj.

dysmaturity, 1. the failure of an organism to develop, ripen, or otherwise achieve maturity in structure or function. **2.** the condition of a fetus or newborn being abnormally small or large for its age of gestation. Kinds of dysmaturity are small for gestational age and large for gestational age. **dysmature,** adj.

dysmelia, an abnormal congenital condition characterized by missing or shortened extremities of the body and associated with abnormalities of the spine in some individuals. It is caused by abnormal metabolism during the development of the embryonic limbs.

dysmenorrhoea, pain associated with menstruation.

dysmetria, an abnormal condition that prevents the affected individual from properly measuring distances associated with muscular acts, and from controlling muscular action. It is associated with cerebellar lesions, and is typically characterized by over- or underestimating the range of motion needed to place the limbs correctly during voluntary movement.

dysmnesic syndrome, a memory disorder characterized by an inability to learn simple new skills, although the person can still perform highly complex skills learnt before the onset of the condition.

dysmorphogenesis, the development of ill-shaped or otherwise malformed body structures.

dysmorphophobia, 1. a fundamental delusion of body image. **2.** the morbid fear of deformity.

dysostosis, an abnormal condition characterized by defective ossification, especially by defects in the normal ossification of fetal cartilages. Kinds of dysostoses include **cleidocranial dysostosis, craniofacial dysostosis, mandibulofacial dysostosis, metaphyseal dysostosis** and **Nager's acrofacial dysostosis.**

dyspareunia, Pain with sexual intercourse.

dyspepsia, a vague feeling of epigastric discomfort, felt after eating. There is an uncomfortable feeling of fullness, heartburn, bloating and nausea. **dyspeptic,** adj.

dysphagia, difficulty in swallowing, commonly associated with obstructive or motor disorders of the oesophagus. Patients with obstructive disorders like oesophageal tumour or lower oesophageal ring are unable to swallow solids but can tolerate liquids. Persons with motor disorders are unable to swallow solids or liquids.

dysphagia lusoria, an abnormal condition characterized by difficulty in swallowing, caused by compression of the oesophagus from an anomalous right subclavian artery that arises from the descending aorta and courses behind or in front of the oesophagus.

dysphasia, an impairment of speech, not as severe as aphasia, which is usually the result of an injury to the speech area in the cerebral cortex of the brain.

dysphonia, any abnormality in the speaking voice, such as hoarseness. Dysphonia puberum identifies the voice changes that occur in adolescent boys.

dysphoria, a disorder of affect characterized by depression and anguish.

dysplasia, any abnormal development of tissues or organs, such as dwarfism or failure to develop sweat glands.

dyspnoea, a shortness of breath or difficulty in breathing that may be caused by certain heart conditions, strenuous exercise or anxiety.   **dyspnoeal, dyspnoeic,** *adj.*

dyspraxia, a partial loss of the ability to perform skilled, coordinated movements in the absence of any associated defect in motor or sensory functions.

dysprosium (Dy), a rare-earth metallic element. Its atomic number is 66 and its atomic weight is 162.50. Radioactive isotopes of dysprosium are used in radioisotope scanning.

dysproteinaemia, an abnormality of the protein content of the blood, usually involving the immunoglobulins.

dysraphia, failure of a raphe to fuse completely, as in incomplete closure of the neural tube.

dysraphic syndrome, a developmental disorder usually involving the spinal cord, such as encephalocoele or myelomenigocoele.

dysreflexia, a condition in which an individual with a spinal cord injury at T7 or above experiences or is at risk of experiencing a life-threatening, uninhibited, sympathetic response of the nervous system to a noxious stimulus. Defining characteristics include paroxysmal hypertension, bradycardia or tachycardia, diaphoresis above the injury, red splotches on the skin above the injury, pallor below the injury, a headache that is a diffuse pain, chilling, conjunctival congestion, blurred vision, chest pain, a metallic taste in the mouth, nasal congestion and pilomotor reflex.   **dysreflexic,** *adj.*

dysrhythmia, any disturbance or abnormality in a normal rhythmic pattern, specifically, irregularity in the brain waves or cadence of speech.

dyssebacea, a skin condition characterized by red, scaly, greasy patches on the nose, eyelids, scrotum and labia.

dyssynergia, any disturbance in muscular coordination, such as in cases of ataxia.

dysthymia, a form of chronic unipolar depression that tends to occur in elderly persons with debilitating physical disorders, multiple interpersonal losses and chronic marital difficulties. Several depressive episodes may merge into a low-grade chronic depressive state.

dystocia, pathological or difficult labour, which may be caused by an obstruction or constriction of the birth passage or an abnormal size, shape, position or condition of the fetus.

dystonia, any impairment of muscle tone. The condition commonly involves the head, neck and tongue, and often occurs as an adverse effect of a medication.

dystonia musculorum deformans, a rare, abnormal condition characterized by intense, irregular torsion muscle spasms that contort the body. The muscles of the trunk, shoulder and pelvis are commonly involved. Muscle power and tone appear normal, but convulsive spasms make the involved muscles relatively useless.

dystonic, referring to an excessive increase in muscle tone, often resulting in postural abnormalities.

dystrophic calcification, the deposition of calcium in abnormal tissues, such as scar tissue or atherotic plaques, but without abnormalities of blood calcium.

dystrophy, any abnormal condition caused by defective nutrition, often applied to a developmental change in muscles that does not involve the nervous system, such as fatty degeneration associated with increased size but decreased strength.   **dystrophic,** *adj.*

dysuria, painful urination, usually the result of a bacterial infection or obstructive condition in the urinary tract. The patient complains of a burning sensation when passing urine, and laboratory examination may reveal the presence of blood, bacteria or white blood cells.

E, symbol for expired gas.

E_1, symbol for monomolecular reaction.

E_2, symbol for bimolecular reaction

ear, the organ of hearing, consisting of the internal, middle, and external ear. The external ear includes the skin-covered cartilaginous auricle visible on either side of the head and the portion of the external auditory canal that is outside the skull. The middle ear contains three very small bones, the malleus, incus and stapes, which transmit vibrations caused by sound waves reaching the tympanic membrane to the oval window of the inner ear. The inner ear contains two separate organs: the vestibular apparatus, which provides the sense of balance, and the organ of Corti, which receives vibrations from the middle ear and translates them into nerve impulses, which are again interpreted by brain cells as specific sounds.

EAR (Estimated Average Requirement), this applies to a group of people and refers to energy, protein, vitamins or minerals. Approximately half the group will require more than the EAR, and half will require less. EAR is taken as the mean of the normal distribution of requirements in a group of individuals for a nuturent.

earache, a pain in the ear, sensed as being sharp, dull, burning, intermittent or constant. The cause is not necessarily a disease of the ear, because infections and other disorders of the nose, oral cavity, larynx and temporomandibular joint can produce referred pain in the ear.

eardrop instillation, the instillation of a medicated solution into the external auditory canal of the ear. The patient is asked to turn the head to the side so that the ear being treated faces upwards. The drops of medicine are directed towards the internal wall of the canal.

eardrops, a topical, liquid form of medication for the local treatment of various conditions of the ear, such as inflammation or infection of the lining of the external auditory canal or impacted cerumen.

eardrum. See tympanic membrane.

ear oximeter, a device placed over the earlobe that transmits a beam of light through the ear tissue to a receiver. It is a non-invasive method of measuring the level of saturated haemoglobin in the blood. The amount of saturated haemoglobin in the blood alters the wavelengths of light transmitted.

earwax. See cerumen.

Eaton agent, an alternative name for *Mycoplasma pneumoniae*, a common cause of atypical pneumonia in humans.

Eaton agent pneumonia. See mycoplasma pneumonia.

Eaton-Lambert syndrome, a form of myasthenia that tends to be associated with lung cancer.

Ebbecke's reaction. See dermatographia.

EBP, abbreviation for epidural blood patch.

EBV, abbreviation for Epstein-Barr virus.

eccentric contraction, a type of muscle contraction that involves lengthening of the muscle fibres, such as when a weight is lowered through a range of motion. The muscle yields to the resistance, allowing itself to be stretched.

eccentric implantation, (in embryology) the embedding of the blastocyst within a fold or recess of the uterine wall, which then closes off from the main cavity.

eccentricity, behaviour that is regarded as odd or peculiar for a particular culture or community, although not unusual enough to be considered pathological.

eccentric jaw relation, (in dentistry) any jaw relation other than centric relation.

ecchondroma, a benign cartilaginous tumour that develops on the surface of a cartilage or under the periosteum of bone.

ecchondrosis. See ecchondroma.

ecchymosis, discolouration of an area of the skin or mucous membrane caused by the extravasation of blood into the subcutaneous tissues as a result of trauma to the underlying blood vessels or by fragility of the vessel walls.

eccrine, of or pertaining to a sweat gland that secretes outwardly through a duct to the surface of the skin.

eccrine gland, one of two kinds of sweat glands in the corium of the skin. Such glands promote cooling by evaporation of their secretion.

ECF, 1. abbreviation for extended care facility. **2.** abbreviation for extracellular fluid.

ECG, 1. abbreviation for electrocardiogram. **2.** abbreviation for electrocardiography.

ecgonine, the principal part of the cocaine molecule.

echinococcosis, an infestation, usually of the liver, caused by the larval stage of a tapeworm of the genus Echinococcus. Humans, especially children, can become infested with larvae by ingesting eggs shed in the stool of infected dogs. Clinical manifestations and prognosis vary, depending upon the tissue invaded and the extent of infestation.

Echinococcus, a genus of small tapeworms that infects primarily canines.

echinocyte. See **burr cell.**

echo beat, a reciprocal heart beat, or one that results from the return of an impulse to an atrium or ventricle to reactivate a contraction.

echocardiography, a diagnostic procedure for studying the structure and motion of the heart. Ultrasonic waves directed through the heart are reflected backwards, or are echoed, when they pass from one type of tissue to another.

echoencephalogram, a recording produced by an echoencephalograph.

echoencephalography, the use of ultrasound to study the intracranial structures of the brain. **echoencephalographic,** adj.

echography. See **ultrasonography.**

echolalia, 1. (in psychiatry) the automatic and meaningless repetition of another's words or phrases, especially as seen in schizophrenia. A kind of echolalia is delayed echolalia. **2.** (in paediatrics) a baby's imitation or repetition of sounds or words produced by others. It occurs normally in early childhood development. **echolalic,** adj.

echopraxia, imitation or repetition of the body movements of another person, a behaviour exhibited by some schizophrenic patients.

echoradiography, a diagnostic procedure using ultrasonography and various devices for the visualization of internal structures of the body.

echo speech. See **echolalia.**

echothiophate iodide, an anticholinesterase used for ophthalmic purposes, such as chronic open-angle glaucoma.

echovirus, a picornavirus associated with many clinical syndromes but not identified as the causative organism of any specific disease. There are several echoviruses, and most are harmless.

eclampsia, the onset of convulsions in a pregnancy complicated by pre-eclampsia. The fits may occur before, during or after labour.

ecological chemistry, the study of chemical compounds synthesized by plants that influence ecology because of their toxic effects.

ecological fallacy, a false assumption that the presence of a pathogenic factor and a disease in a population can be accepted as proof that the agent is the cause of the disease in a particular individual.

ecology, the study of the interaction between living organisms and the various influences of their environment.

econazole, an antifungal agent prescribed in the treatment of tinea and candidiasis.

ecosystem, the sum total of all living and non-living things that support a chain of life events within a particular area.

ecstasy, an emotional state characterized by exultation, rapturous delight or frenzy. **ecstatic,** adj.

ECT, abbreviation for electroconvulsive therapy.

ectasy, methylenedioxymethamphetamine, an abused stimulant drug with no legitimate medical use.

ecthyma, a deep, burrowing form of impetigo characterized by large pustules, crusts and ulcerations surrounded by erythema. Staphylococci and streptococci are the offending bacteria.

ectoderm, the outermost of the three primary cell layers of an embryo. The ectoderm gives rise to the nervous system; the organs of special sense, such as the eyes and ears; the epidermis and epidermal tissue, such as fingernails, hair and skin glands; and the mucous membranes of the mouth and anus. **ectodermal, ectodermic,** adj.

ectodermal cloaca, a part of the cloaca in the developing embryo that lies external to the cloacal membrane and eventually gives rise to the anus and anal canal.

ectomorph, a person whose physique is characterized by slenderness, fragility and a predominance of structures derived from the ectoderm.

ectoparasite, (in medical parasitology) an organism that lives on the outside of the body of the host, such as a louse.

ectopic, 1. (of an object or organ) situated in an unusual place, away from its normal location; for example, an ectopic pregnancy is a pregnancy that occurs outside the uterus. **2.** (of an event) occurring at the wrong time, such as a premature heart beat or premature ventricular contraction.

ectopic foci, cardiac arrhythmias caused by initiation of an excitation impulse at a site other than the sinus node. Ectopic foci may occur in both healthy and diseased hearts.

ectopic myelopoiesis. See **extramedullary myelopoiesis.**

ectopic pregnancy, the embedding of a fertilized ovum outside the uterine cavity. This may occur in the uterine tube (in 95% of cases), on the ovary, in the abdomen or in the cervix.

ectopic teratism, a congenital anomaly in which one or more parts are misplaced, as dextrocardia, palatine teeth and transposition of the great vessels.

ectotoxin. See **exotoxin.**

ectrodactyly, a congenital anomaly characterized by the absence of part or all of one or more of the fingers or toes.

ectrogenic teratism, a congenital anomaly caused by developmental failure in which one or more parts or organs are missing.

ectrogeny, the congenital absence or defect of any organ or part of the body. **ectrogenic,** adj.

ectromelia, the congenital absence or incomplete development of the long bones of one or more of the limbs. Kinds of ectromelia are amelia, hemimelia and phocomelia. **ectromelic,** *adj.,* **ectromelus,** *n.*

ectropion, eversion, most commonly of the eyelid, exposing the conjunctival membrane lining the eyelid and part of the eyeball. The condition may involve only the lower eyelid or both eyelids.

ectrosyndactyly, a congenital anomaly characterized by the absence of some but not all of the digits, with those that are formed being webbed so as to appear fused.

eczema, superficial dermatitis of unknown cause. In the early stage it may be pruritic, erythematous, papulovesicular, oedematous and weeping. **eczematous,** *adj.*

eczema herpeticum, a generalized vesiculopustular skin disease caused by herpes simplex virus or vaccinia virus infection of a pre-existing rash, such as atopic dermatitis.

eczema marginatum. See **tinea cruris.**

eczematous conjunctivitis, conjunctival and corneal inflammation associated with multiple, tiny, ulcerated vesicles.

ED, abbreviation for effective dose.

ED50, symbol for median effective dose, which is the dose sufficient to produce the desired response in half the subjects treated.

edaphon, the composite of organisms that live in the soil. **edaphic,** *adj.*

EDB, abbreviation for ethylene dibromide.

EDC, abbreviation for expected date of confinement.

edentulous, toothless.

edetate (EDTA), one of several salts of edetic acid, including calcium disodium edetate and disodium edetate, used as a chelating agent in treating poisoning with heavy metals.

edetic acid (EDTA). See **edetate.**

edge response function (ERF), the ability of a computed tomography system to reproduce accurately a high-contrast edge, as in the scanning of a structure such as the heart.

edgewise fixed orthodontic appliance, an orthodontic appliance characterized by tooth attachment brackets with a rectangular slot that engages a round or rectangular arch wire. It is used to correct or improve malocclusion.

edrophonium chloride, a cholinesterase inhibitor that acts as an antidote to curare and is used as an aid in the diagnosis of myasthenia gravis.

edrophonium test, a test for myasthenia gravis by the injection of an intravenous solution of edrophonium chloride into a patient.

Edsall's disease {David L. Edsall, American physician, b. 1869}, a cramping condition resulting from excessive exposure to heat.

EDTA, 1. abbreviation for edetate. 2. abbreviation for edetic acid.

educational psychology, the application of psychological principles, techniques and tests to educational problems.

Edwards' syndrome. See **trisomy 18.**

EEE, abbreviation for eastern equine encephalitis. See equine encephalitis.

EEG, 1. abbreviation for electroencephalogram. 2. abbreviation for electroencephalography.

effacement, the 'taking up' of the vaginal portion of the cervix and thinning of its walls as it is stretched and dilated during labour.

effective compliance, the ratio of tidal volume to peak airway pressure.

effective dose (ED), the dosage of a drug that may be expected to cause the desired intensity of effect in the people to whom it is given.

effective dose equivalent, (in radiology) ionising radiation dose received by a given tissue, organ, or the whole body, due to exposure to external radiation.

effective half-life, (in radionuclide imaging) the time taken for a radiopharmaceutical in the body to be reduced to one-half of its original quantity, due to the combination of its radioactive decay half-life and its biological half-life.

effective refractory period, the period after the firing of an impulse during which a fibre may respond at the cellular level to a stimulus but the response will not be propagated.

efferent, directed away from a centre, as certain arteries, veins, nerves and lymphatics.

efferent duct, any duct through which a gland releases its secretions.

efferent nerve, a nerve that transmits impulses away or outwards from a nerve centre, such as the brain or spine, usually resulting in a muscle contraction, release of a glandular secretion, or other activity.

effervescent, producing and releasing gas bubbles.

efficacy, (of a drug or treatment) the maximum ability of a drug or treatment to produce a result, regardless of dosage.

effluent, a liquid, solid or gaseous emission, such as the discharge or outflow from a machine or industrial process.

effleurage, a technique in massage in which long, light or firm strokes are used, usually over the spine and back.

effort syndrome, an abnormal condition characterized by chest pain, dizziness, fatigue and palpitations. This condition is often associated with soldiers in combat but also occurs in other individuals. The symptoms of effort syndrome often mimic angina pectoris but are more closely connected to anxiety states.

effraction, a breaking open or weakening.

effusion, 1. the escape of fluid from blood

vessels because of rupture or seepage, usually into a body cavity. The condition is usually associated with a circulatory or renal disorder and is often an early sign of congestive heart disease. **2.** the outward spread of a bacterial growth.

EFM, abbreviation for electronic fetal monitor.

egest, to discharge or evacuate a substance from the body, especially to evacuate unabsorbed residue of foods from the intestines. **egesta,** *n. pl.,* **egestive,** *adj.*

ego, 1. the conscious sense of the self; those elements of a person, such as thinking, feeling, willing and emotions, that distinguish the person as an individual. **2.** (in psychoanalysis) the part of the psyche that experiences and maintains conscious contact with reality and which tempers the primitive drives of the id and the demands of the superego with the social and physical needs of society.

ego-alien. See **ego-dystonic.**

ego analysis, (in psychoanalysis) the intensive study of the ego, especially the defence mechanisms.

ego boundary, (in psychiatry) a sense or awareness that there is a distinction between the self and others.

egocentric, 1. regarding the self as the centre, object and norm of all experience, and having little regard for the needs, interests, ideas and attitudes of others. **2.** a person possessing these characteristics.

ego-defence mechanism. See **defence mechanism.**

ego-dystonic, describing the elements of a person's behaviour, thoughts, impulses, drives and attitudes that are at variance with the standards of the ego and inconsistent with the total personality.

ego-dystonic homosexuality, a psychosexual disorder in which there is a persistent desire to change sexual orientation from homosexuality to heterosexuality.

ego ideal, the image of the self to which a person aspires both consciously and unconsciously, and against which he measures himself and his performance.

egoism, 1. an overvaluation of the importance of the self, expressed as a willingness to gain an advantage at the expense of others. **2.** the belief that individual self-interest is, or ought to be, the basic motive for all conscious behaviour.

egoist, 1. a person who seeks to satisfy his own interests at the expense of others. **2.** a person who believes in or follows the concept that all conscious action is justifiably motivated by self-interest. **egoistic, egoistical,** *adj.*

ego libido, (in psychoanalysis) concentration of the libido on the self; self-love, narcissism.

egomania, a pathological preoccupation

with the self and an exaggerated sense of one's own importance.

egophony, (in respiratory therapy) a change in the voice sound as heard on auscultation of a patient with pleural effusion.

ego strength, (in psychotherapy) the ability to maintain the ego by a cluster of traits that together contribute to good mental health.

ego-syntonic, those elements of a person's behaviour, thoughts, impulses, drives and attitudes that agree with the standards of the ego and are consistent with the total personality.

egotism, the overvaluation of the importance of the self and undervaluation or contempt of others. **egotistic, egotistical,** *adj.*

egotist, one who places too much importance on the self and is boastful, egocentric and arrogant.

egress, the act of emerging or moving forward.

Egyptian ophthalmia. See **trachoma.**

EHD, abbreviation for electrohaemodynamics.

Ehlers-Danlos syndrome {Edward Ehlers, Danish physician, b. 1863; Henri A. Danlos, French physician, b. 1844}, a hereditary disorder of connective tissue, marked by hyperplasticity of skin, tissue fragility and hypermotility of joints.

eicosanoic acid, a fatty acid containing 20 carbon atoms in a straight chain, such as arachidic acid found in peanut oil, butter and other fats.

eidetic, 1. pertaining to or characterized by the ability to visualize and reproduce accurately the image of objects or events previously seen or imagined. **2.** a person possessing such ability.

eidetic image, an unusually vivid, elaborate and apparently exact mental image resulting from a visual experience, and occurring as a fantasy, dream or memory.

eighth cranial nerve. See **auditory nerve.**

einsteinium (Es) {Albert Einstein, German-born scientist, b. 1879}, a synthetic transuranic metallic element. Its atomic number is 99 and its atomic weight is 254.

ejaculate, the semen discharged in a single emission. **ejaculate,** *v.*

ejaculation, the sudden emission of semen from the male urethra, usually occurring during copulation, masturbation and nocturnal emission. It is a reflex action. The sensation of ejaculation is commonly also called orgasm. **ejaculatory,** *adj.*

ejaculatory duct, the passage through which semen enters the urethra.

ejection, the forceful expulsion of something, such as blood from a ventricle of the heart.

ejection clicks, sharp, clicking sounds from the heart, which may be caused by the sudden swelling of a pulmonary artery, abrupt dilatation of the aorta or forceful opening of the aortic cusps.

ejection fraction (EF), the proportion of blood that is ejected during each ventricular contraction compared with the total ventricular volume.

ejection murmur. See **systolic murmur.**

ejection sounds, sharp, clicking sounds heard early in systole, coinciding with the onset of either right or left ventricular systolic ejection and reflecting either dilatation of the pulmonary artery or aorta or the presence of valvular abnormalities.

Ekbom syndrome. See **restless legs syndrome.**

elaborate, (in endocrinology) a process by which a gland synthesizes a complex substance from simpler substances and secretes it, usually under the stimulation of a tropic hormone from the pituitary gland. **elaboration,** *n.*

elastance, 1. the quality of recoiling or returning to an original form after the removal of pressure. 2. the degree to which an air-filled or fluid-filled organ, such as a lung, bladder or blood vessel, can return to its original dimensions when a distending or compressing force is removed. 3. the measurement of the unit volume of change in such an organ per unit of decreased pressure change. 4. the reciprocal of compliance.

elastic bandage, a bandage of elasticized fabric that provides support and allows movement.

elastic-band fixation, a method of treatment of fractures of the jaw using rubber bands to connect metal splints or wires that are attached to the maxilla and mandible.

elastic cartilage. See **yellow cartilage.**

elasticity, the ability of tissue to regain its original shape and size after being stretched, squeezed or otherwise deformed.

elastic recoil, the difference between intrapleural pressure and alveolar pressure at a given lung volume under static conditions.

elastin, a protein that forms the principal substance of yellow elastic tissue fibres.

elation, an emotional reaction characterized by euphoria, excitement, extreme joyfulness, optimism and self-satisfaction.

elbow, the bend of the arm at the joint that connects the arm and forearm.

elbow bone. See **ulna.**

elbow joint, the hinged articulation of the humerus, ulna and radius. The elbow joint allows flexion and extension of the forearm.

elbow reflex. See **triceps reflex.**

elective, of or pertaining to a procedure that is performed by choice but which is not essential, such as elective surgery.

Electra complex, (in psychiatry) the libidinous desire of a daughter for her father.

electric blood warmer, an electrical device for heating blood before infusions, especially massive transfusions in which cold blood might put the patient into shock.

electric burns, the tissue damage resulting from heat of up to 5000°C generated by an electric current. The point of contact on the skin is burned, and the muscle and subcutaneous tissues may be damaged.

electric cautery. See **electrocautery.**

electric potential gradient, the net difference in electric charge across the membrane of a cell.

electric shock, a traumatic physical state caused by the passage of electric current through the body. It usually involves accidental contact with exposed parts of electrical circuits in home appliances and domestic power supplies, but may also result from lightning or contact with high-voltage wires. The damage electricity does in passing through the body depends on the intensity of the electric current, type of current, and the duration and frequency of current flow. Severe electric shock commonly causes unconsciousness, respiratory paralysis, muscle contractions, bone fractures and cardiac disorders.

electric shock therapy. See **electroconvulsive therapy.**

electric spinal orthosis, an electrical device that helps control curvature of the spine by stimulating back muscles.

electroanaesthesia, the use of an electric current to produce local or general anaesthesia.

electroanalgesia, the use of an electric current applied to the spinal cord or a peripheral nerve to relieve pain.

electroanalytical chemistry, the branch of chemistry concerned with the analysis of compounds using electric current to produce characteristic, observable change in the substance being studied.

electrocardiogram (ECG), a graphic record produced by an electrocardiograph.

electrocardiograph (ECG), a device used for recording the electrical activity of the myocardium to detect abnormal transmission of the cardiac impulse through the conductive tissues of the muscle. Electrocardiography allows diagnosis of specific cardiac abnormalities. **electrocardiographic,** *adj.*

electrocardiographic-auscultatory syndrome. See **Barlow's syndrome.**

electrocardiograph lead, 1. an electrode placed on part of the body and connected to an electrocardiograph. 2. a record, made by the electrocardiograph, that varies depending on the site of the electrode. Electrocardiography is generally performed with the use of three peripheral leads and six leads placed on the precordium. The peripheral or extremity leads are designated I, II and III, and the chest leads are designated V_1, V_2, V_3, V_4, V_5, and V_6 to indicate the points on the precordium on which the electrodes are placed.

electrocautery, the application of a needle or snare heated by electric current for the destruction of tissue, such as for the removal of warts or polyps.

electrocoagulation, a therapeutic, destructive form of electrosurgery in which tissue is hardened by the passage of high-frequency current from an electric cautery device.

electroconvulsive therapy (ECT), the induction of a brief convulsion by passing an electric current through the brain for the treatment of affective disorders. The patient loses consciousness and undergoes tonic contractions for approximately 10 seconds, followed by a somewhat longer period of clonic convulsions accompanied by apnoea; on awakening the individual has no memory of the shock.

electrocution, death caused by the passage of electric current through the body.

electrode, 1. a contact for the induction or detection of electrical activity. **2.** a medium for conducting an electric current from the body to physiological monitoring equipment.

electrodermal audiometry, a method of testing hearing in which a harmless electric shock is used to condition the subject to a pure tone; thereafter, the tone coupled with the anticipation of a shock elicits a brief electrodermal response, which is recorded, and the lowest intensity of the sound producing the skin response is considered the subject's hearing threshold.

electrodesiccation, a technique in electrosurgery in which tissue is destroyed by burning with an electric spark. It is used primarily for eliminating small superficial growths.

electrodynamics, the study of electrostatic charges in motion, as in the flow of electrons in an electric current.

electrodynograph (EDG), an electronic device used to measure pressures exerted in biological activity, such as the pressures exerted by the human foot in walking, running, jogging or climbing stairs.

electroencephalograph, an instrument for receiving and recording the electric potential produced by the brain cells.

electroencephalographer, a person trained in the management of an electroencephalographic laboratory.

electroencephalography (EEG), (historical) radiographic technique to visualize the internal structures of the brain following the introduction of a radiolucent contrast medium. **electroencephalogram,** *n.,* see **endoscopic retrograde cholangiography; cholangiography.**

electrogram, a unipolar or bipolar record of electrical activity of the heart, as recorded from electrodes within the cardiac chambers or on the epicardium. Examples are atrial electrogram (AEG), ventricular electrogram (VEG) and His bundle electrogram (HBE).

electrohydraulic heart, a type of artificial heart in which the ventricles are driven by the alternate pumping of a fluid rather than by compressed air. The device is powered by a compact electrical motor.

electroimmunodiffusion. See **immunodiffusion.**

electrolysis, a process in which electrical energy causes a chemical change in a conducting medium, usually a solution or a molten substance. Electrodes, usually pieces of metal, induce the flow of electrical energy through the medium. Electrons enter the solution through the cathode and leave the solution through the anode. Negatively charged ions, or anions, are attracted to the anode; positively charged ions, or cations, are attracted to the cathode. **electrolytic,** *adj.*

electrolyte, an element or compound that, when melted or dissolved in water or other solvent, dissociates into ions and is able to conduct an electric current. Electrolytes differ in their concentrations in blood plasma, interstitial fluid and cell fluid, and affect the movement of substances between those compartments. Proper quantities of principal electrolytes and balance among them are critical to normal metabolism and function. **electrolytic,** *adj.*

electrolyte balance, the equilibrium between electrolytes in the body.

electrolyte solution, any solution containing electrolytes prepared for oral, parenteral or rectal administration for the replacement or supplementation of ions necessary for homeostasis.

electromagnetic induction, the production in tissue of electric fields and associated eddy currents by magnetic fields generated by coils carrying an electric current.

electromagnetic radiation, every kind of electric and magnetic radiation, regarded as a continuous spectrum of energy that includes energy with the shortest wavelength (gamma rays, with a wavelength of 0.0011 Å) to that with the longest wavelength (long radio waves, with a wavelength of more than 1 million kilometers).

electromagnetic tape. See **magnetic tape.**

electromotive force (EMF), 1. a source of energy that can cause current to flow in an electrical circuit. **2.** the rate at which energy is drawn from the source of energy when unit current flows through the circuit. EMF is measured in volts.

electromyogram (EMG), a record of the intrinsic electrical activity in a skeletal muscle. Such data help in diagnosing neuromuscular problems and are obtained by applying surface electrodes or by inserting a needle electrode into the muscle.

electron, 1. a negatively charged elementary

particle that has a specific charge, mass and spin. The number of electrons circling the nucleus of an atom is equal to the atomic number of the substance. Electrons may be shared or exchanged by two atoms; after the exchange, the atom becomes an ion. **2.** a negative beta particle emitted from a radioactive substance.

electronarcosis, general anaesthesia without the use of anaesthetic gases or drugs. Narcosis is produced by passing an electric current through the brain.

electron capture, a radioactive decay process occurring within certain unstable neuron-deficient nuclei, in which a K shell electron is captured by the nucleus, combining with a proton to form a neutron. The atomic number of the daughter product will be decreased by one.

electroneuromyography, a procedure for testing and recording neuromuscular activity by the electrical stimulation of nerves.

electronic fetal monitor (EFM), a device that allows observation of the fetal heart rate and the maternal uterine contractions. It may be applied externally, in which case the fetal heart is detected by an ultrasound transducer on the abdomen. Internal monitoring of the fetal heart rate is accomplished via an electrode clipped to the fetal scalp.

electronic thermometer, a thermometer that registers temperature rapidly by electronic means.

electron microscope, an instrument, similar to an optic microscope, that scans cell surfaces with a beam of electrons instead of visible light.

electron microscopy, a technique that uses an electron microscope, in which a beam of electrons is focused by an electromagnetic lens and directed onto an extremely thin specimen.

electron scanning microscope. See **scanning electron microscope.**

electron-volt (eV), unit of energy, where 1 electron-volt is the amount of energy gained by an electron accelerated through a potential difference of 1 volt.

electronystagmography, a method of assessing and recording eye movements by measuring the electrical activity of the extraocular muscles.

electrophoresis, the movement of charged suspended particles through a liquid medium in response to changes in an electric field. The pattern of migration can be recorded in bands on an **electrophoretogram.** The technique is widely used to separate and identify serum proteins and other substances. **electrophoretic,** *adj.*

electroporation, a type of osmotic transfection in which an electric current is used to produce holes in cell membranes so the alien DNA molecules can enter the cells.

electroresection, a technique for the re-moval of bladder tumours, by inserting an electrically charged wire through the urethra.

electroshock therapy. See **electroconvulsive therapy.**

electrosleep therapy, a technique designed to induce sleep, especially in psychiatric patients, by administering a low-amplitude pulsating current to the brain. The cathode is placed supraorbitally, and the anode is placed over the mastoid process. The current, which is discharged for 15 to 20 minutes, produces a tingling sensation, but does not always induce sleep.

electrosurgery, surgery performed with various electrical instruments that operate on high-frequency electric current. Kinds of electrosurgery include electrocoagulation, electrodesiccation.

electrotherapy, the treatment of various disorders by electrical means.

electrotonic current, a current induced in a nerve sheath by an action potential within the nerve or an adjacent nerve.

eleidin, a transparent protein substance resembling keratin, found in the stratum lucidum of the epidermis.

element, one of more than 100 primary, simple substances that cannot be broken down by chemical means into any other substance. Each atom of any element contains a specific number of electrons orbiting the nucleus. The nucleus contains a variable number of neutrons and protons. A stable element contains a balanced number of neutrons and protons. A radioactive element has an imbalance of neutrons compared to protons, and will undergo spontaneous decay in order to become more stable.

element 104, a synthetic, radioactive element, the twelfth transuranic element, and the first transactinide element. It is called rutherfordium (Rf).

element 105, a synthetic element, and the thirteenth transuranic element. It is called hahnium (Ha).

element 106, a synthetic element, with a half-life of 0.9 seconds. It was first synthesized in 1974 by scientists working independently in the United States and the USSR.

element 107, an element reportedly synthesized in 1976 by Soviet scientists who bombarded isotopes of bismuth with heavy nuclei of chromium 54. The finding was not confirmed by scientists of other nations.

elephantiasis, the end-stage lesion of filariasis, characterized by tremendous swelling, usually of the external genitalia and the legs. Elephantiasis results from filariasis that has lasted for many years.

elephantoid fever. See **elephantiasis, filariasis.**

eleventh nerve. See **accessory nerve.**

elimination diet, a procedure for identifying a food or foods to which a person is allergic, by successively omitting from the diet certain foods in order to detect those responsible for the symptoms.

ELISA, abbreviation for enzyme-linked immunosorbent assay.

elixir, 1. a clear liquid containing water, alcohol, sweeteners or flavours, used primarily as a vehicle for the oral administration of a drug. **2.** a pharmaceutical product which has a drug incorporated into such a vehicle.

Elliot's position {John W. Elliott, American surgeon, b. 1852}, a supine posture assumed by the patient on the operating table, with a support placed under the lower costal margin to elevate the chest. The position is used in gallbladder surgery.

elliptocyte, an oval red blood cell.

elliptocytosis, a mild abnormal condition of the blood that is characterized by increased numbers of elliptocytes or oval erythrocytes.

Ellis-van Creveld syndrome. See **chondroectodermal dysplasia.**

eluate, a solution or substance that results from an elution process

eluent, a solvent or solution used in the elution process, as in column chromatography.

elution, the removal of an absorbed substance from a porous bed or chromatographic column by means of a stream of liquid or gas, or by the application of heat. The term is also applied to the removal of antibodies or radioactive tracers from erythrocytes.

emaciation, excessive leanness caused by disease or lack of nutrition.

emasculation, a loss of the testes or penis or both.

embalming, the practice of applying antiseptics and preservatives to a corpse so as to retard the natural decomposition of tissues.

Embden-Meyerhof defects {Gustav G. Embden, German biochemist, b. 1874; Otto F. Meyerhof, German biochemist, b. 1884}, a group of hereditary haemolytic anaemias caused by enzyme deficiencies. The most common form of the disorder is a pyruvate kinase deficiency.

Embden-Meyerhof pathway, a sequence of enzymatic reactions in the anaerobic conversion of glucose to lactic acid, producing energy in the form of adenosine triphosphate.

embedded tooth, an unerupted tooth, usually completely covered with bone.

embolectomy, a surgical incision into an artery for the removal of an embolus or clot, performed as emergency treatment for arterial embolism.

embolism, an abnormal circulatory condition in which an embolus travels through the bloodstream and becomes lodged in a blood vessel. Kinds of embolism include air embolism and fat embolism.

embolization agent, a substance used to occlude or drastically reduce blood flow

within a vessel. Examples include vasoconstrictors and silicone beads.

embolized atheroma, an embolized fat particle lodged in a blood vessel.

embolotherapy, a technique of blocking a blood vessel with a balloon catheter. It is used for treating bleeding ulcers and blood vessel defects and, during surgery, to stop blood flow to a tumour.

embolus, *pl.* **emboli,** a foreign object, a quantity of air or gas, a bit of tissue or tumour, or a piece of a thrombus that circulates in the bloodstream until it becomes lodged in a vessel. Kinds of emboli include air embolus and fat embolus. **embolic, emboloid,** *adj.*

embrasure, a normally occurring space formed between adjacent teeth because of variations in positions and contours.

embryatrics. See **fetology.**

embryectomy, the surgical removal of an embryo, most commonly in an ectopic pregnancy.

embryo, 1. any organism in the earliest stages of development. **2.** in humans, the stage of prenatal development between the time of implantation of the fertilized ovum about 2 weeks after conception until the end of the seventh or eighth week. **embryonal, embryonoid, embryonic,** *adj.*

embryoctony, the intentional destruction of the living embryo or fetus in utero.

embryogenesis, the process in sexual reproduction in which an embryo forms from the fertilization of an ovum.

embryological development, the various intrauterine stages and processes involved in the growth and differentiation of the conceptus from the time of fertilization of the ovum until the eighth week of gestation. The stages are related to the biological status of the unborn child and are divided into two distinct periods. The first is embryogenesis, or the formation of the embryo, which occurs during the 10 days to 2 weeks after fertilization until implantation. The second period, organogenesis, involves the differentiation of the various cells, tissues, and organ systems and the development of the main external features of the embryo; it occurs from approximately the end of the second week to the eighth week of intrauterine life. The fetal stage follows these stages, beginning at about the ninth week of gestation.

embryologist, one who specializes in the study of embryology.

embryology, the study of the origin, growth, development and function of an organism from fertilization to birth. Kinds of embryology include comparative embryology, descriptive embryology and experimental embryology. **embryologic, embryological,** *adj.*

embryoma, *pl.* **embryomas, embryomata,**

a tumour arising from embryonic cells or tissues.

embryoma of the ovary. See **dysgerminoma.**

embryomorph, any structure that resembles an embryo, especially a mass of tissue that may represent an aborted conceptus. **embryomorphous,** adj.

embryonal adenomyosarcoma, embryonal adenosarcoma. See **Wilms' tumour.**

embryonal carcinoma, an extremely malignant neoplasm derived from germinal cells, which usually develops in gonads, especially the testes.

embryonal leukaemia. See **stem cell leukaemia.**

embryonate, 1. impregnated; containing an embryo. **2.** of, pertaining to or resembling an embryo.

embryonic anideus, a blastoderm in which the axial elongation of the primitive streak and primitive groove fail to develop.

embryonic blastoderm, the area of the blastoderm that gives rise to the primitive streak from which the embryonic body develops.

embryonic competence, the ability of an embryonic cell to react normally to the stimulation of an inductor, allowing continued, normal growth or differentiation of the embryo.

embryonic disk, the thickened plate from which the embryo develops in the second week of pregnancy.

embryonic layer, one of the three layers of cells in the embryo, the endoderm, the mesoderm and the ectoderm. From these layers of cells arise all of the structures and organs and parts of the body.

embryonic rest, a portion of embryonic tissue that remains in the adult organism. Such tissue may act as organ-specific indicators in certain types of cancer.

embryonic stage, (in embryology) the interval of time from the end of the germinal stage, at 10 days of gestation, to the eighth week.

embryoniform, resembling an embryo.

embryopathy, any anomaly occurring in the embryo or fetus as a result of interference with normal intrauterine development. A kind of embryopathy is rubella embryopathy.

embryoplastic, of or pertaining to the formation of an embryo, usually with reference to cells.

embryoscopy, the examination of an embryo directly by insertion of a lighted instrument through the mother's abdominal wall and uterus.

embryotome, an instrument used in embryotomy.

embryotomy, 1. the dismemberment or mutilation of a fetus for removal from the uterus when normal delivery is not possible.

2. the dissection of an embryo for examination and analysis.

embryulcia, the surgical extraction of the embryo or fetus from the uterus.

emergence, a stage in the process of recovery from general anaesthesia that includes spontaneous respiration, voluntary swallowing and consciousness.

emergency, a serious situation that arises suddenly and threatens the life or welfare of a person or a group of people, as a natural disaster or a medical crisis.

emergency department, (in a health care facility) a section of an institution that is staffed and equipped to provide rapid and varied emergency care, especially for those stricken with sudden and acute illness or those who are the victims of severe trauma.

emergency trolley, a trolley used to carry emergency equipment, such as analgesics, antiseptics, suction devices, sutures, scalpels, surgical needles, sponges, swabs, retractors, haemostats, forceps, trachea tubes, and often a defibrillator. Hospital emergency departments and intensive care units usually have several such trolleys equipped according to prescribed specifications.

emergent evolution, the theory that evolution occurs in a series of major changes at certain critical stages and results from the total rearrangement of existing elements so that completely new and unpredictable characteristics appear within the species.

emetic 1. of or pertaining to a substance that causes vomiting. **2.** an emetic agent, such as apomorphine and syrup of ipecac.

emissary veins, the small vessels in the skull that connect the sinuses of the dura with the veins on the exterior of the skull through a series of anastomoses.

emollient, a substance that softens tissue, particularly the skin and mucous membranes.

emotion, the affective aspect of consciousness as compared with volition and cognition.

emotional abuse, the debasement of a person's feelings so that he perceives himself as inept, uncared for, and worthless.

emotional care of the dying patient, the compassionate, consistent support offered to help the terminally ill patient and the family cope with impending death.

emotional illness. See **mental disorder.**

emotional need, a psychological or mental requirement of intrapsychic origin, usually centring on such basic feelings as love, fear, anger, sorrow, anxiety, frustration, and depression and involving the understanding, empathy, and support of one person for another. Such needs normally occur in everyone but usually are increased during periods of excessive stress or physical and mental illness and during various stages of life, as infancy, early childhood, and old age. If these needs are not routinely met by appropriate, socially accepted means, they can precipitate psychopathological conditions.

emotional response, a reaction to a particular intrapsychic feeling or feelings, accompanied by physiological changes that may or may not be outwardly manifest but that motivate or precipitate some action or behavioural response.

emotional support, the sensitive, understanding approach that helps patients accept and deal with their illnesses, communicate their anxieties and fears, derive comfort from a gentle, sympathetic, caring person, and increase their ability to care for themselves.

empathy, the ability to recognise and to some extent share the emotions and states of mind of another and to understand the meaning and significance of that person's behaviour. It is an essential quality for effective psychotherapy. **empathic,** *adj.*, **empathize,** *v.*

emphysema, an abnormal condition of the pulmonary system, characterised by overinflation and destructive changes of alveolar walls, resulting in a loss of lung elasticity and decreased gases. Acute emphysema may be caused by the rupture of alveoli by severe respiratory efforts, as in acute bronchopneumonia, suffocation, and whooping cough, and occasionally during labour. Chronic emphysema usually accompanies chronic bronchitis, a major cause of which is cigeratte smoking. Emphysema is also seen after asthma or tuberculosis, conditions in which the lungs are overstretched until the elastic fibres of the alveolar walls are destroyed. In old age, the alveolar membranes atrophy and may collapse, resulting in large air-filled spaces with decreased total surface area of the pulmonary membranes.

empiric, of or pertaining to a method of treating disease based on observations and experience without an understanding of the cause or mechanism of the disorder or the way the employed therapeutic agent or procedure effects improvement or cure. The empiric treatment of a new disease may be based on observations and experience gained in the management of analogous disorders. **empirical,** *adj.*

emprosthotonos, a position of the body characterized by a forward, rigid flexure of the body at the waist. The position is the result of a prolonged, involuntary, muscle spasm that is most commonly associated with tetanus infection or strychnine poisoning.

empyema, an accumulation of pus in a body cavity, especially the pleural space, as a result of bacterial infection, as pleurisy or tuberculosis.

emulsify, to disperse a liquid into another liquid, making a colloidal suspension. Bile acts as an emulsifying agent in the digestive tract by dispersing ingested fats into small globules. **emulsification,** *n.*

emulsion, 1. a system consisting of two immiscible liquids, one of which is dispersed in the other in the form of small droplets. **2.** (in photography) a composition sensitive to actinic rays of light, consisting of one or more silver halides suspended in gelatin applied in a thin layer of film.

enalapril maleate, an angiotensin-converting enzyme (ACE) inhibitor, used as an oral antihypertensive drug and as an adjunct to the treatment of congestive cardiac failure.

enamel, a hard white substance that covers the dentin of the crown of a tooth.

enamel hypocalcification, a hereditary dental defect in which the enamel of the teeth is soft and undercalcified in context yet normal in quantity, caused by defective maturation of the ameloblasts.

enamel hypoplasia, a developmental dental defect in which the enamel of the teeth is hard in context but thin and deficient in amount, caused by defective enamel matrix formation with a deficiency in the cementing substance.

enanthema, an eruptive lesion from the surface of a mucous membrane.

enarthrosis. See **ball-and-socket joint.**

ENB, abbreviation for English National Board for Nursing, Midwifery and Health Visiting.

encainide, a sodium channel antagonist used as an antiarrhythmic agent. It is prescribed in the treatment of life-threatening ventricular arrhythmias and other symptomatic ventricular arrhythmias.

encapsulated, (of arteries, muscles, nerves, and other body parts) enclosed in fibrous or membrous sheaths.

encephalitis, an inflammatory condition of the brain. The cause is usually an arbovirus infection transmitted by the bite of an infected mosquito, but it may be the result of lead or other poisoning or of haemorrhage. **Postinfectious encephalitis** occurs as a complication of another infection, such as chickenpox, influenza, or measles, or after smallpox vaccination. Severe inflammation with destruction of nerve tissue may result in a seizure disorder, loss of a special sense or other permanent neurological problem, or death. Usually, the inflammation involves the spinal cord and brain; hence, in most cases, a more accurate term is *encephalomyelitis.*

encephalitis periaxialis diffusa. See **Schilder's disease.**

encephalocele, protrusion of the brain through a congenital defect in the skull; hernia of the brain.

encephalodysplasia, any congenital anomaly of the brain.

encephalogram, a radiograph of the brain made during encephalography.

encephalography, radiographic delineation

of the structures of the brain containing fluid after the cerebrospinal fluid is withdrawn and replaced by a gas, as air, helium, or oxygen. Kinds of encephalography are **pneumoencephalography** and **ventriculography. encephalographic,** *adj.*

encephaloid carcinoma. See **medullary carcinoma.**

encephalomeningocele. See **meningoencephalocele.**

encephalomyelitis, an inflammatory condition of the brain and spinal cord characterized by fever, headache, stiff neck, back pain, and vomiting. Depending on the cause, the age and condition of the person, and the extent of the inflammation and irritation to the central nervous system, seizures, paralysis, personality changes, a decreased level of consciousness, coma, or death may occur.

encephalomyocarditis, an infectious disease of the central nervous system and heart tissue caused by a group of small RNA picornaviruses. Symptoms are generally similar to those of poliomyelitis. Most victims recover promptly without sequelae.

encephalopathy, any abnormal condition of the structure or function of tissues of the brain, especially chronic, destructive, or degenerative conditions, as Wernicke's encephalopathy or Schilder's disease.

encephalotrigeminal angiomatosis. See **Sturge-Weber syndrome.**

enchondroma, *pl.* **enchondromas, enchondromata,** a benign, slowly growing tumour of cartilage cells that arises in the extremity of the shaft of tubular bones, usually in the hands or feet.

enchondromatosis, a congenital disorder characterized by the proliferation of cartilage within the extremity of the shafts of several bones, causing thinning of the cortex and distortion in length.

enchondromatous myxoma, a tumour of the connective tissue, characterized by the presence of cartilage between the cells of connective tissue.

enchondrosarcoma. See **central chondrosarcoma.**

enchondrosis. See **enchondroma.**

enchylema. See **hyaloplasm.**

encode, 1. to translate a message, signal, or stimulus into a code. **2.** to rewrite, manually or automatically, such as by a computer program, information into a form that can be interpreted by a computer.

encoded message, (in communication theory) a message as transmitted by a sender to a receiver.

encopresis, fecal incontinence. **encopretic,** *adj.*

encounter, (in psychotherapy) the interaction between a patient and psychotherapist in which emotional change and personal growth are brought about by the expression of strong feelings by the participants.

encounter group, (in psychology) a small group of people who meet to increase self-awareness, promote personal growth, and improve interpersonal communication.

encyst, to form a cyst or capsule. **encysted,** *adj.*

Endamoeba. See **Entamoeba.**

endarterectomy, the surgical removal of the intimal lining of the artery. The procedure is done to clear a major artery that may be blocked by a clot or accumulation of plaque.

endarteritis, an inflammatory disorder of the inner layer of one or more arteries, which may become partially or completely occluded.

endarteritis obliterans, an inflammatory condition of the lining of the arterial walls in which the intima proliferates, narrowing the lumen of the vessels and occluding the smaller vessels.

end bud, a mass of undifferentiated cells produced from the remnants of the primitive node and the primitive streak at the caudal end of the developing embryo after the formation of the somites is completed. Also called tail bud.

end bulbs of Krause. See **Krause's corpuscles.**

endemic, (of a disease or micro-organism) indigenous to a geographic area or population. See also **epidemic, pandemic.**

endemic goitre, an enlargement of the thyroid gland caused by the dietary intake of inadequate amounts of dietary iodine. Iodine deprivation leads to diminished production and secretion of thyroid hormone by the gland. Initially, the goitre is diffuse; later it becomes multinodular. Endemic goitre occurs occasionally in adolescents at puberty, and widely in population groups in geographic areas in which limited amounts of iodine are present in the soil, water and food. A large goitre may cause dysphagia, dyspnoea, tracheal deviation and cosmetic problems.

endemic typhus. See **murine typhus.**

end-feel, the sensation imparted to the examiner's hands at the end point of the available range of motion. Types of end-feel include capsular, bone-on-bone, spasm and springy block.

endo-, end-, ento-, a combining form meaning 'inward, within': endobiotic, endocranial, endognathion.

endobronchial anaesthesia, a procedure, rarely performed, in which anaesthetic gas is administered into the bronchi.

endocardial cushion defect, any cardiac defect resulting from the failure of the endocardial cushions in the embryonic heart to fuse and form the atrial septum. See also atrial septal defect, congenital cardiac anomaly.

endocardial cushions, a pair of thickened tissue sections in the embryonic atrial canal.

endocardial fibroelastosis, an abnormal condition characterized by hypertrophy of the wall of the left ventricle and the development of a thick, fibroelastic endocardium.

endocarditis, an abnormal condition that affects the endocardium and heart valves, characterized by lesions caused by a variety of diseases. Kinds of endocarditis are bacterial endocarditis, non-bacterial thrombotic endocarditis and Libman-Sacks endocarditis. Untreated, all types of endocarditis are rapidly lethal. See also **bacterial endocarditis, subacute bacterial endocarditis.**

endocardium, pl. **endocardia,** the lining of the heart chambers, containing small blood vessels and a few bundles of smooth muscle. It is continuous with the endothelium of the great blood vessels. Compare epicardium, myocardium.

endocervical, pertaining to the interior of the cervix and uterus.

endocervicitis, an abnormal condition characterized by inflammation of the epithelium and glands of the canal of the uterine cervix. See also **cervicitis.**

endocervix, 1. the membrane lining the canal of the uterine cervix. **2.** the opening of the cervix into the uterine cavity.

endocrine, pertaining to a process in which a group of cells secrete into the blood or lymph circulation a substance that has a specific effect on tissues in another part of the body.

endocrine fracture, any fracture that results from weakness of a specific bone because of an endocrine disorder, such as hyperparathyroidism.

endocrine system, the network of ductless glands and other structures that elaborate and secrete hormones directly into the bloodstream, affecting the function of specific target organs. Glands of the endocrine system include the thyroid and parathyroid, anterior pituitary, posterior pituitary, pancreas, suprarenal glands and gonads. The pineal gland is also considered an endocrine gland because it is ductless. Compare **exocrine.**

endocrine therapy. See **hormone therapy.**

endocrinologist, a medical doctor who specializes in endocrinology.

endocrinology, the study of the anatomy, physiology, and pathology of the endocrine system and the treatment of endocrine problems.

endoderm, (in embryology) the innermost of the cell layers that develop from the embryonic disk of the inner cell mass of the blastocyst. The endoderm comprises the lining of the cavities and passages of the body and the covering for most of the internal organs. Compare **ectoderm, mesoderm.**

endodermal cloaca, a part of the cloaca in the developing embryo that lies internal to the cloacal membrane and gives rise to the bladder and urogenital ducts. Compare ectodermal cloaca. See also **urogenital sinus.**

endodontics, a branch of dentistry that specializes in the diagnosis and treatment of diseases in the dental pulp and its surrounding tissues, including root canal therapy.

endogenous, 1. growing within the body. **2.** originating from within the body or produced from internal causes, such as a disease caused by the structural or functional failure of an organ or system. Compare **exogenous.** endogenic, adj.

endogenous carbon dioxide, carbon dioxide produced within the body by metabolic processes.

endogenous depression, a major affective disorder characterized by a persistent dysphoric mood, anxiety, irritability, fear, brooding, appetite and sleep disturbances, weight loss, psychomotor agitation or retardation, decreased energy, feelings of worthlessness or guilt, difficulty in concentrating or thinking, occasional delusions and hallucinations, and thoughts of death or suicide. Also called major depressive episode. See also **bipolar disorder, depression.**

endogenous infection, an infection caused by the reactivation of previously dormant organisms, as in coccidioidomycosis, histoplasmosis and tuberculosis. Compare germinal infection, mixed infection, retrograde infection, secondary infection.

endogenous obesity, obesity resulting from dysfunction of the endocrine or metabolic systems. Compare **exogenous obesity.** See also **obesity.**

endolymph, the fluid in the membranous labyrinth of the internal ear. Compare **perilymph.**

endolymphatic duct, a labyrinthine passage joining an endolymphatic sac with a utricle and saccule.

endolymphatic hydrops, an obsolete term for **Ménière's disease.**

endometrial, 1. of or pertaining to endometrium. **2.** of or pertaining to the uterine cavity.

endometrial cancer, a malignant neoplastic disease of the endometrium of the uterus, most often occurring in the fifth or sixth decade of life. Some of the factors associated with an increased incidence of the disease are a medical history of infertility, anovulation, administration of exogenous oestrogen, uterine polyps, and a combination of diabetes, hypertension and obesity. Abnormal vaginal bleeding, especially in a postmenopausal woman, is the cardinal symptom. There also may be lower abdominal and low back pain; a large, boggy uterus is often a sign of advanced disease.

endometrial hyperplasia, an abnormal condition characterized by overgrowth of the endometrium resulting from sustained stimulation by oestrogen (of endogenous or exogenous origin) that is not opposed by progesterone. Endometrial hyperplasia often results in abnormal uterine bleeding; such bleeding, particularly in older women, constitutes an indication for biopsy or curettage of the endometrium to establish histopathological diagnosis and to rule out malignancy.

endometrial polyp, a pedunculated overgrowth of endometrium, usually benign. Polyps are a common cause of vaginal bleeding in perimenopausal women, and are often associated with other uterine abnormalities such as endometrial hyperplasia or fibroids.

endometriosis, an abnormal gynaecological condition characterized by ectopic growth and function of endometrial tissue. The most characteristic symptom of endometriosis is pain, particularly dysmenorrhoea and dyspareunia.

endometritis, an inflammatory condition of the endometrium, usually caused by bacterial infection, commonly gonococci or haemolytic streptococci. It is characterized by fever, abdominal pain, malodorous discharge and enlargement of the uterus. It occurs most frequently after childbirth or abortion, and in women fitted with an intrauterine contraceptive device. A kind of endometritis is decidua endometritis. See also **pelvic inflammatory disease.**

endometritis dessicans, obsolete. endometritis characterized by ulceration and shedding of the endometrium of the uterus.

endometrium, the mucous membrane lining of the uterus, consisting of the stratum compactum, stratum spongiosum and stratum basale. The endometrium changes in thickness and structure with the menstrual cycle. Compare **parametrium.**

endomorph, a person whose body build is characterized by a soft, round physique with a large trunk and thighs, tapering extremities, an accumulation of fat throughout the body, and a predominance of structures derived from the endoderm. Compare ectomorph, mesomorph. See also **pyknic.**

endoparasite, (in medical parasitology) an organism that lives within the body of the host, such as a tapeworm.

endophthalmitis, an inflammatory condition of the internal eye in which the eye becomes red, swollen, painful, and, sometimes, filled with pus. This condition may blur the vision and cause vomiting, fever and headache. Also called endophthalmia.

endophthalmitis phacoanaphylactica, an abnormal condition characterized by an acute autoimmune reaction of the eye. It is caused by hypersensitivity of the eye to the protein of the crystalline lens, and commonly occurs after trauma to the crystalline lens

or after a cataract operation. Associated symptoms include swelling and inflammation of the eye, severe pain and blurred vision. Compare **uveitis.**

endophytic, of or pertaining to the tendency to grow inwards, such as an endophytic tumour that grows on the inside of an organ or structure.

endoplasmic reticulum, an extensive network of membrane-enclosed tubules in the cytoplasm of cells. The structure functions in the synthesis of proteins and lipids, and in the transport of these metabolites within the cell.

endorphin, any one of the neuropeptides composed of many amino acids, elaborated by the pituitary gland and acting on the central and the peripheral nervous systems to reduce pain. Endorphins isolated by researchers are alpha-endorphin, beta-endorphin and gamma-endorphin, all chemicals producing pharmacological effects similar to morphine.

endoscope, an illuminated optical instrument for the visualization of the interior of a body cavity or organ. Although the endoscope is generally introduced through a natural opening in the body, it may also be inserted through an incision. See also **fibreoptics. endoscopic,** adj.

endoscopic retrograde cholangiography, (in radiology) a diagnostic procedure for outlining the common bile duct. A flexible fibreoptic duodenoscope is placed in the common bile duct. See also **cholangiography.**

endoscopy, the visualization of the interior of organs and cavities of the body with an endoscope. See also **bronchoscopy, colonoscopy, cystoscopy, oesophagoscopy, fetoscopy, gastroscopy, laparoscopy, laryngoscopy, mediastinoscopy.**

endoskeletal prosthesis, a prosthetic device in which an internal pylon provides the actual support of the body. See also **pylon.**

endosteal hyperostosis, an inherited bone disorder characterized by an overgrowth of the mandible and brow areas. The excessive bone growth can lead to entrapment of cranial nerves. Also called Van Buchem's syndrome.

endothelial myeloma, a malignant myeloma that develops in the bone marrow, occurring most frequently in the long bones. Also called Ewing's tumour.

endothelioma, a combining form meaning 'a tumour of endothelial tissue': haemendothelioma, lymphendothelioma.

endothelium, the layer of squamous epithelial cells that lines the heart, blood and lymph vessels, and the serous cavities of the body.

endotoxin, a toxin contained in the cell walls of some micro-organisms, especially gram-negative bacteria, released when the bacterium dies and is broken down in the body. Compare **exotoxin.**

endotracheal, within or through the trachea.

endotracheal anaesthesia, inhalation anaesthesia, achieved by the passage of an anaesthetic gas or mixture of gases through an endotracheal tube into the respiratory tract.

endotracheal intubation, the management of the patient with an airway catheter inserted into the trachea through the mouth or nose. An endotracheal tube may be used to maintain a patent airway, prevent aspiration of material from the digestive tract in the unconscious or paralysed patient, permit suctioning of tracheobronchial secretions, or administer positive-pressure ventilation that cannot be given effectively by a mask. Endotracheal tubes may be made of rubber or plastic, and usually have an inflatable cuff to maintain a closed system with the ventilator.

endotracheal tube, a large-bore catheter inserted through the mouth or nose and into the trachea to a point above the bifurcation of the trachea proximal to the bronchi. It is used for delivering oxygen under pressure when ventilation must be totally controlled and in general anaesthetic procedures. See also **endotracheal intubation.**

endoxin, an endogenous analogue of digoxin, occurring naturally in humans. It is a hormone that may regulate the excretion of salt.

end-tidal capnography, (in respiratory therapy) the process of continuously recording the percentage of carbon dioxide in expired air. It is used in continuous monitoring of critically ill patients and also in pulmonary function testing.

end-tidal CO$_2$ determination, the concentration of carbon dioxide in a patient's end-tidal breath and arterial blood.

endurance, the ability to continue an activity despite increasing physical or psychological stress. Although endurance and strength are different qualities, weaker muscles tend to have less endurance than strong muscles.

ene, a combining form naming hydrocarbons: ethidene, somnifene, xanthene.

enema, a procedure in which a solution is introduced into the rectum for cleansing or therapeutic purposes. Enemas may be commercially packed disposable units or reusable equipment prepared just before use.

energy, the capacity to do work or to perform vigorous activity. Energy may occur in the form of heat, light, movement, sound or radiation. Human energy is usually expressed as muscle contractions and heat production. Chemical energy refers to the energy released as a result of a chemical reaction. Compare **anergy. energetic,** *adj.*

energy conservation, a principle that energy cannot be created or destroyed, although it can be changed from one form into another, as when heat energy is converted to light energy.

energy cost of activities, the metabolic cost in calories of various forms of physical activity. For example, the average metabolic equivalent of walking at a rate of 3 km/h is 2 METS per minute while the energy cost of walking at a speed of 6 km/h is 5 METs per minute. See also **MET.**

energy-protein malnutrition, a condition resulting from a diet deficient in both calories and proteins. Also called proteincalorie malnutrition. See also **marasmic kwashiorkor, marasmus.**

energy subtraction, (in radiography) a technique in which two different x-ray beams are used alternately to provide a subtraction image resulting from differences in photoelectric interaction.

enervation, 1. the reduction or lack of nervous energy; weakness; lassitude; languor. 2. removal of a complete nerve or of a section of nerve.

en face, "face-to-face"; a position in which the mother's face and the infant's face are approximately 8 inches apart and on the same plane, as when the mother holds the infant up in front of her face or when she holds the child.

enflurane, a non-flammable anaesthetic gas belonging to the ether family, used for induction and maintenance of general anaesthesia in cases where ethers are the drugs of choice.

engagement, fixation of the greatest presenting diameter of the fetus in the materian pelvis; the biparietal diameter.

engorgement, distention or vascular congestion of body tissues, such as the swelling of breast tissue caused by an increased flow of blood and lymph preceding true lactation.

engram, 1. a hypothetical neurophysiological storage unit in the cerebrum that is the source of a particular memory. 2. an interneuronal circuit involving specific neurons and muscle fibres that can be coordinated to perform specific motor activity patterns.

enkephalin, one of two pain-relieving pentapeptides produced in the body. Researchers have isolated enkephalins in the pituitary gland, brain, and GI tract. The encephalins are methionine-enkephalin and isoleucine-enkephalin, each composed of five amino acids, four of which are identical in both compounds. It is believed that these two neuropeptides can depress neurons throughout the central nervous system. Compare **endorphin.**

enol, an organic compound with an alcohol or hydroxyl group adjacent to a double bond.

enophthalmos, backward displacement of the eye in the bony socket, caused by traumatic injury or developmental defect. **enophthalmic,** *adj.*

ensiform process. See **xiphoid process.**

entamoebiasis. See **amoebiasis.**

Entamoeba, a genus of intestinal amoebic parasites of which several species are pathogenic to humans. See also *Entamoeba histolytica.*

Entamoeba histolytica, a pathogenic species of amoeba that causes amoebic dysentery and hepatic amoebiasis in humans. See also **amoebiasis, amoebic dysentery, hepatic amebiasis.**

entamoebiasis. See **amoebiasis.**

enter-. See **entero-.**

enteral nutrition, methods of feeding where nutrients are absorbed through the digestive system. This relates to oral nutrition as well as tube feeding. See **nasogastric, gastrostomy, nasoduodenal, jejunostomy.**

enterectomy, the surgical removal of a portion of intestine.

enteric coating, a coating added to oral medications that are designed to be absorbed from the intestinal tract. The coating resists the effects of stomach juices.

enteric fever. See **typhoid fever.**

enteric infection, a disease of the intestine caused by any infection. Symptoms similar to those caused by pathogens may be produced by chemical toxins in ingested foods, and by allergic reactions to certain food substances. Among bacteria commonly involved in enteric infections are *Escherichia coli, Vibrio cholerae,* and several species of *Salmonella, Shigella* and anaerobic streptococci. Enteric infections are characterized by diarrhoea, abdominal discomfort, nausea and vomiting, and anorexia.

entericoid fever, a typhoid-like, febrile disease characterized by intestinal inflammation and dysfunction. See also **enteric infection, typhoid fever.**

enteritis, inflammation of the mucosal lining of the small intestine, resulting from a variety of causes—bacterial, viral, functional and inflammatory. Involvement of small and large intestine is called enterocolitis. Compare **gastroenteritis.**

entero-, enter-, a combining form meaning 'pertaining to the intestines': enteric, enterobiliary, enteroptosis.

Enterobacter cloacae, a common species of bacteria found in human and animal faeces, dairy products, sewage, soil and water. Also called *Aerobacter aerogenes, Enterobacter aerogenes.*

Enterobacteriaceae, a family of aerobic and anaerobic bacteria that includes both normal and pathogenic enteric micro-organisms. Among the significant genera of the family are *Escherichia, Klebsiella, Proteus* and *Salmonella.*

enterobacterial, of or pertaining to a species of bacteria found in the digestive tract.

enterobiasis, a parasitic infestation with *Enterobius vermicularis,* the common pinworm. The worms infect the large intestine, and the females deposit eggs in the perianal area, causing pruritus and insomnia. Also called oxyuriasis.

Enterobius vermicularis, a common parasitic nematode that resembles a white thread between 0.5 and 1 cm long. Also called **pinworm, seatworm, threadworm.**

enterochromaffin cell. See **argentaffin cell.**

enteroclysis, a radiographic procedure in which a contrast medium is injected into the duodenum to examine the small intestine.

enterococcus, *pl.* **enterococci,** any *Streptococcus* that inhabits the intestinal tract.

enterocolitis, an inflammation involving both the large and small intestines. Also called coloenteritis.

enteroenterostomy, the surgical creation of an artificial connection between two segments of the intestine.

enterohepatic circulation, a route by which part of the bile produced by the liver enters the intestine to be reabsorbed by the liver and recycled back into the intestine. The remainder of the bile is excreted in faeces.

enterokinase, an intestinal juice enzyme that activates the proteolytic enzyme in pancreatic juice by converting trypsinogen to trypsin.

enterolith, a stone or concretion found within the intestine. See also **calculus.**

enterolithiasis, the presence of enteroliths in the intestine.

enteropathy, a disease or other disorder of the intestines.

enterostomy, a surgical procedure that produces an artificial anus or fistula in the intestine by incision through the abdominal wall. Compare **colostomy.**

enterotoxigenic, pertaining to an organism or other agent that produces a toxin causing an adverse reaction by cells of the intestinal mucosa. Examples include bacteria that produce enterotoxins, resulting in intestinal reactions such as vomiting, diarrhoea and other symptoms of food poisoning.

enterotoxin, a toxic substance specific for the cells of the intestinal mucosa, produced usually by certain species of bacteria, such as *Staphylococcus.* See also **enterotoxigenic.**

enterovirus, a virus that multiplies primarily in the intestinal tract. Kinds of enteroviruses are coxsackievirus, echovirus and poliovirus. **enteroviral,** *adj.*

enthesitis, an inflammation of the insertion of a muscle with a strong tendency towards fibrosis and calcification.

entoderm. See **endoderm.**

entrainment, a phenomenon observed in the microanalysis of sound films in which the speaker moves several parts of the body and the listener responds to the sounds by moving in ways that are coordinated with the rhythm of the sounds. Entrainment is thought to be an essential factor in the process of maternal-infant bonding.

entrance block, (in cardiology) a theoretical zone surrounding the heart's natural pacemaker focus, protecting it from discharge by an extraneous impulse that might trigger ectopic ventricular contractions.

entropion, turning inwards or turning towards, usually a condition in which the eyelid turns inwards, towards the eye. Cicatricial entropion can occur in the upper or lower eyelid as a result of scar tissue formation. Spastic entropion results from an inflammation or other factor that affects tissue tone. An inflammation of the eyelid may be the result of an infectious disease or irritation from an inverted eyelash.

entropy, the tendency of a system to go from a state of order to a state of disorder, expressed in physics as a measure of the part of the heat or energy in a thermodynamic system that is not available to perform work.

ENT specialist, a medical doctor who specializes in the treatment of the eye, nose and throat.

enucleation, 1. removal of an organ or tumour in one piece. **2.** removal of the eyeball performed for malignancy, severe infection or extensive trauma, or to control pain in glaucoma.

enuresis, incontinence of urine, especially in bed at night.

environment, all of the many factors, both physical and psychological, that influence or affect the life and survival of a person. **environmental,** adj.

environmental carcinogen, any of several natural or synthetic substances that can cause cancer. Such agents, or oncogens, may be divided into chemical agents, physical agents, and certain hormones and viruses.

environmental control system, control units that regulate various devices for handicapped persons from remote positions such as a bed or wheelchair. Examples include units (often with switches that can be manipulated by the lips, chin or other functional body parts) that control lamps, television, radio, telephone and alarm systems.

environmental services, a housekeeping function of a hospital or other healthcare facility.

enzygotic twins. See **monozygotic twins.**

enzymatic detergent asthma, a type of allergic reaction experienced by persons who have become sensitized to alcalase, an enzyme contained in some laundry detergents.

enzyme, a protein produced by living cells that catalyses chemical reactions in organic matter. Most enzymes are produced in minute quantities and catalyse reactions that take place within the cells.

enzyme-linked immunosorbent assay (ELISA), a laboratory technique for detecting specific antigens or antibodies, using enzyme-labelled immunoreactants and a solid-phase binding support, such as a test tube. ELISA is nearly as sensitive as radioimmunoassay, and more sensitive than complement-fixation, agglutination and other techniques. It is commonly employed in the diagnosis of AIDS infections.

eosin, a group of red, acidic xanthine dyes often used in combination with a blue-purple, basic dye, such as haematoxylin, to stain tissue slides in the laboratory.

eosinophil, a granulocytic, bilobed leukocyte, somewhat larger than a neutrophil, characterized by the large number of coarse, refractile, cytoplasmic granules that stain intensely with the acid dye eosin. **eosinophilic,** adj.

eosinophilia, an increase in the number of eosinophils in the blood, which accompanies several inflammatory conditions. Substantial increases are considered a reflection of an allergic response.

eosinophilic, 1. the tendency of a cell, tissue or organism to be readily stained by the dye eosin. **2.** of or pertaining to an eosinophilic leukocyte.

eosinophilic adenoma. See **acidophilic adenoma.**

eosinophilic enteropathy, a rare form of food allergy that is characterized by nausea, crampy abdominal pain, diarrhoea, urticaria, an elevated eosinophil count in the blood, and eosinophilic infiltrates in the intestine.

eosinophilic granuloma, a growth characterized by numerous eosinophils and histiocytes, usually occurring as a single or multiple lesion in bone.

eosinophilic leukaemia, a malignant neoplasm of leukocytes in which eosinophils are the predominant cells.

eosinophilic pneumonia, inflammation of the lungs, characterized by infiltration of the alveoli with eosinophils and large mononuclear cells, pulmonary oedema, fever, night sweats, cough, dyspnoea, and weight loss.

EP, abbreviation for evoked potential.

ependyma, a layer of ciliated epithelium that lines the central canal of the spinal cord and the ventricles of the brain.

ependymal glioma, a large, vascular, fairly solid glioma in the fourth ventricle.

ependymoblastoma, a malignant neoplasm composed of primitive cells of the ependyma.

ependymoma, a neoplasm composed of differentiated cells of the ependyma.

ephapse, a point of lateral contact between nerve fibres across which impulses may be

of four potent local anesthetics slightly different in chemical structure from the amide group of local anesthetics. Kinds of ester-compound local anesthetics are chloroprocaine, cocaine hydrochloride, and procaine hydrochloride.

estramustine phosphate sodium, a cytotoxic alkylating agent used to treat carcinoma of the prostate.

estrangement, a psychological effect caused by the required separation of a mother from her newborn child when the infant is ill, premature, or has a congenital defect, thereby diverting the mother from establishment of a normal relationship with her child.

état criblé, a condition or state of multiple sievelike perforations in swollen Peyer's patches of the intestine. It is a frequently fatal complication of untreated typhoid fever.

ethacrynate sodium. See **ethacrynic acid.**

ethacrynic acid, a potent diuretic prescribed to relieve the effects of severe oedema and hypertension.

ethambutol hydrochloride, a tuberculostatic antibiotic used in the treatment of tuberculosis.

ethanoic acid. See **acetic acid.**

ethanol, ethyl alcohol.

ethene. See **ethylene.**

ether, a non-halogenated, volatile liquid formerly used as a general anaesthetic. It has an irritating, pungent odour, and is highly flammable and explosive.

ethics, the science or study of moral values or principles, including ideals of autonomy, beneficence, and justice.

ethinyloestradiol, an oestrogen used in the treatment of postmenopausal breast cancer, menstrual cycle irregularities, prostatic cancer and hypogonadism, for contraception, and for relieving menopausal symptoms.

ethionamide, a tuberculostatic antibacterial used to treat tuberculosis.

ethmoidal air cell, one of the numerous, small thin-walled cavities in the ethmoid bone of the skull, rimmed by the frontal maxilla, lacrimal, sphenoidal, and palatine bones.

ethmoid bone, the very light and spongy bone at the base of the cranium, forming most of the walls of the superior part of the nasal cavity.

ethnic group, a population of individuals organized around an assumption of common cultural origin.

ethnocentrism, **1.** a belief in the inherent superiority of the "race" or group to which one belongs. **2.** a proclivity to consider other ethnic groups in terms of one's own racial origins.

ethoheptazine citrate, a non-narcotic analgesic prescribed to relieve mild to moderate pain.

ethology, 1. (in zoology) the scientific study of the behavioural patterns of animals, specifically in their native habitat. **2.** (in psychology) the empirical study of human behaviour, primarily social customs, manners and moral values. **ethologic, ethological,** *adj.,* **ethologist,** *n.*

ethosuximide, an anticonvulsant prescribed in the treatment of epilepsy.

ethyl alcohol. See **alcohol.**

ethyl chloride, a topical anaesthetic for short operations. It is prescribed in the treatment of skin irritations and in minor skin surgery. It is highly flammable.

ethylene, a colourless, flammable gas that is lighter than air and has a slightly sweet odour and taste. It was previously used as a general anaesthetic, being slightly more potent than nitrous oxide.

ethylenediamine, a clear, thick liquid having the odour of ammonia. It is used as a solvent, an emulsifier, and as a stabilizer in aminophylline injections.

ethylene dibromide (EDB), a volatile liquid used as an insecticide and gasoline additive. It has been found to be a cause of cancer in animals.

ethylene dichloride poisoning, the toxic effects of exposure to ethylene dichloride, a hydrocarbon solvent, diluent, and fumigant, and one of the most abundant of all chlorinated organic chemicals. It is an eye, ear, nose, throat, and skin irritant. Inhalation or ingestion can lead to serious illness or death.

ethylene glycol poisoning, the toxic reaction to ingestion of ethylene glycol or diethylene glycol, chemicals used in automobile antifreeze preparations. Symptoms in mild cases may resemble those of alcohol intoxication but without the breath odour of alcoholic beverages. There may also be vomiting, carpopedal spasm, lumbar pain, renal failure, respiratory distress, convulsions, and coma.

ethylene oxide, a gas used to sterilize surgical instruments and other supplies.

ethyl oxide, a colourless, highly volatile liquid solvent similar to diethyl ether. It is widely used in various pharmaceutical processes.

ethynodiol diacetate, a synthetic progestogen used as an oral contraceptive.

etidronate disodium, a bisphosphonate and regulator of calcium metabolism. It is prescribed in the treatment of Paget's disease, in heterotopic ossification caused by injury to the spinal cord, in malignant disease of bone, and in the management of malignant hypercalcaemia.

etomidate, a hypnotic and short-acting, investigational nonbarbiturate intravenous induction agent for general anaesthesia.

etretinate, a synthetic derivative of vitamin A administered by mouth to treat severe recalcitrant psoriasis, including generalized pustular and erythrodermic psoriasis and other skin diseases characterised by abnormal epithelial keratinization.

Eu, symbol for europium.

eucaryon. See **eukaryon.**

eucaryosis. See **eukaryosis.**

eucholia, the normal state of the bile as to the quantity secreted and the condition of the constituents.

euchromatin, that portion of chromosome material that is active in gene expression during cell division. It stains most deeply during mitosis. **euchromatic,** *adj.*

euchromosome. See **autosome.**

eugamy, the union of those gametes that contain the same haploid number of chromosomes. **eugamic,** *adj.*

eugenics, the study of methods for controlling the characteristics of future human populations through selective breeding.

euglobulin, a "true" globulin (a protein insoluble in distilled water). This is one of a number of different properties used to classify proteins.

eugnathic anomaly, (in dentistry) an abnormality of the teeth and their alveolar supports.

eukaryocyte, a cell with a true nucleus, found in all higher organisms and in some microorganisms, as amoebae, plasmodia, and trypanosomes. Also spelt eucaryocyte. **eukaryotic,** *adj.*

eukaryon, 1. a nucleus that is highly complex, organized, and surrounded by a nuclear membrane, usually characteristic of higher organisms. **2.** an organism containing such a nucleus. Also spelt eucaryon.

eukaryosis, the state of having a highly complex, organized nucleus containing organelles surrounded by a nuclear membrane. Also spelt eucaryosis.

eukaryote, an organism having cells that contain a true nucleus. Also spelt eucaryote. **eukaryotic, eucaryotic,** *adj.*

eunuch, a male whose testicles have been destroyed or removed. If this occurs before puberty, secondary sex characteristics fail to develop.

eunuchoidism, deficiency of the function of male hormone or of its formation by the testes. The deficiency leads to sterility and to abnormal tallness, small testes, and deficient development of secondary sexual characteristics, libido, and potency.

euphoretic, 1. (of a substance or event) tending to produce a condition of euphoria. **2.** a substance tending to produce euphoria, as LSD, mescaline, marijuana, and other hallucinogenic drugs.

euphoria, 1. a feeling or state of well-being or elation. **2.** an exaggerated or abnormal sense of physical and emotional well-being not based on reality or truth, disproportionate to its cause, and inappropriate to the situation.

euploid, 1. of or pertaining to an individual, organism, strain, or cell with a chromosome number that is an exact multiple of the normal, basic haploid number characteristic of the species, as diploid, triploid, tetraploid, or polyploid. **2.** such an individual, organism, strain, or cell.

euploidy, the state or condition of having a variation in chromosome number that is an exact multiple of the characteristic haploid number.

European blastomycosis. See **cryptococcosis.**

European typhus. See **epidemic typhus.**

europium (Eu), a rare-earth, metallic element. Its atomic number is 63; its atomic weight is 151.96.

eustachian tube {Bartolomeo Eustachio, Italian anatomist, b. 1520}, a tube, lined with mucous membrane, that joins the nasopharynx and the tympanic cavity, allowing equalization of the air pressure in the inner ear with atmospheric pressure.

eustress, 1. a positive form of stress. **2.** a balance between selfishness and altruism through which an individual develops the drive and energy to care for others.

euthanasia, deliberately bringing about the death of a person who is suffering from an incurable disease or condition, actively, such as by administering a lethal drug, or passively, by allowing the person to die by withholding treatment.

euthenics, the science that deals with improvement of the human species through the control of environmental factors, as pollution, malnutrition, disease, and drug abuse.

euthymism, the characteristic of normal mood responses.

evacuate, 1. to discharge or to remove a substance from a cavity, space, organ, or tract of the body. **2.** a substance discharged or removed from the body. **evacuation,** *n.*

evagination, the turning inside-out or protrusion of a body part or organ.

evaluating, (in the four-step nursing process) a category of nursing behaviour in which a determination is made and recorded regarding the extent to which the established goals of care have been met. To make this judgment, the nurse estimates the degree of success in meeting the goals, evaluates the implementation of nursing measures, investigates the client's compliance with therapy, and records the client's response to therapy. The nurse evaluates effects of the measures used, the need for change in goals of care, the accuracy of the implementation of nursing measures, and the need for change in the client's environment or in the equipment or procedures used.

evaporated milk, homogenized whole milk from which 50% to 60% of the water content has been evaporated. It is fortified with vitamin D, canned, and sterilized.

evaporation, the change of a substance from a solid or liquid state to a gaseous state. The process of evaporation is hastened by an increase in temperature and a decrease in atmospheric pressure. **evaporate,** *v.*

eventration, the protrusion of the intestines from the abdomen.

event-related potential (ERP), a type of brain wave that is associated with a response to a specific stimulus, such as a particular wave pattern observed when a patient hears a clicking sound.

eversion, a turning outward or inside-out.

evisceration, 1. the removal of the viscera from the abdominal cavity; disembowelment. **2.** the removal of the contents from an organ or an organ from its cavity. **3.** the protrusion of an internal organ through a wound or surgical incision, especially in the abdominal wall. **eviscerate,** *v.*

evocation, (in embryology) a specific morphogenetic change within a developing embryo that occurs as a result of the action of a single evocator.

evocator, a specific chemical substance or hormone that is emitted from the organizer part of the embryonic tissue and acts as a morphogenetic stimulus in the developing embryo.

evoked potential (EP), a tracing of a brain wave measured on the surface of the head at various places. The EP, unlike the waves seen on an electroencephalogram, is elicited by a specific stimulus. The stimulus may affect the visual, auditory, or somatosensory pathways, producing a characteristic brain wave pattern. Kinds of evoked potentials include brainstem auditory evoked potential, somatosensory evoked potential, and visual evoked potential.

evoked response audiometry, a method of testing hearing ability at the level of the brainstem and auditory cortex.

evolution, 1. a gradual, orderly, and continuous process of change and development from one condition or state to another. **2.** (in genetics) the theory of the origin and propagation of all plant and animal species, including humans, and their development from lower to more complex forms through the natural selection of variants produced through genetic mutations, hybridization, and inbreeding. Kinds of evolution are convergent evolution, determinant evolution, emergent evolution, organic evolution, orthogenic evolution, and saltatory evolution. **evolutionist,** *n.*

evulsed tooth. See **avulsed tooth.**

Ewing's sarcoma {James Ewing, American pathologist, b. 1866}, a malignant tumour developing from bone marrow, usually in long bones or the pelvis. It is characterized by pain, swelling, fever, and leukocytosis.

exacerbation, an increase in the seriousness of a disease or disorder as marked by greater intensity in the signs or symptoms of the patient being treated.

exanthema, a skin eruption or rash that may have specific diagnostic features of an infectious disease. Chickenpox, measles, roseola infantum, and rubella are usually characterized by a particular type of exanthema. **exanthematous,** *adj.*

exanthem subitum. See **roseola infantum.**

excess mortality, a premature death or one that occurs before the average life expectancy for a person of a particular demographic category.

exchange transfusion in the newborn, the introduction of whole blood in exchange for 75% to 85% of an infant's circulating blood that is repeatedly withdrawn in small amounts and replaced with equal amounts of donor blood. The procedure is performed to improve the oxygen-carrying capacity of the blood in the treatment of erythroblastosis neonatorum by removing Rh and ABO antibodies, sensitized erythrocytes producing haemolysis, and accumulated bilirubin.

excise, to remove completely, as in the surgical excision of the palatine tonsils.

excision, 1. the process of excising or amputating. **2.** (in molecular genetics) the process by which a genetic element is removed from a strand of DNA.

excitability, the property of a cell that enables it to react to irritation or stimulation, such as the reaction of a nerve or myocardial cell to an adequate stimulus.

excitant, a drug or other agent that will arouse the central nervous system or other body system in a particular manner.

excitatory amino acids, amino acids that affect the central nervous system and may in some cases act as neurotoxins. Examples include glutamate and aspartate.

exciting eye, (in sympathetic ophthalmia) the eye that is primarily affected by an injury or infection in a bilateral disorder.

excitement, (in psychiatry) a pathological state marked by emotional intensity, impulsive behaviour, anticipation, and arousal.

excoriation, an injury to the surface of the skin or other part of the body caused by scratching or abrasion.

excreta, any waste matter discharged from the body.

excrete, to evacuate a waste substance from the body.

excretion, the process of eliminating, shedding, or getting rid of substances by body organs or tissues, as part of a natural metabolic activity. Excretion usually begins at the cellular level.

excretory, relating to the process of excretion, often used in combination with a term to identify an object or procedure associated with excretion, as in excretory urography.

excretory duct, a duct that is conductive but not secretory.

excretory urography. See **intravenous urography.**

execute, (of a computer) to follow a set of instructions to complete a program or specified function.

executive physical, a physical examination including extensive laboratory, x-ray, and other tests that is provided periodically to management level personnel at employer expense. Such examinations may be detailed, expensive, and overly complete.

exercise, 1. the performance of any physical activity for the purpose of conditioning the body, improving health, or maintaining fitness or as a means of therapy for correcting a deformity or restoring the organs and bodily functions to a state of health. 2. any action, skill, or manoeuvre that exerts the muscles used in order to develop or strengthen the body or any of its parts. 3. to use a muscle or part of the body in a repetitive way to maintain or develop its strength. Kinds of exercise are active assisted exercise, active exercise, active resistance exercise, aerobic exercise, anaerobic exercise, corrective exercise, isometric exercise, isotonic exercise, muscle-setting exercise, passive exercise, progressive resistance exercise, range of motion exercise, and underwater exercise.

exercise electrocardiogram (exercise ECG), a stress test that is important in the diagnosis of coronary artery disease. An exercise electrocardiogram is recorded as a person walks on a treadmill or pedals a stationary bicycle for a given length of time at a specific rate of speed.

exercise-induced asthma, a form of asthma that produces symptoms after strenuous exercise. The effect may be acute but is reversible.

exercise tolerance, the level of physical exertion an individual may be able to perform before reaching a state of exhaustion. Exercise-tolerance tests are commonly performed on a treadmill under the supervision of a health professional who can stop the test when signs of distress are observed.

exfoliation, peeling and sloughing off of tissue cells. This is a normal process that may be exaggerated in certain skin diseases or after a severe sunburn. **exfoliative,** *adj.*

exfoliative cytology, the microscopic examination of desquamated cells for diagnostic purposes. The cells are obtained from lesions, sputum, secretions, urine, or other material.

exfoliative dermatitis, any inflammatory skin disorder in which there is excessive peeling or shedding of skin.

exhalation. See **expiration.**

exhale, to breathe out or to let out with the breath. **exhalation,** *n.*

exhaustion, a state of extreme loss of physical or mental abilities caused by fatigue or illness.

exhaustion delirium, a delirium that may result from prolonged physical or emotional stress, fatigue, or shock associated with severe metabolic or nutritional problems.

exhibitionism, 1. the flaunting of oneself or one's abilities in order to attract attention. 2. (in psychiatry) a psychosexual disorder occurring in men in which the repetitive act of exposing the genitals to unsuspecting women is a means of achieving sexual excitement and gratification. **exhibitionist,** *n.*

eximer laser, a small laser designed to break up organic molecules, such as cholesterol deposits, without producing intense heat.

existential humanistic psychotherapy, See **humanistic existential therapy.**

existential psychiatry, a school of psychiatry based on the philosophy of existentialism that emphasizes an analytic, holistic approach in which mental disorders are viewed as deviations within the total structure of an individual's existence rather than as caused by any biologicalally or culturally related factors.

existential therapy, a kind of psychotherapy that emphasizes the development of a sense of self-direction through choice, awareness, and acceptance of individual responsibility.

exit block, (in cardiology) the failure of an expected impulse to emerge from its focus of origin and cause a contraction.

exit dose, (in radiotherapy) the amount of radiation at the side of the body opposite the surface to which the beam is directed.

exocoelom. See **extraembryonic coelom.**

exocrine, of or pertaining to the process of secreting outwardly through a duct to the surface of an organ or tissue or into a vessel.

exocrine gland, any one of the two kinds of multicellular glands that open on the surface of the skin through ducts in the epithelium, as the sweat glands and the sebaceous glands.

exogenous, 1. growing outside the body, 2. originating outside the body or an organ of the body or produced from external causes, such as a disease caused by a bacterial or viral agent foreign to the body. **exogenic,** *adj.*

exogenous depression. See **reactive depression.**

exogenous hypertriglyceridaemia. See **hyperlipidaemia type I.**

exogenous obesity, obesity caused by a caloric intake greater than needed to meet the metabolic needs of the body.

exon, (in molecular genetics) the part of a DNA molecule that produces the code for the final messenger RNA.

exonuclease, (in molecular genetics) a

being totally or primarily concerned with what is outside the self. Also spelt extraversion.

extrovert, 1. a person whose interests are directed away from the self and concerned primarily with external reality and the physical environment rather than with inner feelings and thoughts. **2.** a person characterized by extroversion. Also spelt extravert.

extrusion reflex, a normal response in infants to force the tongue outward when touched or depressed. The reflex begins to disappear by about 3 or 4 months of age.

extubation, the process of withdrawing a tube from an orifice or cavity of the body. **extubate,** *v.*

exuberant callus. See **heterotopic ossification.**

exudate, fluid, cells, or other substances that have been slowly exuded, or discharged, from cells or blood vessels through small pores or breaks in cell membranes.

exudative, relating to the exudation or oozing of fluid and other materials from cells and tissues, usually as a result of inflammation or injury.

exudative angina. See **croup.**

exudative enteropathy, diarrhoea seen in diseases characterized by inflammation or destruction of intestinal mucosa.

eye, one of a pair of organs of sight, contained in a bony orbit at the front of the skull, embedded in orbital fat and innervated by one of a pair of optic nerves from the forebrain. Two internal cavities are separated by the crystalline lens. The cavity anterior to the lens is divided by the iris into two chambers, both filled with aqueous humor. The posterior chamber is larger than the anterior chamber and contains the jellylike vitreous body. The outside tunic of the bulb consists of the transparent cornea anteriorly and the opaque sclera posteriorly. The internal tunic of nervous tissue is the retina. Light waves passing through the lens strike a layer of rods and cones in the retina creating impulses that are transmitted by the optic nerve to the brain.

eyebrow, 1. the supraorbital arch of the frontal bone that separates the orbit of the eye from the forehead. **2.** the arch of hairs growing along the ridge formed by the supraorbital arch of the frontal bone.

eyecup, a small vessel, or cup, that is shaped to fit over the eyeball and used to bathe the exposed surface of the organ.

eye dominance, an unconscious preference to use one eye rather than the other for certain purposes, such as sighting a rifle or looking through a telescope.

eyedrops, a liquid medicine that is administered by allowing it to fall in drops onto the conjunctival surface.

eye glasses, transparent devices held in metal or plastic frames in front of the eyes to correct refractive errors or to protect the eyes from harmful electromagnetic waves or flying objects.

eyeground, the fundus of the eye.

eyelash, one of many cilia growing in double or triple rows along the border of the eyelids in front of a row of ciliary glands that are in front of a row of meibomian glands.

eyelid, a movable fold of thin skin over the eye, with eyelashes and ciliary and meibomian glands along its margin. The orbicularis oculi muscle and the oculomotor nerve control the opening and closing of the eyelid.

eye memory. See **visual memory.**

F

f, 1. symbol for breaths per unit time. **2.** symbol for respiratory frequency.

F, 1. abbreviation for **Fahrenheit. 2.** abbreviation for **farad. 3.** symbol for **fluorine. 4.** abbreviation for **frequency.**

F_1, (in genetics) the symbol for the first filial generation; the heterozygous offspring produced by the mating of two unrelated individuals.

F_2, (in genetics) the symbol for the second filial generation; the offspring produced by mating two members of the F_1 generation.

FA, 1. abbreviation for **fatty acid. 2.** abbreviation for **femoral artery. 3.** abbreviation for **folic acid.**

Fabere's test, a test for pain or dysfunction in the hip and sacroiliac joints through overpressure applied at the knee during flexion, abduction and external rotation of the hip.

fabrication, a psychological reaction in which false statements are contrived to mask memory defects.

Fabry's disease, Fabry's syndrome. See **angiokeratoma corporis diffusum.**

FAC, an anticancer drug combination of fluorouracil, doxorubicin and cyclophosphamide.

face, 1. the front of the head from the chin to the brow, including the skin and muscles and structures of the forehead, eyes, nose, mouth, cheeks and jaw. **2.** the visage. **3.** to direct the face toward something. **facial,** *adj.*

face-bow, a device resembling a caliper, used for measuring the relationship of the maxillae to the temporomandibular joints required for the fabrication of denture casts.

facet, 1. (in dentistry) a flattened, highly polished wear pattern on a tooth. **2.** a small, smooth-surfaced process for articulation.

face validity, the apparent validity of a test or measurement device as it is to be used in a particular study.

facial angle, an anthropomorphic expression of the degree of protrusion of the lower face.

facial artery, one of a pair of tortuous arteries that arise from the external carotid arteries, divide into four cervical and five facial branches, and supply various organs and tissues in the head.

facial diplegia, a rare neuromuscular condition characterized by bilateral paralysis of various muscles of the face.

facial hemiplegia, paralysis of the muscles of one side of the face, with the rest of the body not being affected.

facial muscle, one of five groups of facial muscles. They include the muscles of the scalp, the extrinsic muscles of the ear, the muscles of the nose, the muscles of the eyelid and the muscles of the mouth.

facial nerve, either of a pair of mixed sensory and motor cranial nerves that arises from the brainstem at the base of the pons and divides just in front of the ear into its six branches, innervating the scalp, forehead, eyelids, muscles of facial expression, cheeks and jaw.

facial paralysis, an abnormal condition characterized by the partial or the total loss of the functions of the facial muscles or the loss of sensation in the face.

facial perception, the ability to judge the distance and direction of objects through the sensation felt in the skin of the face. The phenomenon is commonly experienced by those who are blind.

facial vein, one of a pair of superficial veins that drain deoxygenated blood from the superficial structures of the face.

facial vision. See **facial perception.**

facies, *pl.* **facies, 1.** the face. **2.** the surface of any body structure, part or organ. **3.** facial expression or appearance.

facilitation, 1. the enhancement or reinforcement of any action or function so that it is carried out with increased ease. **2.** (in neurology) the phenomenon whereby two or more afferent impulses that individually are not strong enough to elicit a response in a neuron can collectively produce a reflex discharge greater than the sum of the separate responses. **3.** (in neurology) the process of lowering the threshold action potential of a neuron by the repeated passage of an impulse along the same pathway.

factitial, artificial or self-induced, such as a factitial dermatitis.

factitial dermatitis, a skin rash caused by the patient, usually for secondary gain or as a manifestation of psychiatric illness.

factitious disorders, conditions marked by disease symptoms caused by deliberate efforts of a person to gain attention. Such attempts to gain attention may be repeated, even when the individual is aware of the hazards involved.

factor I. See **fibrinogen.**

factor II. See **prothrombin.**

factor III. See **thromboplastin.**

factor IV, a designation for calcium as an element in the process of the coagulation of

Ferguson's reflex, a contraction of the uterus after the cervix is stimulated. The reflex is an important function of labour.

fermentation, a chemical change that is brought about in a substance by the action of an enzyme or micro-organism, especially the anaerobic conversion of foodstuffs to certain products. Kinds of fermentation are **acetic, alcoholic, ammoniacal, amylic, butyric, caseous, dextran, diastatic, lactic acid, propionic, storing** and **viscous fermentation.**

fermentative dyspepsia, an abnormal condition characterized by impaired digestion associated with the fermentation of digested food.

fermium (Fm) {Enrico Fermi, Italian physicist, b. 1901}, a synthetic transuranic metallic element. Its atomic number is 100 and its atomic weight is 257.

ferning test, a technique used to determine the presence of oestrogen in the uterine cervical mucus. It is often used as a test for ovulation; high levels of oestrogen cause the cervical mucus to dry on a slide in a fern-like pattern.

ferric, pertaining to a compound of iron in which the metal is trivalent, such as ferric chloride.

ferritin, an iron compound formed in the intestine and stored in the liver, spleen and bone marrow for eventual incorporation into haemoglobin molecules. Serum ferritin levels are used as an indicator of the body's iron stores.

ferromagnetic, pertaining to substances, such as iron, that are strongly affected by magnetism.

ferrous sulphate, a haematinic agent used in the treatment of iron deficiency anaemia.

ferrule, material having a high co-efficient of friction applied to and conforming to the weight-bearing ends of walking aids used to prevent slipping and sliding.

fertile, 1. capable of reproducing or bearing offspring. **2.** of a gamete, capable of inducing fertilization or being fertilized. **3.** prolific; fruitful; not sterile. **fertility,** *n.,* **fertilize,** *v.*

fertile eunuch syndrome, a hypogonadotropic hormonal disorder occurring only in males in which the quantity of testosterone and follicle stimulating hormone is inadequate for the inducement of spermatogenesis and the development of secondary sexual characteristics.

fertile period, the time in the menstrual cycle during which fertilization may occur. Spermatozoa can survive for 48 to 72 hours; the ovum lives for 24 hours. Thus, the fertile period begins 2 to 3 days before ovulation and lasts for 2 to 3 days afterwards.

fertility, the ability to reproduce.

fertility factor. See **F factor.**

fertility rate, the number of births per 1000 women aged 15 through 44.

fertilization, the union of male and female gametes to form a zygote from which the embryo develops. The process takes place in the uterine tube of the female when a spermatozoon, carried in the seminal fluid discharged during coitus, comes in contact with and penetrates the ovum.

fertilization age. See **fetal age.**

fertilization membrane, a viscous membrane surrounding the fertilized ovum that prevents the penetration of additional spermatozoa.

fertilizin, a glycoprotein found on the plasma membrane of the ovum in various species.

festinating gait, a manner of walking in which the speed of the person increases in an unconscious effort to 'catch up' with a displaced centre of gravity. It is a common characteristic of Parkinson's disease.

festoon, a carving in the base material of a denture that simulates the contours of the natural gingival tissues.

fetal advocate, a person who regards the health and well-being of the fetus as a matter of top priority.

fetal age, the age of the conceptus computed from the time elapsed since fertilization.

fetal alcohol syndrome, a congenital abnormality or anomaly resulting from a daily maternal intake of alcohol equivalent to 3 ounces or more of absolute alcohol. It is characterized by typical craniofacial and limb defects, cardiovascular defects, intrauterine growth retardation and retarded development.

fetal alveoli, the terminal pulmonary sacs of a fetus which are filled with fluid before birth.

fetal asphyxia, a condition of hypoxaemia, hypercapnia, and respiratory and metabolic acidosis that may occur in the uterus.

fetal bradycardia, an abnormally slow fetal heart rate, usually below 100 beats per minute.

fetal circulation, the pathway of blood circulation in the fetus. Oxygenated blood from the placenta travels through the umbilical vein to the liver and the ductus venosus, which carries it to the inferior vena cava and right atrium. The blood enters the right atrium at a pressure sufficient to direct the flow across the atrium and through the foramen ovale into the left atrium; thus, oxygenated blood is available for circulation through the left ventricle to the head and upper extremities. The blood is returned to the placenta through the umbilical arteries.

fetal death, the intrauterine death of a fetus, or the death of a fetus weighing at least 500 gm or after 20 or more weeks of gestation.

fetal distress, a compromised condition of the fetus, usually discovered during labour, characterized by a markedly abnormal rate or rhythm of myocardial contraction.

fetal dose, the estimated amount of radiation received by a fetus during an x-ray examination of a pregnant woman.

fetal haemoglobin, haemoglobin F, the major haemoglobin present in the blood of a fetus and neonate.

fetal heart rate (FHR), the number of heartbeats in the fetus occurring in a given unit of time. The FHR varies in cycles of fetal rest and activity and is affected by many factors, including maternal fever, uterine contractions, maternal-fetal hypotension and various drugs. The normal FHR is more than 100 beats per minute and less than 160 beats per minute.

fetal heart tones (fht), the pulsations of the fetal heart heard through the maternal abdomen in pregnancy.

fetal hydantoin syndrome (FHS), a complex of birth defects associated with prenatal maternal ingestion of hydantoin derivatives. Symptoms of FHS include microcephaly, hypoplasia or absence of nails on the fingers or toes, abnormal facies, mental and physical retardation and cardiac defects.

fetal hydrops. See **hydrops fetalis.**

fetal lipoma. See **hibernoma.**

fetal membranes, the structures that protect, support and nourish the embryo and fetus, including the yolk sac, allantois, amnion, chorion, placenta and umbilical cord.

fetal monitor. See **electronic fetal monitor.**

fetal presentation, the part of the fetus that first appears in the pelvis. Normal presentation is cephalic with the vertex presenting. It can also be breech, brow, face or shoulder presentation.

fetal rickets. See **achondroplasia.**

fetal stage, (in embryology) the interval of time from the end of the embryonic stage, at the end of the seventh week of gestation, to birth, 38 to 42 weeks after the first day of the last menstrual period.

fetal tachycardia, a fetal heart rate that continues at 160 or more beats per minute for more than 10 minutes.

feticide. See **embryoctony.**

fetish, 1. any object or idea given unreasonable or excessive attention or reverence. **2.** (in psychology) any inanimate object or any part of the body not of a sexual nature that arouses erotic feelings or fixation. **fetishism,** *n.*

fetishist, a person who believes in or receives erotic gratification from fetishes.

fetochorioni, of or pertaining to the fetus and chorion.

fetofetal transfusion. See **parabiotic syndrome.**

fetology, the branch of medicine concerned with the fetus in utero, including the diagnosis of abnormalities, congenital anomalies, prevention of teratogenic influences and treatment of certain disorders.

fetometry, the measurement of the size of the fetus, especially the diameter of the head and circumference of the trunk.

fetoplacental, of or pertaining to the fetus and the placenta.

fetoprotein, an antigen that occurs naturally in fetuses and occasionally in adults as the result of certain diseases. An increased amount of **alpha fetoprotein** in the fetus is diagnostic for neural tube defects. Leukaemia, hepatoma, sarcoma and other neoplasms are associated with **beta fetoprotein** in the blood of adults.

fetor hepaticus, foul-smelling breath associated with severe liver disease.

fetoscope, a stethoscope for auscultating the fetal heartbeat through the mother's abdomen.

fetoscopy, a procedure in which a fetus may be directly observed in utero, using a fetoscope introduced through a small incision in the abdomen under local anaesthesia.

fetotoxic, pertaining to anything that is poisonous to a fetus.

fetus, the unborn offspring of a viviparous animal after it has attained the particular form of the species; more specifically, the human child in utero after the embryonic period and the beginning of development of the major structural features, usually from the eighth week after fertilization until birth. Kinds of fetuses include **acardius, anideus, lithopedion, mummified fetus, parasitic fetus** and **sirenomelia.** **fetal,** *adj.*

fetus acardiacus, fetus acardius. See **acardius.**

fetus amorphus, a shapeless conceptus in which there are no formed or recognizable parts.

fetus anideus. See **anideus.**

fetus in fetu, a fetal anomaly in which a small, imperfectly formed twin, incapable of independent existence, is contained within the body of the normal twin, the autosite.

fetus papyraceus, a twin fetus that has died in utero early in development and has been pressed flat against the uterine wall by the living fetus.

fetus sanguinolentis, a darkly coloured, partly macerated fetus that has died in utero.

FEV, abbreviation for forced expiratory volume.

fever, an abnormal elevation of the temperature of the body above 37° C (98.6° F) because of disease. Fever results from an imbalance between the elimination and production of heat. Exercise, anxiety and dehydration may increase the temperature of healthy people. Infection, neurological disease, malignancy, pernicious anaemia, thromboembolic disease, paroxysmal tachycardia, congestive heart failure, crushing injury, severe trauma and various drugs may cause fever. Fever has no recognized function in conditions other than infection. It increases metabolic activity by 7% per degree Celsius, requiring a greater intake of food. Kinds of hyperthermia include **habitual fever, intermittent fever** and **relapsing fever.**

fever blister, a cold sore caused by herpesvirus I or II.

fever of unknown origin (FUO), a fever of at least 38.3°C (101° F), that persists for at least 3 weeks without discovery of the cause despite at least 1 week of intensive study.

fever therapy. See **artificial fever.**

fever treatment, the care and management of a person with an elevated temperature.

F factor, (in bacterial genetics) an episome present in conjugating male bacteria but absent in females.

18F-FDG, symbol for {18F}-2-fluoro-2-deoxy-D-glucose, a sugar analogue used in positron emission tomography to determine the local cerebral metabolic rate of glucose as a measure of neural activity in the brain.

FHR, abbreviation for **fetal heart rate.**

FHS, abbreviation for **fetal hydantoin syndrome.**

fht, abbreviation for **fetal heart tones.**

fibre diet, a diet that contains an abundance of fibrous material that resists digestion. Fibrous foods are found mainly in vegetables, fruits and cereals. They add bulk to the diet and reportedly reduce the risk of bowel cancer.

fibreoptic duodenoscope, an instrument for visualizing the interior of the duodenum, consisting of an eyepiece, a flexible tube incorporating bundles of coated glass or plastic fibres with special optic properties, and a terminal light.

fibreoptic endoscopy, the visual examination of the tracheobronchial tree through a fibreoptic endoscope.

fibreoptics, the technical process by which an internal organ or cavity can be viewed, using glass or plastic fibres to transmit light through a specially designed tube and reflect a magnified image. **fibreoptic,** *adj.*

fibrescope, a flexible fibreoptic instrument designed for the examination of particular organs and cavities of the body, as in bronchoscopy, endoscopy and gastroscopy.

fibril, a small filamentous structure that is often a component of a cell, as in a mitotic spindle.

fibrillation, involuntary recurrent contraction of a single muscle fibre or of an isolated bundle of nerve fibres. Fibrillation is usually described by the part that is contracting abnormally, such as atrial or ventricular fibrillation.

fibrin, a stringy, insoluble protein that is a product of the action of thrombin on fibrinogen in the clotting process. It is responsible for the semisolid character of a blood clot.

fibrinase. See **factor XIII.**

fibrindex (fibrinogen index), a test giving a quick estimate of a patient's plasma fibrinogen level, by measuring the time for plasma to clot after thrombin addition; normally 5-12 sec or more if severe.

fibrinogen, a plasma protein essential to the blood clotting process that is converted into fibrin by thrombin in the presence of calcium ions.

fibrinogenopenia, a condition in which there is a deficiency of fibrinogen in the blood.

fibrinokinase, a non-water-soluble enzyme in animal tissue that activates plasminogen.

fibrinolysin, a proteolytic enzyme that dissolves fibrin.

fibrinolysis, the continual process of fibrin decomposition by fibrinolysin that is the normal mechanism for the removal of small fibrin clots. **fibrinolytic,** *adj.*

fibrinopeptide, a product of the action of thrombin on fibrinogen.

fibrin-stabilizing factor. See **factor XIII.**

fibroadenoma, *pl.* **fibroadenomas, fibroadenomata,** a benign tumour composed of dense epithelial and fibroblastic tissue.

fibroangioma. See **angiofibroma.**

fibroareolar tissue. See **areolar tissue.**

fibroblast, a flat, elongated undifferentiated cell in the connective tissue that gives rise to various precursor cells, such as the chondroblast, collagenoblast and osteoblast, that form the fibrous, binding and supporting tissue of the body. **fibroblastic,** *adj.*

fibroblastoma, *pl.* **fibroblastomas, fibroblastomata,** a tumour derived from a fibroblast, now differentiated as a fibroma or a fibrosarcoma.

fibrocarcinoma. See **scirrhous carcinoma.**

fibrocartilage, cartilage that consists of a dense matrix of white collagenous fibres. **fibrocartilaginous,** *adj.*

fibrocartilaginous joint. See **symphysis.**

fibrocystic disease, 1. (of the breast) the presence of single or multiple cysts in the breasts. The cysts are benign and fairly common, yet must be considered potentially malignant and observed carefully for growth or change. **2.** See **cystic fibrosis.**

fibrocyte. See **fibroblast.**

fibroelastic tissue. See **fibrous tissue.**

fibroepithelial papilloma, a benign epithelial tumour containing extensive fibrous tissue.

fibroepithelioma, *pl.* **fibroepitheliomas, fibroepitheliomata,** a neoplasm consisting of fibrous and epithelial components. A kind of fibroepithelioma is **premalignant fibroepithelioma.**

fibroid, 1. having fibres. **2.** *informal.* a fibroma or myoma, particularly of the uterus.

fibroid tumour. See **fibroma.**

fibrolipoma, a fibrous tumour that also contains fatty material.

fibroma, *pl.* **fibromas, fibromata,** a benign neoplasm consisting largely of fibrous or fully developed connective tissue.

fibroma cavernosum, a tumour containing

large vascular spaces, an excessive amount of fibrous tissue and blood or lymph vessels.

fibroma cutis, a fibrous tumour of the skin.

fibroma durum. See **hard fibroma.**

fibroma molle. See **soft fibroma.**

fibroma mucinosum, a fibrous tumour in which there is mucoid material with degeneration.

fibroma myxomatodes. See **myxofibroma.**

fibroma pendulum, a pendulous fibrous tumour of the skin.

fibroma sarcomatosum. See **fibrosarcoma.**

fibroma thecocellulare xanthomatodes. See **theca cell tumour.**

fibromatosis, a gingival enlargement believed to be hereditary, manifesting in the permanent dentition and characterized by a firm hyperplastic tissue that covers the surfaces of the teeth.

fibromyoma uteri. See **leiomyoma uteri.**

fibromyomectomy, a surgical procedure for removal of a uterine fibroma or other type of fibromyoma.

fibromyositis, any one of a large number of disorders in which the common element is stiffness and joint or muscle pain, accompanied by localized inflammation of muscle tissues and fibrous connective tissues. Kinds of fibromyositis include **lumbago, pleurodynia** and **torticollis.**

fibropapilloma. See **fibroepithelial papilloma.**

fibrosarcoma, *pl.* **fibrosarcomas, fibrosarcomata,** a sarcoma that contains connective tissue. It develops suddenly from small nodules on the skin.

fibrosing alveolitis, a severe form of alveolitis characterized by dyspnoea and hypoxia, occurring in advanced rheumatoid arthritis and other autoimmune diseases.

fibrosis, 1. a proliferation of fibrous connective tissue. **2.** an abnormal condition in which fibrous connective tissue spreads over or replaces normal smooth muscle or other normal organ tissue. Fibrosis is most common in the heart, lung, peritoneum and kidney.

fibrositis, an inflammation of fibrous connective tissue, usually characterized by a poorly defined set of symptoms, including pain and stiffness of the neck, shoulder and trunk.

fibrous, consisting mainly of fibres or fibre-containing materials, such as fibrous connective tissue.

fibrous capsule, 1. the external layer of an articular capsule. It surrounds the articulation of two adjoining bones. **2.** the external, tough membranous envelope surrounding some visceral organs, such as the liver.

fibrous dysplasia, an abnormal condition characterized by the fibrous displacement of the osseous tissue within the bones affected. The distinct kinds of fibrous dysplasia are monostotic fibrous dysplasia, polyostotic fibrous dysplasia and polyostotic fibrous dysplasia with associated endocrine disorders. The initial signs may be a limp, pain or fracture on the affected side. Pathological fractures are frequently associated with this process and angulation deformities may follow.

fibrous goitre, an enlargement of the thyroid gland, characterized by hyperplasia of the capsule and connective tissue.

fibrous gold. See **gold foil.**

fibrous histiocytoma. See **dermatofibroma.**

fibrous joint, any one of many immovable joints, such as those of the skull segments, in which a fibrous tissue or a hyaline cartilage connects the bones.

fibrous thyroiditis, a disorder characterized by slowly progressive fibrosis of an enlarged thyroid with replacement of normal thyroid tissue by dense fibrous tissue. Symptoms include a choking sensation, dyspnoea, dysphagia and hypothyroidism, but in some patients the gland functions normally.

fibrous tissue, the fibrous connective tissue of the body, consisting of closely woven elastic fibres and fluid-filled areolae.

fibula, the bone of the leg, lateral to and smaller than the tibia. In proportion to its length, it is the most slender of the long bones.

Fick principle {Adolf E. Fick, German physiologist, b. 1829}, a method for making indirect measurements, based on the law of conservation of mass. It is used specifically to determine cardiac output, in which the amount of oxygen uptake of each unit of blood as it passes through the lungs is equal to the oxygen concentration difference between arterial and mixed venous blood.

Fick's law {Adolf E. Fick}, **1.** (in chemistry and physics) an observed law stating that the rate at which one substance diffuses through another is directly proportional to the concentration gradient of the diffusing substance. **2.** (in medicine) an observed law stating that the rate of diffusion across a membrane is directly proportional to the concentration gradient of the substance on the two sides of the membrane and inversely related to the thickness of the membrane.

fictive kin, people who are regarded as being part of a family even though they are not related.

field, a defined space, area or distance. The field of vision represents the total area that can be seen with one fixed eye. The binocular field is the area that can be seen with both eyes.

Fielder's myocarditis, a rare form of cardiac inflammation that may be due to a viral infection. The pathogen cannot be related to a current or recent disease.

field fever, a form of leptospirosis affecting primarily agricultural workers. It is characterized by fever, abdominal pain, diarrhoea, vomiting, stupor and conjunctivitis.

fiery serpent, an informal term for *Dracunculus medinesis.*

fièvre boutonneuse. See **African tick typhus.**

fifth disease. See **erythema infectiosum.**

fifth nerve. See **trigeminal nerve.**

fight-or-flight. See **flight-or-fight reaction.**

FIGLU, abbreviation for formiminoglutamic acid.

figure 4 test. See **Fabere's test.**

figure-ground relationship, a perceptual field that is divided into a figure, which is the object of focus and a diffuse background.

figure-of-eight bandage, a bandage with successive laps crossing over and around each other like the figure eight.

filament, a fine thread-like fibre. Filaments are found in most tissues and cells of the body and serve various morphological or physiological functions.

filariasis, a disease caused by the presence of filariae or microfilariae in the tissues of the body. Filarial worms are round, long and thread-like, and tend to infest the lymph glands and channels after entering the body as microscopic larvae through the bite of an insect.

filariform, pertaining to a structure or organism that is thread-like.

file, a collection of related data or information kept as a unit.

filial generation, the offspring produced from a given mating or cross in a genetic sequence.

filiform bougie, an extremely thin bougie for passage through a narrow stricture, such as a sinus tract.

filiform catheter, a catheter with a slender, thread-like tip that allows the wider portion of the instrument to be passed through canals that are constricted or irregular.

filiform papilla. See **papilla.**

filling factor, a measure of the geometric relationship of a radiofrequency coil used in NMR imaging and the body.

filling pressure, the pressure in the left ventricle at the end of diastole.

film, 1. a thin sheet or layer of any material, such as a coating of oil on a metal part. **2.** (in photography and radiography) a thin, flexible, transparent sheet of cellulose acetate or similar material coated with a light-sensitive emulsion and used to record images.

film badge, a photographic film packet, sensitive to ionizing radiation, used for estimating the exposure of personnel working with x-rays and other radioactive sources.

film development, the processing of an exposed photographic or x-ray film by immersion in a chemical developer, in order to make the latent image visible. PQ developers consist of phenidone and hydroquinone which act by reducing the exposed silver bromide crystals in the film emulsion to black metallic silver.

film fault, a defect in a photograph or radiograph, usually caused by a chemical, physical or electrical error in its production.

film on teeth, a collection of mucinous deposits adhering to the teeth, which contains micro-organisms, desquamated tissue elements, blood cellular elements and other debris.

film screen mammography. See **mammography.**

filter, 1. a device or material through which a gas or liquid is passed to separate out unwanted matter. **2.** (in radiography) a metal device added to x-ray equipment to remove selectively low-energy x-rays, increase the x-ray quality and reduce patient skin dose.

filtered back projection, a mathematical technique used in magnetic resonance imaging and computed tomography to create images from a set of multiple projection profiles.

filtration, (in radiography and radiotherapy) the addition of sheets of metal into a beam of x-rays, altering the energy spectrum and thus the penetrating ability of the radiation. Filtration is generally provided by aluminum or copper to diagnostic and superficial treatment energies, and by a composite filter of tin, copper and aluminum for orthovoltage beams.

filum, a thread-like structure.

fimbria, any structure forming a border or edge or resembling a fringe. Kinds of fimbria are **fimbria hippocampi, fimbria ovarica** and **fimbriae tubae.**

fimbriae tubae, the branched, finger-like projections at the distal end of each of the fallopian tubes.

fimbria hippocampi, a band of efferent fibres formed by the alveus hippocampi that is continuous with the posterior pillar of the fornix.

fimbria ovarica, the longest of the fimbriae tubae. It extends from the infundibulum to the ovary.

fimbrial tubal pregnancy, a kind of tubal pregnancy in which implantation occurs in the fimbriated distal end of the uterine tube.

fine bore tube, a PVC or polyurethane tube used for feeding. The size generally varies between 5-8 French Gauge with length between 56-156 cm. The tube may have an introducer wire and may be weighted or unweighted. It is used with children and adults for nasogastric or nasoduodenal feeding.

fine bore tube, a PVC or polyurethane tube used for feeding. Size generally varies from 5 French Gauge 8 French Gauge with length 56 cm to 156 cm. The tube may have an introducer wire and may be weighted or unweighted. Used with children and adults for nasogastric or nasoduodenal feeding.

fineness, (in dentistry) a means of grading alloys relative to gold content. The fineness of an alloy is designated in parts per thousand of pure gold.

finger, any of the digits of the hand. The fingers of the hand are composed of a metacarpal bone and three bony phalanges. Some anatomists regard the thumb as a finger.

finger agnosia, a neurological disorder in which a patient is unable to distinguish between stimuli applied to two different fingers without visual clues.

finger percussion. See **percussion.**

finger stick, the act of puncturing the tip of the finger to obtain a small sample of capillary blood.

FiO$_2$, the percentage of inspired oxygen a patient is receiving, usually expressed as a fraction.

first aid, the immediate care that is given to an injured or ill person before treatment. Attention is directed first to the most critical problems: evaluation of airway patency, presence of bleeding and adequacy of cardiac function.

first cuneiform. See **medial cuneiform bone.**

first dentition. See **deciduous tooth.**

first filial generation. See **F$_1$.**

first-generation scanner, an early type of computed tomography device.

first intention. See **intention.**

first metacarpal bone, the metacarpal bone of the thumb.

first nerve. See **olfactory nerve.**

first-order change, a change within a system that itself remains unchanged.

first-order kinetics, a chemical reaction in which the rate of decrease in the number of molecules of a substrate is proportional to the concentration of substrate molecules remaining. The rate of metabolism of most drugs follows the rule of first-order kinetics and is independent of the dose.

first rib, the highest rib of the thoracic cage. It moves about the axis of its neck, raising and lowering the sternum.

Fishberg concentration test, a test of the ability of the kidneys to concentrate urine, developed by American physician Arthur M. Fishberg. The test involves measuring the specific gravity of morning urine samples following overnight deprivation of fluid intake.

fishmeal worker's lung, a type of hypersensitivity pneumonitis that occurs in persons with occupational exposure to fish meal.

fish poisoning, toxic effects caused by ingestion of fish containing substances that may produce symptoms ranging from nausea and vomiting to respiratory paralysis. Scrombroid poisoning usually results from a histamine-like toxin produced by bacterial activity in mackerel, tuna or bonito. Tetraodon poisoning is caused by a toxin in puffer fish.

fish skin disease. See **ichthyosis.**

fish tapeworm infection, an infection caused by the tapeworm *Diphyllobothrium latum*, transmitted to humans when they eat contaminated raw or undercooked freshwater fish.

fission, **1.** the act or process of splitting or breaking up into parts. **2.** a type of asexual reproduction common in bacteria, protozoa and other lower forms of life in which the cell divides into two or more equal components, each of which eventually develops into a complete organism. Kinds of fission are **binary fission** and **multiple fission. 3.** (in physics) the splitting of the nucleus of an atom and subsequent release of energy.

fissiparous, reproduced by fission.

fissural angioma, a tumour composed of a cluster of dilated blood vessels found in an embryonal fissure, especially on lips, face or neck.

fissure, 1. a cleft or groove on the surface of an organ, often marking the division of the organ into parts, such as the lobes of the lung. **2.** a crack-like lesion of the skin, such as an anal fissure. **3.** a lineal fault on a bony surface occurring during the development of a part, such as a fissure in the enamel of a tooth. **fissured,** *adj.*

fissure fracture, any fracture in which a crack extends into the cortex of the bone but not through the entire bone.

fissure-in-ano, a painful linear ulcer at the margin of the anus.

fissure of Bichat. See **transverse fissure.**

fissure of Rolando. See **central sulcus.**

fissure of Sylvius. See **lateral cerebral sulcus.**

fissure sealants, plastic films that are applied to the chewing surfaces of teeth to seal pits and grooves where food and bacteria usually become trapped.

fistula, *pl.* **fistulas, fistulae,** an abnormal passage from an internal organ to the body surface or between two internal organs. **fistulous, fistular, fistulate,** *adj.*

fistula in ano. See **anal fistula.**

fit, 1. *non-technical* a paroxysm or seizure. **2.** the sudden onset of an episode of symptoms, such as a fit of coughing. **3.** the manner in which one surface is aligned to another, such as the fit of a denture to the gingiva and jaw.

Fitzgerald factor, a high molecular weight kinogen that may be required for the interaction of factors XII and XI in the coagulation process.

five-day fever informal, *trench fever.*

five-year survival, a benchmark in the evaluation of response to therapy for cancer patients.

fixating eye, (in strabismus) the normal eye that can be focused.

fixation, (in psychoanalysis) an arrest at a particular stage of psychosexual development, such as anal fixation. **fixate,** *v.,* **fixated,** *adj.*

fixation muscle, a muscle that acts to hold a part of the body in appropriate position.

fixative, 1. any substance used to bind, glue or stabilize. **2.** any substance used to preserve gross or histological specimens of tissue for later examination.

fixed anions, anions that are not part of the body's buffer anions.

fixed bridgework, a dental device incorporating artificial teeth permanently attached in the upper or the lower jaw.

fixed cations, cations that are not part of the body's metabolic buffering system.

fixed coupling, a precise distance between a normal and ectopic beat that is duplicated each time the ectopic beat occurs.

fixed dressing, a dressing usually made of gauze impregnated with a hardening agent, such as plaster of paris, sodium silicate, starch or dextrin, applied to support or immobilize a part of the body.

fixed-drug eruption, well-defined red to purple lesions that appear at the same sites on the skin and mucous membranes each time a particular drug is used.

fixed fulcrum, a tomographic fulcrum that remains at a fixed height.

fixed idea, 1. a persistent, obsessional thought or notion. **2.** in certain mental disorders, especially obsessive-compulsive disorder, a delusional idea that dominates mental activity and persists despite contrary evidence.

fixed interval (FI) reinforcement, (in psychiatry) a specific lapse of time required for reinforcement.

fixed orthodontic appliance, a prosthetic device cemented to the teeth or attached by adhesive material, for changing the relative positions of dentitions.

fixed-performance oxygen delivery system. See **high-flow oxygen delivery system.**

fixed phagocyte. See **phagocyte.**

fixed ratio (FR) reinforcement, (in psychiatry) a specific number of responses required for reinforcement.

fixed vertebrae. See **false vertebrae.**

fixer, a chemical product used in processing photographic or x-ray film. Applied after the developing phase, it neutralizes any developer remaining on the film, removes undeveloped silver halides and hardens the emulsion.

flaccid, weak, soft and flabby; lacking normal muscle tone, such as flaccid muscles. **flaccidity, flaccidness,** *n.*

flaccid bladder, a form of neurogenic bladder caused by interruption of the reflex arc associated with the voiding reflex in the spinal cord.

flaccid paralysis, an abnormal condition characterized by weakening or loss of muscle tone.

flagella, hair-like projections that extend from some unicellular organisms and aid in their movement.

flagellant, a person who receives sexual gratification from the practice of flagellation.

flagellate, a micro-organism that propels itself by waving whip-like filaments or cilia behind its body, such as *Trypanosoma, Leishmania, Trichomonas* and *Giardia.*

flagellation, 1. the act of whipping, beating or flogging. **2.** a type of massage administered by tapping the body with the fingers. See **massage. 3.** a type of sexual deviation in which a person is erotically gratified by being whipped or by whipping another. **4.** the arrangement of flagella on an organism; exflagellation.

flail chest, a thorax in which multiple rib fractures cause instability in part of the chest wall and paradoxical breathing, with the lung underlying the injured area contracting on inspiration and bulging on expiration.

flame photometry, measurement of the wavelength of light rays emitted by excited metallic electrons exposed to the heat energy of a flame, used to identify characteristics in clinical specimens of body fluids.

flange, 1. the part of a denture base that extends from the cervical ends of the teeth to the border of the denture. **2.** a prosthesis with a lateral vertical extension designed to direct a resected mandible into centric occlusion.

flank, the posterior portion of the body between the ribs and the ilium.

flapping tremor. See **asterixis.**

flare, 1. a red blush on the skin at the periphery of an urticarial lesion seen in immediate hypersensitivity reactions. **2.** an expanding skin flush, spreading from an infective lesion or extending from the principal site of a reaction to an irritant. **3.** the sudden intensification of a disease.

flaring of nostrils, a widening of the nostrils during inspiration, a sign of air hunger or respiratory distress.

flashback, 1. a phenomenon experienced by persons who have taken hallucinogenic drugs and unexpectedly re-experience the drug effects. **2.** a phenomenon experienced by persons subjected to extreme stress after which they involuntarily re-experience aspects of the traumatic event.

flask closure, (in dentistry) the joining of two halves of a flask that encloses and forms a denture base.

flat affect, the affect of a patient who does not communicate feelings in verbal or nonverbal responses to events.

Flatau-Schilder disease. See **Schilder's disease.**

flat bone, any of the bones that provide structural contours of the skeleton. Examples include ribs and bones of the skull.

flat electroencephalogram, a graphic chart on which no tracings were recorded during electroencephalography, indicating a lack of brainwave activity.

flatfoot. See **pes planus.**

flatulence, the presence of an excessive amount of air or gas in the stomach and intestinal tract, causing distension of the organs and in some cases mild to moderate pain.

flatus, air or gas in the intestine that is passed through the rectum.

flat wart. See **verruca plana.**

flavoxate hydrochloride, an anticholinergic smooth muscle relaxant used to treat spastic conditions of the urinary tract.

flea {AS}, a wingless, bloodsucking insect of the order *Siphonaptera,* some species of which transmit arboviruses to humans by acting as host or vector to the organism.

flea bite, a small puncture wound produced by a blood-sucking flea. Certain species of fleas transmit plague, murine typhus and probably tularaemia.

flea bites *informal,* erythema toxicum neonatorum.

flea-borne typhus. See **murine typhus.**

flecainide acetate, an antiarrhythmic drug mostly used in the treatment of ventricular arrhythmias.

Fleischner method, a technique for producing lordotic x-ray projections of the lungs. The patient is placed in P-A projection position while leaning backward from the waist to a nearly 45-degree posterior inclination.

Fletcher factor, a prekallikrein blood coagulation substance that interacts with both factor XII and Fitzgerald factor, activating both and accelerating thrombin formation.

flexibilitas cerea. See **cerea flexibilitas.**

flexion, 1. a movement allowed by certain joints of the skeleton that decreases the angle between two adjoining bones, such as bending the elbow. **2.** (in obstetrics) a resistance to the descent of the fetus through the birth canal that causes the neck to flex so that the chin approaches the chest.

flexion jacket, a corset designed to provide spinal immobility.

flexitime, a system of staffing that allows the individualization of work schedules.

flexor carpi radialis, a slender, superficial muscle of the forearm that lies on the ulnar side of the pronator teres. It functions to flex and to help abduct the hand.

flexor carpi ulnaris, a superficial muscle lying along the ulnar side of the forearm. It functions to flex and adduct the hand.

flexor digitorum superficialis, the largest superficial muscle of the forearm, lying on the ulnar side under the palmaris longus. The muscle flexes the second phalanx of each finger and, by continued action, the hand.

flexor retinaculum of the hand. See **retinaculum flexorum manus.**

flexor withdrawal reflex, a common cutaneous reflex consisting of a widespread contraction of physiological flexor muscles and relaxation of physiological extensor muscles. It is characterized by abrupt withdrawal of a body part in response to painful or injurious stimuli.

flexure, a normal bend or curve in a body part, such as the dorsal flexure of the spine.

flight into health, an abnormal but common reaction to an unpleasant physical sensation or symptom in which the person denies the reality of the feeling or observation, insisting that there is nothing wrong.

flight of ideas, (in psychiatry) a continuous stream of talk in which the patient switches rapidly from one topic to another, each subject being incoherent and not related to the preceding one.

flight-or-fight reaction, 1. (in physiology) the reaction of the body to stress, in which the sympathetic nervous system and the adrenal medulla act to increase the cardiac output, dilate the pupils of the eyes, increase the rate of the heartbeat, constrict the blood vessels of the skin, increase the glucose and fatty acids in the circulation, and induce an alert, aroused mental state. **2.** (in psychiatry) a person's reaction to stress by either fleeing from a situation or remaining and attempting to deal with it.

flight to illness, the effort of the patient to convince the therapist that he or she is too ill to terminate therapy and that continued support is needed.

flip angle, in magnetic resonance imaging, the amount of rotation of the macroscopic magnetization vector produced by a radiofrequency pulse with respect to the direction of the static magnetic field.

flip-flop, the binary digit system of semiconductor memory in which data are recorded in one of two states, such as 0 or 1, yes or no, and + or -.

float nurse, a nurse who is available for assignment to duty on an ad hoc basis, usually to assist in times of unusually heavy work loads or assume the duties of absent nursing personnel.

floater, one or more spots that appear to drift in front of the eye, caused by a shadow cast on the retina by vitreous debris. Most floaters are benign and represent remnants of a network of blood vessels that existed prenatally in the vitreous cavity. The sudden onset of several floaters may indicate serious disease. The technical term for floaters is muscae volitantes.

floating kidney, a kidney that is not securely fixed in the usual anatomical location because of congenital malplacement or traumatic injury.

floating rib. See **rib.**

flocculant, an agent or substance that causes flocculation.

flocculation test, a serological test in which a positive result depends on the degree of flocculent precipitation produced in the material being tested. Many tests for syphilis are flocculation tests.

flocculent, clumped or tufted, such as a cloud, or covered with a woolly, fuzzy surface. **flocculate,** *v.*, **flocculation, floccule,** *n.*

flood fever. See **typhus.**

flooding, intense imaginal or in vivo exposure to a feared stimulus. This is a technique used in behaviour therapy for the reduction of anxiety associated with phobia and avoidant behaviours. See **systemic desensitization.**

floppy, floppy disk. See **disk, def. 3**

floppy infant syndrome, a general term for juvenile spinal muscular atrophies, including Werdnig-Hoffmann disease and Wohlfart-Kugelberg-Welander disease.

flora, micro-organisms that live on or within a body to compete with disease-producing micro-organisms and provide a natural immunity against certain infections.

flossing, the mechanical cleansing of tooth surfaces with string-like waxed or unwaxed dental floss.

flotation device, a foam mattress with a gel-like pad located in its centre, designed to protect bony prominences and distribute pressure more evenly against the skin's surface.

flotation therapy, a state of semiweightlessness produced by various types of hospital equipment and used in the treatment and prevention of decubitus ulcers.

flow chart, a graphic representation of a computer programme sequence, an intermediate step between algorithm development and the writing of a computer program.

flowmeter. See **rotameter.**

flow sheet, (in a patient record) a graphic summary of several changing factors, especially the patient's vital signs or weight and the treatments and medications given. In labour, the flow sheet displays the progress of labour.

flow-volume curve, a graphic representation of the instantaneous volumetric flow rates achieved during a forced expiratory vital capacity maneuver. It may be a maximum expiratory flow-volume curve (MEFV) or a partial expiratory flow-volume (PEFV) curve.

flow-volume loop, a pulmonary function test system in which the patient breathes into an electronic spirometer and performs a forced inspiratory and expiratory vital capacity manoeuver. The data are displayed graphically as a loop whose shape indicates lung volume and other data through the complete respiratory cycle.

floxuridine, a cytotoxic antimetabolite agent used experimentally in the treatment of malignant disease of the brain, breast, liver and gallbladder.

flu *informal,* **1.** influenza. **2.** any viral infection, especially of the respiratory or intestinal system.

fluctuant, pertaining to a wave-like motion that is detected when a structure containing a liquid is palpated.

flucytosine, an antifungal prescribed in the treatment of certain serious fungal infections.

fluid, 1. a substance, such as a liquid or gas, that is able to flow and adjust its shape to that of a container because it is composed of molecules that are able to change positions with respect to each other without separating from the total mass. **2.** a body fluid, either intracellular or extracellular, involved in the transport of electrolytes and other vital chemicals to, through and from tissue cells.

fluid balance, a state of equilibrium in which the amount of fluid consumed equals the amount lost in urine, faeces, perspiration and exhaled water vapour.

fluid dram. See **dram.**

fluid ounce, a measure of liquid volume in the apothecaries' system, which is equal to 8 fluidrams or 29.57 ml.

fluid retention, a failure to excrete excess fluid from the body. Causes may include renal, cardiovascular or metabolic disorders.

fluid therapy, the regulation of water balance in patients with impaired renal, cardiovascular or metabolic function by carefully measuring fluid intake against daily losses.

fluid volume deficit, 1. a failure of the body's homeostatic mechanisms that regulate the retention and excretion of body fluids. Defining characteristics include dilute urine, increased output of urine, a sudden loss of body weight, hypotension, increased pulse rate, decreased turgor, increased body temperature, haemoconcentration, weakness and thirst. **2.** the active loss of excessive amounts of body fluid. Defining characteristics include decreased output of urine, high specific gravity of the urine, output of urine that is greater than the intake of fluid, a sudden loss of weight, haemoconcentration, increased serum levels of sodium, increased thirst, alteration in the mental state, dryness of skin and mucous membranes, elevated temperature and an increased pulse rate.

fluid volume excess, a compromised regulatory mechanism of the homeostatic mechanisms that regulate the retention and excretion of body fluids, or of an excess fluid or sodium intake. Defining characteristics include oedema, effusion, weight gain, shortness of breath, third heart sound, pulmonary congestion changes in respiratory pattern, abnormal breath sounds, decreased haemoglobin and haematocrit, blood pressure changes, an alteration in electrolyte balance, restlessness, anxiety and other changes in mental status.

fluke, a parasitic flatworm of the class Trematoda, including the genus *Schistosoma.*

fluocinolone acetonide, a potent topical corticosteroid used as an anti-inflammatory agent.

fluocinonide, a potent, topical, synthetic corticosteroid used to reduce inflammation.

fluorescence, the emission of light of one wavelength (usually ultraviolet) when exposed to light of a different, usually shorter, wavelength. Fluorescence is the principle of the intensifying screen in radiography. **fluoresce,** v., **fluorescent,** *adj.*

fluorescent antibody test (FA test), a test in which a fluorescent dye is used to stain an antibody for identification of clinical specimens. Fluorescent dyes make the dyed organisms glow visibly when examined under a fluorescent microscope. Kinds of fluorescent antibody tests include the FTA-ABS test.

fluorescent microscopy, examination with a fluorescent microscope equipped with a source of ultraviolet light rays, used to study specimens that have been stained with fluorescent dye.

Fluorescent Treponemal Antibody Absorption Test (FTA-ABS test), a serological test for syphilis.

fluoridation, the process of adding fluoride, especially to a public water supply, in order to reduce tooth decay.

fluoride, a salt of hydrofluoric acid introduced into drinking water and applied directly to the teeth to prevent tooth decay.

fluorination, the addition of a fluorine group to a compound, such as those commonly found in topical corticosteroids.

fluorine (F), an element of the halogen family and the most reactive of the non-metals. Its atomic number is 9 and its atomic weight is 19. Small amounts of sodium fluoride are added to the water supply of many communities to harden tooth enamel and decrease dental caries. Excessive amounts of fluoride can mottle tooth enamel and cause osteosclerosis. Acute fluoride poisoning and death can result from the accidental ingestion of insecticides and rodenticides containing fluoride salts.

fluoroacetic acid, a colourless, water-soluble, highly toxic compound that blocks the Krebs' citric acid cycle, causing convulsions and ventricular fibrillation. It is derived from a South African tree and is used in some potent pesticides.

fluorography, a radiographic procedure to record images formed during fluoroscopy.

fluorometry, measurement of fluorescence

emitted by compounds when exposed to ultraviolet or other intense radiant energy. Fluorometry is used to measure urinary oestrogens, triglycerides, catecholamines and other substances. **fluorometric,** *adj.*

fluoroscope, (historical) a device used for the immediate projection of an x-ray image on a fluorescent screen for visual examination. **fluoroscopic,** *adj.*

fluoroscopic compression device, any of several objects that can be placed on a specific area of the patient's abdomen to compress the exterior surface during fluoroscopy.

fluoroscopy, a radiographic technique of dynamic imaging, in which the area of the body being examined is viewed on a television monitor via an image intensifier and television camera.

fluorosis, the condition that results from excessive, prolonged ingestion of fluorine. Severe chronic fluorine poisoning will lead to osteosclerosis and other pathological bone and joint changes in adults.

fluorouracil, a cytotoxic antimetabolite used in the treatment of malignant disease of the skin and internal organs.

fluphenazine, a phenothiazine tranquilizer used in the treatment of psychotic disorders.

flurandrenolone, a moderately potent, topical corticosteroid used as an anti-inflammatory agent.

flurazepam hydrochloride, a benzodiazepine minor tranquilizer used in the treatment of insomnia.

flush, 1. a blush or sudden reddening of the face and neck. **2.** a sudden, subjective feeling of heat. **3.** a prolonged reddening of the face such as may be seen with fever, certain drugs or hyperthyroidism. **4.** a sudden, rapid flow of water or other liquid.

flush device, a device for the accurate transmission of a pressure wave from a catheter to a transducer in an intravenous line.

flutter, a rapid vibration or pulsation that may interfere with normal function.

fly, a two-winged insect of the order Diptera, some species of which transmit arboviruses to humans.

fly bites, bites that may be caused by species of deer, horse or sand flies. Such bites produce a small painful wound with swelling because of substances in the insect's saliva that are injected beneath the surface of the skin.

Fm, symbol for **fermium.**

FMET, abbreviation for **formylmethionine.**

focal illumination. See **illumination.**

focal motor seizure. See **motor seizure.**

focal plane, the plane of tissue that is in focus on a tomogram.

focal seizure, a transitory disturbance in motor, sensory or autonomic function resulting from abnormal neuronal discharges in a localized part of the brain, most frequently motor or sensory areas adjacent to the central sulcus. Focal motor seizures commonly begin as spasmodic movements in the hand, face or foot, and may spread progressively to other muscles to end in a generalized convulsion. Focal seizures may be caused by localized anoxia or a small lesion in the brain.

focal spot. See **real focal spot, apparent focal spot.**

focal zone, (in ultrasonography) the distance along the beam axis of a focused transducer assembly, from the point where the beam area first becomes equal to 4 times the focal area to the point beyond the focal surface where the beam area again becomes equal to 4 times the focal area.

focus, 1. a specific location, such as the site of an infection or the point at which an electrochemical impulse originates. **2.** the point in an x-ray tube or linear accelerator from which x-ray photons are emitted.

focused activity, a therapeutic technique of actively focusing the patient towards adaptive coping abilities and away from maladaptive ones.

focused grid, (in radiography) an x-ray secondary radiation grid consisting of lead strips placed at an angle so that they all point towards a focus at a specific distance.

focus-film distance (FFD), distance from the x-ray tube focus to the imaging medium.

focus-object distance (FOD), distance from the x-ray tube focus to the object being examined.

focus-skin distance (FSD), distance from the x-ray tube or treatment unit focus to the patient's skin.

foil assistant. See **foil holder.**

foil carrier. See **foil passer.**

foil holder, an instrument used for holding a foil pellet in place for various dental restorations.

foil passer, a pointed or forked instrument for carrying pellets of gold foil through an annealing flame or from the annealing tray to a prepared tooth cavity.

foil pellet, a loosely rolled piece of gold foil, used for making various dental restorations such as a permanent tooth cavity filling or tooth crown.

folacin. See **folic acid.**

folate, 1. a salt of folic acid. **2.** any of a group of substances found in some foods and in mammalian cells that act as coenzymes and promote the chemical transfer of single carbon units from one molecule to another.

folate deficiency. See **folic acid.**

Foley catheter {Frederick E. B. Foley, American physician, b. 1891}, a rubber catheter with a balloon tip filled with air or a sterile liquid after it has been placed in the bladder. This kind of catheter is used when continuous drainage of the bladder is required, as in surgery.

folic acid, a yellow, crystalline, water-soluble vitamin of the B complex group essential for cell growth and reproduction. It functions as a coenzyme with vitamins B_{12} and C in the breakdown and utilization of proteins and in the formation of nucleic acids and haeme in haemoglobin. It also increases the appetite and stimulates production of hydrochloric acid in the digestive tract.

folic acid deficiency anaemia, a form of anaemia caused by a lack of folic acid in the diet.

folie, a mental disorder; any of a variety of psychopathological reactions. Kinds of folie include **folie à deux, folie circulaire, folie du doute, folie du pourquoi, folie gemellaire, folie musculaire** and **folie raisonnante.**

folie à deux. See **shared paranoid disorder.**

folie circulaire. See **bipolar disorder.**

folie du doute, an extreme obsessive-compulsive reaction characterized by persistent doubting, vacillation, repetition of behaviour and pathological indecisiveness.

folie du pourquoi, a psychopathological condition characterized by the persistent tendency to ask questions, usually concerning unrelated topics.

folie gemellaire, a psychotic condition occurring simultaneously in twins, sometimes in those not living together or closely associated at the time.

folie musculaire, severe chorea.

folie raisonnante, a delusional form of any psychosis marked by an apparent logical thought process but lacking common sense.

folinic acid, an active form of folic acid.

follicle, a pouch-like depression, such as the dental follicles that enclose the teeth before eruption or the hair follicles within the epidermis. **follicular,** *adj.*

follicle stimulating hormone (FSH), a gonadotropin, secreted by the anterior pituitary gland, that stimulates the growth and maturation of graafian follicles in the ovary and promotes spermatogenesis in the male.

follicular adenocarcinoma, a neoplasm characterized by a follicular arrangement of cells that are usually derived from the thyroid gland. It is not especially malignant but has a greater tendency to metastasize.

follicular cyst, an odontogenic cyst that arises from the epithelium of a tooth bud and dental lamina. The kinds of follicular cysts are dentigerous, primordial and multilocular.

follicular goitre, an enlargement of the thyroid gland characterized by proliferation of the follicles and epithelial tissue.

follicular phase, the first part of the menstrual cycle, when ovarian follicles grow to prepare for ovulation.

folliculitis, inflammation of hair follicles, as in sycosis barbae.

folliculoma. See **granulosa cell tumour.**

folliculosis, a condition characterized by the development of a large number of lymph follicles, which may or may not be associated with an infection.

fomentation, 1. the topical treatment of pain or inflammation with a warm, moist application. **2.** a substance or poultice that is used as a warm, moist application.

fomite, non-living material, such as bed linens, which may convey pathogenic organisms.

Fone's method, a toothbrushing technique that employs large, sweeping, scrubbing circles over occluded teeth, with the toothbrush held at right angles to the tooth surfaces.

fontanelle, a space covered by tough membranes between the bones of an infant's cranium.

food, 1. any substance, usually of plant or animal origin, consisting of carbohydrates, proteins, fats and such supplementary elements as minerals and vitamins, that is ingested or otherwise taken into the body and assimilated to provide energy and promote the growth, repair and maintenance essential for sustaining life. **2.** nourishment in solid form as contrasted with liquid form. **3.** a particular kind of solid nourishment, such as breakfast food or snack food.

food additives, substances that are added to foods to prevent spoilage, improve appearance, enhance the flavour or increase the nutritional value. Most food additives must be approved by the Department of Health after tests to determine if they could be a cause of cancer, birth defects or other health problems.

food allergy, a hypersensitive state resulting from the ingestion of a specific food antigen. Symptoms of sensitivity to specific foods can include allergic rhinitis, bronchial asthma, urticaria, angioneurotic oedema, dermatitis, pruritus, headache, labyrinthitis and conjunctivitis, nausea, vomiting, diarrhoea, pylorospasm, colic, spastic constipation, mucous colitis and perianal eczema. Food allergens are predominantly protein in nature.

food contaminants, substances that make food unfit for human consumption. Examples include bacteria, toxic chemicals, carcinogens, teratogens, and radioactive materials. Also regarded as contaminants are basically harmless substances, such as water, that may be added to food to increase its weight.

food exchange list, a grouping of foods in which the carbohydrate, fat and protein values are equal for the items listed. For example, starchy vegetables are listed as bread exchanges; fish and cheese are meat exchanges.

food poisoning, any of a large group of toxic processes resulting from the ingestion of a food contaminated by toxic substances or by bacteria containing toxins. Kinds of food poisoning include **bacterial food poisoning, ciguatera poisoning, Minamata disease, mushroom poisoning** and **shellfish poisoning.**

foot, the distal extremity of the leg, consisting of the tarsus, the metatarsus and the phalanges.

foot-and-mouth disease, an acute, extremely contagious, rhinovirus infection of cloven-hooved animals. Horses are immune. Uncommonly, the virus is transmitted to humans by direct contact with infected animals, their secretions or with contaminated milk. Symptoms and signs in humans include headache, fever, malaise and vesicles on tongue, oral mucous membranes, hands and feet.

footdrop, an abnormal neuromuscular condition of the lower leg and foot characterized by an inability to dorsiflex, or evert, the foot because of damage to the common peroneal nerve.

footling breech, an intrauterine position of the fetus in which one or both feet are folded under the buttocks at the inlet of the maternal pelvis, one foot presenting in a single footling breech, both feet in a double footling breech.

foramen, *pl.* **foramina,** an opening or aperture in a membranous structure or bone, such as the apical dental foramen and the carotid foramen.

foramen magnum, a passage in the occipital bone through which the spinal cord enters the spinal column.

foramen of Monro, a passage between the lateral and third ventricles of the brain.

foramen ovale, 1. an opening in the septum between the right and left atria in the fetal heart. This opening provides a bypass for blood that would otherwise flow to the fetal lungs. **2.** an oval foramen situated laterally to the foramen rotundum of the sphenoid bone.

foramen rotundum, one of a pair of rounded apertures in the greater wings of the sphenoid bone.

foramen spinosum, a small opening near the posterior angle of the greater wing of the sphenoid bone.

Forbes-Albright syndrome {A. P. Forbes; Fuller Albright, American physician, b. 1900}, an endocrine disease characterized by amenorrhoea, prolactinemia, and galactorrhoea, caused by an adenoma of the anterior pituitary.

Forbes' disease. See **Cori's disease.**

forbidden clone theory, a theory associated with autoimmunity, according to which certain clone cells that can react against the body persist after birth and can be activated by a viral infection or some metabolic change.

force, 1. energy applied in such a way that it

initiates motion, changes the speed or direction of motion, or alters the size or shape of an object. **2.** a push or pull defined as mass times acceleration.

forced expiratory flow (FEF), the average volumetric flow rate during any stated volume interval while a forced expired vital capacity is performed. It is usually expressed as a percentage of vital capacity.

forced expiratory volume (FEV), the volume of air that can be forcibly expelled in 1 second after full inspiration.

forced expired vital capacity (FEVC), a pulmonary function test of the maximal volume of gas that can be forcefully and rapidly exhaled starting from the position of full inspiration.

forced feeding, a rarely used term for a method of administering food by force, such as nasal feeding, to persons who cannot or will not eat.

forced-inhalation abdominal breathing, a respiratory therapy technique in which the patient is trained to inhale through the nose with an effort that is forceful enough to lift small sandbag weights placed on the abdomen.

force platform, an instrument which measures the direction and magnitude of the ground reaction force beneath the foot.

forceps, *pl.* **forceps,** a pair of any of a large variety and number of surgical instruments, all of which have two handles or sides, each attached to a blade, Forceps are used to grasp, handle, compress, pull or join tissue, equipment or supplies.

forceps delivery, an obstetric procedure in which obstetric forceps are used to deliver a baby. It is performed to overcome dystocia and quickly deliver a baby experiencing fetal distress.

forceps tenaculum. See **tenaculum.**

Fordyce-Fox disease, an apocrine gland disorder producing symptoms similar to those of miliaria.

Fordyce's disease, the presence of enlarged oil glands in the mucosal membranes of lips, cheeks, gums and genitalia. It is a common condition and may be symptomless.

forearm, the portion of the upper extremity between elbow and wrist. It contains two long bones, the radius and ulna.

forebrain. See **prosencephalon.**

forefinger, the first, or index, finger.

forefoot, the portion of the foot that includes the metatarsus and toes.

foregut, the cephalic portion of the embryonic alimentary canal.

foreign body, any object or substance found in the body in an organ or tissue in which it does not belong under normal circumstances, such as a particle of dust in the eye.

foreign body obstruction, a disturbance in normal function or a pathological condition caused by an object lodged in a body orifice,

passage or organ. Most cases occur in children who suddenly inhale or swallow a foreign object or insert it in a body opening.

forensic dentistry, the branch of dentistry that deals with the legal aspects of professional dental practices and treatment.

forensic medicine, a branch of medicine that deals with the legal aspects of healthcare.

forensic psychiatry, the branch of psychiatry that deals with legal issues and problems relating to mental disorders, especially the determination of insanity for legal purposes.

foreplay, sexual activities, such as kissing and fondling, that precede coitus.

foreskin, a loose fold of skin that covers the end of the penis or clitoris. Its removal constitutes circumcision.

forewaters, the amniotic fluid between the presenting part and the intact membranes.

formaldehyde, a toxic, colourless, foul-smelling gas that is soluble in water and used in that form as a disinfectant, fixative or preservative.

formalin, a clear solution of formaldehyde in water. A 37% solution is used for fixing and preserving biological specimens for pathological and histological examination.

formation, a cluster of people that occupies and therefore defines a quantum of space.

formative evaluation, judgments made about the effectiveness of nursing interventions as they are implemented.

forme fruste, *pl.* **formes frustes, 1.** an incomplete or atypical form of a disease, or a disease that is spontaneously arrested before it has run its usual course. **2.** (in genetics) an inherited disorder in which there is minimal expression of an abnormal trait.

formic acid, a colourless, pungent liquid found in nature in nettles, ants and other insects.

formiminoglutamic acid (FIGLU), a compound formed in the metabolism of histidine, occurring in urine in elevated levels in folic acid deficiency.

formol. See **formaldehyde.**

formula, a simplified statement, generally using numerals and other symbols, expressing the constituents of a chemical compound, a method for preparing a substance, or a procedure for achieving a desired value or result. **formulaic,** *adj.*

formulary, a listing of drugs intended to include a large enough range of drugs and sufficient information about them to enable health practitioners to prescribe treatment that is medically appropriate. Hospitals maintain formularies that list all drugs commonly stocked in the hospital pharmacy.

formulation, 1. a pharmacological substance prepared according to a formula. **2.** a systematic and precise statement of a problem, theory or method of analysis in research.

formylmethionine (FMET), (in molecular genetics) the first amino acid in a protein sequence.

fornication, (in law) sexual intercourse between two people who are not married to each other.

fornix, *pl.* **fornices,** an arch-like structure or space, such as the fornix cerebri, superior or inferior conjunctival fornices or vaginal fornices.

fornix cerebri, an arch-like body of nerve fibres that lies beneath the corpus callosum of the cranium and serves as the efferent pathway from the hippocampus.

fornix vaginae. See **vaginal fornix.**

Fort Bragg fever. See **pretibial fever.**

fortified milk, pasteurized milk enriched with one or more nutrients, usually vitamin D, which has been standardized at 400 International Units per quart **(fortified vitamin D milk).**

forward-leaning posture, a respiratory therapy technique, intended to reduce or eliminate accessory muscle activity in ambulatory patients with breathing difficulty. It involves walking in a slightly stooped, forward-leaning posture.

fossa, *pl.* **fossae,** a hollow or depression, especially on the surface of the end of a bone, such as the olecranon fossa or coronoid fossa.

foulage. See **pétrissage.**

foundation, 1. a charitable organization usually established to allocate private funds to worthy projects, or to provide other services. **2.** (in dentistry) any device or material added to a remaining tooth structure to enhance the stability and retention of an overlying cast restoration.

fourchette, a band of mucous membranes at the posterior angle of the vagina connecting the posterior ends of the labia minora.

four-handed dentistry, a technique of chairside operating in which four hands simultaneously perform tasks directly associated with dental work being accomplished in the oral cavity of a patient.

Fourier transform (FT) {Jean B. J. Fourier, French mathematician, b. 1768}, (in medical physics) a mathematical procedure that separates out the frequency components of a signal from its amplitudes as a function of time, or vice versa.

Fourier transform imaging, (in MRI) magnetic resonance imaging techniques in which at least one dimension is phase encoded by applying variable gradient pulses along that dimension, before 'reading out' the MRI signal with a gradient magnetic field perpendicular to the variable gradient. The Fourier transform is then used to reconstruct an image from the set of encoded MRI signals.

four-poster cast, a cast to immobilize the cervical vertebrae. It contains four verticle posts or poles on the anterior and posterior lateral sides of the head, and is placed over the shoulders. The head is supported under the chin and occiput, and the posts prevent movement.

four-step nursing process, a nursing process comprising four broad categories of nursing behaviours: assessing, planning, implementing and evaluating.

four-tailed bandage, a narrow piece of cloth with two ties on each end for wrapping a joint, such as an elbow or knee, or a prominence, such as the nose or chin.

fourth-generation scanner, a computed tomography machine in which the x-ray source rotates but the detector assembly does not.

fourth nerve. See **trochlear nerve.**

fourth ventricle, a diamond-shaped cavity of the hindbrain, in front of the cerebellum and behind the pons and the upper part of the medulla oblongata.

fovea centralis, an area at the centre of the retina where cone cells are concentrated and there are no rod cells.

Fox's knife. See **Goldman-Fox knife.**

Fr, symbol for francium.

fractional anaesthesia. See **continuous anaesthesia.**

fractional dilatation and curettage, a diagnostic technique in which each section of the uterus is examined and curetted to obtain specimens of the endometrium from all parts of the uterus.

fractionation, 1. (in neurology) a mechanism within the neural arch of the vertebrae whereby only a portion of the efferent nerves innervating a muscle reacts to a stimulus, even when the reflex requirement is maximal, so that there is a reserve of neurons to respond to additional stimuli. **2.** (in chemistry) the separation of a substance into its basic constituents, by using such procedures as fractional distillation or crystallization. **3.** (in bacteriology) the process of isolating a pure culture by successive culturing of a small portion of a colony of bacteria. **4.** (in histology) the process of isolating the different components of living cells by centrifugation. **5.** (in radiotherapy) the process of administering a dose of radiation over a period of time in smaller units (fractions), in order to achieve maximum damage to the target cells with minimum damage to surrounding normal tissues. Types of fractionation are daily and accelerated hyperfractionation.

fracture, a traumatic injury to a bone in which the continuity of the tissue of the bone is broken. A fracture is classified by the bone involved, the part of that bone, and the nature of the break, such as a comminuted fracture of the head of the tibia. Kinds of fracture include **butterfly fracture, comminuted fracture, complete fracture, compression fracture, displaced fracture, impacted fracture, incomplete fracture, seg-**

mental fracture, spiral fracture and undisplaced fracture.

fracture-dislocation, a fracture involving the bony structures of any joint, with associated dislocation of the same joint.

fragilitas ossium. See **osteogenesis imperfecta.**

fragmented fracture, a fracture that results in multiple bone fragments.

frambesia. See **yaws.**

frame of reference, the personal guidelines of an individual, such as the person's social status, cultural norms and concepts.

Franceschetti's syndrome {Adolphe Franceschetti, Swiss ophthalmologist, b. 1896}, a complete form of mandibulofacial dysostosis.

francium (Fr), a metallic element of the alkali metal group and formed from the decay of actinium. Its atomic number is 87 and its atomic weight is 223.

frank, obvious or clinically evident, such as the unequivocal presence of a condition or a disease.

Frank biopsy guide, a device consisting of a long needle containing a hooked wire used to obtain biopsy samples of breast tissue.

frank breech, an intrauterine position of the fetus in which the buttocks present at the maternal pelvic inlet, the legs are straight up in front of the body, and the feet are at the shoulders.

Frankfort horizontal plane, (in dentistry) a craniometric plane determined by the inferior or borders of the bony orbits and the upper margin of the auditory meatus, passing through the two orbitales and two tragions.

Frankfort-mandibular incisor angle (FMTA), (in dentistry) the precumbency of the mandibular incisor tooth to the Frankfort horizontal plane.

Frank-Starling relationship {Otto Frank, German physiologist, b. 1865; Ernest H. Starling, English physiologist, b. 1866}, an index for determining cardiac output, based on the length of the myocardial fibres at the onset of contraction. The force exerted per beat of the heart is directly proportional to the length or degree of stretch of the myocardial fibre.

fraternal twins. See **dizygotic twins.**

Fraunhofer zone, (in ultrasonography) the zone furthest from the transducer face.

FRC, abbreviation for functional residual capacity.

freckle, a brown or tan macule on the skin, usually resulting from exposure to sunlight. There is an inherited tendency to freckling.

Fredet-Ramstedt's operation. See **pyloromyotomy.**

free-air chamber, (in radiation dosimetry) a device used as a primary standard for calibrating x-ray exposure. It is used in national calibration laboratories throughout the world.

free association, 1. the spontaneous, consciously unrestricted association of ideas, feelings or mental images. **2.** spontaneous verbalization of thoughts and emotions entering the consciousness during psychoanalysis.

freebasing, a chemical process used to increase the stimulating effect of cocaine.

free-floating anxiety, a generalized, persistent, pervasive fear that is not attributable to any specific object, event or source.

free-form foot orthosis, an orthosis moulded directly to a patient's foot.

free gingiva, the unattached coronal portion of the gingiva that encircles a tooth and forms a gingival sulcus.

free gingival groove, a shallow line or depression on the gingival surface at the junction of the free and attached gingivae.

free-induction decay (FID), (in MRI), a signal emitted by a tissue after a radiofrequency (RF) pulse has excited the nuclear spins of the tissue at resonance. The decaying oscillation back to the normal state is the signal from which a magnetic resonance image is made.

free nerve ending, a receptor nerve ending that is not enclosed in a capsule.

free phagocyte. See **phagocyte.**

free radical, a compound with an extra electron or proton. It is unstable and reacts readily with other molecules. Produced in water in body cells following exposure to ionising radiations, it may react with the DNA to cause bond breakages, resulting in cell damage.

free-radical theory of ageing, a concept of ageing based on the premise that the main causative factor is an imbalance between the production and elimination of free chemical radicals in the body tissues.

free thyroxine, the amount of the unbound, active thyroid hormone, thyroxine (T_4), circulating in the blood, measured by special laboratory procedures.

free thyroxine index, the amount of unbound, physiologicalally active thyroxine (T_4) in serum, determined by direct assay or, more frequently, calculated on the basis of an in vitro uptake test.

freeway space, the interocclusal distance or separation between the occlusal surfaces of the teeth when the mandible is in its rest position.

Freiberg's infarction {Albert H. Freiberg, American surgeon, b. 1868}, an abnormal orthopaedic condition characterized by osteochondritis or aseptic necrosis of bone tissue, most commonly affecting the head of the second metatarsal.

Frei test {William S. Frei, German dermatologist, b. 1885}, a test performed to confirm a diagnosis of lymphogranuloma venereum.

Frejka splint, a corrective device consisting of a pillow that is belted between the legs of a baby born with dislocated hips to maintain abduction and articulation of the head of the femur with the acetabulum.

fremitus, a tremulous vibration of the chest wall that can be auscultated or palpated during physical examination. Kinds of fremitus include **bronchial fremitus, coarse fremitus, tactile fremitus** and **vocal fremitus.**

frenectomy, a surgical procedure for excising a frenum or frenulum, such as the excision of the lingual frenum from its attachment into the mucoperiosteal covering of the alveolar process to correct ankyloglossia.

Frenkel exercises, a system of slow repetitive exercises of increasing difficulty, developed to treat ataxia in multiple sclerosis and similar disorders.

frenotomy, a surgical procedure for repairing a defective frenum, such as the cutting or lengthening of the lingual frenum to correct ankyloglossia.

frenulum linguae. See **lingual frenum.**

frenum, *pl.* **frenums, frena,** a restraining portion or structure.

frequency, 1. the number of repetitions of any phenomenon within a fixed period of time, such as the number of heart beats per minute. **2.** (in biometry) the proportion of the number of persons having a discrete characteristic to the total number of persons being studied. **3.** (in electronics) the number of cycles of a periodic quantity that occur in a period of 1 second. Electromagnetic frequencies are expressed in hertz (Hz).

Fresnel zone, (in ultrasonography) the region nearest the transducer face.

freudian {Sigmund Freud, Austrian psychiatrist, b. 1856}, **1.** pertaining to the theories and doctrines of Freud which stress the formative years of childhood as the basis for later psychoneurotic disorders, primarily through the unconscious repression of instinctual drives and sexual desires, and his system of psychoanalysis for treating such disturbances. **2.** pertaining to the school of psychiatry based on Freud's teachings. **3.** pertaining to one who adheres to Freud's school of psychiatry.

freudian fixation, an arrest in psychosexual development characterized by a firm emotional attachment to another person or object. Some kinds of freudian fixation are **father fixation** and **mother fixation.**

freudianism, the school of psychiatry based on the psychoanalytical theories and psychotherapeutic methods of treating psychoneurotic disorders developed by Freud and his followers.

Fricke dosimeter, (in radiation dosimetry) a chemical radiation dosimeter that uses the change of concentration of ferric ions in a solution subject to irradiation, to quantify the amount of dose delivered to the sample.

friction, 1. the act of rubbing one object against another. **2.** a type of massage in which deeper tissues are stroked or rubbed, usually through strong circular movements of the hand.

frictional force, the force component parallel to the surfaces at the point of contact between two objects. It may be increased or decreased by factors such as moisture on a surface.

friction burn, tissue injury caused by abrasion of the skin.

friction rub, a dry, grating sound heard with a stethoscope during auscultation. It is a normal finding when heard over the liver and splenic areas.

Friedländer's bacillus {Carl Friedländer, German pathologist, b. 1847}, a bacterium of the species *Klebsiella pneumonia* which is associated with infection of the respiratory tract, especially lobar pneumonia.

Friedländer's disease, a severe arterial inflammation. There may be swelling and overgrowth of tissue cells lining the blood vessel, leading to complete obstruction of the artery.

Friedman's test {Maurice H. Friedman, American physiologist, b. 1903}, a modification of the Aschheim-Zondek pregnancy test. A sample of urine from a woman is injected into a mature, unmated female rabbit. If, days later, the rabbit ovaries contain fresh corpora lutea or haemorrhaging corpora, the test is positive for pregnancy.

Friedreich's ataxia {Nickolaus Friedreich, German physician, b. 1825}, an abnormal condition characterized by muscular weakness, loss of muscular control, weakness of the lower extremities and an abnormal gait. The primary pathological feature of the disease is pronounced sclerosis of the posterior columns of the spinal cord, with possible involvement of the spinocerebellar tracts and the corticospinal tracts.

frigid, 1. lacking warmth of feeling; unemotional; unimaginative; without passion or ardour and stiff or formal in manner. **2.** a woman who is unresponsive to sexual advances or stimuli, abnormally indifferent or averse to sexual intercourse, or unable to have an orgasm during sexual intercourse. **frigidity,** *n.*

fringe field, (in magnetic resonance imaging) the part of a magnetic field that extends away from the confines of the magnet and cannot be used for imaging. It may affect nearby equipment and personnel.

frit {Fr, fried}, a partially or wholly fused porcelain from which dental porcelain powders are made.

Fröhlich's syndrome. See **adiposogenital dystrophy.**

frôlement, 1. the rustling type of sound often heard on auscultating the chest in diseases of the pericardium. **2.** a kind of massage that uses a light brushing stroke with the hand.

frontal bone, a single cranial bone that forms the front of the skull, from above the orbits, posteriorly to a junction with the parietal bones at the coronal suture.

frontal lobe, the largest of five lobes constituting each of the two cerebral hemispheres. It lies beneath the frontal bone, occupies part of the lateral, medial and inferior surfaces of each hemisphere, and extends posteriorly to the central sulcus and inferiorly to the lateral fissure. Research indicates that the right frontal and right temporal lobes are associated with the non-verbal, specialized activities of the right cerebral hemisphere, and that the left frontal and left temporal lobes are associated with the verbal activities of the left cerebral hemisphere.

frontal lobe syndrome, behavioural and personality changes observed after a neoplastic or traumatic frontal lobe lesion. The patient may become sociopathic, boastful, hypomanic, uninhibited, exhibitionistic and subject to outbursts of irritability or violence. The person may also become depressed, apathetic, lacking in initiative, negligent about personal appearance and inclined to perseverate.

frontal plane, any one of the vertical planes passing through the body from the head to the feet, perpendicular to the sagittal planes, dividing the body into front and back portions.

frontal sinus, one of a pair of small cavities in the frontal bone of the skull that communicates with the nasal cavity. Each sinus opens into the anterior part of the middle meatus through the frontonasal duct.

frontal vein, one of a pair of superficial veins of the face, arising in the plexus of the forehead.

frontocortical aphasia. See **motor aphasia.**

frostbite, traumatic effect of extreme cold on skin and subcutaneous tissues that is first recognized by distinct pallor of exposed skin surfaces, particularly the nose, ears, fingers and toes. Vasoconstriction and damage to blood vessels impair local circulation and result in anoxia, oedema, vesiculation and necrosis. Gentle warming is appropriate first aid treatment.

frostnip. See **frostbite.**

frottage, sexual gratification obtained by rubbing (especially one's genital area) against the clothing of another person, as can occur in a crowd.

frotteur, a person who obtains sexual gratification by the practice of frottage.

frozen section method, (in surgical pathology) a method used in preparing a selected portion of tissue for pathological examination. The tissue is moistened and rapidly frozen, and cut by a microtome in a cryostat.

fructokinase, an enzyme that catalyses the transfer of a phosphate group from adenosine triphosphate to D-fructose.

full blood count (fbc), a determination of the number of red and white blood cells per cubic millimetre of blood.

fructose, a yellowish-to-white, crystalline, water-soluble levorotatory ketose monosaccharide that is sweeter than sucrose and found in honey, several fruits, and combined in many disaccharides and polysaccharides.

fructosuria, presence of fructose in the urine.

fruit sugar. See **fructose.**

frusemide, a diuretic used in the treatment of hypertension, renal failure and oedema.

frustration, a feeling that results from an interference with one's ability to attain a desired goal or satisfaction.

FSH, abbreviation for **follicle stimulating hormone.**

FT, abbreviation for *fast-twitch.* See **fast-twitch fibre.**

FTA-ABS test. See **Fluorescent Treponemal Antibody Absorption Test.**

fuchsin bodies. See **Russell's bodies.**

fugue, a state of dissociative reaction characterized by amnesia and physical flight from an intolerable situation. During the episode, the person appears normal and acts as though consciously aware of what may be very complex activities and behaviour, but after the episode the person has no recollection of the actions or behaviour.

fulcrum, 1. the stable point or position on which a lever, such as the ulna or the femur, turns. Numerous common movements of the body, such as raising the arm and walking, are combinations of lever actions involving fulcrums. **2.** (in radiography) an imaginary pivot point about which the x-ray tube and film move.

fulfilment, a perception of harmony in life that results when an individual has found meaning and leads a purposeful life.

fulguration. See **electrodesiccation.**

full-arch wire, a wire that is attached to the teeth and extends from the molar region of one side of a dental arch to the other.

full diet. See **diet.**

fulminant hepatitis, a rare and frequently fatal form of acute hepatitis in which there is rapid deterioration in the condition of the patient, with hepatic encephalopathy, necrosis of the hepatic parenchyma, blood coagulation disorders, renal failure and coma. The prognosis for adults is generally unfavourable.

fulminating, (of a disease or condition) rapid, sudden, severe, such as an infection, fever or haemorrhage. Also **fulminant. fulminate,** v.

function, 1. an act, process or series of processes that serve a purpose. **2.** to perform an activity or to work properly and normally.

functional ability, the ability to carry out the functions which an individual needs/wishes to perform in the course of daily activity in the usual (or accepted) way.

functional analysis, (in psychiatry) a type of therapy that traces the sequence of events involved in producing and maintaining undesirable behaviour.

functional antagonism, (in pharmacology) a situation in which two agonists interact with different receptors and produce opposing effects.

functional bowel syndrome. See **irritable bowel syndrome.**

functional contracture. See **hypertonic contracture.**

functional differentiation, (in embryology) the specialization or diversification as a result of the particular function of a cell or tissue.

functional disease, 1. a disease that affects function or performance. **2.** a condition marked by signs or symptoms of an organic disease or disorder, although careful examination fails to reveal any evidence of structural or physiological abnormalities. Headache, impotence, certain heart murmurs and constipation may be symptoms of functional disease.

functional dyspepsia, an abnormal condition characterized by impaired digestion caused by an atonic or a neurological problem.

functional imaging, (in radionuclide imaging) a diagnostic procedure in which a sequence of radiographic or scintillation camera images of the distribution of an administered radioactive tracer delineates one or more physiological processes in the body.

functional impotence. See **impotence.**

functional occlusal harmony, an occlusal relationship of opposing teeth in all functional ranges and movements that provides the maximum masticatory efficiency without pathogenic force on the supporting oral structures.

functional overlay, an emotional aspect of an organic disease. It is characterized by symptoms that continue long after clinical signs of the disease have ended.

functional position of the hand, a position for splinting the hand, including the wrist and fingers. The thumb is abducted and in opposition and alignment with the pads of the fingers.

functional progression, a rehabilitative sequence for a musculoskeletal or similar injury. It usually progresses from immobilization for primary healing to endurance and strengthening activities.

functional psychosis, a severe emotional disorder characterized by personality derangement and loss of ability to fnction in reality, but without evidence that the disorder is related to the physical processes of the brain.

functional refractory period, (in cardiology) the shortest interval at which a tissue is capable of conducting consecutive impulses, as measured by the time intervening between the arrival of an initial impulse and the earliest subsequent premature impulse at the distal end of the same conducting tissue.

functional residual capacity, the volume of gas in the lungs at the end of a normal expiration. The functional residual capacity is equal to the residual volume plus the expiratory reserve volume.

fundal height, the height of the fundus, which may be measured in centimetres from the top of the symphysis pubis to the highest point in the midline at the top of the uterus.

fundamental needs of humans, (in nursing education) the 14 basic needs of human beings as described in a curriculum for basic nursing. The needs are respiration; nutrition; elimination; mobility, including posture and locomotion; sleep and rest; clothing; maintenance of normal body temperature; cleanliness; safety; communication; worship, according to the person's faith; work that is satisfying to the person; recreation; and learning and discovery.

fundamentals of nursing, the basic principles and practices of nursing as taught in educational programmes for nurses. The emphasis of this phase of training is the acquisition of the basic skills of nursing.

fundoplication, a surgical procedure involving making tucks in the fundus of the stomach around the lower end of the oesophagus.

fundoscope. See **ophthalmoscope.**

fundoscopy, the examination and study of the fundus of the eye by means of an ophthalmoscope. **fundoscopic,** *adj.*

fundus, *pl.* **fundi,** the base or deepest part of an organ; the portion furthest from the mouth of an organ, such as the fundus of the uterus or the fundus of an eye.

fundus microscopy, examination of the base of the interior of the eye using an instrument that combines an ophthalmoscope and a lens with high magnifying power, for observing minute structures in the cornea and iris.

fundus reflex. See **light reflex.**

fungaemia, the presence of fungi in the blood.

fungal infection, any inflammatory condition caused by a fungus. Most fungal infections are superficial and mild, although persistent and difficult to eradicate. Some kinds of fungal infections are aspergillosis, blastomycosis, candidiasis, coccidioidomycosis and histoplasmosis.

fungicide, an agent that kills fungi.

fungiform papilla. See **papilla.**

fungistatic, having an inhibiting effect on the growth of fungi.

fungus, *pl.* **fungi,** a simple parasitic plant that, lacking chlorophyll, is unable to make its own food and is dependent on other life forms. A simple fungus reproduces by budding; multicellular fungi reproduce by spore formation. **fungal, fungous,** *adj.*

funic souffle, a soft, muffled blowing sound produced by blood rushing through the umbilical vessels and synchronous with the fetal heart sound.

funiculitis, any abnormal inflammatory condition of a cord-like structure of the body, such as the spinal cord or spermatic cord.

funiculus, a division of the white matter of the spinal cord, consisting of fasciculi or fibre tracts.

funiculus umbilicalis. See **umbilical cord.**

funis, a cord-like structure.

funnel chest, a skeletal abnormality of the chest characterized by a depressed sternum. The deformity may not interfere with breathing, but surgical correction is often recommended for cosmetic reasons.

funny bone, a popular name for a point at the lower end of the humerus where the ulnar nerve is near the surface and subject to external pressure, resulting in a tingling sensation.

FUO, abbreviation for **fever of unknown origin.**

furcation, the region of division of the root portion of a tooth.

furrier's lung, a form of occupational hypersensitivity pneumonitis that affects persons who work in the fur industry and are exposed to antigens present in hair and dander of animal pelts.

furrow, a groove, such as the atrioventricular furrow that separates the atria from the ventricles of the heart.

furuncle, a localized, suppurative, staphylococcal skin infection originating in a gland or hair follicle, characterized by pain, redness and swelling. Necrosis deep in the centre of the inflamed area forms a core of dead tissue that extrudes spontaneously, resorbs or is surgically removed. **furunculous,** *adj.*

furunculosis, an acute skin disease characterized by boils or successive crops of boils that are caused by staphylococci or streptococci.

fusiform, a structure that is tapered at both ends.

fusiform aneurysm, a localized dilatation of an artery in which the entire circumference of the vessel is distended.

fusimotor, pertaining to the motor nerve fibres, or gamma efferent fibres, that innervate the intrafusal fibres of the muscle spindle.

fusion, 1. the bringing together into a single entity, as in optic fusion. **2.** the act of uniting two or more bones of a joint. **3.** the surgical joining together of two or more vertebrae, performed to stabilize a segment of the spinal column after severe trauma, a herniated disk or degenerative disease. **4.** (in psychiatry) the tendency of two people experiencing an intense emotion to unite.

fusion beat, (in cardiology) a QRS complex deriving from a collision of impulses within the atria or ventricles as a result of simultaneous activation of those chambers by two foci, usually the sinus node and a ventricular ectopic beat.

fusion-exclusion, (in psychology) a mechanism by which two people can stay in contact with each other and avoid anxiety either by excluding a third person from the relationship or by focusing their energies on a third person.

fusospirochaetal disease, any infection characterized by ulcerative lesions in which both a fusiform bacillus and a spirochaete are found, such as trench mouth or Vincent's angina.

f waves, (in cardiology) waves that represent fibrillation or flutter.

F wave, a wave form recorded in electroneuromyographic and nerve conduction tests. It appears on supramaximal stimulation of a motor nerve, and is caused by antidromic transmission of a stimulus. The F wave is used in studies of motor nerve function in the arms and legs.

g, abbreviation for **gram.**

Ga, symbol for **gallium.**

GA, abbreviation for **general anaesthesia.**

GABA, abbreviation for **gammaamino-butyric acid.**

GABHS, abbreviation for **group A beta-haemolytic streptococcal (skin disease).**

gadolinium (Gd) {Johan Gadolin, Finnish chemist, b. 1760}, a rare earth metallic element. Its atomic number is 64 and its atomic weight is 157.25.

gag reflex, a normal neural reflex elicited by touching the soft palate or posterior pharynx, the response being elevation of the palate, retraction of the tongue and contraction of the pharyngeal muscles.

gait, the manner or style of walking, including rhythm, cadence and speed.

gait determinant, one of a number of the kinetic anatomical factors that govern the locomotion of an individual in the process of walking. Authorities have defined pelvic rotation, pelvic tilt, knee and hip flexion, knee and ankle interaction, and lateral pelvic displacement as the main determinants of gait.

gait disorder, an abnormality in the manner or style of walking, usually as a result of neuromuscular, arthritic or other body changes.

galactokinase, an enzyme that functions in the metabolism of glycogen.

galactokinase deficiency, an inherited disorder of carbohydrate metabolism in which the enzyme galactokinase is deficient or absent. As a result, dietary galactose is not metabolized, galactose accumulates in the blood, and cataracts may develop.

galactophorous duct, a passage for milk in the lobes of the breast.

galactorrhoea, lactation not associated with childbirth or nursing. The condition is sometimes a symptom of a pituitary gland tumour.

galactose, a simple sugar found in the dextrorotatory form in lactose (milk sugar), nerve cell membranes, sugar beets, gums and seaweed and, in the levorotatory form, in flaxseed mucilage.

galactosaemia, an inherited, autosomal recessive disorder of galactose metabolism, characterized by a deficiency of the enzyme galactose-1-phosphate uridyl transferase. Shortly after birth, an intolerance to milk is evident. Hepatosplenomegaly, cataracts and mental retardation develop.

galactosuria, the presence of galactose in the urine.

galactosyl ceramide lipidosis, a rare, fatal, inherited disorder of lipid metabolism, present at birth. Infants become paralysed, blind, deaf and increasingly retarded, and eventually die of bulbar paralysis.

Galant reflex, a normal response in the neonate to move the hips towards the stimulated side when the back is stroked along the spinal cord.

galea aponeurotica. See **epicranial aponeurosis.**

Galeazzi's fracture {Riccardo Galeazzi, Italian surgeon, b. 1866}, a fracture of the distal radius accompanied by dislocation of the radioulnar joint.

Galen's bandage {Claudius Galen, Greek physician, b. 130 AD}, a bandage for the head, consisting of a strip of cloth with each end divided into three pieces.

gall. See **bile.**

gallbladder, a pear-shaped excretory sac lodged in a fossa on the visceral surface of the right lobe of the liver. It serves as a reservoir for bile. About 8 cm long and 2.5 cm wide at its thickest part, it holds about 32 cc of bile. During digestion of fats the gallbladder contracts, ejecting bile through the common bile duct into the duodenum.

gallbladder cancer, a malignant neoplasm of the bile reservoir, characterized by anorexia, nausea, vomiting, weight loss, progressively severe right upper quadrant pain and eventually jaundice. Tumours of the gallbladder are predominantly adenocarcinomas and are often associated with biliary calculi.

gallium (Ga), a metallic element. Its atomic number is 31 and its atomic weight is 69.72. Because of its high boiling point (1983° C; 3602° F), it is used in high-temperature thermometers. Radioisotopes of gallium are used in total body scanning procedures.

gallop {Fr *galop*}, a pathological third or fourth heart sound, which at certain heart rates sometimes mimics the gait of a horse.

gallstone. See **biliary calculus.**

galvanic cautery, galvanocautery. See **electrocautery.**

galvanic electric stimulation {Luigi Galvani, Italian physiologist, b. 1737}, the use of a high-voltage electrical stimulator to treat muscle spasms, oedema of acute injury, myofascial pain and certain other disorders.

galvanometer {Luigi Galvani}, a device

that indicates or measures electrical current by its effects on a needle or coil in a magnetic field. Galvanometers are used in certain diagnostic instruments, such as electrocardiographs.

Gambian trypanosomiasis, a usually chronic form of African trypanosomiasis, caused by the parasite *Trypanosoma brucei gambiense.*

gamete, 1. a mature male or female germ cell that is capable of functioning in fertilization or conjugation and contains the haploid number of chromosomes of the somatic cell. **2.** the ovum or spermatozoon. **gametic,** *adj.*

gamete intrafallopian transfer (GIFT), a human fertilization technique in which male and female gametes are injected through a laparoscope into the fimbriated ends of the uterine tubes.

gametic chromosome, any of the chromosomes contained in the haploid cell, specifically the spermatozoon or ovum, as contrasted to those in the diploid, or somatic cell.

gametocide, any agent that is destructive to gametes or gametocytes, specifically to the malarial gametocytes. **gametocidal,** *adj.*

gametocyte, (in genetics) any cell capable of dividing into or in the process of developing into a gamete, specifically an oocyte or spermatocyte.

gametogenesis, the origin and maturation of gametes, which occurs through the process of meiosis. **gametogenic, gametogenous,** *adj.*

gamma-aminobutyric acid (GABA), an amino acid with neurotransmitter activity found in the brain and also in the heart, lungs, kidneys and certain plants.

gammabenzene hexachloride. See **lindane.**

gamma camera, a device that uses the emission of light from a crystal struck by gamma rays to produce an image of the distribution of radioactive material in a body organ. The light is detected by an array of light-sensitive electronic tubes and is converted to electrical signals for further processing.

gamma efferent fibre, any of the motor nerve fibres that transmit impulses from the central nervous system to the intrafusal fibres of the muscle spindle.

gamma globulin. See **immune gamma globulin.**

gamma-glutamyl transpeptidase, an enzyme that appears in the serum of patients with several types of liver or gallbladder disorders, including drug hepatotoxicity and biliary tract obstruction.

gamma radiation, a high frequency electromagnetic emission of photons from certain radioactive elements in the course of nuclear transition or from nuclear reactions. Gamma radiation is more penetrating than alpha radiation, and beta radiation but has less ion-

izing power and is not deflected in electrical and magnetic fields. The wavelengths of gamma rays emitted by radioactive substances are characteristic of the radioisotopes involved and range from about 4×10^{-10} to 5×10^{-13} m. The depth to which gamma rays penetrate depends on their wavelengths and energy. Gamma radiation and other forms of radiation can injure, distort or destroy body cells and tissue, especially cell nuclei, but controlled radiation is used in the diagnosis and treatment of various diseases. Gamma radiation can penetrate thousands of meters of air and several centimetres of soft tissue and bone.

gamma ray, an electromagnetic radiation of short wavelength emitted by the nucleus of an atom during a nuclear reaction. Composed of high-energy photons, gamma rays lack mass and an electrical charge and travel at the speed of light.

gammopathy, an abnormal condition characterized by the presence of markedly increased levels of gamma globulin in the blood. Monoclonal gammopathy is commonly associated with an electrophoretic pattern showing one sharp, homogenous electrophoretic band in the gamma globulin region. This reflects the presence of excessive amounts of one type of immunoglobulin secreted by a single clone of B cells. Polyclonal gammopathy reflects the presence of a diffuse hypergammaglobulinaemia in which all immunoglobulin classes are proportionally increased.

gamogenesis, sexual reproduction through the fusion of gametes. **gamogenetic,** *adj.*

gamone, a chemical substance secreted by the ova and spermatozoa that supposedly attracts the gametes of the opposite sex to facilitate union. Kinds of gamones are **androgamone** and **gynogamone.**

gampsodactyly. See **pes cavus.**

ganglia. See **ganglion.**

ganglion, *pl.* **ganglia, 1.** a knot or knot-like mass. **2.** one of the nerve cells, chiefly collected in groups outside the central nervous system. The two types of ganglia in the body are the sensory ganglia on the dorsal roots of spinal nerves and sensory roots of the trigeminal, facial, glossopharyngeal and vagus nerves, and the autonomic ganglia of the sympathetic and parasympathetic systems.

ganglionar neuroma, a tumour composed of a solid mass of ganglia and nerve fibres. It is usually found in abdominal tissues and occurs most commonly in children.

ganglionic blockade, the blocking of nerve impulses at synapses of autonomic ganglia, usually by the administration of ganglionic blocking agents.

ganglionic blocking agent, any one of a group of drugs prescribed to produce controlled hypotension, as required in certain surgical procedures or in emergency management of hypertensive crisis. These drugs act by occupying receptor sites on sympathetic and parasympathetic nerve endings of autonomic ganglia.

ganglionic crest. See **neural crest**.

ganglionic glioma, a tumour composed of glial cells and ganglion cells that are nearly mature.

ganglionic neuroma. See **ganglionar neuroma**.

ganglionic ridge. See **neural crest**.

ganglionitis, an inflammation of a nerve or lymph ganglion.

ganglioside, a glycolipid found in the brain and other nervous system tissues. Accumulation of gangliosides because of an inborn error of metabolism results in gangliosidosis or Tay-Sachs disease.

gangliosidosis type I. See **Tay-Sachs disease**.

gangliosidosis type II. See **Sandhoff's disease**.

gangrene, necrosis or death of tissue, usually the result of ischaemia (loss of blood supply), bacterial invasion and subsequent putrefaction. **Dry gangrene** is a late complication of diabetes mellitus that is already complicated by arteriosclerosis in which the affected extremity becomes cold, dry and shriveled, and eventually turns black. **Moist gangrene** may follow a crushing injury or obstruction of blood flow by an embolism, tight bandages or tourniquet. **gangrenous,** *adj.*

gangrenous necrosis. See **necrosis**.

gangrenous stomatitis. See **noma**.

ganja. See **cannabis**.

gantry assembly, mechanical rotating support for certain x-ray or external beam radiotherapy, or radionuclide imaging units.

Ganzfeld effect, a visual field that is patternless, such as a whitewashed surface, producing a sensation of an inability to see.

gap, (in molecular genetics) a short, missing segment in one strand of double-stranded DNA.

gap phenomenon, (in cardiology) a condition in which a premature stimulus encounters a block where an earlier or later stimulus could be conducted.

Gardner-Diamond syndrome, a condition resulting from autoerythrocyte sensitization, marked by large, painful, transient ecchymoses that appear without apparent cause but often accompany emotional upsets, various collagen disorders and abnormalities of protein metabolism.

Gardner's syndrome {Eldon J. Gardner, American geneticist, b. 1909}, familial polyposis of the large bowel, with fibrous dysplasia of the skull, extra teeth, osteomas, fibromas and epidermal cysts.

Gardner-Wells tongs, braces that are attached to the skull of patients immobilized with cervical injuries.

gargle, 1. to hold and agitate a liquid at the back of the throat by tilting the head backwards and forcing air through the solution. **2.** a solution used to rinse the mouth and oropharynx.

gargoylism. See **Hurler's syndrome**.

Gartner's duct {Hermann T. Gartner, Danish anatomist, b. 1785}, one of two vestigial, closed ducts, each one parallel to a uterine tube.

gas, an aeriform fluid possessing complete molecular mobility and the property of indefinite expansion. A gas has no definite shape and its volume is determined by temperature and pressure.

gas chromatography, the separation and analysis of different substances according to their different affinities for a standard absorbent. In the process, a gaseous mixture of the substances is passed through a glass cylinder containing the absorbent which may be dampened with a non-volatile liquid solvent for one or more of the gaseous components.

gas distention. See **flatulence**.

gas embolism, an occlusion of one or more small blood vessels, especially in the muscles, tendons and joints, caused by expanding bubbles of gases. Gas emboli can rupture tissue and blood vessels, causing decompression sickness and death. This phenomenon commonly affects deep-sea divers who rise too quickly to the surface without adequate decompression.

gas exchange, impaired, a condition in which the individual experiences a decreased passage of oxygen and/or carbon dioxide between the alveoli of the lungs and the vascular system. Defining characteristics include confusion, restlessness, irritability, somnolence, hypercapnoea and hypoxia.

gas gangrene, necrosis accompanied by gas bubbles in soft tissue after surgery or trauma. It is caused by anaerobic organisms, such as various species of *Clostridium*. Symptoms include pain, swelling and tenderness of the wound area, moderate fever, tachycardia and hypotension. A characteristic finding is toxic delirium. If untreated, gas gangrene is rapidly fatal.

gas pains. See **flatulence**.

gas-scavenging system, the equipment and procedures used to eliminate anaesthetic gases that escape into the atmosphere of the operating room.

gas therapy, the use of medical gases in respiratory therapy. Kinds of gas therapy include **carbon dioxide therapy, controlled oxygen therapy, helium therapy** and **hyperbaric oxygenation**.

gastrectasia, an abnormal dilatation of the stomach. It may be accompanied by pain, vomiting, rapid pulse and falling body temperature. Causes can include overeating, obstruction of the pyloric valve, or a hernia.

gastrectomy, surgical excision of all or, more commonly, part of the stomach, performed to remove a chronic peptic ulcer, stop the haemorrhage in a perforating ulcer, or remove a malignancy. Preoperatively, a GI series is done and a nasogastric tube is introduced. Under general anaesthesia, one-half to two-thirds of the stomach is removed, including the ulcer and a large area of acid-secreting mucosa.

gastric, of or pertaining to the stomach.

gastric analysis, examination of the contents of the stomach, primarily to determine the quantity of acid present and incidentally to ascertain the presence of blood, bile, bacteria and abnormal cells.

gastric antacid. See **antacid.**

gastric atrophy. See **atrophic gastritis.**

gastric cancer, a malignancy of the stomach with symptoms of vague epigastric discomfort, anorexia, weight loss and unexplained iron deficiency anaemia. Many cases are asymptomatic in the early stages, and metastatic enlargement of the left supraclavicular lymph node may be the first manifestation of a stomach lesion.

gastric dyspepsia, pain or discomfort localized in the stomach.

gastric fistula, an abnormal passage into the stomach, communicating most frequently with an opening on the external surface of the abdomen. A gastric fistula may be created surgically to provide tube feeding for patients with severe oesophageal disorders.

gastric glands, glands in the stomach mucosa that secrete hydrochloric acid, mucin and pepsinogen.

gastric inhibitory polypeptide (GIP), a gastrointestinal hormone found in the mucosa of the small intestine. Release of the hormone, mediated by the presence of glucose or fatty acids in the duodenum, results in the release of insulin by the pancreas and inhibition of gastric acid secretion.

gastric intubation, a procedure in which a small-calibre catheter is passed through the nose into the oesophagus and stomach for the introduction of liquid formulas into the stomach, so as to provide nutrition for unconscious patients or premature or sick newborn infants. Medication or a contrast medium may be instilled for treatment or radiological examination.

gastric juice, digestive secretions of the gastric glands in the stomach, consisting chiefly of pepsin, hydrochloric acid, rennin, lipase and mucin. The pH is strongly acid (0.9 to 1.5).

gastric lavage, the washing out of the stomach with sterile water or a saline solution.

gastric motility, the spontaneous peristaltic movements of the stomach that aid in digestion, moving food through the stomach and out through the pyloric sphincter into the duodenum.

gastric node, a node in one of three groups of lymph glands associated with the abdominal and pelvic viscera supplied by branches of the coeliac artery.

gastric partitioning, a surgical procedure in which a portion of the stomach is closed, reducing its capacity. It is used in the treatment of certain cases of obesity.

gastric ulcer, a circumscribed erosion of the mucosal layer of the stomach that may penetrate the muscle layer and perforate the stomach wall. It tends to recur with stress and is characterized by episodes of burning epigastric pain, belching and nausea, especially when the stomach is empty or after eating certain foods. Characteristically, antacid medication or milk quickly relieves the pain.

gastrin, a polypeptide hormone, secreted by the pylorus, stimulating the flow of gastric juice and contributing to the stimulus that causes secretion of bile and pancreatic enzymes.

gastrinoma, a tumour found usually in the pancreas but sometimes in the duodenum.

gastritis, an inflammation of the lining of the stomach that occurs in two forms. **Acute gastritis** may be caused by severe burns, major surgery, aspirin or other anti-inflammatory agents, corticosteroids, drugs or food allergens, or by the presence of viral, bacterial or chemical toxins. The symptoms…anorexia, nausea, vomiting and discomfort after eating…usually abate after the causative agent has been removed. **Chronic gastritis** is usually a sign of underlying disease, such as peptic ulcer, stomach cancer, Zollinger-Ellison syndrome, or pernicious anaemia. Kinds of gastritis include **antral gastritis, atrophic gastritis, haemorrhagic gastritis** and **hypertrophic gastritis.**

gastrocamera, a small camera that can be lowered into the stomach through the oesophagus and retrieved after recording images of the stomach lining.

gastrocnemius, the most superficial muscle in the posterior part of the leg. It arises by a lateral head and a medial head, and forms the greater part of the calf.

gastrocnemius gait, an abnormal gait associated with a weakness of the gastrocnemius. It is characterized by the dropping of the pelvis on the affected side at the last moment of the stance phase in the walking cycle, accompanied by the lagging or the slowness of forward pelvic movement.

gastrocnemius test, a test of the function of the gastrocnemius muscle by ankle plantar flexion while the patient is in a prone position. The examiner places fingers for palpation on the posterior of the calf while the patient pulls the heel upward.

gastrocoele. See **archenteron.**

gastrocolic omentum. See **greater**

omentum.

gastrocolic reflex, a mass peristaltic movement of the colon that often occurs when food enters the stomach.

gastrodidymus, conjoined, equally developed twins united at the abdominal region.

gastrodisciasis, an infection of trematodes of the genus *Gastrodiscoides,* which are digestive tract parasites.

gastrodisk. See **embryonic disk.**

gastroenteritis, inflammation of the stomach and intestines accompanying numerous GI disorders. Symptoms are anorexia, nausea, vomiting, abdominal discomfort and diarrhoea. The condition may be attributed to bacterial enterotoxins, bacterial or viral invasion, chemical toxins or miscellaneous conditions such as lactose intolerance.

gastroenterologist, a medical doctor who specializes in gastroenterology.

gastroenterology, the study of diseases affecting the GI tract, including the stomach, intestines, gallbladder and bile duct.

gastroenterostomy, surgical formation of an artificial opening between the stomach and small intestine, usually at the jejunum. The operation is performed with a gastrectomy to route food from the remainder of the stomach into the small intestine, or by itself, in the case of a perforating ulcer of the duodenum.

gastroesophageal, of or pertaining to the stomach and oesophagus.

gastroesophageal haemorrhage. See **Mallory-Weiss syndrome.**

gastroesophageal reflux, a backflow of contents of the stomach into the oesophagus that is often the result of incompetence of the lower oesophageal sphincter. Gastric juices are acid and therefore produce burning pain in the oesophagus.

gastrohepatic omentum. See **lesser omentum.**

gastrointestinal (GI), of or pertaining to the organs of the GI tract, from the mouth to the anus.

gastrointestinal allergy, an immediate reaction of hypersensitivity after ingestion of certain foods or drugs. GI allergy differs from food allergy which can affect organ systems other than the digestive system. Characteristic symptoms include itching and swelling of the mouth and oral passages, nausea, vomiting, diarrhoea (sometimes containing blood), severe abdominal pain and, if severe, anaphylactic shock.

gastrointestinal bleeding, any bleeding from the GI tract. The most common underlying conditions are peptic ulcer, oesophageal varices, diverticulitis, ulcerative colitis and carcinoma of the stomach and colon. Vomiting of bright red blood or passage of coffee ground vomitus indicates upper GI bleeding, usually from the oesophagus, stomach or upper duodenum.

gastrointestinal gas. See **flatulence.**

gastrointestinal infection, any infection of the digestive tract caused by bacteria, viruses, parasites or toxins. All may have clinical features of nausea, vomiting, diarrhoea and anorexia in common.

gastrointestinal obstruction, any obstruction of the passage of intestinal contents, caused by mechanical blockage or failure of motility. Blockage may be caused by adhesions resulting from surgery or inflammatory bowel disease, an incarcerated hernia, faecal impaction, tumour, intussusception or volvulus. Failure of motility may follow anaesthesia, abdominal surgery or occlusion of any of the mesenteric arteries to the gut. Symptoms generally include vomiting, abdominal pain and increasing abdominal distention.

gastrointestinal system assessment, an evaluation of the patient's digestive system and symptoms. Discussion of symptoms is encouraged, and information is elicited concerning any changes in eating, bowel habits, the colour, character and frequency of stools and urine, the use of laxatives or enemas, and the occurrence of fatigue, haemorrhoids and oedema of the extremities. Diagnostic aids include a complete blood count, stool examination, prothrombin time and determinations of levels of alkaline phosphatase, serum and urine bilirubin, serum glutamic oxaloacetic transaminase (SGOT), serum glutamic pyruvic transaminase (SGPT), lactic acid dehydrogenase (LDH), blood urea nitrogen, and serum lipase, cholinesterase, calcium, albumin and glucose. Additional laboratory studies for evaluation are total protein level, serum electrolyte profile, serum carotene, delta-xylose tolerance, galactose tolerance, hippuric acid and bromosulphalein tests, albumin-globulin ratio, serum flocculation and thymol turbidity tests, urobilinogen level, the polyvinylpyrrolidone (PVP) test for protein loss, Sulkowitch's test for calcium in urine and Schilling's test for GI absorption of vitamin B_{12}.

gastropore. See **blastopore.**

gastroschisis, a congenital defect characterized by incomplete closure of the abdominal wall with protrusion of the viscera.

gastroscope, a fibreoptic instrument for examining the interior of the stomach. **gastroscopy,** *n.,* **gastroscopic,** *adj.*

gastroscopy, the visual inspection of the interior of the stomach by means of a gastroscope inserted through the oesophagus. **gastroscopic,** *adj.*

gastrostomy, surgical creation of an artificial opening into the stomach through the abdominal wall, performed to feed a patient with cancer of the oesophagus or tracheo-oesophageal fistula, or a patient expected to be unconscious for a prolonged period.

gastrostomy feeding, the introduction of a nutrient solution through a tube that has been surgically inserted into the stomach through the abdominal wall.

gastrothoracopagus, conjoined twins that are united at the thorax and abdomen.

gastrula, the early embryonic stage formed by the invagination of the blastula. The cup-shaped gastrula consists of an outer layer of ectoderm and an inner layer of mesentoderm that subsequently differentiates into the mesoderm and endoderm.

gastrulation, the development of the gastrula in lower animals and formation of the three germ layers in the embryo of humans and higher animals.

gate, a simple electronic circuit, a fundamental building block of a computer.

gate control theory of pain. This theory states that pain signals reaching the nervous system excite a group of small neurons that form a "pain pool." When the total activity of these neurons reaches a minimum level, a theoretic gate opens up and allows the pain signals to proceed to higher brain centres. The areas in which the gates operate are considered to be in the spinal cord dorsal horn and the brainstem. See pain mechanism.

gating, (in MRI) organizing the data so that information used to construct an image comes from the same point in the cycle of a repeating motion, such as a heartbeat.

gating mechanism, (in cardiology) the increasing duration of an action potential from the AV node to a point in the distal Purkinje system, beyond which it decreases again.

Gaucher's disease {Phillipe C. E. Gaucher, French physician, b. 1854}, a rare familial disorder of fat metabolism, caused by an enzyme deficiency and characterized by widespread reticulum cell hyperplasia in the liver, spleen, lymph nodes and bone marrow.

gauntlet bandage, a glove-like bandage covering the hand and the fingers.

gauss {J. K. F. Gauss, German physicist, b. 1777}, a unit of magnetic field strength. It is equal to 1/10,000 of a tesla.

gauze, a transparent fabric of open weave and differing degrees of fineness, most often cotton muslin, used in surgical procedures and for bandages and dressings. It may be sterilized and permeated by an antiseptic or lotion. Kinds of gauze include **absorbable gauze, absorbent gauze** and **petrolatum gauze.**

gavage, the process of feeding a patient through a nasogastric tube.

gay, 1. any person who is homosexual. **2.** of or pertaining to homosexuality.

Gay-Lussac's law {Joseph L. Gay-Lussac, French scientist, b. 1778}, (in physics) a law stating that the volume of a specific mass of a gas will increase as the temperature is increased at a constant rate, determined by the volume of the gas at $0°$ C if the pressure remains constant.

gaze, a fixed stare or state of looking in one direction. A person with normal vision has six basic positions of gaze, each determined by control of different combinations of contractions of extraocular muscles.

gaze palsy, a partial or complete inability to move the eyes to all directions of gaze. A gaze palsy is often named for the absent direction of gaze, such as a right lateral gaze palsy.

GBIA. See **Guthrie test.**

Gd, symbol for **gadolinium.**

GDM, abbreviation for **gestational diabetes mellitus.**

Ge, symbol for **germanium.**

gegenhalten, the involuntary resistance to passive movement of the extremities. The effect may be psychogenic in origin, or a sign of dementia or cerebral deterioration.

Geiger-Müller (GM) counter {Hans Geiger, German physicist, b. 1882; Walther Müller, German physicist}, (in radiation dosimetry) an electronic device used to detect and count ionizing radiations such as beta particles and gamma rays. It cannot discriminate between different types and energies of radiation.

gel, 1. a colloid that is firm even though it contains a large amount of liquid. It is used as a base in various medicines. **2.** (in ultrasonography) an aqueous gel used as a coupling medium between the skin and the transducer, to enable transmission of sound waves.

gelatin buildup, an x-ray film artefact that may appear as a sharp area of either increased or reduced density.

gelatiniform carcinoma. See **mucinous carcinoma.**

gelatinous carcinoma, a former term for **mucinous carcinoma.**

gelatin sponge, an absorbable local haemostatic used to control bleeding in various surgical procedures and in the treatment of epistaxis.

gel diffusion. See **immunodiffusion.**

Gellhorn pessary. See **pessary.**

gemellary, of or pertaining to twins.

gemellipara, a woman who has given birth to twins.

gemellology, the study of twins and the phenomenon of twinning.

gemellus, either of a pair of small muscles arising from the ischium. They rotate the thigh laterally.

gemellus test, a test of the function of the gemellus in hip external rotation while the patient is seated with the knees flexed. The examiner places one hand on the lateral aspect of the knee to prevent flexion or abduction of the hip and the patient rotates the thigh outwards by moving the foot medially.

gemfibrozil, an hypolipidaemic agent used

to treat hyperlipidaemia.

gemistocyte, an astrocyte with an eccentric nucleus and swollen cytoplasm, as seen in areas of nervous tissue affected by oedema or infarction.

gemma, *pl.* **gemmae, 1.** a bud-like projection produced by lower forms of life during the budding process of asexual reproduction. **2.** any budlike or bulblike structure, such as a taste bud or end bulb. **gemmaceous,** *adj.*

gemmate, 1. having buds or gemmae. **2.** to reproduce by budding.

gemmation, the process of cell reproduction by budding.

gemmiferous, having buds or gemmae; gemmiparous.

gemmiform, resembling a bud or gemma.

gemmipara, an animal that produces gemmae or reproduces by budding, such as the hydra. **gemmiparous,** *adj.*

gemmulation. See **gemmation.**

gemmule, 1. the small, asexual reproductive structure produced by the parent during budding that eventually develops into an independent organism. **2.** (according to the early theory of pangenesis) any of the submicroscopic particles containing hereditary elements that are produced by each somatic cell of the parent, and are transmitted through the bloodstream to the gametes.

gender, 1. the classification of the sex of a person into male, female or intersexual. **2.** the particular sex of a person.

gender identity, the sense or awareness of knowing to which sex one belongs.

gender identity disorder, a condition characterized by a persistent feeling of discomfort or inappropriateness concerning one's anatomical sex.

gender role, the expression of a person's gender identity; the image that a person presents to both himself or herself and others demonstrating maleness or femaleness.

gene, the biological unit of genetic material and inheritance. It is considered to be a particular nucleic acid sequence within a DNA molecule that occupies a precise locus on a chromosome and is capable of self-replication by coding for a specific polypeptide chain. Kinds of genes include **complementary genes, dominant gene, lethal gene, mutant gene, operator gene, pleiotropic gene, recessive gene, regulator gene, structural gene, sublethal gene, supplementary genes** and **wild-type gene.**

gene library, (in molecular genetics) a collection of all of the genetic information of a specific species, obtained from cloned fragments.

general adaptation syndrome (GAS), the defence response of the body or psyche to injury or prolonged stress, as described by Hans Selye (1907 1982). It consists of an initial stage of shock or alarm reaction, followed by a phase of increasing resistance or adaptation using the various defence mechanisms of the body or mind, and culminating in either a state of adjustment and healing or exhaustion and disintegration.

general anaesthesia, the absence of sensation and consciousness as induced by various anaesthetic agents, given primarily by inhalation or intravenous injection. Four kinds of nerve blocks attained by general anaesthesia are sensory, voluntary motor, reflex motor and mental. There are several levels of mental block: calmness, sedation, hypnosis, narcosis and complete, potentially lethal depression of all vital regulatory functions of the medulla in the brain.

generalization, the process of reducing or bringing under a general rule or statement, such as classifying items under general categories.

generalized anaphylaxis, a severe reagin-mediated reaction to an allergen characterized by itching, oedema, wheezing respirations, apprehension, cyanosis, dyspnoea, pupillary dilatation, a rapid, weak pulse, and falling blood pressure that may rapidly result in shock and death. Systemic anaphylaxis, the most extreme form of hypersensitivity, may be caused by insect stings, proteins in animal sera, food or certain drugs; parenterally administered penicillin and contrast media containing iodide are frequent causes of anaphylactic shock.

general paresis, an organic mental disorder resulting from chronic syphilitic infection, characterized by degeneration of the cortical neurons; progressive dementia, tremor and speech disturbances; muscular weakness; and ultimately generalized paralysis.

general practitioner (GP), a family practice doctor.

general sales list, a list of medicines that can be sold legally from any retail outlet in the UK.

generation, 1. the act or process of reproduction; procreation. **2.** a group of contemporary individuals, animals or plants that are the same number of life cycles from a common ancestor. **3.** the period of time between the birth of one individual or organism and the birth of its offspring. Kinds of generation include alternate generation, asexual generation, filial generation, parental generation, sexual generation and spontaneous generation.

generative, pertaining to activity that generates new physical or mental growth, such as creative problem solving.

generic, 1. of or pertaining to a genus. **2.** of or pertaining to a substance, product or drug that is not protected by trademark. **3.** of or pertaining to the name of a kind of drug that is also the description of the drug, such as penicillin or tetracycline.

generic equivalent, a pharmaceutical product sold under its generic name, having iden-

gingivitis, a condition in which the gums are red, swollen and bleeding.

gingivoplasty, the surgical contouring of the gingival tissues to maintain healthy gingival tissue.

gingivostomatitis, multiple, painful ulcers on the gums and mucous membranes of the mouth, resulting from a herpesvirus infection.

ginglymus joint. See **hinge joint.**

ginseng, a folk remedy prepared from the root of any species of the genus *Panax*. It is used by some Oriental populations as a heart tonic, aphrodisiac and stimulant.

Giordano-Giovannetti diet, a low-protein, low-fat, high-carbohydrate diet with controlled potassium and sodium intake, used in chronic renal insufficiency and liver failure. Protein is given only in the form of essential amino acids so that the body will use excess blood urea nitrogen to synthesize the nonessential amino acids for the production of tissue protein.

gipoma, a pancreatic tumour that causes changes in secretion of gastric inhibitory polypeptide (GIP).

girdle, any curved or circular structure, such as the hipline formed by the bones and related tissues of the pelvis.

girdle sensation. See **zonaesthesia.**

glabella, a flat triangular area of bone between the two superciliary ridges of the forehead. It is sometimes used as a baseline for cephalometric measurements.

glabrous skin, smooth, hairless skin.

glacial acetic acid, a clear, colourless liquid or crystalline substance (CH_3COOH) with a pungent odour. It is obtained by the destructive distillation of wood, from acetylene and water, or oxidation of ethyl alcohol. Glacial acetic acid is a strong caustic and is potentially flammable with a low flash point. Also called **vinegar acid.**

gland, any one of many organs in the body, comprising specialized cells that secrete or excrete materials not related to their ordinary metabolism. Some glands lubricate; others, such as the pituitary gland, produce hormones; hematopoietic glands take part in the production of blood.

glanders, an infection caused by the bacillus *Pseudomonas mallei,* transmitted to humans from horses and other domestic animals. It is characterized by purulent inflammation of the mucous membranes and the development of skin nodules that ulcerate.

gland of Montgomery. See **areolar gland.**

glands of Zeiss. See **ciliary gland.**

glandular carcinoma. See **adenocarcinoma.**

glandular fever. See **infectious mononucleosis.**

glandula vestibularis major. See **Bartholin's gland.**

glans, *pl.* **glandes, 1.** a general term for a small, rounded mass, or gland-like body. **2.** erectile tissue, as on the ends of the clitoris and penis.

glans of clitoris, the erectile tissue at the end of the clitoris, continuous with the intermediate part of the vaginal vestibular bulbs. It comprises two corpora cavernosa enclosed in a dense, fibrous membrane and connected to the pubis and ischium.

glans penis, the conical tip of the penis that covers the end of the corpora cavernosa penis and corpus spongiosom like a cap. The urethral orifice is normally located at the centre of the distal tip of the glans penis.

Glanzmann's disease. See **thrombasthenia.**

Glasgow Coma Scale, a quick, practical and standardized system for assessing the degree of conscious impairment in the critically ill, and for predicting the duration and ultimate outcome of coma, primarily in patients with head injuries. The system involves three determinants: eye opening, verbal response and motor response, all of which are evaluated independently according to a rank order that indicates the level of consciousness and degree of dysfunction.

glass factor. See **factor XII.**

glaucoma, an abnormal condition of elevated pressure within an eye because of obstruction of the outflow of aqueous humour. Acute (angle-closure, closed-angle or narrow-angle) glaucoma occurs if the pupil in an eye with a narrow angle between the iris and cornea dilates markedly, causing the folded iris to block the exit of aqueous humour from the anterior chamber. Acute glaucoma is accompanied by extreme ocular pain, blurred vision, a red eye and a dilated pupil. Nausea and vomiting may occur. If untreated, acute glaucoma results in complete and permanent blindness within 2 to 5 days. Chronic (open-angle or wide-angle) glaucoma is much more common, often bilateral; it develops slowly and is genetically determined. The obstruction is believed to be within the canal of Schlemm. Chronic glaucoma may produce no symptoms except for gradual loss of peripheral vision over a period of years. Sometimes headaches, blurred vision and dull pain in the eye are present. Cupping of the optic discs may be noted on ophthalmoscopic examination. Halos around lights and central blindness are late manifestations. Both types have elevated intraocular pressure by tonometry. **glaucomatous,** *adj.*

glaucomatocyclitic crisis, a recurrent rise in intraocular pressure in one eye, resembling acute angle-closure glaucoma.

glenohumeral joint, the shoulder joint, formed by the glenoid cavity of the scapula and the head of the humerus.

glia. See **neuroglia.**

gliadin, a protein substance obtained from wheat and rye. Its solubility in diluted alcohol distinguishes gliadin from another grain protein, glutenin.

glibenclam, an oral sulphonylurea antidiabetic drug used as an adjunct to diet in lowering blood glucose levels of patients with non-insulin-dependent diabetes.

gliding, 1. a smooth, continuous movement. 2. the simplest of the four basic movements allowed by various joints of the skeleton. It is common to all movable joints and allows one surface to move smoothly over an adjacent surface, regardless of shape.

gliding joint, a synovial joint in which articulation of contiguous bones allows only gliding movements, as in the wrist and ankle.

gliding zone, an articular cartilage surface area immediately adjacent to a joint space.

glioblastoma. See **spongioblastoma.**

glioblastoma multiforme, a malignant, rapidly growing, pulpy or cystic tumour of the cerebrum, or occasionally of the spinal cord. The lesion spreads with pseudopod-like projections.

glioma, *pl.* **gliomas, gliomata,** any of the largest group of primary tumours of the brain, composed of malignant glial cells. Kinds of gliomas are **astrocytoma, ependymoma, glioblastoma multiforme, medulloblastoma** and **oligodendroglioma.**

glioma multiforme. See **glioblastoma multiforme.**

glioma retinae. See **retinoblastoma.**

glioma sarcomatosum. See **gliosarcoma.**

glioneuroma, *pl.* **glioneuromas, glioneuromata,** a neoplasm composed of nerve cells and elements of their supporting connective tissue.

gliosarcoma, *pl.* **gliosarcomas, gliosarcomata,** a tumour composed of spindle-shaped cells in the delicate supporting connective tissue of nerve cells.

gliosarcoma retinae. See **retinoblastoma.**

glipizide, an oral sulphonylurea drug used as an adjunct to diet in lowering blood glucose levels of patients with non-insulin-dependent diabetes.

glitter cells, white blood cells in which movement of granules is observed in their cytoplasm. They are seen in urine samples in cases of pyelonephritis.

Gln, abbreviation for **glutamine.**

globin, any of a group of globulin protein molecules. They become bound by the iron in haeme molecules to form haemoglobin or myoglobin.

globoid leukodystrophy. See **galactosyl ceramide lipidosis.**

globule, a small spheric mass. Kinds of globules are **dentin globule, Dobie's globule, Marchi's globule, Margagni's globule, milk globule** and **myelin globule.**

globulin, one of a broad category of simple proteins classified by solubility, electrophoretic mobility and size.

globus hystericus, a transitory sensation of a lump in the throat, often accompanying emotional conflict or acute anxiety.

globus pallidus, the smaller and more medial part of the lentiform nucleus of the brain, separated from the putamen by the lateral medullary lamina.

glomangioma, *pl.* **glomangiomas, glomangiomata,** a benign tumour that develops from a cluster of blood cells in the skin.

glomerular, of or pertaining to a glomerulus, especially a renal glomerulus.

glomerular capsule. See **Bowman's capsule.**

glomerular disease, any of a group of diseases in which the glomerulus of the kidney is affected.

glomerular filtration, the renal process whereby fluid in the blood is filtered across the capillaries of the glomerulus and into the urinary space of Bowman's capsule.

glomerular filtration rate (GFR), a measure of kidney function in terms of the amount of blood plasma that can be completely filtered in a fixed time period.

glomerulonephritis, an inflammation of the glomerulus of the kidney, characterized by proteinuria, haematuria, decreased urine production and oedema. Kinds of glomerulonephritis are **acute glomerulonephritis, chronic glomerulonephritis** and **subacute glomerulonephritis.**

glomerulus, *pl.* **glomeruli,** 1. a tuft or cluster. 2. a structure composed of blood vessels or nerve fibres, such as a renal glomerulus.

glomus, *pl.* **glomera,** a small group of arterioles connecting directly to veins and having a rich nerve supply.

glossitis, inflammation of the tongue. Acute glossitis characterized by swelling, intense pain that may be referred to the ears, salivation, fever and enlarged regional lymph nodes, may develop during an infectious disease or after a burn, bite or other injury.

glossitis parasitica. See **parasitic glossitis.**

glossitis rhomboidea mediana. See **median rhomboid glossitis.**

glossodynia, pain in the tongue, caused by acute or chronic inflammation, abscess or ulcer.

glossodynia exfoliativa, a form of chronic glossitis, characterized by pain and sensitivity to spicy foods without any evidence of a pathological condition.

glossoepiglottic, pertaining to the epiglottis and tongue.

glossohyal, of or pertaining to the tongue and horseshoe-shaped hyoid bone at the base of the tongue immediately above the thyroid cartilage.

glossolalia, speech in an unknown "language," as "speaking in tongues" during a state of religious ecstasy.

glossoncus, a local swelling or general enlargement of the tongue.

glossopathy, a pathological condition of the tongue, such as acute inflammation caused by a burn, bite, injury or infectious disease, enlargement resulting from congenital lymphangioma, or a disorder produced by mycotic infection, a malignant lesion or a congenital anomaly.

glossopexy, an adhesion of the tongue to the lip.

glossopharyngeal, of or pertaining to the tongue and pharynx.

glossopharyngeal nerve, either of a pair of cranial nerves essential to the sense of taste, for sensation in some viscera, and for secretion from certain glands.

glossopharyngeal neuralgia, a disorder of unknown origin characterized by recurrent attacks of severe pain in the back of the pharynx, tonsils, base of the tongue, and middle ear.

glossophytia, a condition of the tongue characterized by a blackish patch on which filiform papillae are greatly elongated and thickened like bristly hairs.

glossoplasty, a surgical procedure or plastic operation on the tongue performed to correct a congenital anomaly, repair an injury, or restore a measure of function after excision of a malignant lesion.

glossoptosis, the retraction or downward displacement of the tongue.

glossopyrosis, a burning sensation in the tongue caused by chronic inflammation, exposure to extremely hot or spicy food, or psychogenic glossitis.

glossorrhaphy, the surgical suturing of a wound in the tongue.

glossotrichia, a condition of the tongue characterized by a hair-like appearance of the papillae.

glottis, *pl.* **glottises, glottides, 1.** a slitlike opening between the true vocal cords (plica vocalis). **2.** the phonation apparatus of the larynx, composed of the true vocal cords and the opening between them (rima glottidis). **glottal, glottic,** *adj.*

glow curve, (in radiation dosimetry) the graphic representation of the emitted light intensity that increases with the increasing phosphor temperature.

Glu, abbreviation for glutamic acid.

glucagon, a hormone, produced by alpha cells in the islets of Langerhans, that stimulates the conversion of glycogen to glucose in the liver. Secretion of glucagon is stimulated by hypoglycaemia and growth hormone of the anterior pituitary.

glucagonoma syndrome, a disease associated with a glucagon-secreting tumour of the islet cells of the pancreas, characterized by hyperglycaemia, stomatitis, anaemia, weight loss and a characteristic rash.

glucocorticoid, an adrenocortical steroid hormone that increases glyconeogenesis, exerts an anti-inflammatory effect, and influences many body functions. The most important of the three glucocorticoids is cortisol (hydrocortisone); corticosterone is less active, and cortisone is inactive until converted to cortisol. Glucocorticoids promote the release of amino acids from muscle, mobilize fatty acids from fat stores, and increase the ability of skeletal muscles to maintain contractions and avoid fatigue.

gluconeogenesis, the formation of glycogen from fatty acids and proteins rather than carbohydrates.

glucosan, any of a large group of anhydrous polysaccharides that on hydrolysis yield a hexose, primarily anhydrides of glucose. The glucosans include cellulose, glycogen, starch and the dextrins.

glucose, a simple sugar found in certain foods, especially fruits. It is a major source of energy occurring in human and animal body fluids, and is used to correct energy deficiency and hypoglycaemia.

glucose 1-phosphate, an intermediate compound in carbohydrate metabolism.

glucose 6-phosphate, an intermediate compound in carbohydrate metabolism.

glucose-6-phosphate dehydrogenase (G-6-PD) deficiency, an inherited disorder characterized by red cells partially or completely deficient in glucose-6-phosphate dehydrogenase, a critical enzyme in aerobic glycolysis. The disorder is associated with episodes of acute haemolysis under conditions of stress or in response to certain chemicals or drugs.

glucose tolerance test, a test of the body's ability to metabolize carbohydrates by administering a standard dose of glucose and measuring the blood and urine for glucose at regular intervals thereafter.

glucosuria, abnormal presence of glucose in the urine resulting from the ingestion of large amounts of carbohydrate or from a disease, such as nephrosis or diabetes mellitus. **glucosuric,** *adj.*

glucosyl cerebroside lipidosis. See **Gaucher's disease.**

glue sniffing, the practice of inhaling the vapours of toluene, a volatile organic compound used as a solvent in certain glues.

glutamate, a salt of glutamic acid.

glutamic acid (Glu), a non-essential amino acid occurring widely in a number of proteins. Preparations of glutamic acid are used as aids for digestion.

glutamicacidaemia, an inherited disorder of amino acid metabolism resulting in an excessive level of glutamic acid.

glutamic-oxaloacetic transaminase. See **aspartate aminotransferase.**

glutamic-pyruvic transaminase. See **alanine aminotransferase.**

glutamine (Gln), a non-essential amino acid found in many proteins in the body. It functions as an amino donor for many reactions,

glutargin, arginine glutamate.

glutathione, an enzyme whose deficiency is commonly associated with haemolytic anaemia.

gluteal, pertaining to the buttocks or the muscles that form the buttocks.

gluteal gait. See **Trendelenburg gait.**

gluteal tuberosity, a ridge on the lateral posterior surface of the thigh bone to which the gluteus maximus is attached.

gluten, the insoluble protein constituent of wheat and other grains.

gluten enteropathy. See **coeliac disease.**

gluteus, any of the three muscles that form the buttocks. The **gluteus maximus** acts to extend the thigh. The **gluteus medius** acts to abduct and rotate the thigh. The **gluteus minimus** acts to abduct the thigh.

Gly, abbreviation for **glycine.**

glycerine, a sweet, colourless, oily fluid that is a pharmaceutical preparation of glycerol.

glycerol, an alcohol that is a component of fats. Glycerol is soluble in ethyl alcohol and water.

glycerol kinase, an enzyme in the liver and kidneys that catalyzes the transfer of a phosphate group from adenosin triphosphate to form adenosine diphosphate and L-glycerol-3-phosphate.

glyceryl alcohol. See **glycerine.**

glycine (Gly), a non-essential amino acid occurring widely as a component of animal and plant proteins.

glycocoll. See **glycine.**

glycogen, a polysaccharide that is the major carbohydrate stored in animal cells. It is formed from glucose and stored chiefly in the liver and, to a lesser extent, in muscle cells.

glycogenesis, the synthesis of glycogen from glucose.

glycogenolysis, the breakdown of glycogen to glucose.

glycogenosis. See **glycogen storage disease.**

glycogen storage disease, any of a group of inherited disorders of glycogen metabolism.

glycogen storage disease, type I. See **von Gierke's disease.**

glycogen storage disease, type II. See **Pompe's disease.**

glycogen storage disease, type III. See **Cori's disease.**

glycogen storage disease, type IV. See **Andersen's disease.**

glycogen storage disease, type V. See **McArdle's disease.**

glycogen storage disease, type VI. See **Hers' disease.**

glycolic acid, a substance in bile, formed by glycine and cholic acid, that aids in digestion and absorption of fats.

glycolipid, a compound that consists of a lipid and a carbohydrate, usually galactose, found primarily in the tissue of the nervous system.

glycolysis, a series of enzymatically catalysed reactions by which glucose and other sugars are broken down to yield lactic acid or pyruvic acid, releasing energy in the form of adenosine triphosphate. **Aerobic glycolysis** yields pyruvic acid in the presence of adequate oxygen. **Anaerobic glycolysis** yields lactic acid.

glycoprotein, any of the large group of conjugated proteins in which the non-protein substance is a carbohydrate. These include the mucins, the mucoids and the chondroproteins.

glycopyrronium, an anticholinergic used similarly to atropine in anaesthetic practice.

glycoside, any of several carbohydrates that yield a sugar and a non-sugar on hydrolysis. The plant *Digitalis purpurea* yields a glycoside used in the treatment of heart disease.

glycosphingolipids, compounds formed from carbohydrates and ceramide, a fatty substance, found in tissues of the central nervous system and in erythrocytes.

glycosuria, abnormal presence of a sugar, especially glucose, in the urine. It is a finding most routinely associated with diabetes mellitus. **glycosuric,** *adj.*

glycosuric acid, a compound that is an intermediate product of the metabolism of tyrosine. It forms a melanin-like staining substance in the urine of individuals with alkaptonuria.

glycosylated haemoglobin (Hb A1c), a measure used to monitor diabetic control over weeks or months. Useful in the assessment of people whose diabetes is complicated by other disorders: for example, anorexia nervosa, bulimia nervosa. Routine measurement of blood sugar on a given day may give a misleading indication of a person's overall physiological and psychological health. Measuring the glucose attached to the beta-amino acid chain in haemoglobin allows retrospective monitoring of diabetic control and can be compared with measures of psychological states in order to evaluate interventions.

glycyl alcohol. See **glycerin.**

gm, abbreviation for **gram.** Preferred abbreviation: g.

GMP, abbreviation for **guanosine monophosphate.**

gnathic, of or pertaining to the jaw or cheek.

gnathion, the lowest point in the lower border of the mandible in the median plane. It is a common reference point in the diagnosis and orthodontic treatment of various kinds of malocclusion.

gnathodynamometer, an instrument used for measuring the biting pressure of the jaws of an individual.

gnathodynia, a pain in the jaw, such as that

commonly associated with an impacted wisdom tooth.

gnathology, a field of dental or medical study that deals with the entire masticatory apparatus, including its anatomy, histology, morphology, physiology, pathology and therapeutics.

gnathoschisis, congenital cleft of the upper jaw, as in cleft palate.

gnathostatic cast, a cast of the teeth trimmed so that its occlusal plane is in its normal oral attitude when the cast is set on a plane surface.

gnathostatics, a technique of orthodontic diagnosis based on an analysis of the relationships between the teeth and certain reference points on the skull.

goal, the purpose towards which an endeavour is directed, such as the outcome of diagnostic, therapeutic and educational management of a patient's health problem.

goblet cell, one of the many specialized cells that secrete mucus and form glands of the epithelium of the stomach, intestine and parts of the respiratory tract.

goitre, a hypertrophic thyroid gland, usually evident as a pronounced swelling in the neck. The enlargement may be associated with hyperthyroidism, hypothyroidism or normal levels of thyroid function. The goitre may be cystic or fibrous, containing nodules or an increased number of follicles. See specific goiters. **goitrous,** *adj.*

gold (Au), a yellowish, soft metallic element that occurs naturally as a free metal and as the telluride $AuAgTe_4$. Its atomic number is 79 and its atomic weight is 197. Gold salts, in which gold is attached to sulphur, are often used in the treatment, or chrysotherapy, of patients with rheumatoid arthritis; however, they cause serious toxicity in about 10% of patients and some toxicity in 25% to 50%.

gold 198, a radionuclide which decays by the emission of beta particles and gamma rays, with a half-life of 2.7 days. It may be used in brachytherapy applications, for example in the form of grains implanted into a bladder malignancy.

Goldblatt kidney, an abnormal kidney in which constriction of a renal artery leads to ischaemia and release of renin, a pressor substance associated with hypertension.

gold compound, any drug containing gold salts, usually used with other drugs in rheumatoid arthritis. Gold is potentially toxic and is administered only under the supervision of a specialist.

gold file, (in dentistry) an instrument designed for removing surplus gold from gold restorations. It may be designed and used as either a pull-cut or push-cut file.

gold foil, (in dentistry) pure gold that has been rolled and beaten into a very thin sheet. It is commonly compacted into a retentive tooth cavity form, using gold's property of cold welding.

gold inlay, an intracoronal cast restoration of gold alloy.

gold knife, an instrument that may be contra-angled, with a blade or cutting edge. It is used for trimming excess metal and developing contour in foil restorations.

Goldman-Fox knife, a dental surgical instrument with a sharp cutting edge, designed for the incision and contouring of gingival tissue.

golfer's elbow, a popular term for medial epicondylitis associated with repeated use of the wrist flexors.

Golgi apparatus {Camillo Golgi, Italian anatomist, b. 1844}, one of many small membranous structures found in most cells, composed of various elements associated with the formation of carbohydrate side chains of glycoproteins, mucopolysaccharides and other substances.

Golgi-Mazzoni corpuscles {Camillo Golgi; Vittori Mazzoni, Italian physician, b. 1823}, a number of thin capsules enveloping terminal nerve fibrils in the subcutaneous tissue of the fingers.

Golgi tendon organ, a sensory nerve ending, sensitive to both tension and excessive passive stretch of a skeletal muscle.

gomphosis, *pl.* gomphoses, an articulation by the insertion of a conic process into a socket, such as insertion of a root of a tooth into an alveolus of the mandible or maxilla.

gonad, a gamete-producing gland, such as an ovary or a testis. **gonadal,** *adj.*

gonad dose, a measure of the dose of ionising radiation received by the gonads as a result of x-ray examination or treatment. Radiation dose to the gonads may result in genetic effects observed in the offspring of the person irradiated.

gonad shield, a shaped lead or lead-rubber shield used to protect the gonads of a patient from scattered radiation during certain radiographic procedures.

gonadal dysgenesis, a general designation for a variety of conditions involving anomalies in the development of gonads, such as Turner's syndrome, hermaphroditism and gonadal aplasia.

gonadotrophin, a hormonal substance that stimulates the function of testes and ovaries. The gonadotrophic follicle stimulating hormone and luteinizing hormone are produced and secreted by the anterior pituitary gland. In early pregnancy, chorionic gonadotrophin is produced by the placenta. **gonadotrophic,** *adj.*

gonial angle. See **angle of mandible.**

goniometer, an instrument for measuring ranges of joint movement.

goniometry, a system of testing for various labyrinthine diseases which affect the sense of balance. **goniometric,** *adj.*

gonioscope, an ophthalmoscope used to examine the angle of the anterior chamber of the eye, and demonstrate ocular motility and rotation.

goniotomy, an eye operation performed to remove any obstruction to the flow of aqueous humour in the front chamber of the eye. The procedure is commonly performed in cases of glaucoma.

gonoblast. See **germ cell.**

gonococcal pyomyositis, an acute inflammatory condition of a muscle caused by infection with a *Neisseria gonorrhoeae,* characterized by abscess formation and pain. It is differentiated from sarcoma by the discovery of the gonococcal diplococci within the abscess.

gonococcus, *pl.* **gonococci,** a gram-negative, intracellular diplococcus of the species *Neisseria gonorrhoeae,* the cause of gonorrhoea.

gonocyte. See **germ cell.**

gonorrhoea, a common sexually transmitted disease most often affecting the genitourinary tract and occasionally the pharynx, conjunctiva or rectum. Infection results from contact with an infected person or secretions containing the causative organism *Neisseria gonorrhoeae.* Urethritis, dysuria, purulent, greenish-yellow urethral or vaginal discharge, red or oedematous urethral meatus, and itching, burning, or pain around the vaginal or urethral orifice are characteristic. The vagina may be massively swollen and red, and the lower abdomen may be tense and very tender. As the infection spreads, which is more common in women than in men, nausea, vomiting, fever, and tachycardia may occur as salpingitis, oophoritis or peritonitis develops. Gonococcal ophthalmia involves infection of the conjunctiva and may lead to scarring and blindness. **gonorrhoeal, gonorrhoeic,** *adj.*

gonorrhoeal conjunctivitis, a severe, destructive form of purulent conjunctivitis caused by the gonococcus *Neisseria gonorrhoeae.* Newborn infants receive routine prophylaxis of a topical instillation of 1% solution of silver nitrate or an antibiotic ointment which has largely eradicated the infection in infants.

Gonyaulax catanella, a species of planktonic protozoa that produce a toxin ingested by shellfish along the coasts of North America, resulting in seafood poisoning.

Goodpasture's syndrome {Ernest W. Goodpasture, American pathologist, b. 1886}, a chronic, relapsing pulmonary haemosiderosis, usually associated with glomerulonephritis and characterized by a cough with haemoptysis, dyspnoea, anaemia and progressive renal failure.

gooseflesh. See **pilomotor reflex.**

Gordon's elementary body {Mervyn H. Gordon, English physician, b. 1872}, a particle found in tissues containing eosinophils once thought to be the viral cause of Hodgkin's disease.

Gordon's reflex {Alfred Gordon, American neurologist, b. 1874}, **1.** an abnormal variation of Babinski's reflex elicited by compressing the calf muscles, characterized by extension of the great toe and fanning of the other toes. It provides evidence of disease of the pyramidal tract. **2.** an abnormal reflex, elicited by compressing the forearm muscles, characterized by flexion of the fingers or the thumb and index finger. It is seen in diseases of the pyramidal tract.

Gosselin's fracture {Leon A. Gosselin, French surgeon, b. 1815}, a V-shaped fracture of the distal tibia, extending to the ankle.

GOT, abbreviation for **glutamicoxaloacetic transaminase.**

goundou, a condition characterized by bony exostoses of the nasal and maxillary bones, usually occurring as a late sequela of yaws in people in Africa and Latin America.

gout, a disease associated with an inborn error of uric acid metabolism that increases production or interferes with excretion of uric acid. Excess uric acid is converted to sodium urate crystals that precipitate from the blood and become deposited in joints and other tissues. The condition can result in exceedingly painful swelling of a joint, accompanied by chills and fever. The disorder is disabling and if untreated can progress to the development of tophi and destructive joint changes.

gouty arthritis. See **gout.**

Gowers' muscular dystrophy. See **distal muscular dystrophy.**

GP, abbreviation for general practitioner.

GPT, abbreviation for **glutamic-pyruvic transaminase.** See **alanine aminotransferase.**

graafian follicle {Reijnier de Graaf, Dutch physician, b. 1641}, a mature ovarian vesicle, measuring about 10 to 12 mm in diameter, that ruptures during ovulation to release the ovum. Many primary ovarian follicles, each containing an immature ovum about 35 μ in diameter, are imbedded near the surface of the ovary. Under the influence of the follicle stimulating hormone, one ovarian follicle ripens into a graafian follicle during the proliferative phase of each menstrual cycle. The cavity of the follicle collapses when the ovum is released, and the remaining follicular cells greatly enlarge to become the corpus luteum.

gracile, long, slender and graceful.

gracilis, the most superficial of the five medial femoral muscles. It functions to adduct the thigh and flex the leg, and assists in the medial rotation of the leg after it is flexed.

gradation of activity, therapeutic activities

that are appropriately paced and modified to demand maximal capacities at any point in progression or regression of the patient's condition.

graded exercise test (GXT), a test given a cardiac patient during rehabilitation to assess prognosis and quantify maximal functional capacity.

gradient, 1. the rate of increase or decrease of a measurable phenomenon, such as temperature or pressure. **2.** a visual representation of the rate of change of a measurable phenomenon; a curve.

gradient magnetic field, (in MRI) a magnetic field that changes in strength in a certain given direction. Such fields are used in magnetic resonance imaging to select a region for imaging and also to encode the location of MRI signals received from the object being imaged.

gradient of approach, the inverse relationship between the distance from a positive stimulus and the tendency to approach it.

gradient of avoidance, the inverse relationship between the distance from a negative stimulus and the tendency to avoid it.

graduated resistance exercise. See **progressive resistance exercise.**

graft, a tissue or organ taken from a site or a person and inserted into a new site or person, so as to repair a defect in structure. The graft may be temporary, such as an emergency skin transplant for extensive burns, or permanent, such as the grafted tissue growing to become a part of the body. Skin, bone, cartilage, blood vessel, nerve, muscle, cornea and whole organs, such as the kidney or the heart, may be grafted.

graft-versus-host reaction, a rejection response of certain grafts, especially bone marrow. It involves an incompatibility resulting from a deficiency in the immune response of some patients, and is commonly associated with inadequate immunosuppressive therapy. Characteristic signs may include skin lesions with oedema, erythema, ulceration, scaling and loss of hair.

Graham's law, a law stating that the rate of diffusion of a gas through a liquid (or the alveolar-capillary membrane) is directly proportional to its solubility coefficient and inversely proportional to the square root of its density.

grain (gr), the smallest unit of mass in avoirdupois, troy and apothecaries' weights, being the same in all and equal to 4.79891 mg. The troy and apothecaries' ounces contain 480 grains; the avoirdupois ounce contains 437.5 grains.

grain itch, a skin condition caused by a mite that lives in grain or straw. The lesion consists of an intensely itchy, urticarial papule surmounted by a tiny vesicle.

gram (g, gm), a unit of mass in the metric system equal to 1/1000 of a kilogram,

15.432 grains, and 0.0353 ounce avoirdupois. The preferred abbreviation is g.

gram-equivalent weight (gEq), an equivalent weight of a substance calculated as the gram mass that contains, replaces, or reacts with (directly or indirectly) the Avogadro number of hydrogen atoms.

gram-molecular weight (gmW), an amount in grams equal to the molecular weight of a substance, or the sum of all the atomic weights in its molecular formula.

gram-negative {Hans C. J. Gram, Danish physician, b. 1853}, having the pink colour of the counterstain used in Gram's method of staining micro-organisms. This property is a primary method of characterizing organisms in microbiology.

gram-positive {Hans C. J. Gram}, retaining the violet colour of the stain used in Gram's method of staining micro-organisms. This property is a primary method of characterizing organisms in microbiology.

Gram's stain {Hans C. J. Gram}, the method of staining micro-organisms using a violet stain, followed by an iodine solution, decolourizing with an alcohol or acetone solution and counterstaining with safranin. The retention of either the violet colour of the stain or the pink colour of the counterstain serves as a primary means of identifying and classifying bacteria.

grand mal seizure, an epileptic seizure characterized by a generalized involuntary muscular contraction and cessation of respiration followed by tonic and clonic spasms of the muscles. Breathing resumes with noisy respirations. The teeth may be clenched, the tongue bitten, and control of the bladder lost. As this phase of the seizure passes, the person may fall into a deep sleep for 1 hour or more. Usually, there is no recall of the seizure on awakening. A sensory warning, or aura, usually precedes each grand mal seizure.

grant, an award given to an institution, a project or an individual, usually consisting of a sum of money. A grant is given by a granting agency, the government, a foundation, private enterprise or institution, to provide financial support for research, service or training.

granular, 1. macroscopically looking or feeling like sand. **2.** microscopically appearing to have a few or many particles within or on its surface, such as a stained granular leukocyte. **granularity,** *n.*

granular conjunctivitis. See **trachoma.**

granular endoplasmic reticulum. See **endoplasmic reticulum.**

granularity. See **granular.**

granulation tissue, any soft, pink, fleshy projections that form during the healing process in a wound not healing by first intention, consisting of many capillaries surrounded by fibrous collagen.

granulocyte, one of a group of leukocytes characterized by the presence of cytoplasmic granules. Kinds of granulocytes are **basophil, eosinophil** and **neutrophil.**

granulocyte transfusion, the use of specially prepared leukocytes for the treatment of severe granulocytopenia, and prophylactically for the prevention of serious infection in patients with leukaemia or those receiving cancer chemotherapy.

granulocytic leukaemia. See **acute myeloblastic leukaemia, chronic myeloblastic leukaemia.**

granulocytic sarcoma. See **chloroma.**

granulocytopenia, an abnormal condition of the blood, characterized by a decrease in the total number of granulocytes. **granulocytopenic,** *adj.*

granulocytosis, an abnormal condition of the blood, characterized by an increase in the total number of granulocytes.

granuloma, *pl.* **granulomas, granulomata,** a mass of nodular granulation tissue resulting from inflammation, injury or infection. It is composed of capillary buds and growing fibroblasts.

granuloma annulare, a self-limited, chronic skin disease of unknown cause, consisting of reddish papules and nodules arranged in a ring and most commonly seen on the distal portions of the extremities in children.

granuloma gluteale infantum, a skin condition of the neonate characterized by large, elevated bluish or brownish-red nodules on the buttocks, often occurring as a secondary reaction to the application of strong steroid salves over a period of time.

granuloma inguinale, a sexually transmitted disease characterized by ulcers of the skin and subcutaneous tissues of the groin and genitalia. It is caused by infection with *Calymmatobacterium granulomatis,* a small gram-negative rod-shaped bacillus.

granulomatosis, a condition or disease characterized by the development of granulomas, such as **berylliosis, pulmonary Wegener's granulomatosis** or **Wegener's granulomatosis.**

granulomatous thyroiditis. See **de Quervain's thyroiditis.**

granulosa cell carcinoma. See **granulosa cell tumour.**

granulosa cell tumour, a fleshy ovarian tumour with yellow streaks that originates in cells of the primordial membrana granulosa and may grow to an extremely large size.

granulosa-theca cell tumour, an ovarian tumour composed of either granulosa (follicular) cells or theca cells or both.

granulosis, any disorder characterized by an accumulation of granules in an area of body tissue.

graph, the organization of data consisting of two or more variables along horizontal and vertical axes of a graph to show relationships between specific quantities or other specific factors.

graphospasm. See **writer's cramp.**

grasp reflex, a pathological reflex induced by stroking the palm or sole with the result that the fingers or toes flex in a grasping motion. In young infants the tonic grasp reflex is normal.

grass. See **cannabis.**

Graves' disease {Robert J. Graves, Irish physician, b. 1796}, a disorder characterized by pronounced hyperthyroidism usually associated with an enlarged thyroid gland and exophthalmos. The origin is unknown, but the disease is familial and may be autoimmune; antibodies to thyroglobulin or thyroid microsomes are found in more than 60% of patients with the disorder. Typical signs are nervousness, a fine tremor of the hands, weight loss, fatigue, breathlessness, palpitations, heat intolerance, increased metabolic rate and GI motility. There may be an enlarged thymus, generalized hyperplasia of the lymph nodes, blurred or double vision, localized oedema, atrial arrhythmias and osteoporosis. In patients with inadequately controlled Graves' disease, infection or stress may precipitate a life-threatening thyroid storm.

gravid, pregnant; carrying fertilized eggs or a fetus. **gravidity, gravidness,** *n.*

gravidness. See **gravid.**

gravity, the heaviness or weight of an object resulting from the universal effect of the attraction between any body of matter and any planetary body.

gravity-assisted movement, movement of the body carried in a position where the effects of gravity might provide some assistance.

gravity-eliminated plane, a supported position or plane in which the effect of gravity is absorbed or neutralized. In evaluation of muscle strength, certain tests are conducted in the gravity-eliminated plane.

gray (Gy), the absorption of one joule per kilogram by material exposed to ionizing radiation. One gray equals 100 rad.

great auricular nerve, (in radiation dosimetry) the S.I. unit of absorbed dose; 1 gray is equivalent to 1 joule per kilogram.

great calorie. See **calorie.**

great cardiac vein, one of the five tributaries of the coronary sinus, beginning at the apex of the heart and ascending along the anterior interventricular sulcus to the base of the ventricles. The great cardiac vein drains the blood through its tributaries from the capillaries of the myocardium.

greater multangular. See **trapezium.**

greater omentum, a filmy, transparent extension of the peritoneum, draping the transverse colon and coils of the small intestine. It is attached along the greater curvature of the stomach and the first part of the duodenum; it contains blood vessels and fat pads between its two layers.

greater trochanter, a large projection of the femur to which various muscles are attached, including the gluteus medius, gluteus maximus and obturator internus.

greater vestibular gland. See **Bartholin's gland.**

great saphenous vein, one of a pair of the longest veins in the body, containing 10 to 20 valves along its course through the leg and thigh before ending in the femoral vein. It begins in the medial marginal vein of the dorsum of the foot.

great vessels, the large arteries and veins entering and leaving the heart. They include the aorta, pulmonary arteries and veins, and superior and inferior venae cavae.

green cancer. See **chloroma.**

Greenfield's disease, a disorder of the white matter of the brain tissue, characterized by an accumulation of sphingolipid in both parenchymal and supportive tissues and a diffuse loss of myelination.

Greenough microscope. See **stereoscopic microscope.**

greenstick fracture, an incomplete fracture in which the bone is bent but fractured only on the outer arc of the bend. Children are particularly likely to have greenstick fractures.

grenade-thrower's fracture, a fracture of the humerus caused by violent muscular contraction.

Grenz rays, (in radiotherapy) low energy x-rays of between 10 and 30 kVp, which may be used to treat very superficial skin conditions.

Greulich-Pyle method, a technique for evaluating the bone age of children, using a single frontal radiograph of the left hand and wrist.

grey baby syndrome. See **grey syndrome.**

grey hepatization. See **hepatization.**

grey scale, (in ultrasonograpy) a property of the display in which intensity information is recorded as changes in the brightness of the display.

grey scale display, (in ultrasonography) a signal-processing method of selectively amplifying and displaying the level echoes from soft tissues at the expense of the larger echoes.

grey substance, the grey tissue that makes up the inner core of the spinal column, arranged in two large lateral masses connected across the midline by a narrow commissure. The grey substance splays outwards, forming the posterior and anterior horns of the spinal cord. The horns consist primarily of cell bodies of interneurons and cell bodies of motorneurons. Nuclei in the grey matter of the spinal cord function as centres for all spinal reflexes.

grey syndrome, a toxic condition in neonates, especially premature infants, caused by a reaction to chloramphenicol. The name of the condition comes from a characteristic ashen-grey cyanosis, accompanied by abdominal distention, hypothermia, vomiting, respiratory distress and vascular collapse. The condition is fatal if the drug is continued.

Grey Turner's sign, bruising of the skin of the loin in acute haemorrhagic pancreatitis.

grid (in radiography). See **secondary radiation grid.**

grid cassette. See **x-ray cassette.**

grid cut-off, (in radiography) the fading of a radiographic image at the edges of the film, due to unwated absorption of the primary beam. It is caused by the use of a grid focused at the incorrect distance, or by a mis-aligned grid.

grief, a nearly universal pattern of physical and emotional responses to bereavement, separation or loss. The physical components are similar to those of fear, hunger, rage and pain.

grief reaction, a complex of somatic and psychological symptoms associated with some extreme sorrow or loss, specifically the death of a loved one. Somatic symptoms include feelings of tightness in the throat and chest with choking and shortness of breath, abdominal distress, lack of muscular power and extreme tiredness and lethargy. Psychological reactions involve a generalized awareness of mental anguish and discomfort accompanied by feelings of guilt, anger, hostility, extreme restlessness, inability to concentrate, and lack of capacity to initiate and maintain organized patterns of activities.

grieving, anticipatory, grieving before an actual loss, as contrasted with grief in response to an actual loss. Defining characteristics include the potential loss of something or someone important, expressions of distress, denial of potential loss, anger, guilt or sorrow, and changes in eating habits, sleep patterns, activity level, libido and patterns of communication.

grieving, dysfunctional, an absence or lack of resolution of a grieving response. Defining characteristics include expressions of distress or denial of the loss; grief, anger, sadness and weeping; changes in patterns and habits of sleeping, eating and dreaming; and alterations in libido and activity levels.

griffe des orteils. See **pes cavus.**

grinder's asthma, a condition characterized by asthmatic symptoms caused by inhalation of fine particles produced by industrial grinding processes.

grinder's disease. See **silicosis.**

grinding-in, a clinical corrective grinding of one or more natural or artificial teeth to improve centric and eccentric occlusions.

grip and pinch strength, the measurable

ability to exert pressure with the hand and fingers. A patient forcefully squeezes grip or pinch dynamometers, which may express results in either pounds or kilograms of pressure.

gripes, severe and usually spasmodic pain in the abdominal region caused by an intestinal disorder.

griseofulvin, an antifungal used in the treatment of fungal infections of the skin, hair and nails.

Griswald brace, an orthosis for the control of vertebral body compression fractures. It is designed with two anterior forces with each equal to one-half the posterior force to extend the spine.

groin, each of two areas where the abdomen joins the thighs.

Groünblad-Strandberg syndrome {Ester E. Groünblad, Swedish ophthalmologist, b. 1898; James V. Strandberg, 20th century Swedish dermatologist}, an autosomal recessive disorder of connective tissue characterized by premature ageing and breakdown of the skin, grey or brown streaks on the retina, and haemorrhagic arterial degeneration including retinal bleeding that causes loss of vision. Angina pectoris and hypertension are common; weak pulse, episodic claudication and fatigue with exertion may affect the extremities.

groove, a shallow, linear depression in various structures throughout the body, such as those forming channels for nerves along the bones, those in bones for the insertion of muscles, and those between certain areas of the brain.

gross, 1. macroscopic, as *gross pathology,* from the study of tissue changes without magnification by a microscope. **2.** large or obese.

gross anatomy, the study of the organs or parts of the body large enough to be seen with the naked eye.

Grossman principle, (in radiography) a method of linear tomography.

gross sensory testing, an evaluation procedure that usually precedes motor evaluation of a patient; it includes assessment of passive motion sense in the shoulder, elbow, wrist and fingers, and ability to localize touch stimuli to specific fingers.

gross visual skills, the general ability of a person to track a large, bright object side-to-side or upside-down without jerkiness, nystagmus or convergence, and discriminate among various basic shapes and colours.

ground, 1. (in electricity) a connection between the electrical circuit and the ground, which becomes a part of the circuit. **2.** (in psychology) the background of a visual field that can enhance or inhibit the ability of a patient to focus on an object.

ground itch, pruritic macules, papules and vesicles secondary to penetration of the skin by hookworm larvae, prevalent in tropical and subtropical climates.

ground substance. See **matrix.**

group, (in research) any set of items or groups of people under study. An **experimental group** is studied to determine the effect of an event, substance or technique. A **control group** serves as a standard or reference for comparison with an experimental group. It is similar to the experimental group in number and is identical in specified characteristics, such as sex, age or other factors.

group A beta-haemolytic streptococcal (GABHS) skin disease, a bacterial skin infection that affects mainly meat packers. The source of the bacteria is believed to be freshly butchered meat.

group function, (in dentistry) the simultaneous contacting of opposing teeth in a segment or a group.

group therapy, the application of psychotherapeutic techniques within a small group of emotionally disturbed persons who, usually under the leadership of a psychotherapist, discuss their problems in an attempt to promote individual psychological growth and favourable personality change. A kind of group therapy is **psychodrama.**

growing fracture, a fracture, usually linear, in which consecutive x-ray images show a gradual separation of the fracture edges as the pressure of soft tissues force the edges apart.

growing pains, 1. rheumatism-like pains that occur in the muscles and joints of children or adolescents as a result of fatigue, emotional problems, postural defects and other causes that are not related to growth, and may be symptoms of various disorders. **2.** emotional and psychological problems experienced during adolescence.

growth, 1. an increase in the size of an organism or any of its parts, as measured in increments of weight, volume or linear dimensions, occurring as a result of hyperplasia or hypertrophy. **2.** the normal progressive anatomical, physiological, psychological, intellectual, social and cultural development from infancy to adulthood, as a result of the gradual and normal processes of accretion and assimilation. In childhood, growth is categorized according to the approximate age at which distinctive physical changes usually appear and specific developmental tasks are achieved. **3.** any abnormal localized increase of the size or number of cells, such as in a tumour or neoplasm. **4.** a proliferation of cells, specifically a bacterial culture or mould.

growth and development, altered, a condition in which an individual demonstrates deviations from the norms that apply to his or her age group. Defining characteristics include delay or difficulty in performing skills typical of the age group, altered physical growth, inability to perform self-care or self-control activities appropriate for the age, flat effect, listlessness and decreased responses.

growth failure, a lack of normal physical and psychologic development as a result of genetic, nutritional, pathological or psychosocial factors.

growth hormone (GH), a single-chain peptide secreted by the anterior pituitary gland in response to growth hormone releasing factor (GHRF) from the hypothalamus. Growth hormone promotes protein synthesis in all cells, increases fat mobilization and use of fatty acids for energy, and decreases use of carbohydrate. A deficiency of GH causes dwarfism; an excess results in gigantism or acromegaly.

growth hormone release inhibiting hormone. See **somatostatin.**

growth hormone releasing factor (GHRF), somatotropin releasing factor released by the hypothalamus.

Grünfelder's reflex, an involuntary dorsal flexion of the great toe with a fan-like spreading of the other toes, caused by continued pressure on the posterior lateral fontanel.

grunting, abnormal, short, audible, grunt-like breaks in exhalation that often accompany severe chest pain. The grunt occurs because the glottis briefly stops the flow of air, halting the movement of the lungs and their surrounding or supporting structures.

G-6-PD deficiency, abbreviation for **glucose-6-phosphate dehydrogenase deficiency.**

GTP, abbreviation for **guanosine triphosphate.**

GU, abbreviation for **genitourinary.**

guaiac, a wood resin, commonly used as a reagent in laboratory tests for the presence of occult blood.

guaiacol poisoning. See **phenol poisoning.**

guaiac test, a test, using guaiac as a reagent, performed on faeces and urine for detecting occult blood in the intestinal and urinary tracts.

guaifenesin, glyceryl guaiacolate, an expectorant.

guanase. See **guanine deaminase.**

guanethidine sulphate, an adrenergic neuron blocking drug used in the treatment of moderate and severe hypertension, and in eyedrops for the treatment of glaucoma.

guanine, a major purine base found in nucleotides and a fundamental constituent of DNA and RNA. In free or uncombined form it occurs in trace amounts in most cells, usually as a product of the enzymatic hydrolysis of nucleic acids and nucleotides.

guanine deaminase, an enzyme that catalyses the hydrolysis of guanine to xanthine and ammonia.

guanine deaminase assay, the measurement of an enzyme in the blood that commonly increases in patients with hepatitis and other types of liver disease and mononucleosis.

guanosine, a compound derived from a nucleic acid, composed of guanine and a sugar, D-ribose. It is a major molecular component of DNA and RNA.

guanosine monophosphate (GMP), a nucleotide that plays an important role in various metabolic reactions and in the formation of RNA from DNA templates.

guanosine triphosphate (GTP), a high-energy nucleotide, similar to adenosine triphosphate, that functions in various metabolic reactions, such as the activation of fatty acids and formation of the peptide bond in protein synthesis.

guaranine, caffeine.

Gubbay test of motor proficiency, a screening test for the identification of developmental dyspraxia.

Guedel's signs {Arthur E. Guedel, American anaesthesiologist, b. 1883}, a system for describing the stages and planes of anaesthesia during an operative procedure. **Stage I** (amnesia and analgesia) begins with the administration of an anaesthetic and continues to the loss of consciousness. **Stage II** (delirium or excitement) begins with the loss of consciousness and includes the onset of total anaesthesia. **Stage III** (surgical anaesthesia) begins with establishment of a regular pattern of breathing and total loss of consciousness, and includes the period during which signs of respiratory or cardiovascular failure first appear. This stage is divided into four planes: At *plane 1* all movements cease and respiration is regular and "automatic." At *plane 2* the eyeballs become fixed centrally, conjunctivae lose their luster and intercostal muscle activity diminishes. At *plane 3* intercostal paralysis occurs and respiration becomes solely diaphragmatic. At *plane 4* deep anaesthesia is achieved, with cessation of spontaneous respiration and absence of sensation. **Stage IV** (premortem) signals danger. This stage is characterized by pupils that are maximally dilated and skin that is cold and ashen. Blood pressure is extremely low, often unmeasurable, and the brachial pulse is feeble or entirely absent. Cardiac arrest is imminent.

Guérin's fracture {Alphonse F.M. Guérin, French surgeon, b. 1816}, a fracture of the maxilla.

guided imagery, a therapeutic technique in which a patient is encouraged to concentrate on an image that helps relieve pain or discomfort.

guide plane, 1. a part of an orthodontic appliance that has an established inclined plane for changing the occlusal relation of the maxillary and mandibular teeth, and permitting their movement to normal positions. **2.** a plane developed on the occlusal sufaces of occlusion rims for positioning the mandible in centric relation. **3.** two or more vertically parallel surfaces of abutment teeth shaped to direct the path of placement and removal of a partial denture.

guide-shoe marks, an x-ray image artefact caused by pressure of guide shoes, i.e. curved metal lips that guide x-ray film in automatic developing systems.

Guillain-Barré syndrome {Georges Guillain, French neurologist, b. 1876; Jean A. Barré, French neurologist, b. 1880}, an idiopathic, peripheral polyneuritis occurring between 1 and 3 weeks after a mild episode of fever associated with a viral infection or immunization. Symmetrical pain and weakness affect the extremities, and paralysis may develop. The neuritis may spread, ascending to the trunk and involving the face, arms and thoracic muscles.

guilt, a feeling caused by tension between the ego and superego when one falls below the standards set for oneself.

guilty, (in criminal law) a verdict by the court, finding that to a moral certainty it is beyond reasonable doubt that the defendant committed the crime and is responsible for the offense as charged.

Guinea worm infection. See **dracunculiasis.**

gullet. See **oesophagus.**

gum, **1.** a sticky excretion from certain plants. **2.** See **gingiva.**

gumboil, an abscess of the gingiva and periosteum resulting from injury, infection or dental decay. The gum is characteristically red, swollen and tender.

gum camphor. See **camphor.**

gumma, **1.** a granuloma, characteristic of tertiary syphilis, varying from 1 mm to 1 cm in diameter. It is usually encapsulated and contains a central necrotic mass surrounded by inflammatory and fibrotic zones of tissue. **2.** a soft granulomatous lesion sometimes occurring with tuberculosis.

Gunning's splint {Thomas B. Gunning, American dentist, b. 1813}, a maxillomandibular splint used for supporting the maxilla and mandible in jaw surgery.

gunshot fracture, a fracture caused by a bullet or similar missile.

Gunther's disease {Hans Gunther, German physician, b. 1884}, a rare congenital disorder of porphyrin metabolism associated with sunlight-induced skin lesions.

gurgling rale, an abnormal coarse sound heard during auscultation, especially over large cavities or over a trachea nearly filled with secretions.

Gurvich radiation. See **mitogenetic radiation.**

gustatory organ. See **taste bud.**

gut, **1.** intestine. **2.** *informal.* digestive tract.

3. suture material manufactured from the intestines of sheep.

Guthrie test, a blood test carried out on a newborn (usually by heel prick) for the detection of phenylketonuria. The test is carried out between the 6th and 14th day, when the baby is well-established on milk feeds. The test is deferred if the baby is receiving antibiotics, as this is a bacterial inhibition test.

gutta-percha, the coagulated, rubbery sap of various tropical trees, used for temporarily sealing the dressings of prepared tooth cavities.

gutta-percha point, any of the fine, tapered cylinders of gutta-percha that may be used to fill a root canal.

guttate psoriasis, an acute form of psoriasis consisting of teardrop-shaped, red, scaly patches measuring 3 to 10 mm all over the body.

Guyon tunnel, a fibrosseous tunnel formed in part by the pisohamate ligament of the hand. It contains the ulnar artery and nerve, and may be the site of a compression injury.

gynaecography, a radiographic examination of the uterus and ovaries by means of intraperitoneal carbon dioxide insufflation. **gynaecogram,** *n.*

gynaecoid pelvis, a type of pelvis characteristic of the normal female and associated with the smallest incidence of cephalopelvic disproportion.

gynaecology, a branch of medicine concerned with the healthcare of women, including their sexual and reproductive function and the diseases of their reproductive organs, excluding diseases of the breast. **gynaecological,** *adj.*

gynaecomastia, an abnormal enlargement of one or both breasts in men. The condition is usually temporary and benign. It may be caused by a hormonal imbalance, tumour of the testis or pituitary, medication with oestrogens or steroidal compounds, or failure of the liver to inactivate circulating oestrogen, as in alcoholic cirrhosis.

gynaephobia, an anxiety disorder characterized by a morbid fear of women or a morbid aversion to the society of women.

gynandrous, describing a man or a woman who has some of the physical characteristics usually attributed to the other sex, such as a female pseudohermaphrodite. **gynandry,** *n.*

gynogamone, a gamone secreted by the female gamete.

gypsum, a mineral composed mainly of crushed calcium sulphate hemihydrate. It is used in making plaster of paris surgical casts and impressions for dentures. Gypsum dust has an irritant action on the mucous membranes of the respiratory tract and conjunctiva.

gyrase, an enzyme that enables certain DNA molecules to twist themselves into coils in order to replicate.

gyri cerebri, the convolutions of the outer surface of the cerebral hemisphere, separated from each other by sulci.

gyrus, one of the tortuous convolutions of the surface of the brain caused by infolding of the cortex.

H, symbol for hydrogen.

$_1$H, symbol for deuterium.

$_2$H, symbol for tritium.

habeas corpus, a right retained by all psychiatric patients that enables an individual who claims to be deprived of liberty and detained illegally to be heard.

habilitation, the process of supplying a person with the means to develop maximum independence in activities of daily living through training or treatment.

habit, 1. a customary or particular practice, manner or mode of behaviour. **2.** an involuntary pattern of behaviour or thought. **3.** *archaic,* appearance or physique, as pyknic habit. **4.** the habitual use of drugs or narcotics.

habitat, a natural environment where a species of a plant or animal, including humans, may live and grow normally.

habit spasm, an involuntary twitching or tic usually involving a small muscle group of the face, neck or shoulders, and resulting in movements such as spasmodic blinking or rapid jerking of the head to the side.

habit training, the process of teaching a child how to adjust to the demands of the external world by forming certain habits, primarily those related to eating, sleeping, elimination and dress.

habitual abortion, when three or more consecutive abortions have taken place.

habitual fever. See **habitual hyperthermia.**

habitual hyperthermia, a condition of unknown cause occurring in young females, characterized by body temperatures of 37.2°C to 38°C (99° to 100.5°F) regularly or intermittently for years, associated with fatigue, malaise, vague aches and pains, insomnia, bowel disturbances and headaches.

habituation, 1. an acquired tolerance from repeated exposure to a particular stimulus. **2.** a decline and eventual elimination of a conditioned response by repetition of the conditioned stimulus. **3.** psychological and emotional dependence on a drug, tobacco or alcohol, resulting from the repeated use of the substance but without the addictive, physiological need to increase dosage.

habitus, describing a person's appearance or physique, such as an athletic habitus.

hacking, a form of massage in which the skin is struck using the back of the tips of the three medial fingers.

Haeckel's law. See **recapitulation theory.**

haemadsorption, a process in which a substance or an agent, as certain viruses and bacilli, adheres to the surface of an erythrocyte.

haemagglutination, the coagulation of erythrocytes.

haemagglutinin, a kind of antibody that agglutinates red blood cells. These substances are classified according to the source of cells agglutinated as **autologous** (from the same organism), **homologous** (from an organism of the same species) and **heterologous** (from an organism of a different species).

haemangioblastoma, *pl.* **haemangioblastomas, haemangioblastomata,** a brain tumour composed of a proliferation of capillaries and of disorganized clusters of capillary cells or angioblasts.

haemangioendothelioma, *pl.* **haemangioendotheliomas, haemangioendotheliomata, 1.** a tumour, consisting of endothelial cells, that grows around an artery or a vein. It rarely becomes malignant. **2.** malignant haemangioendothelioma.

haemangioma, *pl.* **haemangiomas, haemangiomata,** a benign tumour consisting of a mass of blood vessels. Kinds of haemangiomas include **capillary haemangioma, cavernous haemangioma** and **nevus flammeus.**

haemangioma simplex. See **capillary haemangioma.**

haemangiosarcoma. See **angiosarcoma.**

haematemesis, vomiting of bright red blood, indicating rapid upper GI bleeding. It is commonly associated with oesophageal varices or peptic ulcer.

haematocoele, a cyst-like accumulation of blood within the tunica vaginalis of the scrotum. It is usually caused by injury.

haematochezia, the passage of red blood through the rectum. The cause is usually bleeding in the colon or rectum, but it can result from loss of blood higher in the digestive tract, depending on the transit time. Cancer, colitis and ulcers are among the causes of haematochezia.

haematocrit, a measure of the packed cell volume of red cells, expressed as a percentage of the total blood volume. The normal range is between 43% and 49% in men, and between 37% and 43% in women.

haematogenic shock, a condition of shock caused by loss of blood or plasma.

haematogenous, originating or transported in the blood.

haematological death syndrome. See **acute radiation exposure.**

haematological effect, (in radiobiology) the

response of blood cells to radiation exposure. In general, all types of blood cells are destroyed by radiation, and the degree of cell depletion increases with increasing dose.

haematologist, a medical specialist in the field of haematology.

haematology, scientific medical study of blood and blood-forming tissues. **haematological,** *adj.*

haematoma, a collection of extravasated blood trapped in the tissues of the skin or in an organ, resulting from trauma or incomplete haemostasis after surgery. Initially, there is frank bleeding into the space; if the space is limited, pressure slows and eventually stops the flow of blood. The blood clots, serum collects, the clot hardens, and the mass becomes palpable to the examiner and is often painful to the patient.

haematomyelia, the appearance of frank blood in the fluid of the spinal cord.

haematopoiesis, the normal formation and development of blood cells in the bone marrow. In severe anaemia and other haematological disorders, cells may be produced in organs outside the marrow (extramedullary haematopoiesis). **haematopoietic,** *adj.*

haematopoietic syndrome, a group of clinical features associated with effects of radiation on the blood and lymph tissues. It is characterized by vomiting, destruction of the bone marrow, and atrophy of the spleen and lymph nodes.

haematospermia, the presence of blood in the semen. Causes may include vascular congestion, infection involving seminal vesicles, coitus interruptus, sexual abstinence or frequent coitus.

haematoxylin-eosin, a stain commonly used to treat tissue sections on microscope slides.

haematuria, abnormal presence of blood in the urine. Haematuria is symptomatic of many renal diseases and disorders of the genitourinary system. **haematuric,** *adj.*

haeme, the pigmented, iron containing, non-protein portion of the haemoglobin molecule. There are four haeme groups in a haemoglobin molecule, each consisting of a cyclic structure of four pyrrole residues, called protoporphyrin, and an atom of iron in the centre.

haemoblastic leukaemia. See **stem cell leukaemia.**

haemochromatosis, a rare disease of iron metabolism, characterized pathologically by excess iron deposits throughout the body.

haemoconcentration, an increase in the number of red blood cells resulting either from a decrease in plasma volume or increased production of erythrocytes.

haemocyanin, an oxygen-carrying protein molecule present in certain lower animals, particularly arthropods and mollusks.

haemocytoblastic leukaemia. See **stem cell leukaemia.**

haemodiafiltration, a technique similar to haemofiltration, used to treat uraemia by convective transport of the solute rather than diffusion.

haemodialysis, a procedure in which impurities or wastes are removed from the blood. It is used in treating renal insufficiency and various toxic conditions. The patient's blood is shunted from the body through a machine for diffusion and ultrafiltration, and then returned to the patient's circulation. Haemodialysis requires access to the patient's bloodstream, a mechanism for the transport of the blood to and from the dialyser, and a dialyser. Access may be achieved by an external shunt or an arteriovenous fistula. The external shunt is constructed by inserting two cannulas through the skin into a large vein and a large artery. An arteriovenous fistula is created by the anastomosis of a large vein to an artery. Dialysis takes from 3 to 8 hours; it may be necessary daily in acute situations, or 2 or 3 times a week in chronic renal failure.

haemodialyser. See **dialyser.**

haemodynamics, the study of the physical aspects of blood circulation, including cardiac function and peripheral vascular physiology.

haemofiltration, a type of haemodialysis in which there is convective transport of the solute through ultrafiltration across the membrane.

haemoglobin (Hb), a complex protein-iron compound in the blood that carries oxygen to the cells from the lungs and carbon dioxide away from the cells to the lungs. Each erythrocyte contains 200 to 300 molecules of haemoglobin, each molecule of haemoglobin contains several molecules of haeme, and each molecule of haeme can carry one molecule of oxygen. A haemoglobin molecule contains four globin polypeptide chains, designated in adults as the alpha (Grk α), beta (Grk β), gamma (Grk γ), and delta (Grk δ) chains. More than 100 haemoglobins with different electrophoretic mobilities and characteristics have been identified and classified, such as S, C, D and O. New haemoglobins are named for the laboratory, town or hospital where they are discovered.

haemoglobin oxygen saturation, a quantitative measure of volume of oxygen per volume of blood, depending on the grams of haemoglobin per decilitre of blood.

haemoglobin saturation, the amount of oxygen combined with haemoglobin in proportion to the amount of oxygen the haemoglobin is capable of carrying.

haemoglobin $_{\text{Seattle}}$, an abnormal haemoglobin in which glutamic acid replaces alanine at position 76 of the β chain.

haemoglobin $_{Yakima}$, an abnormal haemoglobin in which histadine replaces aspartic acid at position 99 in the β chain.

haemoglobin A (Hb A), a normal haemoglobin.

haemoglobin A, a normal haemoglobin that occurs in small amounts in adults, characterized by the substitution of δ chains for β chains.

haemoglobin C, an abnormal type of haemoglobin characterized by the substitution of lysine for glutamic acid at position 6 of the β chain of the haemoglobin molecule.

haemoglobin C (Hb C) disease, a genetic blood disorder characterized by a moderate, chronic haemolytic anaemia and associated with the presence of haemoglobin C, an abnormal form of the red cell pigment.

haemoglobin electrophoresis, a test to identify various abnormal haemoglobins in the blood, including certain genetic disorders such as sickle cell anaemia.

haemoglobinaemia, presence of free haemoglobin in the blood plasma.

haemoglobin F (Hb F), the normal haemoglobin of the fetus, most of which is broken down in the first days after birth and replaced by haemoglobin A. It has an increased capacity to carry oxygen and is present in increased amounts in some pathological conditions.

haemoglobinopathy, any of a group of inherited disorders characterized by variation of the structure of the haemoglobin molecule. Kinds of haemoglobinopathies include haemoglobin C disease, haemoglobin S-C disease and sickle cell anaemia.

haemoglobin S (Hb S), an abnormal type of haemoglobin, characterized by the substitution of the amino acid valine for glutamic acid in the β chain of the haemoglobin molecule.

haemoglobin S-C (Hb S-C) disease, a genetic blood disorder in which two different abnormal alleles, one for haemoglobin S and one for haemoglobin C, are inherited.

haemoglobinuria, an abnormal presence of haemoglobin in the urine, unattached to red blood cells. Kinds of haemoglobinuria include cold haemoglobinuria, march haemoglobinuria and nocturnal haemoglobinuria.

haemoglobin variant, any type of haemoglobin other than haemoglobin A. All variants are characterized by an alteration in the sequence of amino acids in the polypeptide chains of globin contained in the haemoglobin molecule. These variations are genetically determined.

haemogram, a written or graphic record of a differential blood count that emphasizes the size, shape, special characteristics and numbers of the solid components of the blood.

haemolysin, any one of the numerous substances that lyse or dissolve red blood cells.

Haemolysins are produced by strains of many kinds of bacteria, including some of the staphylococci and streptococci. They are also contained in venoms and in certain vegetables.

haemolysis, the breakdown of red blood cells and the release of haemoglobin. It occurs normally at the end of the lifespan of a red cell, but may occur in a variety of other circumstances, including certain antigen-antibody reactions, metabolic abnormalities and mechanical trauma, as in cardiac prosthesis or exposure to snake venoms. haemolytic, adj.

haemolytic anaemia, a disorder characterized by the premature destruction of red blood cells. Anaemia may be minimal or absent, reflecting the ability of the bone marrow to increase production of red blood cells.

haemolytic disease of the newborn. See erythroblastosis fetalis.

haemolytic jaundice, a yellowish discolouration of the skin caused by a breakdown of red blood cells, resulting in excess production of bilirubin.

haemolytic uraemia syndrome, a rare kidney disorder marked by renal failure, microangiopathic haemolytic anaemia and platelet deficiency.

haemoperfusion, the perfusion of blood through a sorbent device, such as activated charcoal or resin beads, rather than through dialysis equipment. Haemoperfusion may be used in treating uraemia, liver failure and certain forms of drug toxicity.

haemopericardium, an accumulation of blood within the pericardial sac surrounding the heart.

haemoperitoneum, the presence of extravasated blood in the peritoneal cavity.

haemophilia, a group of hereditary bleeding disorders in which there is a deficiency of one of the factors necessary for coagulation of the blood. The two most common forms of the disorder are haemophilia A and haemophilia B. Greater than usual loss of blood during dental procedures, epistaxis, haematoma and haemarthrosis are common problems in haemophilia. Severe internal haemorrhage and haematuria are less common. See von Willebrand's disease and specific blood factors. haemophiliac, n., haemophilic, adj.

haemophilia A, a hereditary blood disorder, transmitted as an X-linked recessive trait, caused by a deficiency of coagulation factor VIII. Haemophilia A is considered the classic type of haemophilia.

haemophilia B, a hereditary blood disorder, transmitted as an X-linked recessive trait, caused by a deficiency of factor IX. See coagulation factor, haemophilia.

haemophilia C, a hereditary blood disorder transmitted as an X-linked recessive trait. It is caused by a deficiency of factor XI.

Haemophilus, a genus of gram-negative pathogenic bacteria, frequently found in the respiratory tract of humans and other animals, such as *Haemophilus influenzae,* which causes influenza and one form of meningitis.

Haemophilus influenzae, a small, gram-negative, non-motile, parasitic bacterium that occurs in two forms, encapsulated and non-encapsulated, and in six types, a, b, c, d, e and f. Almost all infections are caused by encapsulated type b organisms.

haemopoietic, related to the process of formation and development of the various types of blood cells.

haemoptysis, coughing up of blood from the respiratory tract. Blood-streaked sputum often occurs in minor upper respiratory infections or bronchitis. More profuse bleeding may indicate Aspergillus infection, lung abcess, tuberculosis, or bronchogenic carcinoma.

haemorrhage, a loss of a large amount of blood in a short period of time, either externally or internally. Haemorrhage may be arterial, venous or capillary. Symptoms of massive haemorrhage are related to hypovolaemic shock: rapid, thready pulse; thirst; cold, clammy skin; sighing respirations; dizziness; syncope; pallor; apprehension; restlessness; and hypotension. If bleeding is contained within a cavity or joint, pain will develop as the capsule or cavity is stretched by the rapidly expanding volume of blood. **haemorrhagic,** *adj.*

haemorrhagic diathesis, an inherited predisposition to any one of a number of abnormalities characterized by excessive bleeding.

haemorrhagic disease of newborn, a bleeding disorder of neonates that is usually caused by a deficiency of vitamin K.

haemorrhagic familial angiomatosis. See **Osler-Weber-Rendu disease.**

haemorrhagic fever, an arbovirus infection characterized by fever, chills, headache, malaise and respiratory or GI symptoms, followed by capillary haemorrhages. Severe infection leads to oliguria, kidney failure, hypotension and possibly death. Many forms of the disease occur in specific geographic areas. Some kinds of haemorrhagic fever are **Argentine haemorrhagic fever, dengue fever** and **Far Eastern haemorrhagic fever.**

haemorrhagic gastritis, a form of acute gastritis usually caused by a toxic agent, such as alcohol, aspirin or other drugs, or bacterial toxins that irritate the lining of the stomach. If bleeding is significant, vasoconstrictors and ice water lavage of the stomach may be necessary.

haemorrhagic lung. See **congestive atelectasis.**

haemorrhagic scurvy. See **infantile scurvy.**

haemorrhagic shock, a state of physical collapse and prostration associated with the sudden and rapid loss of significant amounts of blood. Severe traumatic injuries often cause such blood losses, which in turn produce low blood pressure in affected individuals.

haemorrhoid, a varicosity in the lower rectum or anus caused by congestion in the veins of the haemorrhoidal plexus. Internal haemorrhoids originate above the internal sphincter of the anus. If they become large enough to protude from the anus, they become constricted and painful. Small internal haemorrhoids may bleed with defaecation. External haemorrhoids appear outside the anal sphincter. They are usually not painful, and bleeding does not occur unless a haemorrhoidal vein ruptures or thromboses.

haemosiderin, an iron-rich pigment that is a product of red cell haemolysis. Iron is often stored in this form.

haemosiderosis an increased deposition of iron in a variety of tissues, usually in the form of haemosiderin and without tissue damage.

haemostasis, the termination of bleeding by mechanical or chemical means or by the complex coagulation process of the body, consisting of vasoconstriction, platelet aggregation, and thrombin and fibrin synthesis.

haemostatic, of or pertaining to a procedure, device or substance that arrests the flow of blood. Direct pressure, tourniquets and surgical clamps are mechanical haemostatic measures. Cold applications are haemostatic and include the use of an ice bag on the abdomen to halt uterine bleeding, and irrigation of the stomach with an iced solution to check gastric bleeding. Gelatin sponges, solutions of thrombin and microfibrillar collagen, which causes the aggregation of platelets and formation of clots, are used to arrest bleeding in surgical procedures.

haemothorax, an accumulation of blood and fluid in the pleural cavity, between the parietal and visceral pleura. It is usually the result of trauma. Haemothorax may also be caused by the rupture of small blood vessels as a result of inflammation.

haemotroph, the total nutritive substances supplied to the embryo from the maternal circulation after the development of the placenta. Also spelled **haemotrophe. haemotrophic,** *adj.*

hafnium (Hf), a hard, brittle, silver-grey metallic element of the first transition group. Its atomic number is 72 and its atomic weight is 178.49.

Hagedorn needle {Hans C. Hagedorn, Danish physician, b. 1888}, a flat surgical needle with a cutting edge near its point and a very large eye at the other end.

Hageman factor. See **factor XII.**

Haglund's deformity, a foot disorder characterized by an enlarged posterior-superior lateral aspect of the calcaneus, often associated with an inverted subtalar joint. It is a common cause of posterior Achilles bursitis.

hair, a filament of keratin consisting of a root and a shaft formed in a specialized follicle in the epidermis. There are three stages of hair development: **anagen,** the active growing stage; **catagen,** a short interlude between growth and resting phases; and **telogen,** the resting or club stage before shedding. Scalp hair grows at an average rate of 1 mm every 3 days, body and eyebrow hair at a much slower rate.

hair matrix carcinoma. See **basal cell carcinoma.**

hair pulling. See **trichotillomania.**

hairy-cell leukaemia, an uncommon neoplasm of blood-forming tissues, characterized by pancytopenia, a massively enlarged spleen, and the presence in blood and bone marrow of reticulum cells with many fine projections on their surface. The disease usually appears in the fifth decade, with an insidious onset and a variable course marked by anaemia, thrombocytopenia and spontaneous bruising.

hairy leukoplakia, a form of leukoplakia characterized by raised, white puffy areas on the sides of the tongue.

hairy tongue, a dark, pigmented overgrowth of the filiform papillae of the tongue, a benign and frequent side effect of some antibiotics.

halcinonide, a very potent corticosteroid used topically as an anti-inflammatory agent.

half-life (t), 1. the time taken for the activity of a radionuclide to reduce by one-half. Each radionuclide has a unique half-life, which may be from a fraction of a second to thousands of years. **2.** the amount of time required to reduce a drug level to one-half of its initial value.

half-normal saline, (in respiratory therapy) a solution of 0.45% NaCl used for mucosal hydration. As the fluid tends to evaporate, the saline concentration increases achieving nearly normal saline concentration in the respiratory tract.

half-sibling, one of two or more children who have at least one parent in common; a half-brother or half-sister.

half-value layer (HVL), (in radiation dosimetry) the thickness of a named material required to reduce the intensity of a narrow beam of radiation to one-half of its original value. Also called **half-value thickness (HVT).**

half-value thickness (HVT). See **half-value layer.**

halfway house, a specialized treatment facility, usually for psychiatric patients who no longer require complete hospitalization but who need some care and time to adjust to living independently.

halisteresis, osteomalacia; a loss or lack of calcium salts in bone.

halitosis, offensive breath resulting from poor oral hygiene, dental or oral infections, the ingestion of certain foods, use of tobacco or some systemic diseases, such as the odour of acetone in diabetes and ammonia in liver disease.

Hallervorden-Spatz disease {Julius Hallervorden, German neurologist, b. 1882; H. Spatz, German neurologist, b. 1888}, a progressive neurological disease of children, with symptoms of parkinsonism. It is characterized by rigidity, athetosis and dementia.

Hallpike caloric test, a method for evaluating the function of the vestibule of the ear in patients with vertigo or hearing loss. Irrigation of the ears with cool and warm water or air mimics the stimulus of turning in the vestibular apparatus, causing nystagmus.

hallucination, a sensory perception that does not result from an external stimulus. It can occur in any of the senses and is classified accordingly as auditory, gustatory, olfactory, tactile or visual. Kinds of hallucinations are **hypnagogic hallucination, lilliputian hallucination** and **stump hallucination. hallucinate,** v.

hallucinogen, a substance that causes hallucination, usually accompanied by some or all of the following: mood change, anxiety, sensory distortion, delusion, depersonalization, increased pulse, temperature and blood pressure, and dilatation of the pupils. Hallucinogens include **lysergide, mescaline, peyote, phencyclidine hydrochloride** and **psilocybin.**

hallucinosis, a pathological mental state in which awareness consists primarily or exclusively of hallucinations. A kind of hallucinosis is alcoholic hallucinosis.

hallux, pl. **halluces,** the great toe.

hallux rigidus, a painful deformity of the great toe, limiting motion at the metatarsophalangeal joint.

hallux valgus, a deformity in which the great toe is angulated away from the midline of the body towards the other toes; in some cases the great toe rides over or under the other toes.

halo cast, an orthopaedic device used to help immobilize the neck and head. It incorporates the trunk, usually with shoulder straps, and an apparatus by means of an outrigger within the cast to secure pins to a band around the skull.

halo effect, the beneficial effect of an interview or other encounter, as may occur in the course of a research project or a healthcare visit. It is the result of indefinable interpersonal factors present in the interaction.

halogenated hydrocarbon, a volatile liquid used for general anaesthesia, administered in combination with nitrous oxide, oxygen, or both. Nausea, vomiting, laryngospasm and pharyngeal irritation are less severe and frequent when this anaesthesia is used. Kinds of halogenated hydrocarbons are **enflurane, halothane, isoflurane, methoxyflurane** and **trichloroethylene.**

haloperidol, a butyrophenone tranquillizer used in the treatment of psychotic disorders, as an antiemetic and in the control of Gilles de la Tourette's syndrome.

halothane, an inhalational anaesthetic used for induction and maintenance of general anaesthesia.

halothane-related hepatitis, an adverse reaction of some patients to inhalation of halothane, a general anaesthetic. The reaction is characterized by hepatitis and a severe fever that develops several days after exposure to the anaesthetic.

hamamelis water. See **witch hazel, def 2.**

hamate bone, a carpal bone that rests on the fourth and fifth metacarpal bones and projects a hook-like process, the hamulus, from its palmar surface.

Hamman-Rich syndrome. See **interstitial pneumonia.**

hammertoe, a foot digit permanently flexed at the midphalangeal joint, resulting in a claw-like appearance. The anomaly may be present in more than one digit but is most common in the second toe.

hamstring muscle, any one of three muscles at the back of the thigh; medially the semimembranosus and semitendinosus, and laterally the biceps femoris.

hamstring reflex, a normal deep tendon reflex elicited by tapping one of the hamstring tendons behind the knee, resulting in contraction of the tendon and flexion of the knee.

hamstring tendon, one of the three tendons from the three hamstring muscles in the back of the thigh.

hamular notch. See **pterygomaxillary notch.**

hand, the part of the upper limb distal to the forearm. It is the most flexible part of the skeleton and has a total of 27 bones, 8 forming the carpus, 5 forming the metacarpus and 14 comprising the phalangeal section.

hand condenser, (in dentistry) an instrument for compacting amalgams or gold foil using force applied by the operator.

hand dynamometry, a technique for measuring muscle function. A hand dynamometer is used with the non-dominant arm to measure grip strength. Values obtained are compared with a reference range. Values less than normal may indicate protein malnutrition.

handedness, voluntary or involuntary preference for use of either the left or right hand. The preference is related to cerebral dominance, with left-handedness corresponding to dominance of the right side of the brain and vice versa.

hand-foot-and-mouth disease, a Coxsackie viral infection characterized by the appearance of painful ulcers and vesicles on the mucous membranes of the mouth and on the hands and feet. The disease is highly contagious and affects mainly children.

hand-foot syndrome. See **sickle cell crisis.**

handicapped, referring to a person who has a congenital or acquired mental or physical defect that interferes with normal functioning of the body system or the ability to be self-sufficient in modern society.

handpiece, a device for holding rotary instruments in a dental engine or condensing points in mechanical condensing units.

hanging drop preparation, a technique used for the examination and identification of certain micro-organisms, such as spirochetes or trichomonads. A specimen suspected of containing the micro-organism is diluted with a sterile isotonic solution. A drop of this fluid mixture is placed on a glass cover slip, which is then inverted carefully and placed over the slide so that the drop is hanging from the slip into the concavity in the special slide.

hangman's fracture, a fracture of the posterior elements of the cervical vertebrae with dislocation of C2 or C3.

hangnail, a piece of partially disconnected epidermis of the cuticle or nail fold. Tearing the skin fragment causes a red, painful, easily infected sore.

hangover, a popular term for a group of symptoms, including nausea, thirst, fatigue, headache and irritability, resulting from the use of alcohol and certain drugs.

Hanot's disease {Victor C. Hanot, French physician, b. 1844}, primary biliary cirrhosis.

Hansen's disease. See **leprosy.**

haploid, having only one complete set of non-homologous chromosomes.

hapten, a non-proteinaceous substance that acts as an antigen by combining with particular bonding sites on an antibody. Unlike a true antigen, it does not induce the formation of antibodies.

haptics, the science concerned with studying the sense of touch. **haptic,** *adj.*

haptoglobin, a plasma protein whose only known function is to bind free haemoglobin.

Hara diagnosis, a slow and gentle palpation of the abdomen to identify areas that are tense, relaxed, painful, hard, etc.

hard copy, any readable output from a computer, produced on paper or another permanent medium.

hard data, information about a patient obtained by observation and measurement, including laboratory data, as opposed to information collected by interviewing the patient.

hard disk, a computer data storage medium that consists of a rigid disk with an electromagnetic coating allowing information to be transcribed on it and from it.

hardening of the arteries, arteriosclerosis.

hard fibroma, a neoplasm composed of fibrous tissue in which there are few cells.

hardness of x-rays. See **beam hardening, beam quality.**

hard palate, the bony portion of the roof of the mouth, continuous posteriorly with the soft palate and bounded anteriorly and laterally by the alveolar arches and the gums.

hardware, the tangible parts of a computer, such as chips, boards, wires, transformers and peripheral devices.

hardware bug. See **bug.**

Hardy-Weinberg equilibrium principle {G. H. Hardy, 20th century English mathematician; Wilhelm Weinberg, German physician, b. 1862}, a mathematical relationship between the frequency of genes and the resulting genotypes in populations.

harelip. See **cleft lip.**

hare's eye. See **lagophthalmos.**

harlequin colour, a transient flushing of the skin on the lower side of the body with pallor of the upward side.

harlequin fetus, an infant whose skin at birth is completely covered with thick, horny scales that resemble armour, and are divided by deep red fissures.

Harris tube {Franklin Harris, American surgeon, b. 1895}, a tube used for gastric and intestinal decompression. It is a mercury weighted, single lumen tube passed through the nose and carried through the alimentary tract by gravity. The location of the tube is followed by fluoroscopy.

Hartmann's solution. See **Ringer's lactate solution.**

Hartnup disease {Hartnup, family name of first patients diagnosed in England, 1956}, a recessive genetic metabolic disorder characterized by pellagra-like skin lesions, transient cerebellar ataxia and hyperaminoaciduria, caused by defects in intestinal absorption and renal reabsorption of neutral amino acids.

harvest fever. See **leptospirosis.**

Hashimoto's disease {Hakaru Hashimoto, Japanese surgeon, b. 1881}, an autoimmune thyroid disorder, characterized by the production of antibodies in response to thyroid antigens and replacement of normal thyroid structures with lymphocytes and lymphoid germinal centres. The thyroid, typically enlarged, pale yellow and lumpy on the surface, shows dense lymphocytic infiltration; the remaining thyroid tissue frequently contains small empty follicles. The goitre is usually asymptomatic, but occasionally patients complain of dysphagia and a feeling of local pressure. The thymus is usually enlarged, and regional lymph nodes often show hyperplasia.

hashish. See **cannabis.**

Haverhill fever {Haverhill, Massachusetts, disorder first diagnosed, 1925}, a febrile disease, caused by infection with *Streptobacillus moniliformis,* transmitted by the bite of a rat. The spirochaete-like bacterium is normally present in rat saliva. Characteristically, the wound from the bite heals but within 10 days fever, chills, vomiting, headache, muscle and joint pain and a rash appear.

haversian canal {Clopton Havers, English physician, b. 1650}, one of the many tiny longitudinal canals in bone tissue, averaging about 0.05 mm in diameter. Each contains blood vessels, connective tissue, nerve filaments and, occasionally, lymphatic vessels.

haversian canaliculus, any one of the many tiny passages radiating from the lacunae of bone tissue to larger haversian canals.

haversian system, a circular district of bone tissue, consisting of lamellae in the bone around a central canal.

Hawthorne effect, a general, unintentional, but usually beneficial effect on a person, a group of people, or the function of the system being studied. It is the effect of an encounter, as with an investigator or healthcare provider, or of a change in a programme or facility, as by painting an office or changing the lighting system.

hay fever *informal,* an acute seasonal allergic rhinitis stimulated by tree, grass or weed pollens.

hazard, a condition or phenomenon that increases the probability of a loss arising from some danger that may result in injury or illness. **hazardous,** *adj.*

Hb, abbreviation for **haemoglobin.**

HB, abbreviation for **hepatitis B.**

Hb A, abbreviation for **haemoglobin A.**

Hb A₂, abbreviation for **haemoglobin A₂.**

Hb C, abbreviation for **haemoglobin C.**

HBE, abbreviation for **His bundle electrocardiogram.**

Hb F, abbreviation for **haemoglobin F.**

HBIG, abbreviation for **hepatitis B immune globulin.**

Hb S, abbreviation for **haemoglobin S.**

HBsAG, abbreviation for **hepatitis B surface antigen.**

Hb S-C, abbreviation for **haemoglobin S-C.**

HCG, abbreviation for **human chorionic gonadotrophin.**

HCG radioreceptor assay, a urine test to detect pregnancy or missed abortion, performed by measuring human chorionic gonadotrophin, a chemical found only in the urine of pregnant women or in tumours that produce HCG.

HCl, abbreviation for **hydrochloric acid.**

HDCR, abbreviation for **Higher Diploma of the College of Radiographers.**

H deflection, (in cardiology) an indication on

Hg, symbol for **mercury.**

hiatus, a usually normal opening in a membrane or other body tissue. **hiatal,** *adj.*

hiatus hernia, protrusion of a portion of the stomach upwards through the diaphragm. The major difficulty in symptomatic patients is gastroesophageal reflux, the backflow of acid contents of the stomach into the oesophagus.

Hib disease, an infection caused by Haemophilus influenzae type b (Hib), which affects mainly children in the first 5 years of life. It is a leading cause of bacterial meningitis as well as pneumonia, joint or bone infections, and throat inflammations.

hibakusha, persons who have been exposed to atomic bomb explosions. In 1985, some 370,000 hibakusha still lived in Hiroshima and Nagasaki, more than 40 years after the World War II atomic bomb attacks. Their average age was over 60.

hibernoma, *pl.* **hibernomas, hibernomata,** a benign tumour, usually on the hips or the back, composed of fat cells that are partly or entirely of fetal origin.

hiccough, a characteristic sound produced by the involuntary contraction of the diaphragm, followed by rapid closure of the glottis. Hiccoughs have a variety of causes, including indigestion, rapid eating, certain types of surgery and epidemic encephalitis. Also spelt **hiccup.**

hickory stick fracture. See **greenstick fracture.**

hidradenitis. See **hydradenitis.**

hidrosis, sweat production and secretion. **hidrotic,** *adj.*

high blood pressure. See **hypertension.**

high-calorie diet, a diet that provides 500-1000 or more calories a day beyond what is ordinarily recommended. It may be prescribed for nursing mothers, patients with severe weight loss caused by illness, or persons with abnormally high metabolic rates or energy requirements.

high-density lipoprotein (HDL), a plasma protein containing about 50% protein (apoprotein) with cholesterol and triglycerides. It may serve to stabilize very low-density lipoprotein, and is involved in transporting cholesterol and other lipids from plasma to tissues.

high-energy phosphate compound, a chemical compound containing a high-energy bond between phosphoric acid residues and certain organic substances. When the bond is hydrolysed, a large amount of energy is released.

Higher Diploma of the College of Radiographers (HDCR), post-qualifying diploma awarded by the College of Radiographers, prior to the development of postgraduate diplomas.

highest intercostal vein, one of a pair of veins that drain the blood from the upper two or three intercostal spaces.

high-flow oxygen delivery system, respiratory care equipment that supplies inspired gases at a preset oxygen concentration.

high-frequency ventilation (HFV), a technique for providing ventilatory support to patients by operating at a breathing rate of 60 breaths per minute or more. **High-frequency jet ventilation (HFJV)** is a type using a high-pressure gas source that has a respiratory rate of 100 to 400 cycles per minute. **High-frequency oscillation (HFO)** is a form that forces small impulses of gas in and out of the airway at frequencies of 400 to 4000 per minute.

high labial arch, a labial arch wire adapted to lie gingival to the anterior tooth crowns, having auxiliary springs that extend downwards in contact with the teeth to be moved.

high-potassium diet, a diet that contains foods rich in potassium, including all leafy green vegetables, brussels sprouts, citrus fruits, bananas, dates, raisins, legumes, meats and whole grains. It is indicated for conditions resulting in the loss of extracellular fluid.

high-protein diet, a diet that contains large amounts of protein, consisting largely of meats, fish, milk, legumes and nuts. It may be indicated in protein depletion from any cause.

high-risk infant, any neonate, regardless of birth weight, size or gestational age, who has a greater than average chance of morbidity or mortality, especially within the first 28 days of life, due to preconceptual, prenatal, natal or postnatal conditions or circumstances that interfere with the normal birth process or impede adjustment to extrauterine growth and development.

high-speed handpiece, a rotary or vibratory cutting instrument that operates at high speeds, powered by a conventional dental engine and propelled by gears, a belt drive or turbine.

high-vitamin diet, a dietary regimen that includes a variety of foods that contain therapeutic amounts of all of the vitamins necessary for the metabolic processes of the body. It is often ordered in combination with other therapeutic diets containing larger than usual amounts of protein or calories, especially when treating severe or chronic infection, malnutrition or vitamin deficiency.

hilus, a depression or pit at that part of an organ where vessels and nerves enter.

hindgut, the caudal portion of the embryonic alimentary canal.

hind kidney. See **metanephros.**

hinge axis, the joint where the mandible meets the skull and the point of rotation of the mandible.

hinge axis-orbital plane, a craniofacial plane usually determined by marking three points on the face of the patient. Two of the points, one on each side of the face, are located on the hinge axis. The third point is located on the face at the level of the orbital rim just beneath the eye.

hinged knee, an appliance designed to protect and support the knee during activity. It consists of an elastic sleeve with bars hinged at the axis of the knee joint and stabilized with straps.

hinge joint, a synovial joint providing a connection in which articular surfaces are closely moulded togetl.er in a manner that permits extensive motion in one plane.

hip. See **coxa.**

hipbone. See **innominate bone.**

hip joint. See **coxal articulation.**

hippocampal commissure, a thin, triangular layer of transverse fibres that connects the medial edges of the posterior pillars of the fornix.

hippocampal fissure, a fissure reaching from the posterior aspect of the corpus callosum to the tip of the temporal lobe.

hippocampus, *pl.* **hippocampi,** a curved convoluted elevation of the floor of the inferior horn of the lateral ventricle of the brain.

hippocampus minor. See **calcar avis.**

Hippocrates, a Greek physician born circa 460 BC on the island of Cos. Referred to as the "Father of Medicine," Hippocrates introduced a scientific approach to healing.

Hippocratic oath, an oath, attributed to Hippocrates, that serves as an ethical guide for the medical profession. It is traditionally incorporated into the graduation ceremonies of medical colleges.

hip replacement, replacement of the hip joint with an artificial ball and socket joint, performed to relieve a chronically painful and stiff hip in advanced osteoarthritis, an improperly healed fracture or joint degeneration. Antibiotic therapy is begun preoperatively, and the patient is taught to walk with crutches. The femoral head, neck and part of the shaft are removed, and the contours of the socket are smoothed. A prosthesis of a durable, hard metal alloy or stainless steel is shaped to resemble a femur and head of a femur, and is attached to the femur with screws or an acrylic cement; a metal or a plastic acetablum is implanted.

Hirschberg's reflex, a diagnostic test for pyramidal tract disease. The test result is regarded as positive if inversion of the foot occurs when the sole is stroked at the base of the great toe.

Hirschfeld-Dunlop file, a kind of periodontal file, used with a pull stroke to remove tooth calculus. Various models with different angulations are available for different tooth surfaces.

Hirschfeld's method {Isador Hirschfeld, American dentist, b. 1881}, a toothbrushing technique in which the bristles are placed against the axial surfaces of the teeth at a slight incisal or occlusal angle and in contact with the teeth and gingivae, then vigorously rotated in very small circles.

Hirschsprung's disease {Harald Hirschsprung, Danish physician, b. 1831}, the congenital absence of autonomic ganglia in the smooth muscle wall of the colon, resulting in poor or absent peristalsis in the involved segment of colon, accumulation of faeces and dilatation of the bowel (megacolon). Symptoms include intermittent vomiting, diarrhoea and constipation. The abdomen may become distended to several times its normal size.

hirsutism, excessive body hair in a masculine distribution as a result of heredity, hormonal dysfunction, porphyria or medication. Treatment of the specific cause will usually stop growth of more hair. **hirsute,** *adj.,* **hirsuteness,** *n.*

hirsutoid papilloma of the penis, a condition characterized by clusters of small, white papules on the coronal edge of the glans penis.

His. See **histidine.**

His bundle. See **bundle of His.**

His bundle electrogram (HBE) {Wilhelm His, Jr., German physician, b. 1863}, (in cardiology) a direct recording of the electrical activity in the bundle of His.

His-Purkinje system {Wilhelm His, Jr.; Johannes E. Purkinje, Czechoslovakian physiologist, b. 1787}, the conduction system in the cardiac tissues from the bundle of His to the distal Purkinje fibres.

histamine, a compound found in all cells, produced by the breakdown of histidine. It is released in allergic, inflammatory reactions and causes dilatation of capillaries, decreased blood pressure, increased secretion of gastric juice and constriction of smooth muscles of the bronchi and uterus.

histamine headache, a headache associated with the release of histamine from the body tissues and marked by symptoms of dilated carotid arteries, fluid accumulation under the eyes, tearing or lacrimation and rhinorrhoea.

histidine (His), a basic amino acid found in many proteins, and a precursor of histamine. It is an essential amino acid in infants.

histidinaemia, an inherited metabolic disorder affecting the amino acid histidine. The condition leads to retardation and nervous system disorders.

histiocyte. See **macrophage.**

histiocytic leukaemia. See **monocytic leukaemia.**

histiocytic malignant lymphoma, a lymphoid neoplasm containing undifferentiated primitive cells or differentiated reticulum cells.

histiotypic growth, the uncontrolled proliferation of cells, as occurs in bacterial cultures and moulds.

histocompatibility antigens, a group of genetically determined antigens on the surface of many cells. Histocompatibility antigens are the cause of most graft rejections.

histocompatibility locus, a set of positions on a chromosome occupied by a complex of genes that govern several tissue antigens.

histogram, (in research) a graph showing the values of one or more variables plotted against time or against frequency of occurrence.

histography, the process of describing or creating visualizations of tissues and cells. **histographer,** *n.,* **histographic,** *adj.,* **histographically,** *adv.*

histoid neoplasm, a growth that resembles the tissues in which it originates.

histologist, a medical scientist who specializes in the study of histology.

histology, 1. the science dealing with the microscopic identification of cells and tissue. **2.** the structure of organ tissues, including the composition of cells and their organization into various body tissues. **histological,** *adj.,* **histologically,** *adv.*

histone, any of a group of strongly basic, low molecular weight proteins that are soluble in water, insoluble in dilute ammonia, and combine with nucleic acid to form nucleoproteins. They are found in the cell nucleus.

histoplasma agglutinin, an agglutinin associated with fungal lung infections.

Histoplasma capsulatum, a dimorphic fungal organism that is a single budding yeast at body temperature and a mould at room temperature. It is the causative organism in histoplasmosis.

histoplasmosis, an infection caused by inhalation of spores of the fungus *Histoplasma capsulatum.* **Primary histoplasmosis** is characterized by fever, malaise, cough and lymphadenopathy. Spontaneous recovery is usual; small calcifications remain in the lungs and affected lymph glands. **Progressive histoplasmosis,** a sometimes fatal, disseminated form of the infection, is characterized by ulcerating sores in the mouth and nose, enlargement of the spleen, liver and lymph nodes, and severe and extensive infiltration of the lungs.

history, 1. a record of past events. **2.** a systematic account of the medical and psychosocial occurrences in a patient's life, and factors in family, ancestors and environment that may have a bearing on the patient's condition.

history of present illness, an account obtained during the interview with the patient regarding the onset, duration and character of the present illness, in addition to any acts or factors that aggravate or ameliorate the symptoms.

histotoxin, any substance that is poisonous to the body tissues. It is usually generated from within the body rather than being introduced externally. **histotoxic,** *adj.*

histrionic personality, a personality characterized by behavioural patterns and attitudes that are over-reactive, emotionally unstable, overly dramatic, self-centred and exhibited as a means of attracting attention, whether consciously or unconsciously.

histrionic personality disorder, a disorder characterized by dramatic, reactive and intensely exaggerated behaviour which is typically self-centred. It results in severe disturbance in interpersonal relationships that can lead to psychosomatic disorders, depression, alcoholism and drug dependency.

hives. See **urticaria.**

HLA, abbreviation for **human leukocyte antigen.**

HLA-A, abbreviation for *human leukocyte antigen A.* See **human leukocyte antigen.**

HLA-B, abbreviation for *human leukocyte antigen B.* See **human leukocyte antigen.**

HLA-D, abbreviation for *human leukocyte antigen D.* See **human leukocyte antigen.**

HLH, abbreviation for **human luteinizing hormone.**

HMG-CoA reductase, a rate-controlling enzyme of cholesterol synthesis.

Ho, symbol for **holmium.**

H₂O, symbol for **water.**

Hodgkin's disease {Thomas Hodgkin, English physician, b. 1798}, a malignant disorder characterized by painless, progressive enlargement of lymphoid tissue, usually first evident in cervical lymph nodes; splenomegaly; and the presence of Reed-Sternberg cells, large, atypical macrophages with multiple or hyperlobulated nuclei and prominent nucleoli. Symptoms include anorexia, weight loss, generalized pruritus, low-grade fever, night sweats, anaemia and leukocytosis. Total lymph radiotherapy is the treatment of choice for early stages of the disease; combination chemotherapy is the treatment for advanced disease.

Hoffmann's atrophy. See **Werdnig-Hoffmann disease.**

Hoffmann's reflex {Johann Hoffmann, German neurologist, b. 1857}, an abnormal reflex elicited by sudden, forceful flicking of the nail of the index, middle or ring finger, resulting in flexion of the thumb and the middle and distal phalanges of one of the other fingers.

hoist, a lifting device designed to lift a heavy or dependent person. It is intended to remove the physical strain placed on a carer in performing an unassisted lift. In selecting the appropriate hoist, a thorough assessment of the patient, environment and operator is necessary. Types of hoist include floor-fixed, mobile and ceiling-fixed. Methods of operation include hydraulic, electrical, etc.

holandric, 1. designating genes located on the non-homologous portion of the Y chromosome. **2.** of or pertaining to traits or conditions transmitted only through the paternal line.

holandric inheritance, the acquisition or expression of traits or conditions only through the paternal line, transmitted by genes carried on the non-homologous portion of the Y chromosome.

hold-relax, a technique of proprioceptive neuromuscular facilitation used in treating hypertonicity or motor dysfunction. It is often applied when there is muscle tightness on one side of a joint and when immobility is the result of pain.

holism, a philosophical concept in which an entity is seen as more than the sum of its parts. Also spelt **wholism.**

holistic, of or pertaining to the whole; considering all factors, such as holistic medicine. Also **wholistic.**

holistic counselling, an alternative form of psychotherapy that focuses on the whole person (mind, body and spirit) and health.

holistic medicine, a system of comprehensive or total patient care that considers the physical, emotional, social, economic and spiritual needs of the person, his or her response to the illness, and the impact of illness on the person's ability to meet self-care needs.

Hollenback condenser. See **pneumatic condenser.**

hollow cathode lamp, a lamp consisting of a metal cathode and an inert gas. It emits a line spectrum of specific wavelengths related to the metal of the cathode.

holmium (Ho), a rare earth metallic element. Its atomic number is 67 and its atomic weight is 164.93.

holoacardius, a separate, grossly defective monozygotic twin fetus in which the heart is absent and the circulation in utero is accomplished totally by the heart of the viable twin through a vascular shunt.

holoacardius acephalus, a grossly defective separate twin fetus that lacks a heart, a head and most of the upper portion of the body.

holoacardius acormus, a grossly defective, separate twin fetus in which the trunk is malformed and little more than the head is recognizable.

holoacardius amorphus, a malformed separate twin fetus in which there are no recognizable or formed parts.

holoarthritis, a form of arthritis that involves all or most of the joints.

holoblastic, of or pertaining to an ovum that contains little or no yolk and undergoes total cleavage.

holocephalic, a malformed fetus in which several parts are deficient although the head is complete.

holodiastolic. See **pandiastolic.**

holoenzyme, a complete enzyme-cofactor complex that gives full catalytic activity.

holographic reconstruction, a method of producing three-dimensional images with diagnostic ultrasound equipment.

hologynic, 1. designating genes located on attached X chromosomes. **2.** of or pertaining to traits or conditions transmitted only through the maternal line.

hologynic inheritance, the acquisition or expression of traits or conditions only through the maternal line, transmitted by genes located on attached X chromosomes. The phenomenon is not known to occur in humans.

holoprosencephaly, a congenital defect characterized by multiple midline facial defects, including cyclopia in severe cases. **holoprosencephalic, holoprosencephalous,** *adj.*

holorachischisis. See **complete rachischisis.**

holosystolic. See **pansystolic.**

Holtzman inkblot technique, a modification of the Rorschach test in which many more pictures of inkblots are used, the subject is permitted only one response to each design, and the scoring is predominantly objective rather than subjective.

Homan's sign {John Homan, American surgeon, b. 1877}, pain in the calf with dorsiflexion of the foot, indicating thrombophlebitis or thrombosis.

home adaptations, the architectural, physical or practical alteration made to an individual's place of residence, enabling that individual to remain, function or be cared for in that environment. It is usually carried out to facilitate independent living or an improved care environment; for example, provision of ramps, rails, altered room layout or provision of additional facilities, such as a bathroom, a toilet extension or a lift.

home assessment, 1. the assessment of an individual's ability to function at home. **2.** the collection of information about an individual's home, so as to allow preparation of an appropriate intervention programme linked to the documented needs.

home care, a health service provided in the patient's place of residence for the purpose of promoting, maintaining or restoring health or minimizing the effects of illness and disability. Service may include medical, dental and nursing care, speech and physical therapy, and other services such as the provision of transportation.

homoeodynamics, the constantly changing interrelatedness of body components while maintaining an overall equilibrium.

homoeopathist, a doctor who practices homoeopathy.

homoeopathy, a system of therapeutics based on the theory that "like cures like." The theory was advanced in the late eighteenth century by Dr. Samuel Hahnemann, who believed that a large amount of a particular drug may cause symptoms of a disease and moderate dosage may reduce those symptoms; thus, some disease symptoms could be treated by very small doses of medicine. **homeopathic,** *adj.*

homoeostasis, a relative constancy in the internal environment of the body, naturally maintained by adaptive responses that promote healthy survival. Various sensing, feedback and control mechanisms function to effect this steady state. Some of the functions controlled by homoeostatic mechanisms are the heartbeat, hematopoiesis, blood pressure, body temperature, electrolytic balance, respiration and glandular secretion. **homoeostatic,** *adj.*

homoeotypic, pertaining to or characteristic of the regular or usual type, specifically applied to the second meiotic division of germ cells in gametogenesis as distinguished from the first meiotic division. Also **homoeotypical.**

homoeotypic mitosis, the equational division of chromosomes, as occurs in the second meiotic division of germ cells in gametogenesis.

Home's silver precipitation method, (in dentistry) a technique for depositing silver in enamel and dentine by the application of ammoniac silver nitrate solution and its reduction with formalin or eugenol.

homicide, the death of one human being caused by another human. Homicide is usually intentional and often violent.

hominal physiology, the study of the specific physical and chemical processes involved in the normal functioning of humans; human physiology.

homoiothermal. See **warm-blooded.**

homoiothermic, pertaining to the ability of warm-blooded animals to maintain a relatively stable internal temperature regardless of the temperature of the environment. This ability is not fully developed in newborn humans.

homoblastic, developing from the same germ layer or a single type of tissue.

homochronous inheritance, the appearance of traits or conditions in the offspring at the same age as they appeared in the parents.

homocystinuria, a rare biochemical abnormality characterized by the abnormal presence of homocystine, an amino acid, in the blood and urine, caused by any of several enzyme deficiencies in the metabolic pathway of methionine to cystine. **homocystinuric,** *adj.*

homogenate, a tissue that is or has been made homogenous.

homogeneous, 1. consisting of similar elements or parts. **2.** having a uniform quality throughout. **homogeneity,** *adj.*

homogenesis, reproduction by the same process in succeeding generations so that offspring are similar to the parents.

homogenetic, 1. of or pertaining to homogenesis. **2. homogenous, def. 2.**

homogenized milk, pasteurized milk that has been mechanically treated to reduce and emulsify the fat globules so that the cream cannot separate and the protein is more digestible.

homogenous, 1. homogeneous. **2.** having a likeness in form or structure because of a common ancestral origin. **3.** homoplasty.

homogentisic acid. See **glycosuric acid.**

homogeny, 1. homogenesis. **2.** a likeness in structure or form because of a common ancestral origin.

homograft. See **allograft.**

homolateral, pertaining to the same side of the body.

homolateral limb synkinesis, a condition of hemiplegia in which there appears to be a mutual dependency between the affected upper and lower limbs. Efforts at flexion of an upper extremity cause flexion of the lower extremity.

homologue, 1. any organ corresponding in function, origin and structure to another organ, for example the flippers of a seal corresponding to human hands. **2.** (in chemistry) one of a series of compounds, each formed by an added common element; for example, CO, carbon monoxide, is followed by CO_2 carbon dioxide, with the addition of an oxygen atom. **homologous,** *adj.*

homologous chromosomes any two chromosomes in the diploid complement of the somatic cell that are identical in size, shape and gene loci. In humans there are 22 pairs of homologous chromosomes and one pair of sex chromosomes.

homologous disease. See **graft-versus-host reaction.**

homologous tumour, a neoplasm made up of cells resembling those of the tissue in which it is growing.

homonymous hemianopia, blindness or defective vision in the right or left halves of the visual fields of both eyes.

homoplasty, having a likeness in form or structure acquired through similar environmental conditions or parallel evolution, rather than because of common ancestral origin. **homoplastic,** *adj.*

homopolymer, a compound formed from subunits that are the same, such as a carbohydrate composed of a series of glucose units.

homosexual, 1. of, pertaining to or denoting the same sex. **2.** a person who is sexually attracted to members of the same sex.

homosexual panic, an acute attack of anxiety based on unconscious conflicts concerning gender identity and fear of being homosexual.

homothermal. See **warm-blooded.**

homovanillic acid, an acid produced by normal metabolism of dopamine. It may be elevated in the urine in association with tumours of the adrenal gland.

homozygosis, 1. the formation of a zygote by the union of two gametes that have one or more pairs of identical genes. **2.** the production of purebred organisms or strains through the process of inbreeding.

homozygous, having two identical genes at corresponding loci on homologous chromosomes.

homunculus, *pl.* **homunculi, 1.** a dwarf in which all body parts are proportionally developed, with no deformity or abnormality. **2.** (in early embryological theories of development) a minute and complete human being contained in each of the germ cells that after fertilization grows from microscopic to normal size. **3.** a small anatomical model of the human form; a manekin. **4.** (in psychiatry) an imaginary little man possessing magical powers.

hook grasp, a type of prehension in which an object is grasped with the fingers alone.

hookworm *non-technical,* a nematode of the genera *Ancylostoma, Necator,* or *Uncinaria.* Most hookworm infections in the Western hemisphere are caused by the species *Necator americanus.*

hopelessness, a state in which an individual sees limited or no alternatives or personal choices available, and is unable to mobilize energy on his or her own behalf. Defining characteristics include passivity, decreased verbalization, decreased affect, verbal cues with a despondent content, lack of initiative, decreased response to stimuli, decreased appetite, increased sleep, and lack of involvement in care or passivity in allowing care.

hora somni (hs), (in prescriptions) a Latin phrase meaning "at bedtime."

hordeolum, a furuncle of the margin of the eyelid originating in the sebaceous gland of an eyelash.

horizon, a specific stage of human embryonic development based on the appearance and ultimate formation of certain anatomical characteristics. The classification comprises 23 stages, each lasting 2 to 3 days, beginning with fertilization of the ovum.

horizontal fissure of the right lung, a cleft that marks the separation of the upper and middle lobes of the right lung.

horizontal pursuit, a visual screening test in which the patient is asked to follow with both eyes a target moving in a horizontal plane, while the examiner observes accuracy of alignment and other factors.

horizontal resorption, a pattern of bone reduction in marginal periodontitis, whereby the marginal crest of the alveolar bone between adjacent teeth remains level and the bases of the periodontal pockets are supracrestal.

horizontal transmission, the spread of an infectious agent from one person or group to another, usually through contact with contaminated material, such as sputum or faeces.

hormone, a complex chemical substance produced in one part or organ of the body, initiating or regulating the activity of an organ or a group of cells in another part of the body. Hormones secreted by the endocrine glands are carried through the bloodstream to the target organ.

hormone therapy, the treatment of certain disorders with hormones obtained from endocrine glands or substances that simulate hormonal effects.

horn, a projection or protuberance on a body structure. An example is the iliac horn.

Horner's syndrome {Johann F. Horner, Swiss ophthalmologist, b. 1831}, a neurological condition characterized by miotic pupils, ptosis and facial anhidrosis, resulting from a lesion in the spinal cord, with damage to a cervical nerve.

horny layer. See **stratum corneum.**

horripilation. See **pilomotor reflex.**

horse serum, immunoglobulins prepared from the blood of immunized horses, formerly much used as passive immunizing agents.

horseshoe fistula, an abnormal, semicircular passage in the perianal area with both openings on the surface of the skin.

horseshoe kidney, a relatively common congenital anomaly characterized by an isthmus of parenchymal tissue connecting the two kidneys at the lower poles.

Hortega cells. See **microglia.**

Horton's arteritis. See **temporal arteritis.**

Horton's headache. See **migrainous cranial neuralgia.**

Horton's histamine cephalalgia. See **histamine headache.**

hospice, a system of family-centred care designed to assist the chronically ill person to be comfortable and maintain a satisfactory lifestyle through the terminal phase of illness.

hospital, a healthcare facility that provides inpatient beds, continuous nursing services and an organized medical staff. Diagnosis and treatment are provided for a variety of diseases and disorders, at both medical and surgical level.

hospital-acquired infection. See **nosocomial infection.**

hospitalism, the physical or mental effects of hospitalization or institutionalization on patients, especially infants and children in whom the condition is characterized by social regression, personality disorders and stunted growth.

host, 1. an organism in which another, usually parasitic organism is nourished and harboured. A **primary** or **definitive host** is one in which the adult parasite lives and reproduces. A **secondary** or **intermediate host** is one in which the parasite exists in its nonsexual, larval stage. A **reservoir host** is a primary animal host for organisms that are sometimes parasitic in humans, and from which humans may become infected. **2.** the recipient of a transplanted organ or tissue.

hostility, the tendency of an organism to threaten harm to another or to itself. The hostility may be expressed passively and actively.

hotline, a means of contacting a trained counsellor or specific agency for help with a particular problem, such as rape hotline or battered child hotline. The person needing help calls a telephone number and speaks to a counsellor who remains anonymous.

hot spot, 1. (in molecular genetics) a site in a gene sequence at which mutations occur with an unusually high frequency. **2.** (in radionuclide imaging) an area of increased radionuclide uptake on scan image.

Hounsfield unit, (in computed tomography) the numerical information contained in each pixel. It is used to represent the density of tissue.

house doctor, a medical doctor on call and immediately available in a hospital or other healthcare facility.

housekeeping department, a unit of a hospital staff responsible for cleaning the hospital premises and furnishings.

housemaid's knee, a chronic inflammation of the bursa in front of the kneecap, characterized by redness and swelling. It is caused by prolonged and repetitive pressure of the knee on a hard surface.

house-man, the junior doctors who are employed at a hospital while receiving additional training after graduation from medical college.

house surgeon, a surgeon on call and immediately available on the premises of a hospital.

housewives' eczema *nontechnical,* contact dermatitis of the hands caused and exacerbated by their frequent immersion in water and use of soaps and detergents.

Houston's valves. See **plicae transversales recti.**

Howell-Jolly bodies, spheric and granular inclusions in the erythrocytes observed on microscopic examination of stained blood smears.

HPL, abbreviation for human placental lactogen.

HPV, 1. abbreviation for **human papillomavirus. 2.** abbreviation for **human parvovirus.**

hs, abbreviation for *hora somni.*

HSV, abbreviation for *herpes simplex virus.* See **herpes genitalis, herpes simplex.**

Hubbard tank {Leroy W. Hubbard, American surgeon, b. 1857}, a large tank in which a patient may be immersed to perform underwater exercise.

huffing, a type of forced expiration with an open glottis to replace coughing when pain limits normal coughing.

Huhner test, a test for male fertility in which a semen sample is examined for spermatozoa activity.

human bite, a wound caused by the piercing of skin by human teeth. Bacteria are usually present, and serious infection often follows.

human chorionic gonadotrophin (HCG), a hormone produced by the trophoblast. It is detected in urine from 30 days after conception.

human chorionic somatomammotrophin (HCS), a hormone produced by the syncytiotrophoblast during pregnancy. It regulates carbohydrate and protein metabolism of the mother.

human ecology, the study of interrelationships between individuals and their environments, as well as among individuals within the environment.

human insulin, a biosynthetic product manufactured from two forms of *Escherichia coli* using recombinant DNA technology. An advantage of human insulin is the elimination of allergic reactions that occur with animal insulins.

human leukocyte antigen (HLA), any one of four significant genetic markers identified as specific loci on chromosome 6. They are HLA-A, HLA-B, HLA-C and HLA-D. Each locus has several genetically determined alleles; each of these is associated with certain diseases or conditions.

human natural killer cells, lymphocytes that are able to lyse tumour and virally infected cells, as part of the body's natural defence against malignancy and invasion by pathogens.

human papillomavirus (HPV), a virus that is the cause of common warts of the hands and feet, as well as lesions of the mucous membranes. The virus can be transmitted through sexual contact and is frequently found in women with cancer of the cervix.

human parvovirus (HPV), a small, single-stranded DNA virion that has been associated with several diseases, including erythema infectiosum and aplastic crises of chronic haemolytic anaemias.

human placental lactogen (HPL), a placental hormone that aids growth and development of the breast during pregnancy.

human protein C, an anticoagulant produced by genetically engineered bacteria. It inactivates coagulation cofactors 5 and 8c, and mediates clot lysis by tissue plasminogen activator (t-PA).

human rhinovirus 14, the common cold virus. It has a complex protein coat containing "sticky sites" that help attach the virus to cell receptors in the upper respiratory system. More than 100 strains of the virus are known, making it difficult to devise a vaccine that would protect against all variations.

humanistic existential therapy, a kind of psychotherapy that promotes self-awareness and personal growth by stressing current reality, and by analysing and altering specific patterns of response to help a person realize his or her potential. Kinds of humanistic existential psychotherapy are **client-oriented therapy, existential therapy, Gestalt therapy.**

humanistic nursing model, a conceptual framework in which the nurse-patient relationship is analysed as a human-to-human event rather than a nurse-to-patient interaction.

humanistic psychology, a branch of psychology that emphasizes a person's struggle to develop and maintain an integrated, harmonious personality as the primary motivational force in human behaviour.

humectant, a substance that promotes retention of moisture.

humeral. See **humerus.**

humeral articulation. See **shoulder joint.**

humerus, *pl.* **humeri,** the largest bone of the upper arm, comprising a body, a head and a condyle. The nearly hemispheric head articulates with the glenoid cavity of the scapula. The condyle at the distal end has several depressions into which articulate the radius and ulna. **humeral,** *adj.*

humidification, the process of increasing the relative humidity of the atmosphere around a patient, through the use of aerosol generators or steam inhalators that exert an antitussive effect. Humidification acts by decreasing the viscosity of bronchial secretions.

humoral immunity, one of the two forms of immunity that respond to antigens such as bacteria and foreign tissue. Humoral immunity is the result of circulating antibodies carried in the immunoglobulins IgA, IgB and IgM.

humoral response, one of a broad category of hypersensitivity reactions. Humoral responses are mediated by B cell lymphocytes and occur in type I, type II and type III hypersensitivity reactions.

hung-up reflex, a deep tendon reflex in which, after a stimulus is given and the reflex action takes place, there is a slow return of the limb to its neutral position.

Hunner's ulcer. See **interstitial cystitis.**

Hunter's canal. See **adductor canal.**

Hunter's syndrome {Charles Hunter, 20th century English physician}, a hereditary defect in mucopolysaccharide metabolism affecting only males, characterized by dwarfism, kyphosis, gargoylism and learning disabilities.

Huntington's chorea {George S. Huntington, American physician, b. 1851}, a rare, abnormal hereditary condition characterized by chronic, progressive chorea and mental deterioration that terminates in dementia. An individual afflicted with the condition usually shows the first signs in the fourth decade of life and dies about 15 years later.

Hurler's syndrome {Gertrude Hurler, German physician, b. 1920}, a type of mucopolysaccharidosis transmitted as an autosomal-recessive trait, resulting in severe mental retardation. Facial characteristics include a low forehead and enlargement of the head. Corneal clouding is common, and the neck is short. Marked kyphosis is apparent at the dorsolumbar level, and the hands and fingers are short and broad.

Hürthle cell adenoma {Karl W. Hürthle, German histologist, b. 1860}, a benign tumour of the thyroid gland composed of large cells with granular eosinophilic cytoplasm (Hürthle cells).

Hürthle cell carcinoma, a malignant neoplasm of the thyroid gland composed of Hürthle cells.

Hürthle cell tumour, a neoplasm of the thyroid gland composed of large cells with granular eosinophilic cytoplasm (Hürthle cells); it may be benign (Hürthle cell adenoma) or malignant (Hürthle cell carcinoma).

Hutchinson's freckle {Sir Jonathan Hutchinson, English surgeon, b. 1828}, a tan patch on the skin that grows slowly, becoming mottled, dark, thick and nodular. The lesion is usually seen on one side of the face of an elderly person.

Hutchinson's teeth {Sir Jonathan Hutchinson}, a characteristic of congenital syphilis in which the permanent incisor teeth are peg-shaped, widely spaced and notched at the end with a centrally placed crescent-shaped deformity.

Hutchinson's triad {Sir Jonathan Hutchinson}, interstitial keratitis, notched teeth and deafness, characteristic signs of congenital syphilis.

Hutchison-type neuroblastoma {Sir Robert G. Hutchison, English physician, b. 1871}, a neuroblastoma that has metastasized to the cranium.

HV, abbreviation for **Health Visitor.**

HVA, abbreviation for **Health Visitors Association.**

HV interval (HBE), (in cardiology) the conduction time through the His-Purkinje system, measured from the earliest onset of the His potential to the onset of ventricular activation.

HVL, abbreviation for **half-value layer.**

HVT, abbreviation for **half-value thickness.**

hyaline cartilage, the gristly, elastic connective tissue comprised of specialized cells in a translucent, pearly-blue matrix. Hyaline cartilage thinly covers the articulating ends of bones, connects the ribs to the sternum, and supports the nose, trachea and part of the larynx.

hyaline cast, a transparent cast composed of

mucoprotein.

hyaline membrane disease. See **acute respiratory distress syndrome.**

hyaline thrombus, a translucent, colourless mass consisting of haemolysed erythrocytes.

hyaloid artery, an embryonic blood vessel that branches to supply the vitreous body of the eye. It persists in the adult as a narrow passage through the vitreous body from the optic disc to the posterior surface of the crystalline lens.

hyaloplasm, the portion of the cytoplasm that is clear and more fluid, as opposed to the granular and reticular part.

hyaluronic acid, a mucopolysaccharide formed by the polymerization of acetylglucosamine and glucuronic acid. Known as the cement substance of tissues, it forms a gel in intercellular spaces.

hyaluronidase, an enzyme that hydrolyses hyaluronic acid. It is used to increase the absorption and dispersion of other parenteral drugs, for hypodermoclysis, and for improving resorption of radiopaque x-ray contrast agents.

hybrid, 1. an offspring produced from mating plants or animals from different species, varieties or genotypes. **2.** of or pertaining to such a plant or animal.

hybridization, 1. the process of producing hybrids by crossbreeding. **2.** (in molecular genetics) the process of combining single-stranded nucleic acids whose base composition is identical but whose base sequence is different to form stable double-stranded duplex molecules.

hybridoma, a hybrid cell formed by the fusion of a myeloma cell and an antibody-producing cell. Hybridomas are used in the production of monoclonal antibodies.

hybrid subtraction, a two-step subtraction method for producing digitalized x-ray images, using at least four images.

hybrid vigour. See **heterosis.**

hydantoin, any one of a group of anticonvulsant medications, chemically similar to the barbiturates. They act to limit seizure activity and reduce the spread of the abnormal electrical excitation from the focus of a seizure.

hydatid, a cyst or cyst-like structure usually filled with fluid, especially the cyst formed around the developing scolex of the dog tapeworm *Echinococcus granulosus.* **hydatidiform,** *adj.*

hydatid cyst, a cyst in the liver that contains larvae of the tapeworm *Echinococcus granulosus.* Patients are generally asymptomatic, except for hepatomegaly and a dull ache over the right upper quadrant of the abdomen.

hydatid disease. See **echinococcosis.**

hydatid mole, an intrauterine neoplastic mass of grape-like enlarged chorionic villi. Characteristic signs of the condition are extreme nausea, uterine bleeding, anaemia, hyperthyroidism, an unusually large uterus for the length of pregnancy, absence of fetal heart sounds, oedema and high blood pressure.

hydatidosis, infestation with the tapeworm *Echinococcus granulosus.*

hydradenitis, an infection or inflammation of the sweat glands.

hydralazine hydrochloride, a vasodilator used in the treatment of hypertension.

hydramnios, an abnormal condition of pregnancy characterized by an excess of amniotic fluid.

hydranencephaly, a neurological disorder in which the cerebral hemispheres are lacking although the cerebellum, brainstem and other central nervous system tissues may be normal. The newborn may show normal neurological functions but fails to develop.

hydrargyrism. See **mercury poisoning.**

hydraemic ascites, an abnormal accumulation of fluid within the peritoneal cavity accompanied by haemodilution, as in protein calorie malnutrition.

hydroa, an unusual vesicular and bullous skin condition of childhood that recurs each summer after exposure to sunlight, sometimes accompanied by itching and lichenification.

hydrocarbon, any one of a large group of organic compounds, the molecules of which are composed of hydrogen and carbon. Many of these are derived from petroleum.

hydrocoele, an accumulation of fluid in any sac-like cavity or duct, specifically in the tunica vaginalis testis or along the spermatic cord. The condition is caused by inflammation of the epididymis or testis, or by lymphatic or venous obstruction in the cord.

hydrocephalus, a pathological condition characterized by an abnormal accumulation of cerebrospinal fluid, usually under increased pressure, within the cranial vault and subsequent dilatation of the ventricles. Interference with the normal flow of cerebrospinal fluid may be caused by increased secretion of the fluid, obstruction within the ventricular system (non-communicating or intraventricular hydrocephalus), or defective reabsorption from the cerebral subarachnoid space (communicating or extraventricular hydrocephalus). It results from developmental anomalies, infection, trauma or brain tumours. **hydrocephalic,** *adj., n.*

hydrochloric acid, a compound consisting of hydrogen and chlorine. Hydrochloric acid is secreted in the stomach and is a major component of gastric juice.

hydrochlorothiazide, a diuretic and antihypertensive used in the treatment of hypertension and oedema.

hydrocholeretics, drugs that stimulate the production of bile with a low specific gravity or a minimal proportion of solid constituents.

hydrocortisone, hydrocortisone acetate, hydrocortisone butyrate, hydrocortisone sodium phosphate, hydrocortisone sodium succinate, hydrocortisone is the main glucocorticoid secreted by the adrenal cortex. It is administered as the free alcohol, or as an ester, by mouth or by injection, as replacement therapy in adrenocortical hyposecretion, as an anti-inflammatory where corticosteroids are indicated, and topically in the treatment of inflammatory conditions of the skin and mucous membranes.

hydroflumethiazide, a diuretic and antihypertensive used in the treatment of hypertension and oedema.

hydrogen (H), a gaseous, univalent element. Its atomic number is 1 and its atomic weight is 1.008. It is the simplest and lightest of the elements, and is normally a colourless, odourless, highly inflammable diatomic gas. It occurs in pure form only sparsely in the earth and atmosphere, but is plentiful in the sun and many other stars. Hydrogen is a component of numerous compounds, several many of them produced by the body. As a component of water, hydrogen is crucial in the metabolic interaction of acids, bases, and salts within the body and in the fluid balance necessary for the body to survive. Hydrogen makes it possible for water…which serves as a host to many body functions…to dissolve the many different substances on which the body depends, such as oxygen and food substances. Hydrogen also makes the process of hydrolysis possible, by which compounds unite with water and split into simpler compounds.

hydrogenation. See **reduction.**

hydrogen bonding, the attractive force of compounds in which a hydrogen atom covalently linked to an electronegative element, such as oxygen, nitrogen or sulphur, has a large degree of positive character relative to the electronegative atom, thereby causing the compound to possess a large dipole.

hydrogen ion concentration of blood, a measure of blood pH and its effect on the ability of the haemoglobin molecule to hold oxygen.

hydrogen peroxide, a topical anti-infective used to cleanse open wounds, as a mouthwash, and to aid in the removal of cerumen from the external ear.

hydrolase, an enzyme that cleaves ester bonds by the addition of water.

hydrolysis, the chemical alteration or decomposition of a compound with water.

hydrometer, a device that determines the specific gravity or density of a liquid by a comparison of its weight with that of an equal volume of water. A calibrated, hollow glass device is placed in the liquid being examined, and the depth to which the device settles in the liquid is noted.

hydronephrosis, distention of the pelvis and calyces of the kidney by urine that cannot flow past an obstruction in a ureter. Ureteral obstruction may be caused by a tumour, a calculus lodged in the ureter, inflammation of the prostate gland, or oedema caused by a urinary tract infection. The person may experience pain in the flank and, in some cases, haematuria, pyuria and hyperpyrexia. **hydronephrotic,** *adj.*

hydropenia, lack of water in the body tissues.

hydrophilic, pertaining to the property of attracting water molecules, possessed by polar radicals or ions.

hydrophobia, 1. *nontechnical,* rabies. **2.** a morbid, extreme fear of water.

hydrophobic, pertaining to the property of repelling water molecules or side chains that are more soluble in organic solvents.

hydrophthalmos. See **congenital glaucoma.**

hydrops, an abnormal accumulation of clear, watery fluid in a body tissue or cavity, such as a joint, the abdomen, middle ear or gallbladder. Formerly called dropsy.

hydrops fetalis, massive oedema in the fetus or newborn, usually in association with severe erythroblastosis fetalis. Severe anaemia and effusions of the pericardial, pleural and peritoneal spaces also occur.

hydroquinone, a dermatological bleaching agent used to reduce pigmentation of the skin in certain skin conditions in which an excess of melanin causes hyperpigmentation.

hydrosalpinx, an abnormal condition of the uterine tube in which the tube is cystically enlarged and filled with clear fluid. It is the end-result of an infection that has previously occluded the tube at both ends.

hydrostatic pressure, the pressure exerted by a liquid.

hydrostatic dosimetry, the weighing of a person under water to determine lean to fat body weight.

hydrotherapy, the use of water in the treatment of various disorders such as pain relief, reduction of muscle spasms, and muscle strengthening.

hydrothorax, a non-inflammatory accumulation of serous fluid in one or both plural cavities.

hydrotropism, the tendency of a cell or organism to turn or move in a certain direction under the influence of a water stimulus.

hydrous wool fat. See **lanolin.**

hydroxide, an ionic compound that contains the OH⁻ ion, usually consisting of metals or the metal equivalent of the ammonium cation (NH_4^-) that inactivates an acid.

hydroxyandrosterone, a sex hormone secreted by the testes and adrenal glands. Its normal accumulation in the urine of men after 24-hour collection is 0.1 to 8 mg, and in women it is 0 to 0.5 mg.

hydroxyapatite, an inorganic compound composed of calcium, phosphate and hydroxide. It is found in the bones and teeth in a crystallized lattice-like form that gives these structures rigidity.

hydroxybenzene. See carbolic acid.

hydroxychloroquine sulphate, an antirheumatic drug that is also used as a suppressor of lupus erythematosus. It is has been used as an amoebicide.

17-hydroxycorticosteroid, any of the hormones, such as cortisol, secreted by adrenal glands. They are measured in the urine in a test for determining adrenal function and diagnosing hypo- or hyperadrenalism.

11-hydroxyetiocholanolone, a sex hormone secreted by the testes and adrenal glands.

5-hydroxyindoleacetic acid, an acid produced by serotonin metabolism, measured in the blood and urine to aid in the diagnosis of certain kinds of tumours. It commonly rises above normal levels in whole blood in relation to asthma, diarrhoea, rapid heartbeat and other symptoms, and is also elevated in the urine of patients with carcinoid syndrome.

hydroxyl (OH), a radical compound containing an oxygen atom and a hydrogen atom.

hydroxyprogesterone hexanoate, a progestational steroid used in the treatment of habitual abortion.

hydroxyproline, an amino acid that is elevated in the urine in diseases of the bone and certain genetic disorders, such as Marfan's syndrome.

5-hydroxytryptamine. See serotonin.

hydroxyurea, a cytotoxic drug used in the treatment of a variety of tumours and non-malignant haematological conditions.

hydroxyzine hydrochloride, a sedative antihistamine used for the relief of anxiety and pruritus.

hygrometer, an instrument that directly measures relative humidity of the atmosphere or the proportion of water in a specific gas or gas mixture, without extracting the moisture.

hygroscopic humidifier, a humidifying device attached to the tubing circuit of a mechanical ventilator or anaesthesia gas machine to maintain a constant rate of humidity in the patient's trachea.

hymen, a fold of mucous membrane, skin and fibrous tissue at the introitus of the vagina. It may be absent, small, thin and pliant or, rarely, tough and dense, completely occluding the introitus.

Hymenolepis, a genus of intestinal tapeworms infesting humans. Heavy infestation may cause abdominal pain, bloody stools and disorders of the nervous system. Contaminated food spreads the disease.

hymenotomy, the surgical incision of the hymen.

hyoglossal. See glossohyal.

hyoid bone, a single U-shaped bone suspended from the styloid processes of the temporal bones. The bone attaches to various muscles, such as the hypoglossus and sternohyoideus.

hyoscine, {Giovanni A. Scopoli, Italian naturalist b.1723} an anticholinergic alkaloid obtained from the leaves and seeds of several solanaceous plants. It is a depressant of the central nervous system. It is used to prevent motion sickness and as a antiemetic, a sedative in obstetrics and a cyclopegic and mydriatic.

hypalgesia, the perception of a painful stimulus to a degree that varies significantly from a normal perception of the same stimulus.

hyperacidity, an excessive amount of acidity, as in the stomach.

hyperactivity, any abnormally increased activity involving either the entire organism or a particular organ, such as the heart or thyroid.

hyperadrenalism. See Cushing's disease.

hyperadrenocorticism. See Cushing's syndrome.

hyperaldosteronism. See aldosteronism.

hyperalimentation, 1. overfeeding, ingestion or administration of a greater than optimal amount of nutrients, in excess of the demands of the appetite. **2.** See **total parenteral nutrition.**

hypaesthesia, an abnormal weakness of sensation in response to stimulation of the sensory nerves. Touch, pain, heat and cold are poorly perceived. **hypaesthetic,** adj.

hyperaemia, increased blood in part of the body, caused by increased blood flow, as in the inflammatory response, local relaxation of arterioles or obstruction of the outflow of blood from an area. Skin overlying a hyperaemic area usually becomes reddened and warm. **hyperaemic,** adj.

hyperaesthesia, an extreme sensitivity of one of the body's sense organs, such as pain or touch receptors in the skin.

hyperammonaemia, abnormally high levels of ammonia in the blood. Untreated, the condition leads to asterixis, vomiting, lethargy, coma and death.

hyperbaric oxygen therapy. See **hyperbaric oxygenation.**

hyperbaric oxygenation, the administration of oxygen at greater than normal atmospheric pressure. The procedure is performed in specially designed chambers that permit delivery of 100% oxygen at atmospheric pressure that is three times normal. The technique is employed to overcome the natural limit of oxygen solubility in blood. Hyperbaric oxygenation has been used to treat carbon monoxide poisoning, air embolism, smoke inhalation, acute cyanide poisoning, decompression sickness, clostridial myonecrosis, as well as certain cases of blood loss or anaemia in which increased oxygen transport may compensate in part for the haemoglobin deficiency.

hyperbarism, any disorder resulting from exposure to increased ambient pressure, usually from sudden exposure to or a significant increase in pressure.

hyperbasaemia, elevated arterial bicarbonate concentration, caused by metabolic or non-respiratory factors.

hyperbetalipoproteinaemia, type II hyperlipoproteinaemia, a genetic disorder of lipid metabolism in which there are abnormally high levels of serum cholesterol and xanthomas appear on the tendons of the heels, knees and fingers.

hyperbilirubinaemia, greater than normal amounts of the bile pigment bilirubin in the blood, often characterized by jaundice, anorexia and malaise. Hyperbilirubinaemia is most often associated with liver disease or biliary obstruction, but it also occurs when there is excessive destruction of red blood cells.

hyperbilirubinaemia of the newborn, an excess of bilirubin in the blood of the neonate, resulting from hepatic dysfunction. It is usually caused by a deficiency of an enzyme, resulting from physiological immaturity or increased haemolysis, especially from blood group incompatibility which, in severe cases, can lead to kernicterus.

hypercalcaemia, greater than normal amounts of calcium in the blood, most often resulting from excessive bone resorption and release of calcium, as occurs in hyperparathyroidism, metastatic tumours of bone, Paget's disease and osteoporosis. Clinically, patients with hypercalcaemia are confused and have anorexia, abdominal pain, muscle pain and weakness. **hypercalcaemic,** *adj.*

hypercalciuria, the presence of abnormally great amounts of calcium in the urine, resulting from conditions such as sarcoid, hyperparathyroidism or certain types of arthritis. It is characterized by augmented bone resorption. Concentrated amounts of calcium in the urinary tract may form kidney stones. **hypercalciuric,** *adj.*

hypercapnia, greater than normal amounts of carbon dioxide in the blood.

hyperchloraemia, an excessive level of chloride in the blood.

hyperchlorhydria, the excessive secretion of hydrochloric acid by cells lining the stomach.

hypercholesterolaemia, a condition in which greater than normal amounts of cholesterol are present in the blood. High levels of cholesterol and other lipids may lead to the development of atherosclerosis.

hypercholesterolaemic xanthomatosis. See familial hypercholesterolaemia.

hyperchromic, having a greater density of colour or pigment.

hyperchylomicronaemia, type I hyperlipoproteinaemia, a rare congenital deficiency of an enzyme essential to fat metabolism. Fat accumulates in the blood as chylomicrons. The condition affects children and young adults, who develop xanthomas (fatty deposits) in the skin, hepatomegaly and abdominal pain.

hypercoagulability, a tendency of the blood to coagulate more rapidly than is normal.

hyperdactyly. See polydactyly.

hyperdiploid. See hyperploid.

hyperdynamic syndrome, a cluster of symptoms that signal the onset of septic shock, often including shivering, rapid rise in temperature, flushing of the skin, galloping pulse, and alternating rise and fall of the blood pressure. This is a medical emergency that requires expert medical support in a hospital.

hyperemesis gravidarum, an abnormal condition of pregnancy characterized by severe and persistent vomiting. Its aetiology is not fully understood.

hyperextension, (of a joint) a position of maximum extension.

hyperextension bed, a bed used in paediatric orthopaedics to maintain any correction achieved by suspension of a body part, and to increase the range of motion of the hips after an operative muscle release procedure.

hyperextension suspension, an orthopaedic procedure used in the postoperative positioning of hip muscles. The procedure uses traction equipment, including metal frames, ropes and pulleys to relieve the weight of the lower limbs and position properly the muscles of the hip, without applying traction to the lower limbs involved.

hyperflexia, the forcible overflexion or bending of a limb.

hyperfractionation, a technique in radiotherapy where 2 or 3 smaller than usual fractions are given daily, to achieve an increase in the total dose over the same overall period of time.

hyperfunction, increased function of any organ or system.

hypergenesis, excessive growth or over-development. The condition may involve the entire body, as in gigantism, or any particular part. It may also result in the formation of extra parts, such as the development of additional fingers or toes. **hypergenetic,** *adj.*

hypergenetic teratism, a congenital anomaly in which there is excessive growth of a part or organ or the entire body, as in gigantism.

hypergenitalism, the presence of abnormally large external genitalia. The condition is usually associated with precocious puberty.

hyperglycaemia, a greater than normal amount of glucose in the blood. It is most frequently associated with diabetes mellitus, the condition may occur in newborns, after administration of glucocorticoid hormones, and with an excess infusion of intravenous solutions containing glucose.

hyperglycaemic-glycogenolytic factor. See **glucagon.**

hyperglycaemic-hyperosmolar non-ketotic coma, a diabetic coma in which the level of ketone bodies is normal. It is caused by hyperosmolarity of extracellular fluid and results in dehydration of intracellular fluid, often a consequence of overtreatment with hyperosmolar solutions.

hyperhidrosis, excessive perspiration, often caused by heat, hyperthyroidism, strong emotion, the menopause or infection.

hyperimmune, a characteristic associated with an unusual abundance of antibodies, producing a greater than normal immunity.

hyperinsulinism, an excessive amount of insulin in the body, as may occur when a greater than required dose is administered.

hyperintention, an excessive amount of concentration on an objective, which may result in failure to accomplish the goal.

hyperkalaemia, greater than normal amounts of potassium in the blood. This condition is seen frequently in acute renal failure. Early signs are nausea, diarrhoea and muscle weakness.

hyperkalaemic periodic paralysis. See **adynamia episodica hereditaria.**

hyperkeratosis, overgrowth of the cornified epithelial layer of the skin.

hyperkinesis. See **attention deficit disorder.**

hyperlipaemia, an excessive level of blood fats, usually due to a lipoprotein lipase deficiency or a defect in the conversion of low-density lipoproteins (LDL) to high-density lipoproteins (HDL).

hyperlipidaemia, an excess of lipids in the plasma, including the glycolipids, lipoproteins and phospholipids.

hyperlipidaemia type I, a condition of elevated lipid levels in the blood, characterized by an increase in both cholesterol and triglycerides, and caused by the presence of chylomicrons. It is inherited as an autosomal recessive trait with a low risk of atherosclerosis.

hyperlipidaemia type IIA, hyperlipidaemia type IIB. See **familial hypercholesterolaemia.**

hyperlipidaemia type III. See **broad beta disease.**

hyperlipidaemia type IV, a relatively common form of hyperlipoproteinaemia characterized by a slight elevation in cholesterol levels, a moderate elevation of triglycerides and an elevation of the normal triglyceride carrier protein VLDL. It is sometimes familial and associated with an increased risk factor for coronary atherosclerosis.

hyperlipidaemia type V, a condition of elevated blood lipids characterized by slightly increased cholesterol, greatly increased triglycerides, elevation of the triglyceride carrier protein VLDL and chylomicrons. It is a genetically heterogenous disorder.

hyperlipoproteinaemia, any of a large group of inherited and acquired disorders of lipoprotein metabolism characterized by greater than normal amounts of certain protein-bound lipids and other fatty substances in the blood.

hypermagnesaemia, a greater than normal amount of magnesium in the plasma, found in people with kidney failure and those receiving large quantities of medications containing magnesium, such as antacids. Toxic levels of magnesium cause cardiac arrhythmias and depression of deep tendon reflexes and respiration.

hypermetria, an abnormal condition which is a form of dysmetria, characterized by a dysfunction of the power to control the range of muscular action. It results in movements that overreach the intended goal of the affected individual.

hypermetropia, hypermetropy, See **hyperopia.**

hypermorph, 1. a person whose arms and legs are disproportionately long in relation to the trunk, and whose sitting height is disproportionate to the standing height. 2. (in genetics) a mutant gene that shows an increased activity in the expression of a trait.

hypermotility, an excessive movement of the involuntary muscles, particularly in the GI tract.

hypernatraemia, a greater than normal concentration of sodium in the blood, caused by excessive loss of water and electrolytes. It results from polyuria, diarrhoea, excessive sweating or inadequate water intake. People with hypernatraemia may become mentally confused, have seizures and lapse into coma. Care must be taken to restore water balance slowly, because further electrolyte imbalances may occur.

hyperopia, farsightedness, a condition resulting from an error of refraction in which rays of light entering the eye are brought into focus behind the retina.

hyperornithinaemia, a metabolic disorder involving the amino acid ornithine which tends to accumulate in the tissues, causing seizures and retardation.

hyperosmia, an abnormally increased sensitivity to odours.

hyperosmolarity, a state or condition of abnormally increased osmolarity. **hyperosmolar,** *adj.*

hyperosmotic, pertaining to an increased concentration of osmotically active components.

hyperoxaluria, an excessive level of oxalic acid or oxalates, primarily calcium oxalate, in the urine. An excess of oxalates may lead to the formation of renal calculi.

hyperoxia, a condition of abnormally high oxygen tension in the blood.

hyperoxygenation, the use of high concentrations of inspired oxygen before and after endotracheal aspiration.

hyperparathyroidism, an abnormal endocrine condition characterized by hyperactivity of any of the four parathyroid glands with excessive secretion of parathyroid hormone (PTH). It results in increased resorption of calcium from the skeletal system and increased absorption of calcium by the kidneys and GI system. The condition may be primary, originating in one or more of the parathyroid glands, or secondary, resulting from an abnormal hypocalcaemia-producing condition in another part of the body, causing a compensatory hyperactivity of the parathyroid glands.

hyperphenylalaninaemia, an abnormally high concentration of phenylalanine in the blood. This symptom may be the result of one of several defects in the metabolic process of breaking down phenylalanine.

hyperphoria, the tendency of an eye to deviate upwards.

hyperpigmentation, unusual darkening of the skin. Causes include heredity, drugs, exposure to the sun and adrenal insufficiency.

hyperplasia, an increase in the number of cells of a body part.

hyperploid, 1. of or pertaining to an individual, organism, strain or cell that has one or more chromosomes in excess of the basic haploid number or an exact multiple of the haploid number characteristic of the species. **2.** such an individual, organism, strain or cell.

hyperploidy, any increase in chromosome number that involves individual chromosomes rather than entire sets, resulting in more than the normal haploid number characteristic of the species, as in Down's syndrome.

hyperpnoea, a deep, rapid or laboured respiration. It occurs normally with exercise, and abnormally with pain, fever, hysteria or any condition in which the supply of oxygen is inadequate, such as cardiac and respiratory disease. **hyperpnoic,** *adj.*

hyperprolactinaemia, an excessive amount of prolactin in the blood. The condition is caused by a hypothalamic-pituitary dysfunction. In women it is usually associated with gynaecomastia, galactorrhoea and secondary amenorrhoea; in men it may be a factor in decreased libido and impotence.

hyperptyalism. See ptyalism.

hyperpyrexia, an extremely elevated temperature sometimes occurring in acute infectious diseases, especially in young children. Malignant hyperpyrexia, characterized by a rapid rise in temperature, tachycardia, tachypnoea, sweating, rigidity and blotchy cyanosis, occasionally occurs in patients undergoing general anaesthesia. **hyperpyretic,** *adj.*

hyperreactivity, an abnormal condition in which responses to stimuli are exaggerated.

hyperreflection, a compulsion to devote excessive attention to oneself.

hyperreflexia, a neurological condition characterized by increased reflex reactions.

hypersensitivity, an abnormal condition characterized by an excessive reaction to a particular stimulus. **hypersensitive,** *adj.*

hypersensitivity pneumonitis. an inflammatory form of interstitial pneumonia that results from an immunological reaction in a hypersensitive person. The reaction may be provoked by a variety of inhaled organic dusts, often those containing fungal spores. A wide variety of symptoms may occur, including asthma, fever, chills, malaise and muscle aches, which usually develop 4 to 6 hours after exposure. Kinds of hypersensitivity pneumonitis include **bagassosis** and **farmer's lung.**

hypersensitivity reaction, an inappropriate and excessive response of the immune system to a sensitizing antigen. The antigenic stimulant is an allergen. Hypersensitivity reactions are classified by the components of the immune system involved in their mediation. Humoral reactions, mediated by the circulating B lymphocytes, are immediate and include three types: anaphylactic hypersensitivity, cytotoxic hypersensitivity, and immune system hypersensitivity. Cellular reactions, mediated by the T lymphocytes, are delayed, cell-mediated hypersensitivity reactions.

hypersomnia, 1. sleep of excessive depth or abnormal duration, usually caused by psychological rather than physical factors and characterized by a state of confusion on awakening. **2.** extreme drowsiness, often associated with lethargy. **3.** a condition characterized by periods of deep, long sleep.

hyperspadias. See epispadias.

hypersplenism, a syndrome consisting of splenomegaly and a deficiency of one or more types of blood cells. The numerous causes of this syndrome include lymphomas, the haemolytic anaemias, malaria, tuberculosis and various connective tissue and inflammatory diseases. Patients complain of abdominal pain on the left side, and often experience fullness after little eating because the greatly enlarged spleen is pressing against the stomach.

hypersthenic, 1. pertaining to a condition of excessive strength or tonicity of the body or a body part. **2.** pertaining to a body type characterized by massive proportions.

hypertelorism, a developmental defect characterized by an abnormally wide space between two organs or parts. A kind of hypertelorism is ocular hypertelorism.

hypertension a common, often asymptomatic disorder characterized by elevated blood pressure persistently exceeding 140/90 mm Hg. Essential hypertension, the most frequent kind, has no single identifiable cause, but the risk of the disorder is increased by obesity, a high sodium level in serum, hypercholesterolaemia and a family history of high blood pressure. Known causes of hypertension include adrenal disorders, such as aldosteronism, Cushing's syndrome and phaeochromocytoma, thyrotoxicosis, toxaemia of pregnancy and chronic glomerulonephritis. Persons with mild or moderate hypertension may be asymptomatic or may experience suboccipital headaches especially on rising, as well as tinnitus, lightheadness, easy fatigability and palpitations. Malignant hypertension, characterized by a diastolic pressure higher than 120 mm Hg, severe headaches, blurred vision and confusion, may result in fatal uraemia, myocardial infarction, congestive heart failure or a cerebrovascular accident. Kinds of hypertension are **essential hypertension, malignant hypertension** and **secondary hypertension.**

hypertensive crisis, a sudden severe increase in blood pressure to a level exceeding 200/120 mm Hg, occurring most frequently in untreated hypertension and in patients who have stopped taking prescribed antihypertensive medication. Characteristic signs include severe headache, vertigo, diplopia, tinnitus, nosebleeding, twitching muscles, tachycardia or other cardiac arrhythmia, distended neck veins, narrowed pulse pressure, nausea and vomiting. The patient may be confused, irritable or stuporous, and the condition may lead to convulsions, coma, myocardial infarction, renal failure, cardiac arrest or stroke.

hypertensive encephalopathy, a set of symptoms, including headache, convulsions and coma associated with glomerulonephritis.

hypertetraploid. See **hyperploid.**

hyperthermia, 1. a much higher than normal body temperature induced therapeutically or iatrogenically. **2.** *non-technical,* malignant hyperthermia. **3.** a state in which an individual's body temperature is elevated above the normal range. Defining characteristics include increase in body temperature, flushed skin, skin warm to the touch, increased respiratory rate, tachycardia and seizures or convulsions.

hyperthyroidism, a condition characterized by hyperactivity of the thyroid gland. The gland is usually enlarged, secreting greater than normal amounts of thyroid hormones, and the metabolic processes of the body are accelerated. Nervousness, exophthalmos, tremor, constant hunger, weight loss, fatigue, heat intolerance, palpitations and diarrhoea may develop.

hypertonia, 1. abnormally increased muscle tone or strength. The condition is sometimes associated with genetic disorders. **2.** a condition of excessive pressure, as in the intraocular pressure of glaucoma.

hypertonic, (of a solution) having a greater concentration of solute than another solution, hence exerting more osmotic pressure than that solution, such as a hypertonic saline solution that contains more salt than is found in intracellular and extracellular fluid.

hypertonic contracture, prolonged muscle contraction resulting from continuous nerve stimulation in spastic paralysis.

hypertonic saline, a saline solution that contains 1% to 15% sodium chloride (compared with normal saline at 0.9%). It is used as a bronchial lavage to stimulate sputum production and promote coughing.

hypertonic solution, a solution that increases the degree of osmotic pressure on a semipermeable membrane.

hypertrichosis. See **hirsutism.**

hypertriglyceridaemia. See **hyperchylomicronaemia.**

hypertriploid. See **hyperploid.**

hypertrophic angioma. See **haemangioendothelioma.**

hypertrophic catarrh, a chronic condition characterized by inflammation and discharge from a mucous membrane, accompanied by the thickening of the mucosal and submucosal tissue.

hypertrophic gastritis, an inflammatory condition of the stomach characterized by epigastric pain, nausea, vomiting, and distention. It is differentiated from other forms of gastritis by the presence of prominent rugae (folds), enlarged glands, and nodules on the wall of the stomach. This condition often occurs with peptic ulcer, Zollinger-Ellison syndrome, or gastric hypersecretion.

hypertrophic gingivitis. See **gingivitis.**

hypertrophic obstructive cardiomyopathy. See **idiopathic hypertrophic subaortic stenosis.**

hypertrophic scarring, scarring caused by excessive formation of new tissue in the healing of a wound. It has the appearance of a hard, tumour-like keloid.

hypertrophy, an increase in the size of an organ caused by an increase in the size, rather than the number, of cells. Kinds of hypertrophy include **adaptive hypertrophy, compensatory hypertrophy, Marie's hypertrophy, physiological hypertrophy** and **unilateral hypertrophy. hypertrophic,** *adj.*

hyperuricaemia. See **gout.**

hyperventilation, a pulmonary ventilation rate that is greater than what is metabolically necessary for the exchange of respiratory gases. It is the result of an increased frequency of breathing, increased tidal volume, or a combination of both. It causes excessive intake of oxygen and exhalation of carbon dioxide. Hypocapnia and respiratory alkalosis then occur, leading to chest pain, dizziness, faintness, numbness of the fingers and toes, and psychomotor impairment.

hypervitaminosis, an abnormal condition resulting from excessive intake of toxic amounts of one or more vitamins, especially over a long period of time. Serious effects may result from overdoses of vitamins A, D, E or K, but rarely with the water-soluble B and C vitamins.

hypervolaemia, an increase in the amount of extracellular fluid, particularly in the volume of circulating blood or its components.

hypha, pl. **hyphae,** the thread-like structure of the mycelium in a fungus.

hyphaema, a haemorrhage into the anterior chamber of the eye, usually caused by a blunt or percussive injury. Glaucoma may result from recurrent bleeding.

hypnagogic hallucination, one that occurs in the period between wakefulness and sleep.

hypnagogue, an agent or substance that tends to induce sleep or the feeling of dreamy sleepiness, as occurs before falling asleep. **hypnagogic,** adj.

hypnoanalysis, the use of hypnosis as an adjunct to other techniques in psychoanalysis.

hypnosis, a passive, trance-like state that resembles normal sleep during which perception and memory are altered, resulting in increased responsiveness to suggestion. Susceptibility to hypnosis varies from person to person. Hypnosis is used in some forms of psychotherapy, in behaviour modification programmes, or in medicine to reduce pain and promote relaxation.

hypnotherapy, the use of hypnosis as an adjunct to other techniques in psychotherapy.

hypnotic trance, an artificially induced sleep-like state, as in hypnosis.

hypnotic, a drug used to induce sleep.

hypnotism, the study or practice of inducing hypnosis.

hypnotist, one who practises hypnotism.

hypnotize, 1. to put into a state of hypnosis. **2.** to fascinate, entrance or control through personal charm.

hypoacidity, a deficiency of acid.

hypoactivity, any abnormally diminished activity of the body or its organs, such as decreased cardiac output, thyroid secretion or peristalsis.

hypoadrenalism. See **Addison's disease.**

hypoalbuminaemia, a condition of abnormally low levels of albumin in the blood.

hypoalimentation, a condition of insufficient or inadequate nourishment.

hypobarism, air pressure that is significantly less than sea level normal of 760 mm Hg.

hypobasaemia, reduced arterial bicarbonate concentration caused by metabolic or non-respiratory factors.

hypobetalipoproteinaemia, an inherited disorder in which there are less than normal amounts of beta-lipoprotein in the serum.

hypocalcaemia, a deficiency of calcium in the serum that may be caused by hypoparathyroidism, vitamin D deficiency, kidney failure, acute pancreatitis or inadequate plasma magnesium and protein. Mild hypocalcaemia is asymptomatic. Severe hypocalcaemia is characterized by cardiac arrhythmias and tetany with hyperparaesthesia of the hands, feet, lips and tongue. **hypocalcaemic,** adj.

hypocapnia, an abnormally low arterial carbon dioxide level.

hypochloraemia, a decrease in the chloride level in the blood serum. The condition may occur as a result of prolonged gastric suctioning.

hypochloraemic alkalosis, a metabolic alkalosis resulting from increased blood bicarbonate secondary to loss of chloride from the body.

hypochlorhydria, a deficiency of hydrochloric acid in the stomach's gastric juice.

hypochlorite poisoning, toxic effects of ingestion or skin contact with household or commercial bleaches or similar chlorinated products. Symptoms include pain and inflammation of the mouth and digestive tract, vomiting and breathing difficulty.

hypochlorous acid, a greenish-yellow liquid derived from an aqueous solution of lime.

hypochondria, hypochondriac neurosis. See **hypochondriasis.**

hypochondriac region, the part of the abdomen in the upper zone on both sides of the epigastric region and beneath the cartilages of the lower ribs.

hypochondriasis, 1. a chronic, abnormal concern about the health of the body. **2.** a disorder characterized by extreme anxiety, depression, and an unrealistic interpretation of real or imagined physical symptoms as indications of a serious illness or disease, despite rational medical evidence that no disorder is present. **hypochondriac,** adj., n., **hypochondriac, hypochondriacal,** adj.

hypochondrium. See **hypochondriac region.**

hypochondroplasia, an inherited form of dwarfism that resembles a mild form of achondroplasia.

hypochromic, having less than normal colour, usually describing a red blood cell and characterizing anaemia associated with decreased synthesis of haemoglobin.

hypochromic anaemia, any of a large group of anaemias characterized by a decreased concentration of hemoglobin in the red blood cells.

hypocycloidal motion, (in computed tomography) a circular pattern of movement of the x-ray tube and film that results in blurring of structures outside the focal plane and elimination of ghost images.

hypocytic leukaemia. See **aleukaemic leukaemia.**

hypodermic, of or pertaining to the area below the skin, as a hypodermic injection.

hypodermic needle, a short, thin, hollow needle that attaches to a syringe for injecting a drug or medication under the skin or into vessels, and for withdrawing a fluid, such as blood, for examination.

hypodiploid. See **hypoploid.**

hypofibrinogenaemia, a deficiency of fibrinogen, a blood clotting factor, in the blood. The condition may occur as a complication of abruptio placentae.

hypogammaglobulinaemia, a less than normal concentration of gamma globulin in the blood, usually the result of increased protein catabolism or loss of protein in the urine, as in nephrosis.

hypogastric artery. See **internal iliac artery.**

hypogastrium. See **pubic region.**

hypogenitalism, a condition of retarded sexual development caused by a defect in male or female hormonal production in the testis or ovary.

hypogeusia, reduced taste.

hypoglossal nerve, either of a pair of cranial nerves essential for swallowing and moving the tongue.

hypoglossus, 1. a muscle that retracts and pulls down the side of the tongue. **2.** the hypoglossal nerve.

hypoglycaemia, a less than normal amount of glucose in the blood, usually caused by administration of too much insulin, excessive secretion by the islet cells of the pancreas, or dietary deficiency. The condition may result in weakness, headache, hunger, visual disturbances, ataxia, anxiety, personality changes and, if untreated, delirium, coma and death.

hypoglycaemic agent, any of a large, heterogeneous group of drugs used to decrease the amount of glucose circulating in the blood. Hypoglycaemic agents include insulin, the sulphonylureas and the biguanides. Insulin in its various forms is given parenterally and acts by increasing the use of carbohydrates and metabolism of fats and protein. The sulphonylureas act by stimulating the release of endogenous insulin from the pancreas. The biguanides act by potentiating the action of endogenous insulin, augmenting cellular use of glucose.

hypoglycaemic shock treatment. See **insulin shock treatment.**

hypogonadism, a deficiency in the secretory activity of the ovary or testis. The condition may be primary, caused by a gonadal dysfunction involving the Leydig cells in the male, or secondary to a hypothalamic-pituitary disorder.

hypokalaemia, a condition in which an inadequate amount of potassium, the major intracellular cation, is found in the circulating bloodstream. Hypokalaemia is characterized by abnormal ECG, weakness and flaccid paralysis, and may be caused by starvation, treatment of diabetic acidosis, adrenal tumour or diuretic therapy.

hypokalaemic alkalosis, a pathological condition resulting from the accumulation of base or loss of acid from the body associated with a low level of serum potassium.

hypokinesia, a condition of abnormally diminished motor activity.

hypolipaemia. See **hypolipoproteinaemia.**

hypolipoproteinaemia, a group of defects of lipoprotein metabolism that result in varying complexes of signs. Primary or hereditary, hypolipoproteinaemia factors include abnormal transport of triglycerides in the blood, low levels of high-density lipoproteins, high levels of low-density lipoproteins and abnormal deposition of lipids in the body. Types include **abetalipoproteinaemia, hypobetalipoproteinaemia, lecithincholesterol acyltransferase deficiency** and **Tangier disease.**

hypomagnesaemia, an abnormally low concentration of magnesium in the blood plasma, resulting in nausea, vomiting, muscle weakness, tremors, tetany and lethargy. Mild hypomagnesaemia is usually the result of inadequate absorption of magnesium in the kidney or intestine. A more severe form is associated with malabsorption syndrome, protein malnutrition and parathyroid disease.

hypomania, a psychopathological state characterized by optimism, excitability, a marked hyperactivity and talkativeness, heightened sexual interest, quick anger and irritability, and a decreased need for sleep. **hypomaniac,** *n.,* **hypomanic,** *adj.*

hypometria, an abnormal condition which is a form of dysmetria, characterized by a dysfunction of the power to control the range of muscular action. It results in movements that fall short of the intended goals of the affected individual.

hypomobility, a lack of normal movement of a joint or body part. This may result from an articular surface dysfunction, or from disease or injury affecting a bone or muscle.

hypomorph, 1. a person whose legs are disproportionately short in relation to the trunk and whose sitting height is greater in proportion than the person's standing height. **2.** (in genetics) a mutant allele that has a reduced effect on the expression of a trait but at a level too low to result in abnormal development.

hyponatraemia, a less than normal concentration of sodium in the blood, caused by inadequate excretion of water or excessive water in the circulating bloodstream. In severe cases, the person may develop water intoxication with confusion and lethargy, leading to muscle excitability, convulsions and coma.

hypoparathyroidism, a condition of diminished parathyroid function, which can be caused by primary parathyroid dysfunction or elevated serum calcium levels.

hypopharyngeal, 1. of, pertaining to, or involving the hypopharynx. **2.** situated below the pharynx.

hypopharynx, the inferior portion of the pharynx, between the epiglottis and the larynx. It is a critical dividing point in separating solids and fluids from air entering the region.

hypophoria, a type of strabismus in which the patient may not show signs of ocular muscle imbalance until the affected eye is covered, resulting in a downward deviation.

hypophosphataemic rickets, a rare familial disorder in which there is impaired resorption of phosphate in the kidneys and poor absorption of calcium in the small intestine, resulting in osteomalacia, retarded growth, skeletal deformities and pain.

hypophosphatasia, congenital absence of alkaline phosphatase, an enzyme essential to the calcification of bone tissue.

hypophyseal cachexia. See **panhypopituitarism.**

hypophyseal dwarf. See **pituitary dwarf.**

hypophyseal hormones, hormones associated with body growth and exercise effects, such as luteinizing hormone, growth hormone and antidiuretic hormone.

hypophysectomy, surgical removal of the pituitary gland. It may be performed to slow the growth and spread of endocrine-dependent malignant tumours of the breast, ovary or prostate gland, halt deterioration of the retina in diabetes, or excise a pituitary tumour. **hypophysectomize,** v.

hypophysis cerebri. See **pituitary gland.**

hypopigmentation, unusual lack of skin colour, seen in albinism or vitiligo.

hypopituitarism, an abnormal condition caused by diminished activity of the pituitary gland and marked by excessive deposits of fat and persistence or acquisition of adolescent characteristics.

hypoplasia, incomplete or underdeveloped organ or tissue, usually the result of a decrease in the number of cells. Kinds of hypoplasia are cartilage-hair hypoplasia and enamel hypoplasia. **hypoplastic,** adj.

hypoplasia of the mesenchyme. See **osteogenesis imperfecta.**

hypoplastic anaemia, a broad category of anaemias characterized by decreased production of red blood cells.

hypoplastic dwarf. See **primordial dwarf.**

hypoploid, 1. also hypoploidic, of or pertaining to an individual, organism, strain or cell that has fewer than the normal haploid number, or an exact multiple of the haploid number of chromosomes characteristic of the species. **2.** such an individual, organism, strain or cell.

hypoploidy, any decrease in chromosome number that involves individual chromosomes rather than entire sets, resulting in fewer than the normal haploid number characteristic of the species, as seen in Turner's syndrome.

hypopnoea, shallow or slow respiration. In well-conditioned athletes this is normal and accompanied by a slow pulse; otherwise, it is characteristic of damage to the brainstem, in which case it is a grave sign accompanied by a rapid, weak pulse.

hypopotassaemia, a deficiency of potassium in the blood.

hypoproliferative anaemias, a group of anaemias caused by inadequate production of erythrocytes. The condition is associated with protein deficiencies, renal diesease and myxoedema.

hypoproteinaemia, a disorder characterized by a decrease in the amount of protein in the blood to an abnormally low level, accompanied by oedema, nausea, vomiting, diarrhoea and abdominal pain.

hypoprothrombinaemia, an abnormal reduction in the amount of prothrombin (factor II) in the circulating blood, characterized by poor clot formation, longer bleeding time and possible haemorrhage.

hypoptyalism, a condition in which there is a decrease in the amount of saliva secreted by the salivary glands.

hypopyon, an accumulation of pus in the anterior chamber of an eye, appearing as a grey fluid between the cornea and iris. It may occur as a complication of conjunctivitis, herpetic keratitis or corneal ulcer.

hyporeflexia, a neurological condition characterized by weakened reflex reactions.

hyposalivation, a decreased flow of saliva that may be associated with dehydration, radiation therapy of the salivary gland regions, anxiety, use of drugs, as atropine and antihistamines, vitamin deficiency, various forms of parotitis, or various syndromes such as the Plummer-Vinson syndrome.

hyposensitization. See **immunotherapy.**

hyposmolarity, a state or condition of abnormally reduced osmolarity.

hypospadias, a congenital defect in which the urinary meatus is on the underside of the penis. Incontinence does not occur because the sphincters are not defective.

hypostatic, pertaining to an accumulation of deposits of substances or congestion in a body area. It results from a lack of activity.

hypostatic pneumonia, a type of pneumomia associated with elderly or debilitated persons who remain in the same position for long periods. Gravity tends to accelerate fluid congestion in one area of the lungs, increasing susceptibility to infection.

hyposthenic, 1. pertaining to a lack of strength or muscle tone. 2. pertaining to a body type characterized by a slender build.

hypotelorism, a developmental defect characterized by an abnormally decreased distance between two organs or parts. A kind of hypotelorism is **ocular hypotelorism.**

hypotension, an abnormal condition in which the blood pressure is not adequate for normal perfusion and oxygenation of the tissues. Causes may include an expanded intravascular space, a decreased intravascular volume or a diminished cardiac thrust.

hypotensive anaesthesia. See **deliberate hypotension.**

hypotetraploid. See **hypoploid.**

hypothalamic amenorrhoea, cessation of menses caused by disorders that inhibit the hypothalamus from initiating the cycle of neurohormonal interactions of the brain, pituitary and ovary. This cycle is necessary for ovulation and subsequent menstruation.

hypothalamic hormones, a group of hormones secreted by the hypothalamus, including vasopressin, oxytocin, and the thyrotrophin-releasing and gonadotrophin-releasing hormones.

hypothalamic-pituitary-adrenal axis, the combined system of neuroendocrine units that regulate the body's hormonal activities.

hypothalamus, a portion of the diencephalon of the brain, forming the floor and part of the lateral wall of the third ventricle. It activates, controls and integrates the peripheral autonomic nervous system, endocrine processes and many somatic functions, such as body temperature, sleep and appetite. **hypothalamic,** *adj.*

hypothenar, an eminence or fleshy elevation on the ulnar side of the palm of the hand.

hypothermia, 1. an abnormal and dangerous condition in which the temperature of the body is below 95° F (35° C), usually caused by prolonged exposure to cold. Respiration is shallow and slow, and the heart rate is faint and slow. The person is very pale and may appear to be dead. People most susceptible to hypothermia are those who are very old or very young, those with cardiovascular problems, and those who are hungry, tired or under the influence of alcohol. Treatment includes slowly warming the person. Hospitalization is necessary for evaluating and treating any metabolic abnormalities that may result from hypothermia. 2. the deliberate and controlled reduction of body temperature with cooling mattresses or ice, as used in preparation for some surgical procedures. 3. the state in which an individual's body temperature is reduced below the normal range, but not below 35.5°C (96° F) (rectal). Defining characteristics include mild shivering, cool skin, moderate pallor, slow capillary refill, tachycardia, cyanotic nail beds, hypertension and piloerection.

hypothermia blanket, a covering used to conserve heat in the body of a patient suffering from hypothermia.

hypothermia therapy, the reduction of a patient's body temperature to counteract high prolonged fever caused by an infectious or neurological disease. Less frequently, this is used as an adjunct to anaesthesia in heart or brain surgery. Hypothermia may be produced by placing crushed ice around the patient, immersing the body in ice water, autotransfusing blood after it is circulated through coils submerged in a refrigerant or, most commonly, by applying cooling blankets or vinyl pads containing coils through which cold water and alcohol are circulated by a pump.

hypothesis, (in research) a statement derived from a theory that predicts the relationship among variables representing concepts, constructs or events. Kinds of hypotheses include **causal hypothesis, null hypothesis** and **predictive hypothesis.**

hypothrombinaemia, a deficiency of the clotting factor thrombin in the blood.

hypothyroid dwarf. See **cretin dwarf.**

hypothyroidism, a condition characterized by decreased activity of the thyroid gland. It is caused by surgical removal of all or part of the gland, an overdose of antithyroid medication, decreased effect of thyroid releasing hormone secreted by the hypothalamus, decreased secretion of thyroid stimulating hormone by the pituitary gland, or by atrophy of the thyroid gland itself. Weight gain, sluggishness, dryness of the skin, constipation, arthritis and slowing of the metabolic processes may occur. Untreated, hypothyroidism leads to myxoedema, coma and death.

hypotonic, (of a solution) having a smaller concentration of solute than another solution, hence exerting less osmotic pressure than that solution, such as a hypotonic saline solution that contains less salt than is found in intra- and extracellular fluid. Cells expand in a hypotonic solution.

hypotriploid. See **hypoploid.**

hypoventilation, an abnormal condition of the respiratory system, characterized by cyanosis, clubbing of the fingers, polycythaemia, increased carbon dioxide arterial tension, Cheyne-Stokes breathing and generalized decreased respiratory function. Hypoventilation may be caused by uneven distribution of inspired air (as in bronchitis), obesity, neuromuscular or skeletal disease affecting the thorax, decreased response of the respiratory centre to carbon dioxide, and reduced functional lung tissue, as seen in atelectasis, emphysema and pleural effusion. Hypoventilation results in hypoxia, hypercapnia, pulmonary hypertension with cor pulmonale, and respiratory acidosis.

hypovitaminosis. See **avitaminosis.**

hypovolaemia, an abnormally low circulating blood volume.

hypovolaemic shock, a state of physical collapse and prostration caused by massive blood loss, circulatory dysfunction and inadequate tissue perfusion. The common signs include low blood pressure, feeble pulse, clammy skin, tachycardia, rapid breathing and reduced urinary output. The associated blood losses may stem from GI bleeding, internal or external haemorrhage, or excessive reduction of intravascular plasma volume and body fluids. Disorders that may cause hypovolaemic shock are dehydration from excessive perspiration, severe diarrhoea, protracted vomiting, intestinal obstruction, peritonitis, acute pancreatitis and severe burns, all of which deplete body fluids.

hypoxaemia, an abnormal deficiency of oxygen in the arterial blood. Symptoms of acute hypoxaemia are cyanosis, restlessness, stupor, coma, Cheyne-Stokes breathing, apnoea, increased blood pressure, tachycardia as well as an initial increase in cardiac output that later falls, resulting in hypotension and ventricular fibrillation or asystole. Chronic hypoxaemia stimulates red blood cell production by the bone marrow, leading to secondary polycythaemia.

hypoxia, an inadequate, reduced tension of cellular oxygen, characterized by cyanosis, tachycardia, hypertension, peripheral vasoconstriction, dizziness and mental confusion. The tissues most sensitive to hypoxia are the brain, heart, pulmonary vessels and liver.

hypoxic drive, the low arterial oxygen pressure stimulus to respiration, mediated through the carotid bodies.

hypsibrachycephaly, the condition of having a skull that is high, with a broad forehead. **hypsibrachycephalic,** *adj., n.*

hypsicephaly. See **oxycephaly.**

hysterectomy, surgical removal of the uterus. It is performed to remove fibroid tumours of the uterus, or to treat chronic pelvic inflammatory disease, severe recurrent endometrial hyperplasia, uterine haemorrhage and precancerous or cancerous conditions of the uterus. Types of hysterectomy include **total hysterectomy,** in which the uterus and cervix are removed, and **radical hysterectomy,** in which ovaries, oviducts, lymph nodes and lymph channels are removed with the uterus and cervix. Menstruation ceases after either type is performed. One or both ovaries and oviducts may be removed at the same time. A kind of hysterectomy is **caesarean hysterectomy. hysterectomize,** *v.*

hysteresis, 1. a lagging or retardation of one of two associated phenomena, or failure to act in unison. **2.** the influence of the previous condition or treatment of the body on its subsequent response to a given force.

hysteria, 1. a general state of tension or excitement in a person or group, characterized by unmanageable fear and temporary loss of control over emotions. **2.** *obsolete.* a psychoneurosis, now commonly called **hysterical neurosis.**

hysteric apepsia. See **anorexia nervosa.**

hysterical amaurosis, monocular or, more rarely, binocular blindness occurring after an emotional shock and lasting for hours, days or months.

hysterical personality. See **histrionic personality.**

hysterical trance, a somnambulistic state occurring as a symptom of hysterical neurosis.

hysterosalpingo-oophorectomy, surgical removal of one or both ovaries and oviducts along with the uterus. It is usually performed for the treatment of malignant neoplastic disease of the reproductive tract and chronic endometriosis. To avoid the severe symptoms of sudden menopause, a portion of one ovary is left unless a malignancy is present.

hysterosalpingography, a radiographic technique to visualize the cavity of the uterus and uterine tubes in a non-pregnant woman, following the introduction of radiopaque contrast medium into the cervical canal. **hysterosalpingogram,** *n.*

hysteroscopy, direct visual inspection of the cervical canal and uterine cavity through a hysteroscope. It is used for examination of the endometrium, to secure a specimen for biopsy, remove an intrauterine device or excise cervical polyps. **hysteroscope,** *n.,* **hysteroscopic,** *adj.*

hysterotomy, surgical incision of the uterus, performed as a method of abortion in a pregnancy beyond the first trimester of gestation in which a saline-injection abortion was incomplete, or a tubal sterilization is to be carried out with the abortion.

Hz, abbreviation for **hertz.**

HZV, abbreviation for **herpes zoster virus.** See **chickenpox.**

I

i, a plural-forming element used in native and later scientific Latin words: bacilli, bronchi, plumbi, and in scientific terms derived through Latin from Greek: encephali, pylori, tympani.

I, 1. symbol for **inspired gas. 2.** symbol for **iodine.**

I.A.D.R., abbreviation for **International Association for Dental Research.**

I.C.S., abbreviation for **International Congress of Surgeons.**

I.M.A., abbreviation for **Industrial Medical Association.**

I:E ratio, (in respiratory therapy) the duration of inspiration to expiration. A range of 1:1.5 to 1:2 for an adult is considered acceptable for mechanical ventilation. Ratio increases to 1:1 or 2:1 or higher may cause haemodynamic complications.

iatrogenic caused by treatment or diagnostic procedures. **iatrogenesis,** *n.*

ibuprofen, a non-steroidal anti-inflammatory agent, used as an analgesic and in the treatment of rheumatoid and osteoarthritic conditions.

IC, abbreviation for **inspiratory capacity.**

ice therapy, the local or general application of cold for therapeutic and preventative purposes.

ICD, abbreviation for *International Classification of Diseases.*

Iceland disease, a group of symptoms associated with effects of a viral infection of the nervous system, including muscular pain and weakness, depression, and sensory changes.

ichthammol, a topical anti-infective used for treating certain skin diseases.

ichthyosis, any of several inherited dermatological conditions in which the skin is dry, hyperkeratotic and fissured, resembling fish scales. It usually appears at or shortly after birth and may be part of one of several rare syndromes. **ichthyotic,** *adj.*

ichthyosis congenita, ichthyosis fetalis. See **lamellar exfoliation of the newborn.**

ichthyosis fetus. See **harlequin fetus.**

ichthyosis vulgaris, a hereditary skin disorder characterized by large, dry, dark scales that cover the face, neck, scalp, ears, back and extensor surfaces, but not the flexor surfaces of the body.

ICN, abbreviation for **International Council of Nurses.**

ICP, abbreviation for **intracranial pressure.**

ICSH, abbreviation for **interstitial cell-stimulating hormone.** See **luteinizing hormone.**

ictal, pertaining to a sudden, acute onset, such as convulsions of an epileptic seizure.

icterus index, a liver function test in which the blood serum is compared in intensity of colour with that of potassium dichromate. When an excessive amount of bilirubin is present and jaundice becomes apparent, the index is higher; subnormal values are associated with various anemias.

icterus neonatorum, jaundice of the newborn infant.

icterus. See **jaundice.**

ictus, *pl.* **ictuses, ictus, 1.** a seizure. **2.** a cerebrovascular accident. **ictal, ictic,** *adj.*

ICU, abbreviation for **intensive care unit.**

ID, abbreviation for **infectious disease.**

id, 1. (in psychoanalysis) the part of the psyche functioning in the unconscious that is the source of instinctive energy, impulses and drives. **2.** the true unconscious.

id reaction, the autosensitization resulting from a fungal infection that causes pruritus and vesicular lesions. These secondary lesions, caused by circulating antigens, are usually distant from the primary fungal infection.

IDDM, abbreviation for **insulin-dependent diabetes mellitus.**

idèe fixe. See **fixed idea.**

idea, any thought, concept, intention or impression that exists in the mind as a result of awareness, understanding or other mental activity. Kinds of ideas include autochthonous idea, compulsive idea, dominant idea, fixed idea, idea of influence, idea of persecution and idea of reference.

idea of influence, an obsessive delusion, often seen in paranoid disorders, that external forces or persons are controlling one's thoughts, actions and feelings.

idea of persecution, an obsessive delusion, often seen in paranoid disorders, that one is being threatened, discriminated against or mistreated by other persons or by external forces.

idea of reference, an obsessive delusion that the statements or actions of others refer to oneself, usually taken to be depreciatory, often seen in paranoid disorders.

ideal gas law, a rule that PV = nRT, with the product of pressure (P) and volume (V) equal to the product of the number of moles of gas (n), temperature (T) and a gas constant (R).

idealized image, a self-concept of a person with a compulsive craving for perfection and admiration. It results in high unrealistic and unattainable goals.

ideational apraxia, a condition in which the conceptual process is lost, often because of a lesion in the parietal lobe. The individual is unable to formulate a plan of movement and does not know the proper use of an object because of a lack of perception of its purpose. There is no loss of motor movement.

identical twins. See **monozygotic twins.**

identification, an unconscious defence mechanism by which a person patterns his or her personality on that of another person, assuming the person's qualities, characteristics and actions. Kinds of identification are **competitive identification** and **positive identification.**

identity, a component of self-concept characterized by one's persisting consciousness of being oneself, separate and distinct from others. **Identity confusion** refers to an altered self-concept in which one does not maintain a clear consciousness of a consistent and continuous self. **Identity diffusion** is a lack of clarity and consistency in one's perception of the self, resulting in a high degreee of anxiety.

identity crisis, a period of disorientation concerning an individual's sense of self and role in society, occurring most frequently in the transition from one stage of life to the next. Identity crises are most common during adolescence, when a sudden increase in the strength of internal drives combined with greater peer pressure and adult expectations of more mature behaviour often results in conflicts.

ideomotor apraxia, the inability to translate an idea into motion, resulting from some interference with the transmission of the appropriate impulses from the brain to the motor centers. There is no loss of the ability to perform an action automatically, but the action cannot be performed on request.

idiogram, a diagram or graphic representation of a karyotype, showing the number, relative sizes and morphology of the chromosomes of a species, individual or cell.

idiojunctional rhythm, a heart rhythm emanating from the AV junction but without retrograde conduction to the atria.

idiomere. See **chromomere.**

idiopathic, without a known cause.

idiopathic disease, a disease that develops without an apparent or known cause, although it may have a recognizable pattern of signs and symptoms and may be curable.

idiopathic hypertrophic subaortic stenosis, a cardiomyopathic disorder, usually involving the left ventricle of the heart, that obstructs emptying.

idiopathic multiple pigmented haemorrhagic sarcoma. See **Kaposi's sarcoma.**

idiopathic respiratory distress syndrome.

See **acute respiratory distress syndrome.**

idiopathic scoliosis, an abnormal condition characterized by a lateral curvature of the spine. It is the most common type of scoliosis. The main factors in diagnosing idiopathic scoliosis are the degree, balance, and rotational component of the curvature. The rotational component may contribute to rib cage deformities and impingement on the pulmonary and the cardiac systems. Neurologic deficits are commonly associated with severe curvature and vary according to the extent to which the curvature has impinged on the spinal cord. Some signs of such impingement are reflex, sensation, and motor alterations of the lower extremities.

idiopathic thrombocytopenic purpura (ITP), bleeding into the skin and other organs caused by a deficiency of platelets. **Acute ITP** is a disease of children that may follow a viral infection, lasts a few weeks to a few months, and usually has no residual effects. **Chronic ITP** is more common in adolescents and adults, begins more insidiously and lasts longer. Antibodies to platelets are found in patients with ITP.

idiopathy, any primary disease that arises without an apparent cause. **idiopathic,** *adj.*

idiosyncrasy, 1. a physical or behavioural characteristic or manner that is unique to an individual or a group. **2.** an individual's unique hypersensitivity to a particular drug, food or other substance. **idiosyncratic,** *adj.*

idiot savant, *pl.* **idiot savants, idiots savants,** an individual with severe mental retardation who is nonetheless capable of performing certain unusual mental feats, primarily those involving music, puzzle-solving or the manipulation of numbers.

idiotype, the portion of an immunoglobulin molecule conferring unique character; most often including its binding site.

idioventricular, originating in a ventricle.

IDL (intermediate-density lipoprotein), a lipid-protein complex with a density between VLDL (very-low-density lipoprotein) and LDL (low-density lipoprotein). In a type III hyperlipoproteinaemic person the IDL concentration in the blood is found to be elevated.

idoxuridine, a topical antiviral used for herpes simplex keratitis and other herpetic infections of the body surfaces.

ifosfamide, a cytotoxic anticancer drug that is an analogue of, and used similarly to, cyclophosphamide.

Ig, abbreviation for **immunoglobulin.**

IgA, abbreviation for **immunoglobulin A.**

IgA deficiency, a selective lack of immunoglobulin A, the most common type of immunoglobulin deficiency. Immunoglobulin A is a major protein antibody in the saliva and mucous membranes of the intestines and bronchi. It protects against bacterial and viral infections. A deficiency of immunoglobulin A is associated with heredity and autoimmune abnormalities. The IgA deficiency is common in patients with rheumatoid arthritis and in those with systemic lupus erythematosus. Common symptoms are respiratory allergies associated with chronic sinopulmonary infection.

IgD, abbreviation for **immunoglobulin D.**

IgE, abbreviation for **immunoglobulin E.**

IgG, abbreviation for **immunoglobulin G.**

IgM, abbreviation for **immunoglobulin M.**

IGT, abbreviation for **impaired glucose tolerance.**

Ikwa fever. See **trench fever.**

ILD, abbreviation for **interstitial lung disease.**

Ile, abbreviation for **isoleucine.**

ileal conduit, a method of urinary diversion through intestinal tract tissue. Ureters are implanted in a section of dissected ileum that is then sewed to an ostomy in the abdominal wall, where a collecting device is attached.

ileitis, inflammation of the ileum.

ileo-anal anastomosis, a surgical procedure in which the colon and rectum are removed but the anus is left intact along with the anal sphincter. An anastomosis is formed between the lower end of the small intestine and the anus.

ileocaecal valve, the valve between the ileum of the small intestine and the caecum of the large intestine. The valve consists of two flaps that project into the lumen of the large intestine, just above the vermiform appendix.

ileocaecostomy. See **caecoileostomy.**

ileocolic node, a node in one of three groups of superior mesenteric lymph glands, forming a chain around the ileocolic (mesenteric) artery.

ileocystoplasty, a surgical procedure in which the bladder is reconstructed using a segment of the ileum for the bladder wall.

ileostomate, a person who has undergone an ileostomy.

ileostomy, surgical formation of an opening of the ileum onto the surface of the abdomen, through which faecal matter is emptied. The operation is performed in advanced or recurrent ulcerative colitis, Crohn's disease or cancer of the large bowel. Intestinal antibiotics are given to decrease the bacterial count. A nasogastric or intestinal tube is passed. The diseased portion of the large bowel is removed in a permanent ileostomy; occasionally, the distal and proximal segments of bowel may be reconnected after ulcerated areas have healed. A loop of the proximal ileum is then brought out onto the abdomen and sutured in place, and a stoma is formed. Postoperatively, the patient wears a temporary disposable bag to collect the semiliquid faecal matter, which begins to drain once peristalsis is restored and the tube is removed.

ileum, *pl.* **ilea,** the distal portion of the small intestine, extending from the jejunum to the caecum. It ends in the right iliac fossa, opening into the medial side of the large intestine. **ileac, ileal,** *adj.*

ileus, an obstruction of the intestines, such as an adynamic ileus caused by immobility of the bowel, or a mechanic ileus in which the intestine is blocked by mechanical means.

iliac circumflex node, a node in one of the seven clusters of parietal lymph nodes of the abdomen. This node is one of a group found along the course of the deep iliac circumflex vessels.

iliac fascia, the portion of the endo-abdominal fascia attached with the iliacus to the crest of the ilium; it passes under the inguinal ligament into the thigh.

iliac region. See **inguinal region.**

iliacus, a flat, triangular muscle that covers the inner curved surface of the iliac fossa. It acts to flex and laterally rotate the thigh.

iliofemoral, of or pertaining to the ilium and femur.

ilioinguinal, of or pertaining to the hip and inguinal regions.

iliolumbar ligament, one of a pair of ligaments forming part of the connection between the vertebral column and the pelvis. Each iliolumbar ligament attaches to a transverse process of the fifth lumbar vertebra and passes to the base of the sacrum.

iliopectineal line, a bony ridge on the inner surface of the ilium and pubic bones that divides the true and false pelvises.

iliopsoas, one of the pair of muscle complexes that flexes the thigh and the lumbar vertebral column.

ilium, *pl.* **ilia,** one of the three bones that make up the innominate bone. The ilium forms part of the acetabulum and provides attachment for several muscles, including the obturator internus, gluteals, iliacus and sartorius. **iliac,** *adj.*

illicit, pertaining to an act that is unlawful or otherwise not permitted.

illness, an abnormal process in which aspects of the social, physical, emotional or intellectual condition and function of a person are diminished or impaired, compared with that person's previous condition.

illness prevention, a system of health education programmes and activities directed towards protecting patients from real or potential health threats, minimizing risk factors and promoting healthy behaviour.

illumination, the lighting up of a part of the body or an object under a microscope for the purpose of examination. **illuminate,** *v.*

illusion, a false interpretation of an external sensory stimulus, usually visual or auditory, such as a mirage in the desert or voices in the wind.

IM, abbreviation for **intramuscular.**

image, 1. a representation or visual reproduction of the likeness of someone or something, such as a painting, photograph, radiography or sculpture. **2.** an optical representation of an object, such as that produced by refraction or reflection. **3.** a person or thing that closely resembles another; semblance. **4.** a mental picture, representation, idea or concept of an objective reality. **5.** (in psychology) a mental representation of something previously perceived and subsequently modified by other experiences. Kinds of images include **body image, eidetic image, memory image, mental image, motor image** and **tactile image.**

image acquisition time, the time required to carry out a magnetic resonance imaging procedure comprising only the data acquisition time.

image foreshortening, (in radiology) a distortion of the x-ray image due to the relative angulation of the beam and recording medium.

image format, 1. (in computed tomography) the manner in which an image is stored, such as on a floppy disk, magnetic tape or film. **2.** (in radiography) the arrangement and display parameters of an image.

image intensifier, 1. an electronic device used to produce a fluoroscopic image with a low-radiation exposure. A beam of x-rays is converted into a pattern of electrons. The electrons are accelerated and concentrated onto a small fluorescent screen. **2.** (in radiography) an electronic device used to produce an image using low radiation exposure. The x-ray beam at the input is converted into a pattern of electrons and accelerated to a smaller output phosphor. The intensified image may be viewed via a video camera on a monitor, or recorded on film.

image matrix, 1. (in radiology) an arrangement of columns or rows of imaginary cells, or pixels, forming a digital image. **2.** (in radiography) the selected image format.

imagery, (in psychiatry) the formation of mental concepts, figures, ideas; any product of the imagination. In mentally disturbed persons, these images are often bizarre and delusional.

imagination, 1. the ability to form; the act or process of forming mental images or conscious concepts of things that are not immediately available to the senses. **2.** (in psychology) the ability to reproduce images or ideas stored in the memory by the stimulation or suggestion of associated ideas.

imaging, See **diagnostic imaging.**

imago, (in analytical psychology) an unconscious, usually idealized mental image of a significant individual, such as one's mother, in a person's early, formative years.

imbalance, 1. lack of balance between opposing muscle groups. **2.** an abnormal balance of fluid and electrolytes in the body tissues. **3.** an unequal distribution of sub-

jects in a population group. **4.** a person with mental abilities that are remarkable in one area but deficient in others, such as an idiot savant.

imbricate, to build a surface with overlapping layers of material. Surgeons may imbricate with layers of tissue when closing a wound or other opening in a body part. **imbrication,** *n.*

iminoglycinuria, a benign familial condition characterized by the abnormal urinary excretion of the amino acids glycine, proline and hydroxyproline.

imipenem-cilastatin sodium, a broad spectrum parenteral antibiotic. It is used for the treatment of serious infections caused by susceptible organisms.

imipramine hydrochloride, a tricyclic antidepressant used in the treatment of depression.

immediate auscultation, a method of examining a patient by placing an ear or stethoscope on the skin directly over the body part being studied.

immediate hypersensitivity, an allergic reaction that occurs within minutes after exposure to an allergen.

immediate percussion. See **percussion.**

immediate postoperative fit prosthesis (IPOF), a temporary or preparatory prosthesis, such as a pylon .

immediate post-traumatic automatism, a post-traumatic state in which a person acts spontaneously and automatically without having any recollection of the behaviour.

immersion, placing a body or an object into water or other liquid, so that it is completely covered by the liquid.   **immerse,** *v.*

immersion foot, an abnormal condition of the feet characterized by damage to the muscles, nerves, skin and blood vessels, caused by prolonged exposure to dampness or by prolonged immersion in cold water.

imminent abortion. See **inevitable abortion.**

immiscible, not capable of being mixed, such as oil and water.

immune complex hypersensitivity, an IgG or IgM complement-dependent, immediate acting humoral hypersensitivity to certain soluble antigens. It is seen in serum sickness, Arthus reaction and glomerulonephritis.

immune cytolysis, cell destruction mediated by a particular antibody in conjunction with complement.

immune gamma globulin, one of a variety of passive immunizing agents obtained from pooled, immune human donor plasma. They are used for passive immunization against chickenpox, hepatitis, rabies, measles and tetanus, where immediate protection is required or active immunization is not possible.

immune globulin. See **immune gamma globulin.**

immune human globulin. See **immune gamma globulin.**

immune response, a defence function of the body that produces antibodies to destroy invading antigens and malignancies. Important components of the immune system and response are immunoglobulins, lymphocytes, phagocytes, complement, properdin, the migratory inhibitory factor and interferon. The kinds of immune response are humoral immune response, involving B lymphocytes or B cells, and cell-mediated immune response, involving T lymphocytes or T cells. B cells and T cells derive from the haemopoietic stem cells. The receptor sites on the surface membranes of the B cells are the combining sites of immunoglobulin molecules, identified by letter names, M, G, A, E and D. Immunoglobulin M, the antibody that immature B cells synthesize and incorporate in their cytoplasmic membranes, is the predominant antibody produced. The T cells develop in the thymus gland and proliferate with antigen receptors on their surface membranes. The T cells assist in the antigen-antibody reaction of the B cells and control the cell-mediated response. The cell-mediated response is also effective against fungi, viruses and tumours, and is the major reaction in the rejection of organ transplants.

immune serum globulin. See **chickenpox, immune gamma globulin, immunoglobulin antibody.**

immune serum. See **antiserum.**

immune system, a biochemical complex that protects the body against pathogenic organisms and other foreign bodies. The system incorporates the humoral immune response which produces antibodies to react with specific antigens, and the cell-mediated response which uses T cells to mobilize tissue macrophages in the presence of a foreign body.

immunity, 1. (in civil law) exemption from a duty or an obligation generally required by law, such as exemption from taxation, exemption from penalty for wrongdoing, or protection against liability. **2.** the quality of being insusceptible to or unaffected by a particular disease or condition. Kinds of immunity are active immunity and passive immunity. **immune,** *adj.*

immunization, a process by which resistance to an infectious disease is induced or augmented.

immunoassay, a competitive-binding assay in which the binding protein is an antibody.

immunocompetence, the ability of an immune system to mobilize and deploy its antibodies and other responses to stimulation by an antigen.

immunodeficient, an abnormal condition of the immune system in which cellular or humoral immunity is inadequate and resistance to infection is decreased. Kinds of immunodeficient conditions are hypogammaglobulinaemia and lymphoid aplasia.

immunodiagnosis. See **serological diagnosis.**

immunodiagnostic, pertaining to or characterizing a diagnosis based on an antigen-antibody reaction.

immunodiffusion, a technique for the identification and quantification of any of the immunoglobulins. It is based on the presence of a visible precipitate that results from an antigen-antibody combination under certain circumstances. **Gel diffusion** is a technique that involves evaluation of the precipitin reaction in a clear gel. **Electroimmunodiffusion** is a gel diffusion to which an electric field is applied, accelerating the reaction. **Double gel diffusion** is a technique that permits identification of antibodies in mixed specimens. In an agar plate, each antigen-antibody combination forms a separate line; observation of the location, shape and thickness of a line permits identification and quantification of the antibody.

immunoelectrodiffusion. See **immuno-diffusion.**

immunoelectrophoresis, a technique that combines electrophoresis and immuno-diffusion to separate and allow identification of complex proteins. The proteins in the test serum are spread out in agar and separated by electrophoresis. **immunoelectrophoretic,** *adj.*

immunofluorescence, a technique used for the rapid identification of an antigen by exposing it to known antibodies tagged with the fluorescent dye fluorescein, and observing the characteristic antigen-antibody reaction of precipitation. **immunofluorescent,** *adj.*

immunofluorescence test. See **fluorescent antibody test.**

immunofluorescent microscopy. See **fluorescent microscopy, immunofluorescence.**

immunogen, any agent or substance capable of provoking an immune response or producing immunity. **immunogenic,** *adj.*

immunoglobulin, any of five structurally and antigenically distinct antibodies present in the serum and external secretions of the body. Kinds of immunoglobulins are **IgA, IgD, IgE, IgG** and **IgM.**

immunoglobulin A (IgA), one of the five classes of humoral antibodies produced by the body, and one of the most prevalent. It is found in all bodily secretions, it is the major antibody in the mucous membrane lining the intestines, as well as the bronchi, saliva and tears. IgA combines with a protein in the mucosa and defends body surfaces against invading micro-organisms.

immunoglobulin D (IgD), one of the five classes of humoral antibodies produced by the body. It is a specialized protein found in small amounts in serum tissue. It increases in quantity during allergic reactions to milk, insulin, penicillin and various toxins.

immunoglobulin E (IgE), one of the five classes of humoral antibodies produced by the body. It is concentrated in the lung, skin and the cells of mucous membranes. It reacts with some antigens to release certain chemical mediators that cause Type I hypersensitivity reactions characterized by wheal and flare.

immunoglobulin G (IgG), one of the five classes of humoral antibodies produced by the body. It is a specialized protein synthesized by the body in response to invasions by bacteria, fungi and viruses.

immunoglobulin M (IgM), one of the five classes of humoral antibodies produced by the body, and the largest in molecular structure. It is the first immunoglobulin the body produces when challenged by antigens, and is found in circulating fluids. It is the dominant antibody in ABO incompatibilities.

immunohaematology, the study of antigen-antibody reactions and their effects on blood.

immunological tests, tests based on the principles of antigen-antibody reactions.

immunological theory of ageing, a concept based on the premise that normal cells are unrecognized as such, thereby triggering immune reactions within the individual's own body.

immunologist, a specialist in immunology.

immunology, the study of the reaction of tissues of the immune system of the body to antigenic stimulation.

immunomodulator, a substance that acts to alter the immune response by augmenting or reducing the ability of the immune system to produce specifically modified serum antibodies. Corticosteroids, cytotoxic agents, thymosin and the immunoglobulins are among the immunomodulating substances. **immunomodulation,** *n.*

immunopotency, the ability of an antigen to elicit an immune response.

immunoselection, 1. the survival of certain cells because they lack surface antigens that would otherwise make them vulnerable to attack and destruction by antibodies of an immune system. **2.** the chance of survival of a fetus because its genotype is compatible with that of the mother's immune system.

immunosuppression, 1. the administration of agents that interfere significantly with the ability of the immune system to respond to antigenic stimulation by inhibiting cellular and humoral immunity. Immunosuppression may be deliberate, such as in preparation for transplantation to prevent rejection by the host of the donor tissue, or incidental, as often results from cancer chemotherapy. **2.** an abnormal condition of the immune system characterized by

markedly inhibited ability to respond to antigenic stimuli. **immunosuppressed,** *adj.*

immunosuppressive, 1. of or pertaining to a substance or procedure that lessens or prevents an immune response. **2.** an immunosuppressive agent, such as an immunosuppressive drug used to prevent graft rejection.

immunosurveillance, the continuous detection and protection activity of the immune system in guarding against the presence of "non-self," or foreign proteins in the body tissues.

immunotherapy, a special treatment of allergic responses that administers increasingly large doses of the offending allergens to develop immunity gradually. Immunotherapy is based on the premise that low doses of the offending allergen will bind with IgG to prevent an allergic reaction through damping of the action of IgE by fostering the synthesis of the blocking IgG antibody. **immunotherapeutic,** *adj.*

immunotoxin (IT), a plant or animal toxin attached to a monoclonal antibody and used to destroy a specific target cell.

impacted, tightly or firmly wedged in a limited amount of space. **impact,** *v.,* **impaction,** *n.*

impacted fracture, a bone break in which the adjacent fragmented ends of the fractured bone are wedged together.

impacted tooth, a tooth positioned against another tooth, bone or soft tissue in a way that its complete and normal eruption is impossible or unlikely. It may be further described according to its position, such as mesioangular, distoangular or vertical.

impaction, 1. an obstacle or malposition that prevents a tooth from erupting. **2.** the presence of a large or hard faecal mass in the rectum or colon.

impaired glucose tolerance (IGT), a condition in which fasting plasma glucose levels are higher than normal but lower than those diagnostic of diabetes mellitus.

impairment, any disorder in structure or function resulting from anatomical, physiological or psychological abnormalities that interfere with normal activities.

impedance, a form of electrical resistance observed in an alternating current that is analagous to the classic electrical resistance that occurs in a direct current circuit.

impedance audiometry. See **audiometry.**

impedance plethysmography, a technique for detecting blood vessel occlusion. It determines volumetric changes in the limb by measuring changes in its girth, as indicated by changes in the electric impedance of mercury-containing Silastic tubes in a pressure cuff.

implosive therapy. See **flooding.**

imperative idea. See **compulsive idea.**

imperforate, lacking a normal opening in a body organ or passage. An infant may be born with an imperforate anus.

imperforate anus, any of several congenital, developmental malformations of the anorectal portion of the GI tract. The most common form is anal agenesis, in which the rectal pouch ends blindly above the surface of the perineum. Other forms include anal stenosis, in which the anal aperture is small, and anal membrane atresia, in which the anal membrane covers the aperture, creating an obstruction.

impermeable, (of a tissue, membrane or film) preventing the passage of a substance through it.

impetigo, a streptococcal, staphylococcal or combined infection of the skin, beginning as focal erythema and progressing to pruritic vesicles, erosions and honey-coloured crusts. Lesions usually form on the face and spread locally. The disorder is highly contagious by contact with the discharge from the lesions. impetiginous, adj.

implant. 1. (in radiotherapy) See interstitial therapy. **2.** (in surgery) material inserted or grafted into an organ or structure of the body. The implant may be of tissue, such as in a blood vessel graft, or of an artificial substance, such as in a hip prosthesis, a cardiac pacemaker or a container of radioactive material.

implant restoration, a single- or multiple-tooth implant crown or bridge that replaces a missing tooth or teeth.

implantation, (in embryology) the process involving the attachment, penetration and embedding of the blastocyst in the lining of the uterine wall during the early stages of prenatal development. Kinds of implantation include **eccentric implantation, interstitial implantation** and **superficial implantation.**

implantation dermoid cyst, a tumour derived from embryonal tissues, caused by an injury that forces part of the ectoderm into the body.

implementation, a deliberate action performed to achieve a goal, such as carrying out a plan in caring for a patient. **implement,** v.

implementation mechanism, the means by which innovations are transferred from the planners to the units of service.

implementing, (in four-step nursing process) a category of nursing behaviour in which the actions necessary for accomplishing the healthcare plan are initiated and completed. Implementing includes the performance or assisting in the performance of the patient's activities of daily living; counselling and teaching the patient or the patient's family; providing care to achieve therapeutic goals and optimize the achievement of health goals by the patient; supervising and evaluating the work of staff members; and recording and exchanging information relevant to the patient's continued healthcare.

implosion, 1. inward bursting. **2.** a psychiatric treatment for people disabled by phobias and anxiety in which the person is desensitized to anxiety-producing stimuli by repeated intense exposure in imagination or reality, until the stimuli are no longer stressful. **implode,** v.

impotence, 1. weakness. **2.** inability of the adult male to achieve penile erection or, less commonly, to ejaculate having achieved an erection. **Functional impotence** has a psychological basis. **Anatomical impotence** results from physically defective genitalia. **Atonic impotence** involves disturbed neuromuscular function. **impotent,** adj.

impregnate, 1. to inseminate and make pregnant; to fertilize. **2.** to saturate or mix with another substance. **impregnable,** adj., **impregnation,** n.

impression, 1. (in dentistry and prosthetic medicine) a mould of a part of the mouth or other part of the body from which a replacement or prosthesis may be formed. **2.** (in the medical record) the examiner's diagnosis or assessment of a problem, disease or condition. **3.** a strong sensation or effect on the mind, intellect or feelings.

imprinting, (in ethology) a special type of learning that occurs at critical points during the early stages of development in animals.

imprisonment, (in law) the act of confining, detaining or arresting a person or in any way restraining personal liberty and preventing free exercise of movement.

impulse, 1. (in psychology) a sudden, irresistible, often irrational inclination, urge, desire or action resulting from a particular feeling or mental state. **2.** (in physiology) the electrochemical process involved in neural transmission. **impulsive,** adj.

impulsion, an abnormal, irrational urge to commit an unlawful or socially unacceptable act.

IMV, abbreviation for **intermittent mandatory ventilation.**

In, symbol for indium.

inactivation, a reversible denaturation of a protein.

inactive colon, hypotonicity of the bowel resulting in decreased contractions and propulsive movements, and a delay in the normal 12-hour transit time of luminal contents from caecum to anus. Colonic inactivity may be caused by acquired or congenital megacolon, ageing, anticholinergic drugs, depression, faulty habits of elimination, inadequate fluid intake, lack of exercise, a low-residue or starvation diet, neuroendocrine response to surgical stress, prolonged bed rest, or a neurological disease, such as diabetic visceral neuropathy, multiple sclerosis, parkinsonism and spinal cord lesions. Normal motility of the colon is frequently compromised by the continued use of laxatives.

inadequate personality, a personality characterized by a lack of physical stamina, emotional immaturity, social instability, poor judgment, reduced motivation, ineptness...especially in interpersonal relationships...and an inability to adapt or react effectively to new or stressful situations.

inanimate, not alive; lacking signs of life.

inanition, 1. an exhausted condition resulting from lack of food and water or a defect in assimilation; starvation. **2.** a state of lethargy characterized by a loss of vitality or vigour in all aspects of social, moral and intellectual life.

inanition fever, a temporary, mild, febrile condition of the newborn in the first few days after birth, usually caused by dehydration.

inborn, innate; acquired or occurring during intrauterine life, with reference to both normally inherited traits and developmental or genetically transmitted anomalies.

inborn error of metabolism, one of many abnormal metabolic conditions caused by an inherited defect of a single enzyme or other protein. People with such diseases generally display a large number of physical signs that are characteristic of the genetic trait. Inborn errors of metabolism may be detected in the fetus in utero by the examination of squamous and blood cells obtained by amniocentesis and fetoscopy. Laboratory tests after birth often show higher than normal levels of particular metabolites in the blood and urine, such as phenylpyruvic acid and phenylalanine in PKU and galactose in galactosaemia. Kinds of inborn errors of metabolism include **phenylketonuria, Tay-Sachs disease, Lesch-Nyhan syndrome, galactosaemia,** and **glucose-6-phosphate dehydrogenase deficiency.**

inborn reflex. See **unconditioned response.**

inbreeding, the production of offspring by the mating of closely related individuals, organisms or plants; self-fertilization is the most extreme form, which normally occurs in certain plants and lower animals. The practice of inbreeding provides a greater chance for both desirable and undesirable recessive genes to become homozygous and be expressed phenotypically.

incarcerate, to trap, imprison or confine, such as a loop of intestine in an inguinal hernia.

incentive spirometry, spirometric therapy in which the patient is given special encouragement to achieve a maximum inspiratory capacity.

incest, sexual intercourse between members of the same family who are so closely related as to be legally prohibited from marrying one another by reason of their consanguinity. **incestuous,** *adj.*

incidence, 1. the number of times an event occurs. **2.** (in epidemiology) the number of new cases in a particular period of time.

incident report, a document describing any accident or deviation from policies or orders involving a person on the premises of a health care facility.

incidental additives, food additives caused by the use of pesticides, herbicides or chemicals involved in food processing.

incineration, the removal or reduction of waste materials by burning.

incipient, coming into existence; at an initial stage; beginning to appear, such as a symptom or disease.

incipient dental caries, a dental condition in which a lesion of tooth decay is initially detectable.

incisal angle, the degree of slope between the axis-orbital plane and the discluding surface of the maxillary incisor teeth.

incisal guide, the part of a dental articulator that maintains the incisal guide angle.

incisal guide pin, a metal rod, attached to the upper member of an articulator, that touches the incisal guide table to maintain the established vertical separation of the upper and lower members of the articulator.

incision, 1. a cut produced surgically by a sharp instrument creating an opening into an organ or space in the body. **2.** the act of making an incision.

incisor, one of the eight front teeth, four in each dental arch. Incisors first appear as milk teeth during infancy; they are replaced by permanent incisors during childhood, and last until old age. The crown of the incisor is chisel-shaped and has a sharp cutting edge. The upper incisors are larger and stronger than the lower incisors, and are directed obliquely downwards and forward.

inclusion, 1. the act of enclosing or the condition of being enclosed. **2.** a structure within another, such as inclusions in the cytoplasm of the cells.

inclusion bodies, microscopic objects of various shapes and sizes observed in the nucleus or cytoplasm of blood cells or other tissue cells, depending on the type of disease.

inclusion conjunctivitis, an acute, purulent, conjunctival infection caused by *Chlamydia* organisms. It occurs in two forms: bilateral chemosis, redness and purulent discharge characterize the infection in infants; the adult variety is unilateral, less severe, less purulent and associated with preauricular lymphadenopathy.

inclusion dermoid cyst, a tumour derived from embryonal tissues, caused by the inclusion of a foreign tissue when a developmental cleft closes.

inclusiveness principle, a rule that response to various objects in the environment is proportional to the amount of stimulus provided by each object.

incoherent, 1. disordered; without logical connection; disjointed; lacking orderly continuity or relevance. 2. unable to express one's thoughts or ideas in an orderly, intelligible manner, usually as a result of emotional stress.

incompatible, unable to coexist. A tissue transplant may be rejected because recipient and donor antibody factors are incompatible.

incompetence, lack of ability. Body organs that do not function adequately may be described as incompetent. Kinds of incompetence include **aortic incompetence, ileocaecal incompetence and valvular incompetence. incompetent,** *adj.*

incompetency, a legal status of a person declared to be unable to provide for his or her own needs and protection.

incompetent cervix , (in obstetrics) a condition characterized by dilatation of the cervical os of the uterus before term, without labour or contractions of the uterus. Miscarriage or preterm delivery may result.

incomplete abortion, an abortion in which the products of conception are not entirely expelled or removed, often causing haemorrhage that may require surgical evacuation.

incomplete fistula. See **blind fistula.**

incomplete fracture, a bone break in which the crack in the osseous tissue does not completely traverse the width of the affected bone but may angle off in one or more directions.

incongruent communication, a communication pattern in which the sender gives conflicting messages at verbal and non-verbal levels, and the listener does not know which message to accept.

incontinence, the inability to control urination or defaecation. Urinary incontinence may be caused by cerebral clouding in elderly individuals, infection, lesions in the brain or spinal cord, damage to peripheral nerves of the bladder, or injury to the sphincter or perineal structures, sometimes occurring in childbirth. Stress incontinence precipitated by coughing, straining or heavy lifting occurs more often in women than in men. Faecal incontinence may result from relaxation of the anal sphincter, or due to central nervous system or spinal cord disorders; it may be treated by a programme of bowel training. incontinent, *adj.*

incontinence, functional, an involuntary, unpredictable passage of urine. Defining characteristics include the urge to void or bladder contractions sufficiently strong to result in loss of urine before reaching an appropriate receptacle.

incontinence, reflex, an involuntary loss of urine occurring at somewhat predictable intervals when a specific bladder volume is reached. Defining characteristics include no awareness of bladder filling; no urge to void or feelings of bladder fullness; or uninhibited bladder contractions or spasms at regular intervals.

incontinence, stress, loss of urine of less than 50 ml occurring with increased abdominal pressure. Defining characteristics include reported or observed dribbling with increased abdominal pressure, urinary urgency or urinary frequency (more often than every 2 hours).

incontinence, total, continuous and unpredictable loss of urine. Defining characteristics include a constant flow of urine occurring at unpredictable times without distention or unihibited bladder contractions or spasms, unsuccessful incontinence refractory treatments, nocturia, lack of perineal or bladder awareness, and unawareness of incontinence.

incontinence, urge, involuntary passage of urine occurring soon after a strong sense of urgency to void. Defining characteristics include urinary urgency, frequency (voiding more often than every 2 hours), bladder contractions or spasms, nocturia (urination more than 2 times per night), voiding in small amounts (less than 100 cc) or in large amounts (500 cc), and an inability to reach a toilet in time.

increment, 1. an increase or gain. 2. the act of growing or increasing. 3. the amount of an increase or gain in intrauterine pressure as uterine contractions begin in labour. **incremental,** *adj.*

incrustation, hardened exudate, scale or scab.

incubation period, 1. the time between exposure to a pathogenic organism and the onset of symptoms of a disease. 2. the time required to induce the development of an embryo in an egg, or induce the development and replication of tissue cells or microorganisms in culture media. 3. The time allowed for a chemical reaction or process to proceed.

incubator, an apparatus used to provide a controlled environment, especially a particular temperature.

incudectomy, surgical removal of the incus, performed to treat conductive deafness resulting from necrosis of the tip of the incus. The defective incus is excised and replaced with a bone chip graft so that sound vibrations are again transmitted.

incus, *pl.* **incudes,** one of the three ossicles in the middle ear, resembling an anvil. It communicates sound vibrations from the malleus to the stapes.

indandione derivative, one of a small group of oral anticoagulants for long-term therapeutic use in patients who cannot tolerate other oral anticoagulants.

indemnity insurance, also known as professional liability insurance. This is carried out by healthcare professionals in case there is legal action against them. It aims to redress for acts which have damaged patients or clients. See duty, malpractice.

indentation, a notch, pit or depression in the surface of an object, such as toothmarks on the tongue or skin. **indent,** *v.*

independence, 1. the state or quality of being independent; autonomy; free from the influence, guidance, or control of a person or a group. **2.** a lack of requirement or reliance on another for physical existence or emotional needs. **independent,** *adj.*

independent assortment, (in genetics) a basic principle stating that the members of a pair of genes are randomly distributed in the gametes, independent of the distribution of other pairs of genes.

independent living centres, rehabilitation facilities in which disabled persons can receive special education and training in the performance of all or most activities of daily living with a particular handicap.

independent variable, (in research) a variable controlled by the researcher and evaluated by its measurable effect on the dependent variable or variables.

indeterminate cleavage, mitotic division of the fertilized ovum into blastomeres that have similar developmental potential and, if isolated, can give rise to a complete individual embryo.

index case, (in epidemiology) the first case of a disease as contrasted with the appearance of subsequent cases.

Index Medicus, an index published monthly by the National Library of Medicine, which lists articles from the medical literature from around the world, classified by subject and by author.

index myopia, a kind of nearsightedness caused by a variation in the index of refraction of the media of the eye.

Indian tick fever. See **Marseilles fever.**

indican, a substance (potassium indoxyl sulfate) produced in the intestine by the decomposition of tryptophan, absorbed by the intestinal wall and excreted in the urine.

indication, a reason to prescribe a medication or perform a treatment; for example, a bacterial infection may be an indication for the prescription of a specific antibiotic, or appendicitis is an indication for appendisectomy. **indicate,** *v.*

indicator, a tape, paper, tablet or any other substance used to test for a particular reaction, because of its change in a predictable and visible way. Some kinds of indicators are **autoclave indicator, dipsticks** and **litmus paper.**

indigenous, native to or occurring naturally in a specified area or environment, such as certain species of bacteria in the human digestive tract.

indigestion. See **dyspepsia.**

indirect anaphylaxis, an exaggerated reaction of hypersensitivity to a person's own antigen that occurs because the antigen has been altered in some way.

indirect calorimetry, the measurement of the amount of heat generated in an oxidation reaction, by determining the intake or consumption of oxygen, or measuring the amount of carbon dioxide or the amount of nitrogen released and translating these quantities into a heat equivalent.

indirect division. See **mitosis.**

indirect ophthalmoscope, an ophthalmoscope with a biconvex lens that produces a reversed direct image.

indirect percussion. See **percussion.**

indirect restorative method, the technique for fabricating a restoration on a cast of the original, such as the indirect construction of an inlay.

indirect retainer, a portion of a removable partial denture that resists movement of a distal extension away from its tissue support by means of lever action opposite the fulcrum line of the direct retention.

indium (In), a silvery metallic element with some non-metallic chemical properties. Its atomic number is 49 and its atomic weight is 114.82.

individual immunity, a form of natural immunity not shared by most other members of the race and species.

individual psychology, a modified system of psychoanalysis, developed by Alfred Adler. It views maladaptive behaviour and personality disorders as resulting from a conflict between the desire to dominate and feelings of inferiority.

indoleacetic acid, a major terminal metabolite of tryptophan, present in very small amounts in normal urine and excreted in elevated quantities by patients with carcinoid tumours.

indomethacin, a non-steroidal anti-inflammatory agent used in the treatment of arthritis and certain other inflammatory conditions.

induce, to cause or stimulate the start of an activity, as an enzyme induces a metabolic activity. **inducer, induction,** *n.*

induced fever, a deliberate elevation of body temperature by application of heat or inoculation with a fever-producing organism, in order to kill heat-sensitive pathogens.

induced hypotension. See **deliberate hypotension.**

induced lethargy, a trance-like state produced during hypnosis.

induced trance, a somnambulistic state resulting from hypnotism.

inducer, (in molecular genetics) a substance, usually a molecular substrate of a specific enzyme, that combines with and deactivates the active repressor produced by the regulator gene.

induction, (in embryology) the process of stimulating and determining morphogenetic differentiation in a developing embryo through the action of chemical substances transmitted from one to another of the embryonic parts.

induction of anaesthesia, all portions of the anaesthetic process that occur before attaining the desired level of anaesthesia, including premedication with a sedative, hypnotic, tranquilizer or curariform adjunct to anaesthesia, intubation, administration of oxygen, and administration of the anaesthetic.

Induction of labour, an obstetric procedure in which labour is initiated artificially by means of amniotomy or administration of oxytocics. It is carried out if it is deemed that continuing the pregnancy would affect the health of mother and/or baby.

induction phase, the period of time during which a normal cell becomes transformed into a cancerous cell.

inductive approach, the analysis of data and examination of practice problems within their own context rather than from a predetermined theoretical basis.

inductor, (in embryology) a tissue or cell that emits a chemical substance that stimulates some morphogenetic effect in the developing embryo.

induration, hardening of a tissue, particularly the skin, because of oedema, inflammation or infiltration by a neoplasm. **indurated,** *adj.*

industrial psychology, the application of psychological principles and techniques to the problems of business and industry, including the selection of personnel, motivation of workers, and development of training programs.

indwelling catheter, any catheter designed to be left in place for a prolonged period.

inert, 1. not moving or acting, such as inert matter. **2.** (of a chemical substance) not taking part in a chemical reaction or acting as a catalyst, such as neon or an inert gas. **3.** (of a medical ingredient) not active pharmacologically; serving only as a bulking, binding or other excipient in a medication.

inert gas, a chemically inactive gaseous element. The inert gases are argon, helium, krypton, neon, radon and xenon.

inertia, 1. the tendency of a body at rest to remain at rest unless acted on by an outside force, and the tendency of a body in motion to remain at motion in the direction in which it is moving unless acted on by an outside force. **2.** an abnormal condition characterized by a general inactivity or sluggishness, such as colonic inertia or uterine inertia.

inertial impaction, the deposition of large aerosol particles on the walls of an airway conduit. The impaction caused by inertia tends to occur where the airway direction changes.

inevitable abortion, a condition of pregnancy in which spontaneous abortion is imminent and cannot be prevented. It is characterized by bleeding, uterine cramping, dilatation of the cervix and presentation of the conceptus in the cervical os.

infant, 1. a child who is in the earliest stage of extrauterine life, a time extending from birth to approximately 12 months of age, when the baby is able to assume an erect posture; some extend the period to 24 months of age. **2.** (in law) a person not of full legal age; a minor. **3.** of or pertaining to infancy; in an early stage of development. **infantile,** *adj.*

infant botulism, an intoxication from neurotoxins produced by *Clostridium botulinum* that occurs in children less than 6 months of age. The condition is characterized by severe hypotonicity of all muscles, constipation, lethargy and feeding difficulties, and it may lead to respiratory insufficiency. The botulism neurotoxin is usually found in the GI tract rather than in the blood, indicating that it is probably produced in the gut as opposed to being ingested.

infant death, the death of a live-born infant before 1 year of age.

infant feeding. See **bottle feeding, breast-feeding.**

infant mortality, the statistical rate of infant death during the first year after live birth. It is expressed as the number of such births per 1000 live births in a specific geographic area or institution in a given period of time.

infanticide, 1. the killing of an infant or young child. **2.** one who takes the life of an infant or young child. **infanticidal,** *adj.*

infantile, 1. of, relating to, or characteristic of infants or infancy. **2.** lacking maturity, sophistication or reasonableness. **3.** affected with infantilism. **4.** being in a very early stage of development.

infantile arteritis, a disorder in infants and young children characterized by inflammation of many arteries in which atherosclerotic lesions are rarely present.

infantile autism, a disability characterized by abnormal emotional, social and linguistic development in a child. It may result from organic brain dysfunction, in which case it occurs before 3 years of age, or it may be associated with childhood schizophrenia, in which case the autism occurs later but before the onset of adolescence. The autistic child remains fixed at one of the consecutive stages through which a normal infant passes as it develops. Treatment includes psychotherapy, often accompanied by play therapy.

infantile coeliac disease. See **coeliac disease.**

infantile cerebral sphingolipidosis. See **Tay-Sachs disease.**

infantile cortical hyperostosis, a familial

disorder characterized in infants by bony swellings and tenderness in the affected areas. The mandible is most commonly involved.

infantile dwarf, a person whose mental and physical development is greatly retarded as a result of various causes, such as genetic or developmental defects.

infantile eczema. See **atopic dermatitis.**

infantile hemiplegia, paralysis of one side of the body that may occur at birth from a cerebral haemorrhage, in utero from lack of oxygen, or during a febrile illness in infancy.

infantile paralysis. See **poliomyelitis.**

infantile pellagra. See **kwashiorkor.**

infantile scurvy, a nutritional disease caused by an inadequate dietary supply of vitamin C, most commonly occurring because cow's milk, unfortified with vitamin C, is the principal food in an infant's diet.

infantile spinal muscular atrophy. See **Werdnig-Hoffmann disease.**

infantilism, 1. a condition in which various anatomical, physiological and psychological characteristics of childhood persist in the adult. **2.** a condition, usually of psychological rather than organic origin, characterized by speech and voice patterns in an older child or adult that are typical of very young children.

infarct, a localized area of necrosis in a tissue, vessel, organ or part resulting from tissue anoxia caused by an interruption in the blood supply to the area or, less frequently, by circulatory stasis produced by the occlusion of a vein that ordinarily carries blood away from the area. Kinds of infarct include **anaemic infarct, calcareous infarct, cicatrized infarct, haemorrhagic infarct** and **uric acid infarct. infarcted,** *adj.*

infarct extension, a myocardial infarction that has spread beyond the original area, usually as a result of the death of cells in the ischaemic margin of the infarct zone.

infarction, 1. the development and formation of an infarct. **2.** an infarct. Kinds of infarction include **myocardial infarction** and **pulmonary infarction.**

infect, to transmit a pathogen that may induce development of an infectious disease in another person.

infection, 1. the invasion of the body by pathogenic micro-organisms that reproduce and multiply, causing disease by local cellular injury, secretion of a toxin, or antigen-antibody reaction in the host. **2.** a disease caused by the invasion of the body by pathogenic micro-organisms. **infectious,** *adj.*

infection control, the policies and procedures of a hospital or other health facility to minimize the risk of nosocomial or community-acquired infections spreading to patients or members of staff.

infection control committee, a group of hospital health professionals composed of infection control personnel, with medical, nursing, administrative and occasionally dietary and housekeeping department representatives, who plan and supervise infection control activities.

infection control nurse, a registered nurse who is assigned responsibility for activities of surveillance and infection prevention and control.

infectious, 1. capable of causing an infection. **2.** caused by an infection.

infectious hepatitis. See **hepatitis A**.

infectious mononucleosis, an acute herpesvirus infection caused by the Epstein-Barr virus (EBV). It is characterized by fever, a sore throat, swollen lymph glands, atypical lymphocytes, splenomegaly, hepatomegaly, abnormal liver function and bruising. Rupture of the spleen may occur, requiring immediate surgery and blood transfusion.

infectious myringitis, an inflammatory, contagious condition of the eardrum caused by viral or bacterial infection, characterized by the development of painful vesicles on the drum.

infectious nucleic acid, DNA or, more commonly, viral RNA that is able to infect the nucleic acid of a cell and induce the host to produce viruses.

infectious parotitis. See **mumps.**

infectious polyneuritis. See **Guillain-Barré syndrome.**

infective tubulointerstitial nephritis, an acute inflammation of the kidneys caused by an infection by *Escherichia coli* or other pyogenic pathogen. The condition is characterized by chills, fever, nausea and vomiting, flank pain, dysuria, proteinuria and haematuria. The kidney may become enlarged, and portions of the renal cortex may be destroyed.

infectivity, the ability of a pathogen to spread rapidly from one host to another.

inferior, 1. situated below or lower than a given point of reference, as the feet are inferior to the legs. **2.** of poorer quality or value.

inferior alveolar artery, an artery that descends with the inferior alveolar nerve from the first or mandibular portion of the maxillary artery to the mandibular foramen.

inferior aperture of minor pelvis, an irregular aperture bounded by the coccyx, the sacrotuberous ligaments, part of the ischium, the sides of the pubic arch and the pubic symphysis.

inferior aperture of thorax, an irregular opening bounded by the twelfth thoracic vertebra, eleventh and twelfth ribs, and the edge of the costal cartilages as they meet the sternum.

inferior conjunctival fornix, the space in the fold of conjunctiva created by the reflection of the conjunctiva covering the eyeball and the lining of the lower eyelid.

inferior gastric node, a node in one of two groups of gastric lymph glands, lying between the two layers of the lesser omentum along the pyloric half of the greater curvature of the stomach.

inferior maxillary bone. See **mandible.**

inferior mesenteric node, a node in one of the three groups of visceral lymph glands serving the viscera of the abdomen and the pelvis.

inferior mesenteric vein, the vein in the lower body that returns the blood from the rectum, sigmoid colon and descending colon.

inferior orbital fissure, a groove in the inferolateral wall of the orbit that contains the infraorbital and zygomatic nerves and infraorbital vessels.

inferior phrenic artery, a small, visceral branch of the abdominal aorta, arising from the aorta itself, the renal artery or the coeliac artery.

inferior radioulnar joint. See **distal radioulnar articulation.**

inferior sagittal sinus, one of the six venous channels of the posterior dura mater, draining blood from the brain into the internal jugular vein. It receives deoxygenated blood from several veins from the falx cerebri and, in some individuals, a few veins from the cerebral hemispheres.

inferior subscapular nerve, one of two small nerves on opposite sides of the back that supply the distal part of the subscapularis; it ends in the teres major.

inferior thyroid vein, one of the few veins that arise in the venous plexus on the thyroid gland and form a plexus ventral to the trachea, under the sternothyroideus muscle. The veins receive the oesophageal, tracheal and inferior laryngeal veins.

inferior ulnar collateral artery, one of a pair of branches of the deep brachial arteries carrying blood to the muscles of the forearm.

inferior vena cava, the large vein that returns deoxygenated blood to the heart from parts of the body below the diaphragm. It is formed by the junction of the two common iliac veins at the right of the fifth lumbar vertebra. It ascends along the vertebral column, pierces the diaphragm and opens into the right atrium of the heart.

inferiority complex, 1. a feeling of fear and resentment resulting from a sense of being physically inadequate, characterized by a variety of abnormal behaviours. **2.** (in psychoanalysis) a complex characterized by striving for unrealistic goals because of an unresolved Oedipus complex. **3.** *informal,* a feeling of being inferior.

inferolateral, situated below and to the side.

inferomedial, situated below and towards the centre.

infertile, denoting the inability to produce offspring. This condition may be present in one or both sex partners, and may be temporary and reversible. The condition is classified as primary, where pregnancy has never occurred, and secondary, where there have been one or more pregnancies. **infertility.** *n.*

infest, to attack, invade and subsist on the skin or in the internal organs of a host. Compare infect.

infestation, the presence of animal parasites in the environment, on the skin or in the hair of a host.

infiltration, the process whereby a fluid passes into the tissues, such as when a local anaesthetic is administered.

inflammation, the protective response of the tissues of the body to irritation or injury. Inflammation may be acute or chronic; its cardinal signs are redness (rubor), heat (calor), swelling (tumor) and pain (dolor), accompanied by loss of function. Histamine, kinins and various other substances mediate the inflammatory process.

inflammatory bowel disease. See **ulcerative colitis.**

inflammatory fracture, a fracture of bone tissue weakened by inflammation.

inflammatory response, a tissue reaction to injury or an antigen. The response may include pain, swelling, itching, redness, heat, loss of function or a combination of symptoms.

influenza, a highly contagious infection of the respiratory tract caused by a myxovirus and transmitted by airborne droplet infection. Symptoms include sore throat, cough, fever, muscular pains and weakness. The onset is usually sudden, with chills, fever and general malaise. Treatment is symptomatic and usually involves bed rest, aspirin and drinking of fluids. Fever and constitutional symptoms distinguish influenza from the common cold. Complete recovery between 3 to 10 days is the rule. Three main strains of influenza virus have been recognized: type A, type B and type C. New strains of the virus emerge at regular intervals and are named according to their geographic origin. **Asian flu** is a type A influenza.

influenza vaccine, an active immunizing agent prescribed for immunization against influenza.

informal admission, a type of admission to a psychiatric hospital in which there is no formal or written application and the patient is free to leave at any time.

informed consent, permission obtained from a patient to perform a specific test or procedure. Informed consent is required before performing most invasive procedures and before admitting a patient to a research study.

infraclavicular fossa, a small pocket or indentation just below the clavicle on both sides of the body.

infraction fracture, a pathological fracture characterized by a small radiolucent line; it is most commonly associated with a disorder of metabolism.

infranodal block, a type of atrioventricular (AV) block in which an impairment of the stimulatory mechanism of the heart causes blockage of the impulse in the bundle of His or in both bundle branches after leaving the AV node. The condition is often the result of arteriosclerosis, degenerative diseases, a defect in the conduction system, or a tumour; it is most often seen in older patients. Symptoms include frequent episodes of fainting and a pulse rate of between 20 and 50 beats per minute.

infrapatellar fat pad, an area of palpable soft tissue in front of the joint space on either side of the patellar tendon.

infraradian rhythm, a biorhythm that repeats in patterns greater than 24-hour periods.

infrared radiation, electromagnetic radiation in which the wavelengths are between 10^{-5} m and 10^{-4} m, or longer than those of visible light waves but shorter than those of radio waves. Infrared radiation striking the body surface is perceived as heat.

infrared therapy, treatment by exposure to various wavelengths of infrared radiation. Infrared treatment is performed to relieve pain and stimulate blood circulation.

infrared thermography, measurement of temperature through the detection of infrared radiation emitted from heated tissue.

infundibulum, *pl.* **infundibula,** a funnel-shaped structure or passage, such as the cavity formed by the fimbriae tubae at the distal end of the uterine tubes.

infusate, a parenteral fluid infused into a patient over a specific time period.

infusion, 1. the introduction of a substance, such as a fluid, electrolyte, nutrient or drug, directly into a vein or interstitially by means of gravity flow. **2.** the substance introduced into the body by infusion. **3.** the steeping of a substance, such as a herb, to extract its medicinal properties. **4.** the extract obtained by the steeping process. **infuse,** *v.*

infusion pump, an apparatus designed to deliver measured amounts of a drug through injection over a period of time. Some kinds of infusion pumps can be surgically implanted.

ingrown hair, a hair that fails to follow the normal follicle channel to the surface, with the free end becoming embedded in the skin.

ingrown toenail, a toenail whose free distal margin grows or is pressed into the skin of the toe, causing an inflammatory reaction.

inguinal, of or pertaining to the groin.

inguinal canal, the tubular passage through the lower layers of the abdominal wall that contains the spermatic cord in the male and the round ligament in the female. It is a common site for hernias.

inguinal falx, the inferior terminal portion of the common aponeurosis of the obliquus internus abdominis and the transverse abdominis.

inguinal hernia, a hernia in which a loop of intestine enters the inguinal canal; in the male it sometimes fills the entire scrotal sac.

inguinal node, one of approximately 18 nodes in the group of lymph glands in the upper femoral triangle of the thigh.

inguinal region, the part of the abdomen surrounding the inguinal canal, in the lower zone on both sides of the pubic region.

inguinal ring, either of the two apertures of the inguinal canal, the internal end opening into the abdominal wall and the external end opening into the aponeurosis of the obliquus externus abdominis above the pubis.

INH. See isoniazid.

inhalant, a substance introduced into the body by inhalation.

inhalation administration of medication, the administration of a drug by inhalation of the vapour released from a fragile ampoule packed in a fine mesh that is crushed for immediate administration. The medication is absorbed into the circulation through the mucous membrane of the nasal passages. Vapourized medication is also given by inhalation.

inhalation analgesia, the occasional administration of anaesthetic gas during the second stage of labour to reduce pain. Consciousness is retained to allow the woman to follow instructions, avoiding the adverse effects of general anaesthesia.

inhalation anaesthesia, surgical narcosis achieved by the administration of an anaesthetic gas or a volatile anaesthetic liquid via a carrier gas. Administration of an inhalation anaesthetic is usually preceded by intravenous or intramuscular administration of a short-acting sedative or hypnotic drug, often a barbiturate.

inhalation therapy, a treatment in which a substance is introduced into the respiratory tract with inspired air. Oxygen, water and various drugs may be administered using techniques of inhalation therapy.

inhale, to breathe in or draw in with the breath. **inhalation,** *n.*

inherent, inborn, innate; natural to an environment.

inherent rate, the frequency of impulse formation attributed to a given pacemaker location.

inheritance, 1. the acquisition or expression of traits or conditions by transmission of genetic material from parents to offspring. **2.** the sum total of the genetic qualities or traits transmitted from parents to offspring;

the total genetic make-up of the fertilized ovum. Kinds of inheritance include **alternative, amphigenous, autosomal, blending, codominant, complemental, crisscross, cytoplasmic, holandric, hologynic, homochronous, maternal, mendelism, monofactorial, multifactorial, supplemental** and **x-linked inheritance. inherited,** *adj.* **inherit,** *v.*

inherited disorder, any disease or condition that is genetically determined and involves either a single gene mutation, multifactorial inheritance or a chromosomal aberration.

inhibin, a reproductive system hormone that inhibits activity of the follicle stimulating hormone.

inhibiting hormone. See **hormone.**

inhibition, 1. the act or state of inhibiting or of being inhibited, restrained, prevented or held back. **2.** (in psychology) the unconscious restraint of a behavioural process, usually resulting from the social or cultural forces of the environment. **3.** (in psychoanalysis) the process in which the superego prevents the conscious expression of an unconscious instinctual drive, thought or urge. **4.** (in physiology) restraining, checking, or arresting the action of an organ or cell or the reducing of a physiological activity by an antagonistic stimulation. **5.** (in chemistry) the stopping or slowing down of the rate of a chemical reaction.

inhibition assay, an immunoassay in which an excess of antigens prevents or inhibits the completion of either the initial or indicator phase of the reaction.

inhibitor, a drug or other agent that prevents or restricts a certain action.

inhibitory, tending to stop or slow a process, such as a neuron that suppresses the intensity of a nerve impulse.

inion, the most prominent point of the back of the head, where the occipital bone protrudes the farthest.

initial contact stance stage, one of the five stages in the stance phase of walking or gait, specifically associated with the moment when the foot touches the ground or floor, and the leg prepares to accept the weight of the body.

initial plan of care, a medical plan prepared by a doctor for the care of a patient.

initiation codon, (in molecular genetics) the triplet of nucleotides that code for formylmethionine, the first amino acid in protein sequences.

initiator, a cocarcinogenic factor that causes a usually irreversible genetic mutation in a normal cell and primes it for uncontrolled growth. Examples include radiation, aflatoxins, urethane and nitrosamines.

injection, 1. the act of forcing a liquid into the body by means of a syringe. Injections are designated according to the anatomical site involved; the most common are intraarterial, intradermal, intramuscular, intravenous and subcutaneous. **2.** the substance injected. **3.** redness and swelling observed in the physical examination of a part of the body, caused by dilatation of the blood vessels secondary to an inflammatory or infectious process. **inject,** *v.*

injection cap, a rubber diaphragm covering a plastic cap. It permits needle insertion into a catheter or vial.

injection technique. See **intradermal injection, intramuscular injection, intrathecal injection, intravenous injection, subcutaneous injection,** and **see other specific injection techniques.**

injunction, a court order that prevents a party from performing a particular act.

inlay splint, a casting for fixing or supporting one or more approximating teeth.

inlet, a passage leading into a cavity, such as the pelvic inlet that marks the brim of the pelvic cavity.

in loco parentis, the assumption by a person or institution of the parental obligations of caring for a child without adoption.

innate, 1. existing in or belonging to a person from birth; inborn; hereditary; congenital. **2.** a natural and essential characteristic ·of something or someone; inherent. **3.** originating in or produced by the intellect or the mind.

innate immunity. See **natural immunity.**

inner cell mass, a cluster of cells localized around the animal pole of the blastocyst of placental mammals from which the embryo develops.

inner ear. See **internal ear.**

innervation, the distribution or supply of nerve fibres or nerve impulses to a part of the body.

innervation apraxia. See **motor apraxia.**

innocent, benign, innocuous or functional; not malignant, such as an innocent heart murmur.

innominate, without a name; unnamed. The term is traditionally applied to certain anatomical structures, such as the hipbone.

innominate artery, one of the three arteries that branch from the arch of the aorta.

innominate bone, the hipbone. It consists of the ilium, ischium and pubis, and unites with the sacrum and coccyx to form the pelvis.

innominate vein, a large vein on either side of the neck, formed by the union of the internal jugular and subclavian veins. The two veins drain blood from the head, neck and upper extremities, and unite to form the superior vena cava.

inoculate, to introduce a substance (inoculum) into the body, so as to produce or increase immunity to the disease or condition associated with the substance.

inoculum, *pl.* **inocula,** a substance introduced into the body to cause or increase immunity to a specific disease or condition.

It may be a toxin, a live, attenuated or killed virus or bacterium, or an immune serum.

inorganic, (in chemistry) a chemical compound that does not contain carbon.

inorganic acid, a compound containing no carbon that is made up of hydrogen and an electronegative element, such as hydrochloric acid.

inorganic chemistry, the study of the properties and reactions of all chemical elements and compounds other than hydrocarbons.

inorganic dust, dry, finely powdered particles of an inorganic substance, especially dust, which, when inhaled, can cause abnormal conditions of the lungs.

inorganic phosphorus, phosphorus that may be measured in the blood as phosphate ions.

inosine, a nucleoside derived from animal tissue, especially intestines. It was originally used in food processing and flavouring.

inosine pranobex, a form of inosine used as an antiviral. Its main action is stimulation of the immune system.

inositol, an isomer of glucose that occurs widely in plant and animal cells.

inotropic, pertaining to the force or energy of muscular contractions, particularly contractions of the heart muscle. An inotropic agent increases myocardial contractility.

inpatient, 1. a patient who has been admitted to a hospital or other healthcare facility for at least an overnight stay. **2.** of or pertaining to the treatment or care of such a patient or to a healthcare facility to which a patient may be admitted for 24-hour care.

input, the information or material that enters a system.

input device, a device that allows for the entry of commands or information for processing in a form acceptable to a computer, such as a typewriter, keyboard, tape drive, disk drive, microphone or light pen.

insanity, a severe mental disorder or defect, such as a psychosis, rather than a neurosis. It is used more in legal and social than in medical terminology. When a person is classified as insane, various legal actions can ensue, such as commitment to an institution, appointment of a guardian, or dissolution of a contract.

insect bite, the bite of any parasitic or venomous arthropod such as a louse, flea, mite, tick or arachnid. Many arthropods inject venom that produces poisoning or severe local reaction, saliva that may contain viruses, or substances that produce mild irritation.

insecticide, a chemical agent that kills insects.

insecticide poisoning. See **chlorinated organic insecticide poisoning.**

insemination, injection of semen into the uterine canal. It may involve an artificial process unrelated to sexual intercourse.

insenescence, 1. the process of ageing. **2.** the state of being chronologically old but retaining the vitality of a person with a younger biological age.

insensible perspiration, a small amount of perspiration continually excreted by the sweat glands in the skin, which evaporates before it may be observed.

insertion, 1. (in anatomy) the place of attachment, such as of a muscle to the bone it moves. **2.** The positioning of a dental prosthesis, such as a removable denture in its planned site on the dental arch.

insertion forceps. See **point forceps.**

insertion path, the direction of placement and removal of a removable partial denture on its supporting oval structures; path of insertion.

insertion site, the point in a vein where a needle or catheter is inserted.

in-service education, a programme of instruction or training provided by an agency or institution for its employees.

insidious, of, pertaining to, or describing a development that is gradual, subtle or imperceptible.

insight, 1. the capacity of comprehending the true nature of a situation or of penetrating an underlying truth. **2.** an instance of comprehending an underlying truth, primarily through intuitive understanding. **3.** (in psychology) a type of self-understanding encompassing both an intellectual and emotional awareness of the unconscious nature, origin and mechanisms of one's attitudes, feelings and behaviour.

in situ, 1. in the natural or usual place. **2.** describing a cancer that has not metastasized or invaded neighbouring tissues, such as carcinoma in situ.

insoluble, unable to be dissolved, usually in a specific solvent, such as a substance that is insoluble in water.

insomnia, chronic inability to sleep or remain asleep throughout the night; wakefulness; sleeplessness.

insomniac, 1. a person with insomnia. **2.** pertaining to, causing, or associated with insomnia. **3.** characteristic of or occurring during a period of sleeplessness.

inspiration, the act of drawing air into the lungs in order to exchange oxygen for carbon dioxide, the end-product of tissue metabolism. The major muscle of inspiration is the diaphragm, the contraction of which creates a negative pressure in the chest, causing the lungs to expand and air to flow inwards. Lungs at maximal inspiration have an average total capacity of 5500 to 6000 ml of air.

inspiratory, of, or pertaining to, inspiration.

inspiratory capacity (IC), the maximum volume of gas that can be inhaled from the resting expiratory level.

inspiratory hold, either of two kinds of modification in an intermittent positive pressure breathing (IPPB) pressure waveform. They are: (1) a pressure hold, in which a preset pressure is reached and held for a designated period, and (2) a volume hold, in which a predetermined volume is delivered and then held for a designated period.

inspiratory reserve volume, the maximum volume of gas that can be inspired from the end-tidal inspiratory level.

inspiratory resistance muscle training, respiratory therapy exercises that require inhalation against some type of resisting force, such as abdominal breathing practice with weights on the abdomen.

inspissate, (of a fluid) to thicken or harden through the absorption or evaporation of the liquid portion, such as milk in an inspissated milk duct. **inspissation,** *n*.

instillation, 1. a procedure in which a fluid is slowly introduced into a cavity or passage of the body and allowed to remain for a specific length of time before being drained or withdrawn. 2. a solution thus introduced. **instill,** *v*.

instinct, an inborn psychological representation of a need, such as life instincts of hunger, thirst and sex, and the destructive and aggressive death instincts.

instinctive reflex. See **unconditioned response**.

institutionalize, to place a person in an institution for psychological or physical treatment, or for the protection of the person or society. **institutionalization,** *n*., **institutionalized,** *adj*.

instrument, a surgical tool or device designed to perform a specific function, such as cutting, dissecting, grasping, holding, retracting or suturing. Some kinds of instruments are clamp, needle holder, retractor and speculum.

instrumental conditioning. See **operant conditioning**.

instrumentation, the use of instruments for treatment and diagnosis.

insufficiency, inability to perform a necessary function adequately. Some kinds of insufficiency are **adrenal insufficiency, aortic insufficiency, ileocecal insufficiency, pulmonary insufficiency** and **valvular insufficiency**.

insufflate, to blow a gas or powder into a tube, cavity, or organ to allow visual examination, remove an obstruction or apply medication. **insufflation,** *n*.

insulation, a non-conducting substance that offers a barrier to the passage of heat or electricity.

insulin, 1. a naturally occurring hormone secreted by the beta cells of the islands of Langerhans in the pancreas in response to increased levels of glucose in the blood. The hormone acts to regulate the metabolism of glucose and the processes necessary for the intermediary metabolism of fats, carbohydrates and proteins. Insulin lowers blood glucose levels and promotes transport and entry of glucose into the muscle cells and other tissues. 2. a pharmacological preparation of the hormone administered in treating diabetes mellitus. The various preparations of insulin available for prescription vary in promptness, intensity and duration of action. They are termed rapid-acting, intermediate-acting and long-acting.

insulin kinase, an enzyme, assumed to be present in the liver, that activates insulin.

insulin reaction, the adverse effects caused by excessive levels of circulating insulin. See **hyperinsulinism**.

insulin resistance, a complication of diabetes mellitus characterized by a need for more than 200 units of insulin per day to control hyperglycaemia and ketosis. The cause is associated with insulin binding by high levels of antibody.

insulin shock, hypoglycaemic shock caused by an overdose of insulin, a decreased intake of food or excessive exercise. It is characterized by sweating, trembling, chilliness, nervousness, irritability, hunger, hallucination, numbness and pallor. Uncorrected, it will progress to convulsions, coma and death. Treatment requires an immediate dose of glucose.

insulin shock treatment, a rarely used procedure involving the injection of large doses of insulin, administered as a therapeutic measure in psychoses, especially schizophrenia, and depression.

insulin tolerance test, a test of the body's ability to use insulin, in which insulin is given and blood glucose is measured at regular intervals. It is also used to investigate adenohypophyseal function (of the anterior pituitary).

insulin zinc suspensions, a family of insulin injections in which insulin is complexed with zinc to give insulins of intermediate to long duration of action.

insulin-dependent diabetes mellitus (IDDM), an inability to metabolize carbohydrate caused by an overt insulin deficiency, occurring in children and characterized by polydipsia, polyuria, polyphagia, loss of weight, diminished strength and marked irritability. Insulin-dependent diabetes mellitus tends to be unstable and brittle, with the patients quite sensitive to insulin and physical activity and liable to develop ketoacidosis. Previously called brittle diabetes, juvenile diabetes, juvenile-onset diabetes, JOD, juvenile-onset-type diabetes, ketosis-prone diabetes.

insulinogenic, promoting the production and release of insulin by the islands of Langerhans in the pancreas.

insulinoma, *pl.* **insulinomas, insulinomata,** a benign tumour of the insulin-secreting cells of the islands of Langerhans.

insuloma. See **insulinoma**.

intake, 1. the process in which a person is

admitted to a clinic or hospital, or is signed in for an office visit. The reason for the visit and various identifying data about the patient are noted. **2.** the amount of food or fluids ingested in a given period of time.

intangible elements, psychological factors, such as cognitive ability, knowledge, ability to solve problems, emotions and attitudes.

integral dose, (in radiotherapy) the total amount of energy absorbed by a patient or object during exposure to radiation.

integrating dose meter, (in radiotherapy) an ionization chamber, usually designed to be placed on the patient's skin, with a measuring system for determining the total radiation administered during an exposure.

integration, 1. the act or process of unifying or bringing together. **2.** (in psychology) the organization of all elements of the personality into a coordinated, functional whole that is in harmony with the environment. **integrate,** v.

integration of self, one of the components of high-level well-being. It is characterized by the integration of mind, body and spirit into one harmoniously functioning unit.

integument, a covering or skin. **integumentary,** adj.

integumentary system, the skin and its appendages, hair, nails, and sweat and sebaceous glands.

integumentary system assessment, an evaluation of the general condition of a patient's integument, and of factors or abnormalities that may contribute to the presence of a dermatological disorder. The nurse asks if the patient suffers from itching, pain, rashes, blisters or boils; if the skin usually is dry, oily, thin, rough, bumpy or puffy; if it feels hot or cold, if it peels, changes in colour, or is marked with dark liver (ageing) spots. Observations are made of the intactness, turgor, elasticity, temperature, cleanliness, odour, wetness or dryness, and colour of the skin. The following are then noted: cyanosis of the lips, circumoral area, or mucous membranes, earlobes, or nailbeds; jaundice of the sclera; pale conjunctivae; pigment distribution; and evidence of plethora. The following features are recorded: indications of rashes, oedema, needle marks, insect bites, scabies, acne, sclerema, decubiti, uraemic frost on the beard or eyebrows, and pressure spots over bony prominences. The nails are examined for brittleness, lines, a convex ram's horn or concave spoon shape, and the condition of surrounding tissue, including clubbing of the fingers and toes. A note is made of the existence and characteristics of maculae, papules, vesicles, pustules, bullae, hives, warts, moles, ulcers, scars, keloids, petechiae, lipomas, crusts of dried exudate, flakes of dead epidermis, excoriations, blackheads or a chancre.

intellect, 1. the power and ability of the mind to know and understand, as contrasted with feeling or willing. **2.** a person possessing a great capacity for thought and knowledge. **intellectual,** adj., n.

intellectualization, (in psychiatry) a defence mechanism in which reasoning is used as a means of blocking a confrontation with an unconscious conflict, and the emotional stress associated with it.

intelligence, 1. the potential ability and capacity to acquire, retain and apply experience, understanding, knowledge, reasoning and judgment, in coping with new experiences and solving problems. **2.** the manifestation of such ability. **intelligent,** adj.

intelligence quotient (IQ), a numerical expression of a person's intellectual level, as measured against the statistical average of his or her age group. On several of the traditional scales it is determined by dividing the mental age, derived through psychological testing, by the chronological age and multiplying the result by 100. Average IQ is considered to be 100.

intelligence test, any of a variety of standarized tests designed to determine the mental age of an individual by measuring the relative capacity to absorb information and solve problems. Two kinds of intelligence tests are **Stanford-Binet** and **Wechsler-Bellevue scale.**

intensifying screen, 1. a device consisting of fluorescent material, which is placed in contact with the film in a radiographic cassette. Radiation from a therapeutic process interacts with the fluorescent phosphor, releasing light photons. These expose the film with greater efficiency than radiation alone would achieve. Thus, patient exposure can be reduced. **2.** (in radiography) a base coated with a phosphor, usually a rare earth such as gadolinium oxysulphide, with emits light when irradiated with x-rays. Usually mounted in an x-ray cassette, with the x-ray film sandwiched between, the light emitted by the phosphor exposes the x-ray film with greater efficiency, requiring less radiation dose to the patient.

intensive care, constant, complex, detailed healthcare, as provided in various acute life-threatening conditions, such as multiple trauma, severe burns, myocardial infarction or after certain kinds of surgery.

intensive care unit (ICU), a hospital unit in which patients requiring close monitoring and intensive care are housed for as long as necessary. An ICU contains highly technical and sophisticated monitoring devices and equipment, and members of staff in the unit are trained to provide critical care as required by the patients.

intention, a kind of healing process: Healing by **primary intention** is the primary union of the edges of a wound, progressing to complete healing without scar formation or granulation; healing by **secondary intention** is wound closure in which the edges are separated, granulation tissue develops to fill the gap; finally, epithelium grows over the granulations, producing a scar.

intention tremor, fine, rhythmic, purposeless movements that tend to increase during voluntary movements.

intentional additives, substances that are deliberately added in the manufacture of food or pharmaceutical products to improve or maintain flavour, colour, texture or consistency, or to enhance or conserve nutritional value.

interaction coaching, an attempt to modify disturbed mother-infant interactions. The goal is to improve interactional "fit" between mother and child.

interaction processes, a component of the theory of effective practice. The processes consist of a series of interactions between a nurse and a patient in a sequence of actions and reactions until both patient and nurse understand what is required, so that the desired act is achieved.

interactional model, a family therapy model that views the family as a communication system comprising interlocking subsystems. Family dysfunction occurs when the rules governing family interaction become ambiguous. The therapeutic goal is to help the family clarify their rules.

interactionist theory, an ageing theory that views age-related changes as resulting from the interaction between the individual characteristics of the person, the circumstances in society, and the history of social interaction patterns of the person.

interarticular fibrocartilage, one of four kinds of fibrocartilage, consisting of flattened fibrocartilaginous plates between the articular cartilage of the most active joints, such as the sternoclavicular, wrist and knee joints.

intercalary, occurring between two others, such as the absence of the middle part of a bone with the proximal and distal parts present.

intercalate, to insert between adjacent surfaces or structures. **intercalation,** *n.*

intercapillary glomerulosclerosis, an abnormal condition characterized by degeneration of the renal glomeruli. It is associated with diabetes and often produces albuminuria, nephrotic oedema, hypertension and renal insufficiency.

intercellular, between or among cells.

intercellular bridge, a structure that connects adjacent cells, occurring primarily in the epithelium and other stratified squamous epithelia. It consists of slender strands of cytoplasm that project from the surfaces of adjacent cells.

interchange. See **reciprocal translocation.**

intercondylar fracture, a fracture of the tissue between condyles.

intercostal, of, or pertaining to, the space between two ribs.

intercostal bulging, the visible bulging of the soft tissues of the intercostal spaces that occurs when increased expiratory effort is needed to exhale, as in asthma, cystic fibrosis or obstruction of a respiratory passage by a foreign body.

intercostal muscles, the muscles between adjacent ribs. They are designated as external and internal, and function as secondary ventilatory muscles.

intercostal node, a node in one of three groups of thoracic parietal lymph nodes situated near the dorsal parts of the intercostal spaces, and associated with lymphatic vessels that drain the posterolateral area of the chest.

intercourse *informal,* sexual intercourse. See **coitus.**

intercristal, of, or pertaining to, the space between two crests.

intercurrent disease, a disease that develops in and may alter the course of another disease.

interdental canal, any one of the nutrient channels that pass upwards to the teeth through the body of the mandible.

interdental gingiva, the soft supporting tissue, consisting of prominent horizontal collagen fibres, that normally fills the space between two approximating teeth.

interdental groove, a linear, vertical depression on the surface of the interdental papillae. It functions as a sluiceway for the egress of food from the interproximal areas.

interdental spillway, a sluiceway formed by the interproximal contours of adjoining teeth and their investing tissues.

interference, the effect of a component on the accuracy of measurement of the desired analyte.

interferent, any chemical or physical phenomena that can interfere or disrupt a reaction or process.

interferential current therapy, a form of electrical stimulation therapy, using two or three different currents that are passed through a tissue from surface electrodes. Portions of each current are cancelled by the other, resulting in a different net current applied to the target tissue.

interferon, a natural cellular protein formed when cells are exposed to a virus or other foreign particle of nucleic acid. It induces the production of translation inhibitory protein (TIP) in non-infected cells. TIP blocks translation of viral RNA, thus giving other cells protection against both the original and other viruses. Interferon is species-specific.

interferon alpha, any of a group of naturally occurring compounds with complex actions on the immune system. They are produced commercially by recombinant DNA and tissue culture techniques. They have antiviral and antitumour activities, and are used in the treatment of hepatitis B and a variety of cancers.

interferon nomenclature, a system recommended by the International Interferon Nomenclature Committee for identifying interferon compounds. For a specific isolated product, "interferon" is the first word of the name. It is followed by a Greek letter written in full, an arabic number, and a lower case letter appended by a dash; for example: interferon alpha-2a.

interfibrillar mass of Flemming, interfilar mass. See **hyaloplasm.**

interior mesenteric artery, a visceral branch of the abdominal aorta, arising just above the division into the common iliacs and supplying the left half of the transverse colon, all of the descending and iliac colons, and most of the rectum.

interiorization, the merging of reflex and cognitive processes as a response to the environment.

interkinesis, the interval between the first and second nuclear divisions in meiosis.

interlace mode, (in radiology) a process whereby a conventional television camera tube reads off its target assembly, so that each of two fields represents repeated adjacent active traces and horizontal retraces of the electron beam across a television screen.

interleukin-1 (IL-1), a protein with numerous immune system functions, including activation of resting T cells, endothelial and macrophage cells, mediation of inflammation, and stimulation of synthesis of lymphokines, collagen and collagenases.

interleukin-2 (IL-2), a protein with various immunological functions, including the ability to initiate proliferation of activated T cells. IL-2 is used in the laboratory to grow T cell clones with specific helper, cytotoxic and suppressor functions.

interleukin-3 (IL-3), an immune response protein that supports the growth of pluripotent bone marrow stem cells. It is a growth factor for mast cells.

interleukin-4 (IL-4), an immune response protein that is a growth factor for activated B cells, resting T cells and mast cells.

interlobular duct, any duct connecting or draining the lobules of a gland.

interlocked twins, monozygotic twins positioned in the uterus in a way that the neck of one becomes entwined with the neck of the other during presentation, so that vaginal delivery is not possible.

intermediate cell mass. See **nephrotome.**

intermediate cuneiform bone, the smallest of the three cuneiform bones of the foot, located between the medial and lateral cuneiform bones.

intermediate host, any animal in which the larval or intermediate stages of a parasite

develop. Humans are intermediate hosts for malaria parasites.

intermediate mesoderm. See **nephrotome.**

intermenstrual, of or pertaining to the time between menstrual periods.

intermittent, occurring at intervals; alternating between periods of activity and inactivity, such as rheumatoid arthritis which is marked by periods of signs and symptoms followed by periods of remission.

intermittent assisted ventilation (IAV), (in respiratory therapy) a system in which an assisted rate is combined with spontaneous breathing.

intermittent claudication. See **claudication.**

intermittent fever, a fever that recurs in cycles of paroxysms and remissions, such as in malaria. Kinds of intermittent fever include **bidoutertian malaria, double quartan malaria** and **quartan malaria.**

intermittent mandatory ventilation (IMV), a method of respiratory therapy in which the patient is allowed to breathe independently and at certain prescribed intervals.

intermittent positive pressure breathing. See **IPPB.**

intermittent positive pressure ventilation. See **IPPV.**

intermittent tube feeding, delivery of nutrients into the stomach, duodenum or jejunum. Volume of feed required in a 24-hour period is determined, and a normal feed pattern is stimulated by providing approximately 500 mls per meal. Feeding is controlled by an external feed pump.

internal, within or inside.   **internally,** *adv.*

internal aperture of tympanic canaliculus, the upper opening of the tympanic channel in the temporal bone, leading to the tympanum.

internal carotid artery, each of two arteries starting at the bifurcation of the common carotid arteries, opposite the cranial border of the thyroid cartilage, through which blood circulates to many structures and organs in the head.

internal carotid plexus, a network of nerves on the internal carotid artery, formed by the internal carotid nerve.

internal cervical os, an internal opening of the uterus that corresponds to the slight constriction or isthmus of that organ about midway in its length.

internal cuneiform bone. See **medial cuneiform bone.**

internal ear, the complex inner structure of the ear, communicating directly with the acoustic nerve, transmitting sound vibrations from the middle ear. It has two parts: the osseous labyrinth and membranous labyrinth.

internal fertilization, the union of gametes within the body of the female after insemination.

internal fistula, an abnormal passage between two internal organs or structures.

internal fixation, any method of holding together the fragments of a fractured bone without the use of appliances external to the skin. After open reduction of the fracture, smooth or threaded pins, Kirschner wires, screws, plates attached by screws or medullary nails may be used to stabilize the fragments.

internal iliac artery, a division of the common iliac artery, supplying the walls of the pelvis, the pelvic viscera, genital organs and part of the medial thigh.

internal iliac node, a node in one of seven groups of parietal lymph nodes serving the abdomen and pelvis.

internal iliac vein, one of the pair of veins in the lower body that join the external iliac vein to form the two common iliac veins.

internal jugular vein, one of a pair of veins in the neck. Each vein collects blood from one side of the brain, face and neck, and both unite with the subclavian vein to form the brachiocephalic vein.

internal mammary artery bypass, a surgical procedure to correct a coronary artery obstruction. The internal mammary artery in situ, and still attached to the subclavian artery, is anastomosed to the coronary artery beyond the obstruction.

internal medicine, the branch of medicine concerned with the study of the physiology and pathology of internal organs, and the medical diagnosis and treatment of disorders of these organs.

internal oblique muscle. See **obliquus internus abdominis.**

internal os, the internal opening of the cervical canal.

internal pterygoid muscle. See **pterygoideus medialis.**

internal respiratory nerve of Bell. See **phrenic nerve.**

internal rotation, the turning of a limb towards the midline of the body.

internal standard, an element or compound added in a known amount to yield a signal against which an instrument or an analyte to be measured can be calibrated.

internal strabismus. See **esotropia.**

internal thoracic artery, one of a pair of arteries that arise from the first portions of the subclavian arteries, supplying the pectoral muscles, breasts, pericardium and abdominal muscles.

internal thoracic vein, one of a pair of veins that accompanies the internal thoracic artery, receiving tributaries that correspond to those of the artery.

internalization, the process of adopting within the self, either unconsciously or consciously through learning and socialization, the attitudes, beliefs, values and standards of another person or, more generally, of the society or group to which one belongs.

International Association for Dental Research (IADR), an international organization concerned with research in dentistry and the exchange of information regarding such research.

International Classification of Diseases (ICD), an official list of categories of diseases, physical and mental, issued by the World Health Organization (WHO). It is used primarily for statistical purposes in the classification of morbidity and mortality data.

International Commission on Radiation Protection (ICRP), a non-governmental organization, founded in England in 1928 to provide general guidance on the safe use of radiation sources, including appropriate protective measures and codes of practice for the medical use of ionising radiations. The ICRP was reorganized in 1950 to include effects of nuclear energy.

International Congress of Surgeons (I.C.S.), an international professional organization of surgeons.

International Council of Nurses (ICN), the oldest international health organization. It is a federation of nurses' associations from 93 nations, and was one of the first health organizations to develop strict policies of non-discrimination based on nationality, race, creed, colour, politics, sex or social status. The objectives of the ICN include promotion of national associations of nurses, improvement of standards of nursing and competence of nurses, improvement of the status of nurses within their countries, and provision of an authoritative international voice for nurses. The ICN is active in the World Health Organization (WHO), the United Nations Educational, Scientific and Cultural Organization (UNESCO), and other international organizations.

International Red Cross Society, an international philanthropic organization, based in Geneva, Switzerland. It is concerned primarily with the humane treatment and welfare of victims of war and calamity, and the neutrality of hospitals and medical personnel in times of war.

International System of Units, a system for the standardization of the measurement of certain substances, including some antibiotics, vitamins, enzymes and hormones. An International Unit (IU) of substance is the amount that produces a specific biological result.

International Unit (IU, I.U.), a unit of measure in the International System of Units.

internuncial neuron, a connecting neuron in a neural pathway, usually serving as a link between two other neurons.

interocclusal record, a record of the positional relation of opposing teeth or jaws to each other, made on the occlusal surfaces of occlusal rims or teeth with a plastic material that hardens, such as plaster of paris, wax, zinc oxide-eugenol paste or acrylic resin.

interoceptive, pertaining to stimuli originating from within the body regarding the functioning of the internal organs or the receptors they activate.

interoceptor, any sensory nerve ending located in cells in the viscera that responds to stimuli originating from within the body regarding the function of the internal organs, such as digestion, excretion and blood pressure.

interparietal fissure. See **intraparietal sulcus.**

interperiosteal fracture, an incomplete fracture in which the periosteum is not disrupted.

interpersonal psychiatry, a theory of psychiatry introduced by Sullivan. It stresses that the nature and quality of relationships with significant others as the most critical factor in personality development.

interpersonal therapy, a kind of psychotherapy that views faulty communications, interactions and interrelationships as basic factors in maladaptive behaviour. A kind of interpersonal therapy is **transactional analysis.**

interphase, the metabolic stage in the cell cycle during which the cell is not dividing, the chromosomes are not individually distinguishable, and biochemical and physiological activities such as DNA synthesis occur.

interpolated PVC, a ventricular extrasystole sandwiched between two sinus-conducted beats.

interpolated VPB, a ventricular extrasystole that occurs between two consecutive beats of the dominant heart rhythm.

interpolation, 1. the transfer of tissues, as in plastic surgery or transplants. **2.** in statistics, the introduction of an estimated intermediate value of a variable between known values of the variable.

interpretation, a psychotherapeutic intervention in which the therapist draws the client's attention to features of their relationship. It usually implies that the client's past relationships influence the current one with the therapist. Supervision of an inexperienced therapist's interpretations is usually necessary to ensure that they are not simly the product of countertransference (q.v.). See **transference.**

interproximal film. See **bite wing film.**

interpubic disk, the fibrocartilaginous plate connecting the opposed surfaces of the pubic bones at the pubic symphysis.

interradicular space, the area between the roots of a multirooted tooth, normally occupied by a bony septum, and the periodontal membrane.

intersex, the condition in which an individual has both male and female anatomical characteristics to varying degrees, or where the appearance of the external genitalia is ambiguous or differs from the gonadal or genetic sex. **intersexual,** *adj.*

interspinal ligament, one of many thin, narrow membranous ligaments that connect adjoining spinous processes and extend from the root of each process to the apex.

interspinous, of or pertaining to the space between any spinous processes.

interstitial, of or pertaining to the space between tissues, as interstitial fluid.

interstitial cell-stimulating hormone (ICSH), the luteinizing hormone that also stimulates the production of testosterone by the Leydig, or interstitial, cells of the testis.

interstitial cystitis, an inflammation of the bladder, believed to be associated with an autoimmune or allergic response. The bladder wall becomes inflamed, ulcerated and scarred, causing frequent, painful urination. Haematuria often occurs.

interstitial emphysema, a form of emphysema in which air or gas escapes into the interstitial tissues of the lung after a penetrating injury or as the result of a rupture in an alveolar wall. Since the alveoli must be decompressed, there is danger that the pleura will be torn, resulting in a pneumothorax.

interstitial fluid, an extracellular fluid that fills the spaces between most of the cells of the body and provides a substantial portion of the liquid environment of the body. Formed by filtration through the blood capillaries, it is drained away as lymph.

interstitial growth, an increase in size by hyperplasia or hypertrophy within the interior of a part or structure that is already formed.

interstitial hypertrophic neuropathy. See **Dejerine-Sottas disease.**

interstitial implantation, (in embryology) the complete embedding of the blastocyst within the endometrium of the uterine wall.

interstitial keratitis, an uncommon inflammation within the layers of the cornea, the first symptom of which is a diffuse haziness. Blood vessels may grow into the area and cause permanent opacities. Its causes are syphilis, tuberculosis, leprosy and vascular hypersensitivity.

interstitial lung disease, a respiratory disorder characterized by a dry, unproductive cough and dyspnoea on exertion. X-ray films usually show fibrotic infiltrates in the lung tissue. The fibrosing or scarring of lung tissue is often the result of an immune reaction to an inhaled substance. Interstitial lung disease may also result from infections, uraemic pneumonitis, cancers, congenital or inherited disorders, or circulatory impairment.

interstitial myositis. See **myositis.**

interstitial nephritis, inflammation of the interstitial tissue of the kidney, including the tubules. The condition may be acute or chronic. **Acute interstitial nephritis** is an immunological, adverse reaction to certain drugs, often sulphonamide or methicillin. Acute renal failure, fever, rash and proteinuria are characteristic of this condition. **Chronic interstitial nephritis** is a syndrome of interstitial inflammation and structural changes, sometimes associated with conditions such as ureteral obstruction, pyelonephritis, exposure of the kidney to a toxin, rejection of a transplant and certain systemic diseases. Gradually, renal failure, nausea, vomiting, weight loss, fatigue and anaemia develop. Acidosis and hyperkalaemia may follow.

interstitial plasma cell pneumonia. See **pneumocystosis.**

interstitial pneumonia, a diffuse, chronic inflammation of the lungs beyond the terminal bronchioles. It is characterized by fibrosis and collagen formation in the alveolar walls, and the presence of large mononuclear cells in the alveolar spaces. Symptoms include progressive dyspnoea, clubbing of the fingers, cyanosis and fever. The disease may result from a hypersensitive reaction to drugs. Interstitial pneumonia may also be an autoimmune reaction, since it often accompanies coeliac disease, rheumatoid arthritis, Sjögren's syndrome and systemic sclerosis.

interstitial pregnancy. See **ectopic pregnancy.**

interstitial therapy, (in radiotherapy) the use of sealed radioactive sources placed directly into the area to be irradiated. The radioactive sources may be afterloaded; for example, iridium-192 wires implanted into a malignant tumour of the breast.

interstitial tubal pregnancy, a kind of tubal pregnancy in which implantation occurs in the proximal, interstitial portion of one of the uterine tubes.

intertransverse ligament, one of many fibrous bands connecting the transverse processes of vertebrae.

intertrigo, an erythematous irritation of opposing skin surfaces caused by friction. Common sites are the axillae, the folds beneath large or pendulous breasts, and the inner aspects of the thighs. **intertriginous,** *adj.*

intertrochanteric crest, one of a pair of ridges along the thigh bones, curving obliquely from the greater to the lesser trochanter.

intertrochanteric fracture, a fracture characterized by a crack in the tissue of the proximal femur between the greater and lesser trochanters.

intertrochanteric line, a line that runs across the anterior surface of the thigh bone from the greater to the lesser trochanter, winding around the medial surface and ending in the linea aspera.

intervention, any act performed to prevent harm from occurring to a patient, or to improve the mental, emotional or physical function of a patient. A physiological process may be monitored or enhanced, and a pathological process may be arrested or controlled.

intervertebral, of or pertaining to the space between any two vertebrae, such as the fibrocartilaginous disks.

intervertebral disk, one of the fibrous disks found between adjacent spinal vertebrae, except the axis and the atlas. The disks vary in size, shape, thickness and number, depending on the location in the back and the particular vertebrae they separate.

intervertebral fibrocartilage. See **intervertebral disk.**

intervertebral foramen, any of the passages between adjacent vertebrae through which the spinal nerves and vessels pass.

interview, a communication with a patient initiated for a specific purpose and focused on a specific content area. A **problem-seeking interview** is an enquiry that focuses on gathering data to identify problems that the patient needs to resolve. A **problem-solving interview** focuses on problems that have already been identified by the patient or healthcare professional.

intervillous space, one of several spaces between the chorionic villi of the endometrium of the gravid uterus, beneath the placenta. The intervillous spaces act as small reservoirs for oxygenated maternal blood.

intestinal absorption, the passage of the products of digestion from the lumen of the small intestine into the blood and lymphatic vessels in the wall of the gut. The surface area of the intestine is greatly increased by the presence of finger-like villi, each of which contains capillaries and a lymphatic vessel, or lacteal.

intestinal amoebiasis. See **amoebic dysentery.**

intestinal angina, chronic vascular insufficiency of the mesentery caused by atherosclerosis and resulting ischaemia of the smooth muscle of the small bowel. Abdominal pain or cramping after eating, constipation, melena, malabsorption and weight loss are characteristic of the condition.

intestinal apoplexy, the sudden occlusion of one of the three principal arteries to the intestine by an embolism or thrombus. This condition leads rapidly to necrosis of intestinal tissue, and is often fatal.

intestinal dyspepsia, an abnormal condition characterized by impaired digestion associated with a problem that originates in the intestines.

intestinal fistula, an abnormal passage from

the intestine to an external abdominal opening or stoma, usually created surgically for the exit of faeces after removal of a malignant or severely ulcerated segment of the bowel.

intestinal flu, a viral gastroenteritis, usually caused by infection by an enterovirus. It is characterized by abdominal cramps, diarrhoea, nausea and vomiting.

intestinal infarction. See **intestinal strangulation.**

intestinal juices, the secretions of glands lining the intestine.

intestinal lymphangiectasia. See **hypoproteinaemia.**

intestinal obstruction, any obstruction that results in failure of the contents of the intestine to pass through the lumen of the bowel. The most common cause is a mechanical blockage resulting from adhesions, impacted faeces, tumour of the bowel, hernia, intussusception, volvulus or the strictures of inflammatory bowel disease. Obstruction of the small bowel may cause severe pain, vomiting of faecal matter, dehydration, and eventually a drop in blood pressure. Obstruction of the colon causes less severe pain, marked abdominal distentiona and constipation.

intestinal strangulation, the arrest of blood flow to the bowel, resulting in oedema, cyanosis and gangrene of the affected loop of bowel. This condition is usually caused by a hernia, intussusception or volvulus. Early signs of intestinal strangulation resemble those of intestinal obstruction.

intestinal tonsil, one of a group of lymphatic nodules forming a single layer in the mucous membrane of the ileum opposite the mesenteric attachment.

intestine, the portion of the alimentary canal extending from the pyloric opening of the stomach to the anus. It includes the small and large intestines.   **intestinal,** *adj.*

intima, *pl.* **intimae,** the innermost layer of a structure, such as the lining membrane of an artery, vein, lymphatic or organ.   **intimal,** *adj.*

intoe. See **metatarsus varus.**

intolerance, a condition characterized by an inability to absorb or metabolize a nutrient or medication. Exposure to the substance may cause an adverse reaction.

intoxication, 1. the state of being poisoned by a drug or other toxic substance. **2.** the state of being inebriated because of an excessive consumption of alcohol. **3.** a state of mental or emotional hyperexcitability, usually euphoric.

intoxication amaurosis, loss of vision occurring without the presence of an apparent ophthalmic lesion, caused by a systemic poison such as alcohol or tobacco.

intra-abdominal pressure, the degree of pressure within the abdominal cavity.

intra-aortic balloon pump, a counterpulsation device that provides temporary cardiac assistance in the management of refractory left ventricular failure, as may follow myocardial infarction or occur in preinfarction angina.

intra-arterial, pertaining to a structure or action inside an artery.

intra-articular, within a joint.

intra-articular fracture, a fracture involving the articular surfaces of a joint.

intra-articular injection, the injection of a medication into a joint space, usually to reduce inflammation, such as in bursitis or fibromyositis.

intra-articular ligament, a ligament that forms part of the joints between 16 of the 24 ribs, dividing the joints into two cavities, each containing a synovial membrane.

intra-atrial, within an atrium in the heart.

intra-atrial block, delayed or abnormal conduction within the atria, identified on an electrocardiogram by a prolonged and often notched P wave.

intracanalicular fibroma, a tumour containing glandular epithelium and fibrous tissue, occurring in the breast.

intracanicular papilloma, a benign warty growth in certain glands, especially the breast.

intracapsular fracture, a fracture within the capsule of a joint.

intracardiac catheter. See **cardiac catheter.**

intracardiac lead, 1. an electrocardiographic conductor in which the exploring electrode is placed within one of the cardiac chambers, usually by means of cardiac catheterization. **2.** *informal,* a tracing produced by such a lead on an electrocardiograph.

intracartilaginous ossification. See **ossification.**

intracatheter, a thin, flexible plastic catheter introduced and threaded into a blood vessel to infuse blood, fluid or medication.

intracavitary, pertaining to the space within a body cavity.

intracavitary therapy, 1. a kind of radiotherapy in which one or more radioactive sources are placed, usually with the help of an applicator or holding device, within a body cavity to irradiate the walls of the cavity or adjacent tissues. **2.** (in radiotherapy) the use of sealed radioactive sources placed in a body cavity to irradiate the adjacent area. The radioactive sources may be afterloaded; for example, caesium-137 sources in applicators placed in the uterine canal and lateral vaginal fornices to irradiate a malignant tumour of the cervix.

intracellular fluid, a fluid within cell membranes throughout most of the body, containing dissolved solutes that are essential to electrolytic balance and healthy metabolism.

intracerebral, within the tissue of the brain, inside the bony skull.

intracistroni, within a cistron.

intracoronal retainer, 1. a retainer in which the prepared tooth cavity and its cast restoration lie largely within the body of the coronal portion of a tooth and within the contour of the tooth crown, such as an inlay. **2.** a direct retainer used in the construction of removable partial dentures. It consists of a female portion within the coronal segment of the crown of an abutment, and a fitted male portion attached to the denture proper.

intracranial, within the cranium.

intracranial aneurysm, an aneurysm of any of the cerebral arteries. Characteristics of the condition include sudden severe headache, stiff neck, nausea, vomiting, and sometimes loss of consciousness. Kinds of intracranial aneurysms include **berry aneurysm, fusiform aneurysm** and **mycotic aneurysm.**

intracranial electroencephalography. See **electroencephalography.**

intracranial pressure, pressure that occurs within the cranium.

intractable, having no relief, such as a symptom or a disease that remains unrelieved by the therapeutic measures employed.

intracutaneous, within the layers of the skin.

intracystic papilloma, a benign epithelial tumour formed with a cystic adenoma.

intradermal injection, the introduction of a hypodermic needle into the dermis for the purpose of instilling a substance, such as a serum or vaccine.

intradermal test, injecting a patient with small amounts of extracts of suspected allergens.

intraductal carcinoma, a frequently large neoplasm occurring most often in the breast.

intradural lipoma, a fatty tumour in or beneath the dura mater of the spine or sacrum. It tends to infiltrate the dorsal column and roots of spinal nerves, causing pain and dysfunction.

intraepidermal carcinoma, a neoplasm of squamous epidermal cells that does not proliferate into the basal area and often occurs at many sites simultaneously.

intraepidermal vesicle, a fluid-filled, blister-like cavity within the epidermis.

intraepithelial carcinoma. See **carcinoma in situ.**

intrafusal muscle, the striated muscle tissue within a muscle spindle.

intramembranous ossification. See **ossification.**

intramuscular (IM) injection, the introduction of a hypodermic needle into a muscle to administer a medication.

intraocular, pertaining to structures or substances within the eyeball.

intraocular pressure, the internal pressure of the eye, regulated by resistance to the flow of aqueous humour through the fine sieve of the trabecular meshwork. Contraction or relaxation of the longitudinal muscles of the ciliary body affects the size of the apertures in the meshwork.

intraoperative, pertaining to the period of time during a surgical procedure.

intraoperative ultrasound, a diagnostic technique that uses a portable ultrasound device to scan the spinal cord during spinal surgery. Intraoperative ultrasound can distinguish between syrinxes, or fluid-filled cysts, and neoplastic growths in nervous system tissue.

intraoral orthodontic appliance, an orthodontic device placed inside the mouth to correct or alleviate malocclusion.

intraparietal sulcus, an irregular groove on the convex surface of the parietal lobe that marks the division of the inferior and superior parietal lobules.

intrapartum, from the onset of labour to the completion of the third stage of labour with the expulsion of the placenta.

intraperiosteal fracture, a fracture that does not rupture the periosteum.

intrapsychic conflict, an emotional conflict within oneself.

intrapulmonary shunt, (in respiratory therapy) a condition of perfusion without ventilation, expressed as a ratio of QS/QT, with QS reflecting the difference between end capillary oxygen content and mixed venous oxygen content, and QT representing cardiac output. The condition may occur in atelectasis, pneumonia, pulmonary oedema and adult respiratory distress syndrome (ARDS).

intrarenal haemodynamics, the pattern of blood flow or distribution in the various parts of the kidney. Normally, the renal cortex and outer medulla receive the major portion of renal blood flow.

intrathecal, of or pertaining to a structure, process or substance within a sheath, such as the cerebrospinal fluid within the theca of spinal canal.

intrathecal injection, the introduction of a hypodermic needle into the subarachnoid space, for the purpose of instilling a material for diffusion throughout the spinal fluid.

intrathoracic goitre, an enlargement of the thyroid gland that protrudes into the thoracic cavity.

intrauterine contraceptive device (IUCD), a contraceptive device consisting of a bent strip of radiopaque plastic with a fine monofilament tail that is inserted and left in the uterine cavity for the purpose of altering the physiology of the uterus and uterine tubes to prevent pregnancy.

intrauterine fracture, a fracture that occurs during fetal life.

intrauterine growth curve, a line on a standardized graph representing the mean weight for gestational age through pregnancy to term.

intrauterine growth retardation, an abnormal process in which the development and maturation of the fetus is impeded or delayed by genetic factors, maternal disease or fetal malnutrition caused by placental insufficiency.

intravascular coagulation test, a test for detecting internal coagulation of blood.

intravenous (IV), of or pertaining to the inside of a vein, as of a thrombus or an injection, infusion or catheter.

intravenous alimentation. See **total parenteral nutrition.**

intravenous bolus, a relatively large dose of medication administered IV in a short period of time, usually within 1 to 30 minutes. The IV bolus is commonly used when administration of a medication is needed quickly, such as in an emergency, when drugs are administered that cannot be diluted, such as various cancer chemotherapeutic drugs, and when the therapeutic purpose is to achieve a peak drug level in the bloodstream of the patient.

intravenous cholangiography, (in diagnostic radiology) radiographic technique to visualize the biliary tract following a bolus injection or slow infusion of radiopaque contrast medium.

Intravenous controller, any one of several devices that automatically deliver IV fluid at selectable flow rates, usually between 1 and 69 drops per minute. The controller is commonly equipped with a rate selector, drop sensor, drop indicator and drop alarm. When the infusion does not flow at the prescribed rate, the drop alarm emits a visual and an audible signal.

intravenous DSA (IV-DSA), a form of digital subtraction angiography in which radiopaque contrast medium is injected into a vein in order to visualize arteries in the body.

intravenous fat emulsion, a preparation of 10% fat administered intravenously to help maintain the weight of an adult patient or the weight and growth of a younger patient. Such fat emulsions are prepared from refined soybean oil and egg-yolk phospholipids and may contain such major fatty acids as linoleic, oleic, palmitic and linolenic acids. The IV fat emulsion is isotonic and may be administered into a peripheral vein, but it is not mixed with other solutions employed in parenteral alimentation. IV fat emulsions are often administered when hyperalimentation is not sufficient to maintain adequate treatment of a patient, or when the patient needs calories but cannot tolerate the high percentage of dextrose contained in hyperalimentation solutions.

intravenous feeding, the administration of nutrients through a vein or veins.

intravenous infusion, 1. a solution administered intravenously through an infusion set that includes a plastic or glass vacuum bottle or bag containing the solution and tubing connecting the bottle to a catheter or a needle in the patient's vein. **2.** the process of administering a solution intravenously.

intravenous infusion filter, any one of the numerous devices used in helping to ensure the purity of an IV solution. IV filters strain the IV solution to remove contaminants such as dissolved impurities (detergents, proteins and polysaccharides), extraneous salts, micro-organisms, particles, precipitates and undissolved drug powders. Any such contaminants may complicate the IV therapy and recovery of the patient. Some filters are built into the primary IV tubing; others must be attached.

intravenous infusion therapy, the calculations for determining the delivery rate of IV fluid for the individual patient, and the necessary preparations prior to venepuncture and administration of the fluid.

intravenous injection, a hypodermic injection into a vein for the purpose of instilling a single dose of medication, injecting a contrast medium or beginning an IV infusion of blood, medication or a fluid solution, such as saline or dextrose in water.

intravenous peristaltic pump, any one of several devices for administering IV fluids by exerting pressure on the IV tubing rather than on the fluid itself. Most peristaltic pumps operate with normal IV tubing and deliver fluid at a selectable drop-per-minute rate. This device can typically infuse between 1 and 99 drops of IV fluid per minute, and is equipped with a drop sensor, rate selector, power switch indicator lamp and drop indicator and alarm. The drop indicator flashes whenever a drop of IV fluid passes the drop sensor.

intravenous piston pump, any one of several devices that accurately control the infusion of IV fluids by piston action. Most IV piston pumps can be operated by battery, as well as by electric current, and require special tubing. Some models are portable. IV piston pumps are commonly equipped with controls that allow selectable flow rates and indicators that display flow rates, dose limits and cumulative fluid volumes.

intravenous pump, a pump designed to regulate the rate of flow of a fluid given intravenously through an intracatheter or scalp vein needle.

intravenous push. See **intravenous bolus.**

intravenous pyelography (IVP), See **intravenous urography.**

intravenous syringe pump, any one of several devices that automatically compress a syringe plunger at a controlled rate. Such devices are used with disposable syringes that can deliver blood, medications or nutrients by IV, arterial or subcutaneous routes. They are especially useful in treating ambulatory patients.

intravenous therapy, the administration of fluids or drugs, or both, into the general circulation through a venipuncture.

intravenous urography. radiographic technique to visualize and evaluate the function of the kidneys, ureters and bladder, following intravenous administration of a bolus of radiopaque contrast medium.

intraventricular, of or pertaining to the space within a ventricle.

intraventricular block, the slowed conduction or stoppage of the cardiac excitatory impulse, occurring within the ventricles. The block can occur as a right bundle branch block, a left bundle branch block, or left anterior or posterior fascicular block. The block is identified on an electrocardiogram. Kinds of intraventricular block include **bundle branch block** and **infranodal block.**

intraventricular hydrocephalus. See **hydrocephalus.**

intrinsic, 1. denoting a natural or inherent part or quality. **2.** originating from or situated within an organ or tissue.

intrinsic asthma, a non-seasonal, non-allergic form of asthma, usually first occurring later in life than allergic asthma, that tends to be chronic and persistent rather than episodic. The precipitating factors include inhalation of irritating pollutants in the atmosphere, such as dust particles, smoke, aerosols, strong cooking odours, paint fumes and other volatile substances.

intrinsic factor, a substance secreted by the gastric mucosa that is essential for the intestinal absorption of cyanocobalamin. A deficiency of intrinsic factor results in pernicious anaemia.

intrinsic minus hand deformity, an abnormality that results from interruption of the ulnar and median nerves at the wrist. It results in metacarpophalangeal joint hyperextension and interphalangeal joint flexion.

introitus, an entrance or orifice to a cavity or a hollow tubular structure of the body, such as the vaginal introitus.

introjection, an unconscious mechanism in which an individual incorporates into his or her own ego structure the qualities of another person.

intromission, the insertion of one object into another, such as the introduction of the penis into the vagina.

intron, (in molecular genetics) a sequence of base pairs in DNA that interrupts the continuity of genetic information.

intropretive hyperthermia, hyperthermia delivered to internal sites that have been exposed by a surgical procedure.

introspection, 1. the act of examining one's own thoughts and emotions by concentrating on the inner self. **2.** a tendency to look inwards and view the inner self. **introspective,** *adj.*

introversion, 1. the tendency to direct one's interests, thoughts and energies inwards or towards things concerned only with the self. **2.** the state of being totally or primarily concerned with one's own intrapsychic experience. Also spelt **intraversion.**

introvert, 1. a person whose interests are directed inwards, and who is shy, withdrawn, emotionally reserved and self-absorbed. **2.** to turn inwards or direct one's interests and thoughts towards oneself.

intubation, passage of a tube into a body aperture, specifically the insertion of a breathing tube through the mouth or nose or into the trachea, to ensure a patent airway for the delivery of an anaesthetic gas or oxygen. **Blind intubation** is the insertion of a breathing tube without the use of a laryngoscope. Kinds of intubation are **endotracheal intubation, nasogastric intubation.**

intussusception, prolapse of one segment of bowel into the lumen of another segment. This kind of intestinal obstruction may involve segments of the small intestine, the colon or the terminal ileum and caecum.

inulin, a fructose-derived substance used as a diagnostic aid in tests of kidney function, specifically glomerular filtration. It is not metabolized or absorbed by the body, but is readily filtered through the kidney.

inulin clearance, a test of the rate of filtration of a starch, inulin, in the glomerulus of the kidney. Inulin is given by mouth, and the glomerular filtration rate can be estimated from the length of time needed for the inulin to appear in the urine.

inunction, 1. the rubbing of a drug mixed with an oil or fatty substance into the skin, with absorption of the active ingredient. **2.** any compound thus applied.

inundation fever. See **scrub typhus.**

in utero, inside the uterus.

invagination, 1. a condition in which one part of a structure telescopes into another part, as the intestine during peristalsis. If the invagination is extensive or involves a tumour or polyps, it may cause an intestinal obstruction. **2.** surgery for repair of a hernia by replacing the contents of the hernial sac in the abdominal cavity. **invaginate,** *v.*

invariable behaviour, behaviour that results from physiological response to a stimulus and is not modified by individual experience, such as a reflex.

invasion, the process by which malignant cells move into deeper tissue and through the basement membrane, gaining access to blood vessels and lymphatic channels.

invasion of privacy, (in law) the violation of another person's right to be left alone and free from unwarranted publicity and intrusion.

invasive, characterized by a tendency to

spread, infiltrate and intrude.

invasive carcinoma, a malignant neoplasm composed of epithelial cells that infiltrate and destroy surrounding tissues.

invasive mole. See **chorioadenoma destruens.**

invasive thermometry, measurement of tissue temperature using probes placed directly in the tissue.

inverse anaphylaxis, an exaggerated reaction of hypersensitivity induced by an antibody rather than an antigen.

inverse I:E ratio, an inspiratory/expiratory ratio in which the frequency of inhalations is greater than the rate of exhalations. Such situations occur when there is a need to improve oxygenation.

inverse relationship. See **negative relationship.**

inverse square law, 1. a law stating that the amount of radiation emitted is inversely proportional to the square of the distance between the source and the irradiated surface; for example, a person 2 feet from a patient being treated with radium is exposed to four times more radiation than he or she would be exposed to at 4 feet. **2.** (in radiation dosimetry) a law which states that the intensity of radiation from a point source is inversely proportional to the square of the distance from the source, provided that there is no attenuation of the beam of radiation. For example, if the distance from a source is doubled, then the radiation dose will be one-quarter of its previous value.

inversion, 1. an abnormal condition in which an organ is turned inside out, such as a uterine inversion. **2.** a chromosomal defect in which two or more segments of a chromosome break off and become separated. They rejoin the chromosome in the wrong order.

invert, to turn something upside down or inside out.

invisible differentiation, (in embryology) a fixed determination for specialization and diversification that exists in embryonic cells but is not yet visibly apparent.

in vitro, (of a biological reaction) occurring in laboratory apparatus.

in vitro fertilization (IVF), a method of fertilizing human ova outside the body, by collecting the mature ova and placing them in a dish with a sample of spermatozoa. After the ova are allowed to incubate over a period of 48 to 72 hours, the fertilized ova are injected into the uterus through the cervix. The procedure takes between 2 to 3 days.

in vivo, (of a biological reaction) occurring in a living organism.

in vivo tracer study, (in nuclear medicine) a diagnostic procedure in which a series of radiograms of an administered radioactive tracer passing through a compartment in the patient's body demonstrate normal or abnormal structures or processes.

in vivo tracer study, (in radionuclide imaging) diagnostic technique in which a radiopharmaceutical is injected and a series of dynamic images obtained using a gamma camera.

involucrum, *pl.* **involucra,** a sheath or coating, such as that encasing a sequestrum of necrotic bone.

involuntary, occurring without conscious control or direction.

involuntary muscle. See **smooth muscle.**

involuntary nervous system. See **visceral nervous system.**

involution, 1. a normal process characterized by a decrease in the size of an organ and a decrease in the size of its cells, such as postpartum involution of the uterus. **2.** (in embryology) a developmental process in which a group of cells grows over the rim at the border of the organ or part and, rolling inwards, rejoins the organ or part to form a tube.

involutional melancholia, a state of depression occurring during the climacteric. The disorder begins gradually and is characterized by pessimism, irritability, insomnia, loss of appetite, feelings of anxiety and an increase in motor activity, ranging from mere restlessness to extreme agitation.

inward aggression, destructive behaviour that is directed against oneself.

iodinated, a sterile, buffered isotonic solution containing radioiodinated normal human serum adjusted to provide not more than 1 mCi of radioactivity per millilitre in diagnostic tests of blood volume and cardiac output.

iodine (I), a non-metallic element of the halogen group. Its atomic number is 53 and its atomic weight is 126.90. It is an essential micronutrient or trace element, and almost 80% of the iodine present in the body is in the thyroid gland. Iodine deficiency can result in goitre or cretinism. Radioisotopes of iodine are used in radioisotope scanning procedures and in palliative treatment of cancer of the thyroid.

iodism, a condition produced by excessive amounts of iodine in the body. It is characterized by increased lacrimation and salivation, rhinitis, weakness and a typical skin eruption.

iodize, to treat or impregnate with iodine or an iodide. Table salt is iodized to prevent the occurrence of goitre in areas with insufficient iodine in the drinking water or food.

iododerma, a skin rash caused by a hypersensitivity to ingested iodides. The lesions may be acneiform, bullous or fungating.

iodoform, a topical anti-infective used as an antiseptic.

iodophor, an antiseptic or disinfectant that combines iodine with another agent, such as a detergent.

iodopsin, a photosensitive chemical in the cones of the retina that reacts in association with other chemicals and plays a part in colour vision. Iodopsin is more stable when exposed to bright light than rhodopsin, which is found in the rods of the retina.

ion, an atom or group of atoms that has acquired an electrical charge through the gain or loss of an electron or electrons.

ion exchange chromatography, the process of separating and analysing different substances according to their affinities for chemically stable but very reactive synthetic exchangers, which are composed largely of polystyrene and cellulose. Ion exchange chromatography is often used to separate components of nucleic acids and proteins elaborated by various structures throughout the body.

ion-selective electrode, a potentiometric electrode that develops a potential in the presence of one ion (or class of ions) but not in the presence of a similar concentration of other ions.

ionic bonding, a force that holds atoms together by the transfer of a single valance electron, such as from a cation to an anion. Ionic compounds do not form true molecules, and in aqueous solution break down into their constituent ions.

ionic dissociation, a phenomenon whereby ions in ionic compounds in an aqueous solution are freed from their mutual bonds and distribute themselves uniformly throughout the solvent.

ionic strength, the sum of the concentrations of all ions in a solution, weighted by the squares of their charges.

ionization, the process in which a neutral atom or molecule gains or loses electrons and thus acquires a negative or positive electrical charge.

ionization chamber, 1. a small cavity filled with air that has the capability of collecting the ionic charge liberated during irradiation. **2.** (in radiation dosimetry) an electronic device consisting of an air-filled chamber and central electrode which collects charge when irradiated, in order to measure radiation exposure.

ionize, to cause a neutral atom to gain or lose electrons as in ionization.

ionized calcium, the ionized, unbound, non-complexed fraction of serum calcium that is biologically active.

ionizing energy, the average energy lost by a beam of ionising radiation in air in producing one ion pair.

ionizing radiation, high-energy electromagnetic waves (x-rays and gamma rays) and beams of particles (alpha particles, beta particles, electrons, neutrons, positrons, protons) that produce ionization of the atoms with which they interact. Such ionization can damage cells, usually indirectly, by the ionization of the intracellular water producing free radicals which break DNA chemical bonds.

iontophoretic pilocarpine test, a sweat test used in the diagnosis of cystic fibrosis. Pilocarpine iontophoresis is employed to stimulate production of sweat, which is analysed for concentrations of sodium and chloride electrolytes.

Iowa trumpet, a kind of needle guide used in performing a pudendal block. It consists of a long thin cylinder through which a needle may be passed. A ring is attached to the proximal end of the guide, allowing the operator to hold it securely.

ipecacuanha, an emetic prescribed to cause emesis in certain types of poisoning and drug overdose.

IPOF, abbreviation for **immediate postoperative fit prosthesis.**

IPPB (intermittent positive pressure breathing), a form of assisted or controlled respiration produced by a ventilatory apparatus in which compressed gas is delivered under positive pressure into the person's airways until a preset pressure is reached. Passive exhalation is allowed through a valve.

IPPV (intermittent positive pressure ventilator), a pressure-cycled ventilator for providing a flow of air into the lungs at a predetermined pressure. As the pressure is attained, the flow is stopped, pressure is released and the patient exhales.

IPPV, abbreviation for See **IPPB.**

ipsilateral, pertaining to the same side of the body.

IQ, abbreviation for **intelligence quotient.**

Ir, symbol for **iridium.**

iridectomy, surgical removal of part of the iris of the eye, performed most often to restore drainage of the aqueous humour in glaucoma, or remove a foreign body or a malignant tumour.

iridium (Ir), a silvery-bluish metallic element. Its atomic number is 77 and its atomic weight is 192.2. The radioactive isotope iridium 192 is frequently used in brachytherapy applications.

iridotomy, a surgical incision into the iris of the eye, performed to relieve occlusion of the pupil, enlarge the pupil in cataract extraction, or treat postoperative glaucoma.

iris, a circular, contractile disc suspended in aqueous humour between the cornea and crystalline lens of the eye, and perforated by a circular pupil. The periphery of the iris is continuous with the ciliary body, and is connected to the cornea by the pectinate ligament. The iris divides the space between the lens and the cornea into an anterior and a posterior chamber. Dark pigment cells under the translucent tissue of the iris are variously arranged in different people to produce different coloured irises. **iridic,** *adj.*

iritis, an inflammatory condition of the iris of the eye characterized by pain, lacrimation, photophobia and, if severe, diminished visual acuity. On examination, the eye looks cloudy, the iris bulges and the pupil is contracted.

iron (Fe), a common metallic element essential for the synthesis of haemoglobin. Its atomic number is 26 and its atomic weight is 55.85. It is used as a haematinic in the form of its salts and complexes.

iron-binding capacity, the maximum amount of iron with which protein in serum can combine, normally 4.5-8mmol/litre (250-450 g/ml); increased in iron deficiency.

iron deficiency anaemia, a microcytic, hypochromic anaemia caused by inadequate supplies of iron needed to synthesize haemoglobin. It is characterized by pallor, fatigue and weakness. Iron deficiency may be the result of an inadequate dietary supply of iron, poor absorption of iron in the digestive system or chronic bleeding.

iron dextran, an injectable haematinic prescribed in the treatment of iron deficiency anaemia not responsive to oral iron therapy.

iron lung. See **Drinker respirator.**

iron metabolism, a series of processes involved in the entry of iron into the body through its absorption, its transport and storage throughout the body, its utilization for the formation of haemoglobin and other iron compounds, and its eventual excretion. Iron normally enters the body through the epithelium of the intestinal mucosa, being oxidized from ferrous to ferric iron in the process. Once iron enters the blood, it cycles between the plasma and reticuloendothelial or erythropoietic system. Plasma iron is delivered to the normoblast for haemoglobin synthesis where it remains up to 4 months in the haemoglobin molecules of a mature red cell. When red cells deteriorate and break down, the iron is released from the haemoglobin by the reticuloendothelial system to re-enter the transport pool for recycling.

iron salts poisoning, poisoning caused by overdose of ferric or ferrous salts, characterized by vomiting, bloody diarrhoea, cyanosis, and gastric and intestinal pain.

iron saturation, the capacity of iron to saturate transferrin, measured in the blood to detect iron excess or deficiency.

iron transport, the process whereby iron is carried from its entry point into the body, the intestinal mucosa, to the various sites of utilization and storage. Transferrin binds with free iron and shuttles it to storage and utilization sites.

iron-rich food, any nutrient containing a relatively large amount of iron. The best source of dietary iron is liver, with oysters, clams, heart, kidney, lean meat and tongue

as second choices. Leafy green vegetables are the best plant sources.

irradiation, exposure to any form of radiant energy such as heat, light or x-ray. Radioactive sources of radiant energy, such as x-rays or isotopes of iodine or cobalt, are used diagnostically to examine internal body structures or destroy micro-organisms or tissue cells that have become cancerous. Infrared or ultraviolet light may be used to produce heat in body tissues to relieve pain and soreness, or treat skin ailments. Ultraviolet light is also used to identify certain bacteria and toxic moulds. **irradiate,** *v.*

irreducible, unable to be returned to the normal position or condition; for example, an irreducible hernia.

irrelevance, (in psychiatry) any response, action or statement not pertinent to the existing situation or condition, that is indicative of a neurotic or psychotic condition.

irreversible coma. See **brain death.**

irrigate, to flush with a fluid, usually with a slow, steady pressure on a syringe plunger. It may be carried out to cleanse a wound or clear tubing.

irrigation, the process of washing out a body cavity or wound with a stream of water or other fluid. **irrigate,** *v.*

irrigator, an apparatus with a flexible tube for flushing or washing out a body cavity.

irritable bowel syndrome, abnormally increased motility of the small and large intestines, generally associated with emotional stress. Most of those affected are young adults, who complain of diarrhoea and occasionally pain in the lower abdomen. Pain is usually relieved by moving the bowels. As there is no organic disease present in irritable bowel syndrome, no specific treatment is necessary.

IRV, abbreviation for *inspiratory reserve volume.* See **pulmonary function test.**

ischaemia, decreased blood supply to a body organ or part, often marked by pain and organ dysfunction, as in ischaemic heart disease. **ischaemic,** *adj.*

ischaemic contracture. See **Volkmann's contracture.**

ischaemic heart disease, a pathological condition of the myocardium caused by lack of oxygen reaching the tissue cells.

ischaemic lumbago, a pain in the lower back and buttocks caused by vascular insufficiency, as in occlusion of the abdominal aorta.

ischaemic pain, the unpleasant, often excruciating sensation associated with ischaemia, resulting from peripheral vascular disease, decreased blood flow caused by constricting orthopaedic casts, or insufficient blood flow caused by surgical trauma or accidental injury. Ischaemic pain caused by occlusive arterial disease is often severe and may not be relieved, even with narcotics. The individual with peripheral vascular disease may experience ischaemic pain only while exercising, because the metabolic demands for oxygen cannot be met by the occluded flow of blood.

ischial spines, two relatively sharp bony projections into the pelvic outlet from the ischial bones that form the lower border of the pelvis.

ischium, *pl.* **ischia,** one of the three parts of the hip bone, joining the ilium and pubis to form the acetabulum. The ischium comprises the dorsal part of the hip bone and is divided into the body of the ischium, which forms two fifths of the acetabulum, and the ramus, which joins the inferior ramus of the pubis.

ISG, abbreviation for **immune serum globulin.**

Ishihara colour test {Shinobu Ishihara, Japanese ophthalmologist, b. 1879}, a test of colour vision using a series of plates on which round dots are printed in a variety of colours and patterns. People with normal colour vision are able to discern specific numbers or patterns on the plates; the inability to pick out a given number or shape is symptomatic of a specific deficiency in colour perception.

island fever. See **scrub typhus.**

islands of Langerhans {Paul Langerhans, German pathologist, b. 1847}, clusters of cells within the pancreas that produce insulin, glucagon and pancreatic polypeptide. They form the endocrine portion of the gland; their hormonal secretions released into the bloodstream are balanced, important regulators of sugar metabolism.

islet cell adenoma. See **insulinoma.**

islet cell antibody, an immunoglobulin that reacts with the cytoplasm of all of the cells of the pancreatic islets. These antibodies occur in most of newly diagnosed insulin-dependent diabetic patients.

islet cell tumour, any tumour of the islands of Langerhans.

islets of Langerhans. See **islands of Langerhans.**

isoagglutinin, an antibody that causes agglutination of erythrocytes in other members of the same species that carry an isoagglutinogen on their erythrocytes.

isoagglutinogen, an antigen that causes the agglutination of erythrocytes in others of the same species that carry a corresponding isoagglutinin in their serum.

isoamyl alcohol. See **amyl alcohol.**

isoantibody, an antibody to isoantigens found in other members of the same species.

isoantigen, a substance that interacts with isoantibodies in other members of the same species.

isobar, 1. a line connecting points of equal pressure on a graph. **2.** (in nuclear medicine) one of a group of nuclides having the same total number of neutrons and protons in the nucleus, but proportioned such as to result in different values of the atomic number.

isobutyl alcohol, a clear, colourless liquid that is miscible with ethyl alcohol or ether.

isocapnic, pertaining to a steady level of carbon dioxide in the tissues despite changing levels of ventilation.

isocarboxazid, a monoamine oxidase inhibitor used in the treatment of depression.

isocentre, (in radiography/radiotherapy) point around which all movements of an isocentrically mounted unit rotate.

isochromosome, a chromosome with identical arms on either side of the centromere.

isodose chart, (in radiotherapy) a graphic representation of the distribution of radiation in tissue; lines are drawn through points receiving equal doses.

isodose distribution, (in radiotherapy) graphic representation of the planned radiation dose in an individual patient.

isoelectric, pertaining to the electrical base line of an electrocardiogram.

isoelectric electroencephalogram. See **flat electroencephalogram.**

isoelectric focusing, the ordering and concentration of substances according to their isoelectric points.

isoelectric period, a period in physiological activity, such as nerve conduction or muscle contraction, where there is no variation in electrical potential.

isoelectric point, the pH at which a molecule containing several ionizable groups is electrically neutral. The number of positively charged groups equals the number of negatively charged groups.

isoenzyme, an enzyme that may appear in multiple forms, with slightly different chemical or other characteristics. It may be produced in different organs, although each enzyme performs essentially the same function.

isoflows, (in respiratory therapy) a measure of early small airways dysfunction in a patient made by comparing flow rates between air and helium at fixed points in time.

isogamete, a reproductive cell of the same size and structure as the one with which it unites. **isogametic,** *adj.*

isogamy, sexual reproduction in which there is fusion of gametes of the same size and structure, such as in certain algae, fungi and protozoa. **isogamous,** *adj.*

isogeneic. See **syngeneic.**

isogenesis, development from a common origin and according to similar processes. **isogenetic, isogenic,** *adj.*

isograft, surgical transplantation of histocompatible tissue obtained from genetically identical individuals, such as between a patient and identical twin.

isohaemagglutinin. See **isoagglutinin.**

isohydric shift, the series of reactions in red

blood cells in which CO_2 is taken up and oxygen is released without the production of excess hydrogen ions.

isoimmunization, the development of antibodies against antigens from the same species (isoantigens), such as the development of anti-Rh antibodies in an Rh-negative person.

isokinetic, pertaining to a concentric or eccentric contraction that occurs at a set speed against a force of maximal resistance produced at all points in the range of motion.

isolation, the separation of a seriously ill patient from others, in order to prevent the spread of an infection or protect the patient from irritating environmental factors.

isolation incubator, an incubator bed regularly maintained for premature or other infants who require isolation.

isoleucine (Ile), an amino acid occurring in most dietary proteins. It is essential for the proper growth of infants and nitrogen balance in adults.

isomers, molecules that have the same molecular weight and formula but different structures, resulting in different properties.

isometheptene mucate, an indirectly acting adrenergic agent with vasoconstrictor effects. It is a component of some combination medications used to treat migraine.

isometric, maintaining the same length or dimension.

isometric exercise, a form of active exercise that increases muscle tension by applying pressure against stable resistance. This may be accomplished by opposing different muscles in the same individual, such as by making a limb push or pull against an immovable object. There is no joint movement and the length of the muscle remains unchanged.

isometric growth, an increase in size of different organs or parts of an organism at the same rate.

isoniazid, a tuberculostatic antibacterial used in the treatment of tuberculosis.

iso-osmotic solution, a solution with electrolytes that will exert the same osmotic pressure as another solution.

isopentoic acid. See isovaleric acid.

isophane insulin suspension, a suspension of protamine with insulin. It is a commonly prescribed intermediate-acting insulin.

isoprenaline hydrochloride, a beta-adrenergic stimulant used as a bronchodilator and cardiac stimulant.

isopropanol. See isopropyl alcohol.

isopropyl alcohol, a clear, colourless, bitter aromatic liquid that is miscible with water, ether, chloroform and ethyl alcohol.

isopropylacetic acid. See isovaleric acid.

isopropylaminoacetic acid. See valine.

isoproterenol hydrochloride, a beta-adrenergic stimulant used as a bronchodilator and as a cardiac stimulant.

isosmotic. See isotonic.

isosorbide dinitrate, isosorbide mononitrate, anti-anginal agents used as coronary vasodilators in the treatment of angina pectoris and congestive heart failure.

isotachophoresis, the ordering and concentration of substances of intermediate effective mobilities between an ion of high effective mobility and one of much lower effective mobility, followed by their migration at a uniform velocity.

isotones, atoms that have the same number of neutrons but different numbers of protons.

isotonic, (of a solution) having the same concentration of solute as another solution, hence exerting the same amount of osmotic pressure as that solution. Also isosmotic.

isotonic exercise, a form of active exercise in which the muscle contracts and causes movement. Throughout the procedure, there is no significant change in the resistance so that the force of the contraction remains constant.

isotope, one of two or more forms of a chemical element that have the same number of protons in the atomic nucleus and the same atomic number, but they differ in the number of their nuclear neutrons and atomic weights. Carbon (^{12}C) has six nuclear neutrons, while its isotope ^{14}C has eight.

isotopic tracer, an isotope or artificial mixture of isotopes of an element incorporated into a sample to permit observation of the course of the element, either alone or in combination, through a chemical, physical or biological process.

isotretinoin, an anti-acne agent prescribed for cystic acne.

isovaleric acid, a fatty acid with a pungent taste and disagreeable odour, found in valerian and other plant products, as well as in cheese. It also occurs as a metabolite of the amino acid leucine and is found in the sweat of feet and in the urine of patients with smallpox, hepatitis and typhus.

isovolume pressure-flow curve, a curve on a graph describing the relationship of driving pressure to the resulting volumetric flow rate in the airways at any given lung inflation.

isovolumic contraction, (in cardiology) an early phase of systole in which the left ventricle is generating enough tension to overcome the resistance of the aortic end-diastolic pressure.

isoxsuprine hydrochloride, a myometrial relaxant and peripheral vasodilator, used in the management of premature labour. It has also been used to improve the circulation in peripheral vascular disease.

isthmus, *pl.* **isthmuses, isthmi,** a narrow connection between two larger bodies or parts, such as the isthmus of the auditory tube in the ear.

IT, abbreviation for immunotoxin.

itch, 1. a sensation, usually on the skin, that

makes one want to scratch. **2.** a tingling, annoying sensation on an area of the skin that makes one want to scratch it. **3.** the pruritic condition of the skin caused by infestation with the parasitic mite *Sarcoptes scabiei.* **itchy,** *adj.*

ITP, abbreviation for **idiopathic thrombocytopenic purpura**.

IU, I.U., abbreviation for **International Unit.**

IUCD, abbreviation for **intrauterine contraceptive device.**

IV, 1. abbreviation for **intravenous. 2.** *informal,* equipment consisting of a bottle of fluid, infusion set with tubing and an intracatheter, used in intravenous therapy. **3.** intravenous administration of fluids or medication by injection into a vein.

IV push, a technique in which a bolus of medication or a large volume of IV fluid is given rapidly via IV injection or infusion.

IV-type traction frame, a metal support that holds traction equipment consisting of two metal uprights, one at each end of the bed, which support an overhead metal bar.

IVF, abbreviation for in **vitro fertilization.**

ivory bones. See **osteopetrosis.**

IVP, abbreviation for **intravenous pyelography.**

IVU, addreviation for **intravenous urology.**

Ixodes, a genus of parasitic, hard-shelled ticks associated with the transmission of a variety of arbovirus infections, such as Rocky Mountain spotted fever.

ixodid, of or pertaining to hard ticks of the family *Ixodidae.*

J, abbreviation for **joule.**

J chain, the portion of the IgM molecule possibly holding the structure together, hence "joining chain."

J-pouch, a faecal reservoir formed surgically by folding over the lower end of the ileum in an ileo-anal anastomosis.

Jaccoud's dissociated fever {Sigismond Jaccoud, French physician, b. 1830}, a form of meningitic fever accompanied by a paradoxical slow pulse rate.

jacket, a supportive or confining therapeutic casing or garment for the torso. Types of jacket are **Minerva jacket** and **Sayre's jacket.**

jacknife position, an anatomical position in which the patient is placed on the back in a semisitting position, with the shoulders elevated and the thighs flexed at right angles to the abdomen. Examination and instrumentation of the male urethra is facilitated by this position.

Jackson crib, a removable orthodontic appliance retained in position by crib-shaped wires.

jacksonian epilepsy, See **focal seizure.**

Jacob's membrane {Arthur Jacob, Irish surgeon, b. 1790}, the outermost of the nine layers of the retina, composed of rods and cones interacting directly with the optic nerve.

Jacquemier's sign, blue colouration of the vagina seen from early pregnancy due to increased blood supply.

Jacquemier's sign {Jean M. Jacquemier, French obstetrician, b. 1806}, a deepening of the colour of the vaginal mucosa just below the urethral orifice. It may sometimes be noted after the fourth week of pregnancy.

jactitation, twitchings or spasms of muscles or muscle groups, as observed in the restless body movements of a patient with a severe fever.

jail fever. See **epidemic typhus.**

Jakob-Creutzfeldt disease. See **Creutzfeldt-Jakob disease.**

jamais vu, the sensation of being a stranger with a person one knows or a familiar place.

Janeway's spots, {Edward G. Janeway, American Physician, b. 1841}, a small erythematous or haemorrhagic macule occurring on the palms or soles. It is sometimes diagnostic of subacute bacterial endocarditis.

janiceps a conjoined, twin fetal monster in which the heads are fused, with the faces looking in opposite directions.

Jansen's disease. See **metaphyseal dysostosis.**

Jarisch-Herxheimer reaction {Adolph Jarisch, Austrian dermatologist, b. 1850; Karl Herxheimer, German dermatologist, b. 1861}, a sudden transient fever and exacerbation of skin lesions observed several hours after administration of penicillin or other antibiotics in the treatment of syphilis, leptospirosis or relapsing fever.

Jarvik-7 {Robert K. Jarvik, American physician, b. 1946}, an artificial heart designed by Jarvik for use in humans. The Jarvik-7 was an early model that depended on air pressure to drive the ventricles.

jaundice, a yellow discolouration of the skin, mucous membranes, and sclerae of the eyes, caused by greater than normal amounts of bilirubin in the blood. Persons with jaundice may also experience nausea, vomiting and abdominal pain, and may pass dark urine. Jaundice is a symptom of many disorders, including liver diseases, biliary obstruction and the haemolytic anaemias. Newborns commonly develop physiological jaundice which disappears after a few days. **jaundiced,** *adj.*

jaw, a common term used to describe the maxillae and mandible, as well as the soft tissue that covers these structures.

jaw reflex, an abnormal reflex elicited by tapping the chin with a rubber hammer while the mouth is half-open and the jaw muscles are relaxed.

jaw relationship, any relation of the mandible to the maxillae.

jaw-winking, an involuntary facial movement phenomenon in which the eyelid droops when the jaw is closed but raises when the jaw is moved. The raising of the eyelid often appears exaggerated.

Jefferson fracture, a fracture characterized by bursting of the ring of the atlas.

jejunal feeding tube, a hollow tube inserted into the jejunum for administration of liquified foods.

jejunoileitis. See **Crohn's disease.**

jejunostomy, a surgical procedure to create an artificial opening to the jejunum through the abdominal wall. It may be a permanent or a temporary opening.

jejunum, *pl.* **jejuna,** one of the three portions of the small intestine, connecting proximally with the duodenum and distally with the ileum. The jejunum has a slightly larger diameter, a deeper colour and a thicker wall than the ileum, and contains heavy, circular folds that are absent in the lower part of the ileum. **jejunal,** *adj.*

jellyfish sting, a wound caused by skin contact with a jellyfish, a sea animal with a gelatinous body and tentacles containing stinging structures. In most cases, a tender, red welt develops on the affected skin. In some cases, severe localized pain and nausea, weakness, excessive lacrimation, nasal discharge, muscle spasm, perspiration and dyspnoea may occur.

jet humidifier, a humidifier that increases the surface area for exposure of water to gas by breaking the water into small aerosol droplets. A foaming mixture of liquid and gas is produced. Gas issuing from the unit has a maximum amount of water vapour and a minimum of liquid water particles.

jet lag, a condition characterized by fatigue, insomnia and sluggish body functions, caused by disruption of the normal circadian rhythm and resulting from air travel across several time zones.

jet nebulizer, a respiratory humidifier that uses the Bernoulli effect to convert a source of liquid into a fine mist of aerosol particles.

Jeune's syndrome, a form of lethal, short-limbed dwarfism characterized by constriction of the upper thorax, and occasionally polydactylism. It is inherited as an autosomal recessive trait.

JOD, abbreviation for *juvenile-onset diabetes.* See **insulin-dependent diabetes mellitus.**

Jod-Basedow phenomenon, thyrotoxicosis occurring when dietary iodine is given to a patient with endemic goitre in an area of environmental iodine deficiency. It is presumed that iodine deficiency protects some patients with endemic goitre from developing thyrotoxicosis.

jogger's heel, a painful condition, common among joggers and distance runners. It is characterized by bruising, bursitis, fasciitis or calcaneal spurs, and is caused by repetitive and forceful strikes of the heel on the ground.

joint, any one of the connections between bones. Each is classified according to structure and movability as fibrous, cartilaginous or synovial. Fibrous joints are immovable, cartilaginous joints slightly movable, and synovial joints freely movable. Typical immovable joints are those connecting most of the bones of the skull with a sutural ligament. Typical, slightly movable joints are those connecting the vertebrae and the pubic bones.

joint appointment, 1. a faculty appointment to two institutions within a university or system, pertaining to the schools of nursing and medicine of the same university. **2.** (in academic nursing) the appointment of a member of the faculty of a university to a clinical service of an associated service institution.

joint chondroma, a cartilaginous mass that develops in the synovial membrane of a joint.

joint fracture, a fracture of the articular surfaces of the bony structures of a joint.

joint instability, an abnormal increase in joint mobility.

joint mouse, a small, movable calculus in or near a joint, usually the knee joint.

joint practice, 1. the practice of a doctor and a nurse practitioner, usually private, who work as a team, sharing responsibility for a group of patients. **2.** (in in-patient nursing) the practice of making joint decisions about patient care through the committees of doctors and nurses working on a division.

joint protection, the use of orthotics with therapeutic exercise to prevent damage or deformity of a joint during rehabilitation, so as to restore power and range of motion. An example is a metal ankle-foot orthosis that allows weight-bearing on an extended knee.

jointly exhaustive categories, categories on a research instrument that are sufficiently complete to allow every possible subject, factor or variable to be classified and assigned to a category.

joule {James P. Joule, English physicist, b. 1818}, a unit of energy or work in the MKS (meter-kilogram-second) system; 1 joule is equivalent to 1 newton metre.

judgement, 1. (in law) the final decision of the court regarding the case before it. **2.** the reason given by the court for its decision; an opinion. **3.** an award, penalty or other sentence of law given by the court. **4.** (in psychiatry) the ability to recognize the relationships of ideas and to form correct conclusions from those data as well as from those acquired from experience.

jugular foramen, one of a pair of openings between the lateral part of the occipital bone and petrous part of the temporal bones in the skull.

jugular fossa, a deep depression adjacent to the interior surface of the petrosa of the temporal bone of the skull.

jugular process, a portion of the occipital bone that projects laterally from the squamous part. On its anterior border, a deep notch forms the posterior and medial boundary of the jugular foramen.

jugular pulse, a pulsation in the jugular vein caused by waves transmitted from the right side of the heart by the circulating blood.

jugular venous pressure (JVP), blood pressure in the jugular vein, which reflects the volume and pressure of the venous blood in the right side of the heart. With elevated JVP, the neck veins may be distended as high as the angle of the jaw.

juice, any fluid secreted by the tissues of animals or plants. Kinds of juices include **gastric juice, intestinal juice** and **pancre-**

atic juice.

jumentous, having a strong animal odour, especially that of a horse. It is used to describe the odour of urine during certain disease conditions.

jumpers heel, characterised by variable coalescence of punctate black dots, which appear suddenly on the sides of heels. The condition usually affects jumpers. See also **calcaneal petechiae**.

jumping gene, (in molecular genetics) a unit of genetic information associated with a segment of DNA that can move from one position in the genome to another.

junction lines, (in radiology) vertical lines that appear in the mediastinum on a P-A (posterior-anterior) projection x-ray image.

junction naevus, a hairless, flat or slightly raised, brown skin blemish, arising from pigment cells at the epidermal-dermal junction. Malignant change may be signalled by increase in size, hardness or darkening, bleeding, or the appearance of satellite discolouration around the naevus.

junctional extrasystole, an extrasystole arising from the atrioventricular junction.

junctional rhythm, the cardiac rhythm originating in the atrioventricular junction.

junctional tachycardia, an automatic heart rhythm of greater than 100 beats/minute, emanating from the AV junction.

junctura cartilaginea. See **cartilaginous joint**.

junctura fibrosa. See **fibrous joint**.

junctura synovialis. See **synovial joint**.

jungian psychology. See **analytical psychology**.

Junin fever. See **Argentine haemorrhagic fever**.

juvenile, 1. a young person; youth; child; youngster. 2. of, pertaining to, characteristic of, or suitable for a young person; youthful. 3. physiologically underdeveloped or immature. 4. denoting psychological or intellectual immaturity; childish.

juvenile alveolar rhabdomyosarcoma, a rapidly growing tumor of striated muscle with a grave prognosis, occurring in children and adolescents, chiefly in the extremities.

juvenile angiofibroma. See **nasopharyngeal angiofibroma**.

juvenile delinquency, persistent antisocial, illegal or criminal behaviour by children or adolescents to the degree that it cannot be controlled or corrected by the parents, it endangers others in the community, and becomes the concern of a law enforcement agency. Such behavioural patterns are characterized by aggressiveness, destructiveness, hostility and cruelty, and are more frequently in boys than in girls.

juvenile delinquent, a person who performs illegal acts and who is below the legal age at which he or she can be treated, tried and punished as an adult.

juvenile diabetes. See **insulin-dependent diabetes mellitus**.

juvenile kyphosis. See **Scheuermann's disease**.

juvenile lentigo. See **lentigo**.

juvenile periodontitis, an abnormal condition that may affect the dental alveoli, especially in the anterior and first molar regions of children and adolescents. Formerly called periodontosis.

juvenile rheumatoid arthritis, a form of rheumatoid arthritis, usually affecting the larger joints of children under 16 years of age. As bone growth in children is dependent on the epiphyseal plates of the distal epiphyses, skeletal development may be impaired if these structures are damaged.

juvenile spinal muscular atrophy, a disorder beginning in childhood, in which progressive degeneration of anterior horn and medullary nerve cells leads to skeletal muscle wasting. The condition usually begins in the legs and pelvis.

juvenile xanthogranuloma, a skin disorder characterized by groups of yellow, red or brown papules or nodules on the extensor surfaces of the arms and legs, and in some cases on the eyeball, meninges and testes of children.

juvenile-onset diabetes. See **insulin-dependent diabetes mellitus**.

juxtaglomerular cells, smooth muscle cells lining the glomerular end of the afferent arterioles in the kidney, in opposition to the macula densa region of the early distal tubule. These cells synthesize and store renin.

juxtaposition, the placement of objects end-to-end or side by side.

K, 1. symbol for **kilo**. 2. symbol for Kelvin scale. 3. symbol for potassium.

K$_m$, symbol for **Michaelis-Menten constant**.

Kahn test {Reuben L. Kahn, American bacteriologist, b. 1887}, 1. a serological test for syphilis. The appearance of a white precipitate in a serum sample allowed to stand overnight in a mixture with a sensitized antigen is regarded as a positive reaction. 2. a test for the presence of cancer by measuring the proportion of albumin A in a blood sample.

kakke disease. See **beriberi**.

kakosmia. See **cacosmia**.

kala-azar, a disease caused by the protozoan *Leishmania donovani,* transmitted to humans, particularly to children, by the bite of the sand fly. Kala-azar occurs in Asia, Africa, South and Central American countries, and in the Mediterranean region. The liver and spleen are the main sites of infection; signs and symptoms include anaemia, hepatomegaly, splenomegaly, irregular fever, and emaciation.

kalaemia, the presence of potassium in the blood.

kaliuresis, the excretion of potassium in the urine.

kallikrein-kinin system, a proposed hormonal system that functions within the kidney, with the enzyme kallikrein in the renal cortex mediating production of bradykinin, which acts as a vasodilator peptide.

Kallmann's syndrome {Franz J. Kallman, American psychiatrist, b. 1897}, a condition characterized by the absence of the sense of smell because of agenesis of the olfactory bulbs and by secondary hypogonadism because of the lack of LHRH.

kali mur, (in homeopathy) a biochemical tissue salt normally used for the second stage of all inflammatory conditions.

kali sulph, (in homeopathy) a biochemical tissue salt found in the external layers of the skin, used for the third stage of all inflammatory diseases.

kanamycin sulphate, an aminoglycoside antibiotic used in the treatment of certain severe infections and those resistant to other antibiotics.

Kanner's syndrome. a form of infantile psychosis with an onset in the first 30 months of life. It is characterized by infantile autism. Treatment may include psychotherapy and special education, depending on the intelligence level of the child.

kaolin, an adsorbent used internally to treat diarrhoea, often in combination with pectin, or morphine.

Kaposi's sarcoma (KS) {Moritz J. Kaposi, Austrian dermatologist, b. 1837}, a malignant, multifocal neoplasm of reticuloendothelial cells that begins as soft, brownish or purple papules on the feet and slowly spreads in the skin, metastasizing to the lymph nodes and viscera. It is most often found in people with AIDS or AIDS-related illnesses but is also occasionally associated with other disorders such as diabetes mellitus or malignant lymphoma.

Kaposi's varicelliform eruption. See **eczema herpeticum**.

Kardex a trademark for a card-filing system that allows quick reference to the particular needs of each patient for certain aspects of nursing care.

Kartagener's syndrome an inherited disorder characterized by bronchiectasis, chronic paranasal sinusitis, and transposed viscera, usually dextrocardia.

karyenchyma. See **karyolymph**.

karyogamy, the fusion of cell nuclei, as in conjugation and zygosis. **karyogamic**, *adj.*

karyogenesis, the formation and development of the nucleus of a cell. **karyogenetic**, *adj.*

karyokinesis, the division of the nucleus and equal distribution of nuclear material during mitosis and meiosis. **karyokinetic**, *adj.*

karyoklasis, 1. the disintegration of the cell nucleus or nuclear membrane. 2. the interruption of mitosis. Also spelled **karyoclasis**. **karyoklastic**, **karyoclastic**, *adj.*

karyology, the branch of cytology that concentrates on the study of the cell nucleus, especially the structure and function of the chromosomes. **karyological**, *adj.*, **karyologist**, *n.*

karyolymph, the clear, usually nonstaining, fluid substance of the nucleus. It consists primarily of proteinaceous, colloidal material in which the nucleolus, chromatin, linin, and various submicroscopic particles are dispersed. **karyolymphatic**, *adj.*

karyolysis, the dissolution of the cell nucleus. It occurs normally, both as a form of necrobiosis and during the generation of new cells through mitosis and meiosis.

karyolytic 1. of or pertaining to karyolysis. 2. that which causes the destruction of the cell nucleus.

karyomere, 1. a saclike structure containing an unequal portion of the nuclear material after atypical mitosis. 2. a segment of the chromosome.

karyometry, the measurement of the nucleus of a cell. **karyometric,** *adj.*

karyomit, 1. a single chromatin fibril of the network within the nucleus of a cell. **2.** a chromosome.

karyomitome, the fibrillar chromatin network within the nucleus of a cell.

karyomitosis. See **karyokinesis.**

karyomorphism, the shape or form of a cell nucleus, especially that of the leukocyte. **karyomorphic,** *adj.*

karyon, the nucleus of a cell. **karyontic,** *adj.*

karyophage, an intracellular protozoan parasite that destroys the nucleus of the cell it infects. **karyophagic, karyophagous,** *adj.*

karyoplasm. See **nucleoplasm.**

karyoplasmic ratio. See **nucleocytoplasmic ratio.**

karyopyknosis, the state of a cell in which the nucleus has shrunk and the chromatin has condensed into solid masses. **karyopyknotic,** *adj.*

karyoreticulum. See **karyomitome.**

karyorrhexis, the fragmentation of chromatin and distribution of it throughout the cytoplasm as a result of nuclear disintegration. **karyorrhectic,** *adj.*

karyosome, a dense irregular mass of chromatin filaments in the cell nucleus.

karyospherical, 1. of or pertaining to a nucleus that is spherical in shape. **2.** such a nucleus.

karyostasis, the resting stage of the nucleus between cell division. **karyostatic,** *adj.*

karyotheca, the membrane that encloses a cell nucleus. **karyothecal,** *adj.*

karyotin. See **chromatin.**

karyotype, 1. the total morphological characteristics of the somatic chromosome complement of an individual or species, described in terms of number, form, size, and arrangement within the nucleus, as determined by a microphotograph taken during the metaphase stage of mitosis. **2.** a diagrammatic representation of the chromosome complement of an individual or species, arranged in pairs in descending order of size and according to the position of the centromere. **karyotypical,** *adj.*

Kasabach method (in radiology) a technique for positioning a patient for x-ray examination of the odontoid process.

katadidymus, conjoined twins that are united in the lower portion of the body and separated at the top.

katal (K, kat), an enzyme unit in moles per second defined by the SI system: 1 K = 6.6 × 10⁹ U

Kawasaki disease. See **mucocutaneous lymph node syndrome.**

Kayser-Fleischer ring {Bernhard Kayser, German ophthalmologist, b. 1869; Bruno Fleischer, German ophthalmologist, b. 1874}, a grey-green to red-gold pigmented ring at the outer margin of the cornea, pathognomonic of hepatolenticular degeneration, a rare progressive disease caused by a defect in copper metabolism and transmitted as an autosomal recessive trait.

K capture. See **electron capture.**

K cell. See **null cell.**

Kedani fever. See **scrub typhus.**

keel, (in prosthetics) a device in a stored-energy foot prosthesis that functions as a cantilever spring, bending the foot upward when weight is applied to the toe.

kefir, a slightly effervescent, acidulous beverage prepared from the milk of cows, sheep, or goats through fermentation by kefir grains, which contain yeasts and lactobacilli. Also spelled **kephir.**

Kegel exercises. See **pelvic floor exercises.**

Keith-Flack node. See **sinoatrial node.**

Keith-Wegener-Barker classification system, a method of classifying the degree of hypertension in a patient on the basis of retinal changes. The stages are group 1, identified by constriction of the retinal arterioles; group 2, constriction and sclerosis of the retinal arterioles; group 3, characterized by haemorrhages and exudates in addition to group 2 conditions; and group 4, papilloedema of the retinal arterioles.

Kellgren's syndrome {Henry Kellgren, Swedish physician, b. 1827}, a form of osteoarthritis affecting the proximal and distal interphalangeal joints, the first metatarsophalangeal and carpometacarpal joints, the knees, and the spine.

Kelly clamp {Howard A. Kelly, American gynaecologist, b. 1858}, a curved haemostat without teeth, used primarily in gynaecological procedures for grasping vascular tissue.

keloid, an overgrowth of collagenous scar tissue at the site of a wound of the skin. The new tissue is elevated, rounded, and firm, with irregular, clawlike margins. Also spelled **cheloid. keloidal, cheloidal,** *adj.*

keloidosis, habitual or multiple formation of keloids. Also spelled **cheloidosis.**

Kelvin scale (K) {Lord Kelvin (William Thomson), British physicist, b. 1824}, an absolute temperature scale calculated in Celsius units from the point at which molecular activity apparently ceases, -273° C. To convert Celsius degrees to Kelvin, add 273.

Kennedy classification {Edward Kennedy, American dentist, b. 1883}, a method of classifying edentulous conditions and partial dentures, based on the position of the spaces of the missing teeth in relation to the remaining teeth.

Kenny treatment. See **Sister Kenny's treatment.**

kenogenesis. See **cenogenesis.**

Kent bundle {Albert F. S. Kent, English physiologist, b. 1863}, an accessory pathway between atria and ventricles outside of the conduction system and found on both sides of the heart.

Kenya fever. See **Marseilles fever.**

kephir. See **kefir.**

kerasin, a cerebroside, found in brain tissue, that consists of a fatty acid, galactose, and sphingosine.

keratectomy, surgical removal of a portion of the cornea, performed to excise a small, superficial lesion that does not warrant a corneal graft. Corneal epithelium grows rapidly, filling a small surgical area in about 60 hours.

keratic, 1. of or pertaining to keratin. **2.** of or pertaining to the cornea.

keratic precipitate, a group of inflammatory cells deposited on the endothelial surface of the cornea after trauma or inflammation, sometimes obscuring vision.

keratin, a fibrous, sulphur-containing protein that is the primary component of the epidermis, hair, nails, enamel of the teeth, and horny tissue of animals.

keratinization, a process by which epithelial cells exposed to the external environment lose their moisture and are replaced by horny tissue.

keratinocyte, an epidermal cell that synthesizes keratin and other proteins and sterols. These cells constitute 95% of the epidermis, being formed as undifferentiated, or basal, cells at the dermal-epidermal junction.

keratitis any inflammation of the cornea. Kinds of keratitis include **dendritic keratitis, interstitial keratitis, keratoconjunctivitis sicca,** and **trachoma. keratic,** *adj.*

keratoacanthoma, *pl.* **keratoacanthomas, keratoacanthomata,** a benign, rapidly growing, flesh-coloured papule of the skin with a central plug of keratin. The lesion is most common on the face or the back of the hands and arms.

keratoconjunctivitis, inflammation of the cornea and the conjunctiva. Kinds of keratoconjunctivitis include **eczematous conjunctivitis, epidemic keratoconjunctivitis,** and **keratoconjunctivitis sicca.**

keratoconjunctivitis sicca, dryness of the cornea caused by a deficiency of tear secretion in which the corneal surface appears dull and rough, and the eye feels gritty and irritated. The condition may be associated with erythema multiforme, Sjögren's syndrome, trachoma, and vitamin A deficiency.

keratoconus, a noninflammatory protrusion of the central part of the cornea. More common in females, it may cause marked astigmatism.

keratoderma blennorrhagica, the development of hyperkeratotic skin lesions of the palms, soles, and nails. The condition tends to occur in some patients with Reiter's syndrome.

keratohyalin, a substance in the granules found in keratinocytes of the epidermis.

keratolysis, the loosening and shedding of the outer layer of the skin, which may occur normally by exfoliation or as a congenital condition in which the skin is shed at periodic intervals. **keratolytic,** *adj.*

keratomalacia, a condition, characterized by xerosis and ulceration of the cornea, resulting from severe vitamin A deficiency. Early symptoms include night blindness, photophobia, swelling and redness of the eyelids, and drying, roughness, pain, and wrinkling of the conjunctiva. In advanced deficiency, Bitot's spots appear, the cornea becomes dull, lustreless, and hazy, and, without adequate therapy, it eventually softens and perforates, resulting in blindness.

keratomycosis linguae. See **parasitic glossitis.**

keratopathy, any noninflammatory disease of the cornea.

keratoplasty, a procedure in ophthalmic surgery in which an opaque portion of the cornea is excised.

keratosis, any skin condition in which there is overgrowth and thickening of the cornified epithelium. Kinds of keratosis include **actinic keratosis, keratosis senilis,** and **seborrhoeic keratosis. keratotic,** *adj.*

keratosis follicularis, a name of several skin disorders characterized by keratotic papules that coalesce to form brown or black, crusted, wartlike patches.

keratosis seborrhoeica. See **seborrhoeic keratosis.**

kerion an inflamed, boggy granuloma that develops as an immune reaction to a superficial fungus infection, generally in association with *Tinea capitis* of the scalp.

Kerley lines, (in radiology) lines resembling interstitial infiltrate that appear on chest x-ray images and are associated with certain disease conditions, such as congestive heart failure and pleural lymphatic engorgement.

KERMA, acronym for *kinetic energy released per unit mass of medium,* a quantity that describes the amount of energy transferred from a beam of ionizing radiation to the medium at the point of interaction.

kernicterus, an abnormal toxic accumulation of bilirubin in central nervous system tissues caused by hyperbilirubinaemia.

Kernig's sign {Vladimir M. Kernig, Russian physician, b. 1840}, a diagnostic sign for meningitis marked by a loss of the ability of a seated or supine patient to completely extend the leg when the thigh is flexed on the abdomen.

kerosene poisoning, a toxic condition caused by the ingestion of kerosene or the inhalation of its fumes. Symptoms after ingestion include drowsiness, fever, a rapid heartbeat, tremors, and severe pneumonitis if the fluid is aspirated. Vomiting is not induced.

ketamine hydrochloride, a nonbarbiturate general anaesthetic administered parenterally to achieve dissociative anaesthesia. Ketamine hydrochloride is particularly useful for brief, minor surgical procedures and for the induction of inhalation anaesthesia in paediatric, geriatric, and disturbed patients. It is also abused for its psychotropic effects when it is taken by mouth, and has been known informally as Special K.

ketoacidosis, acidosis accompanied by an accumulation of ketones in the body, resulting from faulty carbohydrate metabolism. It occurs primarily as a complication of diabetes mellitus and is characterized by a fruity odour of acetone on the breath, mental confusion, dyspnoea, nausea, vomiting, dehydration, weight loss, and, if untreated, coma. Emergency treatment includes the administration of insulin and IV fluids and the evaluation and correction of electrolyte imbalance.   **ketoacidotic,** *adj.*

ketoaciduria, presence in the urine of excessive amounts of ketone bodies, occurring as a result of uncontrolled diabetes mellitus, starvation, or any other metabolic condition in which fats are rapidly catabolized. **ketoaciduric,** *adj.*

11-ketoandrosterone, a sex hormone, secreted by the testes and adrenal glands, that may be measured in the urine to assess hormonal and adrenal functions.

ketoconazole, an oral antifungal agent used to treat candidiasis, coccidioidomycosis, histoplasmosis, and other fungal diseases.

11-ketoetiocholanolone, a sex hormone, secreted by the testes and adrenal glands, that may be measured in the urine to assess hormonal and adrenal functions.

ketogenic diet, a diet that is high in fats and low in carbohydrates.

ketonaemia, the presence of ketones, mainly acetone, in the blood. It is characterized by the fruity breath odour of ketoacidosis.

ketone alcohol, an alcohol containing the ketone group.

ketone bodies, the normal metabolic products, ß-hydroxybutyric acid and aminoacetic acid, from which acetone may arise spontaneously. The two acids are products of lipid pyruvate metabolism, via acetyl-CoA in the liver, and are oxidized by the muscles.

ketone group, the chemical carbonyl group with attached hydrocarbons.

ketonuria. See **ketoaciduria.**

ketoprofen, a nonsteroidal antiinflammatory drug with analgesic and antipyretic action. It is used for the treatment of rheumatoid and osteoarthritis and related conditions.

ketose, the chemical form of a monosaccharide in which the carbonyl group is a ketone.

ketosis, the abnormal accumulation of ketones in the body as a result of a deficiency or inadequate utilization of carbohydrates.

Fatty acids are metabolized instead, and the end products, ketones, begin to accumulate. This condition is seen in starvation, occasionally in pregnancy, and, most frequently, in diabetes mellitus. It is characterized by ketonuria, loss of potassium in the urine, and a fruity odour of acetone on the breath. **ketotic,** *adj.*

ketosis-prone diabetes. See **insulin-dependent diabetes mellitus.**

ketosis-resistant diabetes. See **non-insulin-dependent diabetes mellitus.**

17-ketosteroid, any of the adrenal cortical hormones, or ketosteroids, that has a ketone group attached to its seventeenth carbon atom, commonly measured in the blood and urine to aid the diagnoses of Addison's disease, Cushing's syndrome, stress, and endocrine problems associated with precocious puberty, feminization in men, and excessive hair growth.

keV, an abbreviation for *kiloelectron volts,* an energy unit equivalent to 1000 electron volts.

Kew Gardens spotted fever. See **rickettsialpox.**

keypad, a numeric keyboard consisting of the numerals 1 to 9 arranged in three ranks of three keys each and an additional key for zero, as on some calculators.

key pinch. See **lateral pinch.**

key points of control, areas of the body that can be handled by a therapist in a specific manner to change an abnormal pattern to reduce spasticity throughout the body and to guide the patient's active movements. The key points are the shoulder and pelvic girdle.

key ridge, the lowest point of the zygomaticomaxillary ridge.

kg, abbreviation for kilogram.

kidney, one of a pair of bean-shaped urinary organs in the dorsal part of the abdomen, one on each side of the vertebral column, between the level of the twelfth thoracic vertebra, and the third lumbar vertebra. In most individuals, the right kidney is more caudal than the left. Each kidney is about 11 cm long, 6 cm wide, and 2.5 cm thick. The kidneys produce and eliminate urine through a complex filtration network and reabsorption system comprising more than 2 million nephrons, composed of glomeruli and renal tubules that filter blood under high pressure, removing urea, salts, and other soluble wastes from blood plasma and returning the purified filtrate to the blood. More than 2500 pints of blood pass through the kidneys every day.

kidney cancer, a malignant neoplasm of the renal parenchyma or renal pelvis. Factors associated with an increased incidence of disease are exposure to aromatic hydrocarbons or tobacco smoke and the use of drugs containing phenacetin. Characteristic symptoms include haematuria, flank pain, fever, and the detection of a palpable mass.

kidney dialysis. See **haemodialysis.**

kidney disease, any one of a large group of conditions including infectious, inflammatory, obstructive, vascular, and neoplastic disorders of the kidney. Characteristics of kidney disease are haematuria, persistent proteinuria, pyuria, oedema, dysuria, and pain in the flank. Specific symptoms vary with the type of disorder. For example: haematuria with severe, colicky pain suggests obstruction by a kidney stone; haematuria without pain may indicate renal carcinoma; proteinuria is generally a sign of disease in the glomerulus or filtration unit of the kidney; pyuria indicates infectious disease; and oedema is characteristic of the nephrotic syndrome.

kidney failure, *informal.* renal failure.

kidney machine. See **artificial kidney, dialysis, def. 1.**

kidney stone. See **renal calculus.**

Kielland's forceps. See **obstetric forceps.**

Kielland rotation {Christian Kielland, Norwegian obstetrician, b. 1871}, an obstetric operation in which Kielland's forceps are used in turning the head of the fetus from an occipito-posterior or occipito-transverse position to an occipito-anterior position.

Kiesselbach's plexus, a convergence of small, fragile arteries and veins located superficially on the anterosuperior portion of the nasal septum.

killer cell. See **null cell.**

kilobyte (K, Kb), one thousand (or, more precisely, 1024) bytes.

kilocalorie, a large **calorie.**

kilogram (kg), a unit for the measurement of mass in the metric system. One kilogram is equal to 1000 grams or to 2.2046 pounds avoirdupois.

kilovolt (kV), a unit of electric potential equal to 1000 volts.

kilovolt peak (kVp), a measure of the maximum electrical potential in kilovolts across an x-ray tube. Also known as **kilovoltage peak.**

Kimmelstiel-Wilson disease. See **intercapillary glomerulosclerosis.**

kinaesthesia, the perception of one's own body parts, weight, and movement.

kinaesthetic memory, the recollection of movement, weight, resistance, and position of the body or parts of the body.

kinase, 1. an enzyme that catalyses the transfer of a phosphate group or another high-energy molecular group to an acceptor molecule. **2.** an enzyme that activates a preenzyme (zymogen).

kind firmness, (in psychology) a direct, confident approach to a patient in which rules and regulations are calmly cited in response to infractions and requests.

kinematic face-bow, an adjustable caliper-like device, used for precisely locating the axis of rotation of a mandible through the sagittal plane.

kinematics, (in physiology) the geometry of the motion of the body without regard to the forces acting to produce the motion. The most common types of motions studied in kinematics are flexion, extension, adduction, abduction, internal rotation, and external rotation. Kinematics is especially important in orthopaedics and rehabilitation medicine. Also spelled **cinematics.**

kinesic behaviour, nonverbal cues of communication that include expression, gesture, posture and modify verbal cues.

kinesics, the study of body position and movement in relation to communication.

kinesiological electromyography, the study of muscle activity involved in body movements.

kinesiology, the scientific study of muscular activity and of the anatomy, physiology, and mechanics of the movement of body parts.

kinetic analysis, analysis in which the change of the monitored parameter with time is related to concentration, such as change of absorbance per minute.

kinetics, (in physiology) the study of the forces that produce, arrest, or modify the motions of the body. Newton's laws are applicable to the forces produced by muscles of the body that act on joints. The reaction forces of the muscles contribute to the equilibrium and the motion of the body.

kinetochore. See **centromere.**

kinetotherapeutic bath, a bath in which underwater exercises are performed to strengthen weak or partially paralysed muscles.

kin group, family members who are related genetically or by marriage.

kinomere. See **centromere.**

kinship model family group, a family unit comprising the biological parents and their offspring. It is like a nuclear family but is more closely tied to an extended family.

Kirkland knife {Olin Kirkland, American dentist, b. 1876}, a surgical knife with a heart-shaped blade, sharp on all edges, used for a primary gingivectomy incision.

Kirklin staging system, a system for determining the prognosis of colon cancer, based on the extent to which the tumour has penetrated the bowel area.

Kirschner's wire {Martin Kirschner, German surgeon, b. 1879}, a threaded or smooth metallic wire used in internal fixation of fractures or for skeletal traction.

klang association. See **clang association.**

Klebsiella {Theodore A. E. Klebs, German bacteriologist, b. 1834}, a genus of diplococcal bacteria that appear as small, plump rods with rounded ends. Several respiratory diseases, including bronchitis, sinusitis, and some forms of pneumonia, are caused by infection by species of *Klebsiella.*

Klebs-Loeffler bacillus {Theodore A. E. Klebs; Friederich A. J. Loeffler, German bacteriologist, b. 1852}, *Corynebacterium diphtheriae.*

kleeblattschädel deformity syndrome. See **cloverleaf skull deformity.**

Kleihauer test, a test on maternal blood taken after delivery to estimate the number of fetal cells that have passed into the maternal circulation during labour. All Rhesus negative mothers who have Rhesus positive cells in their bloodstream are given anti-D to prevent isoimmunization.

Kleine-Levin syndrome {Willi Kleine, 20th century German psychiatrist; Max Levin, 20th century American neurologist}, a disorder of unknown cause often associated with psychotic conditions, characterized by episodic somnolence, abnormal hunger, and hyperactivity.

kleptolagnia, sexual excitement or gratification produced by stealing.

kleptomania, a neurosis characterized by an abnormal, uncontrollable, and recurrent urge to steal. The objects, taken not for their monetary value, immediate need, or utility but because of a symbolic meaning usually associated with some unconscious emotional conflict, are usually given away, returned surreptitiously, or kept and hidden. Also spelled cleptomania. kleptomaniac, n.

Klinefelter's syndrome {Harry F. Klinefelter, American physician, b. 1912}, a syndrome of gonadal defects, appearing in males, with an extra X chromosome in at least one cell line. Characteristics are small, firm testes, long legs, gynaecomastia, poor social adaptation, subnormal intelligence, chronic pulmonary disease, and varicose veins. The severity of the abnormalities increases with greater numbers of X chromosomes.

Klippel-Feil syndrome. See **congenital short neck syndrome.**

Klumpke's palsy, atrophic paralysis of the forearm. It is present at birth and involves the seventh and eighth cervical nerves and the first thoracic nerve. The condition may be accompanied by Horner's syndrome, ptosis, and miosis because of involvement of sympathetic nerves.

kneading, a grasping, rolling, and pressing movement, as is used in massaging the muscles.

knee, a joint complex that connects the thigh with the lower leg. It consists of three condyloid joints, 12 ligaments, 13 bursae, and the patella.

knee-ankle interaction, one of the five major kinetic determinants of gait, which helps to minimize the displacement of the centre of gravity of the body during the walking cycle. The knee and the foot work simultaneously to lower the centre of gravity of the body. When the heel of the foot is in contact with the ground, the foot is dorsiflexed and the knee is fully extended so that the associated limb is at its maximum length with the centre of gravity at its lower point.

kneecap. See **patella.**

knee-chest position. See **genupectoral position.**

knee-hip flexion, one of the five major kinematic determinants of gait, which allows the passage of body weight over the supporting extremity during the walking cycle. Knee-hip flexion occurs during the stance and the swing phases of the cycle. The knee first locks into extension as the heel of the weight-bearing limb strikes the ground and is unlocked by final flexion and initiation of the swing phase in the walking cycle. Hip flexion is synchronized with these movements, which help to minimize the vertical displacement of the centre of gravity of the body in the act of walking.

knee-jerk reflex. See **patellar reflex.**

knee joint, the complex, hinged joint at the knee, regarded as three articulations in one, comprising condyloid joints connecting the femur and the tibia and a partly arthrodial joint connecting the patella and the femur. The knee joint and its ligaments permit flexion, extension, and, in certain positions, medial and lateral rotation. It is a common site for sprain and dislocation.

knee replacement, the surgical insertion of a hinged prosthesis, performed to relieve pain and restore motion to a knee severely affected by osteoarthritis, rheumatoid arthritis, or trauma.

knee sling, a leg support in sling form used under the knee for Russell's traction.

knife needle, a slender surgical knife with a needle point, used in the discission of a cataract and in other ophthalmic procedures, such as goniotomy and goniopuncture.

knock-knee. See **genu valgum.**

knot, (in surgery) the interlacing of the ends of a ligature or suture so that they remain in place without slipping or becoming detached. The ends of the suture are passed twice around each other before being pulled taut to make a simple surgeon's knot.

knowledge deficit, a term used in nursing care planning to describe a state in which specific information is lacking. Defining characteristics include a statement by the person that the knowledge deficit exists, or that there is a misconception concerning the information, an observed failure to follow through on instructions, the observation of an inadequate performance on a test, a request by the person for information, or the observation of inappropriate or exaggerated behaviour.

Kocher's forceps {Emil T. Kocher, Swiss surgeon, b. 1841}, a kind of surgical forceps with notched jaws, interlocking teeth, and thick, curved or straight, powerful handles.

Koch's postulates {Robert Koch, German bacteriologist, b. 1843}, the prerequisites for establishing that a specific microorganism causes a particular disease. The conditions are the following: (1) the microorganism must be observed in all cases of the disease; (2) the microorganism must be isolated and grown in pure culture; (3) microorganisms from the pure culture, when inoculated into a susceptible animal, must reproduce the disease; (4) the microorganism must be observed in and recovered from the experimentally diseased animal.

Koebner phenomenon {Heinrich Koebner, Polish dermatologist, b. 1838}, the development of isomorphic lesions at the site of an injury occurring in psoriasis, lichen nitidus, lichen planus, and verruca plana.

Kohnstamm's phenomenon. See **after-movement.**

koilonychia, spoon nails; a condition in which nails are thin and concave from side to side.

Kopan's needle, a long biopsy needle used to locate the position of a breast tumour on x-ray film.

Koplik's spots {Henry Koplik, American paediatrician, b. 1858}, small red spots with bluish white centres on the lingual and buccal mucosa, characteristic of measles. The rash of measles usually erupts a day or two after the appearance of Koplik's spots.

Korotkoff sounds {Nickolai Korotkoff, Russian physician, b. 1874}, sounds heard during the taking of blood pressure using a sphygmomanometer and stethoscope. As air is released from the cuff, pressure on the brachial artery is reduced, and the blood is heard pulsing through the vessel.

Korsakoff's psychosis {Sergei S. Korsakoff, Russian psychiatrist, b. 1854}, a form of amnesia often seen in chronic alcoholics, characterized by a loss of short-term memory and an inability to learn new skills. The person is usually disoriented and confabulates to conceal the condition.

kosher, conforming to or prepared in accordance with the dietary or ceremonial laws of Judaism.

Krabbe's disease. See **galactosyl ceramide lipidosis.**

Kraske position {Paul Kraske, Swiss surgeon, b. 1851}, an anatomical position in which the patient is prone, with hips flexed and elevated, head and feet down. The position is used for renal surgery.

kraurosis, a thickening and shrivelling of the skin.

kraurosis vulvae, a skin disease of aged women characterized by dryness, itching, and atrophy of the external genitalia.

Krause's corpuscles {Wilhelm J. F. Krause, German anatomist, b. 1833}, a number of sensory end organs in the conjunctiva of the eye, mucous membranes of the lips and tongue, epineurium of nerve trunks, the pe-

nis, and the clitoris, and the synovial membranes of certain joints. Krause's corpuscles are tiny cylindrical oval bodies a soft, semifluid core in which the axon terminates either in a bulbous extremity or in a coiled mass.

Krebs' citric acid cycle {Hans A. Krebs, English biochemist, b. 1900}, a sequence of enzymatic reactions involving the metabolism of carbon chains of sugars, fatty acids, and amino acids to yield carbon dioxide, water, and high-energy phosphate bonds. The Krebs' cycle provides a major source of adenosine triphosphate energy and also produces intermediate molecules that are starting points for a number of vital metabolic pathways including amino acid synthesis.

Krebs-Henseleit cycle. See **urea cycle.**

Krukenberg's tumour {Georg P. H. Krukenberg, German gynaecologist, b. 1856}, a neoplasm of the ovary that is a metastasis of a GI malignancy, usually stomach cancer.

KS, abbreviation for **Kaposi's sarcoma.**

KUB, abbreviation for *kidney, ureter, and bladder,* a term used in a radiographic examination to determine the location and size of the kidneys.

Kulchitsky cell carcinoma. See **carcinoid.**

Kulchitsky's cell. See **argentaffin cell.**

Küntscher nail {Gerhard Küntscher, German surgeon, b. 1902}, a stainless steel nail used in orthopaedic surgery for the fixation of fractures of the long bones, especially the femur.

Kupffer's cells {Karl W. von Kupffer, German anatomist, b. 1829}, specialized cells of the reticuloendothelial system lining the sinusoids of the liver. They filter bacteria and other small, foreign proteins out of the blood.

kuru, a slow, progressive, fatal viral infection of the central nervous system observed in natives of the New Guinea highlands. Characteristic of kuru are ataxia and decreased coordination progressing to paralysis, dementia, slurring of speech, and visual disturbances. Incidence of the disease has declined with the decline of cannibalism.

Kussmaul breathing. See **Kussmaul respirations.**

Kussmaul respirations {Adolf Kussmaul, French physician, b. 1822}, abnormally deep, very rapid sighing respirations characteristic of diabetic acidosis.

Kussmaul's sign {Adolf Kussmaul}, **1.** a paradoxical rise in venous pressure with distention of the jugular veins during inspiration, as seen in constrictive pericarditis or mediastinal tumour. **2.** conditions of convulsions and coma associated with a GI disorder caused by absorption of a toxic substance.

Kveim reaction {Morton A. Kveim, Norwegian physician, b. 1892}, a reaction used in a diagnostic test for sarcoidosis, based on an intradermal injection of antigen derived from a lymph node known to be sarcoid.

kVp, abbreviation for **kilovolt peak.**

kVp test cassette, (in radiology) a cassette containing a copper filter, a series of step wedges, and an optical attenuator, used to measure the effective kilovoltage peak across an x-ray tube.

kwashiorkor, a malnutrition disease, primarily of children, caused by severe protein deficiency, usually occurring when the child is weaned from the breast. Characteristics include retarded growth, changes in skin and hair pigmentation, diarrhoea, loss of appetite, nervous irritability, oedema, anaemia, fatty degeneration of the liver, necrosis, dermatoses, and fibrosis, often accompanied by infection and multivitamin deficiencies.

Kyasanur forest disease, an arbovirus infection transmitted by the bite of a tick that is harboured by shrews and other animals in India. Characteristics of the infection include fever, headache, muscle ache, cough, abdominal and eye pain, and photophobia.

kymography, a technique for graphically recording motions of body organs, as of the heart and the great blood vessels.

kyphoscoliosis, an abnormal condition characterized by an anteroposterior curvature and a lateral curvature of the spine. **kyphoscoliotic,** *adj.*

kyphosis, an abnormal condition of the vertebral column, characterized by increased convexity in the curvature of the thoracic spine as viewed from the side. Kyphosis may be caused by rickets or tuberculosis of the spine. **kyphotic,** *adj.*

L, l, symbol for **litre.**

La, symbol for **lanthanum.**

label, **1.** a substance with a special affinity for an organ, tissue, cell, or microorganism in which it may become deposited and fixed. **2.** the process of depositing and fixing a substance in an organ, tissue, cell, or microorganism. **3.** an atom or molecule attached to either a ligand or binding protein and capable of generating a signal for monitoring in the binding reaction.

labelled compound, (in radionuclide imaging) a chemical substance in which part of the molecules are labelled with a radionuclide so that observations of the radioactivity or isotopic composition make it possible to follow the compound through physical, chemical, or biological processes.

labelling, **1.** the providing of information on the constituent parts of a drug, food, device, or cosmetic to the purchaser or user. Regulations on labelling are provided by the European Commission. **2.** the assignment of a word or term to a form of behaviour.

labetalol hydrochloride, an antihypertensive drug with alpha- and beta-blocking properties used for the treatment of hypertension.

labia, *sing.* **labium,** **1.** the lips; the fleshy, liplike edges of an organ or tissue. **2.** the folds of skin at the opening of the vagina.

labial bar, a major connector that is installed labial or buccal to the dental arch and joins bilateral parts of a mandibular removable partial denture.

labial flange, the part of a denture flange that occupies the labial vestibule of the mouth.

labial notch, a depression in the denture border that accommodates the labial frenum.

labia majora, sing. labium majus, two long lips of skin, one on each side of the vaginal orifice outside the labia minora. The embryological derivations of the labia majora and the scrotum are homologous.

labia minora, *sing.* **labium minus,** two folds of skin between the labia majora, extending from the clitoris backward on both sides of the vaginal orifice, ending between it and the labia majora.

labile, **1.** unstable; characterized by a tendency to change or to be altered or modified. **2.** (in psychiatry) characterized by rapidly shifting or changing emotions, as in bipolar disorder and certain types of schizophrenia; emotionally unstable. **lability,** *n.*

labioglossolaryngeal paralysis. See **bulbar paralysis.**

labiolingual fixed orthodontic appliance, an orthodontic appliance for correcting or improving malocclusion, characterized by anchorage to the maxillary and mandibular first permanent molars and by labial and lingual arches.

labium See **labia.**

labium majus See **labia majora.**

labium minus. See **labia minora.**

laboratory, **1.** a facility, room, building, or part of a building in which scientific research, experiments, testing, or other investigative activities are carried out. **2.** of or pertaining to a laboratory.

laboratory core. See **core.**

laboratory diagnosis, a diagnosis arrived at after study of secretions, excretions, or tissue through chemical, microscopic, or bacteriological means or by biopsy.

laboratory error, any error made by the personnel in a clinical laboratory in the performance of a test, in the interpretation of the data, or in reporting or recording the results.

laboratory medicine, the branch of medicine in which specimens of tissue, fluid, or other body substance are examined outside of the person, usually in the laboratory. Some fields of laboratory medicine are **chemistry, cytology, haematology, histology,** and **pathology.**

laboratory test, a procedure, usually conducted in a laboratory, that is intended to detect, identify, or quantify one or more significant substances, evaluate organ functions, or establish the nature of a condition or disease.

labour, the time and the processes that occur during parturition from the beginning of cervical dilatation to the delivery of the placenta.

labour partner, a person who acts as a nonprofessional companion to a woman in labour and delivery, giving her emotional support. Such a companion may also be able to help by encouraging the woman to make use of breathing patterns, concentration techniques, body positions, and massage techniques that are taught in many antenatal classes. Usually, the labour partner is the father of the baby or a close friend or relative of the mother.

laboured breathing, abnormal respiration characterized by evidence of increased effort, including use of the accessory muscles of respiration of the chest wall, stridor, grunting, or nasal flaring.

labyrinth. See **internal ear.**

labyrinthine righting, one of the five basic neuromuscular reactions involved in a change of body positions. The change stimulates cells in the semicircular canals of the inner ear causing neck muscle to respond by automatically adjusting the head to the new position.

labyrinthitis, inflammation of the labyrinthine canals of the inner ear, resulting in vertigo.

labyrinthus osseus. See **osseous labyrinth.**

LAC, abbreviation for **linear attenuation coefficient.**

laceration, 1. the act of tearing or lacerating. **2.** a torn, jagged wound. **lacerate,** *v.,* **lacerated,** *adj.*

lachrymal See **lacrimal.**

lachrymation See **lacrimation.**

lacrimal, of or pertaining to tears. Also spelled **lachrymal.**

lacrimal apparatus, a network of structures of the eye that secrete tears and drain them from the surface of the eyeball. These parts include the lacrimal glands, the lacrimal ducts, the lacrimal sacs, and the nasolacrimal ducts.

lacrimal bone, a small, fragile bone of the face, located at the anterior part of the medial wall of the orbit. It unites with the maxilla to form the lacrimal fossa, which contains the lacrimal duct.

lacrimal canaliculi. See **lacrimal duct.**

lacrimal caruncle, the small, reddish, fleshy protuberance that fills the triangular space between the medial margins of the upper and the lower eyelids.

lacrimal duct, one of two channels through which tears pass from the lacrimal lake to the lacrimal sac of each eye.

lacrimal fistula, an abnormal communication from a tear duct or sac to the surface of the eye or eyelid.

lacrimal gland, one of a pair of glands situated superior and lateral to the eye bulb in the lacrimal fossa. The watery secretion from the gland consists of the tears, slightly alkaline and saline, that moisten the conjunctiva.

lacrimal papilla, the small conic elevation on the medial margin of each eyelid, supporting an apex pierced by the punctum lacrimale through which tears emerge to moisten the conjunctiva.

lacrimal sac, the dilated end of each of the two nasolacrimal ducts. The lacrimal sacs fill with tears secreted by the lacrimal glands and conveyed through the lacrimal ducts.

lacrimation, 1. the normal continuous secretion of tears by the lacrimal glands. **2.** an excessive amount of tear production, as in crying or weeping. Also spelled **lachrymation.**

lactalbumin, a simple, highly nutritious protein found in milk. It is similar to serum albumin.

lactase, an enzyme that catalyses the hydrolysis of lactose to glucose and galactose.

lactase deficiency, an inherited abnormality in which the amount of the enzyme lactase is deficient, resulting in the inability to digest lactose. Also called **alactasia.**

lactate dehydrogenase (LDH), an enzyme that is found in the cytoplasm of almost all body tissues, where its main function is to catalyse the oxidation of L-lactate to pyruvate. It is assayed as a measure of anaerobic carbohydrate metabolism and as one of several serum indicators of myocardial infarction and muscular dystrophies.

lactation, the process of the synthesis and secretion of milk from the breasts in the nourishment of an infant or child. See also **breastfeeding.**

lacteal, of or pertaining to milk.

lacteal fistula, an abnormal passage opening into a lacteal duct.

lacteal gland, one of the many central lymphatic capillaries in the villi of the small intestine. It opens into the lymphatic vessels in the submucosa.

lactic, referring to milk and milk products.

lactic acid, a three-carbon organic acid produced by anaerobic respiration. There are three forms: L-lactic acid in muscle and blood is a product of glucose and glycogen metabolism; D-lactic acid is produced by the fermentation of dextrose by a species of micrococcus; DL-lactic acid is a racaemic mixture found in the stomach, in sour milk, and in certain other foods prepared by bacterial fermentation.

lactic acid fermentation, 1. the production of lactic acid from sugars by various bacteria. **2.** the souring of milk.

lactic acidosis, a disorder characterized by an accumulation of lactic acid in the blood, resulting in a lowered pH in muscle and serum. The condition occurs most commonly in tissue hypoxia.

lactiferous, of or pertaining to a structure that produces or conveys milk, such as the tubules of the breasts.

lactiferous duct, one of many channels carrying milk from the lobes of each breast to the nipple.

lactin. See **lactose.**

Lactobacillus, any one of a group of nonpathogenic, gram-positive, rod-shaped bacteria that produce lactic acid from carbohydrates.

lactogen, a drug or other substance that enhances the production and secretion of milk. **lactogenic,** *adj.*

lactogenic hormone. See **prolactin.**

lacto-ovo-vegetarian, one whose diet consists primarily of foods of vegetable origin and also includes some animal products, such as eggs *(ovo),* milk, and cheese *(lacto),* but no meat, fish, or poultry.

lactose, a disaccharide found in the milk of all mammals. On hydrolysis lactose yields the monosaccharides glucose and galactose.

lactose intolerance, a sensitivity disorder resulting in the inability to digest lactose because of a deficiency of or defect in the enzyme lactase. Symptoms of the disorder are bloating, flatus, nausea, diarrhoea, and abdominal cramps.

lactosuria, the presence of lactose in the urine, a condition that may occur in late pregnancy or during lactation.

lacto-vegetarian, one whose diet consists of milk and milk products *(lacto)* in addition to foods of vegetable origin but does not include eggs, meat, fish, or poultry.

lactulose, a nonabsorbable synthetic disaccharide, 4-0-ß-D-galactopyranosyl-D-fructose, $C_{12}H_{22}O_{11}$. It is hydrolysed in the colon by bacteria, and used in the treatment of constipation and hepatic encephalopathy.

lacuna, *pl.* **lacunae, 1.** a small cavity within a structure, especially bony tissue. **2.** a gap, as in the field of vision.

lacunar state, a pseudobulbar disorder characterized by the appearance of small, smooth-walled cavities in the brain tissue. The condition usually follows a series of small strokes, particularly in older adults with arterial hypertension and arteriosclerosis.

lacus lacrimalis, a triangular space separating the medial ends of the upper and the lower eyelids.

LADME, an abbreviation for the time course of drug distribution, representing the terms *liberation, absorption, distribution, metabolism,* and *elimination.*

Laënnec's catarrh {Rene T. H. Laënnec, French physician, b. 1781}, a form of bronchial asthma characterized by the discharge of small, round, viscous, beadlike bodies of sputum. These bodies, **Laënnec's pearls,** are formed in the bronchioles and appear in the asthmatic person's expectorated bronchial secretions.

lagophthalmos, an abnormal condition in which an eye may not be fully closed because of a neurological or muscular disorder.

laity, a nonprofessional segment of the population, as viewed from the perspective of a member of a particular profession. A clergyman may regard a doctor as a member of the laity, and vice versa.

LAK, abbreviation for **lymphokine-activated killer cells.**

laked blood, blood that is clear, red, and homogenous because of haemolysis of the red blood cells, as may occur in poisoning and severe, extensive burns.

laliophobia, a morbid dread of talking caused by fear and anxiety that one will stammer or stutter. **laliophobic,** *adj.*

lallation, 1. babbling, repetitive, unintelligible utterances, like the babbling of an infant, and the mumbled speech of schizophrenics, alcoholics, and people with severe mental retardation. **2.** a speech disorder characterized by a defective pronunciation of words containing the sound /l/.

lamarckism {Jean B. P. de Lamarck, French naturalist, b. 1744}, the theory postulated that organic evolution results from structural changes in plants and animals that are caused by adaptation to environmental conditions and that these acquired characteristics are transmitted to offspring. **lamarckian,** *adj., n.*

Lamaze method, a method of preparation for childbirth developed in the 1950s by a French obstetrician, Fernand Lamaze. It requires attendance at classes, practice at home, and coaching during labour and delivery, often by a trained coach called a "monitrice." The classes, given during pregnancy, teach the physiology of pregnancy and childbirth, exercises to develop strength in the abdominal muscles and control of isolated muscles of the vagina and perineum, and techniques of breathing and relaxation to promote control and relaxation during labour. The kind and rate of breathing changes with the advancing stages of labour.

lambda, 1. the Greek letter signified by the letter L or l. **2.** a posterior fontanelle of the skull marking the point where the sagittal and lambdoidal sutures meet.

lambdacism, a speech disorder characterized by a defective pronunciation of words containing the sound /l/, or by the excessive use of the sound, or by the substitution of the sound /l/ for /r/.

lambdoid, having the shape of the Greek letter lambda.

lambdoidal suture, the serrated connection between the occipital bone and the parietal bones of the skull.

lamella, *pl.* **lamellae, 1.** a thin leaf or plate, as of bone. **2.** a medicated disc, prepared from glycerin and an alkaloid, for insertion under the eyelid, where it dissolves and is absorbed.

lamellar exfoliation of the newborn, a congenital skin disorder transmitted as an autosomal recessive trait in which a parchment-like, scaly membrane that covers the infant peels off within 24 hours of birth.

lamina, *pl.* **laminae,** a thin flat plate, such as the lamina of the thyroid cartilage that overlies the structure on each side.

lamina dura, a sheet of compact alveolar bone that lies adjacent to the periodontal membrane.

lamina propria, a layer of connective tissue that lies just under the epithelium of the mucous membrane.

laminar flow, an airflow that is concentrated

into a narrow pathway.

laminaria, a type of dried seaweed that swells on absorption of water.

laminated thrombus, a thrombus composed of an aggregation of blood platelets, fibrin, clotting factors, and cellular elements, arranged in layers apparently formed at different times.

laminectomy, surgical chipping away of the bony arches of one or more vertebrae, performed to relieve compression of the spinal cord, as caused by a bone displaced in an injury or as the result of degeneration of a disc, or to reach and remove a displaced intervertebral disc. Spinal fusion may be necessary for stability of the spine if several laminae are removed. **laminectomize,** v.

lampbrush chromosome, an excessively large type of chromosome found in the oocytes of many lower animals. It has a hairy, brushlike appearance.

lance, to incise a furuncle or an abscess to release accumulated pus.

Lancefield's classification {Rebecca C. Lancefield, American bacteriologist, b. 1895}, a serological classification of streptococci based on their antigenic characteristics. The bacteria are divided into 13 groups by the identification of their pathological action.

Lancereaux's diabetes {Etienne Lancereaux, French physician, b. 1829}, a chronic disease of carbohydrate metabolism characterized by marked emaciation.

lancet, **1.** *obsolete.* a very small, pointed, surgical knife, sharp on both sides. **2.** a short pointed blade used to obtain a drop of blood for a capillary sample.

lancinating, sharply cutting or tearing, such as lancinating pain.

Landau reflex, a normal response of infants when held in a horizontal prone position to maintain a convex arc with the head raised and the legs slightly flexed.

landmark position, the correct placement of the hands on the chest in cardiopulmonary resuscitation.

Landouzy-Déjérine muscular dystrophy. See **facioscapulohumeral muscular dystrophy.**

Landsteiner's classification {Karl Landsteiner, American pathologist, b. 1868}, the classification of blood groups A, B, AB, and O on the basis of the presence or absence of the two agglutinogens A and B on the erythrocytes in human blood.

Langer's line. See **cleavage line.**

Langhans' layer. See **cytotrophoblast.**

language, **1.** a defined set of characters that when used alone or in combinations form a meaningful set of words and symbols. **2.** a unified, related set of commands or instructions that a computer can accept.

lanolin, a fatlike substance from the wool of sheep. It contains about 25% water as a water-in-oil emulsion and is used as an ointment base and an emollient for the skin.

lanthanum (La), a rare earth metallic element. Its atomic number is 57; its atomic weight is 138.91.

lanugo, 1. the soft, downy hair covering a normal fetus, beginning with the fifth month of life and almost entirely shed by the ninth month. **2.** the fine, soft hair covering all parts of the body except palms, soles, and areas where other types of hair are normally found.

lanulous, downy or covered with short, fine woolly hair, such as the skin of a fetus.

laparoscope, a type of endoscope, consisting of an illuminated tube with an optical system, that is inserted through the abdominal wall for examining the peritoneal cavity. **laparoscopic,** *adj.,* **laparoscopy,** *n.*

laparoscopy, the examination of the abdominal cavity with a laparoscope through a small incision in the abdominal wall.

laparotomy, any surgical incision into the peritoneal cavity, usually performed under general or regional anaesthesia, often on an exploratory basis. Some kinds of laparotomy are **appendectomy, cholecystectomy,** and **colostomy.** **laparotomize,** v.

Laplace's law {Pierre Simon Marquis de Laplace, French physicist, b. 1749}, a principle of physics that the tension on the wall of a sphere is the product of the pressure times the radius of the chamber and the tension is inversely related to the thickness of the wall.

large for gestational age (LGA) infant, an infant whose fetal growth was accelerated and whose size and weight at birth fall above the ninetieth percentile of appropriate for gestational age infants, whether delivered prematurely, at term, or later than term. Factors other than genetic influences that cause accelerated intrauterine growth include maternal diabetes mellitus and Beckwith's syndrome.

large intestine, the portion of the digestive tract comprising the caecum, appendix, the ascending, transverse, and descending colons, and the rectum.

lariat structure, a ring of intron segments that have been spliced out of an mRNA molecule by enzymes. Some introns form a long tail attached to the ring, giving the structure the appearance of a microscopic cowboy lariat.

Larmor frequency {Sir Joseph Larmor, Irish physicist, b. 1857}, the frequency of the precession of a charged particle when its motion comes under the influence of an applied magnetic field and a central force.

larva migrans. See **cutaneous larva migrans, visceral larva migrans.**

laryngeal cancer, a malignant neoplastic disease characterized by a tumour arising from the epithelium of the structures of the larynx. Chronic alcoholism and heavy use of tobacco increase the risk of developing the cancer. Persistent hoarseness is usually the first sign; advanced lesions may cause a sore throat, dyspnoea, dysphagia, and unilateral cervical adenopathy.

laryngeal intubation, the insertion of a catheter into the larynx for the purpose of removing secretions or introducing gases.

laryngeal prominence. See **Adam's apple.**

laryngectomy, surgical removal of the larynx, performed to treat cancer of the larynx. **laryngectomize,** v.

laryngismus, spasm of the larynx. Laryngismus stridulus, a condition characterized by sudden laryngeal spasm with a crowing sound on inspiration and the development of cyanosis, occurs in inflammation of the larynx, in connection with rickets, and as an independent disease.

laryngitis, inflammation of the mucous membrane lining the larynx, accompanied by oedema of the vocal cords with hoarseness or loss of voice, occurring as an acute disorder caused by a cold, by irritating fumes, by sudden temperature changes, or as a chronic condition resulting from excessive use of the voice, heavy smoking, or exposure to irritating fumes. In acute laryngitis, there may be a cough, and the throat usually feels scratchy and painful.

laryngocele, an abnormal air-containing cavity connected to the laryngeal ventricle. It is caused by an evagination of the mucous membrane of the ventricle and may displace and enlarge the false vocal cord, resulting in hoarseness and airway obstruction. Because a laryngocele is also a potential reservoir of infection, it is usually excised.

laryngography. See **laryngopharyngography.**

laryngopharyngitis, inflammation of the larynx and pharynx.

laryngopharyngography, the radiographic examination of the larynx and the pharynx, usually as part of a barium swallow examination.

laryngopharynx, one of the three regions of the throat, extending from the hyoid bone to the oesophagus. **laryngopharyngeal,** adj.

laryngoscope, an endoscope for examining the larynx.

laryngospasm, a spasmodic closure of the larynx.

laryngostasis. See **croup.**

laryngotracheobronchitis (LTB), an inflammation of the major respiratory passages, usually causing hoarseness, nonproductive cough, and dyspnoea. See also **croup.**

larynx, the organ of voice that is part of the air passage connecting the pharynx with the trachea. The larynx forms the caudal portion of the anterior wall of the pharynx and is lined with mucous membrane that is con-

tinuous with that of the pharynx and the trachea. It is composed of three single cartilages and three paired cartilages, connected by ligaments and moved by various muscles. **laryngeal,** adj.

LAS, abbreviation for **lymphadenopathy syndrome.**

laser, acronym for *light amplification by stimulated emission of radiation,* a source of intense radiation of the visible, ultraviolet, or infrared portions of the spectrum. It is produced by exposing a large number of electrons to a high energy level in a gaseous, solid, or liquid medium. The electrons emit very narrow beams of light, all of one wavelength and parallel to each other.

laser bronchoscopy, bronchoscopy that is performed with the aid of a carbon dioxide laser beam directed through fibre optic equipment in the diagnosis and treatment of bronchial disorders.

laser imager, a device to reproduce images on x-ray film using laser scanning techniques of a digital or analogue signal, to give increased resolution.

laser printer, a device which uses a laser scanning technique of a digital signal to produce a paper hardcopy.

Lassa fever, a highly contagious disease caused by a virulent arenavirus. It is characterized by fever, pharyngitis, dysphagia, and ecchymoses. Pleural effusion, oedema and renal involvement, mental disorientation, confusion, and death from cardiac failure often ensue.

late dyspituitary eunuchism. See **acromegalic eunuchoidism.**

latency stage, (in psychoanalysis) a period in psychosexual development occurring between early childhood and puberty when sexual motivation and expression are repressed or transferred, through sublimation, to the feelings and behavioural patterns expected as typical of the age.

latent, dormant; existing as a potential; for example, tuberculosis may be latent for extended periods of time and become active under certain conditions.

latent carcinoma. See **occult carcinoma.**

latent diabetes. See **impaired glucose tolerance, previous abnormality of glucose tolerance.**

latent heart failure, an abnormal condition in which the heart is unable to pump an adequate supply of blood in relation to venous return and the metabolic needs of body tissues and structures.

latent period, (in radiobiology) an interval of seeming inactivity between the time of exposure to an injurious dose of radiation and the response.

latent phase, the early stage of labour that is characterized by irregular, infrequent, and mild contractions and little or no dilatation of the cervix or descent of the fetus.

latent schizophrenia, a form of schizophrenia characterized by the presence of mild symptoms of the disease.

lateral, 1. on the side. 2. away from the midsagittal plane. 3. farther from the midsagittal plane. 4. to the right or left of the midsagittal plane.

lateral abdominal region. See **lateral region.**

lateral aortic node, a lumbar lymph node in any of three clusters of nodes serving the pelvis and abdomen.

lateral aperture of the fourth ventricle, an opening between the end of each lateral recess of the fourth ventricle and the subarachnoid space.

lateral cerebral sulcus, a deep cleft marking the division of the temporal, frontal, and parietal lobes of brain.

lateral condensation method, a technique for filling and sealing tooth root canals. A preselected gutta-percha cone is sealed into the apex of the root; other cones are forced laterally with a spreader until the canal is filled.

lateral cuneiform bone, one of the three cuneiform bones of the foot, located in the centre of the front row of tarsal bones.

lateral geniculate body, one of two elevations of the lateral posterior thalamus receiving visual impulses from the retina via the optic nerves and tracts and relaying the impulses to the calcarine cortex.

lateral humeral epicondylitis, inflammation of the tissue at the lower end of the humerus at the elbow joint, caused by the repetitive flexing of the wrist against resistance. It may result from athletic activity or manual manipulation of tools or other equipment.

lateral incisal guide angle, (in dentistry) the inclination of the incisal guide in the frontal plane.

laterality. See **handedness.**

lateralization, the tendency for certain processes to be more highly developed on one side of the brain than the other, such as development of spatial and musical thoughts in the right hemisphere and verbal and logical processes in the left hemisphere in most persons.

lateral pectoral nerve, one of a pair of branches from the brachial plexus that, with the medial pectoral nerve, supplies the pectoral muscles.

lateral pelvic displacement, one of the five major kinetic determinants of gait. It helps to synchronize the rhythmic movements of walking, and is produced by the horizontal shift of the pelvis or by relative hip abduction.

lateral pinch, a grasp in which the thumb is opposed to the middle phalanx of the index finger.

lateral projection, (in radiography) a position of a patient between the x-ray tube and the film cassette so the beam will travel from the left to the right side of the body, or vice versa.

lateral recumbent position, the posture assumed by the patient lying on the left side with the right thigh and knee drawn up.

lateral region, the part of the abdomen in the middle zone on both sides of the umbilical region.

lateral resolution, (in ultrasonography) the resolution of objects in a plane perpendicular to the axis of the beam. It is a measure of the ability of the system to detect closely separated objects such as adjacent blood vessels.

lateral rocking, a sideways rocking of the body used to move the body forward or backward when normal muscle action is not possible. The technique is used by some handicapped patients to move the body to or from the edge of a chair or to a different sitting position on a bed.

lateral rotation, a turning away from the midline of the body.

lateral umbilical fold, a fold in the peritoneum produced by a slight protrusion of the inferior epigastric artery and the interfoveolar ligament.

late systolic murmur. See **systolic murmur.**

latex fixation test, a serological test used in the diagnosis of rheumatoid arthritis in which antigen-coated latex particles agglutinate with rheumatoid factors in a slide specimen of serum or synovial fluid.

latissimus dorsi, one of a pair of large triangular muscles on the thoracic and lumbar areas of the back. It extends, adducts, and rotates the arm medially, draws the shoulder back and down, and, with the pectoralis major, draws the body up when climbing.

latitude, (in radiography) the ability of an x-ray imaging system to produce acceptable images over a range of exposures. If a system has wide latitude, it is possible to image parts of the body that vary in thickness or density with only one exposure.

LATS, abbreviation for **long-acting thyroid stimulator.**

LATS-P, abbreviation for **long-acting thyroid stimulator protector.**

lattice formation, a three-dimensional cross-linked structure formed by the reaction of multivalent antigens with antibodies.

laughing gas, *informal.* nitrous oxide, a side effect of which is laughter or giggling when administered in less than anaesthetizing amounts.

Laurence-Moon-Bardet-Biedl syndrome {John Z. Laurence, English ophthalmologist, b. 1830; Robert C. Moon, American ophthalmologist, b. 1844; Georges Bardet, French physician, b. 1885; Artur Biedl, Czechoslovakian physician, b. 1869}, an abnormal condition characterized by obesity, hypogenitalism, mental deficiency, polydactylism, and retinitis pigmentosa.

lavage,   **1.** the process of washing out an organ, usually the bladder, bowel, paranasal sinuses, or stomach for therapeutic purposes. **2.** to perform a lavage. Kinds of lavage are **blood lavage, gastric lavage,** and **peritoneal dialysis.** See also **irrigation.**

law, 1. (in a field of study) a rule, standard, or principle that states a fact or a relationship between factors, such as Dalton's law regarding partial pressures of gas. **2.** a rule, principle, or regulation established and promulgated by a government to protect or to restrict the people affected.

law of definite composition, (in chemistry) a law stating that a given compound is always made of the same elements present in the same proportion.

law of dominance, formerly considered as a separate principle of Mendel's laws of inheritance, but in modern genetics it is incorporated as part of the first Mendelian law, the law of segregation.

law of facilitation. See **facilitation.**

law of independent assortment, law of segregation. See **Mendel's laws.**

law of universal gravitation, (in physics) a law stating that the force with which bodies are attracted to each other is directly proportional to the masses of the objects and inversely proportional to the square of the distance by which they are separated. See also **gravity, mass.**

lawrencium (Lw) {Ernest O. Lawrence, American physicist, b. 1901}, a synthetic transuranic metallic element. Its atomic number is 103; its atomic weight is 257.

lax, a condition of relaxation or looseness.

laxative, 1. of or pertaining to a substance that causes evacuation of the bowel **2.** an agent that promotes bowel evacuation.

lay advisers, lay people who are influential in approving or disapproving new ideas and who may serve as consultants because of their expertise in subjects other than medicine.

lazy colon. See **atonia constipation.**

lazy leukocyte syndrome, an immuno-deficiency disease of children characterized by recurrent stomatitis, gingivitis, otitis media, and low-grade fever with severe neutropenia.

LBW, abbreviation for **low birth weight.**

L-carnitine, an amino acid derivative prescribed for the treatment of primary systemic carnitine deficiency.

LCAT, abbreviation for **lecithin-cholesterol acetyltransferase.**

LD, abbreviation for **lethal dose.**

LD50, (in toxicology) the amount of a substance sufficient to kill one half of a population of test subjects.

LDH, abbreviation for **lactate dehydrogenase.**

LDL, abbreviation for **low-density lipoprotein.**

L-dopa. See **levodopa.**

LE, abbreviation for **lupus erythematosus.**

lead (Pb), a common soft, blue-grey, metallic element. Its atomic number is 82; its atomic weight is 207.19. In its metallic form, lead is used as a protective shielding against x-rays. Lead is also poisonous, a characteristic that has led to a reduction in the use of lead compounds.

lead, an electric connection attached to the body to record electric activity, especially of the heart or brain.

lead equivalent, (in radiation protection) the thickness of lead required to achieve the same shielding effect against radiation, under specified conditions, as that provided by a given material.

leadership, the ability to influence others to the attainment of goals.

lead pipe fracture, a fracture that compresses the bony tissue at the point of impact and creates a linear fracture on the opposite side of the bone involved.

lead poisoning, a toxic condition caused by the ingestion or inhalation of lead or lead compounds. Poisoning also occurs from the ingestion of water from lead pipes, lead salts in certain foods and wines, the use of pewter or earthenware glazed with a lead glaze, and the use of leaded gasoline. Inhalation of lead fumes is common in industry. The acute form of intoxication is characterized by a burning sensation in the mouth and oesophagus, colic, constipation, or diarrhoea, mental disturbances, and paralysis of the extremities, followed in severe cases by convulsions and muscular collapse. Chronic lead poisoning is characterized by extreme irritability, anorexia, and anaemia. Encephalopathy must be anticipated in children with lead poisoning.

leakage radiation, radiation, exclusive of the primary beam, which is emitted through the housing of an x-ray tube or radiotherapy unit.

learned helplessness, a behavioural state and personality trait of a person who believes he or she is ineffectual, responses are futile, and control over reinforcers in the environment has been lost.

learning, 1. the act or process of acquiring knowledge or some skill by means of study, practice, or experience. **2.** knowledge, wisdom, or a skill acquired through systematic study or instruction. **3.** (in psychology) the modification of behaviour through practice, experience, or training.

learning disability, faulty or inadequate development of the mental processes. This results in impaired ability to learn, reduced capability for social adjustment and impaired maturation. It is a broad term for a range of conditions which can occur at any time from conception through early childhood.

leather-bottle stomach. See **linitis plastica.**

Leber's congenital amaurosis {Theodor von Leber, German ophthalmologist, b. 1840}, a rare kind of blindness or severely impaired vision caused by a defect transmitted as an autosomal recessive trait and occurring at birth or shortly thereafter. The eyes appear normal externally, but pupillary constriction to light is sluggish or absent and retinal pigment is degenerated.

Leboyer method of delivery, an approach to the delivery of an infant formulated by the French obstetrician Charles Leboyer. It has four aspects: a gentle, controlled delivery in a quiet, dimly lit room, avoidance of pulling on the head, avoidance of overstimulation of the infant's sensorium, and encouragement of maternal-infant bonding. The goal of the method is to minimize the trauma of birth by gently and pleasantly introducing the newborn to life outside the womb.

lecithin, any of a group of phospholipids common in plants and animals. They are essential for the metabolism of fats and are used in the processing of foods, pharmaceutical products, cosmetics, and inks.

lecithin/sphingomyelin ratio, lecithin and sphingomyelin are phospholipids contained in surfactant, which is secreted by the fetal lungs into the amniotic fluid. Before 34 weeks the two exist in equal amounts, a ratio of 1:1. The lecithin rises to 2:1 sharply after that, and is an indication of lung maturity.

lecitho-, a combining form meaning 'of or pertaining to the yolk of an egg, or to the ovum': **lecithoblast, lecithoprotein, lecithovitellin.**

lectin, a protein substance occurring in seeds and other parts of certain plants that binds with glycoproteins and glycolipids on the surface of animal cells causing agglutination.

Lee-Davidsohn test, a heterophil antibody test for infectious mononucleosis using horse red blood cells.

Lee-White method {Roger I. Lee, American physician, b. 1881; Paul D. White, American physician, b. 1886}, a method of determining the length of time required for a clot to form in a test tube of venous blood.

LeFort I fracture. See **Guérin's fracture.**

left atrioventricular valve. See **mitral valve.**

left brachiocephalic vein, a vessel that starts in the root of the neck at the junction of the internal jugular and the subclavian veins on the left side and runs obliquely across the thorax to join the right brachiocephalic vein and form the superior vena cava.

left common carotid artery, the longer of the two common carotid arteries, springing from the aortic arch and having cervical and thoracic portions.

left coronary artery, one of a pair of branches from the ascending aorta, arising in the left posterior aortic sinus, dividing into the left interventricular artery and the circumflex branch, supplying both ventricles and the left atrium.

left-handedness, a natural tendency by some persons to favour the use of the left hand in performing certain tasks.

left-heart failure, an abnormal cardiac condition characterized by the impairment of the left side of the heart and by elevated pressure and congestion in the pulmonary veins and capillaries. Left-heart failure is usually related to right-heart failure, because both sides of the heart are part of a circuit and the impairment of one side will eventually affect the other.

left hepatic duct, the duct that drains the bile from the left lobe of the liver into the common bile duct.

left innominate vein. See **left brachiocephalic vein.**

left lymphatic duct. See **thoracic duct.**

left pulmonary artery, the shorter and smaller of two arteries conveying venous blood from the heart to the lungs, rising from the pulmonary trunk, connecting to the left lung.

left subclavian artery, an artery that arises from the aortic arch dorsal to the left common carotid at the level of the fourth thoracic vertebra, ascends to the root of the neck, arches laterally to the scalenus anterior, and forms six main branches to supply the vertebral column, spinal cord, ear, and brain.

left ventricle, the thick-walled chamber of the heart that pumps blood through the aorta and the systemic arteries, the capillaries, and back through the veins to the right atrium. It has walls about three times thicker than those of the right ventricle and contains a mitral valve with two flaps that controls the flow of blood from the left atrium.

left ventricular failure, heart failure in which the left ventricle fails to contract forcefully enough to maintain a normal cardiac output and peripheral perfusion. Pulmonary congestion and oedema develop from back pressure of accumulated blood in the left ventricle. Signs include breathlessness, pallor, sweating, and peripheral vasoconstriction. The heart is usually enlarged.

legacy, something that is handed down from the past or is intended to be bestowed on future generations.

legal, actions or conditions that are permitted or authorized by law.

leg cylinder cast, an orthopaedic device of plaster of paris or fibreglass used to immobilize the leg in treating fractures in the legs from the ankle to the upper thigh.

Legg-Calvé-Perthes disease. See **Perthes disease.**

Legionella pneumophila, a small, gram-negative, rod-shaped bacterium that is the causative agent in **Legionnaires' disease.**

Legionnaires' disease, an acute bacterial pneumonia caused by infection with *Legionella pneumophila* and characterized by an influenza-like illness followed within a week by high fever, chills, muscle aches, and headache. The symptoms may progress to dry cough, pleurisy, and sometimes diarrhoea. Usually the disease is self-limited, but mortality has been 15% to 20% in a few localized epidemics. Contaminated air conditioning cooling towers and moist soil may be a source of organisms.

leiomyoblastoma. See **epithelioid leiomyoma.**

leiomyofibroma, *pl.* **leiomyofibromas, leiomyofibromata,** a tumour consisting of smooth muscle cells and fibrous connective tissue, commonly occurring in the uterus in middle-aged women.

leiomyoma, *pl.* **leiomyomas, leiomyomata,** a benign smooth muscle tumour most commonly occurring in the stomach, oesophagus, or small intestine.

leiomyoma cutis, a neoplasm of the smooth muscles of the skin. The lesion is characterized by many small, tender, red nodules.

leiomyoma uteri, a benign neoplasm of the smooth muscle of the uterus. The tumour is characteristically firm, well circumscribed, round, and grey-white. Multiple tumours of this kind develop most often in the myometrium and occur most frequently in women between 30 and 50 years of age.

Leishman-Donovan body {Sir William B. Leishman, English pathologist, b. 1865; Charles Donovan, Scottish physician, b. 1863}, the resting stage of an intracellular, nonflagellated protozoan parasite *(Leishmania donovani)* that causes kala-azar, or visceral leishmaniasis as it appears in infected tissue specimens.

Leishmania {Sir William B. Leishman}, a genus of protozoan parasites. These organisms are transmitted to humans by any of several species of sand flies.

leishmaniasis {Sir William B. Leishman}, infection with any species of protozoan of the genus Leishmania. The diseases caused by these organisms may be cutaneous or visceral. Kinds of leishmaniasis are **American leishmaniasis, kala-azar,** and **oriental sore.** See also *Leishmania.* **leishmanial** *adj.*

length of stay (LOS), the period of time a patient remains in a hospital as an inpatient.

lens, 1. a curved transparent piece of plastic or glass that is shaped, moulded, or ground to refract light in a specific way, as in spectacles, microscopes, or cameras. **2.** *informal.* the crystalline lens of the eye. **lenticular** *adj.*

lens capsule, the clear thin elastic capsule that surrounds the lens of the eye.

lens implant, an artifical lens of clear polymethylmethacrylate that is usually implanted at the time of cataract extraction but may also be used for patients with extreme myopia, diplopia, ocular albinism, and certain other abnormalities.

lenticonus, an abnormal spherical or conical protrusion on the lens of the eye. It is a congenital defect found in Alport's syndrome.

lentigo, *pl.* **lentigines,** a tan or brown macule on the skin brought on by sun exposure, usually in a middle-aged or older person. Another variety, called juvenile lentigo, is unrelated to sunlight and appears in children 2 to 5 years of age, before the onset of freckles.

lentigo maligna. See **Hutchinson's freckle.**

lentigo maligna melanoma, a neoplasm developing from Hutchinson's freckle on the face or other exposed surfaces of the skin in elderly people. It is asymptomatic, flat, and tan or brown, with irregular darker spots and frequent hypopigmentation. It is one of the three major clinical types of melanoma.

lentivirus, a member of a subfamily of retroviruses that includes the AIDS virus. Lentiviruses are usually slow viruses, with long incubation periods that may delay the onset of symptoms until several years after exposure.

LE prep, abbreviation for **lupus erythematosus preparation.**

lepromatous leprosy. See **leprosy.**

lepromin test, a skin sensitivity test used to distinguish between the lepromatous and tuberculoid forms of leprosy. The test consists of intradermal injection of lepromin.

leprosy, a chronic, communicable disease, caused by *Mycobacterium leprae,* that may take either of two forms, depending on the degree of immunity of the host. **Tuberculoid leprosy,** seen in those with high resistance, presents as thickening of cutaneous nerves and anaesthetic, saucer-shaped skin lesions. **Lepromatous leprosy,** seen in those with little resistance, involves many systems of the body, with widespread plaques and nodules in the skin, iritis, keratitis, destruction of nasal cartilage and bone, testicular atrophy, peripheral oedema, and involvement of the reticuloendothelial system. Blindness may result. **lepromatous, leprotic, leprous,** *adj.*

leptocyte. See **target cell.**

leptocytosis, a haematological condition in which target cells are present in the blood. Thalassaemia, some forms of liver disease, and absence of the spleen are associated with leptocytosis.

leptomeninges, the arachnoid membrane and the pia mater, two of the three layers covering the spinal cord.

leptonema, the threadlike chromosome formation in the leptotene stage in the first meiotic prophase of gametogenesis before the beginning of synapsis.

Leptospira, a genus of the family Treponemataceae, order Spirochaetales, tightly coiled microorganisms having spirals with hooked ends. The spirochete may cause jaundice, skin haemorrhages, fever, and muscular illness. See also **leptospirosis.**

Leptospira agglutinin, an agglutinin found in the blood of patients with Weil's disease.

leptospirosis, an acute infectious disease caused by several serotypes of the spirochete *Leptospira interrogans*, transmitted in the urine of wild or domestic animals, especially rats and dogs. Human infections arise directly from contact with an infected animal's urine or tissues or indirectly from contact with contaminated water or soil. Clinical symptoms may include jaundice, haemorrhage into the skin, fever, chills, and muscular pain. The most serious form of the disease is called **Weil's disease.**

leptotene, the initial stage in the first meiotic prophase in gametogenesis in which the chromosomes become visible as single thin filaments.

Leriche's syndrome {Rene Leriche, French surgeon, b. 1879}, a vascular disorder marked by gradual occlusion of the terminal aorta, intermittent claudication in the buttocks, thighs, or calves, absence of pulsation in femoral arteries, pallor and coldness of the legs, gangrene of the toes, and, in men, impotence.

lesbian, 1. a female homosexual. **2.** of or pertaining to the sexual preference or desire of one woman for another. **lesbianism,** *n.*

Lesch-Nyhan syndrome {Michael Lesch, American pediatrician, b. 1939; William L. Nyhan, Jr., American pediatrician, b. 1926}, a hereditary disorder of purine metabolism, characterized by mental deficiency, self-mutilation of the fingers and lips by biting, impaired renal function, and abnormal physical development.

lesion, 1. a wound, injury, or pathological change in body tissue. **2.** any visible, local abnormality of the tissues of the skin, such as a wound, sore, rash, or boil. A lesion may be described as benign, cancerous, gross, occult, or primary.

lesser multangular bone. See **trapezoid bone.**

lesser occipital nerve, one of a pair of cutaneous branches of the cervical plexus, arising from the second cervical nerve, curving around the sternocleidomastoideus, and ascending along the side of the head behind the ear to supply the skin.

lesser omentum, a membranous extension of the peritoneum from the peritoneal layers covering the ventral and the dorsal surfaces of the stomach and the first part of the duodenum.

lesser trochanter, one of a pair of conic projections at the base of the neck of the femur, providing insertion of the tendon of psoas major.

let-down, a sensation in the breasts of lactating women that often occurs as the milk flows into the ducts. It may occur when the infant begins to suck or when the mother hears the baby cry or even thinks of feeding the child.

let-down reflex, a normal reflex in a lactating woman elicited by tactile stimulation of the nipple, resulting in release of milk from the glands of the breast.

lethal, capable of causing death.

lethal dose (LD50), (in radiobiology) the amount of radiation that would kill 50% of the individuals of fixed age.

lethal equivalent, any recessive gene carried in the heterozygous state that, if homozygous, would be lethal and result in the death of the individual or organism.

lethal gene, any gene that produces a phenotypic effect that causes the death of the organism at some stage of development from fertilization of the egg to adulthood. The gene may be dominant, incompletely dominant, or recessive.

lethality, the probability that a person threatening suicide will succeed, based on the method described, the specificity of the plan, and the availability of the means.

lethargic encephalitis. See **epidemic encephalitis.**

lethargy, 1. the state or quality of being indifferent, apathetic, or sluggish. **2.** stupor or coma resulting from disease or hypnosis. Kinds of lethargy include **hysterical lethargy, induced lethargy,** and **lucid lethargy. lethargic,** *adj.*

Letterer-Siwe syndrome {Erich Letterer, German pathologist, b. 1895; Sture A. Siwe, Swedish physician, b. 1897}, any of a poorly classified group of malignant neoplastic diseases of unknown origin, characterized by histiocytic elements. Anaemia, haemorrhage, splenomegaly, lymphadenopathy, and localized tumefactions over bones are usually present.

leucine (Leu), a white, crystalline amino acid essential for optimal growth in infants and nitrogen equilibrium in adults. It cannot be synthesized by the body and is obtained by the hydrolysis of protein during pancreatic digestion.

leucinosis, a condition in which the pathways for the degradation of leucine are blocked and large amounts of the amino acid accumulate in body tissue.

leucocyte. See **leukocyte.**

leucovorin. See **folinic acid.**

leucovorin calcium, See **folinic acid.**

leukapheresis, a process by which blood is

withdrawn from a vein, white blood cells are selectively removed, and the remaining blood is reinfused in the donor.

leukaemia, a malignant neoplasm of blood-forming organs characterized by diffuse replacement of bone marrow with proliferating leukocyte precursors, abnormal numbers and forms of immature white cells in circulation, and infiltration of lymph nodes, the spleen, liver, and other sites. The origin of leukaemia is not clear, but it may result from exposure to ionizing radiation, benzene, or other chemicals that are toxic to bone marrow. Leukaemia is classified according to the predominant proliferating cells, the clinical course, and the duration of the disease. Acute leukaemia usually has a sudden onset and rapidly progresses from early signs, such as fatigue, pallor, weight loss, and easy bruising, to fever, haemorrhages, extreme weakness, bone or joint pain, and repeated infections. Chronic leukaemia develops slowly, and signs similar to those of the acute forms of the disease may not appear for years. **leukaemic,** *adj.*

leukaemia cutis, a condition in which yellow-brown, red, or purple nodular lesions and diffuse infiltrations or large accumulations of leukaemic cells develop in the skin.

leukaemic reticuloendotheliosis. See **hairy-cell leukaemia.**

leukaemoid, resembling leukaemia.

leukaemoid reaction, a clinical syndrome resembling leukaemia in which the white blood cell count is elevated in response to an allergy, inflammatory disease, infection, poison, haemorrhage, burn, or other causes of severe physical stress.

leukocyte, a white blood cell, one of the formed elements of the circulating blood system. There are five types of leukocytes, classified by the presence or absence of granules in the cytoplasm of the cell. The agranulocytes are lymphocytes and monocytes. The granulocytes are neutrophils, basophils, and eosinophils. **leukocytic,** *adj.*

leukocyte alkaline phosphatase, an enzyme that is elevated in various diseases, such as cirrhosis and polycythaemia, and in certain infections. It may be measured in the blood to detect these disorders.

leukocythaemia. See **leukaemia.**

leukocytic crystal. See **Charcot-Leyden crystal.**

leukocytopenia. See **leukopenia.**

leukocytosis, an abnormal increase in the number of circulating white blood cells. An increase often accompanies bacterial, but not usually viral, infections. The normal range is 5000 to 10,000 white cells per cubic millimetre of blood. Kinds of leukocytosis include **basophilia,** **eosinophilia,** and **neutrophilia.**

leukoderma, localized loss of skin pigment

caused by any of a number of specific causes.

leukoerythroblastic anaemia, an abnormal condition in which there are large numbers of immature white and red blood cells. It is characteristic of some anaemias that occur as a result of the replacement of normal bone marrow with malignant tumour.

leukonychia, a benign, congenital condition in which white patches appear under the nails. Trauma, infection, and many systemic disorders can cause white spots or streaks on nails. A common cause is the presence of air bubbles under the nails.

leukopenia, an abnormal decrease in the number of white blood cells to fewer than 5000 cells per cubic millimetre. It may be caused by an adverse drug reaction, radiation poisoning, or other pathological conditions and may affect one or all kinds of white blood cells. **leukopenic,** *adj.*

leukopenic leukaemia. See **aleukaemic leukaemia.**

leukophoresis, a laboratory procedure in which white blood cells are separated by electrophoresis for identification and an evaluation of the types of cells and their proportions.

leukoplakia, a precancerous, slowly developing change in a mucous membrane characterized by thickened, white, firmly attached patches that are slightly raised and sharply circumscribed.

leukopoiesis, the process by which white blood cells form and develop. Neutrophils, basophils, and eosinophils are produced in myeloid tissue in the bone marrow. Lymphocytes and monocytes are almost all normally derived from haemocytoblasts in lymphoid tissue, but a few develop in the marrow. **leukopoietic,** *adj.*

leukorrhoea, a white discharge from the vagina.

leukotomy. See **lobotomy.**

leukotoxin, a substance that can inactivate or destroy leukocytes. **leukotoxic,** *adj.*

leukotrienes, a class of biologically active compounds that occur naturally in leukocytes and that produce allergic and inflammatory reactions. They are thought to play a role in the development of allergic and autoallergic disease, such as asthma and rheumatoid arthritis.

levator, *pl.* **levatores,** **1.** a muscle that raises a structure of the body, as the levator ani raises parts of the pelvic diaphragm. **2.** a surgical instrument used to lift depressed bony fragments in fractures of the skull and other bones.

levator ani, one of a pair of muscles of the pelvic diaphragm that stretches across the bottom of the pelvic cavity like a hammock, supporting the pelvic organs. It functions to support and slightly raise the pelvic floor. The pubococcygeus draws the anus toward the pubis and constricts it.

levator palpebrae superioris, one of the three muscles of the eyelid, also considered a muscle of the eye. It is innervated by the oculomotor nerve, raises the upper eyelid, and is the antagonist of the orbicularis oculi.

levator scapulae, a muscle of the dorsal and lateral aspects of the neck. It acts to raise the scapula and pull it toward the midline.

LeVeen shunt, a tube that is surgically implanted to connect the peritoneal cavity and the superior vena cava to drain an accumulation of fluid in the peritoneal cavity in cirrhosis of the liver, right-sided heart failure, or cancer of the abdomen.

level of inquiry, (in nursing research) one of the levels in a rank-ordered system of classification and organization of the questions to be answered in a research study.

levels of care, a classification of health care service levels by the kind of care given, the number of people served, and the people providing the care. Kinds of health care service levels are **primary health care, secondary health care,** and **tertiary health care.**

lever, (in physiology) any one of the numerous bones and associated joints of the body that act together as a lever so that force applied to one end of the bone to lift a weight at another point tends to rotate the bone in the direction opposite from that of the applied force.

Lévi-Lorain dwarf. See **pituitary dwarf.**

Levin tube {Abraham L. Levin, American physician, b. 1880}, a #16 French, plastic catheter, used in gastric intubation, that has a closed, weighted tip and an opening on the side.

levitation, (in psychiatry) a hallucinatory sensation of floating or rising in the air. **levitate,** v.

levobunolol hydrochloride, a topical ophthalmic beta-blocker used for the treatment of chronic open-angle glaucoma and ocular hypertension.

levodopa, an antiparkinsonian used in the treatment of Parkinson's disease, juvenile forms of Huntington's disease, and chronic manganese poisoning.

levulose. See **fructose.**

levulosuria. See **fructosuria.**

lewisite {Winford L. Lewis, American chemist, b. 1878}, 2-chlorovinyl arsine; a poisonous blister gas, used in World War I, that causes irritation of the lungs, dyspnoea, damage to the tissues of the respiratory tract, tears, and pain.

Leyden-Moebius muscular dystrophy, a form of limb-girdle muscular dystrophy that begins in the pelvic girdle.

Leydig cells {Franz von Leydig, German anatomist, b. 1821}, cells of the interstitial tissue of the testes that secrete testosterone.

Leydig cell tumour, a generally benign neoplasm of interstitial cells of a testis that may cause gynaecomastia in adults and precocious sexual development if the lesion occurs before puberty.

LFT, abbreviation for **liver function test.**

LGA, abbreviation for **large for gestational age.**

LGV, abbreviation for **lymphogranuloma venereum.**

LH, abbreviation for **luteinizing hormone.**

LHRH, abbreviation for **luteinizing hormone releasing hormone.**

Lhermitte's sign {Jacques J. Lhermitte, French neurologist, b. 1877}, sudden, transient, electric shock-like sensations spreading down the body when the head is flexed forward, occurring chiefly in multiple sclerosis but also in compression disorders of the cervical spinal cord.

Li, symbol for **lithium.**

liability, 1. something one is obliged to do or an obligation required to be fulfilled by law, usually financial in nature. **2.** the amount of money required to fulfill a financial obligation.

libel, a false accusation written, printed, or typewritten, or presented in a picture or a sign that is made with malicious intent to defame the reputation of a person who is living or the memory of a person who is dead, resulting in public embarrassment, contempt, ridicule, or hatred.

liberation, the process of drug release from the dosage form.

libidinal development. See **psychosexual development.**

libidinous, 1. pertaining to or belonging to the libido. **2.** having or characterized by sexual desire. Also **libidinal. libidinize,** v.

libido, 1. the psychic energy or instinctual drive associated with sexual desire, pleasure, or creativity. **2.** (in psychoanalysis) the instinctual drives of the id. **3.** lustful desire or striving. Kinds of libido are **bisexual libido, ego libido.**

Libman-Sacks endocarditis {Emanuel Libman, American physician, b. 1872; Benjamin Sacks, American physician, b. 1896}, an abnormal condition and the most common manifestation of lupus erythematosus, characterized by verrucous lesions that develop near the heart valves but rarely affect valvular action.

licensing, the granting of permission by a competent authority (usually a government department or local authority) to an organization or individual to engage in a practice or activity that would otherwise be illegal. Kinds of licensing include the issuing of licences for general hospitals or nursing homes, for certain types of professional practice, and for the production or distribution of certain products.

lichenification, thickening and hardening of the skin, often resulting from the irritation caused by repeated scratching of a pruritic lesion. **lichenified,** *adj.*

lichen nitidus, a rare skin disorder characterized by numerous flat, glistening, pale, discrete papules measuring 2 to 3 mm in diameter.

lichen planus, a nonmalignant, chronic, pruritic skin disease of unknown cause, characterized by small, flat, purplish papules or plaques having fine, grey lines on the surface.

lichen sclerosis et atrophicus, a chronic skin disease characterized by white, flat papules with an erythematous halo and black, hard follicular plugs. In advanced cases, the papules tend to coalesce into large, white patches of thin, pruritic skin.

lichen simplex chronicus, a form of neurodermatitis characterized by a patch of pruritic, confluent papules.

lid. See **eyelid.**

lie, the relationship between the long axis of the fetus and the long axis of the mother.

lien. See **spleen.**

lienal vein, a large vein of the lower body that unites with the superior mesenteric vein to form the portal vein. It returns blood from the spleen and arises from about six large tributaries that unite to form the single vessel passing from left to right across the superior, dorsal part of the pancreas.

life costs, the mortality, morbidity, and suffering associated with a given disease or medical procedure.

life expectancy. See **expectation of life.**

life review, 1. (in psychiatry) a progressive return to consciousness of past experiences. **2.** reminiscences that occur in old age as a consequence of the realization of the inevitability of death.

lifesaving measure, any independent, interdependent, or dependent nursing intervention that is implemented when a patient's physical or psychological status is threatened.

life science, the study of the laws and properties of living matter. Some kinds of life science are **anatomy, bacteriology,** and **biology.**

life space, a term introduced by American psychologist Kurt Lewin to describe simultaneous influences that may affect individual behaviour. The totality of the influences make up the life space.

life-style-induced health problems, diseases with natural histories that include conscious exposure to certain health-compromising or risk factors.

lift assessment, the selection of the most appropriate lift method to use when moving a patient, as from the bed to a chair.

ligament, 1. one of many predominantly white, shiny, flexible bands of fibrous tissue binding joints together and connecting various bones and cartilages. Compare **tendon.**

2. a layer of serous membrane with little or no tensile strength, extending from one visceral organ to another, such as the ligaments of the peritoneum. **ligamentous,** *adj.*

ligamenta flava, the bands of yellow elastic tissue connecting the laminae of adjacent vertebrae from the axis to the first segment of the sacrum.

ligamental tear, a complete or a partial tear of a ligamentous structure connecting and surrounding the bones of a joint, caused by an injury to the joint, as by a sudden twisting motion or by a forceful blow. Ligamental tears may occur at any joint but are most common in the knees.

ligament of the neck of the rib, one of five ligaments of each costotransverse joint, consisting of short, strong fibres passing from the neck of the rib to the transverse process of the adjacent vertebra.

ligament of the tubercle of the rib, one of the five ligaments of each costotransverse joint, comprising a short, thick fasciculus passing obliquely from the transverse process of a vertebra to the tubercle of the associated rib.

ligamentum. See **ligament.**

ligamentum latum uteri. See **broad ligament.**

ligamentum nuchae, the fibrous membrane that reaches from the external occipital protuberance and median nuchal line to the spinous process of the seventh vertebra.

ligand, 1. a molecule, ion, or group bound to the central atom of a chemical compound, such as the oxygen molecule in haemoglobin, which is bound to the central iron atom. **2.** an organic molecule attached to a specific site on a surface or to a tracer element.

ligases, a group of enzymes that catalyse the formation of a bond between substrate molecules coupled with the breakdown of a pyrophosphate bond in ATP or a similar donor molecule.

ligation, tying off of a blood vessel or duct with a suture or wire ligature performed to stop or prevent bleeding during surgery, to stop spontaneous or traumatic haemorrhage, or to prevent passage of material through a duct, as in tubal ligation or to treat varicosities. **ligate,** *v.*

ligature, 1. a suture. **2.** a wire, as used in orthodontia.

ligature needle, a long, thin, curved needle used for passing a suture underneath an artery for ligation of the vessel.

light, 1. electromagnetic radiation of the wavelength and frequency that stimulate visual receptor cells in the retina to produce nerve impulses that are perceived as vision. **2.** electromagnetic radiation with wavelengths shorter than ultraviolet light and longer than infrared light, the range of visible light generally in the range of 400 to 800 nm.

light chain, a subunit of an immunoglobulin molecule composed of a polypeptide chain of about 22,000 daltons, or atomic mass units. An example of a light chain is a Bence Jones protein molecule associated with multiple myeloma.

light chain disease, a type of multiple myeloma in which plasma cell tumours produce only monoclonal light chain proteins. Persons with light chain disease may develop lytic bone lesions, hypercalcaemia, impaired kidney function, and amyloidosis.

light diet, a diet suitable for convalescent or bedridden patients taking little or no exercise. It consists of simple, moderate quantities of soft-cooked and easily digested foods, including meats, potatoes, rice, eggs, pasta, some fruits, refined cereals, and breads.

lightening, a subjective sensation reported by many women late in pregnancy as the fetus settles lower in the pelvis, leaving more space in the upper abdomen.

light pen, an electric device, resembling a pen, that may be used with a computer terminal to enter or modify information displayed on the screen.

light reflex, the mechanism by which the pupil of the eye becomes more or less open in response to direct or consensual pupillary stimulation.

ligneous, woody or resembling wood in texture or other characteristics.

ligneous thyroiditis. See **fibrous thyroiditis.**

lignin, a polysaccharide that with cellulose and hemicellulose forms the chief part of the skeletal substances of the cell walls of plants.

lignocaine hydrochloride, a local anaesthetic agent applied topically or injected. It is used parenterally as an antiarrhythmic agent.

lilliputian hallucination, one in which things seem smaller than they actually are.

limb, 1. an appendage or extremity of the body, such as an arm or leg. 2. a branch of an internal organ, such as a loop of a nephron.

limb-girdle muscular dystrophy, a form of muscular dystrophy transmitted as an autosomal recessive trait. The characteristic weakness and degeneration of the muscles begins in the shoulder girdle or in the pelvic girdle. The condition is progressive. Kinds of limb-girdle muscular dystrophy are **Erb's muscular dystrophy, Leyden-Moebius muscular dystrophy.**

limbic system, a group of structures within the rhinencephalon of the brain that are associated with various emotions and feelings, such as anger, fear, sexual arousal, pleasure, and sadness. The structures of the limbic system are the cingulate gyrus, the isthmus, the hippocampal gyrus, the uncus, and the hippocampus. The structures connect with various other parts of the brain.

lime, 1. any of several oxides and hydroxides of calcium. 2. a citrus fruit yielding a juice with a high ascorbic acid content. Lime juice was one of the first effective agents to be used in the treatment of scurvy.

limited fluctuation method of dosing, a method of drug administration in which the dose is not allowed to rise or fall beyond specified maximum and minimum limits.

limiting resolution, (in computed tomography) the spatial frequency at a modulation transfer function (MTF) equal to 0.1. The absolute object size that can be resolved by a scanner is equal to the reciprocal of the spatial frequency.

limp, an abnormal pattern of ambulation in which the two phases of gait are markedly asymmetric.

LINAC, abbreviation for **linear accelerator.**

lindane, gamma-benzene hexachloride, a paraciticide used topically in the treatment of pediculosis and scabies.

Lindau-von Hippel disease. See **cerebroretinal angiomatosis.**

Lindbergh pump, {Charles A. Lindbergh, American technician, b. 1902} a pump used to preserve an organ of the body by perfusing its tissues with oxygen and other essential nutrients, usually during the transport of an organ from a donor to a recipient.

line, a stripe, streak, or narrow ridge, often imaginary, that serves to connect anatomical reference points or to separate various parts of the body, such as the hairline or nipple line.

linea alba, the portion of the anterior abdominal aponeurosis in the middle line of the abdomen, representing the fusion of three aponeuroses into a single tendinous band extending from the xiphoid process to the symphysis pubis. It contains the umbilicus.

linea albicantes, lines, white to pink or grey in colour, that occur on the abdomen, buttocks, breasts, and thighs and are caused by the stretching of the skin and weakening or rupturing of the underlying elastic tissue.

linea arcuata, the curved tendinous band in the sheath of the rectus abdominis below the umbilicus. It inserts into the linea alba.

linea aspera, the posterior crest of the thigh bone, extending proximally into three ridges to which are attached various muscles, including the gluteus maximus, pectineus, and iliacus.

linea nigra, a dark line appearing longitudinally on the abdomen of a pregnant woman during pregnancy. It usually extends from the symphysis pubis to the umbilicus.

linear accelerator (LINAC) an apparatus used to accelerate electrons to very high energies, using microwaves in an evacuated waveguide. May be used in radiotherapy to provide either an electron beam or an x-ray beam.

linear array, (in radiography) a contiguous sequence of identical discrete detectors.

linear attenuation coefficient (LAC), fraction of x-ray photons removed from the beam per unit thickness of a medium, by a given interaction process.

linear energy transfer (LET), (in radiology) the rate at which energy is transferred to matter along the track of an ionizing particle. It is expressed in terms of kiloelectron volts per micrometre (KeV/um).

linear flow velocity, the velocity of a particle carried in a moving stream, usually measured in centimetres per second.

linear fracture, a fracture that extends parallel to the long axis of a bone but does not displace the bone tissue.

linear grid. See **secondary radiation grid**.

linearity, (in radiology) the ability to obtain the same exposure for the same milliampere-seconds (mAs), regardless of mA and exposure time used.

linear regression, a statistical procedure in which a straight line is established through a data set that best represents a relationship between two subsets or two methods.

linear scan, (in ultrasonography) the motion of the transducer at a constant speed along a straight line at right angles to the beam.

linear tomography, (in radiography) tomography that produces a blurring pattern with linear, or unidirectional, motion. The pattern · is caused by elongation of structures outside the focal plane.

linea semilunaris, the slightly curved line on the ventral abdominal wall. It marks the lateral border of the rectus abdominis and can be seen as a shallow groove when that muscle is tensed.

linea terminalis, a hypothetical line dividing the upper, or false, pelvis, from the lower, or true, pelvis.

line compensator. See **mains voltage compensator.**

line of gravity, an imaginary line that extends from the centre of gravity to the base of support.

line pair (lp), (in radiography) a method to evaluate the resolution of an imaging system, using a test tool consisting of lead strips and adjacent equal-sized spaces. The greater the number of line pairs determined per millimetre, the greater the resolution.

line printer, a high-speed printer, driven by a computer, that prints an entire line of text simultaneously.

Lineweaver-Burk transformation {Hans Lineweaver, American chemist, b. 1907; Dean Burk, American scientist, b. 1904}, a method of converting experimental data from studies of enzyme activity so that they can be displayed on a linear plot.

lingua. See **tongue.**

lingual artery, one of a pair of arteries that arises from the external carotid arteries, divides into four branches, and supplies the tongue and surrounding muscles.

lingual bar, a major connector that is installed lingual to the dental arch and joins bilateral parts of a mandibular removable partial denture.

lingual bone. See **hyoid bone.**

lingual crib, an orthodontic appliance consisting of a wire frame suspended lingually to the maxillary incisor teeth. It is used for obstructing undesirable thumb and tongue habits that can produce malocclusions.

lingual flange, the part of a mandibular denture that occupies the space adjacent to the residual ridge and next to the mouth.

lingual frenum, a band of tissue that extends from the floor of the mouth to the inferior surface of the tongue.

lingual goitre, a tumour at the back of the tongue formed by an enlargement of the primordial thyrolingual duct.

lingual papilla. See **papilla.**

lingual rest, a metallic extension onto the lingual surface of an anterior tooth to provide support or indirect retention for a removable partial denture.

lingual tonsil, a mass of lymphoid follicles near the root of the tongue.

lingua villosa nigra. See **parasitic glossitis.**

liniment, a preparation, usually containing an alcoholic, oily, or soapy vehicle, that is rubbed on the skin as a counterirritant.

linin, the faintly staining threads seen in the nuclei of cells, with granules of chromatin attached to the threads.

linitis, inflammation of cellular tissue of the stomach as in linitis plastica, seen frequently in adenocarcinoma of the stomach.

linitis plastica, a diffuse fibrosis and thickening of the wall of the stomach, resulting in a rigid, inelastic organ. The layer of connective tissue of the stomach becomes fibrotic and thick, and the stomach wall becomes shrunken and rigid. Causes of this condition include infiltrating undifferentiated carcinoma, syphilis, and Crohn's disease.

linkage, 1. (in genetics) the location of two or more genes on the same chromosome so that they do not segregate independently during meiosis but tend to be transmitted together as a unit. The closer the loci of the genes, the more likely they are to be inherited as a group and associated with a specific trait. **2.** (in psychology) the association between a stimulus and the response it elicits. **3.** (in chemistry) the bond between two atoms or radicals in a chemical compound.

linkage group, (in genetics) a group of genes located on the same chromosome that tends to be inherited as a unit.

linkage map. See **genetic map.**

linked genes, genes that are located on the same chromosome and whose position is close enough so that they tend to be transmitted as a linkage group.

linker, (in molecular genetics) a small segment of synthetic DNA having a place on its surface that can be ligated to DNA fragments in cloning.

linoleic acid, a colourless to straw-coloured essential fatty acid with two unsaturated bonds, occurring in linseed and safflower oils.

linolenic acid, an unsaturated fatty acid essential for normal human nutrition. It occurs in glycerides of linseed and other vegetable oils.

liothyronine sodium, a synthetic thyroid hormone which produces a more rapid therapeutic response than thyroxine used in the treatment of severe hypothyroidism.

lip, 1. either the upper or lower fleshy structure surrounding the opening of the oral cavity. **2.** any rimlike structure bordering a cavity or groove; labium.

LIP, abbreviation for **lymphoid interstitial pneumonia.**

lipaemia, a condition in which increased amounts of lipids are present in the blood, a normal occurrence after eating.

lipase, any of several enzymes, produced by the organs of the digestive system, that catalyse the breakdown of lipids through the hydrolysis of the linkages between fatty acids and glycerol in triglycerides and phospholipids.

lipectomy, an excision of subcutaneous fat, as from the abdominal wall.

lipid, any of the free fatty acid fractions in the blood. They are stored in the body and serve as an energy reserve, but are elevated in various diseases, such as atherosclerosis. Kinds of lipids are **cholesterol, fatty acids, neutral fat, phospholipids, phospholipid as phosphorus,** and **triglycerides.**

lipidosis, a general term including several rare familial disorders of fat metabolism. The chief characteristic of these disorders is the accumulation of abnormal levels of certain lipids in the body. Kinds of lipidoses are **Gaucher's disease, Krabbe's disease, Niemann-Pick disease,** and **Tay-Sachs disease.**

lipiduria, the presence of lipids (fat bodies) in the urine.

lipoatrophic diabetes, an inherited disease characterized by insulin-resistant diabetes mellitus, loss of body fat, acanthosis nigricans, and hypertrophied musculature. It is associated with a disorder of the hypothalamus resulting in excessive blood levels of growth hormone and ACTH releasing hormones.

lipoatrophy, a breakdown of subcutaneous fat at the site of an insulin injection. It usually occurs after several injections at the same site.

lipocele. See **adipocele.**

lipochondrodystrophy. See **Hurler's syndrome.**

lipodystrophia progressiva, an abnormal accumulation of fat around the buttocks and thighs and a progressive, symmetrical disappearance of subcutaneous fat from areas above the pelvis and on the face.

lipodystrophy, any abnormality in the metabolism or deposition of fats. Kinds of lipodystrophy are **bitrochan teric lipodystrophy, insulin lipodystrophy,** and **intestinal lipodystrophy.**

lipoedema a condition in which fat deposits accumulate in lower extremities, from the hips to the ankles, accompanied by symptoms tenderness in the affected areas.

lip of hip fracture, a fracture of the posterior lip of the acetabulum, often associated with displacement of the hip.

lipofuscin, a class of fatty pigments consisting mostly of oxidized fats that are found in abundance in the cells of adults.

lipogranuloma, pl. **lipogranulomas, lipogranulomata,** a nodule of necrotic, fatty tissue associated with granulomatous inflammation or with a foreign-body reaction around a deposit of injected material containing an oily substance.

lipohypertrophy, a buildup of subcutaneous fat tissue at the site of an insulin injection.

lipoic acid, a bacterial growth factor found in liver and yeast.

lipoid, any substance that resembles a lipid.

lipolysis, the breakdown or destruction of lipids or fats.

lipoma, pl. **lipomas, lipomata,** a benign tumour consisting of mature fat cells. **lipomatous,** adj.

lipoma annulare colli, a diffuse, symmetrical accumulation of fat around the neck, not a true lipoma.

lipoma arborescens, a fatty tumour of a joint, characterized by a treelike distribution of fat cells.

lipoma capsulare, a benign neoplasm characterized by the abnormal presence of fat cells in the capsule of an organ.

lipoma cavernosum. See **angiolipoma.**

lipoma diffusum renis. See **lipomatous nephritis.**

lipoma dolorosa. See **lipomatosis dolorosa.**

lipoma fibrosum, a fatty tumour containing masses of fibrous tissue.

lipoma myxomatodes. See **lipomyxoma.**

lipoma sarcomatodes. See **liposarcoma.**

lipomatosis, a disorder characterized by abnormal tumourlike accumulations of fat in body tissues.

lipomatosis atrophicans. See **lipodystrophia progressiva, lipomatosis.**

lipomatosis dolorosa, a disorder characterized by the abnormal accumulation of painful or tender fat deposits.

lipomatosis gigantea, a condition characterized by massive deposits of fat.

lipomatosis renis. See **lipomatous nephritis.**

lipomatous myxoma, a tumour containing fatty tissue that arises in connective tissue.

lipomatous nephritis, a rare condition in which the renal nephrons are replaced by fatty tissue. Kidney failure may result.

lipomyxoma, *pl.* **lipomyxo mas, lipomyxomata,** a myxoma that contains fat cells.

lipoprotein, a conjugated protein in which lipids form an integral part of the molecule. They are synthesized primarily in the liver, and are classified according to their composition and density. Kinds of lipoproteins are **chylomicrons, high-density lipoproteins, low-density lipoproteins,** and **very low-density lipoproteins.**

liposarcoma, *pl.* **liposarcomas, liposarcomata,** a malignant growth of primitive fat cells.

liposis. See **lipomatosis.**

liposome, a microscopic liquid-walled vesicle. Liposomes are used to sequester drugs, such as amphotericin, in aqueous solutions in order to modify their pharmacol kinetic or pharma codynamic behaviour.

liposuction, a technique for removing adipose tissue from obese patients with a suction-pump device. It is used primarily to remove or reduce localized areas of fat around the abdomen, breasts, legs, face, and upper arms where the skin is contractile enough to redrape in a normal manner.

liquefaction, the process in which a solid or a gas is made liquid.

liquid, a state of matter, intermediate between solid and gas, in which the substance flows freely with little application of force and assumes the shape of the vessel in which it is contained.

liquid diet, a diet consisting only of liquids and foods that liquefy at body temperature. The diet is prescribed after surgery, in some acute infections of short duration, in the treatment of acute GI disorders, and for patients too ill to chew.

liquid glucose, a thick, syrupy, odourless, and colourless or yellowish liquid obtained by the incomplete hydrolysis of starch primarily consisting of dextrose with dextrins, maltose, and water.

liquor, any fluid or liquid, such as liquor amnii, the amniotic fluid.

liquor amnii. See **amniotic fluid.**

liquorice, a dried root of gummy texture from the leguminous plant *Glycyrrhiza glabra.* It has a sweet, astringent taste and is used as a flavouring agent.

Lisfranc's fracture {Jacque Lisfranc, French surgeon, b. 1790}, a fracture dislocation of the foot in which one or all of the proximal metatarsals are displaced.

lisping, the defective pronunciation of one or

more of the sibilant consonant sounds, usually *s* and *z.*

Listeria monocytogenes {Baron Joseph Lister, Scottish surgeon, b. 1827}, a common species of gram-positive, motile bacillus that causes listeriosis.

listeriosis {Baron Joseph Lister}, an infectious disease caused by a genus of gram-positive motile bacteria that are nonsporulating. Transmitted by direct contact from infected animals to humans, by inhalation of dust, or by contact with mud, sewage, or soil contaminated with the organism, it is characterized by circulatory collapse, shock, endocarditis, hepatosplenomegaly, and a dark red rash over the trunk and the legs. Fever, bacteraemia, malaise, and lethargy are commonly seen.

Liston's forceps {Robert Liston, Scottish surgeon, b. 1794}, a kind of bone cutting forceps.

lithiasis, the formation of calculi in the hollow organs or ducts of the body. Calculi are formed of mineral salts and may irritate, inflame, or obstruct the organ in which they form or lodge. Lithiasis occurs most commonly in the gallbladder, kidney, and lower urinary tract. Lithiasis may be asymptomatic, but more often the condition is extremely painful.

lithium (Li), a silvery white alkali metal occurring in various compounds, such as petalite and spodumene. Its atomic number is 3; its atomic weight is 6.94. Lithium is the lightest known metal. Its salts are used in the treatment of manias.

lithium carbonate, an antimanic agent prescribed in the treatment of of manic-depressive disorders.

lithium fluoride (LiF), a compound commonly used for thermoluminescent dosimetry.

lithopaedion, a fetus that has died in utero and has become calcified or ossified.

lithotomy, the surgical excision of a calculus, especially one from the urinary tract.

lithotomy forceps, forceps for the extraction of a calculus, usually from the urinary tract.

lithotomy position, the posture assumed by the patient lying supine with the hips and the knees flexed and the thighs abducted and rotated externally. Also called **dorsosacral position.**

lithotripsy, a technique in wich renal or gallbladder calculi may be destroyed using focused high-frequency soundwaves, or shockwaves.

lithotrite, an instrument for crushing a stone in the urinary bladder. **lithotrity,** *n.*

litigant, (in law) a party to a lawsuit.

litigate, (in law) to carry on a suit or to contest.

litigious paranoia, a form of paranoia in which the person seeks legal redress for delusional events.

litmus paper, absorbent paper coated with litmus, a blue dye, that is used to determine pH. Acid substances or solutions turn blue litmus to red. Alkaline substances or solutions do not cause a colour change in blue litmus.

Little's disease. See **cerebral palsy.**

Litzmann's obliquity. See **asynclitism.**

live birth, the birth of an infant, irrespective of the duration of gestation, that exhibits any sign of life, such as respiration, heartbeat, umbilical pulsation, or movement of voluntary muscles.

livedo, a blue or reddish mottling of the skin, worse in cold weather and probably caused by arteriolar spasm. **Cutis marmorata** is a transient form of livedo.

livedo reticularis, a vasospastic disorder accentuated by exposure to cold and presenting with a characteristic reddish blue mottling with a typical "fishnet" appearance and involving the entire leg and, less often, the arms.

livedo vasculitis. See **segmented hyalinizing vasculitis.**

liver, the largest gland of the body and one of its most complex organs. More than 500 of its functions have been identified. It is divided into four lobes, contains as many as 100,000 lobules, and is served by two distinct blood supplies. The hepatic artery conveys oxygenated blood to the liver, and the hepatic portal vein conveys nutrient-filled blood from the stomach and the intestines. Some of the major functions performed by the liver are the production of bile by hepatic cells, the secretion of glucose, proteins, vitamins, fats, and most of the other compounds used by the body, the processing of haemoglobin for vital use of its iron content, and the conversion of poisonous ammonia to urea.

liver biopsy, a diagnostic procedure in which a special needle is introduced into the liver under local anaesthesia to obtain a specimen for pathological examination.

liver breath. See **fetor hepaticus.**

liver cancer, a malignant neoplastic disease of the liver, occurring most frequently as a metastasis from another malignancy. Risk factors include haemochromatosis, schistosomiasis, exposure to vinyl chloride or arsenic, and possibly nutritional deficiencies. Alcoholism may be a predisposing factor, but nonalcoholic cirrhosis is a greater risk than alcoholic cirrhosis. Aflatoxins in mouldy grain and peanuts appear to be linked to high rates of hepatocellular carcinoma. Characteristics of liver cancer are abdominal bloating, anorexia, weakness, dull upper abdominal pain, ascites, mild jaundice, and a tender enlarged liver; in some cases tumour nodules are palpable on the liver surface.

liver cell carcinoma. See **malignant hepatoma.**

liver disease, any one of a group of disorders of the liver. The most important diseases in this group are cirrhosis, cholestasis, and viral and toxic hepatitis. Characteristics of liver disease are jaundice, anorexia, hepatomegaly, ascites, and impaired consciousness. The exact diagnosis of liver disease is made through a combination of laboratory tests and clinical findings.

liver flap. See **asterixis.**

liver function test (LFT), a test used to evaluate various functions of the liver, for example, metabolism, storage, filtration, and excretion. Kinds of liver function tests include **alkaline phosphatase, bromsulfalein test, prothrombin time, serum bilirubin,** and **serum glutamic pyruvic transaminase.**

liver scan, a method of imaging the liver, using radionuclide imaging or ultrasonography or computerized tomography or magnetic resonance imaging for example.

liver spot, *nontechnical.* a senile lentigo or actinic keratosis.

living will, a written agreement between a patient and doctor to withhold life-saving measures if the patient's condition is found to be irreversible.

livor mortis, a purple discoloration of the skin in some dependent body area following death as a result of blood cell destruction.

lizard, a scaly-skinned reptile with a long body and tail and two pairs of legs. The symptoms of their bites and the recommended treatment are similar to those of the bites from moderately poisonous snakes.

LLD factor. See **cyanocobalamin.**

LMP, abbreviation for **last menstrual period.**

LNRI, abbreviation for **lower reference nutrient intake** for proteins, vitamins and minerals. This represents the lowest intakes which will meet the needs of some individuals in the group. The value is set at 2 standard deviations below the mean EAR and represents 2. 5% of the group. Values below this are inadequate for most individuals.

loading response stance stage, one of the five stages of the stance phase of walking or gait, specifically associated with the moment when the leg reacts to and accepts the weight of the body.

Loa loa, a parasitic worm of western and central Africa that causes loiasis.

lobar bronchus, a bronchus extending from a primary bronchus to a segmental bronchus into one of the lobes of the right or left lung.

lobar pneumonia, a severe infection of one or more of the five major lobes of the lungs that, if untreated, eventually results in consolidation of lung tissue. The disease is characterized by fever, chills, cough, rusty sputum, rapid shallow breathing, cyanosis, nausea, vomiting, and pleurisy. Complications include lung abscess, atelectasis, empyema, pericarditis, and pleural effusion.

lobe, 1. a roundish projection of any structure. **2.** a portion of any organ, demarcated by sulci, fissures, or connective tissue, as the lobes of the brain, liver, and lungs. **lobar, lobular,** *adj.*

lobectomy, a type of chest surgery in which a lobe of a lung is excised, performed to remove a malignant tumour and to treat uncontrolled bronchiectasis, trauma with haemorrhage, or intractable tuberculosis. Some compensatory emphysema is expected as the remaining lung tissue overexpands to fill the new space. **lobectomize** *v.*

lobotomy, a neurosurgical procedure in which the nerve fibres in the bundle of white matter in the frontal lobe of the brain are severed to interrupt the transmission of various affective responses. Severe intractable depression and pain are among the indications for the operation. It is rarely performed, because it has many unpredictable and undesirable effects.

lobster claw deformity. See **bidactyly.**

lobular carcinoma a neoplasm that often forms a diffuse mass and accounts for a small percentage of breast tumours.

lobule, a small lobe, such as the soft, lower, pendulous part of the external ear. **lobular,** *adj.*

local, 1. of or pertaining to a small circumscribed area of the body. **2.** of or pertaining to a treatment or drug applied locally. **3.** *informal.* a local anaesthetic.

local adaptation syndrome (LAS), the localized response of a tissue, organ, or system that occurs as a reaction to stress.

local anaesthesia, the direct administration of a local anaesthetic agent to tissues to induce the absence of sensation in a small area of the body. Brief surgical or dental procedures are the most common indications for local anaesthesia. The anaesthetic may be applied topically to the surface of the skin or membrane or injected subcutaneously through an intradermal weal. The principal drawbacks to the use of local anaesthesia are the incidence of allergic reactions to certain agents. The advantages include low cost, ease of administration, low toxicity, and safety. A conscious patient can cooperate and does not require respiratory support or intubation.

local anaesthetic, a substance used to reduce or eliminate neural sensation, specifically pain, in a limited area of the body. Local anaesthetics act by blocking transmission of nerve impulses. More than 100 drugs are available for local anaesthesia; they are classified as members of the alcohol-ester or the aminoamide family. Any substance sufficiently potent to induce local anaesthesia has potential for causing adverse side effects, ranging from easily reversible dermatitis to lethal anaphylaxis or simultaneous respiratory and cardiac arrest.

local cerebral blood flow (LCBF), (in positron emission tomography) the parametric image of blood flow through the brain. It is expressed in units of millilitres of blood flow per minute.

local cerebral metabolic rate of glucose utilization (LCMRG), (in positron emission tomography) a parametric image of the brain expressed in units of milligrams of glucose utilization per minute per 100 g of brain tissue.

local control, the arrest of cancer growth at a site of treatment.

local hypothermia, the cooling of a local area of tissue mainly used as a preservative, for severed limbs, or donor organs.

localization, (in radiotherapy) a method used to determine the precise size and target volume and sensitive structures, usually with reference to surface landmarks, by means of a treatment simulator and the use of radiography and/or fluoroscopy.

localization film. See **localization.**

localized scleroderma. See **morphea.**

localizer image, (in computed tomography) an image used to localize a specific body part.

localizing symptom, local symptom. See **symptom.**

lochia, the discharge that flows from the vagina after childbirth. During the first 3 or 4 days post partum, the lochia is red (**lochia rubra**) and is made up of blood, endometrial decidua, and fetal lanugo, vernix, and sometimes meconium, small shreds of placental tissue and membranes. After the third day the amount of blood diminishes, the placental site exudes serous material and lymph, and the lochia becomes darker and thinner and then serous (**lochia serosa**) as evacuation of particulate material is completed. During the second week white blood cells and bacteria appear in large numbers along with fatty, mucinous decidual material, causing the lochia to appear yellow. During the third week and thereafter, as endometrial epithelialization progresses, the amount of lochia decreases markedly and takes on a seromucinous consistency and a grey-white colour (**lochia alba**). Cessation of the flow of lochia at about 6 weeks is usual. **lochial,** *adj.*

locked twins. See **interlocked twins.**

lock forceps. See **point forceps.**

locking point, a point on the body at which light pressure can be applied to help a weak or debilitated patient maintain a desired posture or position. A basic locking point is the body's centre of gravity, at the level of the second sacral vertebra, where mild pressure can assist a patient in standing or walking erect.

lockjaw, *informal.* tetanus.

locomotor ataxia. See **tabes dorsalis.**

loculate, divided into small spaces or cavities.

loculus, a small chamber, pocket, or cavity, such as the interior of a polyp.

locum tenens, a temporary substitute for a doctor who is away from the practice. Usually referred to informally simply as a ''locum''.

locus, a specific place or position, such as the locus of a particular gene on a chromosome.

locus of infection, a site in the body where an infection originates.

Löffler's syndrome {Wilhelm Löffler, Swiss physician, b. 1887}, a benign, idiopathic disorder marked by episodes of pulmonary eosinophilia, transient opacities in the lungs, anorexia, breathlessness, fever, and weight loss.

logotherapy, a treatment modality based on the application of humanistic and existential psychology to assist a patient in finding meaning and purpose in life and unique life experiences.

log roll, a manoeuvre used to turn a reclining patient from one side to the other or completely over without flexing the spinal column. The arms of the patient are folded across the chest and the legs extended. A draw sheet under the patient is manipulated by attending nursing personnel to facilitate the procedure.

loiasis, a form of filariasis caused by the worm *Loa loa,* which may migrate for 10 to 15 years in subcutaneous tissue, producing localized inflammation known as Calabar swellings. The disease is acquired through the bite of an infected African deer fly.

loin, a part of the body on each side of the spinal column between the false ribs and the hip bones.

lomustine, a cytotoxic alkylating agent. It is prescribed in the treatment of a variety of malignant conditions.

long-acting drug, a pharmacological agent with a prolonged effect because of a formulation which results in the continued absorption of small amounts of the drug over an extended period, or because of slow elimination of the absorbed drug from the body.

long-acting insulin, a preparation in which insulin is complexed with zinc or protamine to form a suspension which acts as a depot after injection, resulting in a prolonged hypoglyaemic action.

long-acting thyroid stimulator (LATS), an immunoglobulin, probably an autoantibody, that exerts a prolonged stimulatory effect on the thyroid gland, causing rapid growth of the gland and excessive thyroid activity resulting in hyperthyroidism.

long-arm cast, an orthopaedic cast applied to immobilize upper extremities from the hand to the upper arm. Compare **short-arm cast.**

long bones, the bones that contribute to the height or length of an extremity, particularly the bones of the legs and arms.

longitudinal, **1.** a measurement in the direction of the long axis of an object, body, or organ, such as the longitudinal arch of the foot. **2.** a scientific study that is conducted over a long period of time.

longitudinal diffusion, the diffusion of solute molecules in the direction of flow of the mobile phase.

longitudinal dissociation, (in cardiology) the insulation of parallel pathways of impulses from each other, usually in the AV junction.

longitudinal sound waves, pressure waves formed by the oscillation of particles or molecules parallel to the axis of wave propagation. The compression and expansion of such longitudinal waves at high frequencies is the principle on which ultrasonography is based.

long-leg cast, an orthopaedic cast applied to immobilize the leg from the toes to the upper thigh.

long-leg cast with walker, an orthopaedic cast applied to immobilize the lower extremities from the toes to the upper thigh in treating certain fractures of the leg. This type of cast is the same as the long-leg cast but incorporates a rubber walker, allowing the patient to walk while the leg is encased in the cast.

long-term care, the provision of medical, social, and personal care services on a recurring or continuing basis to persons with chronic physical or mental disorders.

long-term memory, the ability to recall sensations, events, ideas, and other information for long periods of time without apparent effort.

long thoracic nerve, one of a pair of supraclavicular branches from the roots of the brachial plexus.

long tract signs, neurological signs, such as clonus, muscle spasticity, or bladder involvement, that usually indicate a lesion in the middle or upper portions of the spinal cord or in the brain.

loop, **1.** a set of instructions in a computer program that causes certain commands to be executed repeatedly if specified criteria are met. **2.** *informal.* intrauterine device.

loop colostomy, a type of temporary colostomy performed as part of the surgical repair of Hirschsprung's disease. To perform the procedure, an intact segment of colon anterior to the repair is brought through an abdominal incision and sutured onto the abdomen. A loop is formed and held in position by placing a piece of glass rod between the segment and the abdomen.

loop diuretic. See **diuretic.**

loop of Henle, {Friedrich G.J. Henle, German

anatomist, b. 1809}, the U-shaped portion of a renal tubule, consisting of a thin descending limb and a thick ascending limb.

loose association. See **loosening.**

loose fibrous tissue, a constrictive, pliable fibrous connective tissue consisting of interwoven elastic and collagenous fibres, interspersed with fluid-filled areolae.

loosening, (in psychiatry) a disturbance of thinking in which the association of ideas and thought patterns become so vague, diffuse, and unfocused as to lack any logical sequences or relationship to any preceding concepts or themes.

loose-pack joint position, a point in the range of motion at which articulating surfaces are the least congruent and the supporting structures are the most lax.

loperamide hydrochloride, an antiperistaltic used in the treatment of diarrhoea.

lorazepam, a benzodiazepine tranquillizer used in the treatment of anxiety and insomnia.

lordosis, **1.** the normal curvature of the lumbar and cervical spine, seen as an anterior concavity if the person is observed from the side. **2.** an abnormal, increased degree of curvature of any part of the back.

LOS, abbreviation **for length of stay.**

lotion, a liquid preparation applied externally to protect the skin or to treat a dermatological disorder.

Lou Gehrig's disease. See **amyotrophic lateral sclerosis.**

Louis-Bar syndrome. See **ataxia-telangiectasia.**

loupe, a magnifying lens mounted in a frame worn on the head, as used to examine the eyes.

louse, *pl.* **lice,** a small, wingless, parasitic insect of the order Anoplura that is the carrier of such diseases as relapsing fever and typhus.

louse bite, a minute puncture wound produced by a louse that may transmit typhus, trench fever, and relapsing fever. Secondary infection may result from scratching the affected area.

louse-borne typhus. See **epidemic typhus.**

Lovset's manoeuvre, a manoeuvre used to deliver the extended arms of a breech. The baby is rotated through a half circle keeping the back uppermost, to bring the arm below the symphysis pubis, then in a half circle the other way to deliver the other arm.

low back pain, local or referred pain at the base of the spine caused by a sprain, strain, osteoarthritis, ankylosing spondylitis, a neoplasm, or a prolapsed intervertebral disk. Low back pain is a common complaint and is often associated with poor posture, obesity, sagging abdominal muscles, or sitting for prolonged periods of time. Pain may be localized and static; it may be accompanied by muscle weakness or spasms; or it may

radiate down the back of one or both legs, as in sciatica. It may be initiated or increased by coughing, sneezing, rising from a seated position, lifting, stretching, bending, or turning. To guard against the pain, the person may decrease the range of motion of the spine. If an intervertebral disc is prolapsed, deep pressure over the interspace generally causes pain, and flexion of the hip elicits sciatic pain when the knee is extended but not when the knee is flexed (Lasègue's sign).

low birth weight (LBW) infant, an infant whose weight at birth is less than 2500 g, regardless of gestational age. Many low birth weight infants have no problems and develop normally, their smallness being genetic or idiopathic, or the problem that caused their slowed growth being mild or brief.

low blood count, informal. anaemia.

low-calcium diet, a diet that restricts the use of calcium and that eliminates most of the dairy foods, all breads made with milk or dry skimmed milk, and deep-green leafy vegetables. It may be prescribed for patients who form renal calculi.

low-calorie diet, a diet that is prescribed to limit the intake of calories, usually to cause a reduction in body weight. Such diets may be designated as 800 calorie, 1000 calorie, or other specific numbers of calories.

low-cholesterol diet, a diet that restricts foods containing animal fats and saturated fatty acids, such as egg yolk, cream, butter, milk, muscle and organ meats, and shellfish, and concentrates on poultry, fish, vegetables, fruits, cottage cheese, and polyunsaturated fats.

low-density lipoprotein (LDL), a plasma protein containing relatively more cholesterol and triglycerides than protein. It is derived in part, if not completely, from the intravascular breakdown of the very low-density lipoproteins.

lower extremity suspension, an orthopaedic procedure used in the treatment of bone fractures and in the correction of orthopaedic abnormalities of the lower limbs. The procedure uses traction equipment, including metal frames, ropes, and pulleys, to relieve the weight of the lower limb involved rather than to exert traction pull.

lower level discriminator (LLD), (in nuclear medicine) a radiation energy-sensitive device used to discriminate against all radionuclide pulses whose heights are below the accepted level.

lower motor neuron paralysis, an injury to or lesion in the spinal cord that damages the cell bodies or axons, or both, of the lower motor neurons, which are located in the anterior horn cells and the spinal and peripheral nerves. If complete transection of the spinal cord occurs, voluntary muscle control is totally lost. In partial transection, function is altered in varying degrees, depending on the areas innervated by the nerves involved.

lower respiratory infection. See **respiratory tract infection.**

lower respiratory tract, a division of the respiratory system that includes the left and the right bronchi and the alveoli where the exchange of oxygen and carbon dioxide occurs during the respiratory cycle. The bronchi divide into smaller bronchioles in the lungs, the bronchioles into alveolar ducts, the ducts into alveolar sacs, and the sacs into alveoli.

lower segment caesarean section (LSCS), a method for surgically delivering a baby through a transverse incision in the thin supracervical portion of the lower uterine segment. This incision bleeds less during surgery and heals with a stronger scar than the higher vertical scar of the classical caesarean section (which now is rarely used).

low-fat diet, a diet containing limited amounts of fat and consisting chiefly of easily digestible foods of high carbohydrate content. It includes all vegetables, lean meats, fish, fowl, pasta, cereals, and whole wheat or enriched bread. The diet may be indicated in gallbladder disease and malabsorption syndromes.

low-fat milk, milk containing 1% to 2% fat, making it an intermediate in fat content between whole and skimmed milk. Also referred to as semi-skimmed milk.

low-flow oxygen delivery system, respiratory care equipment that does not supply all the inspired gases. The patient inhales some room air along with the oxygen being delivered.

low-grade fever, a temperature that is above 37°C but lower than 38°C for 24 hours.

Lown-Ganong-Levine syndrome (LGL) {Bernard Lown, American physician, b. 1921; William F. Ganong, American physiologist, b. 1924; S. A. Levine, American physician, b. 1891}, a disorder of the atrioventricular (AV) conduction system, marked by ventricular preexcitation. Part or all of the AV nodal connection is bypassed by an abnormal AV connection from the atrial muscle to the bundle of His.

low-power field, the low magnification field of vision under a light microscope.

low-residue diet, a diet that will leave a minimal residue in the lower intestinal tract after digestion and absorption. It consists of tender meats, poultry, fish, eggs, white bread, pasta, simple desserts, clear soups, tea, and coffee. The diet is prescribed in cases of GI irritability or inflammation, and before and after GI surgery.

low-salt diet. See **low-sodium diet.**

low-saturated-fat diet. See **low-cholesterol diet.**

low-sodium diet, a diet that restricts the use of sodium chloride plus other compounds containing sodium, such as baking powder or soda, monosodium glutamate, sodium citrate, sodium propionate, and sodium sulphate. It is indicated in hypertension, oedematous states (especially when associated with cardiovascular disease), renal or liver disease, and therapy with corticosteroids. The degree of sodium restriction depends on the severity of the condition.

loxapine, a major tranquillizer prescribed in the treatment of psychoses.

lozenge. a small, oval, round or oblong tablet containing a medicinal agent incorporated in a flavoured, sweetened mucilage or fruit base that dissolves in the mouth, releasing the drug.

lpm, abbreviation **for litres per minute.**

LP, abbreviation for **lumbar puncture.**

Lr, symbol for **lawrencium.**

LSCS, abbreviation for **lower segment caesarean section.**

LSD, abbreviation for **lysergic acid diethylamide.**

L/S ratio, the lecithin/sphingomyelin ratio, used in a test for fetal lung maturity.

LTB, abbreviation for **laryngotracheobronchitis.** See **croup.**

L-thyroxine. See **thyroxine.**

L-thyroxine sodium, a thyroid hormone used in the treatment of hypothyroidism.

Lu, symbol for **lutetium.**

lucid, clear, rational, and able to be understood.

lucid interval, a period of relative mental clarity between periods of irrationality, especially in organic mental disorders, such as delirium and dementia.

lucid lethargy, a mental state characterized by a loss of will; hence, an inability to act, even though the person is conscious and intellectual function is normal.

Ludwig's angina {Wilhelm F. von Ludwig, German surgeon, b. 1790}, acute streptococcal cellulitis of the floor of the mouth. It is treated with penicillin.

Luer-Lok syringe, a syringe for injection having a simple metal lock mechanism that securely holds the needle in place.

lues. See **syphilis.**

luetic aortitis. See **syphilitic aortitis.**

Lugol's solution {Jean G. A. Lugol, French physician, b. 1786}, an aqueous solution of iodine (5%) and potassium iodide (10%).

Lukes-Collins classification, a system of identifying non-Hodgkin's lymphomas according to B cell, T cell, true, and unclassifiable types. B cell types include lymphocytic, plasmacytic, follicular cell lymphomas, and B cell derived immunoblastic sarcoma. T cell types include T cell derived immunoblastic sarcoma and convoluted cell lymphoma. True types are of histiocytic origin.

lumbago, pain in the lumbar region caused by a muscle strain, rheumatoid arthritis, osteoarthritis, or a herniated intravertebral disc. Ischaemic lumbago, characterized by pain in the lower back and buttocks, is caused by vascular insufficiency, as in terminal aortic occlusion.

lumbar, of or pertaining to the part of the body between the thorax and the pelvis.

lumbar nerves, the five pairs of spinal nerves rising in the lumbar region. They become increasingly large the more caudal their location and pass laterally and downward under the cover of the psoas major or between its fasciculi.

lumbar node, a node in one of the seven groups of parietal lymph nodes serving the abdomen and the pelvis.

lumbar plexus, a network of nerves formed by the ventral primary divisions of the first three and the greater part of the fourth lumbar nerves. It is located on the inside of the posterior abdominal wall, either dorsal to the psoas major or among its fibres and ventral to the transverse processes of the lumbar vertebrae.

lumbar puncture (LP), the introduction of a hollow needle and stylet into the subarachnoid space of the lumbar portion of the spinal canal. With the use of strict aseptic technique, it is performed in various therapeutic and diagnostic procedures. Diagnostic indications include measuring of cerebrospinal fluid (CSF) pressure, obtaining CSF for laboratory analysis, evaluating the canal for the pressure of a tumour, and injecting air, oxygen, or a radiopaque substance for radiographic visualization of the structures of the nervous system of spinal canal and meninges and brain. Therapeutic indications for lumbar puncture include removing blood or pus from the subarachnoid space, injecting sera or drugs, withdrawing CSF to reduce intracranial pressure, introducing a local anaesthetic to induce spinal anaesthesia, and placing a small amount of the patient's blood in the subarachnoid space to form a clot to patch a rent or hole in the dura to prevent leak of CSF into the epidural space.

lumbar region. See **lateral region.**

lumbar subarachnoid peritoneostomy, a surgical procedure for draining cerebrospinal fluid in hydrocephalus, usually in the newborn. First a lumbar laminectomy is performed, then a polyethylene tube is passed from the subarachnoid space around the flank and into the peritoneum.

lumbar subarachnoid ureterostomy, a surgical procedure for draining excess cerebrospinal fluid through the ureter to the bladder in hydrocephalus, usually in the newborn. A polyethylene tube is passed from the lumbar subarachnoid space through the paraspinal muscles and into a ureter.

lumbar veins, four pairs of veins that collect blood by dorsal tributaries from the loins and by abdominal tributaries from the walls of the abdomen. They end in the inferior vena cava.

lumbar vertebra, one of the five largest segments of the movable part of the vertebral column, distinguished by the absence of a foramen in the transverse process and by vertebral bodies without facets. The body of each lumbar vertebra is flattened or slightly concave superiorly and inferiorly and is deeply constricted ventrally at the sides.

lumbodorsal fascia. See **fascia thoracolumbalis.**

lumbosacral plexus, the combination of all the ventral primary divisions of the lumbar, the sacral, and the coccygeal nerves. The lumbar and the sacral plexuses supply the lower limb. The sacral nerves also supply the perineum through the pudendal plexus and the coccygeal area through the coccygeal plexus.

lumbrical plus deformity, a complication of rheumatoid arthritis in which the lumbricals (muscles in the hands and feet) become contracted, with a resultant action of extension rather than flexion.

lumen *pl.* **lumina, lumens, 1.** a cavity or the channel within any organ or structure of the body. **2.** a unit of luminous flux that equals the flux emitted in a unit solid angle by a point source of one candle intensity. **lumenal, luminal,** *adj.*

luminescence, the emission of light by a material after excitation by some stimulus.

lumpectomy, surgical excision of a tumour without removal of large amounts of surrounding tissue or adjacent lymph nodes.

lumpy jaw, *nontechnical.* actinomycosis of cows, caused by infection with *Actinomyces bovis* and not communicable to humans.

lunar month, a period of 4 weeks or 28 days, approximately the time required for the moon to revolve around the earth.

lunate bone, the carpal bone in the centre of the proximal row of carpal bones between the scaphoid and triangular bones.

Lundh test, a pancreatic function test in which the pancreas is stimulated by oral intake of a formula diet and lipase values are measured in aspirate from the duodenum.

lung, one of a pair of light, spongy organs in the thorax, constituting the main component of the respiratory system. The two highly elastic lungs are the main mechanisms in the body for inspiring air from which oxygen is extracted for the arterial blood system and for exhaling carbon dioxide dispersed from the venous system. The lungs are composed of lobes that are smooth and shiny on their surface. The right lung contains three lobes; the left lung two lobes. Each lung is composed of an external serous coat, a subserous layer of areolar tissue, and the parenchyma.

The serous coat comprises the thin, visceral pleura. The subserous areolar tissue contains many elastic fibres and invests the entire surface of the organ. The parenchyma is composed of secondary lobules divided into primary lobules, each of which consists of blood vessels, lymphatics, nerves, and an alveolar duct connecting with air spaces.

lung cancer, a pulmonary malignancy attributable to cigarette smoking, asbestos, acronitrile, arsenic, beryllium, chloromethyl ether, chromium, coal products, ionizing radiation, iron oxide, mustard gas, nickel, petroleum, uranium, and vinyl chloride. Lung cancer develops most often in scarred or chronically diseased lungs, and is usually far advanced when detected, because metastases may precede the detection of the primary lesion in the lung. Symptoms of lung cancer include persistent cough, dyspnoea, purulent or blood-streaked sputum, chest pain, and repeated attacks of bronchitis or pneumonia. Epidermoid cancers and adenocarcinomas each account for approximately 30% of lung tumours, about 25% are small or oat cell carcinomas, and 15% are large-cell anaplastic cancers. Epidermoid tumours tend to remain in the thorax, but other lung lesions metastasize widely; oat cell carcinomas usually invade bone marrow, and large-cell cancers frequently metastasize to mediastinal nodes and GI mucosa. Surgery is the most effective treatment, but only one half of the cases are operable at the time of diagnosis.

lung capacities, lung volumes that consist of two or more of the four primary nonoverlapping volumes. Functional residual capacity is the sum of residual volume and expiratory reserve volume. Inspiratory capacity is the sum of the tidal volume and inspiratory reserve volume. Vital capacity is the sum of the expiratory reserve volume, the tidal volume, and the inspiratory reserve volume. Total lung capacity, at the end of maximal inspiration, is the sum of the functional residual capacity and the inspiratory capacity.

lung compliance, a measure of the ease of expansion by the lungs and thorax during respiratory movements. It is determined by pulmonary volume and elasticity, a high degree of compliance indicating a loss of elastic recoil of the lungs, as in old age or emphysema. Decreased compliance of the lungs occurs in conditions when greater pressure is needed for changes of volume, as in atelectasis, oedema, fibrosis, pneumonia, or absence of surfactant.

lung scan, a method of imaging the lungs, such as radionuclide imaging or computerized tomography.

lunula, *pl.* **lunulae,** a semilunar structure, such as the crescent-shaped pale area at the base of the nail of a finger or toe.

lupoid. See **lupus.**

lupoid hepatitis. See **hepatitis.**

lupus, 1. *nontechnical.* lupus erythematosus. **2.** *obsolete.* any chronic skin condition in which ulcerative lesions spread over the body over a long period of time. **lupoid,** *adj.*

lupus erythematosus. See **systemic lupus erythematosus.**

lupus erythematosus preparation (LE prep), a laboratory test for lupus erythematosus in which normal neutrophils are incubated with a specimen of the patient's serum resulting in the appearance of large, spherical, phagocytized inclusions within the neutrophils if the patient has lupus erythematosus.

lupusa vulgaris, a rare cutaneous form of tuberculosis in which areas of the skin become ulcerated and heal slowly, leaving deeply scarred tissue. The disease is not related to lupus erythematosus.

lusus naturae, a congenital anomaly; teratism.

luteal of or pertaining to the corpus luteum or its functions or effects.

luteal phase. See **secretory phase.**

lutein, a yellow-red, crystalline, carotenoid pigment found in plants with carotenes and chlorophylls and also in animal fats, egg yolk, the corpus luteum, or any lipochrome.

luteinizing hormone (LH), a glycoprotein hormone, produced by the anterior pituitary, that stimulates the secretion of sex hormones by the ovary and the testes and is involved in the maturation of spermatozoa and ova. In men, it induces the secretion of testosterone by the interstitial cells of the testes. In females, LH, working together with FSH, stimulates the growing follicle in the ovary to secrete oestrogen.

luteinizing hormone releasing hormone (LHRH), a neurohormone of the hypothalamus that stimulates and regulates the pituitary gland release of the luteinizing hormone (LH).

luteoma, *pl.* **luteomas, luteomata, 1.** a granulosa or theca cell tumour whose cells resemble those of the corpus luteum. **2.** a unilateral or bilateral nodular hyperplasia of ovarian lutein cells, occasionally developing during the last trimester of pregnancy.

luteotropin. See **prolactin.**

lutetium (Lu), a rare earth metallic element. Its atomic number is 71; and its atomic weight is 174.97.

luxated joint, a condition of complete dislocation, with no contact between articular surfaces of the joint.

LVAD, abbreviation for **left ventricular assist device.**

lyases, a group of enzymes that reversibly split carbon bonds with carbon, nitrogen, or oxygen without hydrolysis or oxygen reduction reactions.

lycopene, a red, crystalline, unsaturated hydrocarbon that is the carotenoid pigment in tomatoes and various berries and fruits. It is considered the primary substance from which all natural carotenoid pigments are derived.

Lyme arthritis. See **Lyme disease.**

Lyme disease, an acute, recurrent inflammatory infection, transmitted by a tickborne spirochete, *Borrelia burgdorferi.* The condition was originally described in Lyme, Connecticut. Knees, other large joints, and temporomandibular joints are most commonly involved, with local inflammation and swelling. Chills, fever, headache, malaise, and an expanding annular, erythematous skin eruption often precede the joint manifestations. Occasionally cardiac conduction abnormalities, aseptic meningitis, and Bell's palsy are associated conditions.

lymph, a thin opalescent fluid originating in many organs and tissues of the body that is circulated through the lymphatic vessels and filtered by the lymph nodes. Lymph enters the bloodstream at the junction of the internal jugular and subclavian veins. It contains chyle, a few erythrocytes, and variable numbers of leukocytes, most of which are lymphocytes. It is otherwise similar to plasma.

lymphadenitis, an inflammatory condition of the lymph nodes, usually the result of systemic neoplastic disease, bacterial infection, or other inflammatory condition. The nodes may be enlarged, hard, smooth or irregular, red, and may feel hot.

lymphadenopathy, any disorder of the lymph nodes or lymph vessels.

lymphadenopathy syndrome (LAS), a persistent, generalized swelling of the lymph nodes. It is often a part of the AIDS-related complex.

lymphangiectasia, dilatation of the smaller lymphatic vessels, characterized by diarrhoea, steatorrhoea, and protein malabsorption. It usually results from obstruction in the larger vessels.

lymphangiography, a radiographic technique to visualize the lymph vessels and lymph nodes, following introduction of a radiopaque contrast medium into superficial lymph vessels distal to the area to be imaged. **Lymphography** may be performed 24 hours later. **lymphangiogram,** *n.*

lymphangioma *pl.* **lymphangiomas, lymphangiomata,** a benign, yellowish tan tumour on the skin, composed of a mass of dilated lymph vessels.

lymphangioma cavernosum, a tumour formed by dilated lymphatic vessels and filled with lymph that is often mixed with coagulated blood.

lymphangioma circumscriptum, a benign skin lesion that develops from superficial hypertrophic lymph vessels.

lymphangioma cysticum. See **cystic lymphangioma.**

lymphangioma simplex, a growth formed by moderately dilated lymph vessels in a circumscribed area, chiefly on the skin.

lymphangitis, an inflammation of one or more lymphatic vessels, usually resulting from an acute streptococcal infection of one of the extremities. It is characterized by fine red streaks extending from the infected area to the axilla or groin, and by fever, chills, headache, and myalgia. The infection may spread to the bloodstream.

lymphatic, 1. of or pertaining to the lymphatic system of the body, consisting of a vast network of tubes transporting lymph. **2.** any one of the vessels associated with the lymphatic network.

lymphatic capillary plexus, one of the numerous networks of lymphatic capillaries that collect lymph from the intercellular fluid and constitute the beginning of the lymphatic system. The lymphatic vessels arise from the capillary plexuses, which vary in size and number in different regions and organs of the body.

lymphatic leukaemia. See **acute lymphocytic leukaemia, chronic lymphocytic leukaemia.**

lymphatic nodule. See **malpighian body.**

lymphatic system, a vast, complex network of capillaries, thin vessels, valves, ducts, nodes, and organs that helps to protect and maintain the internal fluid environment of the entire body by producing, filtering, and conveying lymph and by producing various blood cells. The lymphatic network also transports fats, proteins, and other substances to the blood system and restores 60% of the fluid that filters out of the blood capillaries into interstitial spaces during normal metabolism. Small semilunar valves throughout the lymphatic network help to control the flow of lymph and, at the junction with the venous system, prevent venous blood from flowing into the lymphatic vessels. The lymph collected from throughout the body drains into the blood through two ducts situated in the neck. Various body dynamics, such as respiratory pressure changes, muscular contractions, and movements of organs surrounding lymphatic vessels combine to pump the lymph through the lymphatic system. The system also includes specialized lymphatic organs, such as the tonsils, the thymus, and the spleen. Lymph flows into the general circulation through the thoracic duct.

lymph node, one of the many small oval structures that filter the lymph and fight infection, and in which there are formed lymphocytes, monocytes, and plasma cells. The lymph nodes are of different sizes, some as small as pinheads, others as large as lima beans. Each node is enclosed in a capsule, is composed of a lighter coloured cortical portion and a darker medullary portion, and consists of closely packed lymphocytes, reticular connective tissue laced by trabeculae, and three kinds of sinuses, subcapsular, cortical, and medullary. Lymph flows into the node through afferent lymphatic vessels. Most lymph nodes are clustered in (specific) areas, such as the mouth, the neck, the lower arm, the axilla, and the groin.

lymphoblastic lymphoma, lymphoblastic lymphosarcoma, lymphoblastoma. See **poorly differentiated lymphocytic malignant lymphoma.**

lymphocyte, one of two kinds of small, agranulocytic leukocytes, originating from fetal stem cells and developing in the bone marrow. Lymphocytes normally comprise 25% of the total white blood cell count but increase in number in response to infection. They occur in two forms: **B cells** and **T cells.** B cells circulate in an immature form and synthesize antibodies for insertion into their own cytoplasmic membranes. They reproduce mitotically, each of the clones displaying identical antibodies on their surface membranes. When an immature B cell is exposed to a specific antigen, the cell is activated, travelling to the spleen or to the lymph nodes, differentiating, and rapidly producing **plasma cells** and **memory cells.** Plasma cells synthesize and secrete copious amounts of antibody. Memory cells do not secrete antibody, but if reexposure to the specific antigen occurs, they develop into antibody-secreting plasma cells. The function of the B cell is to search out, identify, and bind with specific antigens. T cells are lymphocytes that have circulated through the thymus gland and have differentiated to become thymocytes. When exposed to an antigen, they divide rapidly and produce large numbers of new T cells sensitized to that antigen. T cells are often called "killer cells" because they secrete immunologically essential chemical compounds and assist B cells in destroying foreign protein.

lymphocyte transformation, an in vitro immunity test process in which a patient's lymphocytes are placed in a culture with an antigen. The rate of transformation is measured by the uptake of radioactive thymidine by the lymphocytes, indicating protein synthesis.

lymphocytic choriomeningitis, an arenavirus infection of the meninges and the cerebrospinal fluid, caused by the lymphocytic choriomeningitis virus and characterized by fever, headache, and stiff neck.

lymphocytic leukaemia. See **acute lymphocytic leukaemia, chronic lympho-cytic leukaemia.**

lymphocytic lymphoma, lymphocytic

lymphosarcoma. See **well-differentiated lymphocytic malignant lymphoma.**

lymphocytic thyroiditis. See **Hashimoto's disease.**

lymphocytoma. See **well-differentiated lymphocytic malignant lymphoma.**

lymphocytopenia, a smaller than normal number of lymphocytes in the peripheral circulation, occurring as a primary haematological disorder or in association with nutritional deficiency, malignancy, or infectious mononucleosis.

lymphocytosis, a proliferation of lymphocytes, as occurs in certain chronic diseases and during convalescence from acute infections.

lymphoderma perniciosa. See **leukaemia cutis.**

lymphoedema, a primary or secondary disorder characterized by the accumulation of lymph in soft tissue and swelling, caused by inflammation, obstruction, or removal of lymph channels. Congenital lymphoedema (Milroy's disease) is a hereditary disorder characterized by chronic lymphatic obstruction. Lymphoedema praecox occurs in adolescence, chiefly in females, and causes puffiness and swelling of the lower limbs. Secondary lymphoedema may follow surgical removal of lymph channels in mastectomy, obstruction of lymph drainage caused by malignant tumours, or the infestation of lymph vessels with adult filarial parasites. **lymphoedematous, lymphoedematose,** *adj.*

lymphoepithelioma, a poorly differentiated neoplasm developing from the epithelium overlying lymphoid tissue in the nasopharynx.

lymphogenous leukaemia. See **acute lymphocytic leukaemia, chronic lymphocytic leukaemia.**

lymphogranuloma venereum (LGV) a sexually transmitted disease caused by a strain of the bacterium *Chlamydia trachomatis*. It is characterized by ulcerative genital lesions, marked swelling of the lymph nodes in the groin, headache, fever, and malaise. Ulcerations of the rectal wall occur less commonly.

lymphography, radiographic imaging of the lymph nodes. See also **lymphangiography.**

lymphoid interstitial pneumonia (LIP), a form of pneumonia that involves the lower lobes with extensive alveolar infllitration by mature lymphocytes, plasma cells, and histiocytes. It is associated with AIDS, dysproteinaemia, and Sjögren's syndrome.

lymphoid leukaemia. See **acute lymphocytic leukaemia, chronic lympho-cytic leukaemia.**

lymphoidocytic leukaemia. See **stem cell leukaemia.**

lymphokine, one of the chemical factors produced and released by T lymphocytes that attract macrophages to the site of infection or inflammation and prepare them for attack. Kinds of lymphokines include **chemotactic factor, lymphotoxin, migration inhibiting factor,** and **mitogenic factor.**

lymphokine-activated killer (LAK) cells, nonspecific cytotoxic cells that are generated in the presence of interleukin-2 and in the absence of antigen.

lymphocytosis, cellular destruction of lymphocytes, especially of certain lymphocytes in the process of an immune response. **lympholytic,** *adj.*

lymphoma, *pl.* **lymphomas, lymphomata,** a neoplasm of lymphoid tissue that is usually malignant but, in rare cases, may be benign. The various lymphomas differ in degree of cellular differentiation and content, but the manifestations are similar in all types. Characteristically, the appearance of a painless, enlarged lymph node or nodes in the neck is followed by weakness, fever, weight loss, and anaemia. With widespread involvement of lymphoid tissue, the spleen and liver usually enlarge, and GI disturbances, malabsorption, and bone lesions frequently develop. Kinds of lymphoma include **Burkitt's lymphoma, giant follicular lymphoma, histiocytic malignant lymphoma, Hodgkin's disease, mixed cell malignant lymphoma. lymphomatoid,** *adj*

lymphoma staging, a system for classifying lymphomas according to the stage of the disease for the purpose of appropriate treatment. Stage I is characterized by the involvement of a single lymph node region or one extralymphatic organ or site and stage II by the involvement of two or more lymph node regions on the same side of the diaphragm or a localized involvement of an extra-lymphatic organ or site plus one or more node regions on the same side of the diaphragm. In stage III lymph nodes on both sides of the diaphragm are affected, and there may be involvement of the spleen or localized involvement of an extralymphatic organ or site. Stage IV is typified by diffuse or disseminated involvement of one or more extralymphatic organs or sites with or without associated lymph node involvement.

lymphopathia venereum. See **lymphogranuloma venereum.**

lymphopenia. See **lymphocytopenia.**

lymphoreticulosis, subacute granulomatous inflammation of lymphoid tissue with proliferation of reticuloendothelial cells, occurring most commonly as the result of a cat scratch. The disorder is characterized by the formation of an ulcerated papule at the site of the scratch, and by fever and tender lymphadenopathy, sometimes progressing to suppuration.

lymphosarcoma. See **non-Hodgkin's lymphoma.**

lymphosarcoma cell leukaemia, a malignancy of blood-forming tissues characterized by many lymphosarcoma cells in the peripheral circulation that tend to infiltrate surrounding tissues.

Lyon hypothesis {Mary L. Lyon, English geneticist, b. 1925}, (in genetics) a hypothesis stating that only one of the two X chromosomes in a female is functional, the other having become inactive early in development.

lyonization {Mary L. Lyon} the process of random inactivation of one of the X chromosomes in the female gamete to compensate for the presence of the double X gene complement.

Lyon's ring, a type of congenital uropathy in females in which submeatal or distal urethral stenosis causes enuresis, dysuria, and recurring infections.

lypressin, an antidiuretic and vasoconstrictor used in diabetes insipidus to decrease urinary water loss.

Lys, abbreviation for **lysine.**

lysergide, a semisynthetic derivative of ergot that is abused for its hallucogenic effects.

Lysholm method, (in radiography) any of several techniques for positioning a patient for x-ray examination of the cranial base, the mastoid and petrous regions of the temporal bone, and the optic foramen and orbital fissure.

lysinaemia, a condition caused by an inborn error of metabolism and resulting in the inability to use the essential amino acid lysine because of an enzyme defect or deficiency. It is characterized by muscle weakness and mental retardation.

lysine (Lys), an essential amino acid needed for proper growth in infants and for maintenance of nitrogen balance in adults.

lysine intolerance, a congenital disorder resulting in the inability to use the essential amino acid lysine because of an enzyme deficiency or defect.

lysine monohydrochloride, a salt of the amino acid lysine, used as a dietary supplement.

lysis, 1. destruction or dissolution of a cell or molecule through the action of a specific agent. Cell lysis is frequently caused by a lysin. **2.** gradual diminution in the symptoms of a disease.

lysis of adhesions, surgery performed to free adhesions of tissues.

lysosome, a cytoplasmic, membrane-bound particle that contains hydrolytic enzymes that function in intracellular digestive processes. If the hydrolytic enzymes are released into the cytoplasm, they cause self-digestion of the cell so that lysosomes may play an important role in certain self-destructive diseases characterized by the wasting of tissue, such as muscular dystrophy.

lysozyme, an enzyme with antiseptic actions

that destroys some foreign organisms. It is found in granulocytic and monocytic blood cells and is normally present in saliva, sweat, breast milk, and tears.

lytes, an informal abbreviation of *electrolytes,* especially the levels of potassium, sodium, phosphorus, magnesium, and calci-um in the blood, as determined by laboratory testing.

lytic cocktail, informal name for an anaesthetic compound of chlorpromazine, meperidine, and promethazine that blocks the automatic nervous system, depresses the circulatory system, and induces neuroplegia.

m, 1. abbreviation for **metre. 2.** (in prescriptions) an abbreviation for the Latin words *mane* meaning (in the) "morning" and *misce* meaning "mix".

M, abbreviation for **metastasis** in the TNM (tumour, node, metastasis) system for staging malignant neoplastic disease.

mA, abbreviation for **milliampere.**

M.A., abbreviation for **Master of Arts.**

MAC, 1. abbreviation for **mid-upper arm circumference.** 2. abbreviation for **mass attenuation coefficient.**

MAC AWAKE, the time at which a patient recovering from general anaesthesia is able to respond rationally to questions and verbal instructions.

macerate, to soften something solid by soaking. **maceration,** *n.*

maceration, the softening and breaking down of skin from prolonged exposure to moisture. Occurs when a dead fetus has been retained in utero for more than 24 hours.

machismo, (in psychology) a concept of the male that includes both culturally desirable traits of courage, and the dysfunctional behaviours of heavy drinking, seduction, and abusive spouse behaviour.

Machupo. See **Bolivian haemorrhagic fever.**

macrencephaly, a congenital anomaly characterized by abnormal largeness of the brain. **macrencephalic, macroencephalic,** *adj.*

macrobiotics, (meaning 'large life') an approach to health in which each individual studies how food, exercise and lifestyle affect his or her health and matches them to suit his or her own needs. It is a theraphy based on the principle that outside influences will affect the internal condition on the body and that these effects can be predicted with a good understanding of yin and yang.

macroblepharia, the condition of having abnormally large eyelids.

macrocephaly, a congenital anomaly characterized by abnormal largeness of the head and brain in relation to the rest of the body, resulting in some degree of mental and growth retardation. The head is more than two standard deviations above the average circumference size for age, sex, race, and period of gestation, with excessively wide fontanelles; the facial features are usually normal. There is symmetrical overgrowth at the head without increased intracranial pressure, as differentiated from hydrocephalus in which the lateral, asymmetric growth of the head is caused by excessive accumulation of cerebrospinal fluid, usually under increased pressure. **macrocephalic, macrocephalous,** *adj.,* **macrocephalus,** *n.*

macrocyte, an abnormally large, mature erythrocyte. It is most commonly seen in megaloblastic anaemia.

macrocytic, (of a cell) larger than normal, as the erythrocytes in macrocytic anaemia.

macrocytic anaemia, a disorder of the blood characterized by impaired erythropoiesis and the abnormal presence of large, fragile, red blood cells in the circulation.

macrocytosis, an abnormal proliferation of macrocytes in the peripheral blood.

macrodrip, (in intravenous therapy) an apparatus that is used to deliver measured amounts of IV solutions at specific flow rates based on the size of drops of the solution. The size of the drops is controlled by the fixed diameter of a plastic delivery tube. The drops delivered by a macrodrip are larger than those delivered by a microdrip.

macroelement. See **macronutrient.**

macroencephaly. See **macrencephaly.**

macrogamete, a large, nonmotile female gamete of certain thallophytes and sporozoa, specifically the malarial parasite *Plasmodium.*

macrogametocyte, an enlarged merozoite that undergoes meiosis to form the mature female gamete during the sexual phase of the life cycle of certain thallophytes and sporozoa, specifically the malarial parasite *Plasmodium.*

macrogenitosomia, a congenital condition in which the genitalia are abnormal because of an excess of androgen during fetal development. It is characterized in boys by enlarged external genitalia and in girls by pseudohermaphroditism.

macroglobulinaemia, a form of monoclonal gammopathy in which a large immunoglobulin (IgM) is vastly overproduced by the clones of a plasma B cell in response to an antigenic signal.

macroglossia, a congenital anomaly characterized by excessive size of the tongue, as seen in certain syndromes of congenital defects, including Down's syndrome.

macrognathia, an abnormally large growth of the jaw. **macrognathic,** *adj.*

macrolide, any of a group of antibiotics produced by actinomycetes or their semisynthetic derivatives. They include erythromycin. Macrolides are generally used against gram-positive bacteria and in patients allergic to penicillins, and in the treatment of atypical pneumonia.

macromolecule, a molecule of colloidal size, such as proteins, nucleic acids, or polysaccharides.

macronucleus, 1. a large nucleus. **2.** (in protozoa) the larger of two nuclei in each cell; it governs cell metabolism and growth as opposed to the micronucleus, which functions in sexual reproduction.

macronutrient, a chemical element required in relatively large quantities for the normal physiological processes of the body.

macrophage, any phagocytic cell of the reticuloendothelial system including Kupffer cell in the liver, splenocyte in the spleen, and histocyte in the loose connective tissue.

macroreentry, (in cardiology) reactivation of a tissue involving a large circuit, such as involvement of both bundle branches.

macroscopic anatomy. See **gross anatomy.**

macrosomia. Large body size.

macula, *pl.* **maculae, 1.** a small pigmented area or a spot that appears separate or different from the surrounding tissue. **2.** See macula lutea.

macula cerulea. See **blue spot, def. 1.**

macula lutea, an oval yellow spot at the centre of the retina 2 mm from the optic nerve. It contains a pit, no blood vessels, and the fovea centralis. Central vision occurs when an image is focused directly on the fovea centralis of the macula lutea. Also called (*informal*) macula.

macule, 1. a small, flat blemish or discolouration that is flush with the skin surface. Compare papule. **2.** a grey scar on the cornea that is visible without magnification. **macular,** *adj.*

Madelung's neck. See **lipoma annulare colli.**

mad hatter's disease. See **mercurialism.**

Madura foot, a progressive, destructive, tropical fungal infection of the foot, named after a district in India.

Maffucci's syndrome {Angelo Maffuci, Italian physician, b. 1845}, a condition characterized by enchondromatosis and multiple cutaneous or visceral haemangiomas.

magaldrate, an antacid used in the treatment of heartburn or acid indigestion.

Magendie's law. See **Bell's law.**

magical thinking, (in psychology) a belief that merely thinking about an event in the external world can cause it to occur. It is regarded as a form of regression to an early phase of development.

magic-bullet approach, 1. a therapeutic or diagnostic method that makes use of a specific mechanistic connection between a drug and a disease or organ. **2.** (in clinical medicine) the administration of a specific drug to cure or ameliorate a given disease or condition. **3.** (in nuclear medicine) the adminis-

tration of a specific radionuclide tagged to an appropriate carrier to provide a gamma camera image of a given organ or structure.

magnesaemia, the presence of magnesium in the blood.

magnesium (Mg), a silver-white mineral element. Its atomic number is 12; its atomic weight is 24.32. Magnesium is the second most abundant cation of the intracellular fluids in the body and is essential for many enzyme activities. It is important to neurochemical transmissions and muscular excitability. Excess magnesium also causes vasodilatation by directly affecting the blood vessels and by ganglionic blockade. Hypomagnesaemia can cause changes in cardiac muscles and skeletal muscle and can cause nephrocalcinosis.

magnesium sulphate, a salt of magnesium prescribed parenterally to correct magnesium deficiency, and orally to treat constipation and heartburn.

magnetic moment, a measure of the net magnetic field produced by an elementary particle or an atomic nucleus spinning about its own axis. It is the basis for nuclear magnetic resonance imaging.

magnetic resonance imaging (MRI), method of imaging based on the principle of nuclear magnetic resonance.

magnetic susceptibility, a measure of the ability of a substance to become magnetized.

magnetic tape, a ribbon of plastic tape coated with an electromagnetic compound that allows for the coding of information in the form of positive and negative charges.

magnetization, the magnetic polarization of a material produced by a magnetic field (magnetic moment per unit volume).

magnetotherapy, a system in which magnets are applied to parts of the body as a means of treatment. An approach pioneered by 18th century Swiss born doctor, Franz Mesmer, who studied in Vienna and developed the idea that man is affected by various forces found in the universe. Scientists have found that when exposed to magnetism, many chemical and physical properties of water change; that the sedimentation rate of a fluid (blood) changes; and that a weak electric current is generated when a magnet touches the human body, increasing the number of ions in the blood which has a positive effect on the body as a whole.

magnet reflex, a pathological reflex seen in an animal that has had its cerebellum removed. If the animal is placed on its back and its head is strongly flexed, all four limbs will flex. Then light pressure by a finger on a toepad causes contraction of limb extensor muscles so that if the finger is slowly removed the limb appears to follow the finger.

magnetron, a source of microwave energy used in medical linear accelerators to accelerate electrons to the therapeutic energies.

magnification, 1. (in radiotheraphy) increase in size of an object when views on an image due to diverging nature of x-ray beam. **2.** (in psychology) cognitive distortion in which the effects of one's behaviour are magnified. See also **minimization.**

magnification factor, (in radiology) factor calculated by dividing image size by the object size.

mag tape, *informal.* See **magnetic tape.**

Mahaim fibres, conductive tracts in cardiac tissue running between the AV node or bundle of His and the muscle of the ventricular septum. They conduct early excitation impulses.

main en griffe. See **clawhand.**

mainframe computer, a large general-purpose computer system for high-volume data processing tasks.

main memory, the memory of a computer contained in its circuitry.

mains voltage compensator, an electrical device that monitors electric power and makes automatic adjustments for fluctuations in voltage.

maintenance dose, the amount of drug required to keep a desired mean steady-state concentration in the tissues.

Majocchi's granuloma {Domenico Majocchi, Italian dermatologist, b. 1849}, a rare type of tinea corporis, mainly affecting the lower legs. It is caused by the fungus *Trichophyton*, which infects the hairs of the affected site and raises spongy granulomas.

major affective disorder, any of a group of psychotic disorders characterized by prolonged and persistent disturbances of mood and related thought distortions, and by other symptoms associated with either depressed or manic states, such as occurs in bipolar disorder, depression, and involutional melancholia.

major connector, a metal plate or bar, used for joining the components of one side of a removable partial denture to those on the opposite side of the dental arch.

major depressive episode. See **endogenous depression, unipolar disorder.**

major element. See **macronutrient.**

major renal calyx. See **renal calyx.**

major surgery, any surgical procedure that requires general anaesthesia or respiratory assistance.

mal, an illness or disease, such as grand mal or petit mal.

malabsorption, impaired absorption of nutrients from the gastrointestinal tract. It occurs in coeliac disease, sprue, dysentery, diarrhoea, and other disorders.

malabsorption syndrome, a complex of symptoms resulting from disorders in the intestinal absorption of nutrients, characterized by anorexia, weight loss, bloating of the abdomen, muscle cramps, bone pain, and steatorrhoea. Anaemia, weakness, and fatigue occur because iron, folic acid, and vitamin B_{12} are not absorbed in sufficient quantity.

malacia, 1. a morbid softening or a sponginess in any part or any tissue of the body. **2.** a craving for spicy foods, such as mustard, hot peppers, or pickles. **malacic,** *adj.*

maladaptation, faulty intrapersonal adaptation to stress or change. It may involve a failure to make necessary changes in the desires, values, needs, and attitudes or an inability to make necessary adjustments to the external world.

malaise, a vague feeling of bodily weakness or discomfort, often marking the onset of disease.

malalignment, a failure of parts of the body to align normally, such as the teeth in the dental arch.

malar, of or pertaining to the cheek or the cheek bone.

malaria, a serious infectious illness caused by one or more of at least four species of the protozoan genus *Plasmodium*, characterized by chills, fever, anaemia, an enlarged spleen, and a tendency to recur. The disease is transmitted from human to human by a bite from an infected *Anopheles* mosquito. Malarial infection can also be spread by blood transfusion from an infected patient or by the use of an infected hypodermic needle. *Plasmodium* parasites penetrate the erythrocytes of the human host, where they mature, reproduce, and burst out periodically. Malarial paroxysms occur at regular intervals, coinciding with the development of a new generation of parasites in the body. **malarial,** *adj.*

malarial haemoglobinuria. See **blackwater fever.**

Malassezia, a genus of fungi. *M. furfur* causes tinea versicolor (previous name: *Pityrosporum oviculare*). *M. ovalis* is a nonpathogenic organism found in sebaceous areas (previous name: *Pityrosporum ovale*).

malathion poisoning, a toxic condition caused by the ingestion or absorption through the skin of malathion, an organophosphorus insecticide. Symptoms include vomiting, nausea, abdominal cramps, headache, dizziness, weakness, confusion, convulsions, and respiratory difficulties.

malaxation. See **pétrissage.**

Malayan pit viper venom. See **ancrod.**

mal del pinto. See **pinta.**

mal de mer. See **motion sickness.**

male, 1. of or pertaining to the sex that produces sperm cells and fertilizes the female to beget children; masculine. **2.** a male person.

male reproductive system assessment, an evaluation of the condition of the patient's genitalia, reproductive history, and past and present genitourinary infections and disorders.

male sexual dysfunction, impaired or inadequate ability of a man to carry on his sex life to his own satisfaction. Symptoms, often psychological in origin, include difficulties in starting and maintaining an erection, premature ejaculation, inability to ejaculate, and even loss of desire.

malfeasance, performance of an unlawful, wrongful act.

malformation, an anomalous structure in the body.

Malgaigne's fracture of the pelvis, trauma involving multiple pelvic fractures, including fracture of the wing of the ilium or sacrum and fracture of the ipsilateral pubic rami, with associated upper displacement of the hemipelvis.

malignant, 1. also virulent. tending to become worse and cause death. **2.** (describing a cancer) anaplastic, invasive, and metastatic. **malignancy,** *n.*

malignant ependymoma. See **ependymoblastoma.**

malignant haemangioendothelioma. See **angiosarcoma.**

malignant hepatoma, a malignant tumour of the liver.

malignant hypertension, a lethal form of both essential hypertension and secondary hypertension. It is a fulminating condition, characterized by severely elevated blood pressure, that commonly damages the intima of small vessels, the brain, retina, heart, and kidneys.

malignant hyperthermia (MH), an autosomal dominant trait characterized by often fatal hyperthermia with rigidity of the muscles occurring in affected people exposed to certain anaesthetic agents.

malignant malnutrition. See **kwashiorkor.**

malignant melanoma. See **melanoma.**

malignant mesenchymoma, a sarcoma that contains mesenchymal elements.

malignant mole. See **melanoma.**

malignant neoplasm, a tumour that tends to grow, invade, and metastasize. It usually has an irregular shape and is composed of poorly differentiated cells. If untreated, it may result in the death of the organism. The degree to which a neoplasm is malignant varies with the kind of tumour and the condition of the patient.

malignant neuroma. See **neurosarcoma.**

malignant pustule. See **anthrax.**

malignant tumour, a neoplasm that characteristically invades surrounding tissue, metastasizes to distant sites, and contains anaplastic cells. A malignant tumour may result in the death of the host if remission or treatment does not intervene.

malingering, a wilful and deliberate feigning of the symptoms of a disease or injury to gain some consciously desired end. **malinger,** *v.,* **malingerer,** *n.*

malleolus, *pl.* **malleoli,** a rounded bony process, such as the protuberance on each side of the ankle.

mallet deformity, a flexion abnormality of the distal joint of a finger or toe. It may be caused by severe damage such as rupture of the terminal tendon.

mallet fracture, avulsion fracture of the dorsal base of a distal phalanx of the hand or foot, involving the associated extensor apparatus and causing dropped flexion of the distal segment.

malleus, *pl.* **mallei,** one of the three ossicles in the middle ear, resembling a hammer with a head, neck, and three processes. It is connected to the tympanic membrane and transmits sound vibrations to the incus.

Mallory bodies, {Frank B. Mallory, American pathologist, b 1862} an eosinophilic cytoplasmic inclusion, alcoholic hyalin, found in the liver cells. It is typically, but not always, associated with acute alcoholic liver injury.

Mallory-Weiss syndrome {G. Kenneth Mallory, American pathologist, b. 1926; Soma Weiss, American physician, b. 1899}, a condition characterized by massive bleeding after a tear in the mucous membrane at the junction of the oesophagus and the stomach. The laceration is usually caused by protracted vomiting, most commonly in alcoholics or in persons whose pylorus is obstructed.

malnutrition, any disorder concerning nutrition. It may result from an unbalanced, insufficient, or excessive diet or to the impaired absorption, assimilation, or use of foods.

malocclusion, abnormal contact of the teeth of the upper jaw with the teeth of the lower jaw. See also **occlusion.**

malonic acid, a white, crystalline, highly toxic substance used as an intermediate compound in the production of barbiturates.

malpighian body {Marcello Malpighi, Italian physician, b. 1628}, **1.** the renal corpuscle, which includes a glomerulus with Bowman's capsule. **2.** lymphoid tissue surrounding the arteries of the spleen.

malpighian corpuscle {Marcello Malpighi}, one of a number of small, round, deep-red bodies in the cortex of the kidney, each communicating with a renal tubule. Malpighian corpuscles average about 0.2 mm in diameter, each composed of two parts: a central glomerulus and a glomerular capsule.

malpractice, (in law) professional negligence that is the proximate cause of injury or harm to a patient, resulting from a lack of professional knowledge, experience, or skill that can be expected in others in the profession or from a failure to exercise reasonable care or judgment in the application of professional knowledge, experience, or skill.

malrotation, 1. any abnormal rotation of an

organ or body part, such as the vertebral column or a tooth. **2.** a failure of the intestinal tract or other viscera to undergo normal rotation during embryonic development.

Malta fever. See **brucellosis.**

malt worker's lung, a respiratory disorder acquired by occupational exposure to fungi-laden particles of mouldy barley grain or malt. See also **organic dust.**

malunion, an imperfect union of previously fragmented bone or other tissue.

mammary duct. See **lactiferous duct.**

mammary gland, one of two discoid, hem-ispheric glands on the chest of mature fe-males, present in rudimentary form in chil-dren and in males. Glandular tissue forms a radius of lobes containing alveoli, each lobe having a system of ducts for the passage of milk from the alveoli to the nipple. The pe-riphery is made up mostly of adipose tissue.

mammary papilla. See **nipple.**

mammillary body, either of the two small round masses of gray matter in the hypothalamus located close to one another in the interpeduncular space.

mammography, radiographic technique to visualize the tissues of the breasts. **mammogram,** *n.*

mammoplasty, plastic reshaping of the breasts, performed to reduce or lift enlarged or sagging breasts, to enlarge small breasts, or to reconstruct a breast after removal of a tumour.

mammothermography, a diagnostic proce-dure in which thermography is used to ex-amine the breast to detect abnormal growths.

mandible, a large bone constituting the low-er jaw. It contains the lower teeth and con-sists of a horizontal portion, a body, and two perpendicular rami that join the body at al-most right angles. The body of the mandible is curved, somewhat resembling a horse-shoe, and has two surfaces and two borders. **mandibular,** *adj.*

mandibular canal, (in dentistry) a passage or channel that extends from the mandibular foramen on the medial surface of the ramus of the mandible to the mental foramen. It holds mandibular blood vessels and a por-tion of the mandibular branch of the inferior dental nerve.

mandibular notch, a depression in the infe-rior border of the mandible, anterior to the attachments of the masseter muscle, where the external facial muscles cross the lower border of the mandible.

mandibular sling, the connection between the mandible and the maxilla, formed by the masseter and the pterygoideus at the angle of the mandible.

mandibulofacial dysostosis, an abnormal hereditary condition characterized by antimongoloid slant of the palpebral fis-sures, colomboma of the lower lid, micrognathia and hypoplasia of the

zygomatic arches, and microtia.

mandrel, a shaft secured in a handpiece or lathe to support an object to be rotated, such as a dental polishing disc or cutting device.

manganese (Mn), a common metallic ele-ment found in trace amounts in tissues of the body where it aids in the functions of vari-ous enzymes. Its atomic number is 25; its atomic weight is 54.938.

mania, a mood disorder characterized by an expansive emotional state, extreme excite-ment, excessive elation, hyperactivity, agita-tion, overtalkativeness, flight of ideas, in-creased psychomotor activity, fleeting atten-tion, and sometimes violent, destructive, or self-destructive behaviour. It is manifested in the major affective disorders as the manic phase of bipolar disorder. Kinds of mania include **Bell's mania, dancing mania, epi-leptic mania, hysterical mania, periodic mania, puerperal mania, and religious mania. maniac,** *n.*, *adj.*, **maniacal,** *adj.*

manic depressive, a person with or exhibit-ing the symptoms of bipolar disorder.

manic-depressive psychosis. See **bipolar disorder.**

manipulation, the skillful use of the hands in therapeutic or diagnostic procedures, such as palpation, reducing a dislocation, turning the position of the fetus, or various treatments in physiotherapy and osteopathy.

mannitol, a poorly metabolized sugar used as an osmotic diuretic, and to decrease intraocular and intracranial pressure.

manoeuvre, 1. an adroit or skillful manipu-lation or procedure. **2.** (in obstetrics) a ma-nipulation of the fetus performed to aid in delivery.

manometer, a device for measuring the pressure of a fluid, consisting of a tube marked with a scale and containing a rela-tively incompressible fluid, such as mercu-ry. The level of the fluid in the tube varies with the pressure of the fluid. Kinds of ma-nometers are **anaeroid manometer** and **sphygmomanometer.**

Mansonella ozzardi, a parasitic worm that is indigenous to Latin America and the Carib-bean islands. It is a relatively benign nema-tode that infects humans. The larvae live in the bloodstream and adult worms are found in the visceral mesenteries.

Mantoux test {Charles Mantoux, French physician, b. 1877}, a tuberculin skin test that consists of intradermal injection of a purified protein derivative of the tubercle bacillus. A hardened, raised red area of 8 to 10 mm, appearing 24 to 72 hours after injec-tion, is a positive reaction.

manual afterloading, a brachytherapy tech-nique in which applicators are positioned and verified using dummy sources and sub-sequently loaded with the active sources. The technique allows optimal positioning of applicators with no radiation dose to theatre staff, although the clinician loading (and unloading) the sources and the nursing staff will be exposed to radiation. Suitable shielding around the patient will minimize patient dose.

manubriosternal articulation, the fibrocartilaginous connection between manubrium and the body of the sternum.

manubrium, one of the three bones of the sternum, presenting a broad quadrangular shape that narrows caudally at its articulation with the superior end of the body of the sternum. **manubrial,** *adj.*

manus. See **hand.**

many-tailed bandage, 1. a broad, evenly shaped bandage with both ends split into strips of equal size and number. As the bandage is placed on the abdomen, chest, or limb, the ends may be overlapped. **2.** an irregularly shaped bandage with torn or cut ends that are tied together.

MAO, abbreviation for **monoamine oxidase.**

MAOI, abbreviation for **monoamine oxidase inhibitor.**

MAP, abbreviation for **mean arterial pressure.**

map distance. See **map unit.**

maple syrup urine disease, an inherited metabolic disorder in which an enzyme necessary for the breakdown of the amino acids valine, leucine, and isoleucine is lacking. The disease is recognized by the characteristic maple syrup odour of the urine and by hyperreflexia.

mapping, (in genetics) the process of locating the relative position of genes on a chromosome through the analysis of genetic recombination.

maprotiline hydrochloride, an antidepressant similar to the tricyclics.

map unit, (in genetics) an arbitrary unit of measure used to designate the distance between genes on a chromosome. It is calculated from the percentage of recombinations that occur between specific genes so that 1% of crossing over represents one unit on a genetic map.

marasmic kwashiorkor, a malnutrition disease, primarily of children, resulting from the deficiency of both calories and protein. The condition is characterized by severe tissue wasting, dehydration, loss of subcutaneous fat, lethargy, and growth retardation.

marasmic thrombus, an aggregation of blood platelets, fibrin, clotting factors, and cellular elements formed in infants with marasmus.

marasmus, a condition of extreme malnutrition and emaciation, occurring chiefly in young children, that is characterized by progressive wasting of subcutaneous tissue and muscle. It results from a lack of adequate calories and proteins and is seen in failure to thrive children and in starvation.

marathon encounter group, an intensive group experience that accelerates self-awareness and promotes personal growth and behavioural change through the continuous interaction of group members for a period ranging from 16 to more than 40 hours.

marble bones. See **osteopetrosis.**

Marburg-Ebola virus disease, a serious febrile disease characterized by rash and severe GI haemorrhages. This disease may be transmitted to hospital personnel by improper handling of contaminated needles or from haemorrhagic lesions of patients. The diagnosis is made by serological abnormalities.

march foot, an abnormal condition of the foot caused by excessive use, such as in a long march. The forefoot is swollen and painful, and one or more of the metatarsal bones may be broken.

march fracture. See **metatarsal stress fracture.**

march haemoglobinuria, a rare, abnormal condition, characterized by the presence of haemoglobin in the urine, that occurs after strenuous physical exertion or prolonged exercise, such as marching or distance running.

Marchiafava-Micheli disease {Ettore Marchiafava, Italian physician, b. 1847; F. Micheli, Italian physician, b. 1872}, a rare disorder of unknown origin characterized by episodic haemoglobinuria, occurring usually, but not always, at night.

Marchi's method {Vittoria Marchi, Italian physician, b. 1851}, a laboratory staining procedure for demonstrating degenerated nerve fibres.

Marcus Gunn pupil sign {Robert Marcus Gunn, English ophthalmologist, b. 1850}, paradoxical dilatation of the pupils in an ophthalmological examination in response to afferent visual stimuli. In a dark room a beam of light is moved from one eye to the other. Normal miosis is caused by the consensual pupil reaction when the normal eye is illuminated; but as the light is moved to the opposite, abnormal eye, the direct reaction to light is weaker than the consensual reaction; hence both pupils dilate.

Marcus Gunn syndrome. See **jaw-winking.**

Marfan's syndrome {Bernard-Jean A. Marfan, French paediatrician, b. 1858}, an abnormal condition characterized by elongation of the bones, often with associated abnormalities of the eyes and the cardiovascular system. The disease causes major pathological musculoskeletal disturbances, such as muscular underdevelopment, ligamentous laxity, joint hypermobility, and bone elongation. With Marfan's syndrome pathological alterations of the cardiovascular system appear to produce fragmentation of the elastic fibres in the media of the aorta, which may lead to aneurysm. Ocular changes associated with the disease include a variety of disorders, including dislocation of the lens. The disease affects men and women equally, elongating the limbs so that most adult patients with the disease are over 6 feet tall. The extremities of individuals with Marfan's syndrome are very long and spiderlike, with greatly extended metacarpals, metatarsals, and phalanges.

marginal peptic ulcer, an ulcer that develops postoperatively at the surgical anastomosis of the stomach and jejunum.

marginal rale. See **atelectatic rale.**

marginal ridge, an elevation of enamel that forms the proximal boundary of the occlusal surface of a tooth.

Marie's hypertrophy {Pierre Marie, French neurologist, b. 1853}, chronic enlargement of the joints caused by periostitis.

Marie-Strümpell disease. See **ankylosing spondylitis.**

marijuana. See **cannabis.**

Marin Amat syndrome, an involuntary facial movement phenomenon in which the eyes close when the mouth opens or when the jaws move in mastication. The effect results from a facial nerve paralysis.

mark, any naevus or birthmark.

marker gene. See **genetic marker.**

markers, body language movements that serve as indicators and punctuation marks in interpersonal communication.

marrow. See **bone marrow.**

Marseilles fever {Marseilles, France}, a disease endemic around the Mediterranean, in Africa, in the Crimea, and in India, caused by *Rickettsia conorii* transmitted by the brown dog tick. Symptoms include chills, fever, an ulcer covered with a black crust at the site of the tick bite, and a rash appearing on the second to fourth day.

Marshall-Marchetti operation {Victor F. Marshall, American urologist, b. 1913; Andrew A. Marchetti, American obstetrician, b. 1901}, a surgical procedure performed to correct a condition of stress incontinence. The procedure, a vesicourethropexy, involves a retropubic incision and suturing of the urethra, vesicle neck, and bladder to the posterior surface of the pubic bone.

marsupialize, to form a pouch surgically to treat a cyst when simple removal would not be effective, such as in a pancreatic or a pilonidal cyst.

Martorell's syndrome. See **Takayasu's arteritis.**

masculine, having the characteristics of a male.

masculinization, the normal development or induction of male sex characteristics. **masculinize,** *v.*

mask, 1. to obscure, as in symptomatic treatment that may mask the development of a disease. **2.** to cover, as does a skin-toned cosmetic that may mask a pigmented naevus. **3.** a cover worn over the nose and mouth to prevent inhalation of toxic or irritating materials, to control delivery of oxygen or anaesthetic gas, or (by medical personnel) to shield a patient during aseptic procedures from pathogenic organisms normally exhaled from the respiratory tract.

mask image, (in digital fluoroscopy) an x-ray image made immediately after contrast material has been injected but before it reaches the anatomic site being examined. The initial mask image is then subtracted electronically from a series of additional images. The technique has the effect of enhancing the image of the tissues being studied.

masking, 1. the covering or concealing of a disorder by a second condition, as when a person begins a weight-loss diet while an undiagnosed wasting disease such as cancer has developed. **2.** the unconscious display of a personality trait that conceals a behavioural aberration.

masking agent, a cosmetic preparation for covering naevi, surgical scars, and other blemishes.

mask of pregnancy. See **chloasma.**

Maslow's hierarchy of need {Abraham H. Maslow, American psychiatrist, b. 1908}, (in psychology) a hierarchical categorization of the basic needs of humans. The most basic needs on the scale are the physiological or biological, such as the need for air, food, or water. Of second priority are the safety needs, including protection and freedom from fear and anxiety. The subsequent order of needs in the hierarchic progression are the need to belong, to love, and to be loved; the need for self-esteem; and ultimately, the need for self-actualization.

masochism {Leopold von Sacher-Masoch, Austrian author, b. 1836}, pleasure or gratification derived from receiving physical, mental, or emotional abuse. **masochistic,** *adj.*

masochist {Leopold von Sacher-Masoch}, a person deriving pleasure or gratification from masochistic acts or abuse.

mass, 1. the physical property of matter that gives it weight and inertia. **2.** (in pharmacology) a mixture from which pills are formed. **3.** an aggregate of cells clumped together such as a tumour.

massage, the manipulation of the soft tissue of the body through stroking, rubbing, kneading, or tapping, to increase circulation, to improve muscle tone, and to relax the patient. The procedure is performed either with the bare hands or through some mechanical means, such as a vibrator. The most common sites for massage are the back, knees, elbows, and heels. Kinds of massage are **cardiac massage, effleurage, flagella-**

tion, friction, frôlement, pétrissage, tapotement, and vibration.

mass attenuation coefficient, the fraction of x-rays removed from an x-ray beam of unit cross-sectional area in a medium of unit mass, for a given interaction process.

masseter, the thick, rectangular muscle in the cheek that functions to close the jaw. It is one of the four muscles of mastication.

mass fragment, a degraded portion of a molecule containing one or more charges.

mass number (A), the sum of the number of protons and neutrons in the nucleus of an atom or isotope.

mass reflex, an abnormal condition, seen in patients with transection of the spinal cord, characterized by a widespread nerve discharge, resulting in flexor muscle spasms, incontinence of urine and faeces, priapism, hypertension, and profuse sweating. A mass reflex may be triggered by scratching or other painful stimulus to the skin, overdistention of the bladder or intestines, cold weather, prolonged sitting, or emotional stress.

mass spectrometer, an analytical instrument for identifying a substance by sorting a stream of charged particles (ions) according to their mass.

mass spectrometry, (in chemistry) a technique for the analysis of a substance in which the constituents are identified and quantified using a mass spectrometer.

mass storage device, a secondary memory device capable of storing large amounts of data.

mass transfer, the movement of mass from one phase to another.

mastalgia, pain in the breast caused by congestion or "caking" during lactation, an infection, fibrocystic disease, especially during or before menstruation, or advanced cancer. The early stages of breast cancer are rarely accompanied by pain. **mastalgic,** *adj.*

mast cell, a constituent of connective tissue containing large basophilic granules that bear heparin, serotonin, bradykinin, and histamine.

mast cell leukaemia, a malignant neoplasm of leukocytes characterized by many connective tissue mast cells in circulating blood.

mastectomy, the surgical removal of one or both breasts, performed to remove a malignant tumour. In a simple mastectomy, only breast tissue is removed. In a radical mastectomy, some of the muscles of the chest are removed with the breast with all lymph nodes in the axilla. In a modified radical mastectomy, the large muscles of the chest that move the arm are preserved. Emotional support and counselling are essential.

Master's Degree in Nursing, a postgraduate programme in a faculty of nursing, based in a university setting, that grants the degree Master of Science (MSc) in Nursing to successful candidates.

mastery, being in command or control of a situation, as in learning accomplishment.

mastication, chewing, tearing, or grinding food with the teeth while it becomes mixed with saliva.

masticatory system, the combination of organs, structures, and nerves involved in chewing. It includes but is not limited to the jaws, the teeth and their supporting structures, the mandibular musculature, the mandible, the maxillae, the temporomandibular joints, the tongue, the lips, the cheeks, the oral mucosa, and cranial nerves.

mastitis, an inflammatory condition of the breast, usually caused by streptococcal or staphylococcal infection. **Acute mastitis,** most common in the first 2 months of lactation, is characterized by pain, swelling, redness, axillary lymphadenopathy, fever, and malaise. If untreated or inadequately treated, abscesses may form. **Chronic tuberculous mastitis** is rare; when it occurs, it represents extension of tuberculosis from the lungs and ribs beneath the breast.

mastocytosis, local or systemic overproduction of mast cells, which, in rare instances, may infiltrate liver, spleen, bones, the GI system, and skin.

mastoid, 1. of or pertaining to the mastoid process of the temporal bone. **2.** breast-shaped.

mastoidectomy, surgical excision of a portion of the mastoid part of the temporal bone, performed to treat chronic suppurative otitis media or mastoiditis when systemic antibiotics are ineffective. In a simple mastoidectomy, infected bone cells are removed and the eardrum is incised to drain the middle ear.

mastoid fontanelle, a posterolateral fontanelle that is usually not palpable.

mastoiditis, an infection of one of the mastoid bones, usually an extension of a middle ear infection, characterized by earache, fever, headache, and malaise. The infection is difficult to treat, often requiring antibiotics administered intravenously for several days.

mastoid process, the conic projection of the caudal, posterior portion of the temporal bone, serving as the attachment for various muscles, including the sternocleidomastoideus, splenius capitis, and longissimus capitis.

masturbation, sexual activity in which the penis or clitoris is stimulated, usually to orgasm, by means other than coitus. **masturbate,** *v,* **masturbatic, masturbatory,** *adj.*

matched group. See group.

materia, matter or material, such as materia medica.

materia medica, 1. the study of drugs and other substances used in medicine, their origins, preparation, uses, and effects. **2.** a substance or a drug used in medical treatment.

maternal and child health services, various facilities and programmes organized for the purpose of providing medical and social services for mothers and children. Medical services include antenatal and postnatal care, family planning services, paediatric care, health visitor services and immunization clinics.

maternal-child attachment, the complex process of attachment of a mother to her newborn baby. In the first minutes and hours after birth, a sensitive period occurs during which the baby and the mother become intimately involved with each other through behaviours and stimuli that are complementary and that provoke further interactions. The mother touches the baby and holds it en face to achieve eye-to-eye contact. The infant looks back eye to eye. The mother speaks in a quiet, high-pitched voice. The mother and the baby move in turn to the voice and sounds of the other, a process known as entrainment; it can be likened to a dance. The infant's movements constitute a response to the mother's voice, and she is encouraged to continue the process.

maternal-child separation syndrome. See **separation anxiety.**

maternal deprivation syndrome, a condition characterized by developmental retardation that occurs as a result of physical or emotional deprivation. It is seen primarily in infants. Typical symptoms include lack of physical growth, with weight below the third percentile for age and size, malnutrition, pronounced withdrawal, silence, apathy, and irritability, and a characteristic posture and body language, featuring unnatural stiffness and rigidity with a slow response reaction to others.

maternal effect. See **maternal inheritance.**

maternal-infant bonding. See **maternal-child attachment.**

maternal inheritance, the transmission of traits or conditions controlled by cytoplasmic factors within the ovum that are not self-replicating and are determined by genes within the nucleus.

maternal mortality, the death of a woman during the child bearing cycle, per 1000 registered total births.

mat gold, a noncohesive form of pure gold, which is prepared by electrodeposition and may be used in the base of some dental restorations.

matrifocal family, a family unit composed of a mother and her children. Biological fathers have a temporary place in the family during the first years of the children's lives, but they maintain a more permanent position in their own original families.

matrix, 1. an intercellular substance, **2.** a basic substance from which a specific organ or kind of tissue develops. **3.** a form used in shaping a tooth surface in dental procedures.

matrix retainer, a mechanical device used to secure the ends of a matrix around a tooth and help compact a restoration in a tooth cavity.

matter, 1. anything that has mass and occupies space. **2.** any substance not otherwise identified as to its constituents, such as grey matter, pus, or serum exuding from a wound.

Matthews Duncan expulsion of the placenta, the placenta is delivered maternal side first, during the third stage of labour with a heavier blood loss.

maturation, 1. the process or condition of attaining complete development. In humans it is the unfolding of full physical, emotional, and intellectual capacities that enable a person to function at a higher level of competency and adaptability within the environment. **2.** the final stages in the meiotic formation of germ cells in which the number of chromosomes in each cell is reduced to the haploid number characteristic of the species. **3.** suppuration. **maturate,** v.

maturational crisis, a transitional or developmental period within a person's life, such as puberty, when his or her psychological equilibrium is upset.

mature, 1. to become fully developed; to ripen. **2.** fully developed or ripened.

mature cell leukaemia. See **polymorphocytic leukaemia.**

maturity, 1. a state of complete growth or development, usually designated as the period of life between adolescence and old age. **2.** the stage at which an organism is capable of reproduction.

maturity-onset diabetes. See **non-insulin-dependent diabetes mellitus**

Mauriceau-Smellie-Viet manoeuvre, a method of delivering the aftercoming head of a breech; it combines jaw flexion and shoulder traction. The baby is straddled across one arm, the middle finger is inserted into the baby's mouth and the other two fingers rest on the baby's malar bones. The other hand rests on the baby's shoulders with the middle finger on the occiput in order to aid flexion.

maxilla, *pl.* **maxillae,** one of a pair of large bones that form the upper jaw, consisting of a pyramidal body and four processes: the zygomatic, frontal, alveolar, and palatine.

maxillary artery, either of two larger terminal branches of the external carotid arteries that rise from the neck of the mandible near the parotid gland and divide into three branches, supplying the deep structures of the face.

maxillary fossa. See **canine fossa.**

maxillary sinus, one of the pair of large air cells forming a pyramidal cavity in the body of the maxilla.

maxillary vein, one of a pair of deep veins of the face, accompanying the maxillary artery. Each maxillary vein is a tributary of the internal jugular and the external jugular veins.

maxillofacial prosthesis, a prosthetic replacement for part, or all, of the upper jaw, nose, or cheek. It is applied when surgical repair alone is inadequate.

maxillomandibular fixation, stabilization of fractures of the face or jaw by temporarily connecting the maxilla and mandible by wires, elastic bands, or metalsplints.

maximal breathing capacity (MBC), the amount of gas exchanged per minute with maximal rate and depth of respiration.

maximal diastolic membrane potential, (in cardiology) the greatest degree of negative transmembrane potential achieved by a cell during diastole.

maximal expiratory flow rate (MEFR), the rate of the most rapid flow of gas from the lungs during the expiratory phase of respiration.

maximal midexpiratory flow rate, the average volumetric rate of gas flow during the middle half (in terms of volume) of a forced expiratory vital capacity manoeuvre.

maximal voluntary ventilation, the maximal volume of gas that a person can ventilate by voluntary effort per unit of time breathing as quickly and deeply as possible.

maximum diastolic potential. See **maximal diastolic membrane potential.**

maximum inspiratory pressure (MIP), the maximum pressure within the alveoli of the lungs that occurs during the inspiratory phase of respiration.

maximum oxygen uptake, the greatest amount of oxygen that can be transported from the lungs to the working muscle tissue.

maximum permissible dose (MPD), (historical) See **dose limit.**

Mayer's reflex {Karl Mayer, Austrian neurologist, b. 1862}, a normal reflex elicited by grasping the ring finger and flexing it at the metacarpophalangeal joint of a person whose hand is relaxed with thumb abducted. The normal response is adduction and apposition of the thumb.

May-Hegglin anomaly {Richard May, German physician, b. 1863; Robert M. P. Hegglin, 20th century Swiss physician}, an inherited haematological condition characterized by leukopenia, giant platelets, and Döhle bodies.

Mayo scissors. See **scissors.**

mazindol, an appetite supressant formerly used in the treatment of obesity.

MBC, abbreviation for **maximal breathing capacity.**

MBD, abbreviation for **minimal brain dysfunction.** See **attention deficit disorder.**

mC, abbreviation for **millicoulomb.**

McArdle's disease {Brian McArdle, 20th century English neurologist}, an inherited metabolic disease marked by an absence of myophosphorylase B and abnormally large amounts of glycogen in skeletal muscle. It is milder than other glycogen storage diseases.

McBurney's point {Charles McBurney, American surgeon, b. 1845}, a site of extreme sensitivity in acute appendicitis, situated in the normal area of the appendix about 2 inches from the right anterior superior spine of the ilium, on a line between that spine and the umbilicus.

McBurney's sign, a reaction of the patient indicating severe pain and extreme tenderness when McBurney's point is palpated. Such a reaction indicates appendicitis.

mcg, abbreviation for **microgram.**

MCH, abbreviation for **mean corpuscular haemoglobin.**

MCHC, abbreviation for **mean corpuscular haemoglobin concentration.**

mCi, abbreviation for **millicurie.**

McMurray's sign {Thomas P. McMurray, English surgeon, b. 1887}, an audible click heard when rotating the tibia on the femur, indicating injury to meniscal structures.

MCTD, abbreviation for **mixed connective tissue disease.**

MCV, abbreviation for **mean corpuscular volume.**

Md, symbol for **mendelevium.**

M.D., abbreviation for *Doctor of Medicine* a postgraduate qualification.

m.d., m.d.u., (in prescriptions) abbreviations for the Latin phrase *'more dicto utendus, a, um'* maining 'to be used as directed'.

MDCR, abbreviation for *Management Diploma of the College of Radiographers.*

Me, abbreviation for the methyl radical CH_3.

Meals on Wheels, a programme designed to deliver hot meals to elderly, physically disabled, or other persons who lack the resources to provide themselves with nutritionally adequate warm meals on a regular basis. This is sometimes administered by the local Department of Social Services but more usually by voluntary groups such as the Women's Royal Voluntary Service.

Mean, occupying a position midway between two extremes of a set of values or data. The **arithmetic mean** is a value that is derived by dividing the total of a set of values by the number of items in the set. The **geometric mean** is a value that is between the first and last of a set of values organized in a geometric progression.

mean arterial pressure (MAP), the arithmetical mean of the blood pressure in the arterial portion of the circulation.

mean corpuscular diameter (MCD), the average diameter of a red corpuscle in micrometers (μm), normally 7.2 (6.6-7.7) μm increased in pernicious anaemia, often reduced in iron deficiency.

mean corpuscular haemoglobin (MCH), an estimate of the amount of haemoglobin in an average erythrocyte, derived from the ratio between the amount of haemoglobin and the number of erythrocytes present in a specimen.

mean corpuscular haemoglobin concentration (MCHC), an estimation of the concentration of haemoglobin in grams per 100 ml of packed red blood cells, derived from the ratio of the haemoglobin to the haematocrit.

mean corpuscular volume (MCV), an evaluation of the average volume of each red cell, derived from the ratio of the volume of packed red cells (the haematocrit) to the total number of red blood cells.

measles, an acute, highly contagious, viral disease involving the respiratory tract and characterized by a spreading maculopapular cutaneous rash that occurs primarily in young children who have not been immunized. Measles is caused by a paramyxovirus and is transmitted by direct contact with droplets spread from the nose, throat, and mouth of infected persons, usually in the prodromal stage of the disease. Indirect transmission by uninfected persons or by contaminated articles is unusual. An incubation period of 7 to 14 days is followed by the prodromal stage, characterized by fever, malaise, coryza, cough, conjunctivitis, photophobia, anorexia, and the pathognomonic Koplik's spots, which appear 1 to 2 days before onset of the rash. Pharyngitis and inflammation of the laryngeal and tracheobronchial mucosa develop, the temperature may rise to 39.5° or 40° C and there is marked granulocytic leukopenia. The papules of the rash first appear as irregular brownish-pink spots around the hairline, the ears, and the neck, then spread rapidly, within 24 to 48 hours, to the trunk and extremities, becoming red, maculopapular, and dense, giving a blotchy appearance. Within 3 to 5 days, the fever subsides, and the lesions flatten, turn a brownish colour, and begin to fade, causing a fine desquamation, especially over heavily affected areas.

measles immune globulin. See **immune gamma globulin.**

measles mumps rubella vaccine (MMR), a combined, live vaccine used for simultaneous active immunization against measles, mumps, and rubella.

measles vaccine, active immunization against measles, now largely replaced by **measles mumps rubella vaccine (MMR).**

measurement, the determination, expressed numerically, of the extent or quantity of a substance, energy, or time.

meatorrhaphy, the suturing of the cut end of the urethra to the glans penis after surgery to enlarge the urethral meatus.

meatoscopy, the visual examination of any meatus, especially the urethra, usually performed with the aid of a speculum.

meatus, *pl.* **meatuses, meatus,** an opening or tunnel through any part of the body, as the external acoustic meatus that leads from the external ear to the tympanic membrane.

mebendazole, an anthelmintic prescribed in the treatment of threadworm, whipworm, roundworm, and hookworm infestations.

MEC, abbreviation for *minimum effective concentration.* A drug is effective at any level above this threshold value at its site of action.

mechanical advantage, (in physiology) the ratio of the output force developed by the muscles to the input force applied to the body structures that the muscles move.

mechanical condenser, a device that delivers automatically controlled impacts for condensing restorative material in the filling of tooth cavities.

mechanical vector. See **vector.**

mechanism, 1. an instrument or process by which something is done, results, or comes into being. **2.** a machine or machine-like system. **3.** a stimulus-response system. **4.** a habit or drive.

mechanism of labour. sequence of passive movements made by the fetus in order to pass through the birth canal during labour.

mechanoreceptor, any sensory nerve ending that responds to mechanical stimuli, such as touch, pressure, sound, and muscular contractions.

Meckel's diverticulum {Johann F. Meckel, German anatomist, b. 1781}, an anomalous sac protruding from the wall of the ileum. It is congenital, resulting from the incomplete closure of the yolk stalk.

meclozine hydrochloride, an antihistamine prescribed in the prevention and treatment of motion sickness.

mecocephaly. See **scaphocephaly.**

meconium, a material that collects in the intestines of a fetus and forms the first stools of a newborn. It is thick and sticky in consistency, usually greenish to black in colour, and composed of secretions of the intestinal glands, some amniotic fluid, and intrauterine debris, such as bile pigments, fatty acids, epithelial cells, mucus, lanugo, and blood.

meconium aspiration, the inhalation of meconium by the fetus or newborn, which can block the air passages and result in failure of the lungs to expand or cause other pulmonary dysfunction.

meconium ileus, obstruction of the small intestine in the newborn caused by impaction of thick, dry, tenacious meconium, usually at or near the ileocecal valve. Symptoms include abdominal distention, vomiting, failure to pass meconium within the first 24 to 48 hours after birth, and rapid dehydration with associated electrolyte imbalance.

meconium plug syndrome, obstruction of

the large intestine in the newborn caused by thick, rubbery meconium that may fill the entire colon and part of the terminal ileum. Symptoms include failure to pass meconium within the first 24 to 48 hours after birth, abdominal distention, and vomiting if complete intestinal blockage occurs.

MED, abbreviation for **minimal effective dose.**

medial, 1. situated or oriented toward the midline of the body. **2.** pertaining to the tunica media, the middle layer of a blood vessel wall. Also **mesial.**

medial antebrachial cutaneous nerve, a nerve of the arm that arises from the medial cord of the brachial plexus, medial to the axillary artery.

medial arteriosclerosis. See **Mönckeberg's arteriosclerosis.**

medial brachial cutaneous nerve, a nerve of the arm arising from the medial cord of the brachial plexus and distributed to the medial side of the arm.

medial cuneiform bone, the largest of three cuneiform bones of the foot, situated on the medial side of the tarsus, between the scaphoid bone and the first metatarsal.

medial geniculate body, either of the two areas on the posterior dorsal thalamus, relaying auditory impulses from the lateral lemniscus to the auditory cortex.

medial pectoral nerve, a branch of the brachial plexus that, with the lateral pectoral nerve, supplies the pectoral muscles.

medial rotation, a turning toward the midline of the body.

median, (in statistics) the number representing the middle value of the scores in a sample. In an odd number of scores arrayed in ascending order, it is the middle score; in an even number of scores so arrayed, it is the average of the two central scores.

median antebrachial vein, one of the superficial veins of the upper limb that drains the venous plexus on the palmar surface of the hand.

median aperture of fourth ventricle, an opening between the lower part of the roof of the fourth ventricle and the subarachnoid space.

median atlantoaxial joint, one of three points of articulation of the atlas and the axis. It allows rotation of the axis and the skull, the extent of rotation limited by the alar ligaments.

median basilic vein, one of the superficial veins of the upper limb, often formed as one of two branches from the median cubital vein. It is commonly used for venipuncture, phlebotomy, or intravenous infusion.

median effective dose (ED_{50}), the dose of a drug that may be expected to cause a specific intensity of effect in one half of the patients to whom it is given.

median glossitis. See **median rhomboid glossitis.**

median jaw relation, (in dentistry) any jaw relation that exists when the mandible is in the median sagittal plane.

median lethal dose (MLD, LD_{50}), (in radiotherapy) the see lethal dose.

median nerve, one of the terminal branches of the brachial plexus that extends along the radial portions of the forearm and the hand and supplies various muscles and the skin of these parts.

median palatine suture, the line of junction between the horizontal portions of the palatine bones that extends from both sides of the skull to form the posterior part of the hard palate.

median plane, a vertical plane that divides the body into right and left halves and passes approximately through the sagittal suture of the skull.

median rhomboid glossitis, a red, depressed, diamond-shaped area on the dorsum of the tongue, frequently irritated by alcohol, hot drinks, or spicy foods.

median sternotomy, a chest surgery technique in which an incision is made from the suprasternal notch to below the xiphoid process. The sternum is then opened with a saw. Closure requires reunion of the sternum with stainless steel sutures.

median toxic dose (TD_{50}), the dosage that may be expected to cause a toxic effect in one half of the patients to whom it is given.

mediastinitis, an inflammation of the mediastinum.

mediastinum, *pl.* **mediastina,** a portion of the thoracic cavity in the middle of the thorax, between the pleural sacs containing the two lungs. It extends from the sternum to the vertebral column and contains all the thoracic viscera, except the lungs. It is enclosed in a thick extension of the thoracic subserous fascia. **mediastinal,** *adj.*

mediate, 1. to cause a change to occur, as in stimulation by a hormone. **2.** to settle a dispute, as in collective bargaining. **3.** situated between two places, things, parts, or terms. **4.** (in psychology) an event that follows one process or event and precedes another; for example, in the process of cognition, perception follows stimulation and precedes thinking. **mediating,** *adj.*, **mediator,** *n.*

medical care, the provision by a doctor of services related to the maintenance of health, prevention of illness, and treatment of illness or injury.

medical centre, 1. a health care facility. **2.** a hospital, especially one staffed and equipped to care for many patients and for a large number of kinds of diseases and dysfunctions, using sophisticated technology.

medical consultation, a procedure whereby, on request by one doctor, another doctor reviews a patient's medical history, examines the patient, and makes recommendations as to care and treatment. The medical consultant often is a specialist with expertise in a particular field of medicine.

medical decision level, a concentration of analyte at which some medical action is indicated for proper patient care.

medical director, a doctor who is usually employed by a hospital or other organization to serve in a medical and administrative capacity as head of the organized medical staff.

medical engineering, a field of study that involves biomedical engineering and technologic concepts to develop equipment and instruments required in health care delivery.

medical examiner. See **coroner.**

medical genetics. See **clinical genetics.**

medical history. See **health history.**

medical illustrator, an artist qualified by special training in preparing illustrations of organs, tissues, and medical phenomena in normal and abnormal states.

medical laboratory technician, a person who, under the supervision of a pathologist, physician, or other medical scientist performs microscopic and bacteriological tests of human blood, tissue, and fluids for diagnostic and research purposes.

medical model, the traditional approach to the diagnosis and treatment of illness in which the doctor focuses on the defect, or dysfunction, within the patient. The medical history and the physical examination and diagnostic tests provide the basis for the identification and treatment of a specific illness.

medical physicist, a health scientist who directs research, training and management of programmes in which patients and health professionals are exposed to potential hazards associated with the use of diagnostic and therapeutic equipment, such as radioactive materials.

medical physics, the study of the effects of ionizing radiation on the body and the methods for protecting people from the undesirable effects of radiation.

medical record administrator, a person who maintains records of patients' medical histories, diagnoses, treatment, and outcome, in a condition that meets medical, administrative, legal, ethical, regulatory, and institutional requirements.

medical secretary, a person who prepares and maintains medical records and performs related secretarial duties.

medical staff, all doctors and health professionals responsible for providing health care in a hospital or other health care facility.

medical staff, honorary, doctors and other health professionals, usually retired, who are recognized by the hospital medical staff for their noteworthy contributions but who may

not admit patients to the hospital or participate in medical staff activities.

medical-surgical nursing, the nursing care of patients whose conditions or disorders are treated pharmacologically or surgically.

medical technician. See **medical laboratory technician.**

Medical Women's International Association (M.W.I.A.), an international professional organization of women doctors.

medicated bath, a therapeutic bath in which medication is dispersed in water, usually in the treatment of dermatological disorders.

medicated enema, a medication administered via an enema. It is usually used preoperatively with patients scheduled for bowel surgery.

medication, 1. a drug or other substance that is used as a medicine. **2.** the administration of a medicine.

medicinal treatment, therapy of disorders based chiefly on the use of appropriate pharmacological agents.

medicine, 1. a drug or a remedy for illness. **2.** the art and science of the diagnosis, treatment, and prevention of disease and the maintenance of good health. **3.** the art or technique of treating disease without surgery. Some of the many branches of medicine include **environmental medicine, forensic medicine, general practice, internal medicine,** and **preventive medicine. medical,** *adj.*

medicolegal, of or pertaining to both medicine and law. Medicolegal considerations, decisions, definitions, and policies provide the framework for informed consent, professional liability, and many other aspects of current practice in the health care field.

meditation, a state of consciousness in which the individual eliminates environmental stimuli from awareness so the mind can focus on a single thing, producing a state of calmness and relief from stress.

meditation therapy, a method of achieving relaxation and consciouness expansion by focusing on a mantra, or a key word, sound, or image while eliminating outside stimuli from one's awareness.

Mediterranean anaemia. See **thalassaemia.**

Mediterranean fever. See **brucellosis.**

medium, *pl.* **media,** a substance through which something moves or through which it acts. A **contrast medium** is a substance that has a density different from that of body tissues, permitting visual comparison of structures when used with imaging techniques such as x-ray film. A **culture medium** is a substance that provides a nutritional environment for the growth of microorganisms or cells. A **dispersion medium** is the substance in which a colloid is dispersed. A **refractory medium** is the transparent tissues and fluid of the eye that refract light.

medium-chain triglyceride (MCT), a glycerine ester combined with an acid and distinguished from other triglycerides by having 8 to 10 carbon atoms. MCTs in foods are usually high in calories and easily digested.

MEDLINE, a computer data base from the National Library of Medicine in the United States that covers approximately 600,000 references to biomedical journal articles published currently and in the 2 preceding years. The files duplicate the contents of the *Unabridged Index Medicus,* also published by the National Library of Medicine, which indexes medical reports from 3000 professional journals in more than 70 countries.

medroxyprogesterone acetate, a progestogen used in the treatment of menstrual disorders caused by hormone imbalance, and in the treatment of certain hormone dependent cancers including renal cell, endometrial and breast carcinomas.

medulla, *pl.* **medullas, medullae, 1.** the most internal part of a structure or organ, such as the spinal medulla. See also **marrow. 2.** *informal.* medulla oblongata.

medulla oblongata, the most vital part of the entire brain, continuing as the bulbous portion of the spinal cord just above the foramen magnum. The medulla contains the cardiac, the vasomotor, and the respiratory centres of the brain, and medullary injury or disease often proves fatal.

medullary, 1. of or pertaining to the medulla of the brain. **2.** of or pertaining to the bone marrow. **3.** of or pertaining to the spinal cord and central nervous system.

medullary carcinoma, a soft, malignant neoplasm of the epithelium containing little or no fibrous tissue.

medullary cystic disease, a chronic familial disease of the kidney, characterized by the slow onset of uraemia. The disease appears in young children or adolescents, who pass large volumes of dilute urine with greater than normal amounts of sodium.

medullary fold. See **neural fold.**

medullary groove. See **neural groove.**

medullary plate. See **neural plate.**

medullary sponge kidney, a congenital defect of the kidney, leading to cystic dilatation of the collecting tubules. Persons with this defect often develop a kidney stone or an infection of the kidney caused by urinary stasis.

medullary tube. See **neural tube.**

medulla spinalis. See **spinal cord.**

medullated neuroma. See **fascicular neuroma.**

medulloblastoma, a poorly differentiated malignant neoplasm composed of tightly packed cells of spongioblastic and neuroblastic lineage. The tumour usually arises in the cerebellum.

medulloepithelioma. See **neurocytoma.**

mefenamic acid, a nonsteroidal anti-inflammatory agent and analgesic used in the treatment of mild to moderate pain.

mefloquine, an antimalarial used in the prophylaxis and treatment of chloroquine-resistant falciparum and vivax malaria.

MEFR, abbreviation for **maximal expiratory flow rate.**

megabladder. See **megalocystis.**

megabyte (Mb), one million bytes, or 1000 kilobytes.

megacaryocyte, an extremely large bone marrow cell having a nucleus with many lobes. Megacaryocytes are essential for the production and proliferation of platelets in the marrow and are normally not present in the circulation blood. **megacaryocytic,** *adj.*

megacolon, massive, abnormal dilatation of the colon that may be congenital, toxic, or acquired. **Congenital megacolon** (Hirschsprung's disease) is caused by the absence of autonomic ganglia in the smooth muscle wall of the colon. **Toxic megacolon** is a grave complication of ulcerative colitis and may result in perforation of the colon, septicaemia, and death. **Acquired megacolon** is the result of a chronic refusal to defecate, usually occurring in children who are psychotic or mentally retarded. The colon becomes dilated by an accumulation of impacted faeces. See also **Hirschsprung's disease.**

megakaryocytic leukaemia, a rare malignancy of blood-forming tissue in which megakaryocytes proliferate abnormally in the bone marrow and circulate in the blood in relatively large numbers.

megalencephaly, a condition characterized by pathological parenchymal overgrowth of the brain. In some cases generalized cerebral hyperplasia is associated with mental deficiency or a brain disorder. **megalencephalic, megalencephalous,** *adj.*

megaloblast, an abnormally large nucleated immature erythrocyte that develops in large numbers in the bone marrow and is plentiful in the circulation in many anaemias associated with deficiency of vitamin B_{12}, folic acid, or intrinsic factor. **megaloblastic,** *adj.*

megaloblastic anaemia, a haematological disorder characterized by the production and peripheral proliferation of immature, large, and dysfunctional erythrocytes. Megaloblasts are usually associated with severe pernicious anaemia or folic acid deficiency anaemia.

megalocephaly. See **macrocephaly.**

megalocystis, an abnormal condition characterized by an enlarged and thin-walled bladder. Also called **megabladder.**

megalomania, an abnormal mental state characterized by delusions of grandeur in which one believes oneself to be a person of great importance, power, fame, or wealth.

See also **mania.**

megaloureter, an abnormal condition characterized by marked dilatation of one or both ureters, resulting from dysfunctional peristaltic action of the smooth muscle in the ureters. Treatment may include surgical resection.

megaoesophagus, abnormal dilatation of the lower segments of the oesophagus caused by distention resulting from the failure of the cardiac sphincter to relax and allow the passage of food into the stomach.

megavitamin therapy, a type of treatment that involves the administration of large doses of certain vitamins and minerals.

megestrol acetate, a progestational agent used to treat endometrial and breast cancer.

megrim. See **migraine.**

meibomian cyst. See **chalazion.**

meibomian gland {Heinrich Meibom, German physician, b. 1638}, one of several sebaceous glands that secrete sebum from their ducts on the posterior margin of each eyelid. The glands are embedded in the tarsal plate of each eyelid.

Meigs' syndrome {Joseph V. Meigs, American gynaecologist, b. 1892}, ascites and hydrothorax associated with a fibroma of the ovaries or other pelvic tumour.

meiocyte, any cell undergoing meiosis.

meiogenic, producing or causing meiosis.

meiosis, the division of a sex cell, as it matures, into two, then four gametes, the nucleus of each receiving one half of the number of chromosomes present in the somatic cells of the species. **meiotic,** *adj.*

Meissner's corpuscle. See **tactile corpuscle.**

melaena, abnormal, black, tarry stool containing digested blood. It usually results from bleeding in the upper GI tract and is often a sign of peptic ulcer or small bowel disease.

melancholia, 1. extreme sadness; melancholy. 2. *obsolete.* the major affective depressive disorder.

melanin, a black or dark brown pigment that occurs naturally in the hair, skin, and in the iris and choroid of the eye. See also **melanocyte.**

melanocyte, a body cell capable of producing melanin. Such cells are distributed throughout the basal cell layer of the epidermis and form melanin pigment from tyrosine, an amino acid.

melanocyte stimulating hormone (MSH), a polypeptide hormone, secreted by the anterior pituitary gland, that controls the intensity of pigmentation in pigmented cells.

melanoderma, any abnormal darkening of the skin caused by increased deposits of melanin or by the salts of iron or silver.

melanoma, any of a group of malignant neoplasms, primarily of the skin, that are composed of melanocytes. Most melanomas develop from a pigmented naevus over a period of several months or years and occur most commonly in fair-skinned people having light-coloured eyes. Any black or brown spot having an irregular border, pigment appearing to radiate beyond that border, a red, black, and blue coloration observable on close examination, or a nodular surface is suggestible of melanoma and is usually excised for biopsy. Kinds of melanoma are **amelanotic melanoma, benign juvenile melanoma, lentigo maligna melanoma, nodular melanoma, primary cutaneous melanoma,** and **superficial spreading melanoma.** Compare **blue naevus.** See also **Hutchinson's freckle.**

melanosis coli, an abnormal condition in which the mucous membrane of the colon is pigmented with melanin.

melanotrichia linguae. See **parasitic glossitis.**

melasma. See **chloasma.**

melatonin, the only hormone secreted into the bloodstream by the pineal gland. The hormone appears to inhibit numerous endocrine functions, including the gonadotropic hormones, and to decrease the pigmentation of the skin.

melioidosis, an infection that is uncommon in humans and is caused by the gram-negative bacillus *Malleomyces pseudomallei.* **Acute melioidasis** is fulminant and usually characterized by pneumonia, empyema, lung abscess, septicaemia, and liver or spleen involvement. **Chronic melioidosis** is associated with osteomyelitis, multiple abscesses of the internal organs, and the development of fistulas from the abscesses. The disease is acquired by direct contact with infected animals.

membrana tectoria, 1. also called **occipitoaxial ligament.** the broad, strong ligament covering the dens and helping to connect the axis to the occipital bone of the skull. Compare **alar ligament, apical dental ligament. 2.** a spiral membrane projecting from the vestibular lip of the cochlea over the organ of Corti.

membrana tympani. See **tympanic membrane.**

membrane, a thin layer of tissue that covers a surface, lines a cavity, or divides a space, such as the abdominal membrane that lines the abdominal wall. The principal kinds of membranes are **mucous membrane, serous membrane, synovial membrane,** and **cutaneous membrane.**

membrane conductance, (in cardiology) the degree of permeability of a cellular membrane to certain ions.

membrane diffusion coefficient, a component of total pulmonary diffusing capacity. It includes qualitative and quantitative characteristics of the functioning alveolar-capillary membrane.

membrane responsiveness, (in cardiology) the relationship between the membrane potential at the time of stimulation and the maximal rate of depolarization of the action potential.

membranous labyrinth, a network of three fluid-filled, membranous, semicircular ducts suspended within the bony semicircular canals of the inner ear, associated with the sense of balance.

membranous stomatitis. See **pseudomembranous stomatitis.**

memory, **1.** the mental faculty or power that enables one to retain and to recall, through unconscious associative processes, previously experienced sensations, impressions, ideas, concepts, and all information that has been consciously learned. **2.** the reservoir of all past experiences and knowledge that may be recollected or recalled at will. **3.** the recollection of a past event, ideas, sensations, or previously learned knowledge. Kinds of memory include **affect memory, anterograde memory, kinesthetic memory, long-term memory, screen memory, short-term memory,** and **visual memory.**

memory cell. See **lymphocyte.**

menadiol sodium diphosphate, a water-soluble analogue of vitamin K.

menarche, the first menstruation and the commencement of cyclic menstrual function.

mendelevium (Md) {Dimitri I. Mendeleyev, Russian chemist, b. 1834}, a synthetic element in the actinide group. Its atomic number is 101. The atomic weight of its most stable isotope is 256. It is the ninth transuranic element.

mendelian genetics. See **Mendel's laws**.

mendelism {Gregor J. Mendel, Austrian geneticist, b. 1822}, the concept of inheritance derived from the application of Mendel's laws. **mendelian,** *adj.*

Mendel's laws {Gregor J. Mendel}, the basic principles of inheritance based on breeding experiments of garden peas. These are usually stated as two laws, commonly called the law of segregation and the law of independent assortment. According to the first, each characteristic of a species is represented in the somatic cells by a pair of units, now known as genes, which separate during meiosis so that each gamete receives only one gene for each trait. According to the second law, the members of a gene pair on different chromosomes segregate independently from other pairs during meiosis, so that the gametes show all possible combinations of factors.

Mendelson's syndrome {Curtis L. Mendelson, American obstetrician, b. 1913}, a respiratory condition caused by the chemical pneumonia resulting from the aspiration of acid gastric contents into the lungs. It usually occurs when a person vomits when inebriated, when stuporous from anaesthesia, or when unconscious, such as during a seizure.

Ménétrier's disease. See **giant hypertrophic gastritis.**

Ménière's disease {Prosper Ménière, French physician, b. 1799}, a chronic disease of the inner ear characterized by recurrent episodes of vertigo, progressive unilateral nerve deafness, and tinnitus. The cause is unknown although occasionally the condition follows middle ear infection or trauma to the head. There also may be associated nausea, vomiting, and profuse sweating. Attacks last from a few minutes to several hours. Also called **Ménière's syndrome, paroxysmal labyrinthine vertigo.**

meningeal hydrops. See **pseudotumour cerebri.**

meninges, *sing.* **meninx,** any one of the three membranes that enclose the brain and the spinal cord, comprising the dura mater, the pia mater, and the arachnoid. **meningeal,** *adj.*

meningioma, *pl.* **meningiomas, meningiomata,** a mesenchymal fibroblastic tumour of the membranes enveloping the brain and spinal cord. The tumours may be nodular, plaquelike, or diffuse lesions that invade the skull, causing bone erosion and compression of brain tissue.

meningism, an abnormal condition characterized by irritation of the brain and the spinal cord and by symptoms that mimic those of meningitis. In meningism, however, there is no actual inflammation of the meninges.

meningitis, *pl.* **meningitides,** any infection or inflammation of the membranes covering the brain and spinal cord. It is usually purulent and involves the fluid in the subarachnoid space. It is characterized by severe headache, vomiting, and pain and stiffness in the neck. The most common causes are bacterial infection with *Streptococcus pneumoniae, Neisseria meningitidis,* or *Haemophilus influenzae.* Aseptic meningitis may be caused by other kinds of bacteria, by chemical irritation, by neoplasm, or by viruses. Many of these diseases are benign and self-limited, such as meningitis caused by strains of coxsackievirus or echovirus. Others are more severe, such as those involving arboviruses, herpesviruses, or poliomyelitis viruses. Yeasts such as *Candida* and fungi such as *Cryptococcus* may cause a severe, often fatal, meningitis. Tuberculous meningitis, invariably fatal if untreated, may result in a variety of neurological abnormalities even with the best treatment available. A kind of meningitis is **tuberculous meningitis.**

meningocele, a saclike protrusion of either the cerebral or spinal meninges through a congenital defect in the skull or the vertebral column. It forms a hernial cyst that is filled with cerebrospinal fluid but does not contain neural tissue. The anomaly is designated a cranial meningocele or spinal meningocele, depending on the site of the defect; it can be easily repaired by surgery.

meningococcal polysaccharide vaccine, a polysaccharide vaccine used as an active immunizing agent against group A and group C meningococcal organisms, which cause meningococcal meningitis.

meningococcaemia, a disease caused by *Neisseria meningitidis* in the bloodstream. Onset is sudden, with chills, pain in the muscles and joints, headache, petechiae, sore throat, and severe prostration. Tachycardia is present, respirations and pulse rate are increased, and fever is intermittent.

meningococcus, *pl.* **meningococci,** a bacterium of the genus *Neisseria meningitidis*, a nonmotile, gram-negative diplococcus, frequently found in the nasopharynx of asymptomatic carriers, that may cause septicaemia or epidemic cerebrospinal meningitis. **meningococcal,** *adj.*

meningoencephalocele, a saclike cyst containing brain tissue, cerebrospinal fluid, and meninges that protrudes through a congenital defect in the skull.

meningomyelocele. See **myelomeningocele.**

meniscectomy, surgical excision of one of the crescent-shaped cartilages of the knee joint, performed when a torn cartilage results in chronic pain and in instability or locking of the joint.

meniscocystosis. See **sickle cell anaemia.**

meniscus, 1. the interface between a liquid and air. 2. a lens with both convex and concave aspects. 3. a curved, fibrous cartilage in the knees and other joints.

Menkes' kinky hair syndrome {John H. Menkes, American neurologist, b. 1928}, a familial disorder affecting the normal absorption of copper from the intestine, characterized by the growth of sparse, kinky hair. Infants with the syndrome suffer cerebral degeneration, retarded growth, and early death.

menopause, strictly, the cessation of menses, but commonly used to refer to the period of the female climacteric. Menses stop naturally with the decline of cyclical hormonal production and function between 45 and 60 years of age but may stop earlier in life. As the production of ovarian oestrogen and pituitary gonadotropins decreases, ovulation and menstruation become less frequent and eventually stop. Fluctuations in the circulating levels of these hormones occur as the levels decline. Hot flushes are the only nearly universal symptom of the menopause. Occasionally, heavy irregular bleeding occurs at this time, usually associated with

myomata (fibroids) or other uterine pathological conditions.

menorrhagia, abnormally heavy or long menstrual periods. Menorrhagia occurs occasionally during the reproductive years of most women's lives. If the condition becomes chronic, anaemia from recurrent excessive blood loss may result. Abnormal bleeding after menopause always warrants investigation to rule out malignancy. **menorrhagic,** *adj.*

menorrhoea, the normal discharge of blood and tissue from the uterus.

menostasis, an abnormal condition in which the products of menstruation cannot escape the uterus or vagina because of stenosis, an occlusion of the cervix, or the introitus of the vagina. An imperforate hymen is a rare cause of menostasis. **menostatic,** *adj.*

menotrophin, a preparation of gonadotrophin extracted from the urine of postmenopausal women. It is prescribed with chorionic gonadotrophin to induce ovulation, in the treatment of female infertility and to stimulate spermatogenesis in the treatment of male infertility.

menses, the normal flow of blood and decidua that occurs during menstruation. The first day of the flow of the menses is the first day of the menstrual cycle.

menstrual age, the age of an embryo or fetus as calculated from the first day of the last menstrual period.

menstrual cycle, the recurring cycle of change in the endometrium during which the decidual layer of the endometrium is shed, then regrows, proliferates, is maintained for several days, and sheds again at menstruation. The average length of the cycle, from the first day of bleeding of one cycle to the first of another, is 28 days. The length, duration, and character vary greatly among women. Menstrual cycles begin at menarche and end with menopause. The three phases of the cycle are the **proliferative phase, secretory phase,** and **menstrual phase.**

menstrual phase, the final of the three phases of the menstrual cycle in which menstruation occurs. The necrotic mucosa of the endometrium is shed, and bleeding, primarily from the spiral arteries, occurs. The average blood loss is 30 ml. For convenience, the days of the menstrual cycle are counted from the first day of tne menstrual phase.

menstruation, the periodic discharge through the vagina of a bloody secretion containing tissue debris from the shedding of the endometrium from the nonpregnant uterus. The average duration of menstruation is 4 to 5 days, and it recurs at approximately 4-week intervals throughout the reproductive life of nonpregnant women. Kinds of menstruation are **anovular menstruation, retrograde menstruation,** and

vicarious menstruation.   **menstruate,** *v.*

mental[1,] **1.** of, relating to, or characteristic of the mind or psyche. **2.** existing in the mind; performed or accomplished by the mind. **3.** of, relating to, or characterized by a disorder of the mind.

mental[2,] of or pertaining to the chin.

mental age (MA), the age level at which one functions intellectually, as determined by standardized psychological and intelligence tests and expressed as the age at which that level is average.

mental deficiency. See **learning disability.**

mental disorder, any disturbance of emotional equilibrium, as manifested in maladaptive behaviour and impaired functioning, caused by genetic, physical, chemical, biological, psychological, or social and cultural factors.

mental handicap. See **learning disability.**

mental health, a relative state of mind in which a person who is healthy is able to cope with and adjust to the recurrent stresses of everyday living.

mental health nursing. See **psychiatric nursing.**

mental health service, any one of a group of government, professional, or lay organizations operating at a community, state, national, or international level to aid in the prevention and treatment of mental disorders.

mental illness. See **mental disorder.**

mental image, any concept or sensation produced in the mind through memory or imagination.

mentality, **1.** the functional power and the capacity of the mind. **2.** intellectual character.

mental retardation. See **Learning disability.**

mental ridge, (in dentistry) a dense elevation that extends from the symphysis to the premolar area on the anterolateral aspect of the body of the mandible.

mental state, the degree of competence shown by a person in intellectual, emotional, psychological, and personality functioning as measured by psychological testing with reference to a statistical norm.

mentation, any mental activity, including conscious and unconscious processes.

menthol, a topical antipruritic with a cooling effect that relieves itching. It is an ingredient in many topical creams and ointments, and is also used in many cold remedies for its aromatic properties which help to relieve congestion.

mentholated camphor, a mixture of equal parts of camphor and menthol, used as a local counterirritant.

menton, the most inferior point on the chin in the lateral view. It is a cephalometric landmark.

mentor, an older, trusted adviser or counsellor who offers helpful guidance to younger colleagues.

mentum, **1.** the chin, especially of the fetus. **2.** a fetal reference point in designating the position of the fetus with respect to the maternal pelvis, as left mentum anterior (LMA) indicates the fetal chin is presenting in the left anterior quadrant of the pelvis.

menu, a list of optional computer applications displayed for selection by the operator, who indicates the next action to be taken by signalling through the keyboard or another device a choice of the options.

mepenzolate bromide, an anticholinergic agent prescribed in the treatment of GI hypermotility.

mephenesin, a curare-like skeletal muscle relaxant sometimes prescribed in the relief of muscle spasm.

meprobamate, a sedative prescribed in the treatment of anxiety and tension and as a muscle relaxant.

mEq, abbreviation for **milliequivalent.**

meralgia, the presence of pain in the thigh.

meralgia paraesthetica, a condition characterized by pain, paraesthesia, and numbness on the lateral surface of the thigh in the region supplied by the lateral femoral cutaneous nerve. The cause of the condition is ischaemia of the nerve caused by its entrapped position in the inguinal ligament.

mercaptopurine, an antimetabolite with cytotoxic and immunosuppressive actions used in the treatment of a variety of malignant diseases, including acute lymphocytic leukaemia, and sometimes as an immunosuppressant.

mercurial, **1.** of or pertaining to mercury, particularly a medicine containing the element mercury. **2.** an adverse effect associated with the administration of a mercurial medication, such as a mercurial tremor caused by mercury poisoning.

mercurial diuretic, any one of several diuretic agents that contain mercury in an organic chemical form. Mercurial diuretics inhibit tubular reabsorption of sodium and chloride and the excretion of potassium but do not produce diuresis in patients who are in metabolic alkalosis. They have been replaced almost completely by less toxic drugs.

mercurialism. See **mercury poisoning.**

mercury (Hg), a metallic element. Its atomic number is 80; its atomic weight is 200.6. It is the only common metal that is liquid at room temperature, and it occurs in nature almost entirely in the form of its sulphide, cinnabar. Mercury is produced commercially and is used in dental amalgams, thermometers, barometers, and other measuring instruments. It forms many poisonous compounds. Elemental mercury is only mildly toxic when ingested, because it is poorly absorbed. The vapour of elemental mercury, however, is readily absorbed through the lungs and enters the brain before it is oxidized. The kidneys retain mercury longer than any of the other body tissues.

mercury poisoning, a toxic condition caused by the ingestion or inhalation of mercury or a mercury compound. The chronic form, resulting from inhalation of the vapours or dust of mercurial compounds or from repeated ingestion of very small amounts, is characterized by irritability, excessive saliva, loosened teeth, gum disorders, slurred speech, tremors, and staggering. Symptoms of acute mercury poisoning appear in a few to 30 minutes and include a metallic taste in the mouth, thirst, nausea, vomiting, severe abdominal pain, bloody diarrhoea, and renal failure that may result in death.

mercy killing. See **euthanasia.**

merergasia, a mild mental incapacity characterized by some emotional instability and some anxiety. **merergastic,** *adj.*

meridians, energy pathways, similar to blood and lymph vesels; detected by certain electronic appliances. There are a total of 26 in the body linked to a particular organ or function of the body.

merisis, an increase in size as a result of cell division and the addition of new material rather than of cell expansion.

meroblastic, pertaining to or characterizing an ovum that contains a large amount of yolk and in which cleavage is restricted to a part of the cytoplasm.

meromelia, a general designation for the congenital absence of any part of a limb. It is used in reference to such conditions as adactyly, hemimelia, or phocomelia.

merozoite, an organism produced from segmentation of a schizont during the asexual reproductive phase of the life cycle of a sporozoan, specifically the malarial parasite *Plasmodium.* See also *Plasmodium.*

merozygote, an incomplete zygote that contains only part of the genetic material of one of the parents. It occurs in bacterial genetics.

Merrifield's knife, a surgical knife with a long, narrow, triangular blade set into a shank, used for gingivectomy incisions.

mesangial IgA nephropathy. See **Berger's disease.**

mesangium, a cellular network in the renal glomerulus that helps support the capillary loops.

mescaline, a psychoactive, poisonous alkaloid derived from a colourless alkaline oil in the flowering heads of the cactus *Lophophora williamsii.* Closely related chemically to adrenaline, mescaline causes heart palpitations, sweating, pupillary dilatation, and anxiety. The drug, taken in capsules or dissolved in a drink, produces visual hallucinations.

mesencephalon, one of the three parts of the brainstem, lying just below the cerebrum and just above the pons. It consists primarily of white substance with some grey substance around the cerebral aqueduct. A red nucleus lies within the reticular formation of the mesencephalon and contains the terminations of fibres from the cerebellum and the frontal lobe of the cerebral cortex. Deep within the mesencephalon are nuclei of the third and the fourth cranial nerves and the anterior part of the fifth cranial nerve. The mesencephalon also contains nuclei for certain auditory and certain visual reflexes. **mesencephalic,** *adj.*

mesenchymal chondrosarcoma, a malignant cartilaginous tumour that develops in many sites.

mesenchyme, a diffuse network of tissue derived from the embryonic mesoderm. It consists of stellate cells embedded in gelatinous ground substance with reticular fibres.

mesenchymoma, a mixed mesenchymal neoplasm composed of two or more cellular elements not usually associated and fibrous tissue.

mesenteric adenitis. See **adenitis.**

mesenteric node, a node in one of three groups of superior mesenteric lymph glands serving parts of the intestine.

mesentery proper, a broad, fan-shaped fold of peritoneum connecting the jejunum and the ileum with the dorsal wall of the abdomen. The root of the mesentery proper is connected to certain structures ventral to the vertebral column. The intestinal border of the mesentery proper separates to enclose the intestine. The cranial part of the mesentery suspends the small intestine and various nerves and arteries.

MESH, an acronym derived from *Medical Subject Headings,* the list of medical terms used by the U.S. National Library of Medicine (NLM) for its computerized system of storage and retrieval of published medical reports. Also spelled **MeSH.**

mesial. See **medial.**

mesiocclusion, an occlusal relationship in which the lower teeth are positioned mesially.

mesiodens, a supernumerary erupted or unerupted tooth that develops between two maxillary central incisors.

mesioversion, 1. a condition in which one or more teeth are closer than normal to the midline. **2.** a condition in which the maxillae or mandible is postioned more anteriorly than normal.

mesocolic node, a node in one of three groups of superior mesenteric lymph glands, proliferating between the layers of the transverse mesocolon, close to the transverse colon.

mesocolopexy, suspension or fixation of the mesocolon.

mesoderm, (in embryology) the middle of

the three cell layers of the developing embryo. It lies between the ectoderm and the endoderm. Bone, connective tissue, muscle, blood, vascular and lymphatic tissue, and the pleurae of the pericardium and peritoneum are all derived from the mesoderm.

mesoglia, See **microglia.**

mesometritis, See **myometritis.**

mesomorph, a person whose physique is characterized by a predominance of muscle, bone, and connective tissue, structures that develop from the mesodermal layer of the embryo.

mesonephric duct, (in embryology) a duct that, in the male, gives rise to the ducts of the reproductive system (ductus epididymidis, ductus deferens, seminal vesicle, ejaculatory duct). In the female, it persists vestigially as **Gartner's duct.**

mesonephric tubule, any of the embryonic renal tubules comprising the mesonephros. They function as excretory structures during the early embryonic development of humans and other mammals but are later incorporated into the reproductive system. In males the tubules give rise to the efferent and aberrant ductules of the testes, the appendix epididymis, and paradidymis, and in females to the epoophoron, paroophoron, and vesicular appendices. All of the structures are vestigial except the efferent ductules of the testes.

mesonephros, *pl.* **mesonephroi, mesonephra,** the second type of excretory organ to develop in the vertebrate embryo. It consists of a series of twisting tubules that arise from the nephrogenic cord caudal to the pronephros and that at one end form the glomerulus and at the other connect with the excretory mesonephric duct. **mesonephric, mesonephroid,** *adj.*

mesosalpinx, the cephalic, free border of the broad ligament in which the uterine tubes lie.

mesothelioma, *pl.* **mesotheliomas, mesotheliomata,** a rare, malignant tumour of the mesothelium of the pleura or peritoneum, associated with earlier exposure to asbestos.

mesothelium, a layer of cells that lines the body cavities of the embryo and continues as a layer of squamous epithelial cells covering the serous membranes of the adult.

messenger RNA (mRNA), (in molecular genetics) an RNA fraction that transmits information from DNA to the protein-synthesizing ribosomes of cells.

mestranol, an oestrogen used in hormone replacement therapy for relief of menopausal symptoms.

Met, abbreviation for **methionine.**

MET, abbreviation for **metabolic equivalent.**

metabolic, of or pertaining to **metabolism.**

metabolic acidosis, acidosis in which excess acid is added to the body fluids or bicarbo-

nate is lost from them. In starvation and in uncontrolled diabetes mellitus, glucose is not present or is not available for oxidation for cellular nutrition. The plasma bicarbonate of the body is used up in neutralizing the ketones that result from the breakdown of body fat for energy that occurs in compensation for the lack of glucose. Metabolic acidosis also occurs when oxidation takes place without adequate oxygen, as in heart failure or shock. Severe diarrhoea, renal failure, and lactic acidosis also may result in metabolic acidosis. Hyperkalaemia often accompanies the condition.

metabolic alkalosis, an abnormal condition characterized by the significant loss of acid in the body or by increased levels of base bicarbonate. The reduction of acid may be caused by excessive vomiting, insufficient replacement of electrolytes, hyperadrenocorticism, and Cushing's disease. A decrease in base bicarbonate may be caused by various problems, such as the ingestion of excessive bicarbonate of soda and other antacids during the treatment of peptic ulcers, and by the administration of excessive intravenous fluids containing high concentrations of bicarbonate. Severe, untreated metabolic alkalosis can lead to coma and death. Signs and symptoms of metabolic alkalosis may include apnoea, headache, lethargy, irritability, nausea, vomiting, and atrial tachycardia.

metabolic component, the bicarbonate component of plasma.

metabolic disorder, any pathophysiological dysfunction that results in a loss of metabolic control of homeostasis in the body.

metabolic equivalent (MET), a unit of measurement of heat production by the body. One MET is equal to 50 kilogram calories (kcal) per hour per square metre of body surface of a resting individual.

metabolic rate, the amount of energy liberated or expended in a given unit of time. Energy is stored in the body in energy-rich phosphate compounds (adenosine triphosphate, adenosine monophosphate, and adenosine diphosphate) and in proteins, fats, and complex carbohydrates.

metabolic respiratory quotient (R), the ratio of production of CO_2 to the corresponding consumption of O_2. The values of R change according to the fuel being burned; thus, because fat contains relatively little O_2 compared with glucose, the R of fat is lower than that of glucose, whereas the R of protein is between that of glucose and fat.

metabolism, the aggregate of all chemical processes that take place in living organisms, resulting in growth, generation of energy, elimination of wastes, and other bodily functions as they relate to the distribution of nutrients in the blood after digestion. Metabolism takes place in two steps: anabolism, the constructive phase, in which smaller molecules (as amino acids) are converted to larger molecules (as proteins); and catabolism, the destructive phase, in which larger molecules (as glycogen) are converted to smaller molecules (as pyruvic acid). The metabolic rate is customarily expressed (in calories) as the heat liberated in the course of metabolism.

metabolite, a substance produced by metabolic action or necessary for a metabolic process. An essential metabolite is one required for a vital metabolic process.

metacarpus, the middle portion of the hand, consisting of five slender bones numbered from the thumb side, metacarpals I through V. Each metacarpal consists of a body and two extremities.   **metacarpal,** *adj., n.*

metacentric, pertaining to a chromosome in which the centromere is located near the centre so that the arms of the chromatids are of approximately equal length.

metacommunication, communication that indicates how verbal communication should be interpreted. It may support or contradict verbal communication.

metagenesis, the regular alternation of sexual with asexual methods of reproduction within the same species.   **metagenetic, metagenic,** *adj.*

metal, any element that conducts heat and electricity, is malleable and ductile, and forms positively charged ions (cations) in solution.

metal fume fever, an occupational disorder caused by the inhalation of fumes of metallic oxides and characterized by symptoms similar to those of influenza.

metamodel, (in neurolinguistics), a theory that language is a representation of experience, as in a map or model, rather than an experience in itself.

metamorphopsia, a defect in vision in which objects are seen as distorted in shape, resulting from disease of the retina or imperfection of the media.

metamorphosis, a change in shape or structure, especially a change from one stage of development to another, such as the transition from the larval to the adult stage.

metamyelocyte, a stage in the development of the granulocyte series of leukocytes. It is intermediate between the myelocyte stage and the mature granulocyte.

metanephrine, one of the two principal urinary metabolites of adrenaline and noradrenaline in the urine, the other being vanillylmandelic acid.

metanephrogenic, capable of forming the metanephros, or fetal kidney.

metanephros, *pl.* **metanephroi, metanephra,** the third, and permanent, excretory organ to develop in the vertebrate embryo. It consists of a complex structure of secretory and collecting tubules that develop into the kidney.

metaphase, the second of the four stages of nuclear division in mitosis and in each of the two divisions of meiosis, during which the chromosomes become arranged in the equatorial plane of the spindle to form the equatorial plate, with the centromeres attached to the spindle fibres in preparation for separation.

metaphyseal dysostosis, an abnormal condition that affects the skeletal system and is characterized by a disturbance of the mineralization of the metaphyseal area of the bones, resulting in dwarfism. Metaphyseal dysostosis is classified as the Gansen type, Schmidt type, Spahar-Hartmann type, or cartilage-hair hypoplasia. The Gansen type is characterized by metaphyseal alterations similar to those of achondroplasia but not involving the skull or the epiphyses of the long bones. The Schmidt type of metaphyseal dysostosis is characterized by developmental changes from the weight-bearing age to approximately 5 years of age. The Spahar-Hartmann type is characterized by skeletal changes and severe genu varum. Cartilage-hair hypoplasia is characterized by severe dwarfism and hair that is sparse, short, and brittle.

metaphyseal dysplasia, an abnormal condition characterized by disordered modelling of the long cylindrical bones.

metaphysis, a region of bone in which diaphysis and epiphysis converge.

metaplasia, the conversion of normal tissue cells into an abnormal form in response to chronic stress or injury.

metaraminol bitartrate, an adrenergic vasopressor prescribed in the treatment of hypotension and shock.

metarubricyte, a red blood cell possessing a nucleus. Such cells, usually normoblasts in their final stage, are not normally found in the blood of adults.

metastasis, *pl.* **metastases, 1.** the process by which tumour cells are spread to distant parts of the body. Because malignant tumours have no enclosing capsule, cells may escape and be transported by the lymphatic circulation or the bloodstream to other organs far from the primary tumour. **2.** a tumour that develops in this way.   **metastatic,** *adj.,* **metastasize,** *v.*

metastasizing mole. See **chorioadenoma destruens.**

metastatic calcification, the pathological process whereby calcium salts accumulate in previously healthy tissues.

metastatic ophthalmia. See **sympathetic ophthalmia.**

metatarsal, 1. of or pertaining to the metatarsus of the foot. **2.** any one of the five bones comprising the metatarsus.

metatarsalgia, a painful condition around the metatarsal bones caused by an abnormal-

metatarsal stress fracture, a break or rupture of a metatarsal bone, resulting from prolonged running or walking. The condition is often difficult to diagnose with x-ray films.

metatarsus, a part of the foot, consisting of five bones numbered I to V, from the medial side. Each bone has a long, slender body, a wedge-shaped proximal end, a convex distal end, and flattened, grooved sides for the attachment of ligaments. Kinds of metatarsus include **metatarsus valgus** and **metatarsus varus. metatarsal,** *adj.*

metatarsus adductus. See **metatarsus varus.**

metatarsus valgus, a congenital deformity of the foot in which the forepart rotates outward away from the midline of the body and the heel remains straight.

metatarsus varus, a congenital deformity of the foot in which the forepart rotates inward toward the midline of the body and the heel remains straight.

metathalamus, one of five parts of the diencephalon. It is composed of a medial geniculate body and a lateral geniculate body on each side. The medial geniculate body acts as a relay station for nerve impulses between the inferior brachium and the auditory cortex. The lateral geniculate body accommodates the terminal ends of the fibres of the optic tract. **metathalamic,** *adj.*

metazoa, a category of multicellular animals whose cells have become differentiated into tissues and organs, particularly those possessing a digestive tract.

Metchnikoff's theory {Elie Metchnikoff, Russian-French biologist, b. 1845} a theory that living cells ingest microorganisms, as seen in the process of phagocytosis and the ingestion of injurious microbes by leukocytes.

meteorism, accumulation of gas in the abdomen or the intestine, usually with distention.

meteorotropism, a reaction to meteorological influences shown by various biological occurrences, such as sudden death, attacks of arthritis, and angina. **meteorotropic,** *adj.*

methadone hydrochloride, an opiate analgesic used as a substitute for heroin, as part of a maintenance programme or to permit withdrawal without development of acute abstinence syndrome. Methadone does not produce marked euphoria, sedation, or narcosis. It is also used as a cough suppressant.

methamphetamine hydrochloride, a central nervous system stimulant not used legitimately in the United Kingdom but produced illicitly for recreational use.

methandriol, an anabolic hormone used as adjunctive therapy in senile and postmenopausal osteoporosis.

methanol, a clear, colourless, toxic, liquid distillate of wood miscible with water, alcohol, and ether. It is widely used as a solvent and in the production of formaldehyde. Ingestion of methanol paralyses the optic nerve and may cause death.

methanol extractable residue, an immunotherapeutic substance, prepared from a methanol extracted fraction of the Bacillus Calmette-Guérin (BCG). It is given to prevent or delay recurrences of Stage II malignant melanoma after surgery and to prolong drug-induced remissions in acute myelocytic leukaemia.

methaemoglobin, a form of haemoglobin in which the iron component has been oxidized from the ferrous to the ferric state. Methaemoglobin cannot carry oxygen and so contributes nothing to the oxygen transporting capacity of the blood.

methaemoglobinaemia, the presence of methaemoglobin in the blood, causing cyanosis because of the red cell's inability to release oxygen.

methenamine hippurate, see **hexamine hippurate.**

methionine (Met), an essential amino acid needed for proper growth in infants and for maintenance of nitrogen balance in adults. It is a source for methyl groups and sulphur in the body.

methocarbamol, a skeletal muscle relaxant prescribed in the treatment of skeletal muscle spasm.

method, a technique or procedure for producing a desired effect, such as a surgical procedure, a laboratory test, or a diagnostic technique.

methodology, **1.** a system of principles or methods of procedure in any discipline, as education, research, diagnosis, or treatment. **2.** the section of a research proposal in which the methods to be used are described.

methohexital sodium, an intravenous barbiturate prescribed for the induction of anaesthesia in short surgical procedures as a supplement to other anaesthetics.

methotrexate, a cytotoxic and immunosuppressant drug used in the treatment of severe psoriasis, rheumatoid arthritis, and a variety of malignant diseases.

methoxamine hydrochloride, an adrenergic drug that acts as a vasoconstrictor, used to maintain blood pressure during anaesthesia.

methoxsalen, a psoralen compound which sensitizes the skin to UV light, and which is used in the photochemotherapy of psoriasis.

3-methoxy-4-hydroxymandelic acid, a product of metabolism that may be measured in the urine to determine the levels of the catecholamines (adrenaline and noradrenaline). Increased concentrations of this acid may raise the blood pressure, indicate the presence of tumours, muscular dystrophy, or myasthenia gravis.

methyl (Me), the chemical radical -CH_3.

methyl alcohol. See **methanol.**

methyldopa, an antihypertensive used to reduce blood pressure levels.

methylene blue, a bluish-green crystalline substance used as a histology stain and as a laboratory indicator. It is also used in the treatment of cyanide poisoning and methaemoglobinaemia.

methylergometine maleate, a synthetic ergot alkaloid prescribed as an oxytocic to prevent or to treat postpartum haemorrhage.

methylphenidate hydrochloride, a central nervous system stimulant used in the treatment of hyperkinesis in children and in the treatment of narcolepsy in adults.

methylphenobarbitone, an anticonvulsant, similar phenobarbitone, used in the treatment of epilepsy.

methylprednisolone, a glucocorticoid prescribed in the treatment of inflammatory conditions, including rheumatic fever, rheumatoid arthritis, and chronic obstructive airways disease.

methyltestosterone, an androgen prescribed in the treatment of testosterone deficiency, and as an anabolic steroid to stimulate growth, weight gain, and red blood cell production.

methysergide maleate, a vasoconstrictor used for the prevention of migraine and cluster headache.

metoclopramide hydrochloride, a dopamine and serotonin antagonist used as an antiemetic and to stimulate GI motility.

metolazone, a diuretic and antihypertensive used for the treatment of oedema and high blood pressure.

metopic, of or pertaining to the forehead.

metoprolol tartrate, a beta-blocker used in the treatment of hypertension, angina, cardiac arrhythmias, thyrotoxicosis, and in the prophylaxis of migraine.

metralgia, tenderness or pain in the uterus.

metre, a metric unit of length equal to 39.37 inches.

metred dose inhaler, a device designed to deliver a measured dose of an inhalation drug. It consists usually of a canister of aerosol spray, mist, or fine powder that releases a specific dose each time the canister is pushed against a dispensing valve. It is intended to reduce the risk of overmedication by the person.

metric, of or pertaining to a system of measurement that uses the metre as a basis.

metric equivalent, any value in metric units of measurement that equals the same value in English units, such as 2.54 cm equal 1 inch or 1 L equals 1.0567 quarts.

metric system, a decimal system of measurement based on the metre as the unit of length, on the gram as the unit of weight or mass, and, as a derived unit, on the litre as the unit of volume.

metritis, inflammation of the walls of the uterus.

metrodynia. See **metralgia.**

metronidazole, an antimicrobial prescribed in the treatment of amoebiasis, trichomoniasis, and anaerobic bacterial infections.

metronoscope, 1. a device that exposes a small amount of reading matter to the eyes for brief preset time periods. It is used in testing and to help increase reading speed. **2.** an apparatus that exercises the eyes rhythmically to improve binocular coordination.

metrorrhagia, excessive uterine bleeding other than that caused by menstruation. It may be caused by uterine lesions and may be a sign of a urogenital malignancy.

metyrapone, a diagnostic test drug. It is used to test hypothalamicopituitary function.

metyrosine, a catecholamine synthesis inhibitor used in the treatment of phaeochromocytoma.

Meuse fever. See **trench fever.**

MeV, abbreviation for *mega electronvolts.*

mevalonate kinase, an enzyme in the liver and in yeast that catalyses the transfer of a phosphate group from adenosine triphosphate to produce adenosine diphosphate and 5-phosphomevalonate.

mexiletine hydrochloride, an antiarrhythmic drug used for the treatment of symptomatic ventricular dysrhythmias.

Meynet's node, any one of the numerous nodules that may develop within the capsules surrounding joints and in tendons affected by rheumatic diseases, especially in children.

mezlocillin sodium, a semisynthetic penicillin antibiotic used for serious infections caused by susceptible strains of bacteria.

mfd, abbreviation for **microfarad.**

mg, abbreviation for **milligram.**

Mg, symbol for **magnesium.**

MI, abbreviation for **myocardial infarction.**

micellar chromatography, a method of monitoring minute quantities of drugs in whole body fluids by using micellar or colloidial compounds to keep proteins in solution. The technique eliminates the need to remove proteins that usually interfere with chromatographic analysis of blood serum, urine, or saliva.

miconazole nitrate, an antifungal used topically in the treatment of fungal infections of the skin and vagina and parenterally to treat systemic fungal infections.

micrencephalia. See **microcephaly.**

micrencephalon, 1. an abnormally small brain. See also **microcephaly. 2.** *obsolete.* the cerebellum. **micrencephalic,** *adj.,* n.

micrencephaly. See **microcephaly.**

microaerophile, a microorganism that requires free oxygen for growth but at a lower concentration than that contained in the atmosphere. **microaerophilic,** *adj.*

microampere, one millionth of an ampere.

microaneurysm, a microscopic aneurysm characteristic of thrombotic purpura.

microangiopathy, a disease of the small blood vessels, such as diabetic microangiopathy, in which the basement membrane of capillaries thickens, or thrombotic microangiopathy, in which thrombi form in the arterioles and the capillaries.

microbe, a **microorganism. microbial,** *adj.*

microbiology, the branch of biology concerned with the study of microorganisms, including algae, bacteria, viruses, protozoa, fungi, and rickettsiae.

microbrachia, a developmental defect characterized by abnormal smallness of the arms. **microbrachius,** *n.*

microcentrum. See **centrosome.**

microcephaly, a congenital anomaly characterized by abnormal smallness of the head in relation to the rest of the body and by underdevelopment of the brain, resulting in some degree of mental retardation. The head is more than two standard deviations below the average circumference size for age, sex, race, and period of gestation. The facial features are generally normal. **microcephalic, microcephalous,** *adj.,* **microcephalic, microcephalus,** *n.*

microcheiria, a developmental defect characterized by abnormal smallness of the hands. The condition is usually associated with other congenital malformations or with bone and muscle disorders. Also spelled **microchiria.**

microcirculation, the flow of blood throughout the system of smaller vessels of the body, those with a diameter of 100 μm or less.

microcomputer, a complete multiuse electronic digital computer system consisting of a central processing unit, storage facilities, I/O ports, and high-speed internal storage.

microcurie (μCi, μc) {Marie and Pierre Curie}, (historical) a unit of radiation equal to one millionth (10^{-6}) of a curie.

microcyte, an abnormally small erythrocyte, often occurring in iron deficiency and other anaemias.

microcytic, (of a cell) smaller than normal, such as the erythrocytes in microcytic anaemia.

microcytic anaemia, a haematological disorder characterized by abnormally small erythrocytes, usually associated with chronic blood loss or a nutritional anaemia.

microcytosis, a haematological condition characterized by erythrocytes that are smaller than normal. Microcytosis and hypochromatosis are usual in iron deficiency anaemia. **microcytic,** *adj.*

microdactyly, a developmental defect characterized by abnormal smallness of the fingers and toes. The condition is usually associated with bone and muscle disorders.

microdrepanocytic, pertaining to a blood disorder marked by the presence of both microcytes and drepanocytes, such as occurs in sickle cell-thalassaemia.

microdrip, (in intravenous therapy) an apparatus for delivering relatively small, measured amounts of intravenous solutions at specific flow rates. A microdrip is usually used to deliver small volumes of solution over a long time. With a microdrip, 60 drops deliver 1 ml of solution.

microelement. See **micronutrient.**

microencapsulation, a laboratory technique used in the bioassay of hormones in which certain antibodies are encapsulated with a perforated membrane. The antibodies cannot escape through the tiny perforations, but hormones that bind with the antibodies may enter the structure to bind with them.

microfarad (mfd), a unit of capacity that equals one millionth (10^{-6}) of a farad.

microfiche, a sheet of microfilm that contains several separate photographic reproductions. The sheet is a convenient size for filing and enables large amounts of data to be stored in a relatively small space. See also **microfilm.**

microfilament, any of the submicroscopic cellular filaments, such as the tonofibrils, found in the cytoplasm of most cells, that function primarily as a supportive system.

microfilaria, *pl.* **microfilariae,** the prelarval form of any filarial worm.

microfilm, a strip of 16 mm or 35 mm film that contains photographic reproductions of pages of books, documents, or other library or medical records in greatly reduced size. The film is viewed through special machines that enlarge the photographic images.

microfluorometry. See **cytophotometry.**

microgamete, the small, motile male gamete of certain thallophytes and sporozoa, specifically the malarial parasite *Plasmodium.* It corresponds to the sperm of the higher animals.

microgametocyte, an enlarged merozoite that undergoes meiosis to form the mature male gamete during the sexual phase of the life cycle of certain thallophytes and sporozoa.

microgenitalia, a condition characterized by abnormally small external genitalia.

microglia, small migratory interstitial cells that form part of the central nervous system. They serve as phagocytes that collect waste products of the nerve tissue of the body.

micrognathia, underdevelopment of the jaw, especially the mandible. **micrognathic,** *adj.*

microgram (mg, μg), a unit of measurement of mass equal to one millionth (10^{-6}) of a gram.

microgyria, a developmental defect of the brain in which the convolutions are abnormally small, resulting in structural malformation of the cortex. The condition is usually associated with mental retardation and physical defects.

microgyrus, *pl.* **microgyri,** an underdeveloped, malformed convolution of the brain.

microhm, a unit of electric resistance equal to one millionth of an ohm.

microinvasive carcinoma, a squamous epithelial neoplasm that has penetrated the basement membrane, the first stage in invasive cancer.

microlitre (μL), a unit of liquid volume equal to one millionth of a litre.

microlith, a small rounded mass of mineral matter or calcified stone.

micromelic dwarf, a dwarf whose limbs are abnormally short.

micrometer, an instrument used for measuring small angles or distances on objects being observed through a microscope or telescope.

micrometre, a unit of measurement, commonly referred to as a *micron*, that is, one thousandth (10^{-3}) of a millimetre.

micromyeloblastic leukaemia, a malignant neoplasm of blood-forming tissues, characterized by the proliferation of small myeloblasts distinguishable from lymphocytes only by special staining techniques and microscopic examination.

micron (μ or mu), **1.** a metric unit of length equal to one millionth of a metre; micrometre **2.** (in physical chemistry), a colloidal particle with a diameter of between 0.2 and 10 microns.

micronucleus, 1. a small or minute nucleus. **2.** (in protozoa) the smaller of two nuclei in each cell; it functions in sexual reproduction as opposed to the macronucleus, which governs cell metabolism and growth. **3.** See **nucleolus.**

micronutrient, an organic compound, such as a vitamin, or a chemical element, such as zinc or iodine, essential only in minute amounts for the normal physiological processes of the body.

microorganism, any tiny, usually microscopic entity capable of carrying on living processes. Kinds of microorganisms include **bacteria, fungi, protozoa,** and **viruses.**

micropenis. See **microphallus.**

microphage, a neutrophil capable of ingesting small things, such as bacteria. **microphagic,** *adj.*

microphallus, an abnormally small penis. When observed in the newborn, the nurse examines the child for other signs of ambiguous genitalia.

microphthalmos, a developmental anomaly characterized by abnormal smallness of one or both eyes. When the condition occurs in the absence of other ocular defects, it is called pure microphthalmos or nanophthalmos. **microphthalmic,** *adj.*

microplasia. See **dwarfism.**

micropodia, a developmental anomaly characterized by abnormal smallness of the feet. The condition is often associated with other congenital malformations or with bone and skeletal disorders.

microprosopus, a fetus in which the face is abnormally small or underdeveloped.

micropsia, a condition of vision by which a person perceives objects as smaller than they really are. **microptic,** *adj.*

microreentry, (in cardiology) an impulse reentry involving a very small circuit, such as within Purkinje fibres.

microscopic, 1. of or pertaining to a microscope. **2.** very small; visible only when magnified and illuminated by a microscope.

microscopic anatomy, the study of the microscopic structure of the tissues and cells. Kinds of microscopic anatomy are **cytology** and **histology.**

microscopy, a technique for observing minute materials using a microscope. Kinds of microscopy include **darkfield microscopy, electron microscopy,** and **immunofluorescent microscopy.**

microshock, the passage of current directly into the cardiac tissue.

microsomal enzymes, a group of enzymes associated with a certain particulate fraction of liver homogenate that plays a role in the metabolism of many drugs.

microsomia, the condition of having an abnormally small and underdeveloped yet otherwise perfectly formed body with normal proportionate relationships of the various parts.

Microsporum, a genus of dermatophytes of the family Moniliaceae. The type species is *M. audouinii,* which causes epidemic tinea capitis in children. Formerly called *Microsporon.*

microthermy, a form of therapy in which heat generated by radio wave conversion is used in physiotherapy.

microtome, a device that cuts specimens of tissue prepared in paraffin blocks into extremely thin slices for microscopic study by a surgical pathologist.

microvascular, pertaining to the portion of the circulatory system that is composed of the capillary network.

microwave interstitial system, a microwave-generated hyperthermia system that creates a heat field in certain accessible tumours no more than 5 cm beneath the skin. The microwaves produce a temperature of about 43° C to destroy the tumour cells. The treatment can be monitored on a video terminal that shows location of the tumour and heat applicators.

microwaves, electromagnetic radiation in the frequency range of 300 to 2450 MHz.

microwave thermography, measurement of temperature through the detection of microwave radiation emitted from heated tissue.

micturate, micturition. See **urination.**

micturating urethrography. See **urethro-**

graphy.

micturition reflex, a normal reaction to a rise in pressure within the bladder, resulting in contraction of the bladder wall and relaxation of the urethral sphincter. Voluntary inhibition normally prevents incontinence.

midarm muscle circumference, an indication of muscle wasting in the upper arm calculated by subtracting the triceps skin fold (TSF) from the midupper arm circumference (MAC) measurement.

midaxillary line, an imaginary vertical line that passes midway between the anterior and posterior axillary folds.

midazolam hydrochloride, a parenteral benzodiazapine with sedative, hypnotic, anxiolytic and amnesiac properties. It is used for preoperative sedation and impairment of memory of preoperative events, for conscious sedation before short diagnostic or endoscopic procedures, and in terminal care.

midbody, 1. the middle of the body, or the midregion of the trunk. **2.** a mass of granules that appears in the middle of the spindle during mitotic anaphase.

midbrain. See mesencephalon.

midclavicular line, (in anatomy) an imaginary line that extends downward over the trunk from the midpoint of the clavicle, dividing each side of the anterior chest into two parts.

middle cardiac vein, one of the five tributaries of the coronary sinus that drains blood from the capillary bed of the myocardium. It receives tributaries from both ventricles, and ends in the right extremity of the coronary sinus.

middle costotransverse ligament. See ligament of the neck of the rib.

middle cuneiform bone. See intermediate cuneiform bone.

middle ear, the tympanic cavity and the auditory ossicles contained in an irregular space in the temporal bone. It is separated from the external ear by the tympanic membrane and from the inner ear by the oval window. The auditory tube carries air from the posterior pharynx into the middle ear.

middle kidney. See mesonephros.

middle lobe syndrome, localized atelectasis of the middle lobe of the right lung, characterized by chronic infection, cough, dyspnoea, wheezing, and obstructive pneumonitis. Asymptomatic obstruction of the bronchus may occur. The condition is caused by enlargement of the surrounding cuff of lymphatic glands.

middle mediastinum, the widest part of the mediastinum containing the heart, ascending aorta, lower half of the superior vena cava, pulmonary trunk, and phrenic nerves.

middle plate. See nephrotome.

middle sacral artery, a small, visceral branch of the abdominal aorta, descending to the fourth and fifth lumbar vertebrae, the sacrum, and the coccyx.

middle suprarenal artery, one of a pair of small, visceral branches of the abdominal aorta, arising opposite the superior mesenteric artery, and supplying the suprarenal gland.

middle temporal artery, one of the branches of the superficial temporal artery on each side of the head.

middle umbilical fold, the fold of peritoneum over the urachal remnant within the abdomen.

midgut, the middle portion of the embryonic alimentary canal. It consists of endodermal tissue, is connected to the yolk sac during early prenatal development, and eventually gives rise to some of the small intestine and part of the large intestine.

MIDIRS, abbreviation for the *Midwives Information and Resource Service.*

midlife transition, a period between early adulthood and middle adulthood that occurs between 40 and 45 years of age.

midline, an imaginary line that divides the body into right and left halves.

midline episiotomy. See episiotomy.

midplane dose (MPD), (in radiotherapy) the dose prescribed to the midpoint when using two beams directly opposed to one another.

midposition, the end-expiratory or end-tidal level or position of the lung-chest system under any given conditions, defining the patient's functional residual capacity.

midsagittal plane. See median plane.

midstance, one of the five stages in the stance phase of walking, or gait, directly associated with the period of single-leg support of body weight or the period during which the body advances over the stationary foot.

midstream specimen of urine (MSU), a urine specimen collected during the middle of a flow of urine, after the urinary opening has been carefully cleaned.

midupper arm circumference (MAC), an indication of upper arm muscle wasting based on measurement of the circumference of the arm at a midpoint between the tip of the acromial process of the scapula and olecranon process of the ulna.

midwife, 1. A person who practises midwifery. Among the responsibilities of the midwife are supervision of normal pregnancy, labour and delivery, to conduct deliveries on her own responsibility and to care for both mother and baby in the first six weeks postpartum. **2.** in traditional use) a (female) person who assists women in childbirth. See also **registered midwife.**

migraine, a recurring vascular headache characterized by a prodromal aura, unilateral onset, and severe pain, photophobia, and autonomic disturbances during the acute phase, which may last for hours or days. The disorder occurs more frequently in women than in men, and a predisposition to migraine may be inherited. The head pain is related to dilatation of extracranial blood vessels, which may be the result of chemical changes that cause spasms of intracranial vessels. An impending attack may be heralded by visual disturbances, such as flashing lights or wavy lines, or by a strange taste or odour, numbness, tingling, vertigo, tinnitus, or a feeling that part of the body is distorted in size or shape. The acute phase may be accompanied by nausea, vomiting, chills, polyuria, sweating, facial oedema, irritability, and extreme fatigue.

migrainous cranial neuralgia, a variant of migraine, characterized by closely spaced episodes of excruciating, throbbing, unilateral headaches often accompanied by dilatation of temporal blood vessels, flushing, sweating, lacrimation, nasal congestion or rhinorrhoea, ptosis, and facial oedema. Repeated episodes usually occur in clusters within a few days or weeks and may be followed by a relatively long remission period. A typical attack begins abruptly without prodromal signs, as a burning sensation in an orbit or temple.

migration, the passage of the ovum from the ovary into a uterine tube and then into the uterus.

migratory gonorrhoeal polyarthritis. See **migratory polyarthritis.**

migratory ophthalmia. See **sympathetic ophthalmia.**

migratory polyarthritis, arthritis progressively affecting a number of joints and finally settling in one or more, occurring in patients with gonorrhoea and developing a few days to a few weeks after the onset of gonorrhoeal urethritis. The patient usually has a moderate fever. Large joints are most affected; after the swelling subsides, the overlying skin may peel.

migratory thrombophlebitis, an abnormal condition in which multiple thromboses appear in both superficial and deep veins. It may be associated with malignancy, especially carcinoma of the pancreas, often preceding other evidence of cancer by several months.

Mikulicz's syndrome {Johann von Miculicz-Radecki, Polish surgeon, b. 1850}, an abnormal bilateral enlargement of the salivary and lacrimal glands, found in a variety of diseases, including leukaemia, tuberculosis, and sarcoidosis.

mild, gentle, subtle, or of low intensity, such as a mild infection.

milia neonatorum, a nonpathological skin condition characterized by minute epidermal cysts consisting of keratinous debris that occur on the face and, occasionally, the trunk of the newborn.

miliaria, minute vesicles and papules, often with surrounding erythema, caused by occlusion of sweat ducts during times of exposure to heat and high humidity.

miliary, describing a condition marked by the appearance of very small lesions the size of millet seeds, such as miliary tuberculosis, which is characterized by tiny tubercules throughout the body.

miliary carcinosis, a condition characterized by the presence of numerous cancerous nodules resembling miliary tubercules.

miliary tuberculosis, extensive dissemination by the bloodstream of tubercle bacilli. In children it is associated with high fever, night sweats, and, often, meningitis, pleural effusions, or peritonitis. A similar illness may occur in adults but with a less abrupt onset and, occasionally, with weeks or months of nonspecific symptoms, such as weight loss, weakness, and low-grade fever. Multiple small opacities resembling millet seeds may be evident on chest x-ray films.

milieu, *pl.* **milieus, milieux,** the environment, surroundings, or setting.

milieu extérieur, the external or physical surroundings of an organism, including the social environment, especially the home, school, and recreational facilities, that plays a dominant role in personality development.

milieu intérieur, a basic concept in physiology that multicellular organisms exist in an aqueous internal environment composed of the blood, lymph, and interstitial fluid that bathes all cells and provides a medium for the elementary exchange of nutrients and waste material. All fundamental processes necessary for the maintenance and life of the tissue elements depend on the stability and balance of this environment.

milieu therapy, a type of psychotherapy in which the total environment is used in treating mental and behavioural disorders. It is primarily conducted in a hospital or other institutional setting where the entire facility acts as a therapeutic community.

milium, *pl.* **milia,** a minute, white cyst of the epidermis caused by obstruction of hair follicles and eccrine sweat glands. One variety is seen in newborn infants and disappears within a few weeks. Another type is found primarily on the faces of middle-aged women.

milk, a liquid secreted by the mammary glands or udders of animals that suckle their young. After breast feeding, people consume the milk of the cow, as well as that of many other animals, including the goat. Milk is a basic food containing carbohydrate (in the form of lactose), protein (mainly casein, with small amounts of lactalbumin, and lactoglobulin), suspended fat, the minerals calcium and phosphorus, the vitamins A, riboflavin, niacin, thiamine, and, when the milk is fortified, vitamin D. It is a valuable nutrient for adults and nearly a complete food for infants.

milk-alkali syndrome, a condition of alkalosis caused by the excessive ingestion of milk, antacid medications containing calcium, or other sources of absorbable alkaline substances. The condition results in hypercalcaemia, hypocalciuria, and calcium deposits in the kidneys and other tissues.

milk ejection reflex. See **let-down reflex.**

milker's nodule, a smooth, brownish-red papilloma of the fingers or palm that begins as a macule and progresses through a vesicular stage to become a nodule. The disease is acquired from pustular lesions on the udder of a cow infected with poxvirus.

milk globule, a spherical droplet of fat in milk that tends to separate out as cream.

milking, a procedure used to express the contents of a duct or tube, to test for tenderness, or to obtain a specimen for study. The examiner compresses the structure with a finger and moves the finger firmly along the duct or tube to its opening.

Milkman's syndrome, a form of osteomalacia characterized by multiple, bilateral, symmetric absorption stripes, indicating pseudofractures, in hypocalcified long bones and the pelvis and scapula.

milk of magnesia, a laxative and antacid containing magnesium hydroxide prescribed to relieve constipation and acid indigestion.

milkpox. See **alastrim.**

milk sugar. See **lactose.**

milk tooth. See **deciduous tooth.**

milky ascites. See **chylous ascites.**

Miller-Abbott tube {Thomas G. Miller, American physician, b. 1886; William O. Abbott, American physician, b. 1902}, a long, small-caliber, double-lumen catheter, used in intestinal intubation for decompression. It has several openings on the side of its tip.

milliampere (mA) {Andre Ampere}, a unit of electric current that is one thousandth (10^{-3}) of an ampere.

milliampere seconds (mAs), the product obtained by multiplying the electric current in milliamperes by the time in seconds.

millicoulomb (mC) {Charles A. de Coulomb}, a unit of electric charge that is one thousandth of a coulomb.

millicurie (mCi) {Marie and Pierre Curie}, a unit of radioactivity that is equal to one thousandth of a curie, or 3.70×10^7 disintegrations per second.

milliequivalent (mEq), 1. the number of grams of solute dissolved in 1 ml of a normal solution. **2.** one thousandth of a gram equivalent.

milliequivalent per litre (mEq/L), one thousandth of 1 gram of a specific substance dissolved in 1 L of plasma.

milligram (mg), a metric unit of weight equal to one thousandth (10^{-3}) of a gram.

millilitre (ml), a metric unit of volume that is one thousandth (10^{-3}) of a litre.

millimetre (mm), a metric unit of length equal to one thousandth (10^{-3}) of a metre.

millimole (mmol), a unit of metric measurement of mass that is equal to one thousandth (10^{-3}) of a mole.

milliosmol, a unit of measure representing the concentration of an ion in a solution, expressed in milligrams per liter divided by atomic weight. **milliosmolar,** *adj.*

millipede, a many-legged, wormlike arthropod. Certain species squirt irritating fluids that may cause dermatitis.

milliroentgen (mR) {William von Roentgen}, a unit of radiation that is equal to one thousandth (10^{-3}) of a roentgen.

millivolt (mV) {Alessandro Volta}, a unit of electromotive force equal to one thousandth of a volt.

Milwaukee brace {Milwaukee, Wisconsin}, an orthotic device that helps immobilize the torso and the neck of a patient in the treatment or correction of scoliosis, lordosis, or kyphosis. It is usually constructed of strong but light metal and fibreglass supports lined with rubber to protect against abrasion.

mimic spasm, involuntary, stereotyped movements of a small group of muscles, as of the face. The spasm is usually psychogenic and may be aggravated by stress or anxiety but is generally controllable. Also called tic.

min, abbreviation for **minim.**

Minamata disease, a severe, degenerative, neurological disorder caused by the ingestion of grain or of seafood contaminated by soluble mercuric salts. The term is derived from a tragedy involving Japanese who ate seafood from Minamata Bay. Symptoms may not appear for several weeks or months; they include paraesthesia of the mouth and extremities, tunnel vision, difficulties with speech, hearing, muscular coordination, and concentration, weakness, emotional instability, and stupor.

mind, 1. the part of the brain that is the seat of mental activity and that enables one to know, reason, understand, remember, think, feel, and to react and adapt to surroundings and all external and internal stimuli. **2.** the totality of all conscious and unconscious processes of the individual that influence and direct mental and physical behaviour. **3.** the faculty of the intellect or understanding in contrast to emotion and will.

mine damp. See **damp.**

mineral, 1. an inorganic substance occurring naturally in the earth's crust, having a characteristic chemical composition and (usually) crystalline structure. **2.** (in nutrition) a mineral usually referred to by the name of a metal, nonmetal, radical, or phosphate rather than by the name of the compound of which it is a part.

mineral deficiency, the inability to use one or more of the mineral elements essential in human nutrition because of a genetic defect, malabsorption dysfunction, or the lack of that mineral in the diet. Minerals act as catalysts in nerve response, muscle contraction, and the metabolism of nutrients in foods. They also regulate electrolyte balance and hormonal production, and strengthen skeletal structures. See also **specific minerals.**

mineralization, the addition of any mineral to the body.

mineralocorticoid, a hormone, secreted by the adrenal cortex, that maintains normal blood volume, promotes sodium and water retention, and increases urinary excretion of potassium and hydrogen ions. Aldosterone, the most potent mineralocorticoid in regard to electrolyte balance, and corticosterone, a glucocorticoid and a mineralocorticoid, act on the distal tubules of the kidneys to enhance the reabsorption of sodium into the plasma.

mineral soap. See **bentonite.**

miner's cramp. See **heat cramp.**

miner's elbow, an inflammation of the olecranon bursa, caused by resting the weight of the body on the elbow, as in some coal mining activities. The condition is sometimes seen in school children who lean on their elbows.

miner's pneumoconiosis. See **anthracosis.**

Minerva cast, an orthopaedic cast applied to the trunk and the head, with spaces cut out for the face area and the ears. The section encasing the trunk extends to the sternum and the distal rib border anteriorly and across the distal rib border posteriorly. The cast is used for immobilizing the head and part of the trunk in the treatment of torticollis, cervical and thoracic injuries, and cervical spinal infections.

minicomputer, a medium-sized computer, intermediate in size and processing capacity between a microcomputer and a mainframe computer.

minim (min) a measurement of volume in the apothecaries' system, originally one drop (of water). Sixty minims equal 1 fluid dram. One minim equals 0.06 ml.

minimal bactericidal concentration. See **minimal inhibitory concentration.**

minimal brain dysfunction. See **attention deficit disorder.**

minimal inhibitory concentration, the lowest concentration of an antibiotic medication in the blood that is effective against an infection, determined by injecting infected venous blood into a culture medium containing various concentrations of a proposed antibiotic.

minimal occlusive volume (MOV), the volume of endotracheal cuff inflation that still permits a minimum airway leak during the inspiratory phase of ventilation.

mini-mental state examination, a brief psychological test designed to differentiate between dementia, psychosis, and affective disorders. It may include ability to identify common objects such as a pencil and a watch, write a sentence, and demonstrate orientation by identifying the day, month, and year, as well as town and country.

minimization, (in psychology) cognitive distortion in which the effects of one's behaviour are minimized.

minimum alveolar concentration (MAC), the smallest amount of a gas detected and measured in the alveoli of the lungs.

Minnesota Multiphasic Personality Inventory (MMPI), a psychological test that includes 550 statements for interpretation by the subject, used clinically for evaluating personality and for detecting various disorders, such as depression and schizophrenia.

minocycline hydrochloride, a tetracycline antibiotic active against bacteria, rickettsia, and other organisms. It is prescribed in the treatment of a variety of infections, including acne vulgaris.

minor, (in law) a person not of legal age; a person beneath the age of majority.

minor connector, (in dentistry) a device that links the major connector or base of a removable partial denture to other denture units, such as rests and retainers.

minor element. See **micronutrient.**

minor renal calyx. See **renal calyx.**

minor surgery, any surgical procedure that does not require general anaesthesia or respiratory assistance.

minoxidil, a vasodilator prescribed in the treatment of severe refractory hypertension, and applied topically to encourage hair growth in alopecia.

minute ventilation, the total ventilation per minute measured by expired gas collection for a period of 1 to 3 minutes.

miosis, 1. contraction of the sphincter muscle of the iris, causing the pupil to become smaller. **2.** an abnormal condition characterized by excessive constriction of the sphincter muscle of the iris, resulting in very small, pinpoint pupils.

miotic, 1. of or pertaining to miosis. **2.** causing constriction of the pupil of the eye. **3.** any substance or pharmaceutic that causes constriction of the pupil of the eye. Such agents are used in the treatment of glaucoma.

MIP, abbreviation for **maximum inspiratory pressure.**

miracidium, *pl.* **miracidia,** the ciliated larva of a parasitic trematode that hatches from an egg and can survive only by penetrating and further developing within a host snail, whereupon the larva further develops into a maternal sporocyte that produces more larvae.

mirage, an optical illusion caused by the

refraction of light through air layers of different temperatures, such as the illusionary sheets of water that seem to shimmer over stretches of hot sand and pavement.

MIRIAD, the *Midwifery Research Database* produced by the Midwifery Research Initiative from Oxford, England. Updates are produced on an annual basis.

mirror speech, abnormal speech characterized by the reversal of the order of syllables in a word.

misanthropy, an aversion to men, sometimes understood as an aversion to all human beings.

miscarriage. See **spontaneous abortion.**

miscible, able to be mixed or mingled with another substance.

misogamy, an aversion to marriage. **misogamic, misogamous,** *adj.,* **misogamist,** *n.*

misogyny, an aversion to women. **misogynist,** *n.,* **misogynistic,** *adj.*

misopaedia, an aversion to children. **misopaedic,** *adj.,* **misopaedist,** *n.*

misophobia. See **mysophobia.**

missed abortion, a condition in which a dead, immature embryo or fetus is not expelled from the uterus for 2 or more months. The uterus diminishes in size, and symptoms of pregnancy abate; infection and disorders of the clotting of the mother's blood may follow. Also known as **carneous mole.**

missile fracture, a penetration fracture caused by a projectile, such as a bullet or a piece of shrapnel.

mistura, any of a number of mixtures of drugs, often suspensions of insoluble substances intended for internal use.

mite {AS}, a minute arachnid with a flat, almost transparent body and four pairs of legs. Many species of these relatives of ticks and spiders are parasitic, including the chigger and *Sarcoptes scabiei,* which cause localized pruritus and inflammation.

mite typhus. See **scrub typhus.**

mithramycin. See **plicamycin.**

mithridatism. See **tachyphylaxis.**

mitleiden psychosomatic symptoms sometimes experienced by expectant fathers.

mitochondrion, *pl.* **mitochondria,** a small rodlike, threadlike, or granular organelle, within the cytoplasm, that functions in cellular metabolism and respiration and occurs in varying numbers in all living cells except bacteria, viruses, blue-green algae, and mature erythrocytes. Mitochondria provide the principal source of cellular energy through oxidative phosphorylation and adenosine triphosphate synthesis. They also contain the enzymes involved with electron transport and the citric and fatty acid cycles. **mitochondrial,** *adj.*

mitogen, an agent that triggers mitosis. **mitogenic,** *adj.*

mitogenesia, the production by or formation resulting from mitosis.

mitogenesis, the induction of mitosis in a cell. **mitogenetic,** *adj.*

mitogenetic radiation, the force or specific energy that is supposedly given off by cells undergoing division.

mitogenic factor, a kind of lymphokine that is released from activated T lymphocytes and stimulates the production of normal unsensitized lymphocytes.

mitogenic radiation. See **mitogenetic radiation.**

mitome, the reticular network sometimes observed within the cytoplasm and nucleoplasm of fixed cells.

mitomycin, a cytotoxic antibiotic used in the treatment of a variety of malignant diseases.

mitosis, a type of cell division that occurs in somatic cells and results in the formation of two genetically identical daughter cells containing the diploid number of chromosomes characteristic of the species. Mitosis is the process by which the body produces new cells for both growth and repair of injured tissue. Kinds of mitosis are **heterotypical mitosis, homeotypical mitosis, multipolar mitosis,** and **pathologic mitosis. mitotic,** *adj.*

mitotane, a cytotoxic drug that destroys normal and neoplastic adrenal cortical cells. It is prescribed in the treatment of carcinoma of the adrenal cortex.

mitotic figure, any chromosome or chromosome aggregation during any of the stages of mitosis.

mitotic index, the number of cells per unit (usually 1000) undergoing mitosis during a given time. The ratio is used primarily as an estimation of the rate of tissue growth.

mitral, 1. of or pertaining to the mitral valve of the heart. **2.** shaped like a mitre.

mitral gradient, the difference in pressure in the left atrium and left ventricle during diastole.

mitral regurgitation, a lesion of the mitral valve that allows the flow of blood from the left ventricle into the left atrium. The condition may result from congenital valve abnormalities, rheumatic fever, mitral valve prolapse, endocardial fibroelastosis, dilatation of the left ventricle because of severe anemia, myocarditis, or myocardiopathy. Symptoms include dyspnoea, fatigue, intolerance to exercise, and heart palpitations. Congestive heart failure may ultimately occur.

mitral stenosis. See **mitral valve stenosis.**

mitral valve, one of the four valves of the heart, situated between the left atrium and the left ventricle; the only valve with two, rather than three, cusps. The mitral valve allows blood to flow from the left atrium into the left ventricle but prevents blood from flowing back into the atrium. Ventricular contraction in systole forces the blood against the valve, closing the two cusps and assuring the flow of blood from the ventricle into the the aorta.

mitral valve prolapse (MVP), protrusion of one or both cusps of the mitral valve back into the left atrium during ventricular systole, resulting in incomplete closure of the valve and the backflow of blood. Most patients are asymptomatic, although some may experience chest pain, palpitations, fatigue, or dyspnoea. The condition may lead to mitral regurgitation, resulting in enlargement of the left atrium and ventricle.

mitral valve stenosis, an obstructive lesion in the mitral valve of the heart caused by adhesions on the leaflets of the valve, usually the result of recurrent episodes of rheumatic endocarditis. Hypertrophy of the left atrium develops and may be followed by right-sided heart failure and pulmonary oedema (cor pulmonale).

mittelschmerz, abdominal pain in the region of an ovary during ovulation, which usually occurs midway through the menstrual cycle. Present in many women, mittelschmerz is useful for identifying ovulation, thus pinpointing the fertile period of the cycle.

Mittendorf's dot, an eye anomaly characterized by the presence of a small dense floating opacity behind the posterior lens capsule. It is a remnant of the hyaloid artery that was present in the eye during embryonic development. The object usually does not affect vision.

mixed anaesthesia. See **balanced anaesthesia.**

mixed aneurysm. See **compound aneurysm.**

mixed cell malignant lymphoma, a lymphoid neoplasm containing lymphocytes and histiocytes (macrophages).

mixed cell sarcoma, a tumour consisting of two or more cellular elements, excluding fibrous tissue.

mixed connective tissue disease (MCTD), a systemic disease characterized by the combined symptoms of various collagen diseases, such as synovitis, polymyositis, scleroderma, and systemic lupus erythematosus.

mixed culture, a laboratory culture that contains two or more different strains of organisms.

mixed dentition, a phase of dentition during which some of the teeth are permanent and some are deciduous.

mixed glioma, a tumour, composed of glial cells, that contains more than one kind of cell, the most common being nonneural cells of ectodermal origin.

mixed infection, an infection by several microorganisms, as in some abscesses, pneumonia, and infections of wounds. Numerous combinations of bacteria, viruses, and fungi may be involved.

mixed leukaemia, a malignancy of blood-forming tissues characterized by the proliferation of eosinophilic, neutrophilic, and basophilic granulocytes, in contrast to one predominant cell line.

mixed lymphocyte culture (MLC) reaction, an assay of the function of the T cell lymphocytes, primarily used for histocompatibility testing before grafting.

mixed porphyria. See **variegate porphyria.**

mixed sleep apnoea, a condition marked by signs and symptoms of both central sleep apnoea and obstructive sleep apnoea. Mixed sleep apnoea often begins as central sleep apnoea and is followed by development of the obstructive form.

mixed tumour, a growth composed of more than one kind of neoplastic tissue, especially a complex embryonal tumour of local origin.

mixed venous blood, blood that is composed of the venous blood from the heart and all systemic tissues in proportion to their venous returns. In the absence of abnormalities, mixed venous blood is present in the main pulmonary artery.

mixture, 1. a substance composed of ingredients that are not chemically combined and do not necessarily occur in a fixed proportion. **2.** (in pharmacology) a liquid containing one or more medications in suspension. The proportions of the ingredients are specific to each mixture.

ml, abbreviation for **millilitre.**

MLC, abbreviation for **mixed lymphocyte culture.** See **mixed lymphocyte culture reaction.**

MLD, abbreviation for **minimum lethal dose.**

mm, abbreviation for **millimetre.**

MMEF, abbreviation for *maximal mid-expiratory flow.*

M-mode, abbreviation for *motion mode,* a variation of B-mode ultrasound scanning. It is used in echocardiography.

mmol, abbreviation for **millimole.**

MMPI, abbreviation for **Minnesota Multiphasic Personality Inventory.**

MMR, abbreviation for **measles, mumps,** and **rubella vaccine.**

Mn, symbol for **manganese.**

Mo, symbol for **molybdenum.**

mobile arm support, a forearm support device that enables persons with upper extremity disabilities to fulfil some activities of daily living, such as by helping to position the hand properly for self-feeding. The orthotic device may be mounted on a wheelchair.

mobility, the velocity a particle or ion attains for a given applied voltage and a relative measure of how quickly an ion may move in an electric field.

mobility, impaired physical, an inability to achieve a functional level of mobility in the environment, combined with one or more of the following: a reluctance to move, a limited range of motion of the limbs or extremities, a decrease in the strength or control of the musculoskeletal system, abnormal or impaired ability to coordinate movements, or any of a large number of imposed restrictions on movement, such as medically required bed rest or traction.

mobilizations, a form of passive movement but its rhythm and grade are such that the patient or model can prevent it being formed.

Mobitz I heart block {Woldemar Mobitz, German physician, b. 1889}, second degree or partial atrioventricular (AV) block in which the PR interval increases progressively until the propagation of an atrial impulse does not occur and the corresponding ventricular beat drops out. After the pause, the progressive shortening of the PR interval begins again. Symptoms include fatigue, dizziness, and, in some cases, syncope. Mobitz I heart block is caused by abnormal conduction of the cardiac impulse in the AV node.

Mobitz II heart block, second degree or partial atrioventricular block, characterized by the sudden nonconduction of an atrial impulse and a periodic dropped beat without prior lengthening of the PR interval. This kind of block usually results from impaired conduction in the bundle branches and may be caused by anterior myocardial infarction, myocarditis, drug toxicity, electrolyte disturbances, rheumatoid nodules, and various degenerative diseases. Long-term therapy requires the implantation of a pacemaker.

Möbius' syndrome {Paul J. Möbius, German neurologist, b. 1853}, a rare developmental disorder characterized by congenital bilateral facial palsy usually associated with oculomotor and other neurological dysfunctions, speech disorders, and various anomalies of the extremities.

mode, a value or term in a set of data that occurs more frequently than other values or terms.

model, (in nursing theory) a conceptual framework or theory that explains a phenomenon and allows predictions to be made. Examples include Orem's *Self-care Model*, Roy's *Adaptation Model* and King's *Interaction Model*.

model of human occupation, a conceptual framework for occupational therapists. Developed by Kielhofner.

modelling, a technique used in behaviour therapy in which a person learns a desired response by observing it performed.

modem, MODEM, abbreviation for *modulate/demodulate*. It is a device for transforming serial binary numbers into an audible tone, and vice versa, for transmission over a telephone line to another computer. Common rates of data transfer are 300 and 1200 baud.

moderator band, a thick bundle of muscle in the central part of the right ventricle of the heart. Also called **trabecula septomarginalis.**

modified milk, cow's milk in which the protein content has been reduced and the fat content increased to correspond to the composition of breast milk.

modified radical mastectomy, a surgical procedure in which a breast is completely removed with the underlying pectoralis minor and some of the adjacent lymph nodes. The pectoralis major is not excised. The operation is performed in treating early and well-localized malignant neoplasms of the breast.

modified release, see **sustained release.**

modulation transfer function (MTF), a quantitative measure of the ability of an imaging system to reproduce patterns that vary in spatial frequency.

Moeller's glossitis {Julius O. L. Moeller, German surgeon, b. 1819}, a form of chronic glossitis, characterized by burning or pain in the tongue and an increased sensitivity to hot or spicy foods.

mohel, an ordained Jewish circumciser.

MOHO, abbreviation for **model of human occupation.**

moiety, a part of a molecule that exhibits a particular set of chemical and pharmacological characteristics.

moist gangrene. See **gangrene.**

mol. See **mole².**

molality, the numbers of moles of solute per kilogram of water or other solvent.

molar, 1. any one of the 12 molar teeth, six in each dental arch, three located posterior to the premolar teeth. The crown of each molar is nearly cubical, convex on its buccal surface and its lingual surface and flattened on its surfaces of contact. It is surmounted by four or five cusps separated by cruciate depressions and has a large rounded neck. **2.** of or pertaining to the gram molecular weight of a substance.

molarity, the number of moles of solute per litre of water or other solvent.

molar pregnancy, pregnancy in which a hydatid mole develops from the trophoblastic tissue of the early embryonic stage of development. The signs of pregnancy are all exaggerated: the uterus grows more rapidly than is normal, morning sickness is often severe and constant, blood pressure is likely to be elevated, and blood levels of chorionic gonadotropins are extremely high.

molar solution, a solution that contains one mole of solute per litre of solution.

mole¹, *informal.* **1.** a pigmented naevus. **2.** (in obstetrics) a hydatidiform mole.

mole², the standard unit used to measure the amount of a substance. A mole of a substance is the amount containing the same number of elementary particles (atoms, electrons, ions, molecules, or other particles) as there are atoms in 12 g of carbon 12. Also spelled **mol.** **molar,** *adj.*

molecular genetics, the branch of genetics that focuses on the chemical structure and the functions, replication, and mutations of the molecules involved in the transmission of genetic information, such as DNA and RNA.

molecular lesion. See **point lesion.**

molecular weight, the total of the atomic weights of the atoms in a molecule.

molecule, the smallest unit that exhibits the properties of an element or compound. A molecule is composed of two or more atoms that are chemically combined.

mole percent, a percentage calculation expressed in terms of moles of a substance in a mixture or solution rather than in terms of molecular weight.

mole volume, the volume occupied by one mole of a substance, which may be a solid, liquid, or gas. It is numerically equal to the molecular weight divided by the density.

molluscum, any skin disease having soft, rounded masses or nodules.

molluscum contagiosum, a disease of the skin and mucous membranes, caused by a poxvirus. It is characterized by scattered white papules. Palms of the hands and soles of the feet are not affected. The disease most frequently occurs in children and in adults with an impaired immune response. It is transmitted from person to person by direct or indirect contact.

molybdenum (Mo), a greyish metallic element. Its atomic number is 42; its atomic weight is 95.94. Molybdenum is poisonous if ingested in large quantities.

molybdenum 99, radionuclide which is the parent of technetium-99. Used in radio-nuclide imaging in a generator which is eluted with saline to obtain molybdenum-free technetium-99m.

Mönckeberg's arteriosclerosis {Johann G. Mönckeberg, German pathologist, b. 1877}, a form of arteriosclerosis in which extensive calcium deposits are found in the media of the artery with little obstruction of the lumen.

Monge's disease. See **altitude sickness.**

Mongolian spot, a benign, bluish-black macule occurring over the sacrum and on the buttocks of some newborns. It usually disappears during early childhood.

mongolism. See **Down's syndrome.**

Monilia. See *Candida albicans.*

monilial vulvovaginitis, moniliasis. See **candidiasis.**

monitor, 1. to observe and evaluate a function of the body closely and constantly. **2.** a mechanical device that provides a visual or audible signal or a graphic record of a particular function, such as a cardiac monitor or a fetal monitor.

monoamine, an amine containing one amine group.

monoamine oxidase (MAO), an enzyme that catalyses the oxidation of amines.

monoamine oxidase inhibitor (MAOI), any of a chemically heterogeneous group of drugs used primarily in the treatment of depression resistant to less toxic treatments. These drugs also exert an antianxiety effect, especially in anxiety associated with phobia. MAOIs interact with many drugs and with foods containing large amounts of the amino acid tyromine, to produce a life-threatening hypertensive crisis. By inhibiting the enzyme monoamine oxidase, these drugs prevent the breakdown of amine neurotransmitters in the brain causing them to accumulate; this probably explains their clinical effects. Selective inhibitors of monamine oxidase type B selectively inhibit the breakdown of dopamine and are used in the treatment of Parkinsons disease.

monobasic acid, an acid with only one replaceable hydrogen atom, such as hydrochloric acid (HCl).

monoblast. a large, immature monocyte. Certain of the leukaemias are characterized by greatly increased production of monoblasts in the marrow and by the abnormal presence of these forms in the peripheral circulation. **monoblastic,** *adj.*

monoblastic leukaemia, a progressive malignancy of blood-forming organs, characterized by the proliferation of monoblasts and monocytes.

monocephalus. See **syncephalus.**

monochorial twins, monochorionic twins. See **monozygotic twins.**

monoclonal, of, pertaining to, or designating a group of identical cells or organisms derived from a single cell.

monoclonal gammopathy. See **gammopathy.**

monocyte, a large mononuclear leukocyte with an ovoid or kidney-shaped nucleus, containing lacy, linear chromatin material and grey-blue cytoplasm filled with fine, reddish, and azurophilic granules. See also **monocytosis.**

monocytic leukaemia, a malignancy of blood-forming tissues in which the predominant cells are monocytes. The disease has an erratic course characterized by malaise, fatigue, fever, anorexia, weight loss, splenomegaly, bleeding gums, dermal petechiae, anaemia, and unresponsiveness to therapy. There are two forms: **Schilling's leukaemia,** in which most of the cells are monocytes that probably arise from the reticuloendothelial system, and the more common **Naegeli's leukaemia,** in which a large number of the cells resemble myeloblasts.

monocytosis, an increased proportion of monocytic white blood cells in the circulation.

monoethanolamine, an amino alcohol formed by the decarboxylation of serine. It is used as a surfactant in pharmaceutical products.

monofactorial inheritance, the acquisition or expression of a trait or condition that depends on the transmission of a single specific gene.

monohybrid, pertaining to or describing an individual, organism, or strain that is heterozygous for only one specific trait or that is heterozygous for the single trait or gene locus under consideration.

monohybrid cross, the mating of two individuals, organisms, or strains that have different gene pairs for only one specific trait or in which only one particular characteristic or gene locus is being followed.

monohydric alcohol, an alcohol containing one hydroxyl group.

monomer, a molecule that repeats itself to form a polymer, such as the molecules of fibrin monomer that polymerize to form fibrin in the blood-clotting process. **monomeric,** *adj.*

monomolecular reaction (E^1), a first-order chemical kinetic reaction in which only one substance is involved in the reaction.

monomphalus, conjoined twins that are united at the umbilicus.

mononeuritis multiplex. See **multiple mononeuropathy.**

mononeuropathy, any disease or disorder that affects a single nerve trunk. Some common causes of disorders involving single nerve trunks are electric shock, radiation, and fractured bones that may compress or lacerate nerve fibres. Casts and tourniquets that are too tight may also damage a nerve by compression or by ischaemia.

mononuclear cell, a leukocyte, including lymphocytes and monocytes, with a round or oval nucleus.

mononucleosis, 1. an abnormal increase in the number of mononuclear leukocytes in the blood. **2.** See **infectious mononucleosis.**

monooctanoin, a gallstone dissolving agent used to dissolve cholesterol gallstones.

monoovular. See **uniovulvar.**

monophasic, having one phase, part, aspect, or stage.

monoploid, haploid. Also **monoploidic.**

monopodial symmelia. See **sympus monopus.**

monopus, a fetus or individual with the congenital absence of a foot or leg.

monorchid, a male who has monorchism.

monorchism, a condition in which only one testicle has descended into the scrotum. **monorchidic,** *adj.*

monosaccharide, a carbohydrate consisting of a single basic unit with the general formula $C_n (H_2O)_n$, with n ranging from 3 to 8.

monosome, 1. an unpaired X or Y sex chromosome. **2.** the single, unpaired chromosome in monosomy.

monosomy, a chromosomal aberration characterized by the absence of one chromosome from the normal diploid complement. **monosomic,** *adj.*

monosomy X. See **Turner's syndrome.**

monospecific, an antibody that will react with only one type of antigen.

monounsaturated fatty acid. See **unsaturated fatty acid.**

monovular. See **uniovular.**

monovulatory, routinely releasing one ovum during each ovarian cycle.

monozygotic (MZ), pertaining to or developed from a single fertilized ovum, or zygote, such as occurs in identical twins. **monozygosity,** *n.*, **monozygous,** *adj.*

monozygotic twins, two offspring born of the same pregnancy and developed from a single fertilized ovum that splits into equal halves during an early cleavage phase in embryonic development, giving rise to separate fetuses. Such twins are always of the same sex, have the same genetic constitution, possess identical blood groups, and closely resemble each other in physical, psychologic, and mental characteristics. Monozygotic twins may have single or separate placentas and membranes, depending on the time during development when division occurred.

Monson curve {George S. Monson, American dentist, b. 1869}, the curve of occlusion in which each tooth cusp and incisal edge conform to a segment of the surface of a sphere 8 inches (20 cm) in diameter, with its centre in the region of the glabella.

monstrosity, 1. the state or condition of having severe congenital defects. **2.** anything that deviates greatly from the normal; a monster or teras.

mons veneris, a pad of fatty tissue and coarse skin that overlies the symphysis pubis in the woman. Also called **mons pubis.**

Monteggia's fracture {Giovanni B. Monteggia, Italian physician, b. 1762}, fracture of the proximal third of the ulna, associated with radial dislocation or rupture of the annular ligament and resulting in the angulation or over-riding of ulnar fragments.

Montercaux fracture, a fracture of the neck of the fibula associated with the diastasis of ankle mortise.

Montgomery's gland. See **Montgomery's tubercle.**

Montgomery's tubercles {William F. Montgomery, Irish gynaecologist, b. 1797}, small papillae on the surface of nipples and aerolas that secrete a fatty, lubricating substance. Also called **Montgomery's gland.**

mood, a prolonged emotional state that influences one's whole personality and life functioning. See also **affect.**

mood-congruent psychotic features, the characteristics of a psychosis in which the content of hallucinations or delusions is consistent with an elevated, expansive mood or with a depression.

moon face, a condition characterized by a rounded, puffy face, occurring in people treated with large doses of corticosteroids, such as those with rheumatoid arthritis or acute childhood leukaemia.

Moore's fracture {Edward M. Moore, American surgeon, b. 1814}, a fracture of the distal radius with associated dislocation of the ulnar head, resulting in the securement of the styloid process under the annular ligaments of the wrist.

MOPP, an abbreviation for a combination drug regimen used in the treatment of cancer, containing three antineoplastics, Mustine, Oncovin (vincristine sulphate), Procarbazine hydrochloride, and prednisolone (a glucocorticoid). MOPP is used in the treatment of Hodgkin's disease.

morbid anatomy. See **pathological anatomy.**

morbidity, 1. an illness or an abnormal condition or quality. **2.** (in statistics) the rate at which an illness or abnormality occurs, calculated by dividing the entire number of people in a group by the number in that group who are affected with the illness or abnormality. **3.** the rate at which an illness occurs in a particular area or population.

morbid physiology. See **pathological physiology.**

morbilli. See **measles.**

morbilliform, describing a skin condition that resembles the erythematous, maculopapular rash of measles.

Morgagni's globule {Giovanni B. Morgagni, Italian anatomist, b. 1682}, a minute opaque sphere that may form from fluid coagulation between the eye lens and its capsule, especially in cataract.

Morgagni's tubercle {Giovanni B. Morgagni}, one of several small, soft nodules on the surface of each of the areola in women. The tubercles are produced by large sebaceous glands just under the surface of the areolae.

morgan {Thomas H. Morgan, American biologist, b. 1896}, (in genetics) a unit of measure used in mapping the relative distances between genes on a chromosome.

morgue, a unit of a hospital with facilities for the storage and autopsy of dead persons.

Morita therapy, an alternative therapy that has as its focus the neurotic symptoms of the patient. The goal of the therapy is to enable the patient to live responsibly and constructively, even if the symptoms persist.

morning after pill, *informal.* A large dose of an oestrogen given orally, over a short period of time, to a woman within 24 to 72 hours after unprotected sexual intercourse to prevent conception, as an emergency measure.

morning dip, a significant decline in respiratory function observed in some asthmatic persons during the early morning hours.

morning sickness. See **nausea and vomiting of pregnancy.**

moron, *obsolete.* a retarded person having an IQ between 50 and 70 and incapable of developing beyond the mental age of 12 years.

Moro reflex {Ernst Moro, German pediatrician, b. 1874}, a normal mass reflex in a young infant elicited by a sudden loud noise, such as by striking the table next to the child, resulting in flexion of the legs, an embracing posture of the arms, and usually a brief cry.

morphea, localized scleroderma consisting of patches of yellowish or ivory-coloured, rigid, dry, smooth skin.

morphine sulphate, an opiate analgesic used to control severe pain.

morphogenesis, the development and differentiation of the structures and the form of an organism, specifically the changes that occur in the cells and tissue during embryonic development. Also called **morphogeny.**

morphogeny. See **morphogenesis.**

morphology, the study of the physical shape and size of a specimen, plant, or animal. **morphological,** *adj.*

Morquio's disease {Luis Morquio, Uruguayan physician, b. 1867}, a familial form of mucopolysaccharidosis that results in abnormal musculoskeletal development in childhood. Dwarfism, hunchback, enlarged sternum, and knock-knees may occur.

mortality, 1. the condition of being subject to death. **2.** the death rate, which reflects the number of deaths per unit of population in any specific region, age group, disease, or other classification, usually expressed as deaths per 1000, 10,000, or 100,000.

mortar, a cup-shaped vessel in which materials are ground or crushed by a pestle in the preparation of drugs.

Morton's foot, See **metatarsalgia.**

Morton's neuroma, See **metatarsalgia.**

Morton's plantar neuralgia {Thomas G. Morton, American surgeon, b. 1835}, a severe throbbing pain that affects the anastomotic nerve branch between the medial and the lateral plantar nerves.

Morton's toe. See **metatarsalgia.**

morula, *pl.* **morulas, morulae,** a solid, spherical mass of cells resulting from the cleavage of the fertilized ovum in the early stages of embryonic development. **morular,** *adj.*

Morton' toe, a form of syringomyelia with tissue changes in the extremities, such as paraesthesia of the forearms and hands, and progressive painless ulceration of the fingertips.

mosaic, 1. (in genetics) an individual or organism that developed from a single zygote but that has two or more kinds of genetically different cell populations. Such a condition results from a mutation, crossing-over, or, more commonly in humans, nondisjunction of the chromosomes during early embryogenesis, which causes a variation in the number of chromosomes in the cells. 2. (in embryology) a fertilized ovum that undergoes determinate cleavage.

mosaic bone, bone tissue appearing to be made up of many tiny pieces cemented together, as seen on microscopic examination of an x-ray film of the affected bone. It is characteristic of Paget's disease of the bone.

mosaic cleavage. See **determinate cleavage.**

mosaic development, a kind of embryonic development occurring in the blastocyst. The fertilized ovum undergoes determinate cleavage, developing according to a precise, unalterable plan in which each blastomere has a characteristic position, limited developmental potency, and is a precursor of a definite part of the embryo.

mosaicism, (in genetics) a condition in which an individual or an organism that develops from a single zygote has two or more cell populations that differ in genetic constitution.

mosaic wart, a group of contiguous plantar warts.

mosquito bite, a bite of a bloodsucking arthropod of the subfamily Culicidae that may result in a systemic allergic reaction in a hypersensitive person, an infection, or, most often, a pruritic wheal.

mosquito forceps, a small haemostatic forceps.

Mössbauer spectrometer {Rudolf L. Mössbauer, German physicist, b. 1929}, an instrument that can detect small changes between an atomic nucleus and its environment, such as caused by changes in temperature, pressure, or chemical state.

mother fixation, an arrest in psychosexual development characterized by an abnormally persistent, close, and often paralysing emotional attachment to one's mother.

motile, capable of spontaneous but unconscious or involuntary movement. **motility,** *n.*

motion sickness, a condition caused by erratic or rhythmic motions in any combination of directions, such as in a boat or a car. Severe cases are characterized by nausea, vomiting, vertigo, and headache, mild cases by headache and general discomfort.

motivational conflict, a conflict resulting from the arousal of two or more motives that direct behaviour toward incompatible goals. Kinds of motivational conflict include **approach-approach conflict, approach-avoidance conflict,** and **avoidance-avoidance conflict.**

motor, 1. of or pertaining to motion, the body apparatus involved in movement, or the brain functions that direct purposeful activities. **2.** of or pertaining to a muscle, nerve, or brain centre that produces or subserves motion.

motor aphasia, the inability to utter remembered words, caused by a cerebral lesion in the inferior frontal gyrus (Broca's motor speech area) of the left hemisphere in right-handed individuals. The condition most commonly is the result of a stroke. The patient knows what to say but cannot articulate the words.

motor apraxia, the inability to carry out planned movements or to handle small objects, although the proper use of the object is recognized. The condition results from a lesion in the premotor frontal cortex on the opposite side of the affected limb.

motor area, a portion of the cerebral cortex that includes the precentral gyrus and the posterior part of the frontal gyri and that causes the contraction of the voluntary muscles on stimulation with electrodes. Normal voluntary activity requires associations between the motor area and other parts of the cortex; removal of the motor area from one cerebral hemisphere causes paralysis of voluntary muscles, especially of the opposite side of the body.

motor coordination, the coordination of body functions that involve movement, including gross motor, fine motor, and motor planning.

motor dysfunction, any type of disorder found in learning disabled children that has a motor component.

motor end plate, a broad band of terminal fibres of the motor nerves of the voluntary muscles. Motor nerves derived from the cranial and spinal nerves enter the sheaths of striated muscle fibres, lose their myelin sheaths, and ramify like the roots of a tree. The neurilemma of the nerve fibre merges with the sarcolemma of the muscle, and the axon synapses with the muscle fibres.

motor fibre, one of the fibres in the spinal nerves that transmit impulses to muscle fibres.

motor image, a visual concept of one's bodily movements, real or imagined.

motor lag, a prolonged latent period between the reception of a stimulus and the initiation of a motor response.

motor nerve. See **motor neuron.**

motor neuron, one of various efferent nerve cells that transmit nerve impulses from the brain or from the spinal cord to muscular or glandular tissue. Also called **motoneuron.**

motor neuron disease, a fatal degenerative disease of the central nervous system involving progressive degeneration of the motor nuclei of cranial nerves, the anterior cells in the spinal cord, and the corticospinal tracts. It tends to affect middle-age men and there is no known cause.

motor neuron paralysis, an injury to the spinal cord that causes damage to the motor neurons and results in various degrees of functional impairment depending on the site of the lesion. See **lower motor neuron paralysis, upper motor neuron paralysis.**

motor planning, the ability to plan and execute skilled nonhabitual tasks.

motor point, 1. a point at which a motor nerve enters the muscle it innervates. **2.** a point at which electrical stimulation will cause contraction of a muscle.

motor seizure, a transitory disturbance in brain function caused by abnormal neuronal discharges that arise initially in a localized motor area of the cerebral cortex. The manifestations depend on the site of the abnormal electric activity, such as tonic contractures of the thumb, caused by excessive discharges in the motor area of the cortex controlling the first digit.

motor sense, the feeling or perception enabling a person to accomplish a purposeful movement, presumably achieved by evoking a sensory engram or memory of the pattern for that specific movement.

motor unit, a functional structure consisting of a motor neuron and the muscle fibres it innervates.

mould, 1. a fungus. **2.** a growth of fungi. **3.** a plastic shell used to keep the head or other body part immobile during radiotherapy. **4.** a hollow form for casting or shaping an object, as a prosthesis.

moulding, the natural process by which a baby's head is shaped during labour as it is squeezed into and through the birth passage by the uterine contractions. The head may become quite elongated, and the bones of the skull may be caused to overlap slightly at the suture lines. Most of the changes caused by moulding resolve themselves during the first few days of life.

mountain fever, mountain tick fever. See **Rocky Mountain spotted fever.**

mourning, a psychological process of reaction activated by an individual to assist in overcoming a great personal loss. The process is finally resolved when a new object relationship is established.

mouse, a hand-controlled cursor movement device. Rolling the device on a flat surface causes the cursor to move in the same direction on a computer screen.

mouse-tooth forceps, a kind of dressing forceps that has one or more fine sharp points on the tip of each blade. The tips turn in, and the delicate teeth interlock.

mouth, 1. the nearly oval oral cavity at the anterior end of the digestive tube, bounded anteriorly by the lips and containing the tongue and the teeth. It consists of the vestibule and the mouth cavity proper. The vestibule, situated in front of the teeth, is bounded externally by the lips and the cheeks, internally by the gums and the teeth. The vestibule receives the secretion from the parotid salivary glands and communicates, when the jaws are closed, with the mouth cavity proper by an aperture on each side behind the molar teeth and by narrow clefts between opposing teeth. The mouth is roofed by the hard and the soft palates. The tongue forms the greater part of the floor of the cavity. **2.** an orifice.

mouthstick, a device that can be manipulated with the mouth and can be used to type, push buttons, turn pages, or operate power wheelchairs and other equipment for paralysed patients.

mouth-to-mouth resuscitation, a procedure in artificial resuscitation, performed most often with cardiac massage. The victim's nose is sealed by pinching the nostrils closed, the head is extended, and air is breathed by the rescuer through the mouth into the lungs.

mouth-to-nose resuscitation, a procedure in artificial resuscitation in which the mouth of the victim is covered and held closed and air is breathed through the victim's nose.

MOV, abbreviation for **minimal occlusive volume.**

movement decomposition, a distortion in voluntary movement in which the movement occurs in a distinct sequence of isolated steps, rather than in a normal, smooth, flowing pattern.

moving grid, (in radiography) a secondary radiation grid that is continuously moved or oscillated during a radiographic exposure.

moxibustion, a method of producing analgesia or altering the function of a system of the body by igniting moxa, wormwood, or other combustible, slow-burning substance and holding it as near the point on the skin as possible without causing pain or burning. It is also sometimes used in conjunction with acupuncture.

MPD, 1. abbreviation for **maximum permissible dose. 2.** (in radiotherapy) abbreviation for **mid-plane dose.**

MPS, abbreviation for **mucopolysaccharidosis.**

mR, abbreviation for **milliroentgen.**

MRC, abbreviation for **Medical Research Council.**

MRCGP, abbreviation for **Member of the Royal College of General Practitioners.**

MRCOG, abbreviation for **Member of the Royal College of Obstetricians and Gynaecologists.**

MRCP, abbreviation for **Member of the Royal College of Physicians.**

MRCPath, abbreviation for **Member of the Royal College of Pathologists.**

MRCS, abbreviation for **Member of the Royal College of Surgeons.**

MRPharmS, abbreviation for **Member of**

the **Royal Pharmaceutical Society of Great Britain.** Membership is dependent upon qualifications, post-graduate training, and passing a registration exam and is a prerequisite to practising as a pharmacist in the UK.

MS, abbreviation for **multiple sclerosis.**

M.Sc., abbreviation for **Master of Science.** See **Master's Degree Programme in Nursing.**

MSH, abbreviation for melanocyte stimulating hormone.

Much's granules {Hans C. Much, German physician, b. 1880}, granules and rods, found in tuberculosis sputum, that stain with gram stain but not by the usual methods for acid-fast bacilli.

mucin, a mucopolysaccharide, the chief ingredient in mucus. Mucin is present in most glands that secrete mucus and is the lubricant protecting body surfaces from friction or erosion.

mucinoid, resembling mucin.

mucinous adenocarcinoma. See **mucinous carcinoma.**

mucinous carcinoma, an epithelial neoplasm with a sticky gelatinous consistency caused by the copious mucin secreted by its cells.

mucocutaneous, of or pertaining to the mucous membrane and the skin.

mucocutaneous lymph node syndrome (MLNS), an acute, febrile illness, primarily of young children, characterized by inflamed mucous membranes of the mouth, "strawberry tongue," cervical lymphadenopathy, polymorphous rash on the trunk, and oedema, erythema, and desquamation of the skin on the extremities. Other commonly associated findings include arthralgia, diarrhoea, otitis, pneumonia, photophobia, meningitis, and electrocardiographic changes.

mucoepidermoid carcinoma, a malignant neoplasm of glandular tissues, especially the ducts of the salivary glands.

mucogingival junction, the scalloped linear area of the gums that separates the gingivae from the alveolar mucosa.

mucoid, 1. resembling mucus. 2. also **mucinoid.** a group of glycoproteins, including colloid and ovomucoid, similar to the mucins, the primary difference being in solubility.

mucolytic, 1. exerting a destructive effect on the mucus. 2. any agent that dissolves or destroys the mucus.

mucomembranous, of or pertaining to a mucous membrane, such as that of the small intestine or the bladder.

mucopolysaccharidosis (MPS), *pl.* **mucopolysaccharidoses,** one of a group of genetic disorders characterized by greater than normal accumulations of mucopolysaccharides in the tissues, with other symp-

toms specific to each type. The disorders are numbered MPS I through MPS VII, and each type has a specific eponym. In all types there is pronounced skeletal deformity (especially of the face), mental and physical retardation, and decreased life expectancy. Kinds of mucopolysaccharidosis include **Hunter's syndrome (MPS II), Hurler's syndrome (MPS I),** and **Morquio's disease (MPS IV).**

mucoprotein, a compound, present in all connective and supporting tissue, that contains polysaccharides combined with protein and is relatively resistant to denaturation.

mucopurulent, characteristic of a combination of mucus and pus.

mucormycosis. See **zygomycosis.**

mucosa, *pl.* **mucosae, mucous membrane. mucosal,** *adj.*

mucositis, any inflammation of a mucous membrane, such as the lining of the mouth and throat.

mucous. See **mucus.**

mucous colitis. See **irritable bowel syndrome.**

mucous membrane, any one of four major kinds of thin sheets of tissue that cover or line various parts of the body. Mucous membranes line cavities or canals of the body that open to the outside, such as the linings of the mouth, the digestive tube, the respiratory passages, and the genitourinary tract. It consists of a surface layer of epithelial tissue covering a deeper layer of connective tissue and protects the underlying structure, secretes mucus, and absorbs water, salts, and other solutes.

mucous plug, See **operculum.**

mucous shreds. See **shreds.**

mucous tumour. See **myxoma.**

mucoviscidosis. See **cystic fibrosis.**

mucus, the viscous, slippery secretions of mucous membranes and glands, containing mucin, white blood cells, water, inorganic salts, and exfoliated cells. **mucoid, mucous,** *adj.*

mucus trap suction apparatus, a catheter containing a trap to prevent mucus being aspirated from the nasopharynx and trachea of a newborn infant and entering the mouth of the person operating the device.

mud bath, the application of warm mud to the body for therapeutic purposes.

mulibrey nanism, a rare genetic disorder characterized by dwarfism, constrictive pericarditis, muscular hypotonia, anomalies of the skull and face, and characteristic yellow dots in the ocular fundus. The name of the condition is an acronym composed of the first two letters of the anatomical sites of the principal defects: *muscle, liver, brain,* and *eyes.*

müllerian duct {Johannes P. Müller, German physiologist, b. 1801}, one of a pair of embryonic ducts that become the fallopian tubes, uterus, and vagina in females and that atrophy in males.

Müller's manoeuvre {Johannes P. Müller}, an inspiratory effort against a closed airway or glottis. The effort decreases intrapulmonary and intrathoracic pressures and expands pulmonary gas.

multicentric mitosis. See **multipolar mitosis.**

multidisciplinary health care team, a group of health care workers who are members of different disciplines, each one providing specific services to the patient.

multifactorial, of, pertaining to, or characteristic of any condition or disease resulting from the interaction of many factors, specifically the interaction of several genes, usually polygenes, with or without the involvement of environmental factors. Many disorders, such as spina bifida, are considered to be multifactorial.

multifactorial inheritance, the tendency to develop a physical appearance, disease, or condition that is a condition of many genetic and environmental factors, such as stature and blood pressure.

multifocal, an action, such as the transmission of an impulse, that arises from more than two foci.

multiform, an organ, tissue, or other object that may appear in more than one shape.

multigenerational model, a model of family therapy that focuses on reciprocal role relationships over a period of time. The family is viewed as an emotional system where patterns of interacting and coping can be passed from one generation to the next and can cause stress to the members on whom they are projected. The goal is to help the family members attain a higher level of differentiation.

multigenerational transmission process, the repetition of relationship patterns, including divorce, suicide, or alcoholism, associated with emotional dysfunction that can be traced through several generations of the same family.

multigravida, a woman who has been pregnant more than once.

multiinfarct dementia, a form of organic brain disease characterized by the rapid deterioration of intellectual function, caused by vascular disease. Symptoms include emotional lability, disturbances in memory, abstract thinking, judgement, and impulse control, and focal neurological impairment, such as abnormalities of gait, pseudobulbar palsy, and paraesthesia.

multilocular cyst, one of three kinds of follicular cyst, containing many spaces and not associated with a tooth.

multipara, *pl.* **multiparae,** a woman who has delivered more than one viable infant.

multipenniform, (of a bodily structure)

having a shape resembling a pattern of many feathers.

multiphasic screening, a technique of screening populations for diseases in which there is combined use of a battery of screening tests. The technique serves to identify any of several diseases being screened for in a population.

multiple benign cystic epithelioma. See **trichoepithelioma.**

multiple cartilaginous exostoses. See **diaphyseal aclasis.**

multiple enchondromatosis. See **enchondromatosis.**

multiple endocrine adenomatosis. See **adenomatosis.**

multiple factor. See **polygene.**

multiple family therapy, psychotherapy in which four or five families meet weekly to confront and deal with problems or issues that they have in common.

multiple fission, cell division in which the nucleus first divides into several equal parts followed by the division of the cytoplasm into as many cells as there are nuclei.

multiple fracture, 1. a fracture extending several fracture lines in one bone. 2. the fracture of several bones at one time or from the same injury.

multiple gene. See **polygene.**

multiple idiopathic haemorrhagic sarcoma. See **Kaposi's sarcoma.**

multiple impact therapy, psychotherapy in which families come together for intensive work meetings over a 3-day weekend or weeklong encounter.

multiple lipomatosis, a rare, inherited disorder characterized by discrete, localized, subcutaneous deposits of fat in the tissues of the body.

multiple mononeuropathy, an abnormal condition characterized by dysfunction of several individual nerve trunks. It may be caused by various diseases.

multiple myeloma, a malignant neoplasm of the bone marrow. The tumour, composed of plasma cells, destroys osseous tissue, especially in flat bones, causing pain, fractures, and skeletal deformities.

multiple myositis. See **polymyositis.**

multiple neuroma. See **neuromatosis.**

multiple peripheral neuritis, acute or subacute disseminated inflammation or degeneration of symmetrically distributed peripheral nerves, characterized initially by numbness, tingling in the extremities, hot and cold sensations, and slight fever, progressing to pain, weakness, diminished reflexes, and in some cases flaccid paralysis. The disorder may be caused by toxic substances, such as antimony, arsenic, carbon monoxide, copper, lead, mercury, nitrobenzol, organophosphates, and thallium, or various drugs.

multiple personality, an abnormal condition in which the organization of the personality is fragmented. It is characterized by the presence of two or more distinct subpersonalities.

multiple personality disorder, a dissociative disorder characterized by the existence of two or more distinct, clearly differentiated personality structures within the same individual, any of which may dominate at a particular time. The various subpersonalities are usually dramatically different from one another and may or may not be aware of the existence of the others. Transition from one subpersonality to another is usually sudden and associated with psychosocial stress.

multiple plasmacytoma of bone. See **multiple myeloma.**

multiple pregnancy, a pregnancy in which there is more than one fetus in the uterus at the same time.

multiple sclerosis (MS), a progressive disease characterized by disseminated demyelination of nerve fibres of the brain and spinal cord. The first signs are paraesthesias, or abnormal sensations in the extremities or on one side of the face. Other early signs are muscle weakness, vertigo, and visual disturbances, such as nystagmus, diplopia (double vision), and partial blindness. Later in the course of disease there may be extreme emotional lability, ataxia, abnormal reflexes, and difficulty in urinating.

multiple self-healing squamous epithelioma. See **keratoacanthoma.**

multiplicative growth. See **merisis.**

multipolar mitosis, cell division in which the spindle has three or more poles and results in the formation of a corresponding number of daughter cells.

multisynaptic, pertaining to a nervous process or system of nerve cells requiring a series of synapses.

multivalent, 1. (in chemistry) denoting the capacity of an element to combine with three or more univalent atoms. **2.** (in immunology) able to act against more than one strain of organism.

mummification, a dried-up state, such as occurs in dry gangrene or a dead fetus in utero.

mummified fetus, a fetus that has died in utero and has shrivelled and dried up.

mumps, an acute viral disease, characterized by a swelling of the parotid glands, caused by a paramyxovirus. It is most likely to affect children between 5 and 15 years of age, but it may occur at any age. In adulthood the infection may be severe. The incidence of mumps is highest during the late winter and early spring. The mumps paramyxovirus lives in the saliva of the affected individual and is transmitted in droplets or by direct contact. The virus is present in the saliva from 6 days before to 9 days after the onset of the swelling of the parotid gland. The

prognosis in mumps is good, but the disease sometimes involves complications, such as arthritis, pancreatitis, myocarditis, oophoritis, and nephritis. About one half of the men with mumps-induced orchitis suffer some atrophy of the testicles, but because the condition is usually unilateral, sterility rarely results. The common symptoms include anorexia, headache, malaise, and low-grade fever, followed by earache, parotid gland swelling and a temperature of 38.3° to 40° C. The patient also experiences pain when drinking acidic liquids or when chewing. The salivary glands may also become swollen.

mumps vaccine, a live viral vaccine used for active immunization against mumps.

Munchausen's syndrome {Baron von Munchausen, legendary sixteenth century confabulator}, an unusual condition characterized by habitual pleas for treatment and hospitalization for a symptomatic but imaginary acute illness. The affected person may logically and convincingly present the symptoms and history of a real disease.

mural, something that is found on or against the wall of a cavity, as a mural thrombus on an interior wall of the heart.

Murchison fever. See **Pel-Ebstein fever.**

murine typhus, an acute arbovirus infection caused by *Rickettsia typhi* and transmitted by the bite of an infected flea. The disease is similar to epidemic typhus but less severe. It is characterized by headache, chills, fever, myalgia, and rash. A dull-red, maculopapular rash, mainly on the trunk, appears about the fifth day and lasts for 4 to 8 days.

murmur, a low-pitched fluttering or humming sound, such as a heart murmur.

muromonab-CD3 (orthoclone OKT3), a parenteral monoclonal antibody used as an immunosuppressant in the control of acute organ transplant rejection.

Murphy's sign, a test for gallbladder disease in which the patient is asked to inspire while the examiner's fingers are held under the liver border at the bottom of the rib cage. The inspiration causes the gallbladder to descend onto the fingers, producing pain if the gallbladder is inflamed.

Murray Valley encephalitis, an acute inflammatory disease of the brain, once epidemic in Australia's Murray Valley, characterized by convulsions, muscle rigidity, high fever, mental confusion, and coma.

muscae volitantes. See **floater.**

muscarinic, stimulating the postganglionic parasympathetic receptor.

muscle, a kind of tissue composed of fibres that are able to contract, causing and allowing movement of the parts and organs of the body. Muscle fibres are richly vascular, irritable, conductive, and elastic. There are two basic kinds, striated muscle and smooth muscle. Striated muscle, which comprises all skeletal muscles except for the myocardium, is long and voluntary; it responds very quickly to stimulation and is paralysed by interruption of its innervation. Smooth muscle, which comprises all visceral muscles, is short and involuntary; it reacts slowly to all stimuli and does not entirely lose its tone if innervation is interrupted. The myocardium is sometimes classified as a third (cardiac) kind of muscle, but it is basically a striated muscle that does not contract as quickly as the striated muscle of the rest of the body, and it is not completely paralysed if it loses its neural stimuli.

muscle albumin, albumin present in muscle.

muscle bridge, a band of myocardial tissue over one or more of the large epicardial coronary vessels. It may cause constriction of the artery during systole.

muscle of expression. See **facial muscle.**

muscle reeducation, the use of physical therapeutic exercises to restore muscle tone and strength after an injury or disease.

muscle relaxant, a drug that reduces the contractility of muscle fibres. Curare derivatives and succinylcholine compete with acetylcholine and block neural transmission at the myoneural junction. Quinine sulphate reduces muscle tension by increasing the refractory period of muscle fibres and by decreasing the excitability of the motor end plate. Baclofen inhibits monosynaptic and polysynaptic reflexes at the spinal level. The benzodiazepines reduce muscle tension, chiefly by acting on reticular neuronal mechanisms that control muscle tone. Dantrolene apparently achieves its effect by interfering with the release of calcium from the sarcoplasmic reticulum of muscle.

muscle-setting exercise, a method of maintaining muscle strength and tonality by alternately contracting and relaxing a skeletal muscle or any group of muscles without moving the associated part of the body.

muscle testing, a method of evaluating the contractile unit, including the muscle, tendons, and associated tissues, of a moving part of the body by neurological or resistance testing. The tests may include range of motion ability, isokinetic measurement of muscle strength, and functional tests, such as specific agility drills, as well as other medical tests.

muscle tone, a normal state of balanced muscle tension.

muscular, 1. of or pertaining to a muscle. **2.** characteristic of well-developed musculature.

muscular atrophy, a condition of motor unit dysfunction, usually the result of a loss of efferent innervation.

muscular branch of the deep brachial artery, one of several similar branches of the deep brachial artery, supplying certain arm muscles, such as the coracobrachialis, biceps brachii, and brachialis.

muscular dystrophy, a group of genetically transmitted diseases characterized by progressive atrophy of symmetrical groups of skeletal muscles without evidence of involvement or degeneration of neural tissue. In all forms of muscular dystrophy there is an insidious loss of strength with increasing disability and deformity, although each type differs in the groups of muscles affected, the age of onset, the rate of progression, and the mode of genetic inheritance. The main types of the disease are pseudohypertrophic (Duchenne) muscular dystrophy, limb-girdle muscular dystrophy, and facioscapulohumeral (Landouzy-Déjérine) muscular dystrophy. Rarer forms include Becker's muscular dystrophy, distal muscular dystrophy, ocular myopathy, and myotonic muscular dystrophy.

muscular sarcoidosis, sarcoidosis of the skeletal muscles in which there is interstitial inflammation, fibrosis, atrophy, and damage of the muscle fibres as sarcoid tubercles form within and replace normal muscle cells.

muscular system, all of the muscles of the body, including the smooth, cardiac, and striated muscles, considered as an interrelated structural group.

muscular tumour. See **myoma.**

musculature, the arrangement and condition of the muscles.

musculocutaneous nerve, one of the terminal branches of the brachial plexus. It is formed on each side by division of the lateral cord of the plexus into two branches. Various branches and filaments supply different structures, such as the biceps, the brachialis, the humerus, and the skin of the forearm.

musculoskeletal, of or pertaining to the muscles and the skeleton.

musculoskeletal system, all of the muscles, bones, joints, and related structures, such as the tendons and connective tissue, that function in the movement of the parts and organs of the body.

musculoskeletal system assessment, an evaluation of the condition and functioning of the patient's muscles, joints, and bones and of factors that may contribute to abnormalities in these body structures.

musculospiral nerve. See **radial nerve.**

mush bite, a procedure used in making dental impressions for the construction of full or partial dentures. The patient brings his upper and lower jaws together into a block of softened wax, thus supplying a spatial relationship between the maxilla and mandible.

mushroom, the fruiting body of the fungus of the class Basidomycetes, especially edible members of the order Agaricales, known as the field mushrooms or meadow mushrooms. Mushrooms are composed largely of water and are of limited nutritional value.

Fungal poisoning is caused by ingestion of mushrooms of the genus *Amanita*, in particular *A. muscaria* and *A. phalloides*.

mushroom poisoning, a toxic condition caused by the ingestion of certain mushrooms, particularly two species of the genus *Amanita*. Muscarine in *Amanita muscaria* produces intoxication in from a few minutes to 2 hours. Symptoms include lacrimation, salivation, sweating, vomiting, laboured breathing, abdominal cramps, diarrhoea, and, in severe cases, convulsions, coma, and circulatory failure. Atropine is usually administered in treatment. More deadly but slower-acting phalloidine in *A. phalloides* and *A. verna* causes similar symptoms, as well as liver damage, renal failure, and death in 30% to 50% of the cases.

music therapy, a form of adjunctive psychotherapy in which music is used as a means of recreation and communication, especially with autistic children, and as a means to elevate the mood of depressed and psychotic patients.

mustard gas, a poisonous gas used in chemical warfare during World War I. It causes corrosive destruction of the skin and mucous membranes, often resulting in permanent respiratory damage and death.

mustine hydrochloride, a cytotoxic alkylating agent used in the treatment of a variety of cancers, especially Hodgkin's disease.

mutacism, mimmation, or the incorrect use of /m/ sounds.

mutagen, any chemical or physical environmental agent that induces a genetic mutation or increases the mutation rate. **mutagenic,** *adj.,* **mutagenicity,** *n.*

mutagenesis, the induction or occurrence of a genetic mutation.

mutant, 1. any individual or organism with genetic material that has undergone mutation. **2.** relating to or produced by mutation.

mutant gene, any gene that has undergone a change, such as the loss, gain, or exchange of genetic material, that affects the normal transmission and expression of a trait. Kinds of mutant genes are **amorph, antimorph, hypermorph, hypomorph.**

mutase, any enzyme that catalyses the shifting of a chemical group or radical from one position to another within the same molecule or, occasionally, from one molecule to another.

mutation, an unusual change in genetic material occurring spontaneously or by induction. The alteration changes the original expression of the gene. Genes are stable units, but when a mutation occurs, it often is transmitted to future generations. **mutate,** *v.,* **mutational,** *adj.*

mutism, the inability or refusal to speak. The condition may result from an unconscious response to emotional conflict and confu-

sion and is most commonly observed in patients who are catatonic, stuporous, hysterical, or depressed. A kind of mutism is **akinetic mutism.**

muton, (in molecular genetics), the smallest DNA segment whose alteration can result in a mutation.

mutually exclusive categories, categories on a research instrument that are sufficiently precise to allow each subject, factor, or variable to be classified in only one category.

mutual support group, a type of group in which members organize to solve their own problems. They are led by the group members themselves who share a common goal and use their own strengths to gain control over their lives.

mv, abbreviation for **millivolt.**

MV, abbreviation for **megavolt.**

mVO$_2$, symbol for **myocardial oxygen consumption.**

MVV, abbreviation for *maximal voluntary ventilation.* See **maximal breathing capacity.**

M.W.I.A., abbreviation for **Medical Women's International Association.**

MX gene, a human gene that helps the body resist viral infections. When exposed to interferon, the MX gene inhibits the production of viral protein and nucleic acid necessary for the proliferation of new viral particles.

myaesthesia, perception of any sensation in a muscle, such as touch, direction, proprioception, contraction, relaxation, or extension.

myalgia, diffuse muscle pain, usually accompanied by malaise, occurring in many infectious diseases, such as brucellosis, dengue, influenza, leptospirosis, measles, malaria, relapsing fever, rheumatic fever, salmonellosis, tick-borne haemorrhagic fevers, toxoplasmosis, trichinosis, tularaemia, and poliomyelitis. Myalgia occurs in arteriosclerosis obliterans, fibrositis, fibromyositis, Guillain-Barré syndrome, hyperparathyroidism, hypoglycaemia, hypothyroidism, muscle tumour, myoglobinuria, myositis, and renal tubular acidosis. Various drugs may also cause **myalgia. myalgic,** *adj.*

Myalgic encephalopathy (ME), a debilitating condition believed instigated by exposure to viral infection or other agents which, in some cases, result in a chronic, continuing disease process. Documented symptoms include brain malfunction, fatigue, nerve pain and muscle pain.

myasthenia, a condition characterized by an abnormal weakness of a muscle or a group of muscles that may be the result of a systemic myoneural disturbance, as in myasthenia gravis, or myasthenia laryngis involving the vocal cord tensor muscles. **myasthenic,** *adj.*

myasthenia gravis, an abnormal condition characterized by the chronic fatigue and weakness of muscles, especially in the face and throat, as a result of a defect in the conduction of nerve impulses at the myoneural junction. Muscular fatigue in myasthenia gravis is caused by the inability of receptors at the myoneural junction to depolarize because of a deficiency of acetylcholine; hence the diagnosis may be made by administering an anticholinesterase drug and observing improved muscle strength and stamina. The onset of symptoms is usually gradual, with ptosis of the upper eyelids, diplopia, and weakness of the facial muscles. The weakness may then extend to other muscles innervated by the cranial nerves, particularly the respiratory muscles. Muscular exertion aggravates the symptoms.

myasthenia gravis crisis, acute exacerbation of the muscular weakness characterizing the disease, triggered by infection, surgery, emotional stress, or an overdose or insufficiency of anticholinesterase medication. Typical signs and symptoms include respiratory distress progressing to periods of apnoea, extreme fatigue, increased muscular weakness, dysphagia, dysarthria, and fever. The patient may be anxious, restless, irritable, unable to move the jaws or to raise one or both eyelids.

myasthenic crisis, an acute episode of muscular weakness.

mycelium, *pl.* **mycelia,** a mass of interwoven, branched, threadlike filaments that make up most fungi. Also called **hypha.**

mycetismus, mushroom poisoning.

mycetoma, a serious fungal infection involving skin, subcutaneous tissue, fascia, and bone. One kind of mycetoma is **Madura foot.**

mycobacteria, acid-fast microorganisms belonging to the genus *Mycobacterium.* **mycobacterial,** *adj.*

mycobacteriosis, a tuberculosislike disease caused by mycobacteria other than *Mycobacterium tuberculosis.*

Mycobacterium, a genus of rod-shaped, acid-fast bacteria having two significant pathogenic species: *Mycobacterium leprae* causes leprosy; *M. tuberculosis* causes tuberculosis.

mycology, the study of fungi and fungoid diseases. **mycological,** *adj.,* **mycologist,** *n.*

mycomyringitis. See **myringomycosis.**

mycophenolic acid, a bacteriostatic and fungistatic crystalline antibiotic obtained from *Pencillium brevi compactum* and related species.

Mycoplasma, a genus of ultramicroscopic organisms lacking rigid cell walls and considered to be the smallest free-living organisms. Some are saprophytes, some are parasites, and many are pathogens.

mycoplasma pneumonia, a contagious disease of children and young adults caused by *Mycoplasma pneumoniae,* characterized by a 9- to 12-day incubation period and followed by symptoms of an upper respiratory infection, dry cough, and fever.

mycosis, any disease caused by a fungus. Some kinds of mycoses are **athlete's foot, candidiasis,** and **coccidioidomycosis. mycotic,** *adj.*

mycosis fungoides, a rare, chronic, lymphomatous skin malignancy resembling eczema or a cutaneous tumour that is followed by microabscesses in the epidermis and lesions simulating those of Hodgkin's disease in lymph nodes and viscera.

mycotic, pertaining to a disease caused by a fungus.

mycotic aneurysm, a localized dilatation in the wall of a blood vessel caused by the growth of a fungus, usually occurring as a complication of bacterial endocarditis.

mycotoxicosis, a systemic poisoning caused by toxins produced by fungal organisms.

mydriasis, 1. dilatation of the pupil of the eye caused by contraction of the dilator muscle of the iris, a muscular sheath that radiates outward like the spokes of a wheel from the centre of the iris around the pupil. **2.** an abnormal condition characterized by contraction of the dilator muscle, resulting in widely dilated pupils. **mydriatic,** *adj.*

mydriatic and cycloplegic agent, any one of several ophthalmic preparations that dilate the pupil and paralyse the ocular muscles of accommodation. Mydriatics stimulate the sympathetic nerve fibres or block parasympathetic nerve fibres of the eye, temporarily paralysing the iris sphincter muscle. Cycloplegics temporarily paralyse accommodation while relaxing the ciliary muscle. Some drugs may cause both mydriasis and cycloplegia, whereas others are designed to produce a single effect. These drugs are used in diagnostic ophthalmoscopic and refractive examination of the eye.

myelacephalus, a fetus, usually a separate monozygotic twin, whose form and parts are barely recognizable; a slightly differentiated amorphous mass. **myelacephalous,** *adj.*

myelatelia, any developmental defect involving the spinal cord.

myelauxe, a developmental anomaly characterized by hypertrophy of the spinal cord.

myelencephalon, the lower part of the embryonic hindbrain from which the medulla oblongata develops.

myelin, a substance constituting the sheaths of various nerve fibres throughout the body. It is largely composed of fat, which gives the fibres a white, creamy colour. **myelinic,** *adj.*

myelinated, (of a nerve) having a myelin sheath.

myelination, the process of furnishing or

taking on myelin.

myelin globule, a fatlike droplet found in some sputum.

myelinic, of or pertaining to myelin.

myelinic neuroma, a neuroma neoplasm composed of myelinated nerve fibres.

myelinization, development of the myelin sheath around a nerve fibre.

myelinolysis, a pathological process that dissolves the myelin sheaths around certain nerve fibres, such as those of the pons in alcoholic and undernourished people who are afflicted with central pontine myelinolysis.

myelin sheath, a segmented, fatty lamination composed of myelin that wraps the axons of many nerves in the body. In myelinated peripheral nerves, the sheaths are composed of Schwann cells. The myelin sheaths around the central nerve fibres are composed of oligodendroglia. Their lipoid content gives these coverings a whitish appearance. Various diseases, such as multiple sclerosis, can destroy these myelin wrappings.

myelitis, an abnormal condition characterized by inflammation of the spinal cord with associated motor or sensory dysfunction. Some kinds of myelitis are **acute transverse myelitis, leukomyelitis,** and **poliomyelitis. myelitic,** *adj.*

myeloblast, one of the earliest precursors of the granulocytic leukocytes. The cytoplasm appears light blue, scanty, and nongranular when seen in a stained blood smear through a microscope. **myeloblastic,** *adj.*

myeloblastaemia. See **myeloblastosis.**

myeloblastic leukaemia, a malignant neoplasm of blood-forming tissues, characterized by many myeloblasts in the circulating blood and tissues.

myeloblastomatosis, abnormal, localized clusters of myeloblasts in the peripheral circulation.

myeloblastosis, the abnormal presence of myeloblasts in the circulation.

myelocele, a saclike protrusion of the spinal cord through a congenital defect in the vertebral column.

myeloclast. a cell that breaks down the myelin sheaths of nerves of the central nervous system.

myelocyst, any benign cyst that is formed from the rudimentary medullary canals that give rise to the vertebral canal during embryonic development.

myelocystocele, a protrusion of a cystic tumour containing spinal cord substance through a defect in the vertebral column.

myelocystomeningocele, a protrusion of a cystic tumour containing both spinal cord substance and meninges through a defect in the vertebral column.

myelocyte, an immature white blood cell normally found in the bone marrow, being the first of the maturation stages of the granulocytic leukocytes. These cells appear in the circulating blood only in certain forms of leukaemia. **myelocytic,** *adj.*

myelocythaemia, an abnormal presence of myelocytes in the circulating blood, such as in myelocytic leukaemia.

myelocytic leukaemia, a disorder characterized by the unregulated and excessive production of myelocytes of the granulocytic series.

myelocytoma, a localized cluster of myelocytes in the peripheral vasculature that may occur in myelocytic leukaemia.

myelocytosis. See **myelocythaemia.**

myelodiastasis, disintegration and necrosis of the spinal cord.

myelodysplasia, a general designation for the defective development of any part of the spinal cord.

myelofibrosis. See **myeloid metaplasia.**

myelogenesis, 1. the formation and differentiation of the nervous system during prenatal development. **2.** the development of the myelin sheath around the nerve fibre.

myelogenous, pertaining to the cells produced in bone marrow or to the tissue from which such cells originate. Also **myelogenetic, myelogenic.**

myelogenous leukaemia. See **acute myelocytic leukaemia, chronic myelocytic leukaemia.**

myelogeny, the formation and differentiation of the myelin sheaths of nerve fibers during the prenatal development of the central nervous system.

myelogram, 1. an x-ray film taken by the process known as **myelography. 2.** a graphic representation of a count of the different kinds of cells in a stained preparation of bone marrow.

myelography, a radiographic technique to visualize the spinal cord and the subarachnoid space are following intrathecal administration, usually via a lumbar puncture, of a radiopaque contrast medium. **myleographic,** *adj.*

myeloid, 1. of or pertaining to the bone marrow. **2.** of or pertaining to the spinal cord. **3.** of or pertaining to myelocytic forms that do not necessarily originate in the bone marrow.

myeloid leukaemia. See **acute myelocytic leukaemia, chronic myelocytic leukaemia.**

myeloid metaplasia, a disorder in which bone marrow tissue develops in abnormal sites. The primary form is also called **agnogenic myeloid metaplasia, myelofibrosis.**

myeloidosis, an abnormal condition characterized by general hyperplasia of the myeloid tissue.

myeloma, an osteolytic neoplasm consisting of a profusion of cells typical of the bone marrow. It may develop simultaneously in many sites, causing extensive areas of patchy destruction of the bone. Kinds of myeloma are **endothelial myeloma, extramedullary myeloma, giant cell myeloma, multiple myeloma,** and **osteogenic myeloma.**

myelomalacia, abnormal softening of the spinal cord, caused primarily by inadequate blood supply.

myelomatosis. See **multiple myeloma.**

myelomeningocele, a developmental defect of the central nervous system in which a hernial sac containing a portion of the spinal cord, its meninges, and cerebrospinal fluid protrudes through a congenital cleft in the vertebral column. The condition is caused primarily by the failure of the neural tube to close during embryonic development, although in some instances it may result from the reopening of the tube from an abnormal increase in cerebrospinal fluid pressure.

myelomere, any of the embryonic segments of the brain or spinal cord during prenatal development.

myelomonocytic leukaemia. See **monocytic leukaemia.**

myelopathic anaemia. See **myelophthisic anaemia.**

myelopathy, 1. any disease of the spinal cord. 2. any disease of the myelopoietic tissues.

myelophthisic anaemia, a disorder attributed to several pathological processes that displace the haemopoietic tissues of the bone marrow.

myelopoiesis, the formation and development of the bone marrow or the cells that originate from it. A kind of myelopoiesis is **extramedullary myelopoiesis. myelopoietic,** adj.

myeloradiculodysplasia, any developmental abnormality of the spinal cord and spinal nerve roots.

myeloschisis, a developmental defect characterized by a cleft spinal cord that results from the failure of the neural plate to fuse and form a complete neural tube.

myelosuppression, the inhibition of the process of production of blood cells and platelets in the bone marrow.

myiasis, infection or infestation of the body by the larvae of flies, usually through a wound or an ulcer, but, rarely, through the intact skin.

myitis. See **myositis.**

mylohyoideus, one of a pair of flat triangular muscles that form the floor of the cavity of the mouth.

myocardial infarction (MI), an occlusion of a coronary artery, caused by atherosclerosis or an embolus resulting from a necrotic area in the vasculature myocardium. The onset of MI is characterized by a crushing, vicelike chest pain that may radiate to the left arm, neck, or epigastrium and sometimes simulates the sensation of acute indigestion or a gallbladder attack. The patient usually becomes ashen, clammy, short of breath, faint, and anxious and often feels that death is imminent. Typical signs are tachycardia, a barely perceptible pulse, low blood pressure, an elevated temperature, cardiac arrhythmia, and electrocardiographic evidence of elevation of the ST segment and Q wave. Laboratory studies usually show an increased sedimentation rate, leukocytosis, and elevated serum levels of creatine phosphokinase, lactic dehydrogenase, and glutamic-oxaloacetic transaminase. Potential complications in MI are pulmonary or systemic embolism, pulmonary oedema, shock, and cardiac arrest.

myocardiopathy, any disease of the myocardium.

myocarditis, an inflammatory condition of the myocardium caused by viral, bacterial, or fungal infection, serum sickness, rheumatic fever, or chemical agent, or as a complication of a collagen disease. Myocarditis most frequently occurs in an acute viral form and is self-limited, but it may lead to acute heart failure.

myocardium, a thick, contractile, middle layer of uniquely constructed and arranged muscle cells that forms the bulk of the heart wall. The myocardium contains a minimum of other tissue, except for the blood vessels, and is covered interiorly by the endocardium. The contractile tissue of the myocardium is composed of fibres with the characteristic cross-striations of muscular tissue. The fibres, which are about one third as large in diameter as those of skeletal muscle and contain more sarcoplasm, branch frequently and are interconnected to form a network that is continuous except where the bundles and the laminae are attached at their origins and insertions into the fibrous trigone of the heart. Most of the myocardial fibres function to contract the heart. Contraction involves the action of calcium ions and sodium ions and a complex electrochemical process. **myocardial,** adj.

myoclonus, a spasm of a muscle or a group of muscles. **myoclonic,** adj.

myodiastasis, an abnormal condition in which there is separation of muscle bundles.

myoedema, pl. **myoedemas, myoedemata, muscle oedema.**

myofacial pain dysfunction syndrome. See **temporomandibular joint pain dysfunction syndrome.**

myofibril, a slender striated strand of muscle tissue. Myofibrils occur in groups of branching threads running parallel to the cellular long axis.

myogelosis, a condition in which there are hardened areas or nodules within muscles, especially the gluteal muscles.

myogenic, pertaining to muscles, particularly cardiac and smooth muscles that do not require nerves to initiate and maintain contractions.

myoglobin, a ferrous globin complex consisting of one haem molecule containing one iron molecule attached to a single globin chain. Myoglobin is found in muscle and is responsible for the red colour of that tissue and for its ability to store oxygen.

myoglobinuria, the presence of myoglobin, a respiratory pigment of muscle tissue, in the urine.

myokinase. See **adenylate kinase.**

myoma, *pl.* **myomas, myomata,** a common, benign fibroid tumour on the uterine muscle. Menorrhagia, backache, constipation, dysmenorrhoea, dyspareunia, and other symptoms develop proportionate to the size, location, and rate of growth of the tumour.

myoma praevium. See **leiomyoma uteri.**

myoma striocellulare. See **rhabdomyoma.**

myomectomy, the surgical removal of muscle tissue.

myomere. See **myotome.**

myometritis, an inflammation or infection of the myometrium of the uterus.

myometrium, *pl.* **myometria,** the muscular layer of the wall of the uterus. The fibres of the myometrium course around the uterus horizontally, vertically, and diagonally.

myonecrosis, the death of muscle fibres. **Progressive** or **clostridial myonecrosis** is caused by the anaerobic bacteria of the genus *Clostridium.* Seen in deep wound infections, progressive myonecrosis is accompanied by pain, tenderness, a brown serous exudate, and a rapid accumulation of gas within the tissue of the muscle.

myoneural, of or pertaining to a muscle and its associated nerve, especially to nerve endings in muscles.

myoneural junction. See **neuromuscular junction.**

myopathy, an abnormal condition of skeletal muscle characterized by muscle weakness, wasting, and histological changes within muscle tissue, as seen in any of the muscular dystrophies. **myopathic,** *adj.*

myope, an individual who is nearsighted or afflicted with myopia.

myophosphorylase deficiency glycogenosis. See **McArdle's disease.**

myopia, a condition of nearsightedness caused by the elongation of the eyeball or by an error in refraction so that parallel rays are focused in front of the retina. Some kinds of myopia are **chronic myopia, curvature myopia, index myopia,** and **pathological myopia. myopic,** *adj.*

myorrhaphy, suturing of a wound in a muscle.

myorrhexis, a tearing in any muscle. **myorrhectic,** *adj.*

myosarcoma, a malignant tumour of muscular tissue.

myosin, a cardiac and skeletal muscle protein that makes up close to one half of the proteins that occur in muscle tissue. The interaction of myosin and actin is essential for muscle contraction.

myositis, inflammation of muscle tissue, usually of the voluntary muscles. Causes of myositis include infection, trauma, and infestation by parasites. Kinds of myositis include **epidemic myositis, interstitial myositis, parenchymatous myositis, polymyositis,** and **traumatic myositis.**

myositis fibrosa, an uncommon inflammation of the muscles, characterized by abnormal formation of connective tissue.

myositis ossificans, a rare, inherited disease in which muscle tissue is replaced by bone. It begins in childhood, with stiffness in the neck and back and progresses to rigidity of the spine, trunk, and limbs.

myositis purulenta, any bacterial infection of muscle tissue. This condition may result in the formation of an abscess or multiple abscesses.

myositis trichinosa, inflammation of the muscles resulting from infection by the parasite *Trichinella spiralis.*

myostasis, an abnormal condition of weakened muscle in which there is a relatively fixed length of muscle fibers in the relaxed state. **myostatic,** *adj.*

myostroma, the framework of muscle tissue.

myotatic reflex. See **deep tendon reflex.**

myotenotomy, surgical division of the whole or part of a muscle by cutting through its main tendon.

myotome, 1. The muscle plate of an embryonic somite that develops into a voluntary muscle. **2.** a group of muscles innervated by a single spinal segment. **3.** an instrument for cutting or dissecting a muscle.

myotomic muscle, any of the numerous muscles of the trunk of the body, derived from the myotomes and divided into the deep muscles of the back and the thoracoabdominal muscles.

myotomy, the cutting of a muscle, performed to gain access to underlying tissues or to relieve constriction in a sphincter, as in severe oesophagitis or pyloric stenosis.

myotonia, any condition in which a muscle or a group of muscles does not readily relax after contracting. **myotonic,** *adj.*

myotonia atrophica. See **myotonic muscular dystrophy.**

myotonia congenita, a rare, mild, and nonprogressive form of myotonic myopathy evident early in life. The only effects of the disorder are hypertrophy and stiffness of the muscles.

myotonic muscular dystrophy, a severe form of muscular dystrophy marked by ptosis, facial weakness, and dysarthria. Weakness of the hands and feet precedes that in the shoulders and hips. Myotonia of the hands is usually present.

myotonic myopathy, any of a group of disorders characterized by increased skeletal muscle tone and decreased relaxation of muscle after contraction. Kinds of myotonic myopathy include **myotonia congenita, myotonic muscular dystrophy.**

myringa. See **tympanic membrane.**

myringectomy, excision of the tympanic membrane.

myringitis, inflammation or infection of the tympanic membrane.

myringomycosis, a fungal infection of the tympanic membrane.

myringoplasty, surgical repair of perforations of the eardrum with a tissue graft, performed to correct hearing loss. The openings in the eardrum are enlarged, and the grafting material is sutured over them.

myringotomy, surgical incision of the eardrum, performed to relieve pressure and release pus from the middle ear. The drum is incised, and cultures are taken; fluid is gently suctioned from the middle ear. Ear drops may be instilled to improve drainage.

mysophobia, an anxiety disorder characterized by an overreaction to the slightest uncleanliness, or an irrational fear of dirt, contamination, or defilement. Also spelled **misophobia. mysophobic, misophobic,** *adj.*

myxoedema, the most severe form of hypothyroidism. It is characterized by swelling of the hand, face, feet, and periorbital tissues. At this stage, the disease may lead to coma and death.

myxofibroma, a fibrous tumour that contains myxomatous tissue.

myxoid. See **mucoid,** def. **1.**

myxoma, a neoplasm of the connective tissue, characteristically composed of stellate cells in a loose mucoid matrix crossed by delicate reticulum fibres. These tumours may grow to enormous size and are usually pale grey, soft, and jellylike. Some have exceeded 30 cm in diameter. **myxomatous,** *adj.*

myxoma fibrosum. See **myxofibroma.**

myxoma sarcomatosum. See **myxosarcoma.**

myxopoiesis, the production of mucus.

myxosarcoma, a sarcoma that contains some myxomatous tissue.

myxovirus, any of a group of medium-size RNA viruses that are further divided into orthomyxoviruses and paramyxoviruses. Some kinds of myxoviruses are the viruses that cause influenza, mumps, and parainfluenza.

MZ, abbreviation for **monozygotic.**

n., (in prescriptions) an abbreviation for nocte, a Latin word meaning at 'night'.

n, 2n, 3n, 4n, symbols for the haploid, diploid, triploid, and tetraploid number of chromosomes in a cell, organism, strain, or individual.

N, symbol for **nitrogen.**

Na, chemical symbol for **sodium.**

nabothian gland {Martin Naboth}, one of many small, mucus-secreting glands of the uterine cervix.

NADH, abbreviation for *nicotine adenine dinucleotide, reduced.*

nadir, the lowest point, such as the blood count after it has been depressed by chemotherapy.

nadolol, a beta-adrenergic blocking agent used for long-term management of angina pectoris, hypertension, and thyrotoxicosis, and in migraine prophylaxis.

NADPH, abbreviation for *nicotine adenine disphosphonucleotide, reduced.*

Naegeli's leukaemia. See **monocytic leukaemia.**

Naegeli's obliquity. See **asynclitism.**

Naegeli's pelvis {Franz K. Naegele, German obstetrician, b. 1778}, a rare abnormality of the pelvis whereby one sacral ala has not developed resulting in an asymmetrical pelvis.

Naegeli's rule {Franz K. Naegele}, a method for calculating the estimated date of delivery based on a mean length of gestation. Three months are subtracted from the first day of the last normal menstrual period, and 1 year plus 7 days are added to that date.

naevoid amentia. See **Sturge-Weber syndrome.**

naevoid neuroma, a tumour of nerve tissue that contains numerous small blood vessels.

naevus, a pigmented, congenital skin blemish that is usually benign but may become cancerous.

naevus flammeus, a flat, capillary haemangioma that is present at birth and often varies in colour from pale red to deep reddish purple. These lesions are most often seen on the face. The depth of colour depends on whether the superficial, middle, or deep dermal vessels are involved.

naevus vascularis. See **capillary haemangioma.**

Nager's acrofacial dysostosis {F. R. Nager, 20th century Swiss physician}, an abnormal congenital condition characterized by limb deformities, such as radioulnar synostosis, hypoplasia, and the absence of the radius or of the thumbs.

Nahrungs-Einheit-Milch (nem) a nutritional unit in Pirquet's system of feeding that is equivalent to 1 g of breast milk.

nail, 1. a flattened, elastic structure with a horny texture at the end of a finger or a toe. Each nail is comprised of a root, body, and free edge at the distal extremity. The root fastens the nail to the finger or the toe by fitting into a groove in the skin and is closely moulded to the surface of the corium. The nail matrix beneath the body and the root projects longitudinal vascular ridges. The matrix firmly attaches the body of the nail to the underlying connective tissue. The whitish lunula near the root contains irregularly arranged papillae that are less firmly attached to the connective tissue than the rest of the matrix. The cuticle is attached to the surface of the nail just ahead of the root. **2.** any of various metallic nails used in orthopaedics to fasten together bones or pieces of bone.

nalidixic acid, an antibacterial used in the treatment of urinary tract infections.

naloxone hydrochloride, an opiate antagonist used for the reversal of opiate-induced CNS depression.

naltrexone hydrochloride, an oral opiate antagonist used to block the effects of opiate analgesics, including heroin, morphine, and methadone in patients recovering from addiction.

named nurse, a health care system in which one nurse is assigned to a single patient for delivery of total nursing care.

NANB, abbreviation for **non-A, non-B hepatitis.**

NANDA, abbreviation for **North American Nursing Diagnosis Association.**

nandrolone decanoate, a long-acting androgen used in the treatment of osteoporosis and breast cancer, and to stimulate growth, weight gain, and the production of red blood cells.

nandrolone phenylpropionate, an anabolic steroid with androgenic properties. It is prescribed in the treatment of osteoporosis, in certain anaemias, and in metastatic breast cancers.

nanism, an abnormal smallness or underdevelopment of the body; dwarfism. Kinds of nanism are **mulibrey nanism, Paltauf's nanism, pituitary nanism, renal nanism, senile nanism,** and **symptomatic nanism.** Also called **nanosomia.**

nanocephalic dwarf. See **bird-headed**

dwarf.

nanocephaly, a developmental defect characterized by abnormal smallness of the head. **nanocephalous,** *adj.,* **nanocephalus,** *n.*

nanocormia, abnormal disproportionate smallness of the trunk of the body in comparison to the head and limbs. **nanocormus,** *n.*

nanocurie (nC), a unit of radioactivity equal to one billionth of a curie.

nanogram (ng), a unit of weight equal to one billionth of a gram.

nanomelia, a developmental defect characterized by abnormally small limbs in comparison to the size of the head and trunk. **nanomelous,** *adj.,* **nanomelus,** *n.*

nanometer (nm), a unit of length equal to one billionth of a metre.

nanophthalmos, the condition in which one or both eyes are abnormally small, although other ocular defects are not present.

nanosomus, a person of very short stature; a dwarf.

nanukayami, an acute, infectious disease caused by one of the serotypes of the spirochete *Leptospira* that is indigenous to Japan.

nanus, 1. a dwarf. **2.** a pygmy. **nanoid,** *adj.*

nape, the back of the neck.

naphazoline hydrochloride, an adrenergic vasoconstrictor prescribed in the treatment of nasal congestion and as an ophthalmic vasoconstrictor.

naphthalene poisoning, a toxic condition, caused by the ingestion of naphthalene or paradichlorobenzene, that may cause nausea, vomiting, headache, abdominal pain, spasm, and convulsions.

naphthol camphor, a syrupy mixture of two parts of camphor and one part betanaphthol, used externally as an antiseptic.

naphthol poisoning. See **phenol poisoning.**

nappy rash, a maculopapular and occasionally excoriated eruption in the nappy area of infants caused by irritation from faeces moisture, heat or ammonia produced by bacterial decomposition of urine. Secondary infection by *candida albicans* is common.

napkin ring tumour, a tumour that encircles a tubular structure of the body, usually impairing its function and constricting its lumen to some degree.

napping, periods of sleep, usually during the day, which may last from 15 to 60 minutes without attaining the level of deep sleep.

naproxen, a nonsteroidal antiinflammatory analgesic used for the relief of pain and inflammatory symptoms in arthritis and other conditions.

narcissism, 1. an abnormal interest in oneself, especially in one's own body and sexual characteristics; self-love. **2.** (in psychoanalysis) sexual self-interest that is a normal characteristic of the phallic stage of psychosexual development, occurring as the infantile ego acquires a libido.

narcissistic personality, a personality characterized by behaviour and attitudes that indicate an abnormal love of the self.

narcissistic personality disorder, a condition characterized by an exaggerated sense of self-importance and uniqueness, an abnormal need for attention and admiration, preoccupation with grandiose fantasies concerning the self, and disturbances in interpersonal relationships, usually involving the exploitation of others and a lack of empathy for them. Symptoms include depression, egocentricity, self-consciousness, inconsiderateness, inconsistency, preoccupation with grooming and remaining youthful, and intense concern with psychosomatic pains and illnesses.

narcoanalysis, an interview conducted while the patient is deeply sedated with medication so that inhibitions are reduced and responses will be more truthful.

narcoanaesthesia. See **basal anaesthesia.**

narcolepsy, a syndrome characterized by sudden sleep attacks, cataplexy, sleep paralysis, and visual or auditory hallucinations at the onset of sleep. Persons with narcolepsy experience an uncontrollable desire to sleep, sometimes many times in one day. Episodes may last from a few minutes to several hours. Momentary loss of muscle tone occurs during waking hours (cataplexy), or while the person is asleep.

narcoleptic, 1. of or pertaining to a condition or substance that causes an uncontrollable desire for sleep. **2.** a narcoleptic drug. **3.** a person suffering from narcolepsy.

narcosis, a state of insensibility or stupor caused by narcotic drugs.

narcotic, 1. of or pertaining to a substance that produces insensibility or stupor. **2.** a narcotic drug. Narcotic analgesics, derived from opium or produced synthetically, alter perception of pain; induce euphoria, mood changes, mental clouding, and deep sleep; depress respiration and the cough reflex; constrict the pupils; and cause smooth muscle spasm, decreased peristalsis, emesis, and nausea. Repeated use of narcotics may result in physical and psychological dependence.

narcotic analgesic. See **analgesic.**

narcotic antagonist. See **opiate antagonist.**

narcotic antitussive. See **antitussive.**

nares, *sing.* **naris,** the pairs of anterior openings and posterior openings in the nose that allow the passage of air from the nose to the pharynx and the lungs during respiration.

narrow-angle glaucoma. See **glaucoma.**

nasal, of or pertaining to the nose and the nasal cavity. **nasally,** *adv.*

nasal airway, a flexible, curved piece of rubber or plastic, with one wide, trumpetlike end and one narrow end that can be inserted through the nose into the pharynx.

nasal cannula, a device for delivering oxygen by way of two small tubes that are inserted into the nares.

nasal cavity, one of a pair of cavities that open on the face through the pear-shaped anterior nasal aperture and communicate with the pharynx.

nasal decongestant, a drug that provides temporary relief of nasal symptoms in acute and chronic rhinitis and sinusitis. Most are over-the-counter products and contain a vasoconstrictor, such as ephedrine or phenylephrine.

nasal drip, a method of slowly infusing liquid into a dehydrated infant by means of a catheter inserted through the nose down the oesophagus.

nasal fossa, one of the pair of approximately equal chambers of the nasal cavity that are separated by the nasal septum and open externally through the nostrils and internally into the nasopharynx through the choanae. Each fossa is divided into an olfactory region, consisting of the superior nasal concha and part of the septum, and a respiratory region, constituting the rest of the chamber.

nasal glioma, a neoplasm characterized by the ectopic growth of neural tissue in the nasal cavity.

nasal instillation of medication, the instillation of a medicated solution into the nostrils by drops from a dropper or by an atomized spray from a squeeze bottle. Drops are instilled in each nostril as the patient's neck is hyperextended and the head tilted back over the edge of the bed. Nasal spray is administered to the patient in a sitting position.

nasalis, one of the three muscles of the nose, divided into a transverse part and an alar part. The transverse part serves to depress the cartilaginous portion of the nose and to draw the alar toward the septum. The alar part serves to dilate the nostril.

nasal polyp, a rounded, elongated bit of boggy, dependent mucosa that projects into the nasal cavity.

nasal septum, the partition dividing the nostrils. It is composed of bone and cartilage covered by mucous membrane.

nasal sinus, any one of the numerous cavities in various bones of the skull, lined with ciliated mucous membrane continuous with that of the nasal cavity. The nasal sinuses are divided into frontal sinuses, ethmoidal air cells, sphenoidal sinuses, and maxillary sinus.

nascent, 1. just born; beginning to exist; incipient. 2. (in chemistry) pertaining to any substance liberated during a chemical reaction, which, because of its uncombined state, is more reactive.

nascent oxygen, oxygen that has just been liberated from a chemical compound.

nasion, 1. the anthropometric reference point at the front of the skull where the midsagittal plane intersects a horizontal line

tangential to the highest points in the superior palpebral sulci. 2. the depression at the root of the nose that indicates the junction of the intranasal and the frontonasal sutures.

nasoduodenal tube, a fine bore tube passed via the nose through the stomach into the duodenum. This is an alternative method of providing nutrients. See also **enteral nutrition, gastrostomy, nasogastric feeding.**

nasogastric feeding, the process of introducing nutrients in a liquid form directly into the stomach via a nasogastric tube.

nasogastric intubation, the placement of a nasogastric tube through the nose into the stomach to relieve gastric distention by removing gas, gastric secretions, or food; to instil medication, food, or fluids; or to obtain a specimen for laboratory analysis. After surgery and in any condition in which the person is able to digest food but not eat it, the tube may be introduced and left in place for tube feeding until the ability to eat normally is restored.

nasogastric tube, any tube passed into the stomach through the nose. See **nasogastric intubation.**

nasojejunal tube, a mercury-weighted tube inserted through the nose to allow natural peristaltic movement from the pylorus into the jejunum.

nasolabial reflex, a sudden backward movement of the head, arching of the back, and extension and stretching of the limbs that occurs in infants in response to a light touch to the tip of the nose with an upward sweeping motion.

nasolacrimal, of or pertaining to the nasal cavity and associated lacrimal ducts.

nasolacrimal duct, a channel that carries tears from the lacrimal sac to the nasal cavity.

nasomandibular fixation, a type of maxillomandibular fixation to stabilize fractures of the jaw by using maxillomandibular splints connected to a wire through a hole drilled in the anterior nasal spine of the maxillary bone.

nasopharyngeal angiofibroma, a benign tumour of the nasopharynx, consisting of fibrous connective tissue with many vascular spaces. Typical signs are nasal and eustachian tube obstruction, adenoidal speech, and dysphagia.

nasopharyngeal cancer, a malignant neoplastic disease of the nasopharynx. Depending on the site of a nasopharyngeal tumour, there may be nasal obstruction, otitis media, hearing loss, sensory or motor nerve damage, bony destruction of the skull, or deep cervical lymphadenopathy. Squamous cell and undifferentiated carcinomas are the most common lesions.

nasopharyngeal fibroangioma. See **nasopharyngeal angiofibroma.**

nasopharyngography, radiographic imaging and examination of the nasopharynx.

nasopharyngoscopy, a technique in physical examination in which the nose and throat are visually examined using a laryngoscope, a fibreoptic device, a flashlight, and a dilator for the nares. **nasopharyngoscopic,** *adj.*

nasopharynx, one of the three regions of the throat, situated behind the nose and extending from the posterior nares to the level of the soft palate. Swollen or enlarged pharyngeal tonsils can fill the space behind the posterior nares and may completely block the passage of air from the nose into the throat. **nasopharyngeal,** *adj.*

nasotracheal tube, a catheter inserted into the trachea through the nasal cavity and the pharynx. It is commonly used in respiratory therapy.

natal, of or pertaining to birth.

nates, See **buttock.**

National Childbirth Trust (NCT), a charitable organization that offers information and support to women and their partners during pregnancy and early parenthood.

National Health Service (NHS), the provision of health care facilities and services in the UK financed through taxation and national insurance programmes and free to the user at the point of delivery.

National Pharmaceutical Association (NPA), a trade association for independent community pharmacists.

National Union of Students, a national organization of students in all subject areas.

natriuresis, the excretion of greater than normal amounts of sodium in the urine, as from the administration of natriuretic diuretic drugs or from various metabolic or endocrine disorders.

natriuretic, 1. of or pertaining to the process of natriuresis. **2.** a substance that inhibits the resorption of sodium ions from the glomerular filtrate in the kidneys, thus allowing more sodium to be excreted with the urine.

natural childbirth, labour and parturition accomplished by a mother with little or no medical intervention.

natural dentition, the entire array of natural teeth in the dental arch at any given time, consisting of deciduous or permanent teeth or a mixture of the two. See also **tooth.**

natural family planning method, any one of several methods of family planning that does not rely on a medication or a device for effectiveness in avoiding pregnancy. Some of the methods are also used to pinpoint the time of ovulation to increase the chance of fertilization when artificial insemination or extraction of an oocyte for in vitro fertilization is to be performed. Kinds of natural family planning include **basal body temperature method of family planning, calendar method, ovulation method of family planning,** and **symptothermal method of family planning.**

natural immunity, a usually innate and permanent form of immunity to a specific disease. Kinds of natural immunity include **individual immunity, racial immunity,** and **species immunity.**

naturalistic illness, an illness thought to be caused by impersonal factors, such as the Hispanic model of hot and cold forces.

natural law, a doctrine that holds there is a natural moral order or natural moral law inherent in the structure of the universe.

naturally acquired immunity. See **acquired immunity.**

natural pacemaker, any cardiac pacing site in the heart tissues.

natural radiation, radioactivity that emanates from the soil and rocks or particles and rays that reach the earth from cosmic sources, as actinic radiation from the sun.

natural selection, the natural evolutionary processes by which those organisms best suited for adaptation to the environment tend to survive and propagate the species, whereas those unfit are eliminated.

nature versus nurture, a name given to a longstanding controversy as to the relative influences of nature versus the environment in the development of personality. Nature is represented by innate factors and nurture by social influences.

naturopath, a person who practises naturopathy.

naturopathy, a system of therapeutics based on natural foods, light, warmth, massage, fresh air, regular exercise, and the avoidance of medications. Advocates believe that illness can be healed by the natural processes of the body.

nausea, a sensation often leading to the urge to vomit. Common causes are seasickness and other motion sicknesses, early pregnancy, intense pain, emotional stress, gallbladder disease, food poisoning, and various enteroviruses. **nauseate,** *v.,* **nauseous,** *adj.*

nausea and vomiting of pregnancy, a common condition of early pregnancy, characterized by recurrent or persistent nausea, often in the morning. The causes of the condition are poorly understood. It usually does not begin before the sixth week after the last menstrual period and ends by the twelfth to the fourteenth week of pregnancy.

navel. See **umbilicus.**

navicular, having the shape of a boat, such as the navicular bone in the wrist.

navicular bone. See **scaphoid bone.**

Nb, symbol for **niobium.**

nC, abbreviation for **nanocurie.**

Nd, abbreviation for **neodymium.**

Ne, symbol for **neon.**

near drowning, a pathological state in which the victim has survived exposure to circumstances that usually cause drowning.

Cardiopulmonary resuscitation is performed immediately; hospitalization is always indicated.

nearest neighbour analysis, (in molecular genetics) a biochemical method used to estimate the frequency with which pairs of bases are located next to one another.

nearsightedness. See **myopia.**

nebula, *pl.* **nebulae, 1.** a slight corneal opacity or scar that seldom obstructs vision and that can be seen only by oblique illumination. **2.** a murkiness in the urine. **3.** an oily concoction that is applied with an atomizer.

nebulization, a method of administering a drug by spraying it into the respiratory passages of the patient.

nebulize, to vaporize or disperse a liquid in a fine spray.

nebulizer, a device for producing a fine spray. Intranasal medications are often administered by a nebulizer.

NEC, abbreviation for **necrotizing enterocolitis.**

Necator, a genus of nematode that is an intestinal parasite and causes hookworm disease.

neck, a constricted section, such as the part of the body that connects the head with the trunk. Other such constrictions are the neck of the humerus and the neck of the femur.

neck dissection, surgical removal of the cervical lymph nodes, performed to prevent the spread of malignant tumours of the head and neck.

neck righting reflex, 1. an involuntary response in newborns in which turning the head to one side while the infant is supine causes rotation of the shoulders and trunk in the same direction. The reflex enables the child to roll over from the supine to prone position. **2.** any tonic reflex associated with the neck that maintains body orientation in relation to the head.

necrobiosis lipoidica, a skin disease characterized by thin, shiny, yellow to red plaques on the shins or forearms. Telangiectases, crusting, and ulceration of these plaques may occur.

necrolysis, disintegration or exfoliation of dead tissue. **necrolytic,** *adj.*

necrophilia, 1. a morbid liking for being with dead bodies. **2.** a morbid desire to have sexual contact with a dead body, usually of men to perform a sexual act with a dead woman. **necrophile, necrophiliac,** *n.*

necropsy, necroscopy. See **autopsy.**

necrosis, localized tissue death that occurs in groups of cells in response to disease or injury. In **coagulation necrosis,** blood clots block the flow of blood, causing tissue ischaemia distal to the clot; in **gangrenous necrosis,** ischaemia combined with bacterial action causes putrefaction to set in.

necrotic, pertaining to the death of tissue in response to disease or injury.

necrotizing angiitis. See **periarteritis nodosa.**

necrotizing enteritis, acute inflammation of the small and the large intestine by the bacterium *Clostridium perfringens,* characterized by severe abdominal pain, bloody diarrhoea, and vomiting.

necrotizing enterocolitis (NEC), an acute inflammatory bowel disorder that occurs primarily in preterm or low-birth-weight neonates. It is characterized by ischaemic necrosis of the GI mucosa that may lead to perforation and peritonitis. The cause of the disorder is unknown, although it appears to be a defect in host defences with infection resulting from normal GI flora rather than from invading organisms.

necrotizing vasculitis, an inflammatory condition of blood vessels, characterized by necrosis, fibrosis, and proliferation of the inner layer of the vascular wall, in some cases resulting in occlusion and infarction. Necrotizing vasculitis may occur in rheumatoid arthritis and is common in systemic lupus erythematosus, periarteritis nodosa, and progressive systemic sclerosis.

need-fear dilemma, an approach-avoidance conflict related to the need to experience closeness coupled with fear of the experience.

needle biopsy, the removal of a segment of living tissue for microscopic examination by inserting a hollow needle through the skin or the external surface of an organ or tumour and rotating it within the underlying cellular layers.

needle filter, a device, usually made of plastic, used for filtering medications that are drawn into a syringe before administration.

needle holder, a surgical forceps used to hold and pass a suturing needle through tissue.

NEEP, abbreviation for **negative end-expiratory pressure.**

negative, 1. (of a laboratory test) indicating that a substance or a reaction is not present. **2.** (of a sign) indicating on physical examination that a finding is not present, often meaning that there is no pathological change. **3.** (of a substance) tending to carry or carrying a negative chemical charge.

negative adaptation. See **habituation.**

negative anxiety, (in psychology) an emotional and psychological condition in which anxiety prevents a person's normal functioning and interrupts the person's ability to perform the usual activities of daily living.

negative catalysis, a decrease in the rate of any chemical reaction caused by a substance that is neither part of the process itself nor consumed nor affected by the reaction.

negative end-expiratory pressure (NEEP), a technique used to counterbalance the increase in mean intrathoracic pressure caused by intermittent positive pressure breathing (IPPB) in an effort to return negative intrathoracic pressure for venous return to the right atrium. Generally, the negative pressure is applied to the circuit on exhalation by using a jet or Venturi system and the resulting subatmospheric pressure is applied to the patient's airways.

negative feedback, (in physiology) a decrease in function in response to a stimulus; for example, the secretion of follicle-stimulating hormone decreases even as the amount of circulating oestrogen increases.

negative identity, the assumption of an identity that is at odds with the accepted values and expectations of society.

negative pi meson (pion). See **pi-mesons.**

negative pressure, less than ambient atmospheric pressure, such as in a vacuum, at an altitude above sea level, or in a hypobaric chamber.

negative punishment, a form of behaviour modification in which the removal of something following an operant (behaviour) decreases the probability of the operant's recurrance.

negative reinforcer, (in psychology) an event that, when it occurs immediately following occurrence of a particular behaviour, will decrease the rate of that behaviour. If it precedes a particular behaviour and is terminated by that behaviour, it will increase it.

negative relationship, (in research) an inverse relationship between two variables; as one variable increases, the other decreases.

negativism, a behavioural attitude characterized by opposition, resistance, the refusal to cooperate with even the most reasonable request, and the tendency to act in a contrary manner.

neglect, a condition that occurs when a parent or guardian is unable to or fails to provide minimal physical and emotional care for a child or other dependent person.

negligence, (in law) the commission of an act that a prudent person would not have done or the omission of a duty that a prudent person would have fulfilled, resulting in injury or harm to another person.

Neisseria gonorrhoeae {Albert L. S. Neisser, Polish dermatologist, b. 1855}, a gramnegative, nonmotile, diplococcal bacterium usually seen microscopically as flattened pairs within the cytoplasm of neutrophils. It is the causative organism of gonorrhoea.

Neisseria meningitidis. See **meningococcus.**

Nelson's syndrome {Donald H. Nelson, American physician, b. 1925}, an endocrine disorder that may follow adrenalectomy for Cushing's disease. It is characterized by a marked increase in the secretion of ACTH and MSH by the pituitary gland.

nem, abbreviation for **Nahrungs-Einheit-Milch.**

nematocide, a chemical employed to kill nematode worms.

nematode, a multicellular, parasitic animal of the phylum Nematoda. All species of roundworms belong to the phylum.

neoantigen, a new specific antigen that develops in a cell infected by oncogenic virus; it appears after infection by SV40.

neobehaviourism, a school of psychology based on the general principles of behaviourism but broader and more flexible in concept. It stresses experimental research and laboratory analyses in the study of overt behaviour and in various subjective phenomena that cannot be directly observed and measured.

neobehaviourist, a member of the school of neobehaviourism.

neoblastic, of or pertaining to a new tissue or development within a new tissue.

neocerebellum, those parts of the cerebellum that receive input via the corticopontocerebellar pathway.

neodymium (Nd), a rare earth element. Its atomic number is 60; its atomic weight is 144.27.

neoglottis, a vibrating structure that replaces the glottis in alaryngeal speech, as after a laryngectomy.

neologism, 1. a newly coined word or term. **2.** (in psychiatry) a word coined by a psychotic or delirious patient that is meaningful only to the patient.

neomycin sulphate, an aminoglycoside antibiotic prescribed in the treatment of infections of the intestine, in hepatic coma, and, topically, in the treatment of skin infections. It is not significantly absorbed from the GI tract and is toxic if administered parenterally.

neon (Ne), a colourless, odourless gaseous element and one of the inert gases. Its atomic number is 10; its atomic weight is 20.2. Neon has no compounds and occurs in the atmosphere in the ratio of about 18 parts per million.

neonatal, the period of time covering the first 28 days after birth.

Neonatal Behaviour Assessment Scale, a scale for evaluating and assessing an infant's alertness, motor maturity, irritability, consolability, and interaction with people. It is used as a tool for the evaluation of the neurological condition and the behaviour of a newborn infant.

neonatal breathing, respiration in newborn infants that begins when pulmonary fluid in the lungs is expelled by mechanical compression of the thorax during delivery and by resorption from the alveoli into the bloodstream and lymphatics. As air enters the lungs, the chest and lungs recoil to a resting position, but forceful inspirations are necessary to keep the lungs inflated.

neonatal conjunctivitis. See **ophthalmia neonatorum.**

neonatal death, the death of a live-born infant during the first 28 days after birth.

Early neonatal death is usually considered to be one that occurs during the first 7 days.

neonatal developmental profile, an evaluation of the developmental status of a newborn infant based on three examinations: a gestational age inventory, a neurological examination, and a Neonatal Behaviour Assessment score.

neonatal hyperbilirubinaemia. See hyperbilirubinaemia of the newborn.

neonatal intensive care unit. See special care baby unit (SCBU).

neonatal jaundice. See hyperbilirubinaemia of the newborn.

neonatal mortality, the statistic rate of infant death during the first 28 days after live birth, expressed as the number of such deaths per 1000 live births in a specific geographical area or institution in a given time.

neonatal period, the interval from birth to 28 days of age. It represents the time of greatest risk to the infant.

neonatal pustular melanosis, a transient skin condition of the neonate characterized by vesicles present at birth that become pustular. The lesions contain neutrophils rather than eosinophils and they disappear within 72 hours.

neonatal thermoregulation, the regulation of the body temperature of a newborn infant, which may be affected by evaporation, conduction, radiation, and convection.

neonatal tyrosinaemia. See tyrosinaemia.

neonatal unit. See special care baby unit (SCBU).

neonate, an infant from birth to 4 weeks of age.

neonatology, the branch of medicine that concentrates on the care of the neonate and specializes in the diagnosis and treatment of the disorders of the newborn infant. **neonatal,** *adj.,* **neonatal paediatrician,** *n.*

neoplasia, the new and abnormal development of cells that may be benign or malignant. **neoplastic,** *adj.*

neoplasm, any abnormal growth of new tissue, benign or malignant. **neoplastic,** *adj.*

neoplastic fracture, a fracture resulting from weakened bone tissue caused by neoplasm or by a malignant growth.

neostigmine bromide, a cholinesterase inhibitor used in the treatment of myasthenia gravis.

nephelometer, a photometric apparatus used to determine the concentration of solids suspended in a liquid or a gas, as may be used to determine the number of bacteria in a specimen.

nephelometry, a technique of determining the concentration of solids suspended in a liquid or a gas by use of a nephelometer. **nephelometrical,** *adj.*

nephrectomy, the surgical removal of a kidney, performed to remove a tumour, drain an abcess, or treat hydronephrosis.

nephritic calculus. See renal calculus.

nephritic gingivitis, a kind of stomatitis and gingivitis associated with kidney function failure, accompanied by pain, ammoniac odour, and increased salivation.

nephritis, any one of a large group of diseases of the kidney characterized by inflammation and abnormal function. Kinds of nephritis include **acute nephritis, glomerulonephritis, hereditary nephritis, interstitial nephritis, parenchymatous nephritis,** and **suppurative nephritis.**

nephroangiosclerosis, necrosis of the renal arterioles, associated with hypertension. Early signs of the condition are headaches, blurring of vision, and a diastolic blood pressure greater than 120 mm Hg. Examination of the retina reveals haemorrhages, vascular exudates, and papilloedema. The heart is usually enlarged, especially the left ventricle. Proteins and red blood cells are found in the urine. Heart failure and kidney failure may occur if the disease remains untreated.

nephroblastoma. See Wilms' tumour.

nephrocalcinosis, an abnormal condition of the kidneys in which deposits of calcium form in the parenchyma at the site of previous inflammation or degenerative change.

nephrogenic, 1. generating kidney tissue. **2.** originating in the kidney.

nephrogenic ascites, the abnormal presence of fluid in the peritoneal cavity of patients undergoing haemodialysis for renal failure. The cause of this type of ascites is unknown.

nephrogenic cord, either of the paired longitudinal ridges of tissue that lie along the dorsal surface of the coelom in the early developing vertebrate embryo. It gives rise to the structures comprising the embryonic urogenital system.

nephrogenic diabetes insipidus, an abnormal condition in which the kidneys do not concentrate the urine, resulting in polyuria, polydipsia, and very dilute urine.

nephrogenous, of or pertaining to the formation and development of the kidneys.

nephrogram, a radiographic image of renal tubules opacified by contrast medium obtained almost immediately following injection, during intravenous urography for example.

nephrolith, a calculus formed in a kidney. **nephrolithic,** *adj.*

nephrolithiasis, a disorder characterized by the presence of calculi in the kidney.

nephrology, the study of the anatomy, physiology, and pathology of the kidney. **nephrological,** *adj.*

nephrolytic, of or pertaining to the destruction of the structure and function of a kidney.

nephromere. See nephrotome.

nephron, a structural and functional unit of the kidney, resembling a microscopic funnel with a long stem and two convoluted sections. Each kidney contains about 1.25 million nephrons, each consisting of the renal corpuscle, the loop of Henle, and the renal tubules. Each renal corpuscle consists of the glomerulus of renal capillaries enclosed within Bowman's capsule.

nephronophthisis. See **medullary cystic disease.**

nephropathy, any disorder of the kidney, including inflammatory, degenerative, and sclerotic conditions.

nephropexy, a surgical operation to fixate a floating or ptotic kidney.

nephroptosis, a downward displacement or dropping of a kidney.

nephrorrhaphy, an operation that sutures a floating kidney in place.

nephrosclerosis. See **nephroangiosclerosis.**

nephroscope, a fibreoptic instrument that is used specifically for the disintegration and removal of renal calculi. The nephroscope is inserted percutaneously, and the calculi are located through use of x-ray films of the renal pelvis. An ultrasonic probe emitting high-frequency sound waves breaks up the calculi, which are removed by suction through the scope.

nephrosis. See **nephrotic syndrome.**

nephrostoma, pl. **nephrostomas, nephrostomata,** the funnel-shaped ciliated opening of the excretory tubules into the coelom of the early developing vertebrate embryo. **nephrostomic,** adj.

nephrostomy, a surgical procedure in which an incision is made on the flank of the patient so that a catheter can be inserted into the kidney pelvis for the purpose of drainage.

nephrotic syndrome, an abnormal condition of the kidney characterized by proteinuria, hypoalbuminaemia, and oedema. It occurs in glomerular disease, thrombosis of a renal vein, and as a complication of many systemic diseases, diabetes mellitus, amyloidosis, systemic lupus erythematosus, and multiple myeloma.

nephrotome, a zone of segmented mesodermal tissue in the developing vertebrate embryo. It is the primordial tissue for the urogenital system and gives rise to the nephrogenic cord.

nephrotomography, sectional radiographic examination of the kidneys.

nephrotomy, a surgical procedure in which an incision is made in the kidney.

nephrotoxic, toxic or destructive to a kidney.

nephrotoxin, a toxin with specific destructive properties for the kidneys.

nephroureterolithiasis, the presence of calculi in the kidneys and ureters.

neptunium (Np), a transuranic, metallic element. Its atomic number is 93; its atomic weight is 237.

Nernst equation, {Hermann W. Nernst, German physicist, b. 1864} (in cardiology) an expression of the relationship between the electric potential across a membrane and the concentration ratio between permeable ions on either side of the membrane.

nerve, one or more bundles of impulse-carrying fibres that connect the brain and the spinal cord with other parts of the body. Nerves transmit afferent impulses from receptor organs toward the brain and the spinal cord and efferent impulses peripherally to the effector organs. Each nerve consists of an epineurium enclosing fasciculi of nerve fibres, each fasciculus surrounded by its own sheath of connective tissue.

nerve accommodation, the ability of nerve tissue to adjust to a constant source and intensity of stimulation so that some change in either intensity or duration of the stimulus is necessary to elicit a response beyond the initial reaction.

nerve block anaesthesia. See **conduction anaesthesia.**

nerve compression, a pathological event that causes harmful pressure on one or more nerve trunks, resulting in nerve damage and muscle weakness or atrophy. Any nerve that passes over a rigid prominence is vulnerable, and the degree of damage depends on the magnitude and the duration of the compressive force.

nerve entrapment, an abnormal condition and type of mononeuropathy, characterized by nerve damage and muscle weakness or atrophy. Nerves that pass over rigid prominences or through narrow bony and fascial canals are particularly prone to entrapment. The common signs of this disorder are pain and muscular weakness. One of the most common types of entrapment is **carpal tunnel syndrome.**

nerve fibre, a slender process of a neuron, usually the axon. Each fibre is classified as myelinated or unmyelinated. Myelinated fibres are further designated as A or B fibres; C fibres are unmyelinated. The A fibres are somatic, 1 to 20 μm in diameter, and have a conduction velocity of 5 to 120 metres per second. B fibres are more finely myelinated than A fibres and have a diameter up to 3 μm and a conduction rate of 3 to 15 metres per second. They are both afferent and efferent and are mainly associated with visceral innervation. The unmyelinated C fibres have a diameter of 0.3 to 1.3 μm and a conduction rate of 0.6 to 2 metres per second. They are efferent postganglionic autonomic fibres and afferent fibres that conduct impulses of prolonged, burning pain sensation from the viscera and periphery.

nerve growth factor (NGF), a protein resembling insulin whose hormonelike action affects differentiation, growth, and maintenance of neurons.

nerve impulse. See **impulse.**

nervous breakdown, *informal.* any mental condition that markedly interferes with and disrupts normal functioning.

nervous system, the extensive, intricate network of structures that activates, coordinates, and controls all the functions of the body. It is divided into the central nervous system, composed of the brain and the spinal cord, and the peripheral nervous system, which includes the cranial nerves and the spinal nerves. These morphological subdivisions combine and communicate to innervate the somatic and the visceral parts of the body with the afferent and the efferent nerve fibres. Afferent fibres carry sensory impulses to the central nervous system; efferent fibres carry motor impulses from the central nervous system to the muscles and other organs. The somatic fibres are associated with the bones, the muscles, and the skin. The visceral fibres are associated with the internal organs, the blood vessels, and the mucous membranes.

nervus abducens. See **abducens nerve.**

nervus accessorius. See **accessory nerve.**

nervus facialis. See **facial nerve.**

nervus glossopharyngeus. See **glossopharyngeal nerve.**

nervus hypoglossus. See **hypoglossal nerve.**

nervus oculomotorius. See **oculomotor nerve.**

nervus olfactorius. See **olfactory nerve.**

nervus opticus. See **optic nerve.**

nervus terminalis. See **terminal nerve.**

nervus trigeminus. See **trigeminal nerve.**

nervus trochlearis. See **trochlear nerve.**

nervus vagus. See **vagus nerve.**

nettle rash, a fine, urticarial eruption resulting from skin contact with stinging nettle, a common weed with leaves containing histamine.

network, a system of interconnected computer terminals and peripheral equipment in which each user has some access to others using the system while sharing data, memories, and other capabilities.

networking, 1. (in psychiatric nursing) the process of developing a set of agencies and professional personnel that are able to create a system of communication and support for psychiatric patients, usually those newly discharged from inpatient psychiatric facilities. **2.** a network of supportive contacts or services.

network therapy, a type of psychotherapy conducted in the home of the patient with participation by all persons interested or invested in a particular problem or crisis.

Neufeld nail {Alonzo J. Neufeld. American surgeon, b. 1906}, an orthopaedic nail with a V-shaped tip and shank used for fixating an intertrochanteric fracture. The nail is driven into the neck of the femur until it reaches a round metal plate screwed onto the side of the femur.

neural, of or pertaining to nerve cells and their processes.

neural canal. See **neurocoele.**

neural crest, the band of ectodermally derived cells that lies along the outer surface of each side of the neural tube in the early stages of embryonic development.

neural ectoderm, the part of the embryonic ectoderm that develops into the neural tube.

neural fold, either of the paired longitudinal elevations resulting from the invagination of the neural plate in the early developing embryo. The folds unite to enclose the neural groove and form the neural tube.

neuralgia, an abnormal condition characterized by severe stabbing pain, caused by a variety of disorders affecting the nervous system. **neuralgic,** *adj.*

neural groove, the longitudinal depression that occurs between the neural folds during the invagination of the neural plate to form the neural tube in the early stages of embryonic development.

neural impulse. See **impulse.**

neural plate, a thick layer of ectodermal tissue that lies along the central longitudinal axis of the early developing embryo and gives rise to the neural tube and subsequently to the brain, spinal cord, and other tissues of the central nervous system.

neural tube, the longitudinal tube, lying along the central axis of the early developing embryo, that gives rise to the brain, spinal cord, and other neural tissue of the central nervous system.

neural tube defect, any of a group of congenital malformations involving defects in the skull and spinal column that are caused primarily by the failure of the neural tube to close during embryonic development. In some instances, the cleft results from an abnormal increase in cerebrospinal fluid pressure on the closed neural tube during the first trimester of development.

neural tube formation, the various processes and stages involved in the embryonic development of the neural tube, which subsequently differentiates into the brain, the spinal cord, and other neural tissue of the central nervous system.

neurapraxia, the interruption of nerve conduction without loss of continuity of the axon.

neurasthenia, 1. an abnormal condition characterized by nervous exhaustion and a vague functional fatigue that often follows depression. **2.** (in psychiatry) a stage in the recovery from a schizophrenic experience, during which the patient is listless and apparently unable to cope with routine activities and relationships. **neurasthenic,** *adj.*

neurenteric canal, a tubular passage between the posterior part of the neural tube and the archenteron in the early embryonic development of lower animals.

neurilemma, a layer of cells composed of one or more Schwann cells that encloses the segmented myelin sheaths of peripheral nerve fibres. Each myelinated nerve fibre has a neurilemma cell for each internodal segment between the nodes of Ranvier. The nerve fibres of the brain and the spinal cord are not enclosed by neurilemma. Also spelled **neurolemma. neurilemmal, neurilemmatic, neurilemmatous,** *adj.*

neurilemoma. See **schwannoma.**

neurinoma, *pl.* **neurinomas, neurinomata,**
1. a tumour of the nerve sheath. It is usually benign but may undergo malignant change. A kind of neurinoma is acoustic neurinoma. **2.** a neuroma.

neuritis, *pl.* **neuritides,** an abnormal condition characterized by inflammation of a nerve. Some of the signs of this condition are neuralgia, hyperthesia, anaesthesia, paralysis, muscular atrophy, and defective reflexes.

neuroarthropathy, a condition in which a disease of a joint is secondary to a disease of the nervous system.

neuroblast, any embryonic cell that develops into a functional neuron; an immature nerve cell. **neuroblastic,** *adj.*

neuroblastoma, *pl.* **neuroblastomas, neuroblastomata,** a highly malignant tumour composed of primitive ectodermal cells derived from the neural plate during embryonic life. Symptoms may include an abdominal mass, respiratory distress, and anaemia, depending on the site of the primary tumour and metastases, and hormonally active adrenal lesions may cause irritability, flushing, sweating, hypertension, and tachycardia. A kind of neuroblastoma is Pepper's syndrome.

neurocele. See **neurocoele.**

neurocentral, pertaining to the centrum and the developing vertebrae in the early stages of embryology.

neurocentrum, the embryonic mesodermal tissue that subsequently gives rise to the vertebrae.

neuro check, *nontechnical,* a brief neurological assessment, usually performed in the triage of patients in an emergency situation or on admission to an emergency service. The level of consciousness is evaluated as alert and oriented, lethargic, stuporous, or comatose.

neurocirculatory asthenia, a psychosomatic disorder characterized by nervous and circulatory irregularities, including dyspnoea, palpitation, giddiness, vertigo, tremor, precordial pain, and increased susceptibility to fatigue.

neurocoele, a system of cavities in the central nervous system of humans and other vertebrate animals. It consists of the ventricles of the brain and the central canal of the spinal cord. Also spelled **neurocele,** neurocoel.

neurocytoma, a tumour composed of undifferentiated nerve cells that are usually ganglionic.

neuroderm. See **neuroectoderm.**

neurodermatitis, a nonspecific, pruritic skin disorder seen in anxious, nervous individuals. Excoriations and lichenification are found on easily accessible, exposed areas of the body such as the forearms and forehead. Sometimes loosely (and incorrectly) applied to **atopic dermatitis.**

neurodevelopmental adaptation, a type of therapy that emphasizes the inhibition/integration of primitive postural patterns and promotes the development of normal postural reactions and achievement of normal tone. The therapy is employed in the treatment of children with cerebral palsy.

neuroectoderm, the part of the embryonic ectoderm that gives rise to the central and peripheral nervous systems, including some glial cells. **neuroectodermal,** *adj.*

neuroepithelioma, an uncommon neoplasm of neuroepithelium in a sensory nerve.

neurofibroma, *pl.* **neurofibromas, neurofibromata,** a fibrous tumour of nerve tissue resulting from the abnormal proliferation of Schwann cells.

neurofibromatosis, a congenital condition characterized by numerous neurofibromas of the nerves and skin, by café-au-lait spots on the skin, and, in some cases, by developmental anomalies of the muscles, bones, and viscera. Many large, pedunculated soft-tissue tumours may develop, as exemplified by the famous case of the "Elephant Man" in nineteenth-century England.

neurogen, a substance within the early developing embryo that stimulates the primary organizer to initiate the formation of the neural plate, which gives rise to the primary axis of the body.

neurogenesis, the development of the tissue of the nervous system. **neurogenetic,** *adj.*

neurogenic, 1. pertaining to the formation of nervous tissue. **2.** the stimulation of nervous energy. **3.** originating in the nervous system.

neurogenic arthropathy, an abnormal condition associated with neural damage, characterized by the gradual and usually painless degeneration of a joint.

neurogenic bladder, dysfunctional urinary bladder caused by lesion of the nervous system. Treatment is aimed at enabling the bladder to empty completely and regularly, preventing infection, controlling incontinence, and preserving kidney function. Kinds of neurogenic bladder are **spastic bladder, reflex bladder,** and **flaccid bladder.**

neurogenic fracture, a fracture associated with the destruction of the nerve supply to a specific bone.

neurogenic shock, a form of shock that results from peripheral vascular dilatation as a result of neurological injury.

neuroglia, the supporting or connective tissue cells of the central nervous system. Kinds of neuroglia include **astrocytes, oligodendroglia,** and **microglia. neuroglial,** *adj.*

neurography, the study of the action potentials of the nerves.

neurohormonal regulation, regulation of the function of an organ or a gland by the combined effect of neurological and hormonal activity.

neurohumour, one of the chemical substances, formed and transmitted by a neuron, that is essential for the activity of adjacent neurons or nearby organs or muscles. Kinds of neurohumoral substances are **acetylcholine, dopamine, adrenaline, noradrenaline,** and **serotonin. neurohumoral,** *adj.*

neurohypophyseal hormone, any of a group of hormones secreted by the posterior pituitary gland; these include oxytocin and vasopressin.

neurohypophysis, the posterior lobe of the pituitary gland that is the source of antidiuretic hormone (ADH) and oxytocin. Nervous stimulation controls the release of both substances into the blood. The neurohypophysis releases ADH when stimulated by the hypothalamus by an increase in the osmotic pressure of extracellular fluid in the body. The neurohypophysis releases oxytocin under appropriate stimulation from the hypothalamus.

neuroimmunology, the study of relationships between the immune and nervous systems, as autoimmune activity in neurological diseases.

neurolemma. See **neurilemma.**

neurolepsis, an altered state of consciousness, as induced by a neuroleptic agent, characterized by quiescence, reduced motor activity, anxiety, and indifference to the surroundings. Sleep may occur, but usually the person can be aroused and can respond to commands.

neurolept. See **neuroleptic.**

neuroleptanalgesia, a form of analgesia achieved by the concurrent administration of a neuroleptic and an analgesic. Anxiety, motor activity, and sensitivity to painful stimuli are reduced; the person is quiet and indifferent to the environment and surroundings. Sleep may or may not occur, but the patient is not unconscious and is able to respond to commands.

neuroleptanaesthesia, a form of anaesthesia achieved by the administration of a neuroleptic agent, a narcotic analgesic, and nitrous oxide in oxygen. Induction of anaesthesia is slow, but consciousness returns quickly after the inhalation of nitrous oxide is stopped.

neuroleptic, 1. of or pertaining to neurolepsis. **2.** a drug that causes neurolepsis, such as the butyrophenone derivative, droperidol.

neurolinguistic programming, a communication approach based on a conceptualization of levels of experience within the person and levels of the self. It involves both verbal and nonverbal messages, sensory experience, awareness or perception through patterns of behaviour that can be observed and perceived.

neurological assessment, an evaluation of the patient's neurological status and symptoms. If alert and oriented, the patient is asked about instances of weakness, numbness, headaches, pain, tremors, nervousness, irritability, or drowsiness. Information is elicited regarding loss of memory, periods of confusion, hallucinations, and episodes of loss of consciousness. The patient's general appearance, facial expression, attention span, responses to verbal and painful stimuli, emotional status, coordination, balance, cognition, and ability to follow commands are noted. If the patient is disoriented, stuporous, or comatose, demonstrated signs of these states are recorded.

neurological examination, a systematic examination of the nervous system, including an assessment of mental status, of the function of each of the cranial nerves, of sensory and neuromuscular function, of the reflexes, and of proprioception and other cerebellar functions.

neurologist, a physician who specializes in neurology.

neurology, the field of medicine that deals with the nervous system and its disorders. **neurological,** *adj.* **neurologist,** *n.*

neuroma, *pl.* **neuromas, neuromata,** a benign neoplasm composed chiefly of neurons and nerve fibres, usually arising from a nerve tissue. It may be relatively soft or extremely hard and vary in size. Pain radiating from the lesion to the periphery of the affected nerve is usually intermittent but may become continuous and severe. Kinds of neuromas include **acoustic neuroma, cystic neuroma, false neuroma, multiple neuroma, myelinic neuroma, neuroma cutis, naevoid neuroma,** and **traumatic neuroma.**

neuroma cutis, a neoplasm in the skin that contains nerve tissue and that may be extremely sensitive to painful stimuli.

neuroma telangiectodes. See **naevoid neuroma.**

neuromatosis, a neoplastic disease characterized by numerous neuromas.

neuromodulator, a substance that alters transmission of nerve impulses.

neuromuscular, of or pertaining to the nerves and the muscles.

neuromuscular blockade, the inhibition of

a muscular contraction activated by the nervous system, possibly resulting in muscle weakness or paralysis.

neuromuscular blocking agent, a chemical substance that interferes locally with the transmission or reception of impulses between motor nerves and skeletal muscles. Neuromuscular blocking agents are used to induce muscle relaxation in anaesthesia, endotracheal intubation, and electroconvulsive therapy and as adjuncts in the treatment of tetanus, encephalitis, and poliomyelitis.

neuromuscular junction, the area of contact between the ends of a large myelinated nerve fibre and a fibre of skeletal muscle.

neuromuscular spindle, any one of a number of small bundles of delicate muscular fibres, enclosed by a capsule, in which sensory nerve fibres terminate. The nerve fibres end as naked axons encircling the intrafusal fibres with flattened expansions or ovoid discs.

neuromyal transmission, the passage of excitation from a motor neuron to a muscle fibre at the myoneural junction.

neuromyelitis, an abnormal condition characterized by inflammation of the spinal cord and peripheral nerves.

neuron, the basic nerve cell of the nervous system, containing a nucleus within a cell body and extending one or more processes. Neurons are classified according to the direction in which they conduct impulses and according to the number of processes they extend. Sensory neurons transmit nerve impulses toward the spinal cord and the brain. Motor neurons transmit nerve impulses from the brain and the spinal cord to the muscles and the glandular tissue. Multipolar neurons have one axon and several dendrites, as do most of the neurons in the brain and the spinal cord. Bipolar neurons have only one axon and one dendrite. Unipolar neurons are embryonic structures that originate as bipolar bodies but fuse dendrites and axons into a single fibre that stretches for a short distance from the cell body before separating again into the two processes. As the carriers of nerve impulses, neurons function according to electrochemical processes involving positively charged sodium and potassium ions and the changing electric potential of the extracellular and the intracellular fluid of the neuron. Also spelled **neurone.**

neuronitis, an abnormal condition characterized by inflammation of a nerve or a nerve cell, especially the cells and the roots of the spinal nerves.

neuropathic bladder. See **neurogenic bladder.**

neuropathic joint disease, a chronic, progressive, degenerative disease of one or more joints, characterized by swelling, instability of the joint, haemorrhage, heat, and atrophic and hypertrophic changes in the bone. The disease is the result of an underlying neurological disorder, such as tabes dorsalis from syphilis, diabetic neuropathy, leprosy, or congenital absence or depression of pain sensation.

neuropathy, any abnormal condition characterized by inflammation and degeneration of the peripheral nerves, as that associated with lead poisoning. **neuropathic,** *adj.*

neuroplegia, nerve paralysis caused by disease, injury, or the effect of neuroleptic drugs, administered to achieve **neuroleptanalgesia or neuroleptanaesthesia.**

neuropore, the opening at each end of the neural tube during early embryonic development. Kinds of neuropores are **anterior neuropore** and **posterior neuropore.**

neurosarcoma, a malignant neoplasm composed of nerve tissue, connective tissue, and vascular tissue.

neurosis, 1. any faulty or inefficient way of coping with anxiety or inner conflict, usually involving the use of an unconscious defence mechanism, that may ultimately lead to a neurotic disorder. **2.** *informal.* an emotional disturbance other than psychosis.

neurosurgery, any surgery involving the brain, spinal cord, or peripheral nerves. Brain surgery is performed to treat a wound, remove a tumour or foreign body, relieve pressure in intracranial haemorrhage, excise an abcess, treat parkinsonism, or relieve pain. Kinds of brain surgery include craniotomy, lobotomy, hypophysectomy. Surgery of the spine is performed to correct a defect, remove a tumour, repair a ruptured intervertebral disc, or relieve pain. Kinds of spinal surgery include fusion and laminectomy. Surgery on the peripheral nerves is performed to remove a tumour, relieve pain, or reconnect a severed nerve. One kind of nerve surgery is **sympathectomy.**

neurosyphilis, infection of the central nervous system by syphilis organisms, which may invade the meninges and cerebrovascular system. **neurosyphilitic,** *adj.*

neurotendinous spindle, a capsule containing enlarged tendon fibres, found chiefly near the junctions of tendons and muscles.

neurotic, 1. of or pertaining to neurosis or to a neurotic disorder. **2.** pertaining to the nerves. **3.** one who is afflicted with a neurosis. **4.** *informal.* an emotionally unstable person.

neurotic disorder, any mental disorder characterized by a symptom or group of symptoms that a person finds distressing, unacceptable, and alien to the personality, such as severe anxiety, obsessional thoughts, and compulsive acts, and that produces psychological pain or discomfort disproportionate to the reality of the situation. Although the person's ability to function may be markedly impaired, the behaviour generally remains within acceptable social norms and the perception of reality is unaffected. There is no proof of organic cause. Kinds of neurotic disorders include **anxiety neurosis, obsessive-compulsive neurosis, psychosexual disorder,** and **somatoform disorder.** See also **neurosis, neurotic process.**

neurotic illness. See **neurotic disorder.**

neurotic process, (in psychology) a process in which unconscious conflicts lead to feelings of anxiety. Defence mechanisms are employed to avoid these uncomfortable feelings, and personality disturbance and the symptoms of neurosis ensue.

neurotmesis, a peripheral nerve injury in which the nerve is completely disrupted by laceration or traction.

neurotoxic, having a poisonous effect on nerves and nerve cells, as when ingested lead degenerates peripheral nerves.

neurotoxin, a toxin that acts directly on the tissues of the central nervous system, travelling along the axis cylinders of the motor nerves to the brain. The toxin may be in the venom of snakes, on the spines of a shell or in the flesh of fish or shellfish, or produced by bacteria.

neurotransmitter, any one of numerous chemicals that modify or result in the transmission of nerve impulses between synapses. Neurotransmitters are released from synaptic knobs into synaptic clefts and bridge the gap between presynaptic and postsynaptic neurons. When a nerve impulse reaches a synaptic knob, neurotransmitter molecules squirt into the synaptic cleft and bind to specific receptors. This flow allows an associated diffusion of potassium and sodium ions that causes an action potential. Kinds of neurotransmitters include **acetylcholine chloride, gamma-aminobutyric acid,** and **noradrenaline.**

neurula, *pl.* **neurulas, neurulae,** an early embryo during the period of neurulation when the nervous system tissue begins to differentiate.

neurulation, the development of the neural plate and the processes involved with its subsequent closure to form the neural tube during the early stages of embryonic development.

neutral, the state exactly between two opposing values, qualities, or properties; for example, in electricity a neutral state is one in which there is neither a positive nor a negative charge.

neutralization, the interaction between an acid and a base that produces a solution that is neither acidic nor basic. The usual products of neutralization are a salt and water.

neutral rotation, the position of a limb that is turned neither toward nor away from the body's midline.

neutral thermal environment, an environment created by any method or apparatus to maintain the normal body temperature to minimize oxygen consumption and caloric expenditure, as in an incubator for a premature infant.

neutron, (in physics) an elementary particle that is a constituent of the nuclei of all elements except hydrogen. It has no electric charge and is approximately the same size as a proton. Neutron beams may be used for external beam therapy.

neutron activation analysis, the analysis of elements in a specimen, performed by exposing it to neutron irradiation to convert many elements to a radioactive form in which they can be identified by measuring their emissions of radiation.

neutropenia, an abnormal decrease in the number of neutrophils in the blood. Neutropenia is associated with acute leukaemia, infection, rheumatoid arthritis, vitamin B12 deficiency, and chronic splenomegaly.

neutrophil, a polymorphonuclear granular leukocyte that stains easily with neutral dyes. Neutrophils are the circulating white blood cells essential for phagocytosis and proteolysis in which bacteria, cellular debris, and solid particles are removed and destroyed.

neutrophil alkaline phosphatase. See **leukocyte alkaline phosphatase.**

neutrophilic leukaemia. See **polymorphocytic leukaemia.**

newborn, 1. recently born. **2.** a recently born infant; a neonate.

newborn intrapartum care, care of the newborn in the delivery area during the time after birth before the mother and infant are transferred to the postnatal ward. The nasopharynx and mouth may be suctioned to remove excess mucus as the head is born. Depending on the preference and the condition of the mother, the baby may then be placed on the mother's abdomen and covered with a warm, dry blanket or taken by the midwife to an infant warmer. Apgar scores are assigned at 1 minute of age, at 5 minutes of age and at 10 minutes of age. The baby is handled gently and quietly; bright lights are often avoided, and maternal contact is encouraged.

new growth, a neoplasm or tumour.

Newman, Margaret A., a nursing theorist who contributed to the study of nursing theories and models by defining three approaches to the discovery of nursing theory. They are: "borrowing" of theories from related disciplines, analyzing nursing practice situations in search of conceptual relationships, and creating new conceptual systems from which theories can be derived.

New World typhus. See **murine typhus.**

Nezelof's syndrome {C. Nezelof, 20th century French physician}, an abnormal condition characterized by absent T cell function, deficient B cell function, fairly normal immunoglobulin levels, and little or no specific antibody production. Nezelof's syndrome causes progressively severe, recurrent, and eventually fatal infections. Signs that often appear in infants or in children up to 4 years of age include recurrent pneumonia, otitis media, chronic fungal infections, upper respiratory tract infections, diarrhoea, and hepatosplenomegaly. The disease may also enlarge the lymph nodes and the tonsils. Involved patients may also develop a tendency toward malignancy. Infection may cause sepsis, which is the usual cause of death. Symptoms that often suggest Nezelof's syndrome also include weight loss and poor eating habits.

NGF, abbreviation for **nerve growth factor.**

NGU, abbreviation for **nongonococcal urethritis.**

NHS, abbreviation for **National Health Service.**

Ni, symbol for **nickel.**

niacin. See **nicotinic acid.**

niacinamide. See **nicotinamide**.

nibble, a computer word size representing four bits, or one half of a byte.

nick, (in molecular genetics) a fissure or split in a single strand of DNA that can be made with the enzyme deoxyribonuclease or with ethidium bromide.

nickel (Ni), a silvery-white metallic element. Its atomic number is 28; its atomic weight is 58.71. Many people are allergic to nickel.

nickel dermatitis, an allergic contact dermatitis caused by the metal, nickel. Exposure comes usually from jewellery, wristwatches, metal clasps, and coins. Sweating increases the degree of rash.

nick translation, a method of labeling DNA in the laboratory by using the enzyme DNA polymerase.

nicotinamide, a B complex vitamin. It is closely related to niacin but has no vasodilating action.

nicotine {Jean Nicot Villemain, French ambassador to Portugal, b. 1530}, a colourless, rapidly acting toxic substance in tobacco that is one of the major contributors to the ill effects of smoking. It is used as an insecticide in agriculture and as a parasiticide in veterinary medicine. Ingestion of large amounts causes salivation, nausea, vomiting, diarrhoea, headache, vertigo, slowing of the heartbeat, and, in acute cases, paralysis of respiratory muscles.

nicotine poisoning, poisoning from intake of nicotine. Nicotine poisoning is characterized by stimulation of the central and autonomic nervous systems followed by depression of these systems. In fatal cases, death occurs from respiratory failure.

nicotine resin complex, a source of nicotine used in the formulation of nicotine chewing gum and transdermal nicotine patches used as aids to smoking cessation.

nicotinic acid, a white, crystalline, water-soluble vitamin of the B complex group usually occurring in various plant and animal tissues as nicotinamide. It functions as a coenzyme necessary for the breakdown and use of all major nutrients and is essential for a healthy skin, normal functioning of the GI tract, maintenance of the nervous system, and synthesis of the sex hormones. Symptoms of deficiency include muscular weakness, general fatigue, loss of appetite, various skin eruptions, halitosis, stomatitis, insomnia, irritability, nausea, vomiting, recurring headaches, tender gums, tension, and depression. Severe deficiency results in pellagra.

nicotinyl alcohol, an alcohol used as a vasodilator, in the form of its tartrate salt, in the treatment of peripheral vascular disease, vascular spasm, varicose ulcers, decubital ulcers, chilblains, Ménière's disease, and vertigo.

nidation, the process by which an embryo burrows into the endometrium of the uterus.

NIDDM, abbreviation for **non-insulin-dependent diabetes mellitus.**

nidus, a point or origin, focus, or nucleus of a disease process.

Niemann-Pick disease {Albert Niemann, German paediatrician, b. 1880; Ludwig Pick, German pediatrician, b. 1868}, an inherited disorder of lipid metabolism in which there are accumulations of sphingomyelin in the bone marrow, spleen, and lymph nodes. The disease is characterized by enlargement of liver and spleen, anaemia, lymphadenopathy, and progressive mental and physical deterioration.

nifedipine, a calcium channel blocker used for the treatment of angina pectoris and hypertension.

night blindness. See **nyctalopia.**

Nightingale, Florence (1820-1910), the founder of modern nursing. After limited formal training in nursing, she became superintendent in 1853 of a hospital in London. Her success in reorganizing the hospital led to a request by the British government to head a mission to the Crimea, where Britain was fighting a war with Russia. She arrived in November 1854, with 38 nurses to find 5000 wounded men lacking adequate food and medical supplies. Working many hours on the wards and sending letters to England to obtain money and supplies and to mobilize the government to act, she brought order out of chaos. After her return to England, in 1856, she founded a training school for nurses at St. Thomas' Hospital, whose graduates became matrons of the most important hospitals in Great Britain, thus raising the standards of nursing around the world. Although later bedridden, she carried on her work on the sanitary reform of India, conducted a study of midwifery, helped establish visiting nurse services, and proposed separate institutions for the sick, the insane, the incurable, and children. After Longfellow wrote *Santa Filomena*, she became known as "The Lady with The Lamp." The Nightingale Pledge, named after her, embodies her ideals and has inspired thousands of nurses.

Nightingale ward, a kind of hospital ward, designed by Florence Nightingale, that revolutionized hospital design. The number of beds allowed in a ward of given size was limited to permit the circulation of air and for general cleanliness and the comfort of patients. Three sides of the ward were windowed to admit light and fresh air.

nightmare, a dream occurring during rapid eye movement sleep that arouses feelings of intense, inescapable fear, terror, distress, or extreme anxiety and that usually awakens the sleeper.

night vision, a capacity to see dimly lit objects. It stems from a chemophysical phenomenon associated with the retinal rods. The rods contain the highly light-sensitive chemical rhodopsin, or visual purple, which is essential for the conduction of optic impulses in subdued light.

nigrities linguae. See **parasitic glossitis.**

nihilistic delusion, a persistent denial of the existence of particular things or of everything, including oneself, as seen in various forms of schizophrenia.

Nikolsky's sign {Pyotr V. Nikolsky, Polish dermatologist, b. 1855}, easy separation of the stratum corneum layer of the epidermis from the basal cell layer by rubbing apparently normal skin areas; found in pemphigus and a few other bullous diseases.

90-90 traction. See **traction, 90-90.**

ninth nerve. See **glossopharyngeal nerve.**

niobium (Nb), a silver-grey metallic element. Its atomic number is 41; its atomic weight is 92.906. Formerly called **columbium.**

nipple, a small cylindrical, pigmented structure that projects just below the centre of each breast. The tip of the nipple has about 20 tiny openings to the lactiferous ducts. The skin of the nipple is surrounded by the lighter pigmented skin of the areola. Stimulation of the nipple in men and women causes the structure to become erect through the contraction of radiating smooth muscle bundles in the surrounding areola.

nipple cancer, an inflammatory malignant neoplasm of the nipple and areola that is usually associated with carcinoma in deeper breast structures. It represents only a small percentage of breast cancers.

nipple shield, a device to protect the nipples of a lactating woman. The shield is usually made of soft latex and has a tab on one side with which the mother may hold it. The baby suckles from a teat at the centre of the shield. It is most often used to allow sore or cracked nipples to heal while maintaining lactation.

nirvanic state, (in Zen meditation) a state in which mental processes cease, leading to a radical and lasting alteration of the personality.

Nissl body {Franz Nissl, German neurologist, b. 1860}, any one of the large granular structures in the cytoplasm of nerve cells that stains with basic dyes and contains ribonucleoprotein.

nit, the egg of a parasitic insect, particularly a louse. It may be found attached to human or animal hair or to clothing fibre.

nitrazine paper, an absorbent strip of paper that turns specific colours when exposed to solutions of varied acidity or alkalinity.

nitric acid, a colourless, highly corrosive liquid that may give off suffocating brown fumes of nitrogen dioxide on exposure to air. Commercially prepared nitric acid is a powerful oxidizing agent used in the manufacture of drugs, and, occasionally, as a cauterizing agent for the removal of warts.

nitrite, an ester or salt of nitrous acid, used as a vasodilator, antispasmodic, and antidote to cyanide poisoning. The most widely used nitrites in medicine are amyl nitrite and sodium nitrite.

nitritoid reaction, a group of adverse effects, including hypotension, flushing, lightheadedness, and fainting, produced by administration of arsenicals or gold. The reaction is similar to that caused by administration of nitrites.

nitrobenzene poisoning, a toxic condition caused by the absorption into the body of nitrobenzene, a pale yellow, oily liquid used in the manufacture of aniline, shoe dyes, soap, perfume, and artificial flavours. Exposure in industry is usually by inhalation of the fumes or by absorption through the skin. Symptoms of acute poisoning include headache, drowsiness, nausea, ataxia, cyanosis, and, in extreme cases, respiratory failure.

nitrofuran, one of a group of synthetic antimicrobials used to treat infections caused by protozoa or bacteria.

nitrofurantoin, a urinary antibacterial used in the treatment of urinary tract infections.

nitrogen (N), a gaseous, nonmetallic element. Its atomic number is 7; its atomic weight is 14.008. Nitrogen constitutes approximately 78% of the atmosphere and is a component of all proteins and a major component of most organic substances. Compounds of nitrogen are essential constituents of all living organisms, the proteins and the nucleic acids being especially basic to all life forms.

nitrogen balance, the relationship between the nitrogen taken into the body, usually as food, and the nitrogen excreted from the body in urine and faeces. Positive nitrogen balance, which occurs when the intake of nitrogen is greater than its excretion, implies tissue formation. Negative nitrogen balance indicates wasting or destruction of tissue.

nitrogen fixation, the process by which free nitrogen in the atmosphere is converted by biological or chemical means to ammonia and to other forms usable by plants and animals.

nitrogen mustard. See **mustine hydrochloride.**

nitrogen narcosis, a condition of depressed central nervous system functions by high partial pressure of nitrogen.

nitrogen washout curve, a graphic curve obtained by plotting the concentration of nitrogen in expired alveolar gas during oxygen breathing as a function of time. As a person begins to inhale pure oxygen after breathing ambient air, the nitrogen concentration decreases so that after 4 minutes healthy subjects have a nitrogen concentration in expired alveolar gas of less than 2%.

nitroprusside sodium. See **sodium nitroprusside.**

nitrosamines, potentially carcinogenic compounds produced by reactions of nitrites with amines or amides normally present in the body. Nitrites are produced by bacteria in saliva, and in the intestine from nitrates normally present in vegetables and in nitrate-treated fish, poultry, and meats.

nitrosourea, any one of a group of cytotoxic alkylating drugs used in the chemotherapy of brain tumours, multiple myeloma, Hodgkin's disease, adenocarcinomas, hepatomas, chronic leukaemias, lymphomas, myelomas, and cancers of the breast and ovaries.

nitrous oxide, a gas used as an anaesthetic in dentistry, surgery, and childbirth. It provides light anaesthesia and is delivered in various concentrations with oxygen. Nitrous oxide alone does not provide deep enough anaesthesia for major surgery, for which it is supplemented with other anaesthetic agents.

NMR, abbreviation for **nuclear magnetic resonance.**

NMR imaging. See **magnetic resonance imaging.**

No, symbol for **nobelium.**

N$_2$O, symbol for **nitrous oxide.**

nobelium (No) {Alfred Nobel Institute, Stockholm, Sweden}, a synthetic, transuranic metallic element. Its atomic number is 102. The atomic weight of its most stable isotope is 259.

noble gas. See **inert gas.**

Nocardia, a genus of gram-positive aerobic bacteria, some species of which are pathogenic, as *Nocardia asteroides* which causes maduromycosis.

nocardiosis {Edmund I. E. Nocard}, infection with *Nocardia asteroides,* an aerobic gram-positive species of actinomycetes, characterized by pneumonia, often with cavitation, and by chronic abscesses in the brain and subcutaneous tissues. The organism enters via the respiratory tract and spreads by the bloodstream, especially in Cushing's syndrome.

nociceptive, pertaining to a neural receptor for painful stimuli.

nociceptor, somatic and visceral free nerve endings of thinly myelinated and unmyelinated fibres. They usually react to tissue injury but may also be excited by endogenous chemical substances.

noctambulation. See **somnambulism.**

nocte, (in prescriptions) a Latin word meaning at 'night'.

nocturia, urination, particularly excessive urination at night. Whereas it may be a symptom of renal disease, it may occur in the absence of disease in persons who drink excessive amounts of fluids, particularly alcohol or coffee, before bedtime or in people with prostatic disease.

nocturnal, 1. pertaining to or occurring during the night. 2. describing an individual or animal that is active at night and sleeps during the day.

nocturnal emission, involuntary emission of semen during sleep, usually in association with an erotic dream.

nocturnal paroxysmal dyspnoea, an abnormal condition of the respiratory system, characterized by sudden attacks of shortness of breath, profuse sweating, tachycardia, and wheezing that awaken the person from sleep.

nodal bradycardia. See **bradycardia.**

nodal event, an occurrence that may cause anxiety, such as birth, death, divorce, marriage, or a child leaving home.

node, 1. a small rounded mass. 2. a lymph node. 3. a single computer terminal in a network of terminals and computers.

nodular, (of a structure or mass) small, firm, and knotty.

nodular circumscribed lipomatosis, a condition in which many circumscribed, encapsulated lipomas are distributed around the neck symmetrically, randomly, or like a collar.

nodular cutaneous angiitis, an inflammatory condition of small arteries accompanied by lesions of the skin.

nodular melanoma, a melanoma that is uniformly pigmented, usually bluish-black and nodular and sometimes surrounded by an irregular halo of pale, unpigmented skin.

nodule, 1. a small node. 2. a small nodelike structure.

noise pollution, a noise level in an environment that is uncomfortable for the inhabitants.

noma, an acute, necrotizing ulcerative process involving mucous membranes of mouth or genitalia. There is rapid spreading and painless destruction of bone and soft tissue accompanied by a putrid odour.

nomenclature, a consistent, systematic method of naming used in a scientific discipline to denote classifications and to avoid ambiguities in names, such as binomial nomenclature in biology and chemical nomenclature in chemistry.

Nomina Anatomica, the book of official international nomenclature for anatomy as designated by the International Congress of Anatomists.

nomogram, 1. a graphic representation, by any of various systems, of a numeric relationship. **2.** a graph on which a number of variables is plotted so that the value of a dependent variable can be read on the appropriate line when the values of the other variables are given.

nonadhesive skin traction, one of two kinds of skin traction in which the therapeutic pull of traction weights is applied with foam-backed traction straps that do not stick to the skin over the body structure involved. The straps spread the traction pull over a wide area of skin surface, thus decreasing the vulnerability of the patient to skin breakdown.

non-A, non-B (NANB) hepatitis, viral hepatitis that is caused by a virus antigenically separate from the serological strains that cause hepatitis A or hepatitis B. NANB hepatitis is usually milder than types A or B but is otherwise clinically indistinguishable from them.

nonbacterial thrombic endocarditis, one of the three main types of endocarditis, characterized by various kinds of lesions that affect the heart valves. Some studies indicate that this disease may be the first step in the development of bacterial endocarditis and that the lesions involved cause peripheral arterial embolisms resulting in death.

noncohesive gold foil, a thin sheet of pure gold, used for making dental restorations, such as crowns, that will not cohere at room temperature because of a protective surface coating.

noncommunicating hydrocephalus. See **hydrocephalus.**

noncompetitive inhibition, (in pharmacology) a form of inhibition in which a substance occupies a receptor and cannot be displaced from the receptor by increasing the number of other molecules competing with it in binding the receptor.

noncompliance, lack of adherence, on the part of a client, to a therapeutic regimen because of a health belief, a cultural or spiritual value, or a problem in the relationship between the provider of the recommendation and the client. Defining characteristics of noncompliance include objective tests that show noncompliance, observation of physical or psychological signs that demonstrate lack of compliance, or a failure to keep appointments.

non compos mentis, a legal term applied to a person declared to be mentally incompetent.

nondirective therapy, a psychotherapeutic approach in which the psychotherapist refrains from giving advice or interpretation as the client is helped to identify conflicts and to clarify and understand feelings and values.

nondisjunction, failure of homologous pairs of chromosomes to separate during the first meiotic division or of the two chromatids of a chromosome to split during anaphase of mitosis or the second meiotic division. The result is an abnormal number of chromosomes in the daughter cells.

nonfeasance, a failure to perform a task, duty, or undertaking that one has agreed to perform or that one had a legal duty to perform.

nongonococcal urethritis (NGU), an infectious condition of the urethra in males that is characterized by mild dysuria and a scanty to moderate amount of penile discharge. The discharge may be white or clear, thin or mucoid, or, less often, purulent. The infection is often caused by the obligate intracellular parasite *Chlamydia trachomatis.* Nearly 50% of all cases of urethritis are nongonococcal.

non-Hodgkin's lymphoma, any kind of malignant lymphoma except Hodgkin's disease.

nonimpact printer, a computer printer that produces an image on a medium, such as paper, by ink jet, or by thermal, electomagnetic, or xerographic means.

nonionic, pertaining to compounds without a net negative or positive charge.

non-insulin-dependent diabetes mellitus (NIDDM), a type of diabetes mellitus in which patients are not insulin-dependent or ketosis prone although they may use insulin for correction of symptomatic or persistent hyperglycaemia, and they can develop ketosis under special circumstances, such as infection or stress. About 60% to 90% are obese; in these patients glucose tolerance is often improved by weight loss. Previously called adult-onset diabetes, ketosis-resistant diabetes, maturity-onset diabetes, maturity-onset-type diabetes, MOD, stable diabetes.

noninvasive, pertaining to a diagnostic or therapeutic technique that does not require the skin to be broken or a cavity or organ of the body to be entered, such as obtaining a blood pressure reading by auscultation with a stethoscope and sphygmomanometer.

nonionizing radiation, radiation for which the mechanism of action in tissue does not directly ionize atomic or molecular systems through a single interaction.

nonosteogenic fibroma, a common bone

lesion in which there is degeneration and proliferation of the medullary and cortical tissue, usually near the ends of the diaphyses of the large long bones.

nonparametric test of significance, (in statistics) one of several tests that use a qualitative approach to analyse rank order data and incidence data that cannot be assumed to have a normal distribution. Kinds of nonparametric tests of significance include chi-square, Spearman's rho.

nonpolar, pertaining to molecules that have a hydrophobic affinity, are "water hating." Nonpolar substances tend to dissolve in nonpolar solvents.

nonproductive cough, a sudden, noisy expulsion of air from the lungs that may be caused by irritation or inflammation and does not remove sputum from the respiratory tract. Intratracheal suctioning may be necessary when secretions cause severe respiratory difficulty and coughing is unproductive.

nonprotein nitrogen (NPN), the nitrogen in the blood that is not a constituent of protein, such as the nitrogen associated with urea, uric acid, creatine, and polypeptides.

eye movement. See **sleep.**

nonreflex bladder. See **flaccid bladder.**

nonreversible inhibitor, an effector substance that binds irreversibly to an active site of an enzyme, inhibiting the normal catalytic activity of the enzyme.

nonsense mutation. See **amber mutation.**

nonsexual generation. See **asexual generation.**

nonshivering thermogenesis, a natural method by which newborns can produce body heat by increasing their metabolic rate.

nonspecific urethritis (NSU), inflammation of the urethra not known to be caused by a specific organism. Onset of symptoms is often related to sexual intercourse. The condition is noted by urethral discharge in men and by reddening of the urethral mucosa in women.

nonstress test (NST), an evaluation of the fetal heart rate response to natural contractile activity or to an increase in fetal activity.

nonthrombocytopenic purpura, a disorder characterized by purplish or reddish skin areas although the condition does not involve a decrease in the number of platelets.

nontoxic, not poisonous. Also **atoxic.**

nontropical sprue, a malabsorption syndrome resulting from an inborn inability to digest foods that contain gluten.

nonulcerative blepharitis, a form of blepharitis characterized by greasy scales on the margins of the eyelids around the lashes and hyperaemia and thickening of the skin. Nonulcerative blepharitis is often associated with seborrhoea of the scalp, eyebrows, and the skin behind the ears.

nonverbal communication, the transmission of a message without the use of words. It may involve any or all of the five senses.

Noonan's syndrome {Jacqueline A. Noonan, American cardiologist, b. 1921}, a hypergonadotropic disorder, occurring only in males, characterized by short stature, low-set ears, webbing of the neck, and cubitus valgus. Testicular function may be normal, but fertility is often decreased. The number and morphology of the chromosomes are normal. The cause is unknown.

noradrenaline, an adrenergic hormone that acts to increase blood pressure by vasoconstriction but does not affect cardiac output. It is synthesized naturally by the adrenal medulla and is available also as a drug, levarterenol, given to maintain the blood pressure in acute hypotension secondary to trauma, heart disease, or vascular collapse.

noradrenaline acid tartrate, an adrenergic vasoconstrictor nd cardiac stimulant used in the treatment of cardiac arrest and in certain acute hypotensive states.

norepinephrine. See **noradrenaline.**

no response (NR), the condition for which the maximum decrease in treated tumour volume is less than 50%.

norethistrone, a progestogen prescribed in the treatment of abnormal uterine bleeding and endometriosis. It is also a component in many oral contraceptive medications.

norfloxacin, a 4-quinolone antibacterial drug prescribed for the treatment of urinary tract and ophthalmic infections.

norm, a measure of a phenomenon generally accepted as the ideal standard performance against which other measures of the phenomenon may be measured.

norma basalis, the inferior surface of the base of the skull with the mandible removed, formed by the palatine bones, the vomer, the pterygoid processes, and parts of the sphenoid and temporal bones.

normal, 1. describing a standard, average, or typical example of a set of objects or values. 2. describing a chemical solution in which 1 L contains 1 g of a substance or the equivalent in replaceable hydrogen ions. 3. persons in a nondiseased population. 4. a gaussian distribution.

normal dental function, the correct and healthy action of opposing teeth during mastication.

normal diet. See **regular diet.**

normal human serum albumin. See **albumin (human).**

normal hydrogen electrode (NHE), a reference electrode that is assigned a value of 0 volts.

normal phase, a chromatographic mode in which the mobile phase is less polar than the stationary phase.

normoblast, a nucleated cell that is the normal precursor of the adult circulating erythrocyte. After the extrusion of the nucleus of the normoblast, the young erythrocyte becomes known as a reticulocyte. **normoblastic,** *adj.*

normochromic, pertaining to a blood cell having normal colour, usually because it contains an adequate amount of haemoglobin.

normocyte, an ordinary, normal, adult red blood cell of average size having a diameter of 7 μm. **normocytic,** *adj.*

normoglycaemic, pertaining to a normal blood glucose level.

normotensive, pertaining to the condition of having normal blood pressure. **normotension,** *n.*

normoventilation, the alveolar ventilation rate that produces an alveolar carbon dioxide pressure of about 40 torr at any metabolic rate.

normoxia, an ambient oxygen pressure of about 150 (plus or minus 10) torr, or the partial pressure of oxygen in atmospheric air at sea level.

North American Nursing Diagnosis Association (NANDA), a professional organization of North American registered nurses created in 1982. The purpose of the organization is "to develop, refine, and promote a taxonomy of nursing Diagnostic terminology of general use to the professional".

North Asian tick-borne rickettsiosis, an infection, acquired in the Eastern Hemisphere, caused by *Rickettsia siberica,* and transmitted by ticks. Usual findings include a generalized maculopapular rash involving palms and soles, fever, and lymph node enlargement.

North Asian tick typhus. See **Siberian tick typhus.**

Northern blot test, an electrophoretic test for identifying the presence or absence of particular mRNA molecules and nucleic acid hybridization.

Norton Scale (Norton, McLaren, Exton-Smith), a risk assessment scale for pressure sores mainly used in the care of elderly patients.

nortriptyline, a tricyclic antidepressant prescribed in the treatment of depression.

nose, the structure that protrudes from the anterior portion of the skull and serves as a passageway for air to and from the lungs. The nose filters the air, warming, moistening, and chemically examining it for impurities that might irritate the mucous lining of the respiratory tract. The nose also contains the organ of smell, and it aids the faculty of speech. The external portion is considerably smaller than the internal portion, which lies over the roof of the mouth. The hollow interior portion is separated into a right and a left cavity by a septum. Each cavity is divided into the superior, middle, and inferior meati by the projection of nasal conchae.

The external portion of the nose is perforated by two nostrils and the internal portion by two posterior nares.

nosebleed, a haemorrhage from the nose. Emergency responses to nosebleed include seating the patient upright with the head thrust forward to prevent swallowing of blood. Pressure with both thumbs directly under the nostril and above the lips may block the main artery supplying blood to the nose. Alternatively, pressure with both forefingers on each side of the nostril often slows bleeding by blocking the main arteries and their branches. Continued bleeding may require the insertion of cotton or other absorbent material within the nostril and reapplication of pressure. Cold compresses on the nose, lips, and the back of the head may help control bleeding. Continued bleeding may require cautery.

nosocomial, of or pertaining to a hospital.

nosocomial infection, an infection acquired during hospitalization, often caused by *Candida albicans, Escherichia coli,* hepatitis viruses, herpes zoster virus, *Pseudomonas,* or *Staphylococcus.*

nosology, the science of classifying diseases.

nostrils. See **anterior nares.**

notch, an indentation or a depression in a bone or other organ, such as the auricular notch or the cardiac notch.

notifiable, pertaining to certain conditions, diseases, and events that must, by law, be reported to a governmental agency, such as birth, death, certain communicable diseases, and certain violations of public health regulations.

notochord, an elongated strip of mesodermal tissue that originates from the primitive node and extends along the dorsal surface of the developing embryo beneath the neural tube, forming the primary longitudinal skeletal axis of the body of all chordates. **notochordal,** *adj.*

notochordal canal, a tubular passage that extends from the primitive pit into the head process during the early stages of embryonic development in mammals.

notochordal plate. See **head process.**

notogenesis, the formation of the notochord. **notogenetic,** *adj.*

notomelus, a congenital malformation in which one or more accessory limbs are attached to the back.

nourish, to furnish or supply the essential foods or nutrients for maintaining life.

nourishment, 1. the act or process of nourishing or being nourished. **2.** any substance that nourishes and supports the life and growth of living organisms.

nourish, harmful, injurious, or detrimental to health.

Np, symbol for **neptunium.**

NPA, an abbreviation for **National Pharmaceutical Association.**

NPN, abbreviation for **nonprotein nitrogen.**

N-propyl alcohol, a clear, colourless liquid used as a solvent for resins.

NREM, abbreviation for **nonrapid eye movement.** See **sleep.**

NSU, abbreviation for **nonspecific urethritis.**

nucha, *pl.* **nuchae,** the nape, or back of the neck. **nuchal,** *adj.*

nuchal rigidity, a resistance to flexion of the neck, a condition seen in patients with meningitis.

Nuck's canal, Nuck's diverticulum. See **processus vaginalis peritonei.**

nuclear agenesis. See **Möbius' syndrome.**

nuclear family, a family unit consisting of the biological parents and their offspring. Dissolution of a marriage results in dissolution of the nuclear family.

nuclear family emotional system, the organization of patterns of interaction between family members and the degree to which these patterns promote fusion.

nuclear fission. See **fission.**

nuclear hyaloplasm. See **karyolymph.**

nuclear isomer. See **isomers.**

nuclear magnetic resonance (NMR), 1. principle of **magnetic resonance imaging;** a phenomenon in which the atomic nuclei of certain materials placed in a strong, static magnetic field will absorb radio waves supplied by a transmitter at particular frequencies. 2. spectra emitted by phosphorus in body tissues as measured and imaged on phosphorus nuclear magnetic resonance instruments.

nuclear medicine, a medical discipline that uses radioactive isotopes in the diagnosis and treatment of disease.

nuclear problem, (in psychology) an underlying reason for an individual's reaction to a precipitating event.

nuclear sap. See **karyolymph.**

nuclear spin, an intrinsic form of angular momentum possessed by atomic nuclei containing an odd number of nucleons (protons or neutrons).

nucleic acid, a polymeric compound of high molecular weight composed of nucleotides, each consisting of a purine or pyrimidine base, a ribose or deoxyribose sugar, and a phosphate group. Nucleic acids are involved in energy storage and release and in the determination and transmission of genetic characteristics. Kinds of nucleic acid are **deoxyribonucleic acid** and **ribonucleic acid.**

nucleocapsid, a viral enclosure consisting of a capsid or protein coat that encloses nucleic acid.

nucleochylaema, the ground substance of the nucleus, as distinguished from that of the cytoplasm.

nucleochyme. See **karyolymph.**

nucleocytoplasmic, of or relating to the nucleus and cytoplasm of a cell.

nucleocytoplasmic ratio, the ratio of the volume of a nucleus of a cell to the volume of the cytoplasm. The proportion is usually constant for a specific cell type.

nucleohistone, a complex nucleoprotein that consists of deoxyribonucleic acid and a histone. It is the basic constituent of the chromatin in the cell nucleus.

nucleolar organizer, a part of the nucleus of the cell, thought to consist of heterochromatin, that is responsible for the formation of the nucleolus.

nucleolus, *pl.* **nucleoli,** any one of the small, dense structures composed largely of ribonucleic acid and situated within the cytoplasm of cells. Nucleoli are essential in the formation of ribosomes that synthesize cell proteins.

nucleon, a collective term applied to protons and neutrons within the nucleus.

nucleophilic, a property of some molecules, particularly nucleic acids and proteins, having electrons that can be shared and thus form bonds with alkylating agents.

nucleoplasm, the protoplasm of the nucleus as contrasted with that of the cell. **nucleoplasmic,** *adj.*

nucleoplasmic ratio. See **nucleocytoplasmic ratio.**

nucleoside monophosphate kinase, a liver enzyme that catalyses the transfer of a phosphate group from adenosine triphosphate, producing adenosine diphosphate and a nucleoside diphosphate.

nucleosome, any one of the repeating nucleoprotein units consisting of histones forming a complex with deoxyribonucleic acid that appear as the beadlike structures at distinct intervals along the chromosome.

5-nucleotidase, a nonlipid enzyme, elevated in some liver disorders and measured in the blood to distinguish between certain liver and bone diseases. The normal accumulations in serum are 0.1 to 6 units.

nucleotide, any one of the compounds into which nucleic acid is split by the action of nuclease. A nucleotide consists of a phosphate group, a pentose sugar, and a nitrogenous base.

nucleus, 1. the central controlling body within a living cell, usually a spherical unit enclosed in a membrane and containing genetic codes for maintaining life systems of the organism and for issuing commands for growth and reproduction. 2. a group of nerve cells of the central nervous system having a common function, such as supporting the sense of hearing or smell. 3. the centre of an atom about which electrons rotate. 4. the central element in an organic chemical compound or class of compounds. **nuclear,** *adj.*

nucleus pulposus, the central portion of each intervertebral disc, consisting of a pulpy elastic substance that loses some of its resilience with age.

nuclide, a species of atom characterized by the constitution of its nucleus, in particular by the number of protons and neutrons. Thus, Co-59 and Co-60 are both isotopes of cobalt and are each nuclides but have a different number of neutrons.

Nuhn's gland {Anton Nuhn, German anatomist, b. 1814}, an anterior lingual gland in tissues on the inferior surface and near the apex and midline of the tongue.

null cell, a lymphocyte that develops in the bone marrow and lacks the characteristic surface markers of the B and T lymphocytes. Stimulated by the presence of antibody, cells of this kind can apparently attack certain cellular targets directly and are known as "killer," or K cells. Compare B cell, T cell.

null hypothesis (HO), (in research) a hypothesis that predicts that no difference or relationship exists among the variables studied that could not have occurred by chance alone.

nulligravida, a woman who has never been pregnant.

nullipara, *pl.* **nulliparae,** a woman who has not been delivered of a viable infant. The designation "para 0" indicates nulliparity. **nulliparity,** *n.,* **nulliparous,** *adj.*

numbness, a partial or total lack of sensation in a part of the body, resulting from any factor that interrupts the transmission of impulses from the sensory nerve fibres.

nummular dermatitis, a skin disease characterized by coin-shaped, vesicular, or scaling eczema-like lesions on the forearms and the front of the calves.

Nuremberg tribunal, an international tribunal planned and implemented by the United Nations War Crimes Commission to detect, apprehend, try, and punish persons accused of war crimes. The principle and practice of informed consent was reinforced by the precedent set in the trials in which Nazi physicians were declared guilty of crimes against humanity in performing experiments on human beings who were not volunteers and did not consent.

nurse, 1. a person educated and qualified in the profession of nursing; one whose professional details are held on the UKCC's Professional Register. The practice of the nurse includes health education and promotion, assessment of patient need, planning and implementation of nursing care, and evaluation of such care. The nurse may be a generalist or a specialist and, as a professional, is ethically and legally accountable for the nursing activities performed and for the actions of others to whom the nurse has delegated responsibility. **2.** to provide nursing care.

nurse-client interaction, any process in which a nurse and a client exchange or share information, verbally or nonverbally. It is fundamental to communication and is an essential component of the nursing assessment.

nurse-client relationship, a therapeutic relationship between a nurse and a client built on a series of interactions and developing over time. During the first phase, the phase of establishment, the nurse establishes the structure, purpose, timing, and context of the relationship and expresses an interest in discussing this initial structure with the client. During the middle, developmental, phase of the relationship, the nurse and the client get to know each other better and test the structure of the relationship to be able to trust one another. The last phase, termination, ideally occurs when the goals of the relationship have been accomplished, when both the client and the nurse feel a sense of resolution and satisfaction.

nurse educator, a registered nurse, with an additional teaching qualification, whose primary area of interest, competence, and professional practice is the education of nurses.

nurse manager, a registered nurse who coordinates and manages the activities of nursing personnel engaged in specific nursing services, as care of the elderly or surgery, for two or more patient care units.

nurse practitioner, a nurse who by advanced training and clinical experience in a branch of nursingk, has acquired expert knowledge in the special branch of practice.

nurses' observation scale for inpatient evaluation (NOSIE), a systematic, objective behavioural rating scale, developed in North America and applied by nurses to patient behaviour.

nurses' station, an area in a clinic, ward, or unit in a health care facility that serves as the administrative centre for nursing care for a particular group of patients. It is usually centrally located and may be staffed by a ward secretary or clerk who assists with paperwork and telephone and other communication. Before going on duty, nurses usually meet there to hear the ward report and receive daily assignments.

nurse therapist model, (in psychiatric nursing research) a theoretic framework to clarify the role of the mental health nurse. Techniques from traditional and contemporary modes of treatment, including transactional analysis and crisis intervention, may be used singly or in various combinations.

nursing, 1. the practice in which a nurse assists "the individual, sick or well, in the performance of those activities contributing to health or its recovery (or to a peaceful death) that he would perform unaided if he had the necessary strength, will or knowledge. And to do this in such a way as to help him gain independence as rapidly as possible." (Virginia Henderson) **2.** the professional practice of a nurse. **3.** the process of acting as a nurse, of providing care that encourages and promotes the health of the person being served.

nursing assessment, an identification by a nurse of the needs, preferences, and abilities of a patient. Assessment follows an interview with and observation of a patient by the nurse and considers the symptoms and signs of the condition, the patient's verbal and nonverbal communication, medical and social history, and any other information available. Among the physical aspects assessed are vital signs, skin colour and condition, motor and sensory nerve function, nutrition, rest, sleep, activity, elimination, and conciousness.

nursing audit, a thorough investigation designed to identify, examine, or verify the performance of certain specified aspects of nursing care using established criteria. A **concurrent nursing audit** is performed during ongoing nursing care. A **retrospective nursing audit** is performed after discharge from the care facility, using the patient's record. Often, a nursing audit and a medical audit are performed collaboratively, resulting in a **joint audit.**

nursing care plan, a plan for the nursing care of a particular patient based on the nurse's assessment of that patient's specific needs and circumstances. It has four essential components: identification of the nursing care problems and a statement of the nursing approach to solve those problems; the statement of the expected benefit to the patient; the statement of the specific actions by the nurse that reflect the nursing approach and achieve the goals specified; and the evaluation of the patient's response to nursing care and the readjustment of that care as required.

nursing diagnosis, a statement of a health problem or of a potential problem in the client's health status that a nurse is competent to treat. Four steps are required in the formulation of a nursing diagnosis: A data base is established by collecting information from all available sources, including interviews with the client and the client's family, a review of any existing records of the client's health, observation of the response of the client to any alterations in health status, a physical assessment, and a conference or consultation with others concerned in the care of the client. The second step includes an analysis of the client's responses to the problems, healthy or unhealthy, and a classification of those responses as psychological, physiological, spiritual, or sociological. The third step is the organization of the data so that a tentative diagnostic statement can be made that summarizes the pattern of problems discovered. The last step is the confirmation of the sufficiency and accura-

cy of the data base by evaluation of the appropriateness of the diagnosis to nursing intervention and by the assurance that, given the same information, most other qualified practitioners would arrive at the same nursing diagnosis.

nursing goal, a general goal of nursing involving activities that are desirable but difficult to measure, such as self-care, good nutrition, and relaxation.

nursing history, data collected about a patient's level of wellness, changes in life patterns, sociocultural role, and mental and emotional reactions to illness.

nursing home. See **registered nursing home.**

nursing intervention, any act by a nurse that implements the nursing care plan or any specific objective of that plan, such as turning a comatose patient to avoid the development of decubitus ulcers.

nursing intervention model, (in nursing research) a conceptual framework used to determine appropriate nursing interventions. The model is a holistic representation of the client and the health care system. The goal is to learn what nursing interventions would be most effective for the particular problem within the particular health care system.

nursing objective, a specific aim planned by a nurse to decrease a person's stress, or improve the ability to adapt, or both. A nursing objective may be physical, emotional, social, or cultural and may involve the person's family, friends, and other patients.

nursing observation, an objective, holistic evaluation made by a nurse of the various aspects of a client's condition. It includes the person's general appearance, emotional affect, and nutritional status, habits, and preferences, as well as body temperature, skin condition, and any obvious abnormal processes.

nursing orders, specific instructions for implementing the nursing care plan, including the patient's preferences, timing of activities, details of health education necessary for the particular patient, role of the family, and plans for care after discharge.

nursing process, the process that serves as an organizational framework for the practice of nursing. It encompasses all of the steps taken by the nurse in caring for a patient: assessment (including history taking), planning, implementation of the planned care, and evaluation.

nursing process model, a conceptual framework in which the nurse-patient relationship is the basis of the nursing process. The nursing process is represented as dynamic and interpersonal, the nurse and the patient being affected by each other's behaviour and by the environment around them. Each successful two-way communication is termed a "transaction" and can be analysed to discover the factors that promote transactions.

nursing research, a detailed process in which a systematic study of a problem in the field of nursing is performed. One basic approach requires the following steps: formulation of the problem; review of the literature; development of a theory; formation of a hypothesis or hypotheses; definition of variables; determination of a method for weighting and counting variables; selection of a research design; choice of a population; plan for the analysis of the data; determination of interpretation; and plan for promulgation of the results.

nursing specialty, a nurse's particular professional field of practice, such as surgical, paediatric, or psychiatric nursing.

nursing theory, an organized framework of concepts and purposes designed to guide the practice of nursing.

nurture, to feed, rear, foster, or care for, as in the nourishment, care, and training of growing children.

nutation, the act of nodding, especially involuntary nodding as occurs in some neurological disorders.

nutcracker oesophagus. See **symptomatic oesophageal peristalsis.**

nutrient, a substance that provides nourishment and affects the nutritive and metabolic processes of the body.

nutrient artery of the humerus, one of a pair of branches of the deep brachial arteries, arising near the middle of the arm and entering the nutrient canal of the humerus.

nutrient canal. See **interdental canal.**

nutriment, any substance that nourishes and aids the growth and the development of the body.

nutrition, 1. nourishment. **2.** the sum of the processes involved in the taking in of nutrients and in their assimilation and use for proper body functioning and maintenance of health. **3.** the study of food and drink as related to the growth and maintenance of living organisms.

nutritional alcoholic cerebellar degeneration. See **alcoholic-nutritional cerebellar degeneration.**

nutritional anaemia, a disorder characterized by the inadequate production of haemoglobin or erythrocytes caused by a nutritional deficiency of iron, folic acid, or vitamin B12, or other nutritional disorders.

nutritional assessment, clinically this usually refers to the body's complement of fat, protein, vitamins, minerals and water. It also includes an assessment of food intake. See also **dietary assessment.**

nutritional care, the substances, procedures, and setting involved in assuring the proper intake and assimilation of nutrients, especially for the hospitalized patient. Patients who are unable to feed themselves are assisted, and abnormal intake of food is recorded

and reported. Supplemental nourishment when indicated and fluids are offered between meals.

nutrition, altered: less than body requirements, an inability of an individual to ingest or to digest food or to absorb nutrients in sufficient quantity for the maintenance of normal health, because of psychological, biological, or economic factors. Defining characteristics include loss of weight, reported intake of less food than is recommended, evidence or report of a lack of food, lack of interest in food, aversion to eating, alteration in the taste of food, feelings of fullness immediately after eating small quantities, abdominal pain with no other explanation, sores in the mouth, diarrhoea or steatorrhoea, pallor, weakness, and loss of hair.

nutrition, altered: more than body requirements, an excessive intake of food in relation to the metabolic needs of the body. Defining characteristics include a weight gain of 20% greater than the ideal for the height and body build of the client, sedentary activity level, and dysfunctional eating habits, including eating in response to internal cues than hunger.

nutrition, altered: potential for more than body requirements, the perceived risk that an individual's intake of nutrients will exceed metabolic needs. Defining characteristics include obesity in one or both parents, rapidly increasing percentiles in measurement of an infant's or child's weight as compared with others of the same age, the use of solid foods as a significant part of the diet before 5 months, the use of food as a reward, an observed increase in the baseline weight at the onset of each pregnancy, or dysfunctional eating patterns.

nutritionist, one who studies and applies the principles and science of nutrition.

nyctalopia, poor vision at night or in dim light resulting from decreased synthesis of rhodopsin, vitamin A deficiency, retinal degeneration, or a congenital defect. **nyctalopic,** *adj.*

nyctophobia, an anxiety reaction characterized by an obsessive, irrational fear of darkness.

nycturia. See **nocturia.**

nystagmus, involuntary, rhythmic movements of the eyes; the oscillations may be horizontal, vertical, rotary, or mixed. Jerking nystagmus, characterized by faster movements in one direction than in the opposite direction, may be a sign of barbiturate intoxication or of labyrinthine vestibular, vascular, or neurological disease. Labyrinthine vestibular nystagmus, most frequently rotary, is usually accompanied by vertigo and nausea. Vertical nystagmus is considered pathognomonic of disease of the brainstem's tegmentum, and nystagmus occurring only in the abducting eye is said to be a sign of multiple sclerosis. Seesaw nystagmus, in which one eye moves up and the other down, may be seen in bilateral hemianopia. Pendular nystagmus occurs in albinism, various diseases of the retina and refractive media, and in miners, after many years of working in darkness; in miners, the eye movements are very rapid, increase on upward gaze, and are often associated with vertigo, head tremor, and photophobia. **nystagmic,** *adj.*

nystatin, an antifungal used in the treatment of fungal infections of the GI tract, vagina, and skin. It is not absorbed from the GI tract nor administered parenterally.

nystaxis. See **nystagmus.**

O, symbol for **oxygen atom.**

O₂, symbol for **oxygen molecule.**

oat cell carcinoma, a malignant, usually bronchogenic epithelial neoplasm consisting of small, tightly packed, round, oval, or spindle-shaped epithelial cells. Tumours produced by these cells do not form bulky masses but usually spread along submucosal lymphatics. One third of all malignant tumours of the lung are of this type.

obesity, an abnormal increase in the proportion of fat cells, mainly in the viscera and subcutaneous tissues of the body. **Hyperplastic obesity** is caused by an increase in the number of fat cells in the increased adipose tissue mass. **Hypertrophic obesity** results from an increase in the size of the fat cells in the increased adipose tissue mass.

object, (in psychology) that through which an instinct can achieve its goal.

objective, 1. a goal. **2.** of or pertaining to a phenomenon or clinical finding that is observed; not subjective.

objective data collection, the process in which data relating to the client's problem are obtained by an observer through direct physical examination, including observation, palpation, and auscultation, and by laboratory analyses and radiological and other studies.

objective lens, 1. (in radiotherapy) a lens that accepts light from the output phosphor of an image-intensifier tube and converts it into a parallel beam for recording the image on film. **2.** (in pathology) the term is used for the lower lens on a microscope.

object permanence, a capacity to perceive that something exists even when it is not seen.

object relations, a term from psychoanalytical theory whose meaning varies with the theoretical orientation of the practitioner. 'Object' is the term used for the representation of significant others with whom a person has had a relationship at whatever stage of life. Relationships during infancy are thought to be especially important, and the term object is used to designate the pre-verbal stage of these representations in an infant's consciousness. Object relations refers to the supposed mental relationship of the unconsciousness as well as of the conscious self to these representations.

obligate aerobe, an organism that cannot grow in the absence of oxygen.

obligate anaerobe, an organism that cannot grow in the presence of oxygen, such as

Clostridium tetani, C. botulinum, and *C. perfringens.*

oblique, a slanting direction or any variation from the perpendicular or the horizontal.

oblique bandage, a circular bandage applied spirally in slanting turns, usually to a limb.

oblique fibre, (in dentistry) any one of the collagenous fibres that are bundled together obliquely in the periodontal ligament.

oblique fissure of the lung, 1. the groove marking the division of the lower and middle lobes in the right lung. **2.** the groove marking the division of the upper and the lower lobes in the left lung.

oblique fracture, a fracture that cracks a bone at an oblique angle.

oblique illumination. See **illumination.**

obliquus externus abdominis, one of a pair of muscles that are the largest and the most superficial of the five anterolateral muscles of the abdomen. A broad, thin, four-sided muscle that arises by eight fleshy digitations from the lower eight ribs and inserts in the iliac crest and the linea alba. It acts to compress the contents of the abdomen and assists in micturition, defaecation, emesis, parturition, and forced expiration. Both sides acting together serve to flex the vertebral column. One side alone functions to bend the vertebral column laterally and to rotate it, drawing the shoulder of the same side forward.

obliquus internus abdominis, one of a pair of anterolateral muscles of the abdomen, lying under the obliquus externus abdominis in the lateral and ventral part of the abdominal wall. It functions to compress the abdominal contents and assists in micturition, defecation, emesis, parturition, and forced expiration. Both sides acting together serve to flex the vertebral column. One side acting alone acts to bend the vertebral column laterally and rotate it, drawing the shoulder of the opposite side downward.

observation, 1. the act of watching carefully and attentively. **2.** a report of what is seen or noted, such as a nursing observation.

obsession, a persistent thought or idea with which the mind is continually and involuntarily preoccupied and which suggests an irrational act. **obsessive,** *adj.*

obsessional personality, a type of personality in which persistent, intrusive, irrational, uncontrollable, and unwanted thoughts lead to compulsive actions.

obsessive-compulsive, 1. characterized by or relating to the tendency to perform repetitive acts or rituals, usually as a means of releasing tension or relieving anxiety. **2.** describing a person who has an obsessive-compulsive neurosis.

obsessive-compulsive neurosis, a neurotic condition characterized by the inability to resist or stop the intrusion of persistent, irrational, and uncontrollable urges, ideas, thoughts, or fears contrary to the person's standards or judgments.

obsessive-compulsive personality, a type of personality in which there is an uncontrollable need to perform certain acts or rituals. This behaviour is manifested in many forms and may range from mildly stylized personal habits, such as repeating certain words before undertaking a particular act, to more serious compulsive acts, such as the continuous washing of hands.

obsessive-compulsive reaction. See **obsessive-compulsive neurosis.**

obstetric anaesthesia, any of various procedures used to provide anaesthesia for childbirth. It includes local anaesthesia for episiotomy or episiotomy repair, regional anaesthesia for labour or delivery, such as by paracervical block or pudendal block, or, for a wider block, epidural.

obstetric forceps, forceps used to assist delivery of the fetal head. The several styles of forceps are designed to assist in various clinical situations. Kinds of obstetric forceps include **Kielland's forceps, Neville Barnes forceps** and **Wrigleys forceps.**

obstetrician, a doctor who specializes in obstetrics.

obstetrics, the branch of medicine concerned with pregnancy and childbirth, including the study of the physiological and pathological function of the female reproductive tract and the care of the mother and fetus throughout pregnancy, childbirth, and the immediate postpartum period. **obstetric, obstetrical,** *adj.*

obstruction, 1. something that blocks or clogs. **2.** the act of blocking or preventing passage. **3.** the condition of being obstructed or clogged. **obstruct,** *v.,* **obstructive,** *adj.*

obstructive airways disease, any clinically important obstruction of the respiratory tract that may be associated with symptoms of chronic bronchitis, abnormalities of the bronchi, and emphysema.

obstructive anuria, an abnormal urological condition characterized by an almost complete absence of urination and caused by an obstruction of the urinary tract.

obstructive jaundice. See **cholestasis.**

obstructive sleep apnoea, a form of sleep apnoea involving a physical obstruction in the upper airways. The condition is usually marked by recurrent sleep interruptions, and gasping spells on awakening.

obstructive uropathy, any pathological condition that results in obstruction of the flow of urine. The condition may lead to impairment of kidney function and an increased risk of urinary infection.

obturator, 1. a device used to block a passage or a canal or to fill in a space, such as a prosthesis implanted to bridge the gap in the roof of the mouth in a cleft palate. **2.** nontechnical. an obturator muscle or membrane.

obturator externus, the flat, triangular muscle covering the outer surface of the anterior wall of the pelvis. It functions to rotate the thigh laterally.

obturator foramen, a large opening on each side of the lower portion of the hip bone, formed posteriorly by the ischium.

obturator internus, a muscle that covers a large area of the inferior aspect of the lesser pelvis, where it surrounds the obturator foramen. It arises from the superior and the inferior rami of the pubis, the ischium, and the obturator membrane and inserts into the greater trochanter of the femur. It functions to rotate the thigh laterally and to extend and abduct the thigh when it is flexed.

obturator membrane, a tough fibrous membrane that covers the obturator foramen of each side of the pelvis.

occipital, 1. of or pertaining to the occiput. **2.** situated near the occipital bone, such as the occipital lobe of the brain.

occipital artery, one of a pair of tortuous braces from the external carotid arteries that divides into six branches and supplies parts of the head and scalp.

occipital bone, the cuplike bone at the back of the skull, marked by a large opening, the foramen magnum, the communicates with the vertebral canal. Its inner surface is divided into four fossae. The occipital bone articulates with the tow parietal bones, the two temporal bones, the sphenoid, and the atlas.

occipital lobe, one of the five lobes of each cerebral hemisphere, occupying a relatively small pyramidal portion of the occipital pole. The occipital lobe lies beneath the occipital bone and presents medial, lateral, and inferior surfaces.

occipital sinus, the smallest of the cranial sinuses and one of six posterior superior venous channels associated with the dura mater.

occipitofrontalis, one of a pair of thin, broad muscles covering the top of the skull, consisting of an occipital belly and a frontal belly connected by an extensive aponeurosis. It is the muscle that draws the scalp and raises the eyebrows.

occipitoparietal fissure. See **pariotooccipital sulcus.**

occiput, *pl.* **occiputs, occipita,** the back part of the head.

occluded, closed, plugged, or obstructed, as (in dentistry) an occluded root canal.

occlusal adjustment, (in dentistry) the grinding of the occluding surfaces of teeth to improve the occlusion or relationship between opposing tooth surfaces, their supporting structures, the muscles of mastication, and the temporomandibular joints.

occlusal contouring, the modification by grinding of irregularities of occlusal tooth forms, such as uneven marginal ridges, and extruded or malpositioned teeth.

occlusal form, the shape of the occluding surfaces of a tooth, a row of teeth, or any dentition.

occlusal harmony, a combination of healthy and nondisruptive occlusal relationships between the teeth and their supporting structures, the associated neuromuscular mechanisms, and the temporomandibular joints.

occlusal lug. See **occlusal rest.**

occlusal radiograph, an intraoral radiograph made with the film placed on the occlusal surfaces of one of the arches.

occlusal recontouring, the reshaping of an occlusal surface of a natural or artificial tooth.

occlusal relationship, the relationship of the mandibular teeth to the maxillary teeth when in a defined occlusal contact position.

occlusal rest, a support placed on the occlusal surface of a posterior tooth.

occlusal rest angle, (in dentistry) the angle formed by the occlusal rest with the upright minor connector.

occlusal rim, an artificial dental structure with occluding surfaces attached to temporary or permanent denture bases, used for recording the relation of the maxilla to the mandible and for positioning the teeth.

occlusal spillway, a natural groove that crosses a cusp ridge or a marginal ridge of a tooth.

occlusal trauma, injury to a tooth and surrounding structures caused by malocclusive stresses, including trauma, temporomandibular joint dysfunction, and bruxism.

occlusion, 1. (in anatomy) a blockage in a canal, vessel, or passage of the body. **2.** (in dentistry) any contact between the incising or masticating surfaces of the maxillary and mandibular teeth. **occlude,** *v.,* **occlusive,** *adj.*

occlusive, pertaining to something that effects an occlusion or closure, such as an occlusive dressing.

occlusive dressing, a dressing that prevents air from reaching a wound or lesion and that retains moisture, heat, body fluids, and medication. It may consist of a sheet of thin plastic affixed with transparent tape.

occult, hidden or difficult to observe directly, such as occult prolapse of the umbilical cord or occult blood.

occult blood, blood that appears from a nonspecific source, with obscure signs and symptoms. It may be detected by means of a chemical test or by microscopic or spectroscopic examination.

occult carcinoma, a small carcinoma that does not cause overt symptoms. It may remain localized and be discovered only incidentally at autopsy after death resulting from another cause, or it may metastasize and be discovered in the diagnostic study of the resulting metastatic disease.

occult fracture, a fracture that cannot be initially detected by radiographic examination but may be evident radiographically weeks later. It is accompanied by the usual signs of pan and trauma and may produce soft tissue oedema.

occupancy, the ratio of average daily hospital census to the average number of beds maintained during the reporting period.

occupancy factor (T), the level of occupancy of an area adjacent to a source of radiation, used to determine the amount of shielding required in the walls. T is rated as full, for an office or laboratory next to an x-ray facility; partial, for corridors and toilets; and occasional, for stairways, lifts, cupboards, and outside areas.

occupational accident, an accidental injury to an employee that occurs in the workplace. Occupational accidents account for over 95% of occupational disabilities.

occupational disability, a condition in which a worker is unable to perform the functions required to complete a job satisfactorily because of an occupational disease or an occupational accident.

occupational disease, a disease that results from a particular employment, usually from the effects of long-term exposure to specific substances or of continuous or repetitive physical acts.

occupational health, the ability of a worker to function at an optimum level of well-being at a worksite as reflected in terms of productivity, work attendance, disability compensation claims, and employment longevity.

occupational history, a portion of the health history in which questions are asked about the person's occupation, source of income, effects of the work on worker's health or the worker's health on the job, the duration of the job, and to what degree the occupation satisfies the person.

occupational lung disease, any one of a group of abnormal conditions of the lungs caused by the inhalation of dusts, fumes, gases, or vapors in an environment where a person works.

occupational medicine, a field of preventive medicine concerned with the medical problems and practices relating to occupations and especially to the health of workers in various industries.

occupational neurosis, a neurotic disorder in which various symptoms occur that prevent the activities required by the occupation.

occupational performance, the ability to perform selected activities to a known or specified level or standard in the appropriate environment and within the accepted or stated timescale.

occupational performance tasks, activities that can be used to measure the potential ability or actual proficiency in the handling of certain objects and use of skills related to a given occupation.

occupational socialization, the adaptation of an individual to a given set of job-related behaviours, particularly the expected behaviour that accompanies a specific job.

occupational therapist, a person who practices occupational therapy and who is qualified and registered through the appropriate national body.

occupational therapy, the use of purposeful activity with individuals who are limited by physical injury or illness, psychosocial dysfunction, developmental or learning disabilities, or the aging process to maximize independence, prevent disability, and maintain health.

occupational therapy process, the process or series of steps in which the occupational therapist engages following receipt of the initial referral through to discharge of the patient from the service. It is based upon a problem solving approach.

ochre mutation. See **amber mutation.**

ochronosis, a condition characterized by the deposition of brown-black pigment in connective tissue and cartilage, often caused by alkaptonuria or poisoning with phenol. The urine may be dark-coloured.

ocontic pressure. See **colloid osmotic pressure.**

OCR, abbreviation for **optical character recognition.**

octaploid, octaploidic. See **polyploid.**

ocular, 1. of or pertaining to the eye. 2. an eyepiece of an optic instrument.

ocular dysmetria, a visual disorder in which the eyes are unable to fix the gaze on an object or follow a moving object with accuracy.

ocular hypertelorism, a developmental defect involving the frontal region of the cranium, characterized by an abnormally widened bridge of the nose and increased distance between the eyes.

ocular hypotelorism, a developmental defect involving the frontal region of the cranium, characterized by a narrowing of the bridge of the nose and an abnormal decrease in the distance between the eyes, with resulting convergent strabismus.

ocular myopathy, slowly progressive weakness of ocular muscles, characterized by decreased mobility of the eye and drooping of the upper lid. The disorder may be unilateral or bilateral and may be caused by damage to the oculomotor nerve, an intracranial tumour, or a neuromuscular disease.

ocular spot, an abnormal opacity in the eye. A shower of red and black dots may be seen in the eye after haemorrhage of a retinal vessel; opacities in the crystalline lens are characteristic in cataracts.

oculocephalic reflex, a test of the integrity of brainstem function. When the patient's head is quickly moved to one side and then the other, the eyes will normally lag behind the head movement and then slowly assume the midline position. Failure of the eyes to either lag properly or revert back to the midline indicates a lesion on the ipsilateral side at the brainstem level.

oculogyric crisis, a paroxysm in which the eyes are held in a fixed position, usually up and sideways, for minutes or several hours, often occurring in postencephalitic patients with signs of parkinsonism, or induced by an antidopaminergic drug.

oculomotor nerve, either of a pair of cranial nerves essential for eye movements, supplying certain extrinsic and intrinsic eye muscles.

O.D., abbreviation for **oculus dexter,** a Latin phrase meaning "right eye."

odontectomy, the extraction of a tooth.

odontiasis, the eruption of teeth.

odontitis, inflammation of tooth pulp; pulpitis.

odontodysplasia, an abnormality in the development of the teeth, characterized by deficient formation of enamel and dentin.

odontoid process, the toothlike projection that rises perpendicularly from the upper surface of the body of the second cervical vertebra or axis, which serves as a pivot point for the rotation of the atlas, or first cervical vertebra, enabling the head to turn.

odontogenesis imperfecta. See **dentinogenesis imperfecta.**

odontogenic fibroma, a benign neoplasm of the jaw derived from the embryonic part of the tooth germ, dental follicle, or dental papilla or developing later from the periodontal membrane.

odontogenic fibrosarcoma, a malignant neoplasm of the jaw that develops in a mesenchymal component of a tooth or tooth germ.

odontogenic myxoma, a rare tumour of the jaw; it may develop from the mesenchyme of the tooth germ.

odontoid ligament. See **alar ligament.**

odontology, the scientific study of the anatomy and physiology of the teeth and of the surrounding structures of the oral cavity.

odontoma, an anomaly of the teeth that resembles a hard tumour, such as dens in dente, enamel pearl, and complex or composite odontoma.

odour, a scent or smell. The sense of smell is activated when airborne molecules stimulate receptors of the first cranial nerve.

Odstock wire, a tool measuring the range of movement at the finger joints, normally used in part of a hand assessment. It consists of solder wire encased in polythene tubing which is placed in close contact with the digit in a specified position.

ODTS, abbreviation for **organic dust toxic syndrome.**

odynophagia, a severe sensation of burning, squeezing pain while swallowing, caused by irritation of the mucosa or a muscular disorder of the oesophagus, such as gastroesophageal reflux, bacterial or fungal infection, tumour, achalasia, or chemical irritation.

oedema, the abnormal accumulation of fluid in interstitial spaces of tissue, such as in the pericardial sac, intrapleural space, peritoneal cavity or joint capsules. **oedematous, oedematose,** adj.

Oedipus complex, 1. (in psychoanalysis) a child's desire for a sexual relationship with the parent of the opposite sex, usually with strong negative feelings for the parent of the same sex. **2.** a son's desire for a sexual relationship with his mother.

OER, abbreviation for **oxygen enhancement ratio.**

oesophageal atresia, an abnormal oesophagus that ends in a blind pouch or narrows to a thin cord and thus fails to provide a continuous passage to the stomach.

oesophageal cancer, a malignant neoplastic disease of the oesophagus. Risk factors associated with the disease are heavy consumption of alcohol, smoking, betel-nut chewing, Plummer-Vinson syndrome, hiatus hernia, and achalasia. Oesophageal cancer does not often cause any symptoms in the early stages but in later stages causes painful dysphagia, anorexia, weight loss, regurgitation, cervical adenopathy, and, in some cases, a persistant cough. Left vocal cord paralysis and haemoptysis indicate an advanced state of the disease.

oesophageal dysfunction, any disturbance, impairment or abnormality that interferes with the normal functioning of the oesophagus, such as dysphagia, oesophagitis, or sphincter incompetence. The condition is one of the primary symptoms of scleroderma.

oesophageal lead, 1. an electrocardio-graphic conductor in which the exploring electrode is placed within the lumen of the oesophagus. It is used to identify cardiac arrhythmias. **2.** informal. a tracing produced by such a lead on an electrocardiograph.

oesophageal obturator airway, an emergency airway device that consists of a large tube that is inserted into the mouth through an airtight face mask. Because of the design, air passes only into the trachea.

oesophageal varices, a complex of longitudinal, tortuous veins at the lower end of the oesophagus, enlarged and swollen as the result of portal hypertension.

oesophageal web, a thin membrane that may develop across the lumen of the oesophagus, usually near the level of the cricoid cartilage, and associated with iron-deficiency anaemia.

oesophagectomy, a surgical procedure in which all or part of the oesophagus is removed, as may be required to treat severe, recurrent, bleeding oesophageal varices.

oesophagitis, inflammation of the mucosal lining of the oesophagus, caused by infection, irritation from a nasogastric tube, or backflow of gastric juice from the stomach.

oesophagoscopy, an examination of the oesophagus with an endoscope.

oesophagus, the muscular canal, about 24 cm long, extending from the pharynx to the stomach. It is the narrowest part of the digestive tube and is most constricted at its commencement and at the point where it passes through the diaphragm. It is composed of a fibrous coat, a muscular coat, and a submucous coat and is lined with mucous membrane. **oesophageal,** adj.

oestradiol, the most potent, naturally occurring human oestrogen.

oestriol, a relatively weak, naturally occuring human oestrogen, found in high concentrations in urine.

oestrogen, any one of a group of hormonal steroid compounds that promote the development of female secondary sex characteristics. Human oestrogen is elaborated in the ovaries, adrenal cortices, testes, and fetoplacental unit. During the menstrual cycle oestrogen renders the female genital tract suitable for fertilization, implantation, and nutrition of the early embryo. Oestrogens used therapeutically include **conjugated oestrogens, ethinyloestradiol,** and **oestrone. oestrogenic,** adj.

oestrus, the cyclical period of sexual activity in mammals other than primates.

off-centre grid, (in radiotherapy) a focused grid that is perpendicular to the central-axis x-ray bream but shifted laterally, resulting in a cutoff across the entire grid.

off-focus radiation, (in radiotherapy) x-ray production caused by stray electrons that interact at positions on the anode at points other than the focal spot.

off-line, access to computer information of equipment not part of an operating computer system, such as a drive not connected to the computer, a disk not connected to the computer, a disk not mounted on a drive, or a data printout sheet.

ofloxacin, an antibiotic of the 4-quinolone type.

OH, symbol for **hydroxyl.**

OHF, abbreviation for **Omsk haemorrhagic fever.**

ohm, a unit of measurement of electric resistance. One ohm is the resistance of a conductor in which an electric potential of 1 V produces a current of 1 ampere.

Ohm's law, the principle that the strength or intensity of an unvarying electric current is directly proportional to the electromotive force. The constant of proportionality is the resistance in the circuit.

-oi, -i, a pleural-forming element in borrowings from Greek: *auloi, catenephroi, mesonephroi.*

oil, any of a large number of greasy liquid substances not miscible in water. Oils may be fixed or volatile and are derived from animal, vegetable, or mineral matter.

oil retention enema, an enema containing about 200 to 250 ml of an oil-based solution given to soften a faecal mass.

ointment, a semisolid, greasy, externally applied preparation, usually containing a drug. Various ointments are used as local analgesic, anaesthetic, antiinfective, astringent, depigmenting, irritant, and keratolytic agents.

olecranon, a proximal projection of the ulna that forms the point of the elbow and fits into the olecranon fossa of the humerus when the forearm is extended.

olecranon bursa, the bursa of the elbow.

olecranon fossa, the depression in the posterior surface of the humerus that receives the olecranon of the ulna when the forearm is extended.

olecranon process. See **olecranon.**

olefin, any of a group of unsaturated aliphatic hydrocarbons containing one or more double bonds in the carbon chain. The group is represented by the general formula C_nH_{2n}.

oleic acid, a colourless, liquid, monounsaturated fatty acid occurring in almost all natural fats.

oleometer, a device for measuring the purity of oils.

olfactory, of or pertaining to the sense of smell. **olfaction,** *n.*

olfactory centre, the part of the brain responsible for the subjective appreciation of odours, a complex group of neurons located near the junction of the temporal and parietal lobes.

olfactory foramen, one of several openings in the cribiform plate of the ethmoid bone.

olfactory nerve, one of a pair of nerves associated with the sense of smell. The olfactory nerve is cranial nerve I and is composed of numerous fine filaments that ramify in the mucous membrane of the olfactory area. The area in which the olfactory nerves arise is situated in the most superior portion of the mucous membrane that covers the superior nasal concha. The olfactory nerves connect with the olfactory bulb and the olfactory tract, which are components of the portion of the brain associated with the sense of smell.

oligaemia, a condition of hypovolaemia or reduced circulating intravascular volume.

oligoclonal banding, a process by which cerebrospinal fluid IgG is distributed, following electrophoresis, in discrete bands. Approximately 90% of multiple sclerosis patients show oligoclonal banding.

oligodactyly, a congenital anomaly characterized by the absence of one or more of the fingers or toes. **oligodactylic,** *adj.*

oligodendroblastoma. See **oligodendroglioma.**

oligodendrocyte, a type of neuroglial cell with dendritic projections that coil around axons of neural cells.

oligodendroglia, central nervous system cells that produce myelin.

oligodendroglioma, *pl.* **oligodendrogliomas, olidodendrogliomata,** an uncommon brain tumour composed of nonneural ectodermal cells that usually form part of the supporting connective tissue around nerve cells.

oligodontia, a genetically determined dental defect characterized by the development of fewer than the normal number of teeth.

oligogenic, of or pertaining to hereditary characteristics produced by one or only a few genes.

oliogohydramnios, an abnormally small amount or absence of amniotic fluid.

oligomeganephronia, a type of congenital renal hypoplasia associated with chronic renal failure in children. **oligomeganephronic,** *adj.*

oligomenorrhoea, abnormally light or infrequent menstruation. **oligomenorroeic,** *adj.*

oligopnoea. See **bradypnoea.**

oligospermia, insufficient spermatozoa in the semen.

oliguria, a diminished capacity to form and pass urine, less than 500 ml in every 24 hours, so that the end products of metabolism cannot be excreted efficiently. **oliguric,** *adj.*

olivopontocerebellar, of or pertaining to the olivae, the middle peduncles, and the cerebellum.

olivopontocerebellar atrophy (OPCA), a group of hereditary ataxias characterized by mixed clinical features of pure cerebellar ataxia, dementia, parkinson-like symptoms, spasticity, choreoathetosis, retinal degeneration, myelophaty, and peripheral neuropathy.

Ollier's disease. See **enchondromatosis.**

Ollier's dyschondroplasia {Louis Ollier, French surgeon, b. 1830}, a rare disorder of bone development; the epiphyseal tissue responsible for growth spreads through the bones, causing abnormal irregular growth and, eventually, deformity. A kind of dyschondroplasia is **hereditary multiple exostoses.**

omalgia, pain in the shoulder.

omarthritis, inflammation of the shoulder joint.

ombudsman, a person who investigates and mediates patients' problems and complaints in relation to a hospital's or health centre's services.

omental bursa, a cavity in the peritoneum behind the stomach, the lesser omentum, and the lower border of the liver and in front of the pancreas and duodenum.

omentum, *pl.* **omenta, omentums,** an extension of the peritoneum that enfolds one or more adjacent organs in the stomach. **omental,** *adj.*

omission, (in law) intentional or unintentional neglect to fulfill a duty required by law.

omnipotence, (in psychology) an infantile perception that the outside world is part of the organism, which leads to a primitive feeling of all-powerfulness. This feeling normally becomes limited as the ego and a sense of reality develop, but it is still found in disturbed individuals who lose contact with reality.

omphalic, pertaining to the umbilicus.

omphalitis, an inflammation of the umbilical stump, marked by redness, swelling, and purulent exudate in severe cases.

omphaloangiopagus. See **allantoidoangiopagus.**

omphalocele, congenital herniation of intra-abdominal viscera through a defect in the abdominal wall around the umbilicus.

omphalodidymus. See **gastrodidymus.**

omphalogenesis, the formation of the umbilicus or yolk sac during embryonic development. **omphalogenetic,** *adj.*

omphalomesenteric artery. See **vitelline artery.**

omphalomesenteric circulation. See **vitelline circulation.**

omphalomesenteric duct. See **yolk stalk.**

omphalomesenteric vein. See **vitelline vein.**

omphalopagus. See **monomphalus.**

omphalosite, the underdeveloped parasitic member of unequal conjoined twins united by the vessels of the umbilical cord.

OMR, abbreviation for **optic mark recognition.**

Omsk haemorrhagic fever (OHF), an acute infection, seen in regions of the former Soviet Union, caused by an arbovirus transmitted by the bite of an infected tick or by handling infected muskrats. The disease is characterized by fever, headache, epistaxis, GI and uterine bleeding, and other haemorrhagic manifestations.

onanism. See **masturbation.**

onchocerciasis, a form of filariasis common in Central and South America and in Africa, characterized by subcutaneous nodules, pruritic rash, and eye lesions. It is transmitted by the bites of black flies that deposit *Onchocerca volvulus* microfilariae under the skin. The microfilariae migrate to the subcutaneous tissue and eyes, and fibrous nodules develop around the developing adult worms. Hypersensitive reactions to the dying microfilaria include extreme pruritus, a cellulitis-like rash, lichenification, depigmentation, and rarely, elephantiasis.

oncofetal protein, a protein produced by or associated with a tumour cell, particularly an embryological tumour. An example is alpha-fetoprotein.

oncogene, a potential cancer-including gene. Under normal conditions, such genes play a role in the growth and proliferation of cells, but when altered in some way by a cancer-causing agent, they may cause the cell to be transformed to a malignant state.

oncogenesis, the process initiating and promoting the development of a neoplasm through the action of biological, chemical, or physical agents. **oncogenic,** *adj.*

oncogenic virus, a virus that is able to cause the development of a malignant neoplastic disease. Over 100 oncogenic viruses have been identified.

oncologist, a doctor who specializes in the study and treatment of neoplastic disease, particularly cancer.

oncology, 1. the branch of medicine concerned with the study of tumours. 2. the study of cancerous malignancies.

oncotic pressure gradient, the pressure difference between the osmotic pressure of blood and that of tissue fluid or lymph. It is an important force in maintaining balance between blood and surrounding tissues.

oncovirus, a member of a family of viruses associated with leukemia and sarcoma in animals and, possibly, in humans.

Ondine's curse, apnoea caused by loss of automatic control of respiration. A defect in the central chemoreceptor responsiveness to carbon dioxide leaves the patient with hypercapnia and hypoxaemia, although fully able to breathe voluntarily.

one-and-a-half spica cast, an orthopaedic cast used for immobilizing the trunk of the body cranially to the nipple line, one leg caudally as far as the toes, and the other leg caudally as far as the knee.

one-to-one care. See **primary nursing.**

one-to-one relationship, a mutually defined, collaborative goal-directed patient therapist relationship for the purpose of psychotherapy.

onlay, 1. a cast type of restoration retained by friction and mechanical forces in a prepared tooth for restoring one or more cusps and adjoining occlusal surfaces of a tooth. 2. an occlusal set portion of a removable partial denture, extended to cover the occlusal surface of a tooth.

on-line, access to information or equipment that is part of an operating computer system linked to a central processing unit.

onset of action, the time required after administration of a drug for a response to be observed.

ontogenesis. See **ontogeny.**

ontogenetic, 1. of, relating to, or acquired during ontogeny. **2.** an association based on visible morphological characteristics and not necessarily indicative of a natural evolutionary relationship.

ontogeny, the life history of one organism from a single-celled ovum to the time of birth, including all phases of differentiation and growth.

onychia, inflammation of the nail bed.

onychocryptosis, a nail whose free distal margin grows or is pressed into the skin, causing an inflammatory reaction. See **ingrown toenail.**

onychogryphosis, thickened, curve, claw-like overgrowth of fingernails or toenails.

onycholysis, separation of a nail from its bed, beginning at the free margin, associated with psoriasis, dermatitis of the hand, fungal infection, *Pseudomonas* infection, and many other conditions.

onychomadesis, separation of the nail plate from the nail bed beginning proximally. The condition is usually associated with trauma.

onychomysis, any fungal infection of the nails.

onychophosis, thickening of the nail groove.

onychorrhexis, longitudinal ridges and depressions occurring in the nail bed reflected in the nail plate.

ooblast, the female germ cell from which the mature ovum is developed.

oocentre, See **ovocentre.**

oocyesis, an ectopic ovarian pregnancy.

oocyst, a stage in the development of any sporozoan in which after fertilization a zygote is produced that develops about itself an enclosing cyst wall.

oocyte, a primordial or incompletely developed ovum.

oocytin, the substance in a spermatozoon that stimulates the formation of the fertilization membrane after penetration of an ovum.

oogamy, 1. sexual reproduction by the fertilization of a large, nonmotile female gamete by a smaller, actively motile male gamete, such as occurs in certain algae and the malarial parasite *Plasmodium*. **2.** heterogamy. **oogamous,** *adj.*

oogenesis, the process of the growth and maturation of the female gametes, or ova. **oogenetic,** *adj.*

oogonium, *pl.* **oogonia,** the precursor cell from which an oocyte develops in the fetus during intrauterine life.

ookinesis, the mitotic phenomena occurring in the nucleus of the egg cell during maturation and fertilization. **ookinetic,** *adj.*

ookinete, the motile elongated zygote that is formed by the fertilization of the macrogamete during the sexual reproductive phase of the life cycle of a sporozoan, spe-cifically the malarial parasite Plasmodium.

oophoralgia, pain affecting the ovary

oolemma. See **zona pellucida.**

oophorectomy, the surgical removal of one or both ovaries, performed to remove a cyst or tumour, excise an abscess, treat endometriosis, or, in breast cancer, remove the source of oestrogen, which stimulates some kinds of cancer. In premenopausal women one ovary or a portion of one ovary may be left intact unless a malignancy is present. The operation often accompanies a hysterectomy.

oophoritis, an inflammatory condition of one or both ovaries, usually occurring with salpingitis.

oophorocystectomy, the removal of an ovarian cyst.

oophorosalpingectomy, the surgical removal of one or both ovaries and the corresponding oviducts, performed to remove a cyst or tumour, excise an abscess, or treat the condition of endometriosis. In a bilateral procedure the patient becomes sterile and menopause is induced.

ooplasm, the cytoplasm of the egg, or ovum, including the yolk in lower animals.

oosperm, a fertilized ovum; the cell resulting from the union of the pronuclei of the spermatoon and the ovum after fertilization; a zygote.

opacity, pertaining to an opaque quality of a substance or object, such as cataract opacity.

opaque, 1. of or pertaining to a substance or surface that neither transmits nor allows the passage of light. **2.** neither transparent nor translucent.

open amputation, a kind of amputation in which a straight, guillotine cut is made without skin flaps. Open amputation is performed if an infection is probable or developing or has been recurrent.

open-angle glaucoma. See **glaucoma.**

open-bite, an abnormal dental condition in which the anterior teeth do not occlude in any mandibular position.

open-circuit breathing system, a type of breathing system used in cardiopulmonary therapy in which rebreathing does not occur. Gas is inspired through a breathing branch that is connected to a gas source or open to the ambient atmosphere and then expired into a reservoir or vented back into the atmosphere.

open drainage. See **drainage.**

open-drop anaesthesia, the oldest and simplest anaesthetic technique. A volatile liquid anaesthetic agent is dripped, one drop at time, onto a porous cloth or mask held over the patient's face.

open fracture. See **compound fracture.**

opening pressure, the amount of pressure measured in a manometer following insertion of a spinal needle into the subarachnoid space.

open operation, a surgical procedure that provides a full view of the structures or organs involved through membranous or cutaneous incisions.

open system, a system that interacts with our environment.

operant, any act or response occurring without an identifiable stimulus.

operant conditioning, a form of learning used in behaviour therapy in which the person undergoing therapy is rewarded for the correct response and punished for the incorrect response.

operant level, the frequency or form of a performance under baseline conditions before any systematic conditioning procedures are introduced.

operating microscope, a binocular microscope used in delicate surgery, especially surgery of the eye or ear. The operating microscope that attaches to a surgeon's head has interchangeable oculars for different magnifications.

operating suite, a suite of rooms or an area in a hospital or clinic in which patients are prepared for surgery, undergo surgical procedures, and recover from the anaesthetic procedures required for the surgery.

operating theatre, a room in a hospital or clinic in which surgical procedures requiring anaesthesia are performed.

operating system (OS), the main system programs of a computer that manage the hardware and logical resources of a system including scheduling and file management.

operation, any surgical procedure, such as appendectomy or a hysterectomy.

operationalization of behaviour, (in psychology) the stating of a patient's complaints or problems in specific, observable behavioural terms.

operative cholangiography, (in diagnostic radiology) a radiographic technique to visualize the biliary tree during surgery by the introduction of a radiopaque contrast medium directly into the cystic duct.

operator gene, (in molecular genetics) a genetic unit that regulates the transcription of structural genes in its operon.

operculum, *pl.* **opercula, operculums,** (in obstetrics) a collection of thick mucus in the uterine cervix, that is often expelled at the onset of dilatation of the cervix, just before labour begins or in its early hours; informally known as the "show". **opercular,** *adj.*

operon, (in molecular biology) a segment of DNA consisting of an operator gene and one or more structural genes with related functions controlled by the operator gene in conjunction with a regulator gene.

OPG, abbreviation for **orthopantogram.**

ophthalmia, severe inflammation of the conjunctiva or of the deeper parts of the eye. Some kinds of ophthalmia are **ophthalmia neonatorum, sympathetic ophthalmia,** and **trachoma.**

ophthalmia neonatorum, a purulent conjunctivitis and keratitis of the newborn resulting from exposure of the eyes to chemical, chlamydial, bacterial, or viral agents. Chemical conjunctivitis usually occurs as a result of the instillation of silver nitrate in the eyes of a newborn to prevent a gonococcal infection.

ophthalmic, of or pertaining to the eye.

ophthalmic administration of medication, the administration of a drug by instillation of a cream, ointment or liquid preparation into the conjunctival sac. The medication is placed in the sac as the patient looks away from the point of instillation. The dispenser should not touch the eye, and the medication is not placed directly on to the cornea.

ophthalmic herpes zoster. See **herpes zoster ophthalmicus.**

ophthalmitis, inflammation of the eye ball.

ophthalmologist, a doctor who specializes in ophthalmology.

ophthalmology, the branch of medicine concerned with the study of the physiology, anatomy, and pathology of the eye and the diagnosis and treatment of disorders of the eye. **ophthalmological,** *adj.*

ophthalmometer, an instrument for measuring corneal astigmatism.

ophthalmoplegia, an abnormal condition characterized by paralysis of the motor nerves of the eye. Bilateral ophthalmoplegia of rapid onset is associated with acute myasthenia gravis, acute inflammatory cranial polyneuropathy. Ophthalmoplegia is also associated with ocular dystrophy.

ophthalmoscope, a device for examining the interior of the eye. It includes a light, a mirror with a single hole through which the examiner may look, and a dial holding several lenses of varying strengths.

ophthalmoscopy, the technique of using an ophthalmoscope to examine the eye.

opiate, 1. a narcotic drug that contains opium, derivatives of opium, or any of several semisynthetic or synthetic drugs with opium-like activity. **2.** *informal.* any soporific or narcotic drug. **3.** of or pertaining to opium or opium derivatives.

opiate analgesic. See **analgesic.**

opiate antagonist, a drug that is used primarily in the treatment of opiate-induced respiratory depression. Naxolone is usually adminstered parenterally, in emergency situations. Naltrexone is administered orally in the treatment of opiate addicts to reduce the temptation to take opiates by blocking their effect.

opisthorchiasis, infection with one of the species of Opisthorchis liver flukes commonly found in the Philippines, India, Thailand, and Laos.

opisthorchis sinensis. See **clonorchis sin-**

ensis.

opisthotonos, a prolonged severe spasm of the muscles causing the back on the neck, the heels to bend back on the legs, and the arms and hands to flex rigidly at the joints.

opium, a milky exudate from the unripe capsules of *Papaver somniferum* and *Papaver album* yielding 9.5% or more of anhydrous morphine. It is a narcotic analgesic, and contains several alkaloids, including codeine, morphine, and papaverine.

opium alkaloid, one of several alkaloids isolated from the milky exudate of the unripe seed pods of Papaver somniferum, a species of poppy indigenous to large areas of Asia and the Middle East. Three of the alkaloids, codeine, papaverine, and morphine, are used clinically for the relief of pain. Morphine is the standard against which the analgesic effect of newer drugs is measured. The opium alkaloids have several other effects on the body: coughing is suppressed; the pupils constrict; respiration is depressed; the secretory activity and motility of the GI tract are diminished; and biliary and pancreatic secretions are reduced. All have the potential to produce physical and psychological addiction.

opium tincture, an analgesic and antidiarrhoeal prescribed in the treatment of intestinal hyperactivity, cramping, and diarrhoea.

Oppenheim reflex {Herman Oppenheim, German neurologist, b. 1858}, a variation of Babinski's reflex, elicited by firmly stroking downward on the anterior and medial surfaces of the tibia, characterized by extension of the great toe and fanning of other toes. It is a sign of pyramidal tract disease.

opportunistic infection, 1. an infection caused by normally nonpathogenic organisms in a host whose resistance has been decreased by such disorders as diabetes mellitus or cancer or by a surgical procedure. **2.** an unusual infection with a common pathogen, such as cellulitis, meningitis, or otitis media.

opsonin, an antibody or complement split product that, on attaching to foreign materials, microorganism, or other anigen, enhances phagocytosis of that substance by leukocytes and other macrophages. **opsonize,** *v.*

opsonization, the process whereby opsonins render bacteria more susceptible to phagocytosis by leukocytes.

optic, optical, of or pertaining to the eyes or to sight.

optical atrophy, wasting of the optic disc resulting from degeneration of fibres of the optic nerve and optic tract. Optic atrophy may be caused by a cogenitial defect, inflammation, occlusion of the central retinal artery or internal carotid artery, alcohol, arsenic, lead, tobacco, or other toxic substances. Degeneration of the disc may accompany arteriosclerosis, diabetes, glaucoma, hydrocephalus, pernicious anaemia, and various neurological disorders.

optical character recognition (OCR), any of various systems whereby graphic information is input directly into a computer by means of an optical device.

optical coupling, a method of attaching the crystal window of a scintillator to the window of a photomultiplier tube so there is a minimum loss of light transmitted from the scintillator to the interior of the photomultiplier tube.

optical density, a number describing the blackening of an x-ray film in any specified location.

optical glioma, a tumour composed of glial cells. It develops slowly on the optic nerve or in the optic chiasm, causing loss of vision, and is often accompanied by secondary strabismus, exophthalmos, and ocular paralysis.

optic cup, a two-layered embryonic cavity that develops in early pregnancy. The cells of the optic cup differentiate to form the retina that first develops its layers of rod and cones in the central portion of the cup.

optician, a person who grinds and fits eyeglasses and contact lenses by prescription from an optometrist.

optic mark recognition (OMR), a system whereby marks inpredetermined positions on a specially prepared from are input directly into a computer by means of an optical device.

optic master. See *laser.*

optic nerve, either of a pair of cranial nerves consisting mainly of coarse, myelinated fibres that arise in the retinal ganglionic layer, traverse the thalamus, and connect with the visual cortex. At the optic chiasm the fibres from the inner or nasal half of the retina cross to the optic tract of the temporal or outer half of each retina are uncrossed and pass to the visual cortex on the same side.

optic papilla. See *papilla.*

optic righting, one of the five basic neuromuscular reactions that enable a person to change body positions. It involves a reflex that automatically orients the head to a new optical or visual fixation point, depending on the body position change.

optics, 1. (in physics} a field of study that deals with the electromagnetic radiation of wavelengths shorter than radio waves but longer than x-rays. **2.** (in physiology) a field of study that deals with vision and the process by which the functions of the eye and the brain are integrated in the perception of shape, patterns, movements, spatial relationships, and colour.

optic stalk, one of a pair of slender embryonic structures that become the optic nerve.

optic thermometer, a temperature measuring device in which the properties of transmission and reflection of visible light are temperature dependent, and whose detection can be related to tissue temperature.

optometrist, a person who practices **optometry.**

optometry, the practice of testing the eyes for visual acuity, prescribing corrective lenses, and recommending eye exercises.

oral, of or pertaining to the mouth.

oral administration of medication, the administration of a tablet, capsule, elixir, solution or other form of medication by mouth. Oral administration of medication includes **buccal administration of medication** and **sublingual administration of medication.**

oral airway, a curved tubular device of rubber, plastic, or metal placed in the oropharynx during general anaesthesia to maintain free passage of air and keep the tongue from falling back and obstructing the trachea.

oral cancer, a malignant neoplasm on the lip or in the mouth, occurring at an average age of 60 with a frequency eight times higher in men than in women. Predisposing factors in the cause of the disease are heavy use of tobacco, alcoholism, poor oral hygiene, ill-fitting dentures, syphilis, Plummer-Vinson syndrome, betel nut chewing, and, in lip cancer, overexposure to sun and wind. Premalignant leukoplakia or erythroplakia or a painless nonhealing ulcer may be the first sign of oral cancer; localized pain usually appears later, but lymph nodes may be involved early in the course. Almost all oral tumours are epidermoid carcinomas; adenocarcinomas occur occasionally, whereas sarcomas and metastatic lesions from other sites are rare.

oral character, (in psychoanalysis) a kind of personality exhibiting patterns of behaviour originating in the oral phase of infancy, characterized by optimism, self-confidence, and carefree generosity reflecting the pleasurable aspects of the stage, or pessimism, futility, anxiety, and sadism as manifestations of frustrations or conflicts occurring during the period.

oral contraceptive, oral steroid medication used for contraception. Oral contraceptives usually contain a progestogen alone or a combination of a progestogen and an oestrogen. The steroids act by inhibiting the production of gonadotrophin-releasing hormone by the hypothalamus, and hence the pituitary secretion of gonadotrophins which normally stimulates ovulation. Oral contraceptives result in the endometrium of the uterus thinning and the cervical mucus thickening, thus preventing the penetration of sperm and the implanting of ova.

oral dosage, pertaining to the administration of a medicine by mouth.

oral eroticism, (in psychoanalysis) libidinal fixation at or regression to the oral stage of psychosexual development, often reflected

in such personality traits as passivity, insecurity, and oversensitivity.

oral herpes. See **herpes simplex.**

oral hygiene, the condition or practice of maintaining the tissues and structures of the mouth. Oral hygiene includes brushing the teeth to remove food debris, bacteria, and plaque; massaging the gums with a toothbrush, dental floss, or water irrigator to stimulate circulation and remove foreign matter; application of flouride; and cleansing of dentures and ensuring their proper fit to prevent irritation.

oral mucous membrane, altered, disruptions in the tissue layers of the oral cavity. Defining characteristics include oral pain or discomfort, coated tongue, xerostomia (dry mouth), stomatitis, oral lesions or ulcers, lack of or decreased salivation, leukoplakia, oedema, hypaeremia, oral plaque, desquamation, vesicles, haemorrhagic gingivitis, carious teeth, and halitosis.

oral poliomyelitis vaccine. See **poliomyelitis vaccine.**

oral sadism, (in psychoanalysis) a sadistic form of oral eroticism, manifested by such behaviour as biting, chewing, and other aggressive impulses associated with eating habits.

oral stage, (in psychoanalysis) the initial stage of psychosexual development, occurring in the first 12 to 18 months of life when the feeding experience and other oral activities are the predominant source of pleasurable stimulation. Experiences encountered during this stage determined to a great extent later attitudes concerning food, love, acceptance and rejection, and many other aspects of interpersonal relationships and behavioural patterns.

orbicularis ciliaris, one of the two zones of the ciliary body of the eye, extending from the ora serrata of the retina to the ciliary processes at the margin of the iris.

orbicularis oculi, the muscular body of the eyelid comprising the palpebra, orbita, and lacrimal muscles. The palpebral muscle functions to close it more energetically, such as in winking.

orbicularis oris, the muscle surrounding the mouth, consisting partly of fibres derived from other facial muscles, such as the buccinator, that are inserted into the lips and partly of fibres proper to the lips. It serves to close and purse the lips.

orbicularis palperbrarum. See **orbicularis oculi.**

orbicularis pupillary reflex, a normal phenomenon elicited by forceful closure of the eyelids or attempting to close them while they ate held apart, resulting first in constriction and then dilatation of the pupil.

orbit, one of a pair of bony conical cavities in the skull that accommodate the eyeballs and associated structures, such as the eye muscles, the nerves, and the blood vessels. **orbital,** adj.

orbital aperture, an opening in the cranium to the orbit of the eye.

orbital fat, a semifluid cushion of fat that lines the bony orbit supporting the eye. Traumatic loss of the fat causes a sunken appearance of the eye.

orbital hypertelorism. See **ocular hypertelorism.**

orbital hypotelorism. See **ocular hypotelorism.**

orbital pseudotumour, a specific inflammatory reaction of the orbital tissues of the eye, characterized by exophthalmos and oedematous congestion of the eyelids. The cause is unknown.

orbitomeatal line, a positioning line used in radiography that passes through the outer canthus of the eye and the center of the external auditory meatus.

orchidectomy, a surgical procedure to remove one or both testes. It may be indicated for serious disease or injury to the testis or to control cancer of the prostate by removing a source of androgenic hormones.

orchietomy. See **orchidectomy.**

orchiopexy, an operation to mobilize an undescended testis, bring it into the scrotum, and attach it so that it will not retract.

orchis. See **testis.**

orchitis, inflammation of one or both of the testes, characterized by swelling and pain, often caused by mumps, syphilis, or tuberculosis, **orchitic,** adj.

ordered paris, pertaining to graph coordinates in which the first number of the pari represents a distance along the x (horizontal) axis and the second number is plotted along the y (vertical) axis.

Orem, Dorthea E., author of the Self-Care Nursing Model, a nursing theory introduced in 1959. The theory describes the role of the nurse in giving assistance to a person experiencing inabilities in self-care. The goal of the system is to meet the patient's self-care demands until the family is capable of providing care. The process is divided into three categories: Universal, which consists of self-care to meet physiological and psychosocial needs; Developmental, the self-care required when one goes through developmental stages; and Health Deviation, the self-care required when one has a deviation from a healthy status.

orexigenic, a substance that increases or stimulates the appetite.

oreximania, a condition characterized by a greatly increased appetite and excessive eating resulting from an unrealistic or exaggerated fear of becoming thin.

orf, a viral skin disease acquired from sheep, characterized by painless vesicles that may progress to red, weeping nodules and, finally, to crusting and healing.

organ, a structural part of a system of the body that is comprised of tissues and cells that enable it to perform a particular function, such as the liver, spleen, digestive organs, reproductive organs, or organs of special sense.

organ albumin, albumin characteristic of a particular organ.

organelle, 1. any one of various particles of living substance bound within most cells, such as the mitochondria, the Golgi complex, the endoplastic reticulum, the lysosomes, and the centrioles. **2.** any one of the tiny organs of protozoa associated with locomotion, metabolism, and other processes.

organic, 1. any chemical compound containing carbon. **2.** of or pertaining to an organ.

organic brain syndrome. See **organic mental disorder.**

organic chemistry, the branch of chemistry concerned with the composition, properties, and reactions of chemical compounds containing carbon.

organic dust, dried particles of plants, animals, fungi, or bacteria that are fine enough to be windborne.

organic evolution, the theory that all existing forms of animal and plant life have descended with modification from previous, simpler forms or from a single cell; the origin and perpetuation of species.

organic foods, foods that have been produced and processed without the use of commercial chemicals, such as fertilizers, pesticides, or synthetic substances that enhance colour or flavour.

organic mental disorder, any psychological or behavioural abnormality associated with transient or permanent brain dysfunction caused by a disturbance of the physiological functioning of the brain tissue, such as may occur with cerebral arteriosclerosis, lead poisoning, or many other pathological conditions.

organic motivation. See **physiological motivation.**

organism, an individual living animal or plant able to carry on life functions through mutually dependent organs or organelles.

organization centre, a focal point within the developing embryo from which the organism grows and differentiates.

organizer, (in embryology) any part of the embryo that induces morphological differentiation in some other part. Kinds of organizers include **nucleolar organizer, primary organizer.**

organ of Corti {Alfonso Corti, Italian anatomist, b. 1822}, the true organ of hearing, a spiral structure within the cochlea containing hair cells that are stimulated by sound vibrations into nerve impulses that are transmitted by the auditory nerve to the brain.

organ of Giraldes. See **paradidymis.**

organ of Golgi. See **neurotendinous spindle.**

organogenesis, (in embryology) the formation and differentiation of organs and organ systems during embryonic development. In humans the period extends from approximately the end of the second week through the eighth week of gestation. **organogenetic,** *adj.*

organophosphates, a class of anticholinesterase chemicals used in certain pesticides and medications. They act by causing irreversible inhibition of cholinesterase.

organ specificity, a substance or activity that is identified with a specific organ, such as enzymes that function in particular organ systems.

orgasm, the sexual climax, a series of strong, involuntary contractions of the muscles of the genitalia experienced as exceedingly pleasurable, set off by sexual excitation of critical intensity. **orgasmic,** *adj.*

orgasmic maturity, the physiological maturity of the reproductive system that enables the individual to complete the adult sexual response cycle.

orgasmic platform, congestion of the lower vagina during sexual intercourse.

orientate, 1. to make someone aware of new surroundings, including people and their roles, the layout of a facility, and its routines, rules, and services. **2.** to help a person become aware of a situation or simply of reality, such as when a patient recovers from anaesthesia. **orientation,** *n.,* **oriented,** *adj.*

orientation, 1. (in molecular genetics) the insertion of a fragment of genetic material into a vector so that the placement of the fragment is in the same direction as the genetic map of the vector (the n orientation) of in the opposite direction (the u orientation). **2.** (in psychiatry) the awareness of one's physical environment with regard to time, place, and the identity of other persons.

orifice, the entrance or the outlet of any cavity in the body. **orificial,** *adj.*

ori gene, (in molecular genetics) the site or region in which DNA replication starts.

origin, the more fixed end of a muscle attachment.

ornithine, an amino acid, not a constituent of proteins, that is produced as an important intermediate substance in the urea cycle.

ornithine carbamoyl transferase, an enzyme in the blood that increases in patients with liver and other diseases. Its normal concentrations in serum are 8 to 20 mIU/ml.

ornithine cycle. See **urea cycle.**

Ornithodoros, a genus of ticks, some species of which are vectors for the spirochetes of relapsing fevers.

ornithosis. See **psittacosis.**

oropharynx, one of the three anatomical divisions of the pharynx. It extends behind the mouth from the soft palate above to the level of the hyoid bone below and contains the palatine tonsils and the lingual tonsils. **oropharyngeal,** *adj.*

Oroya fever. See **bartonellosis.**

orphenadrine citrate, a skeletal muscle relaxant with anticholinergic and antihistaminic activity used in the treatment of muscle spasm.

orphenadrine hydrochloride, an anticholinergic agent prescribed in the treatment of Parkinson's disease and drug induced parkinsonism.

orthoclase ceramic feldspar, a plentiful clay in the solid crust of the earth, used as a filler and to give body to fused dental porcelain.

orthodontia. See **orthodontics.**

orthodontic appliance, any device used to modify tooth position. Kinds of such appliances are fixed, movable, active, retaining, intraoral, and extraoral.

orthodontic band, a thin metal ring, usually made of stainless steel, fitted over a tooth for securing orthodontic attachments to a tooth.

orthodontics, the specialty of dentistry concerned with the diagnosis and treatment of malocclusion and irregularities of the teeth.

orthodromic conduction, the conduction of a neural impulse in the normal direction, from a synaptic junction or a receptor forward along an axon to its termination with depolarization.

orthogenesis, the theory that evolution is controlled by intrinsic factors within the organism and progresses according to a predetermined course rather than in several directions as a result of natural selection and other environmental factors. **orthogenetic,** *adj.*

orthogenic, 1. of or pertaining to orthogenesis; orthogenetic. **2.** of or pertaining to the treatment and rehabilitation of children who are mentally or emotionally disturbed.

orthogenic evolution, change within an animal or plant induced solely by an intrinsic factor, independent of any environmental elements.

orthomyxovirus, a member of a family of viruses that includes several organisms responsible for human influenza infection.

orthopaedic nurse, a nurse whose primary area of interest, competence, and professional practice is in orthopaedic nursing.

orthopaedics, the branch of medicine devoted to the study and treatment of the skeletal system, its joints, muscles, and associated structures.

orthopaedic surgeon, a surgeon specializing in orthopaedics.

orthopaedic traction, a procedure in which a patient is maintained in a device attached by ropes and pulleys to weights that exert a pulling force on an extremity or body part while counteraction is maintained. Traction is applied most often to reduce and immobilize fractures, but it also is used to overcome muscle spasm, to stretch adhesions, to correct certain deformities, and to help release arthritic contractures.

orthopantography, a radiographic technique to give a panoramic view of the total dentition, mandible and temperomandibular joints. **orthopantogram (OPG),** *n.*

orthopnoea, an abnormal condition in which a person must sit or stand in order to breathe deeply or comfortably, It occurs in many disorders of the cardiac and respiratory systems, such as asthma, pulmonary oedema, emphysema, pneumonia, and angina pectoris. **orthopnoeic,** *adj.*

orthoptic, 1. of or pertaining to normal binocular vision. **2.** of or pertaining to a procedure or technique for correcting the visual axes of eyes improperly coordinated for binocular vision.

orthoptic examination, an ophthalmoscopic examination of the binocular function of the yes. A stereoscopic instrument presents a slightly different picture to each eye. The examiner notes the degree to which the pictures are combined by the normal process of fusion. If the person has diplopia, separate pictures are seen.

orthoptist, a suitably qualified person who, under the supervision of an ophthalmologist, tests eye muscles and teaches exercise programmes designed to correct eye coordination defect.

orthosis, a force system designed to control, correct, or compensate for a bone deformity, deforming forces, or forces absent from the body. Orthosis often involves the use of special braces. **orthotic,** *adj., n.*

orthostatic, pertaining to an erect or standing position.

orthostatic albuminuria. See **orthostatic proteinuria.**

orthostatic hypotension, abnormally low blood pressure occurring when an individual assumes the standing posture.

orthostatic proteinuria, presence of protein in the urine of some people, especially teenagers, who have been standing. It disappears when they recline and is of no pathological significance.

orthotist, a person who designs, fabricates, and fits braces or other orthopaedic appliances prescribed by doctors or physiotherapists.

orthotonos, a straight, rigid posture of the body caused by a tetanic spasm, usually resulting from strychnine poisoning or tetanus infection. The neck and all other parts of the body are in a position of extension but not as severely as in opisthotonos.

orthovoltage {Court Alessandro Volta}, (in radiotherapy) x-ray energy range of approximately 200 to 500 KeV.

Ortolani's test {Marius Ortolani, 20th century Italian surgeon}, a procedure used to evaluate the stability of the hip joints in newborns and infants. The baby is placed on his back, the hips and knees are flexed at right angles and abducted until the lateral aspects of the knees are touching the table. Internal and external rotation are attempted, and symmetry of mobility is evaluated. A click or a popping sensation (Ortolani's sign) may be felt if the joint is unstable.

os. See **bone.**

Os, symbol for **osmium.**

os calcis. See **calcaneus.**

os capitatum. See **capitate bone.**

oscillator, an electric or other device that produces oscillations, vibrations, or fluctuations, such as an alternating electric current generator.

oscilloscope, an instrument that displays a visual representation of electric variations on the fluorescent screen of a cathode ray tube. The graphic representation is produced by a beam of electrons focused or directed by a magnetic field that is influenced in turn by a source such as an amplified current produced by heart contractions.

os coxae. See **innominate bone.**

os cubiodeum. See **cuboid bone.**

Osgood-Schlatter disease, {Robert B. Osgood, American surgeon, b. 1873; Carl Schlatter, Swiss surgeon, b. 1864}, inflammation or partial separation of the tibial tubercle caused by chronic irritation, usually as a result of overuse of the quadriceps muscle. The condition is characterized by swelling and tenderness over the tibial tubercle that increase with exercise or any activity that extends the leg.

os hamatum. See **hamate bone.**

os hyoideum. See **hyoid bone.**

Osler's disease. See **Osler-Weber-Rendu syndrome, polycythaemia.**

Osler's nodes {Sir William Osler, American-British physician, b. 1849}, tender, reddish or purplish subcutaneous nodules of the soft tissue on the ends of fingers or toes, seen in subacute bacterial endocarditis and usually lasting only 1 or 2 days.

Osler-Weber-Rendu syndrome {Sir William Osler; Frederick P. Weber, British physician, b. 1863; Henri J.L.M. Rendu, French physician, b. 1844}, a vascular anomaly, inherited as a autosomal dominant trait, characterized by haemorrhagic telangiectasia of skin and mucosa. Small red-to-violet lesions are found on the lips, the oral and nasal mucosa, the tongue, and the tips of fingers and toes. The thin, dilated vessels may bleed spontaneously or as a result of only minor trauma, and this condition becomes progressively severe.

os lunatum. See **lunate bone.**

os magnum. See **capitate bone.**

osemehesia, the ability to perceive and distinguish odours; the sense of smell.

osmium (Os) a hard, greyish, pungent-smelling metallic element. Its atomic number is

76; its atomic weight is 190.2.

osmoceptors, receptors in the hypothalamus that respond to osmotic pressure, thereby regulating production of the antidiuretic hormone.

osmolal gap, a difference between the observed and calculated osmolalities in serum analysis. The calculated osmolar values include sodium concentration multiplied by 2, plus glucose and blood urea nitrogen.

osmolality, the osmotic pressure of a solution expressed in osmols or milliosmols per kilogram of water.

osmolar, of or pertaining to the osmotic characteristics of a solution of one or more molecular substances, ionic substances, or both, expressed in osmoles or milliosmoles.

osmolarity, the osmotic pressure of a solution expressed in osmoles or milliosmoles per kilogram of the solution.

osmole, the quantity of a substance in solution in the form of molecules, ions, or both (usually expressed in grams) that has the same osmotic pressure as one mole of an ideal nonelectrolyte. Also **osmol. osmolal,** *adj.*

osmometry, a field of study that deals with the phenomenon of osmosis and the measurement of osmotic forces. **osmometric,** *adj.*

osmosis, the movement of a pure solvent, such as water, through a semipermeable membrane from a solution that has a lower solute concentration to one that has a higher solute concentration. Movement across the membrane continues until the concentrations of the solutions equalize.

osmotic diarrhoea, a form of diarrhoea associated with water retention in the bowel resulting from an accumulation of nonabsorbable water-soluble solutes, such as hexitols, sorbitol, and mannitol (used as sugar substitutes).

osmotic diuresis, diuresis resulting from the presence of certain nonabsorbable substances in tubules of the kidney, such as mannitol, urea, or glucose.

osmotic fragility, a sensitivity to change in osmotic pressure characteristic of red blood cells. Exposed to a hypotonic concentration of sodium in a solution, red cells take in increasing quantities of water, swell until the capacity of the cell membrane is exceeded, and burst. Exposed to a hypertonic concentration of sodium in a solution, red cells give up intracellular fluid, shrink, and break up.

osmotic pressure, 1. the pressure of exerted on a semipermeable membrane separating a solution form a solvent, the membrane being impermeable to the solutes in the solution and permeable only to the solvent. **2.** the pressure exerted on a semipermeable membrane by a solution containing one or more solutes that cannot penetrate the membrane, which is permeable only by the solvent surrounding it.

osmotic transfection, a method of inserting foreign DNA molecules into cells by putting cells into a dilute solution that causes them to rupture. The alien DNA is added to the fluid and is absorbed into the cell nuclei. The cell membranes quickly repair themselves. The foreign DNA can be detected in the cells as a transfection marker.

os naviculare pedis. See **scaphoid bone.**

osphresis, olfaction; the sense of smell.

osseous labyrinth, the bony portion of the internal ear, composed of three cavities; the vestibule, the semicircular canals, and the cochlea, transmitting sound vibrations from the middle ear to the acoustic nerve. All three cavities contain perilymph, in which a membranous labyrinth is suspended.

ossicle, a small bone, such as the malleus, the incus, or the stapes, ossicles of the inner ear. **ossicular,** *adj.*

ossification, the development of bone. **Intramembranous ossification** is that preceded by membrane, such as in the process initially forming the roof and the sides of the skull. **Intracartilaginous ossification** is that preceded by rods of cartilage, such as that forming the bones of the limbs.

ossifying fibromaa, a slow-growing, benign neoplasm of bone, occurring most often in the jaws, especially the mandible.

ostealgia, any pain that is associated with an abnormal condition within a bone, such as **osteomyelitis. ostealgic,** *adj.*

osteanagenesis. See **osteoanagenesis.**

osteitis, an inflammation of bone, caused by infection, degeneration, or trauma. Swelling, tenderness, dull aching pain, and redness in the skin over the affected bone are characteristic of the condition. Some kinds of osteitis are osteitis deformans and osteitis fibrosa cystica.

osteitis fibrosa cystica, an inflammatory degenerative condition in which normal bone is replaced by cysts and fibrous tissue.

osteitis fibrosa disseminata. See **Albright's syndrome.**

ostembryon. See **lithopaedion.**

osteoarthritis, a form of arthritis in which one or may joints undergo degenerative changes, including subchondral bony sclerosis, loss of articular cartilage, and proliferation of bone and cartilage in the joint, forming osteophytes. Inflammation of the synovial membrane of the joint is common late in the disease. The most common form of arthritis, its causes may include chemical, mechanical, genetic, metabolic, and endocrine factors. Emotional stress often aggravates the condition. The condition usually begins with pain after exercise or use of the joint. Stiffness, tenderness to the touch, crepitus, and enlargement develop, and deformity, subluxation, and synovial effusion may eventually occur.

osteoarthropathy, a disorder affecting bones and joints.

osteoblast, a cell that originates in the embryonic mesenchyme and, during the early development of the skeleton, differentiates from a fibroblast to function in the formation of bone tissue.   **osteoblastic,** *adj.*

osteoblastoma, *pl.* **osteoblastomas, osteoblastomata,** a small, benign, fairly vascular tumor of poorly formed bone and fibrous tissue. The lesion causes pain, erosion, and resorption of native bone.

osteochondrodystrophy. See **Morquio's disease.**

osteochondroma, a benign tumour made of bone and cartilage.

osteochondrosis, a disease affecting the ossification centers of bone in children, initially characterized by degeneration and necrosis, followed by regeneration and recalcification. Kinds of osteochondrosis include **Legg-Calve-Perthes disease, Osgood-Schlatter disease,** and **Scheuermann's disease.**

osteoclasia, 1. the destruction and absorption of bony tissue by osteoclasts, such as during growth or the healing of fractures. **2.** the degeneration of bone through disease.

osteoclasis, the intentional surgical fracture of a bone to correct a deformity. **osteoclastic,** *adj.*

osteoclast, 1. a large type of multinucleated bone cell that functions in the development and periods of growth or repair, such as the breakdown and resorption of osseous tissue. During bone healing of fractures, or during certain disease processes, osteoclasts excavate passages through the surrounding tissue by enzymatic action. **2.** a surgical instrument used in the fracturing or refracturing of bones for therapeutic purposes, such as correction of a deformity.

osteoclastic, 1. pertaining to or of the nature of osteoclasts. **2.** destructive to bone.

osteoclastoma, *pl.* **osteoclastomas, osteoclastomata,** a giant cell tumour of the bone, occurring most frequently at the end of a long bone and appearing as a mass surrounded by a thin shell of new, periosteal bone. The lesion may be benign but is more often malignant. It causes local pain, loss of function, and, in some cases, weakness followed by pathological fracture.

osteoclasty. See **osteoclasis.**

osteocyte, a bone cell; a mature osteoblast that has become embedded in the bone matrix. It occupies a small cavity and sends out protoplasmic projections that anastomose with those of other osteoblasts to form a system of minute canals within the bone matrix.   **osteocytic,** *adj.*

osteodystrophy, any generalized defect in bone development, usually associated with disturbances in calcium and phosphorus metabolism and renal insufficiency, such as in renal osteodystrophy.

osteogenesis, the origin and development of bone tissue. **osteogenetic, osteogenic,** *adj.*

osteogenesis imperfecta, a genetic disorder involving defective development of the connective tissue. It is inherited as an autosomal dominant trait and is characterized by abnormally brittle and fragile bones that are easily fractured by the slightest trauma. In its most severe form, the disease may be apparent at birth, when it is known as **osteogenesis imperfecta congenita.** The newborn has multiple fractures that have occurred in utero and is usually severely deformed, because of imperfect formation and mineralization of bone. If the disease has a later onset, it is called **osteogenesis imperfecta tarda** and usually runs a milder course. Symptoms generally appear when the child begins to walk, but they become less severe with age. There is a broad expressivity of the disease so that the number and extent of pathological features may range from minimal to severe involvement.

osteogenic, composed of or originating from any tissue involved in the development, growth, or repair of bone. Also **osteogenous.**

osteogenic sarcoma. See **osteosarcoma.**

osteolysis, the degeneration and dissolution of bone, caused by disease, infection, or ischaemia. The condition commonly affects the terminal bones of the hands and feet, such as in acroosteolysis.   **osteolytic,** *adj.*

osteoma, *pl.* **osteomas, osteomata,** a tumour of bone tissue.

osteomalacia, an abnormal condition of the lamellar bone, characterized by a loss of calcification of the matrix resulting in softening of the bone, accompanied by weakness, fracture, pain, anorexia, and weight loss. The condition is the result of an inadequate amount of phosphorus and calcium available in the blood for mineralization of the bones and may be caused by a diet lacking these minerals or vitamin D, or by a lack of exposure to sunlight.

osteomyelitis, local or generalized infection of bone and bone marrow, usually caused by bacteria introduced by trauma or surgery, by direct extension from a nearby infection, or via the bloodstream. Staphylococci are the most common causative agents. The long bones in children and the vertebrae in adults are the commonest sites of infection as a result of haematogenous spread. Persistent, severe, and increasing bone pain, tenderness, guarding on movement, regional muscle spasm, and fever, suggest this diagnosis. **osteomyelitic,** *adj.*

osteon, the basic structural unit of compact bone, consisting of the haversian canal and its concentric rings of 4 to 20 lamellae.

osteonecrosis, the destruction and death of bone tissue, such as from ischaemia, infection, malignant neoplastic disease, or trauma. **osteonecrotic,** *adj.*

osteopaedion. See **lithopaedion.**

osteopath, a qualified practitioner of osteopathy.

osteopathy, a therapeutic approach to the recognition and correction of structural problems using manipulation. Osteopathy places greater emphasis on the role of the relationship of the organs and the musculoskeletal system than is usual in conventional medicine. **osteopathic,** *adj.*

osteopenia, a condition of subnormally mineralized bone, usually the result of a failure of the rate of bone matrix synthesis to compensate for the rate of bone lysis.

osteopetrosis, an inherited disorder characterized by a generalized increase in bone density, probably caused by faulty bone resorption resulting from a deficiency of osteoclasts. In its most severe form, there is obliteration of the bone marrow cavity, causing severe anaemia, marked deformities of the skull, and compression of the cranial nerves, which may result in deafness and blindness and lead to an early death. **osteopetrotic,** *adj.*

osteophage. See **osteoclast.**

osteoplast. See **osteoblast.**

osteopoikilosis, an inherited condition of the bones, characterized by multiple areas of dense calcification throughout the osseous tissue, producing a mottled appearance on x-ray examination. **osteopoikilotic,** *adj.*

osteoporosis, a disorder characterized by abnormal rarefaction of bone, occurring most frequently in postmenopausal women, in sedentary or immobilized individuals, and in patients on long-term steroid therapy. The disorder may cause pain, especially in the lower back, pathological fractures, loss of stature, and various deformities. Osteoporosis may be idiopathic or secondary to other disorders, such as thyrotoxicosis or the bone demineralization caused by hyperparathyroidism.

osteopsathyrosis. See **osteogenesis imperfecta.**

osteosarcoma, a malignant bone tumour composed of anaplastic cells derived from mesenchyme.

osteosclerosis, an abnormal increase in the density of bone tissue. The condition is commonly associated with ischaemia, chronic infection, and tumour formation, and may be caused by faulty bone resorption as a result of some abnormality involving the osteoclasts. **osteosclerotic,** *adj.*

osteosclerosis fragilis congenita. See **osteopoikilosis.**

osteotome, a surgical instrument for cutting through bone.

osteotomy, the sawing or cutting of a bone. Kinds of osteotomy include block osteotomy, in which a section of bone is excised, cuneiform osteotomy to remove a bone wedge, and displacement osteotomy, in which a bone is redesigned surgically to alter the alignment or weightbearing stress areas.

ostium. See **orifice.**

ostium primum defect, ostium secundum defect. See **atrial septal defect.**

os trapezium. See **trapezium.**

os trapezoideum. See **trapezoid bone.**

os triquetrum. See **triangular bone.**

OT, abbreviation for **occupational therapist, occupational therapy.**

otalgia, pain in the ear. Also called **otodynia, otoneuralgia.**

OTC, abbreviation for **over the counter.**

Othello syndrome, a psychopathological condition, characterized by suspicion of a spouse's infidelity and by morbid jealousy. This condition may be accompanied by rage and violence and is frequently associated with paranoia.

other type of diabetes, a condition that is secondary to other syndromes, such as pancreatic or endocrine or drug-induced diseases, insulin receptor anomalies, or genetic conditions. Previously called **secondary diabetes.**

otic, of or pertaining to the ear. Also **auricular.**

otitic barotrauma, See **barotrauma.**

otitis, inflammation or infection of the ear. Kinds of otitis are otitis externa and otitis media.

otitis externa, inflammation or infection of the external canal or the auricle of the external ear. Major causes are allergy, bacteria, fungi, viruses, and trauma. Allergy to nickel or chromium in earrings and to chemicals in hair sprays, cosmetics, hearing aids, and medications is common. *Staphylococcus aureus, Pseudomonas aeruginosa,* and *Streptococcus pyogenes* are common bacterial causes. Herpes simplex and herpes zoster viruses are frequently implicated. Eczema, psoriasis, and seborrhoeic dermatitis also may affect the external ear.

otitis interna. See **labyrinthitis.**

otitis media, inflammation or infection of the middle ear, a common affliction of childhood. Acute otitis media is most often caused by *Haemophilus influenzae* or *Streptococcus pneumoniae.* Chronic otitis media is usually caused by gram-negative bacteria, such as *Proteus, Klebsiella,* and *Pseudomonas.* Allergy, *Mycoplasma,* and several viruses also may be causative factors. Otitis media is often preceded by an upper respiratory infection. Organisms gain entry to the middle ear through the eustachian tube. Obstruction of the eustachian tube and accumulation of exudate may increase pressure within the middle ear, forcing infection into the mastoid bone or rupturing the tympanic membrane.

Symptoms of acute otitis media include a sense of fullness in the ear, diminished hearing, pain, and fever. Usually only one ear is affected. Squamous epithelium may grow in the middle ear through a rupture in the tympanic membrane, and development of a cholesteatoma and deafness may occur. Pneumococcal otitis media may spread to the meninges.

otocephalus, a fetus with otocephaly.

otocephaly, a congenital malformation characterized by the absence of the lower jaw, defective formation of the mouth, and union or close approximation of the ears on the front of the neck. See also **agnathocephaly. otocephalic, otocephalous,** *adj.*

otodynia. See **otalgia.**

otolaryngologist, a doctor who specializes in the diagnosis and treatment of diseases and injuries of the ears, nose, and throat.

otolaryngology, a branch of medicine dealing with the diagnosis and treatment of diseases and disorders of the ears, nose, and throat, and adjacent structures of the head and neck.

otolith righting reflex, an involuntary response in newborns in which tilting of the body when the infant is in an erect position causes the head to return to the upright position.

otologist, a doctor trained in the diagnosis and treatment of diseases and other disorders of the ear.

otology, the study of the ear, including the diagnosis and treatment of its diseases and disorders.

otoneuralgia. See **otalgia.**

otoplasty, a common procedure in reconstructive plastic surgery in which, for cosmetic reasons, some of the cartilage in the ears is removed to bring the auricle and pinna closer to the head.

otorrhoea, any discharge from the external ear. Otorrhea may be serous, sanguinous, purulent, or contain cerebrospinal fluid. **otorrhoeal, otorrhoeic, otorrhetic,** *adj.*

otosclerosis, a hereditary condition of unknown cause in which irregular ossification in the bony labyrinth of the inner ear, especially of the stapes, occurs, causing tinnitus, then deafness. Also called **otospongiosis.**

otoscope, an instrument used to examine the external ear, the eardrum, and, through the eardrum, the ossicles of the middle ear. It consists of a light, a magnifying lens, and a device for insufflation.

ototoxic, (of a substance) having a harmful effect on the eighth cranial nerve or the organs of hearing and balance. Common ototoxic drugs include the aminoglycoside antibiotics, aspirin, frusemide, and quinine.

OU, abbreviation for *oculus uterque,* a Latin phrase meaning "each eye."

Ouchterlony double diffusion {Orjan T.G. Ouchterlony, Swedish bacteriologist, b. 1914}, a form of gel diffusion technique in which antigen and antibody in separate cells are allowed to diffuse toward each other.

ounce (oz) a unit of weight equal to $^1/_{16}$ of a pound avoirdupois.

outcome, the condition of a client at the end of therapy or of a disease process, including the degree of wellness and the need for continuing care, medication, support, counselling, or education.

outcome criteria, criteria that focus on observable or measurable results of nursing and other health service activities.

outcome data, data collected to evaluate the capacity of a client to function at a level described in the outcome statement of a nursing care plan or in standards for client care.

outcome measure, a measure of the quality of medical care, the standard on which is made the assessment of the expected end result of the intervention employed.

outlet, an opening through which something can exit, such as the pelvic outlet.

outlet forceps, often referred to as Wrigley's forceps, a type of **obstetric forceps.**

outline form, the shape of the cavosurface of a prepared tooth cavity.

outpatient, 1. a patient, not hospitalized, who is being treated at a clinic or surgery. **2.** of or pertaining to a health care facility for patients who are not hospitalized or to the treatment or care of such a patient.

output, 1. the total of any and all measurable liquids lost from the body, including urine, vomitus, diarrhoea, and drainage from wounds, from fistulas, and removed by suction equipment. The output is recorded as a means of monitoring a patient's fluid and electrolyte balance. **2.** the end product of a system.

output device, any device that converts information from a computer into a form that is readable by humans or another machine, such as a printer or CRT.

outreach, a term used to describe the extension of the services and human resources of clinics or inpatient psychiatric facililties to the homes of their clients and patients.

ova and parasites test, a microscopic examination of faeces for detecting parasites, such as amoebas or worms and their ova, which are indicators of parasitic disorders.

ovale malaria. See **tertian malaria.**

ovalocytes, oblong or oval-shaped red blood cells with pale centres that are found occasionally in patients with haemolytic anaemias, certain other anaemias, thalassaemias, and hereditary elliptocytosis. See also **elliptocytosis.**

ovalocytosis. See **elliptocytosis.**

ovarian, of or pertaining to the ovary.

ovarian artery, a slender branch of the abdominal aorta, arising caudal to the renal arteries, and supplying an ovary.

ovarian cancer, a malignant neoplastic disease of the ovary, occurring most frequently in women between 40 and 60 years of age and occasionally in young adolescents.

ovarian carcinoma, a malignant neoplasm of the ovaries rarely detected in the early stage and usually far advanced when diagnosed. Risk factors of the disease are infertility, nulliparity, or low parity, delayed childbearing, repeated spontaneous abortion, endometriosis, Group A blood type, previous irradiation of pelvic organs, and exposure to chemical carcinogens, such as asbestos and talc. After an insidious onset and asymptomatic period, the tumour may become evident as a palpable mass accompanied by irregular or excessive menses or postmenopausal bleeding. In advanced cases the patient may have ascites, oedema of the legs, and pain in the abdomen and the backs of the legs.

ovarian cyst, a globular sac filled with fluid or semisolid material that develops in or on the ovary. It may be transient and physiological or pathological. Kinds of ovarian cysts include **chocolate cyst, corpus luteum cyst,** and **dermoid cyst.**

ovarian pregnancy, a rare type of ectopic pregnancy in which the conceptus is implanted within the ovary.

ovarian seminoma. See **dysgerminoma.**

ovarian varicocele, a varicose swelling of the veins of the uterine broad ligament.

ovarian vein, one of a pair of veins that emerge from convoluted plexuses in the broad ligament near the ovaries and the uterine tubes. The right ovarian vein opens into the inferior vena cava, the left ovarian vein into the renal vein.

ovariectomy. See **oophorectomy.**

ovary, one of the pair of female gonads found on each side of the lower abdomen, beside the uterus, in a fold of the broad ligament. At ovulation, an egg is extruded from a follicle on the surface of the ovary under the stimulation of the gonadotrophic hormones, follicle-stimulating hormone (FSH), and luteinizing hormone (LH). The mature ovarian follicle secretes the hormones oestrogen and progesterone that regulate the menstrual cycle by a negative feedback system in which an increase in oestrogen decreases the secretion of FSH by the pituitary gland and an increase in progesterone decreases the secretion of LH. Each ovary is normally firm and smooth and resembles an almond in size and shape. The ovaries are homologous to the testes.

overbite, vertical overlapping of lower teeth by upper teeth, usually measured perpendicularly to the occlusal plane.

overclosure, an abnormal condition in which the mandible rises too far before the teeth make contact, caused by the loss of occlusal vertical dimension.

overcompensation, an exaggerated attempt to overcome a real or imagined physical or psychological deficit. The attempt may be conscious or unconscious.

overdenture, a complete or partial removable denture supported by retained roots to provide improved support, stability, and tactile and proprioceptive sensation and to reduce ridge resorption.

overdrive suppression, the inhibitory effect of a faster cardiac pacemaker on a slower one.

overdriving, the delivery of excess compressed air to an artificial heart's ventricle during systole.

overhang, an excess of dental filling material that projects beyond the margin of the associated tooth cavity.

overhydration, an excess of water in the body.

overinclusiveness, a type of association disorder observed in some schizophrenia patients. The individual is unable to think in a precise manner because of an inability to keep irrelevant elements outside perceptual boundaries.

overjet, a horizontal projection of upper teeth beyond the lower teeth, usually measured parallel to the occlusal plane.

overload, 1. a burden greater than the capacity of the system designed to move or process it. 2. (in physiology) any factor or influence that stresses the body beyond its natural limits and may impair its health.

overoxygenation, an abnormal condition in which the oxygen concentration in the blood and other tissues of the body is greater than normal, and the carbon dioxide concentration is less than normal. The condition is characterized by a fall in blood pressure, decreased vital capacity, fatigue, errors in judgment, paraesthesia of the hands and feet, anorexia, nausea and vomiting, and hyperaemia.

over the counter (OTC), (of a drug) available to the consumer without a prescription.

overweight, more than normal in body weight after adjustment for height, body build, and age.

oviduct. See **uterine tube.**

oviferous, bearing or capable of producing ova (egg cells).

oviparous, giving birth to young by laying eggs.

oviposition, the act of laying or depositing eggs by the female member of oviparous animals.

ovipositor, a specialized organ, found primarily in insects, for depositing eggs on plants or in the soil.

ovocentre, the centrosome of a fertilized ovum. Also called **oocentre.**

ovoflavin, a riboflavin derived from the yolk of eggs.

ovogenesis. See **oogenesis.**

ovoglobulin, a globulin derived from the white of eggs.

ovogonium. See **oogonium.**

ovoid arch, a dental arch that curves smoothly from the molars on one side to those on the opposite side to form half an oval.

ovo-lacto-vegetarian. See **lacto-vegetarian.**

ovomucin, a glycoprotein derived from the white of eggs.

ovomucoid, of or pertaining to a glycoprotein, similar to mucin, derived from the white of eggs.

ovoplasm. See **ooplasm.**

ovotestis, a gonad that contains both ovarian and testicular tissue; a hermaphroditic gonad. **ovotesticular,** *adj.*

ovovitellin. See **vitellin.**

ovoviviparous, bearing young in eggs that are hatched within the body, such as some reptiles and fishes.

ovulation, expulsion of an ovum from the ovary on spontaneous rupture of a mature follicle as a result of cyclical ovarian and pituitary endocrine function. It usually occurs on the fourteenth day after the first day of the last menstrual period and often causes brief, sharp lower abdominal pain on the side of the ovulating ovary. **ovulate,** *v.*

ovulation method of family planning (Billings), a natural method of family planning that uses observation of changes in the character and quantity of cervical mucus as a means of determining the time of ovulation during the menstrual cycle. The cyclical changes in gonadotropic hormones, especially oestrogen, cause changes in the quantity and character of cervical mucus. In the first days after menstruation, scant thick mucus is secreted by the cervix. These "dry days" are "safe days." The quantity of mucus then increases; it is pearly-white and sticky, becoming clearer and less sticky as ovulation approaches; these "wet days" are "unsafe days." During and just after ovulation the mucus is clear, slippery, and elastic; it resembles the uncooked white of an egg. The day on which this sign is most apparent is the "peak day," probably the day before ovulation. The 4 days after the "peak day" are "unsafe": Fertilization might occur. Effectiveness of the method in identifying the most fertile days of the cycle is augmented by using the basal body temperature method.

ovum, *pl.* **ova,** **1.** an egg. **2.** a female germ cell extruded from the ovary at ovulation.

oxaluric acid, a compound derived from uric acid or from parabonic acid, which occurs in normal urine.

oxazepam, a benzodiazepine used to relieve anxiety.

oxidation, **1.** any process in which the oxygen content of a compound is increased. **2.** any reaction in which the positive valence of a compound or a radical is increased because of a loss of electrons. **oxidize,** *v.*

oxidation-reduction reaction, a chemical change in which electrons are removed (oxidation) from an atom or molecule, accompanied by a simultaneous transfer of electrons (reduction) to another.

oxidative phosphorylation, an ATP generating process in which oxygen serves as the final electron acceptor. The process occurs in mitochondria and is the major source of ATP generation in aerobic organisms.

oxidative water, water produced by the oxidation of molecules of food substances, such as the conversion of glucose to water and carbon dioxide.

oxidize, (of an element or compound) to combine or cause to combine with oxygen, to remove hydrogen, or to increase the valence of an element through the loss of electrons. **oxidation,** *n.*, **oxidizing,** *adj.*

oxidizing agent, a compound that readily gives up oxygen and attracts hydrogen from another compound. In chemical reactions an oxidizing agent acts as an acceptor of electrons, thereby increasing the valence of an element.

oxidoreductase, an enzyme that catalyses a reaction in which one substance is oxidized while another is reduced. An example is alcohol dehydrogenase.

oximeter, any of several devices used to measure oxyhaemoglobin in the blood.

oxpentifylline, an agent which reduces blood viscosity and has been used for the treatment of intermittent claudication associated with chronic occlusive arterial disease.

oxybenzene. See **carbolic acid.**

oxybutynin chloride, an anticholinergic prescribed in the treatment of neurogenic bladder, urinary frequency and incontinence, and nocturnal enuresis.

oxycephaly, a congenital malformation of the skull in which premature closure of the coronal and sagittal sutures results in accelerated upward growth of the head, giving it a long, narrow appearance with the top pointed or conic in shape.

oxycodone pectinate, an opiate analgesic, only available in suppository form, used to treat moderate to severe pain.

oxygen (O_2) a tasteless, odourless, colourless gas essential for human respiration. Its atomic weight is 16; its atomic number is 8. In anaesthesia, oxygen functions as a carrier gas for the delivery of anaesthetic agents to the tissues of the body. In respiratory therapy, oxygen is administered to increase its amount and thus to decrease the amount of other gases circulating in the blood. Overdose of oxygen can cause irreversible toxicity in people with pulmonary abnormalities, especially when complicated by chronic carbon dioxide retention. See also **oxygen toxicity.**

oxygenation, the process of combining or

treating with oxygen. **oxygenate,** *v.*

oxygen capacity of blood, the maximum amount of oxygen that can be made to combine chemically with hemoglobin in a unit of blood, excluding physically dissolved oxygen.

oxygen concentration in blood, the concentration of oxygen in a blood sample, including both oxygen combined with haemoglobin and oxygen physically dissolved in blood.

oxygen consumption, the amount of oxygen in milliliters per minute required by the body for normal aerobic metabolism.

oxygen cost of breathing, the rate at which the respiratory muscles consume oxygen as they ventilate the lungs.

oxygen debt, the quantity of oxygen taken up by the lungs during recovery from a period of exercise or apnoea that is in excess of the quantity needed for resting metabolism during the preexercise period.

oxygen enhancement ratio (OER), (in radiobiology) a measure of tumour sensitivity to the presence or absence of oxygen, expressed as the ratio of radiation dose required to produce a given effect with no oxygen present to the dose required to produce the same effect in one atmosphere of air.

oxygen half-saturation pressure of haemoglobin, the oxygen pressure necessary for 50% saturation of haemoglobin at body temperature and at pH 7.4 or 40 torr carbon dioxide pressure. The value is commonly used as a measure of the affinity between oxygen and haemoglobin.

oxygen mask, a device used to administer oxygen. It is shaped to fit snugly over the mouth and nose and may be secured in place with a strap or held with the hand.

oxygen saturation, the fraction of a total haemoglobin (HB) in the form of HbO_2 at a defined P.

oxygen store, the total quantity of oxygen normally stored in the various body compartments, including the lungs, arterial and venous blood, and tissues.

oxygen tension, the force with which oxygen molecules that are physically dissolved in blood are constantly trying to escape, expressed as partial pressure (PO_2). The tension at any instant is related to the amount of oxygen physically dissolved in plasma; the larger amount carried in chemical combination with haemoglobin serves as a reservoir that releases oxygen molecules to physical solution when the tension decreases and that stores additional molecules of the gas when the tension increases.

oxygen therapy, any procedure in which oxygen is administered to a patient to relieve hypoxia.

oxygen tolerance, an increased capacity to withstand the toxic effects of hyperoxia as a result of any adaptive change occurring within an organism.

oxygen toxicity, a condition of oxygen overdosage that can result in pathological tissue changes, such as retrolental fibroplasia or bronchopulmonary dysplasia.

oxygen transport, the process by which oxygen is absorbed in the lungs by the haemoglobin in circulating deoxygenated red cells and carried to the peripheral tissues. This process is made possible by a special characteristic of haemoglobin, that is, the ability to combine with large quantities of oxygen present at a high concentration, such as in the lungs, and to release this oxygen when the concentration is low, such as in the peripheral tissues.

oxygen uptake, the amount of oxygen an organism removes from the environment, including the amount of oxygen that the lungs remove from the ambient atmosphere, the amount that the blood removes from the alveolar gas in the lungs, or the rate at which an organ or tissue removes oxygen from the blood perfusing it.

oxyhaemoglobin, the product of the combining of haemoglobin with oxygen. It is a loosely bound complex that dissociates easily when there is a low concentration of oxygen.

oxyhaemoglobin dissociation curve, a graphic expression of the affinity between oxygen and haemoglobin, or the amount of oxygen chemically bound at equilibrium to the haemoglobin in blood as a function of oxygen pressure. To define the curve completely, it should also include the pH, temperature, and carbon dioxide pressure.

oxyhaemoglobin saturation, the amount of oxygen actually combined with haemoglobin, expressed as a percentage of the oxygen capacity of that haemoglobin.

oxymetazoline, a nasal decongestant.

oxymetholone, an androgen prescribed in the treatment of testosterone deficiency, and for the stimulation of growth, weight gain, and red blood cell production.

oxyopia, unusual acuteness of vision. A person with normal (6/6) vision when standing 6 metres from the standard Snellen eye chart can read the seventh line of letters, each of which is an eighth of an inch high, while an individual with oxyopia can read smaller letters at that distance. Also called **oxyopy.**

oxytetracycline, a tetracycline antibiotic usd in the treatment of bacterial and rickettsial infections.

oxytocic, 1. of or pertaining to a substance that is similar to the hormone oxytocin. **2.** any one of numerous drugs that stimulate the smooth muscle of the uterus to contract. These drugs are often used to initiate labour at term. Oxytocic agents commonly used include oxytocin, certain prostaglandins, and the ergot alkaloids.

oxytocin, an oxytocic prescribed to stimulate contractions in inducing or augmenting labour, and to contract the uterus to control postpartum bleeding.

oxytocin challenge test, a stress test for the assessment of intrauterine function of the fetus and the placenta. It is performed to evaluate the ability of the fetus to tolerate continuation of pregnancy or the anticipated stress of labour and delivery. A dilute intravenous infusion of oxytocin is begun, monitored by a meter or regulated by an infusion pump. The uterine activity is monitored with a tocodynamometer, and the fetal heart rate is monitored with an ultrasonic sensor as the uterus is stimulated to contract by the oxytocin. Decelerations of the fetal heart rate in certain repeating patterns may indicate fetal distress.

oxyuriasis. See **enterobiasis.**

Oxyuris vermicularis. See *Enterobius vermicularis.*

ozena, a condition of the nose characterized by atrophy of the nasal chonchae and mucous membranes. Symptoms include crusting of nasal secretions, discharge, and, especially, a very offensive odour.

ozone, a form of oxygen characterized by molecules having three atoms. Ozone is formed when oxygen is electrically charged, as might occur in a lightning storm.

ozone shield, the layer of ozone that hangs in the atmosphere from 20 to 40 miles above the surface of the earth and protects the earth from excessive ultraviolet radiation.

ozone sickness, an abnormal condition caused by the inhalation of ozone that may seep into jet aircraft at altitudes over 40,000 feet. It is characterized by headaches, chest pains, itchy eyes, and sleepiness. Exactly why and how ozone causes this condition is not known. It is more prevalent early in the year and occurs more often over the Pacific Ocean.

P, 1. symbol for **phosphorus. 2.** symbol for *gas partial pressure.*

P1, (in genetics) symbol for **parental generation.**

P50, the partial pressure of oxygen at which haemoglobin is half saturated with bound oxygen.

PABA, abbreviation for **paraaminobenzoic acid.**

pabulum, any substance that is food or nutrient.

pacemaker, 1. the sinoatrial node of specialized nervous tissue located at the junction of the superior vena cava and the right atrium. It originates the contractions of the atria, which transmit the impulse on to the atrioventricular node, thereby initiating the contraction of the ventricles. **2.** an electric apparatus used for maintaining a normal sinus rhythm of myocardial contraction by electrically stimulating the heart muscle. A pacemaker may be permanent, emitting the stimulus at a constant and fixed rate, or it may fire only on demand, when the heart does not spontaneously contract at a minimum rate.

pacemaker current, a time-dependent decrease in outward potassium current that is peculiar to the pacemaking cell and causes it to reach threshhold potential.

pacemaker installation fluoroscopy, the fluoroscopic monitoring of the insertion of an artificial pacemaker, used as an aid for correct installation of the device.

pachometer. See **pachymeter.**

pachycephaly, an abnormal thickness of the skull, as in acromegaly. **pachycephalic, pachycephalous,** *adj.*

pachydactyly, an abnormal thickening of the fingers or the toes. **pachydactylic, pachydactylous,** *adj.*

pachyderma alba, an abnormal state of the buccal mucosa in which the appearance is suggestive of whitened elephant hide.

pachyderma oralis, an abnormal state of the buccal mucosa in which the appearance is suggestive of elephant hide.

pachymeter, an instrument used to measure thickness, especially of thin structures, such as a membrane or a tissue.

pachynema, the postsynaptic tetradic chromosome formation that occurs in the pachytene stage of the first meiotic prophase of gametogenesis.

pachyonychia congenita, a congenital deformity characterized by abnormal thickening and raising of the nails on the fingers and the toes, and hyperkeratosis of the palms of the hands and the soles of the feet.

pachytene, the third stage in the first meiotic prophase of gametogenesis in which the paired homologous chromosomes form tetrads. The bivalent pairs become short and thick and intertwine so that four chromatids are visible.

pacifier, 1. an agent that soothes or comforts. **2.** a "dummy" used by infants and children for sucking.

pacini's corpuscles {Filippo Pacini, Italian anatomist, b. 1812}, a number of special sensory end organs resembling tiny white bulbs, each attached to the end of a single nerve fibre in the subcutaneous, submucous, and subserous connective tissue of many parts of the body, especially the palm of the hand, sole of the foot, genital organs, joints, and in the pancreas. They are pressure sensitive, and in cross section resemble an onion.

pack, 1. the act of applying a dressing or dental cement to a surgical wound. **2.** a surgical dressing to cover a wound or to fill the cavity left from a tooth extraction, especially an extraction of a wisdom tooth.

package insert, a leaflet that must be placed inside the package of prescription drugs. In it, the manufacturer is required to describe the drug, to state its generic name, and to give the applicable indications, contraindications, warnings, precautions, adverse effects, form, dosage, and administration.

packed cells, a preparation of blood cells separated from liquid plasma, often administered in severe anaemia to restore adequate levels of haemoglobin and red cells without overloading the vascular system with excess fluids.

PaCO$_2$, abbreviation for **partial pressure of carbon dioxide in arterial blood.**

pad, 1. a mass of soft material used to cushion shock, prevent wear, or absorb moisture, such as the abdominal pads used to absorb discharges from abdominal wounds. **2.** (in anatomy) a mass of fat that cushions various structures, such as the infrapatellar pad lying below the patella.

paederosis. See **paedophilia.**

paediatric anaesthesia, a subspecialty of anaesthetics dealing with the anaesthesia of neonates, infants, and children up to 12 years of age.

paediatric dosage, the determination of the correct amount, frequency, and total number of doses of a medication to be administered to a child or infant. Various formulae have been devised to calculate paediatric dosage from a standard adult dose, although the most reliable method is to use the proportional amount of body surface area to body weight, based on one of the formulae.

paediatric hospitalization, the confinement of a child or infant in a hospital for diagnostic testing or therapeutic treatment.

paediatrician, a doctor who specializes in the care of sick children.

paediatric nurse, a nurse who has specialized in the study of the care of sick children thereby gaining the RN (paediatrics) or equivalent qualification (formerly the RSCN qualification).

paediatric nursing, the branch of nursing concerned with the care of infants and children.

paediatric nutrition, the maintenance of a proper, well-balanced diet, consisting of the essential nutrients and the adequate calorie intake necessary to promote growth and sustain the physiological requirements at the various stages of development. Nutritional needs vary considerably with age, level of activity, and environmental conditions, and they are directly related to the rate of growth.

paediatrics, a branch of medicine concerned with the development and care of children. Its specialties are the particular diseases of children and their treatment and prevention. **paediatric,** *adj.*

paediatric surgery, the special preparation and care of the child undergoing surgical procedures for injuries, deformities, or disease. In addition to the usual fears and emotional trauma of illness and hospitalization, the child may be especially concerned about being anaesthetized.

paedodontics, a field of dentistry devoted to the diagnosis and the treatment of dental problems affecting children.

paedogenesis, the production of offspring by young or larval forms of animals, often by parthenogenesis, as in certain amphibians. **paedogenetic,** *adj.*

paedophilia, 1. an abnormal interest in children. **2.** (in psychiatry) a psychosexual disorder in which the fantasy or act of engaging in sexual activity with prepubertal children is the preferred or exclusive means of achieving sexual excitement and gratification. Also called **pederosis. paedophilic,** *adj.*

paeds, *informal,* paediatrics.

Paget's disease {Sir James Paget, English surgeon, b. 1814}, a common, nonmetabolic disease of bone of unknown cause, usually affecting middle-aged and elderly people, characterized by excessive bone destruction and unorganized bone repair. Most cases are asymptomatic or mild; however, bone pain may be the first symptom. Bowed tibias (sabre shins), kyphosis, and frequent

fractures are caused by the soft, abnormal bone in this condition. Enlargement of the head, headaches, and warmth over involved areas caused by increased vascularity are additional features. The x-ray picture of areas of decreased bone density adjacent to sites of increased density is characteristic. Radioactive bone scans help locate regions of active disease. Complications include fractures, kidney stones if the patient is immobilized, heart failure, deafness or blindness caused by pressure from bony overgrowth, and osteosarcoma.

Paget's disease of the nipple. See **nipple cancer.**

pagophagia, an abnormal condition characterized by a craving to eat enormous quantities of ice. It is associated with a lack of nutrient iron. **pagophagic, pagophagous,** *adj.*

PAHA, abbreviation for **paraaminohippuric acid.**

PAHA sodium clearance test, a test for detecting kidney damage or certain muscle diseases. The test uses the sodium salt of paraaminohippuric acid for determining the rate at which the kidneys remove this salt from the blood and urine.

pain, an unpleasant sensation caused by noxious stimulation of the sensory nerve endings. It is a cardinal symptom of inflammation and is valuable in the diagnosis of many disorders and conditions. Pain may be mild or severe, chronic, acute, piercing, burning, dull, or sharp, precisely or poorly localized, or referred. See also **referred pain.**

pain assessment, an evaluation of the factors that alleviate or exacerbate a patient's pain, used as an aid in the diagnosis and the treatment of disease and trauma. Responses to pain vary widely among individuals and depend on many different physical and psychological factors, such as specific diseases and injuries and the health, pain threshold, fear and anxiety, and cultural background of the individual involved, as well as the way different individuals express their pain experiences. The patient is asked to describe the cause of the pain, if known, its intensity, location, and duration, the events preceding it, and the pattern usually followed for handling pain. Severe pain causes pallor, cold perspiration, piloerection, dilated pupils, and increases in the pulse, respiratory rate, blood pressure, and muscle tension. When brief, intense pain subsides, the pulse may be slower and the blood pressure lower than before the pain began. If pain occurs frequently or is prolonged, the pulse rate and blood pressure may not increase markedly.

pain, chronic, pain that continues for more than 6 months in duration. Defining characteristics include a verbal report or observed evidence of pain experienced for more than 6 months, fear of reinjury, altered ability to continue previous activities, anorexia, weight changes, changes in sleep patterns, facial mask, and guarded movements.

pain management, the relief of the painful sensations experienced in suffering the physiological and psychological effects of disease and trauma. The most common method of pain management is the administration of narcotics, such as morphine, but many authorities support the use of pain-killing drugs with psychological support. Acute pain, occurring in the first 24 to 48 hours after surgery, is often difficult to relieve, and narcotics seldom relieve all such pain. Mild pain may best be relieved by comfort measures and the distraction afforded by television, visitors, reading, and other passive activities. Moderate pain may best be relieved by a combination of comfort measures and drugs. Intervention to relieve severe pain often includes the administration of narcotics, purposeful interaction between the patient and attending hospital personnel, reduction of environmental stimuli, increased comfort measures, and "waking imagined analgesia," in which the patient is encouraged to concentrate on and become distracted by former pleasant experiences.

pain mechanism, the psychosomatic network that communicates unpleasant sensations and the perceptions of noxious stimuli throughout the body, most commonly in association with physical disease and trauma involving tissue damage. Some theories about the pain mechanism that have evolved are the **gate control theory** and **the pattern theory.**

pain receptor, any one of the many free nerve endings throughout the body that warn of potentially harmful changes in the environment, such as excessive pressure or temperature. The free nerve endings constituting most of the pain receptors occur chiefly in the epidermis and in the epithelial covering of certain mucous membranes. The terminal ends of pain receptors consist of unmyelinated nerve fibres that often anastomose into small knobs against the epithelial cells.

pain spot, any spot on the skin where a stimulus can produce pain.

paint, 1. to apply a medicated solution to the skin, usually over a wide area. **2.** a medicated solution that is applied in this way. Kinds of paint include **antiseptics, germicides,** and **sporicides.**

PA interval (HBE), a measurement of intraatrial conduction time measured from the onset of the P wave on a standard ECG, or from the atrial deflection of the high right atrial electrogram to the A wave on the His bundle electrogram (HBE).

pain threshold, the point at which a stimulus, usually one associated with pressure or temperature, activates pain receptors and produces a sensation of pain. Individuals with low pain thresholds experience pain much sooner and faster than individuals with higher pain thresholds.

pair production, the process of x-ray interaction with matter in which the incident x-ray photon is completely absorbed. The process only occurs where the photon has an nenergy of at least 1.02 MeV, and is important in high energy external beam radiotherapy.

PAL (physical activity level), a ration of daily expenditure to basal metabolic rate (BMR). Values range from 1.4 (person with light work energy expenditure, non-active leisure pursuits) to 1.9 (energy-demanding work and active leisure pursuits).

palatal, 1. of or pertaining to the palate. **2.** of or pertaining to the lingual surface of a maxillary tooth.

palate, a structure that forms the roof of the mouth. It is divided into the hard palate and the soft palate. **palatal, palatine,** *adj.*

palatine arch, the vault-shaped muscular structure forming the soft palate between the mouth and the nasopharynx.

palatine bone, one of a pair of bones of the skull, forming the posterior part of the hard palate, part of the nasal cavity, and the floor of the orbit of the eye.

palatine ridge, any one of the four to six transverse ridges on the anterior surface of the hard palate.

palatine suture, one of a number of thin wavy lines marking the joining of the palatine processes that form the hard palate.

palatine tonsil, one of a pair of almond-shaped masses of lymphoid tissue between the palatoglossal and the palatopharyngeal arches on each side of the fauces.

palatitis, an inflammation of the hard palate.

palatomaxillary, of or pertaining to the palate and the maxilla.

palatonasal, of or pertaining to the palate and the nose.

paleogenesis. See **palingenesis.**

paleogenetic, 1. a trait or structure of an organism or species that originated in a previous generation. **2.** relating to the development of such a trait or structure.

palilalia, an abnormal condition characterized by the increasingly rapid repetition of the same word or phrase, usually at the end of a sentence.

palindrome, (in molecular genetics) a segment of DNA in which identical, or almost identical, sequences of bases run in opposite directions.

palingenesis, 1. the regeneration of a lost part. **2.** the hereditary transmission of ancestral structural characteristics. **palingenetic, palingenic,** *adj.*

palladium (Pd), a hard, silvery metallic element. Its atomic number is 46; its atomic weight is 106.4. Highly resistant to tarnish and corrosion, palladium is used in high-grade surgical instruments and in dental inlays, bridgework, and orthodontic appliances.

palliate, to soothe or relieve.   **palliation,** n, **palliative,** adj.

palliative care, therapy designed to relieve or reduce intensity of uncomfortable symptoms but not to produce a cure.

pallidum. See **globus pallidus.**

pallium. See **cerebral cortex.**

pallor, an unnatural paleness or absence of colour in the skin.

palm, the lower side of the hand, between the wrist and the bases of the fingers, when the hand is held horizontal with the thumb in medial position.   **palmar,** adj.

palmar aponeurosis, fascia surrounding the muscles of the palm.

palmar crease, a normal groove across the palm of the hand.

palmar erythema, an inflammatory redness of the palms of the hands.

palmar fascia. See **palmar aponeurosis.**

palmaris longus, a long, slender, superficial, fusiform muscle of the forearm. It functions to flex the hand.

palmar metacarpal artery, one of several arteries arising from the deep palmar arch, supplying the fingers.

palmar pinch, a thumbless grasp in which the tips of the other fingers are pressed against the palm of the hand.

palmar reflex, a reflex that curls the fingers when the palm of the hand is tickled.

palmature, an abnormal condition in which the fingers are webbed.

palm-chin reflex. See **palmomental reflex.**

palmityl alcohol. See **cetyl alcohol.**

palmomental reflex, an abnormal neurological sign, elicited by scratching the palm of the hand at the base of the thumb, characterized by contraction of the muscles of the chin and corner of the mouth on the same side of the body as the stimulus.

palpable, perceivable by touch.

palpate, to use the hands or fingers to examine.

palpation, a technique used in physical examination in which the examiner feels the texture, size, consistency, and location of certain parts of the body with the hands.

palpatory percussion, a technique in physical examination in which the vibrations produced by percussion are evaluated by using light pressure of the flat of the examiner's hand.

palpebra. See **eyelid.**

palpebral commissure. See **canthus.**

palpebral conjunctiva. See **conjunctiva.**

palpebral fissure, the opening between the margins of the upper and lower lids.

palpebral gland. See **meibomian gland.**

palpebra superior, pl. **palpebrae superiores,** the upper eyelid, larger and more movable than the lower eyelid and furnished with an elevator muscle.

palpebrate, 1. to wink or blink. **2.** having eyelids.

palpitate, to pulsate rapidly, as in the unusually fast beating of the heart under various conditions of stress and in patients with certain heart problems.

palpitation, a pounding or racing of the heart, associated with normal emotional responses or with certain heart disorders.

palsy, an abnormal condition characterized by paralysis.

Paltauf's dwarf. See **pituitary dwarf.**

Paltauf's nanism {Arnold Paltauf, Czechoslovakian physician, b. 1860}, dwarfism associated with excessive production or growth of lymphoid tissue.

PAMP, abbreviation for **pulmonary arterial mean pressure.**

pampiniform, having the shape of a tendril.

pampiniform body. See **epoophoron.**

panacea 1. a universal remedy. **2.** an ancient name for a herb or a liquid potion with healing properties.

panacinar emphysema, a form of emphysema that affects all lung areas by causing dilatation and atrophy of the alveoli and by destroying the vascular bed of the lung. Also called **panlobular emphysema.**

panarthritis, an abnormal condition characterized by the inflammation of many joints of the body.   **panarthritic,** adj.

pancake kidney, a congenital anomaly in which the left and right kidneys are fused into a single mass in the pelvis. The fused kidney has two collecting systems and two ureters.

pancarditis, an abnormal condition characterized by inflammation of the entire heart, including the endocardium, myocardium, and pericardium.

Pancoast's syndrome {Henry K. Pancoast, American radiologist, b. 1875}, **1.** a combination of various signs associated with a tumour in the apex of the lung. The signs include neuritic pain in the arm, an x-ray shadow at the apex of the lung, atrophy of the muscles of the arm and the hand, and Horner's syndrome. **2.** an abnormal condition caused by osteolysis in the posterior part of one or more ribs, sometimes involving associated vertebrae.

Pancoast's tumour. See **pulmonary sulcus tumour.**

pancolectomy, the excision of the entire colon, requiring also an ileostomy.

pancreas, a fish-shaped, greyish pink nodular gland that stretches transversely across the posterior abdominal wall in the epigastric and hypochondriac regions of the body and secretes various substances, such as digestive enzymes, insulin, and glucagon. A compound racemose gland composed of exocrine and endocrine tissue, it contains a main duct that runs the length of the organ, draining smaller ducts and emptying into the duodenum.

pancreatectomy, the surgical removal of all or part of the pancreas, performed to remove a cyst or tumour, treat pancreatitis, or repair trauma.

pancreatic cancer, a malignant neoplastic disease of the pancreas, characterized by anorexia, flatulence, weakness, dramatic weight loss, epigastric or back pain, jaundice, pruritus, a palpable abdominal mass, the recent onset of diabetes, and clay-coloured stools if the pancreatic ducts are obstructed. Insulin-secreting tumours of islet cells cause hypoglycaemia, especially in the morning. Nonfunctioning islet cell lesions produce gastrin, causing symptoms of peptic ulcer, or, in some cases, acute diarrhoea and hypokalaemia, and achlorhydria, the result of the lesion's elaboration of secretin.

pancreatic diverticulum, one of a pair of membranous pouches arising from the embryonic duodenum.

pancreatic duct, the primary secretory channel of the pancreas.

pancreatic enzyme, any one of the enzymes secreted by the pancreas in the process of digestion. The most important are trypsin, chymotrypsin, steapsin, and amylopsin.

pancreatic hormone, any one of several chemical compounds secreted by the pancreas, associated with the regulation of cellular metabolism. Major hormones secreted by the pancreas are insulin, glucagon, and pancreatic polypeptide.

pancreatic insufficiency, a condition characterized by inadequate production and secretion of pancreatic hormones or enzymes, usually occurring secondary to a disease process destructive of pancreatic tissue. Nutritional malabsorption, anorexia, poorly localized upper abdominal or epigastric pain, malaise, and severe weight loss often occur.

pancreatic juice, the fluid secretion of the pancreas, produced by the stimulation of food in the duodenum. The juice is essential in breaking down proteins into their amino acid components, in reducing dietary fats to glycerol and fatty acids, and in converting starch to simple sugars.

pancreaticolienal node, a node in one of three groups of lymph glands associated with branches of the abdominal and the pelvic viscera that are supplied by branches of the coeliac artery.

pancreatin, a concentrate of pancreatic enzymes from pigs or beef cattle. It is used as an aid to digestion to replace endogenous pancreatic enzymes in cystic fibrosis and after pancreatectomy.

pancreatitis, an inflammatory condition of the pancreas that may be acute or chronic. **Acute pancreatitis** is generally the result of damage to the biliary tract, as by alcohol, trauma, infectious disease, or certain drugs.

It is characterized by severe abdominal pain radiating to the back, fever, anorexia, nausea, and vomiting. There may be jaundice if the common bile duct is obstructed. The causes of **chronic pancreatitis** are similar to those of the acute form. When the cause is alcohol abuse, there may be calcification and scarring of the smaller pancreatic ducts. There is abdominal pain, nausea, and vomiting, as well as steatorrhoea and creatorrhoea, caused by the diminished output of pancreatic enzymes.

pancreatoduodenectomy, a surgical procedure in which the head of the pancreas and the loop of duodenum that surrounds it are excised.

pancreatography. See **cholangiopancreatography.**

pancreatolith, a stone or calculus in the pancreas.

pancuronium bromide, a non-depolarizing skeletal muscle relaxant used as an adjunct to anaesthesia and mechanical ventilation.

pancytopenia, an abnormal condition characterized by a marked reduction in the number of all of the cellular elements of the blood, the red blood cells, white blood cells, and platelets. See also **anaemia, aplasia. pancytopenic,** *adj.*

pandemic, (of a disease) occurring throughout the population of a country, a people, or the world.

pandiastolic, of or pertaining to the complete diastole.

panencephalitis, inflammation of the entire brain characterized by an insidious onset, a progressive course with deterioration of motor and mental functions, and evidence of a viral cause. Subacute sclerosing panencephalitis is an uncommon childhood disease thought to be caused by a "slow" latent measles virus after recovery from a previous infection. The disease results in ataxia, myoclonus, atrophy, cortical blindness, and mental deterioration. Rubella panencephalitis, a rare disease of adolescents, follows a chronic progressive course marked by motor and mental deterioration and sometimes resembles juvenile paresis.

panendoscope, a cystoscope that allows a wide view of the interior of the bladder.

panaesthesia, the total of all sensations experienced by an individual at one time.

pangenesis, a darwinian theory that every cell and particle of a parent reproduces itself in progeny.

panhypopituitarism, generalized insufficiency of pituitary hormones, resulting from damage to or deficiency of the gland. **Prepubertal panhypopituitarism** a rare disorder usually associated with a suprasellar cyst or craniopharyngioma, is characterized by dwarfism with normal body proportions, subnormal sexual development, and insufficient thyroid and adrenal function. Postpubertal panhypopituitarism may be caused by postpartum pituitary necrosis, resulting from thrombosis of pituitary circulation during or after delivery. Characteristic signs of the disorder are failure to lactate, amenorrhoea, weakness, cold intolerance, lethargy, and loss of libido and of axillary and pubic hair.

panhysterectomy. See **total hysterectomy.**

panic, an intense, sudden, and overwhelming fear or feeling of anxiety that produces terror and immediate physiological changes that result in paralysed immobility or senseless, hysterical behaviour.

panivorous, of or pertaining to the practice of subsisting exclusively on bread. **panivore,** *n.*

panlobular emphysema. See **panacinar emphysema.**

Panner's disease, a rare form of osteochondrosis in which there is abnormal bony growth in the capitulum of the humerus.

panniculus, *pl.* **panniculi,** a membranous layer, the many sheets of fascia covering various structures in the body.

pannus, an abnormal condition of the cornea, which has become vascularized and infiltrated with granular tissue just beneath the surface.

panophthalmitis, an inflammation of the entire eye, usually caused by virulent pyogenic organisms, such as strains of meningococci, pneumococci, streptococci, anthrax bacilli, and clostridia. Initial symptoms are pain, fever, headache, drowsiness, oedema, and swelling. As the infection progresses, the iris appears muddy and grey, the aqueous humour becomes turbid, and precipitates form on the posterior surface of the cornea.

panphobia, an anxiety disorder characterized by an irrational, vague fear or apprehension of some pervading or unknown evil; a generalized fear. **panphobic,** *adj.*

pansystolic, of or pertaining to the entire systole. Also **holosystolic.**

pansystolic murmur. See **systolic murmur.**

panthenol, an alcohol converted in the body to pantothenic acid, a vitamin in the B complex.

panting, a ventilatory pattern characterized by rapid, shallow breathing with small tidal volume.

pantograph, 1. a jointed device for copying a plane figure to any desired scale. **2.** a device that incorporates a pair of face bows fixed to the jaws, used for inscribing centrically related points and arcs leading to them on segments relatable to the three craniofacial planes.

pantomography, a radiographic technique to give a panoramic view of the facial bones, dental arches and associated structures. **pantomogram,** *n.*

pantothenic acid, a member of the vitamin B complex. It is widely distributed in plant and animal tissues and may be an important element in human nutrition.

pantothenyl alcohol. See **panthenol.**

PaO₂, symbol for arterial partial pressure of oxygen.

papain, an enzyme from the fruit of *Carica papaya,* the paw paw tree. It has been used for enzymatic debridement of wounds and promotion of healing.

Papanicolaou test {George N. Papanicolaou, American physician, b. 1883}, a simple smear method of examining stained exfoliative cells. It is used most commonly to detect cancers of the cervix, but it may be used for tissue specimens from any organ. A smear is usually obtained during a routine pelvic examination. The findings are usually reported descriptively and grouped into the following classes: Class I, only normal cells seen; Class II, atypical cells consistent with inflammation; Class III, mild dysplasia; Class IV, severe dysplasia, suspicious cells; Class V, carcinoma cells seen.

papaverine hydrochloride, a smooth muscle relaxant used in the treatment of cardiovascular or visceral spasms, and by direct injection into the corpus cavernosus of the penis in the diagnosis and treatment of impotence.

paper chromatography, the separation of a mixture into its components by filtering it through a strip of special paper.

paper-doll fetus. See **fetus papyraceus.**

paper radioimmunosorbent test (PRIST), a technique for determining total IgE levels in patients with type I hypersensitivity reactions.

papilla, *pl.* **papillae, 1.** a small nipple-shaped projection, such as the conoid papillae of the tongue and the papillae of the corium that extend from collagen fibres, the capillary blood vessels, and sometimes the nerves of the dermis. **2.** the optic papilla, a round white disc in the fundus oculi, which corresponds to the entrance of the optic nerve.

papilla duodeni major. See **hepatopancreatic ampulla.**

papilla of Vater. See **hepatopancreatic ampulla.**

papillary, of or pertaining to a papilla.

papillary adenocarcinoma, a malignant neoplasm characterized by small papillae of vascular connective tissue covered by neoplastic epithelium that projects into follicles, glands, or cysts.

papillary adenocystoma lymphomatosum, an unusual tumour, consisting of epithelial and lymphoid tissues, that develops in the area of the parotid and submaxillary glands.

papillary adenoma, a benign epithelial tumour in which the membrane lining the glandular tissue forms papillary processes that project into the alveoli or grow out of the surface of a cavity.

papillary carcinoma, a malignant neoplasm characterized by many fingerlike projections. It is the most common type of thyroid tumour.

papillary duct, any one of the thousands of straight collecting renal tubules that descend through the medulla of the kidney and join with others to form the common ducts opening into the renal papillae.

papillary muscle, any one of the rounded or conical muscular projections attached to the chordae tendineae in the ventricles of the heart. The papillary muscles are associated with the atrioventricular valves that they help open and close.

papillary tumour. See **papilloma.**

papillate, marked by papillae or nipplelike prominences.

papilliform, shaped like a papilla.

papillitis, 1. an abnormal condition characterized by the inflammation of a papilla, such as the lacrimal papilla. 2. an abnormal condition characterized by the inflammation of a renal papilla.

papilloedema, *pl.* **papilloedemas, papilloedemata,** swelling of the optic disc caused by increased intracranial pressure. The meningeal sheaths that surround the optic nerves from the optic disc are continuous with the meninges of the brain; therefore, increased intracranial pressure is transmitted forward from the brain to the optic disc in the eye to cause the swelling.

papilloma, a benign epithelial neoplasm characterized by a branching or lobular tumour. Kinds of papillomas are **basal cell papilloma, cockscomb papilloma, cutaneous papilloma, fibroepithelial papilloma, hirsutoid papilloma of the penis, intracanalicular papilloma, intracystic papilloma,** and **villous papilloma.** Also called **papillary tumour.**

papillomatosis, an abnormal condition in which there is widespread development of nipplelike growths.

papillomatosis coronae penis. See **hirsutoid papilloma of the penis.**

papillomavirus, the virus that causes warts in humans.

papilloretinitis, an inflammatory occlusion of a retinal vein.

papovavirus, one of a group of small DNA viruses, some of which may be potentially cancer-producing. The human wart is caused by a kind of papovavirus. Kinds of papovaviruses are **papilloma papovavirus, polyoma papovavirus,** and **SV-40 papovavirus.**

pappataci fever. See **phlebotomus fever.**

pappus, the first growth of beard, characterized by downy hairs.

Pap smear {George N. Papanicolaou}, *informal* ,a specimen of exfoliated, epithelial cells and cervical mucus collected during a pelvic examination for cytological evaluation according to the Papanicolaou cytological classification.

Pap test. See **Papanicolaou test.**

papular scaling disease, any of a group of skin disorders in which there are discrete, raised, dry, scaling lesions. Some kinds of papular scaling diseases are **lichen planus, pityriasis rosea,** and **psoriasis.**

papulation, the development of papules.

papule, a small, solid, raised skin lesion less than 1 cm in diameter, such as the lesions of lichen planus and nonpustular acne. Compare **macule. papular,** *adj.*

papulosquamous disease. See **papular scaling disease.**

papyraceous, having a paperlike quality.

papyraceous fetus. See **fetus papyraceus.**

par, a pair, specifically a pair of cranial nerves, as the par nonum or the ninth pair.

PAR, abbreviation for **pulmonary arteriolar resistance.**

paraaminobenzoic acid (PABA), a substance often occurring in association with the vitamin B complex, found in cereals, eggs, milk, and meat and present in detectable amounts in blood, urine, spinal fluid, and sweat. It is widely used as a sunscreen.

paraaminohippuric acid (PAHA, PHA), the N-acetic acid of paraaminobenzoic acid. Its sodium salt is used for measuring the effective renal plasma flow and for determining kidney function.

paraaminosalicylic acid (PAS, PASA), a bacteriostatic agent prescribed for the treatment of tuberculosis when first-line treatments cannot be used.

parabiotic syndrome, a blood transfer condition that can occur between identical twin fetuses because of placental vascular anastomoses. One twin may become anaemic and the other plethoric.

paracentesis, a procedure in which fluid is withdrawn from a cavity of the body. Paracentesis is most commonly performed to remove excessive accumulations of ascitic fluid from the abdomen.

paracervical, pertaining to tissues adjacent to the cervix.

paracervical block, a form of regional anaesthesia in which a local anaesthetic is injected into the area on each side of the uterine cervix that contains the plexus of nerves innervating the uterine cervix.

paracetamol, an analgesic and antipyretic drug prescribed for mild to moderate pain and fever.

paracetamol poisoning, a toxic reaction to the ingestion of excessive doses of paracetamol. In adults doses exceeding 10 to 15 g can produce liver failure, and doses above 25 g can be fatal. Large amounts of paracetamol metabolites can overwhelm the glutathione-detoxifying mechanism of the liver, resulting in progressive necrosis of the liver within 5 days. The onset of symptoms may be marked by nausea and vomiting, profuse sweating, pallor, and oliguria.

paracoccidioidomycosis, a chronic, occasionally fatal, fungal infection caused by *Paracoccidioides brasiliensis,* characterized by ulcers of the oral cavity, larynx, and nose. Other effects include large, draining lymph nodes, cough, dyspnoea, weight loss, and skin, genital, and intestinal lesions. The disease is acquired by inhalation of spores of the fungus.

paradichlorobenzene poisoning. See **naphthalene poisoning.**

paradidymal, 1. pertaining to the paradidymis. **2.** beside the testis.

paradidymis, *pl.* **paradidymides,** a rudimentary structure in the male, situated on the spermatic cord of the epididymis, that consists of vestigial remains of the caudal part of the embryonic mesonephric tubules. A similar vestigial structure, the paroophoron, is found in the female.

paradigm, a pattern that may serve as a model or example.

paradoxical agitation, a period of unexpected excitability that sometimes follows administration of analeptic medications.

paradoxical breathing, a condition in which a part of the lung deflates during inspiration and inflates during expiration. The condition usually is associated with a chest trauma, such as an open chest wound or rib cage damage.

paradoxical bronchospasm, a constriction of the airways after treatment with a sympathomimetic bronchodilator.

paradoxical intention, paradoxical intervention, a psychotherapeutic strategy designed to draw clients' attention to ways in which they may be resisting or avoiding change. The therapist directs the client to perform an action which appears to contradict a commonsense approach to a stated problem; e.g. a client who rarely initiates activities independently of other family members might be directed to undertake no independent activity of any kind whatsoever.

paradoxical pulse. See **pulsus paradoxus.**

paraesthesia, any subjective sensation, experienced as numbness, tingling, or a "pins and needles" feeling. When experienced in the extremities, it is sometimes identified as acroparaesthesia.

paraffin method, (in surgical pathology) a method used in preparing a selected portion of tissue for pathology examination. The tissue is fixed, dehydrated, and infiltrated and embedded in paraffin, forming a block that is cut with a microtome into slices.

parafollicular C cell, a calcitonin-secreting cell located between follicles.

paraganglion, *pl.* **paraganglia,** any one of the small groups of chromaffin cells associated with the ganglia of the sympathetic

nerve trunk and situated outside the adrenal medulla. The paraganglia secrete the hormones adrenaline and noradrenaline.

paragonimiasis, chronic infection with the lung fluke *Paragonimus westermani.* It is characterized by haemoptysis, bronchitis, and, occasionally, abdominal masses, pain and diarrhoea, or cerebral involvement with paralysis, ocular pathological conditions, or seizures. The disease is acquired by ingesting cysts in infected freshwater crabs or crayfish, the intermediate hosts.

parainfluenza virus, a myxovirus with four serotypes, causing respiratory infections in infants and young children and, less commonly, in adults. Types 1 and 2 parainfluenza viruses may cause laryngotracheobronchitis or croup; type 3 is a cause of croup, tracheobronchitis, bronchiolitis, and bronchopneumonia in children; types 1, 3, and 4 are associated with pharyngitis and the common cold.

paraldehyde, a clear, colourless, strong-smelling liquid obtained by the polymerization of acetaldehyde with a small amount of sulphuric acid. Paraldehyde is used as a solvent and may be administered orally, intravenously, intramuscularly, or rectally to induce hypnotic states or sedation.

parallel grid, (in radiography) a secondary radiation grid consisting of parallel lead strips.

parallelogram condenser, (in dentistry) an instrument with a face shaped like a rectangle or parallelogram, used for compacting amalgams in filling teeth.

parallel play, a form of play among a group of children, primarily toddlers, in which each one engages in an independent activity that is similar to but not influenced by or shared with the others.

parallel talk, a form of speech used during children's play therapy in which the clinician verbalizes activities of the child without requiring answers to questions.

Paralympics, an acronym formed from *paraplegic* and *Olympics;* an international competitive wheelchair sports event, usually held in association with the official quadrennial Olympic Games.

paralysis, *pl.* **paralyses,** an abnormal condition characterized by the loss of muscle function or the loss of sensation, or both. It may be caused by a variety of problems, such as trauma, disease, and poisoning. Paralyses may be classified according to cause, muscle tone, distribution, or the part of the body affected. **paralytic,** *adj.*

paralysis agitans. See **Parkinson's disease.**

paralytic dementia. See **paresis, def. 2.**

paralytic ileus, a decrease in or absence of intestinal peristalsis that may occur after abdominal surgery or peritoneal injury or in connection with severe pyelonephritis, ureteral stone, fractured ribs, myocardial infarction, extensive intestinal ulceration, heavy metal poisoning, porphyria, retroperitoneal haematomas, especially those associated with fractured vertebrae, or any severe metabolic disease. Paralytic ileus is characterized by abdominal tenderness and distention, absence of bowel sounds, lack of flatus, and nausea and vomiting. There may be fever, decreased urinary output, electrolyte imbalance, dehydration, and respiratory distress.

paramedical personnel, health care workers who have special training in the performance of supportive health care tasks.

paramesonephric duct, one of a pair of embryonic ducts that develops into the uterus and the uterine tubes.

parameter, 1. a value or constant used to describe or measure a set of data representing a physiological function or system. 2. a statistical value of a population group. 3. *informal.* limits or boundary.

parametric imaging, (in nuclear medicine) a diagnostic procedure in which an image of an administered radioactive tracer is derived according to a mathematical rule, as by the division of one image by another.

parametric statistics, statistics that assume a population has a symmetrical, such as gaussian or log normal, distribution.

parametritis, an inflammatory condition of the tissue of the structures around the uterus.

parametrium, *pl.* **parametria,** the lateral extension of the uterine subserous connective tissue into the broad ligament.

paramitome. See **hyaloplasm.**

paramnesia, 1. a disorder of memory in which one believes one remembers events and circumstances that never actually occurred. 2. a condition in which words are remembered and used without the comprehension of their meaning.

paramyxovirus, a member of a family of viruses that includes the organisms that cause parainfluenza, mumps, and some respiratory infections.

paranasal, situated near or alongside the nose, as the paranasal sinuses.

paranasal sinus, one of the air cavities in various bones around the nose, as the frontal sinus in the frontal bone lying deep to the medial part of the superciliary ridge and the maxillary sinus within the maxilla between the orbit, the nasal cavity, and the upper teeth.

parangi. See **yaws.**

paranoia, (in psychiatry) a disorder characterized by an elaborate system of thinking with delusions of persecution and grandeur usually centered on one major theme. The delusional system typically develops slowly and progressively over a period of months or years, becoming intricate, logical, and highly organized, with the result that it can be most convincing. The person may appear perfectly normal in conduct, conversation, thinking patterns, and emotional responses aside from the delusions. Kinds of paranoia include **acute hallucinatory paranoia, alcoholic paranoia, litigious paranoia,** and **querulous paranoia.**

paranoiac, 1. a person afflicted with or exhibiting characteristics of paranoia. 2. of or pertaining to paranoia.

paranoia hallucinatoria. See **acute hallucinatory paranoia.**

paranoia quaerula. See **querulous paranoia.**

paranoid, 1. pertaining to or resembling paranoia. 2. a person afflicted with a paranoic disorder. 3. *informal.* a person, or pertaining to a person, who is overly suspicious or exhibits persecutory trends or attitudes.

paranoid disorder, any of a large group of mental disorders characterized by an impaired sense of reality and persistent delusions. Kinds of paranoid disorders include **acute paranoid disorder, paranoia,** and **shared paranoid disorder.**

paranoid ideation, an exaggerated, sometimes grandiose, belief or suspicion, usually not of a delusional nature, that one is being harassed, persecuted, or treated unfairly.

paranoid personality, a personality characterized by paranoia.

paranoid personality disorder, a disorder characterized by extreme suspiciousness and distrust of others to the degree that one blames them for one's mistakes and failures and goes to abnormal lengths to validate prejudices, attitudes, or biases.

paranoid reaction, a psychopathological condition associated with ageing and characterized by the gradual formation of delusions, usually of a persecutory nature and often accompanied by related hallucinations.

paranoid schizophrenia, a form of schizophrenia characterized by persistent preoccupation with delusions, usually of a persecutory, grandiose, or jealous nature, accompanied by related hallucinations.

paranoid state, a transitory abnormal mental condition characterized by illogical thought processes and generalized suspicion and distrust, with a tendency toward persecutory ideas or delusions.

paranuclear body. See **centrosome.**

parapertussia, an acute bacterial respiratory infection caused by *Bordetella parapertussis,* having symptoms closely resembling those of pertussis. It is usually milder than pertussis, although it can be fatal.

parapharyngeal abscess, a suppurative infection of tissues adjacent to the pharynx, usually a complication of acute pharyngitis or tonsillitis. Infection may spread to the jugular vein where it may cause thrombophlebitis and septic emboli.

paraphilia, sexual perversion or deviation; a condition in which the sexual instinct is expressed in ways that are socially prohibited or unacceptable or are biologically undesirable, such as the use of an inanimate object for sexual arousal. Kinds of paraphilia include **exhibitionism, fetishism, paedophilia, transvestitism, voyeurism,** and **zoophilia. paraphiliac,** *adj., n.*

paraphimosis, a condition characterized by an inability to replace the foreskin in its normal position after it has been retracted behind the glans penis. Caused by a narrow or inflamed foreskin, the condition may lead to gangrene. Circumcision may be required.

paraplasm, any abnormal growth or malformation. **paraplasmic,** *adj.*

paraplastic, 1. misshapen or malformed. **2.** showing abnormal formative power; of the nature of a paraplasm.

paraplegia, an abnormal condition characterized by motor or sensory loss in the lower limbs. This condition may or may not involve the back and abdominal muscles and may cause either complete or incomplete paralysis. Such injuries commonly occur as the result of car or motorcycle accidents, sporting accidents and falls. Paraplegia less commonly results from nontraumatic lesions, such as scoliosis, spina bifida, and alcoholism. The signs and symptoms of paraplegia may develop immediately from trauma and include the loss of sensation, motion, and reflexes below the level of the lesion. Depending on the level of the lesion and whether damage to the spinal cord is complete or incomplete, the patient may lose bladder and bowel control and develop sexual dysfunctions. An incomplete spinal cord injury does not usually inhibit circumanal sensation, voluntary toe flexion, or sphincter control. **paraplegic,** *adj., n.*

paraprotein, any of the incomplete monoclonal immunoglobins that occur in plasma cell disorders.

parapsoriasis, a group of chronic skin diseases resembling psoriasis, characterized by maculopapular, erythematous, scaly eruptions without systemic symptoms. Parapsoriasis is resistant to all treatment.

parapsychology, a branch of psychology concerned with the study of alleged psychic phenomena, such as clairvoyance, extrasensory perception, and telepathy.

paraquat poisoning, a toxic condition caused by the ingestion of paraquat dichloride, a highly poisonous pesticide. Characteristically, progressive pulmonary fibrosis and damage to the oesophagus, kidneys, and liver develop several days after ingestion. Once fibrosis begins, death is inevitable, usually within 3 weeks.

parasite, 1. an organism living in or on and obtaining nourishment from another organism. A **facultative parasite** may live on a host but is capable of living independently. An **obligate parasite** is one that depends entirely on its host for survival. **2.** See **parasitic fetus. parasitic,** *adj.*

parasitaemia, the presence of parasites in the blood.

parasitic fetus, the smaller, usually malformed member of conjoined, unequal, or asymmetrical twins that is attached to and dependent on the more normal fetus for growth and development.

parasitic fibroma, a pedunculated uterine fibroid deriving part of its blood supply from the omentum.

parasitic glossitis, a mycosis of the tongue, characterized by a black or brown furry patch on the posterior dorsal surface composed of hypertrophied filiform papillae that measure about 1 cm in length and are easily broken.

parasitic thrombus, an aggregation of bodies and spores of malarial parasites formed in the vessels of the brain in cerebral malaria.

parasuicide, deliberately self-damaging behaviour that does not result in death. The term is used to distinguish such behaviour from attempted suicide which implies an intention to cause death. Both parasuicidal behaviour and attempted suicide are associated with eventual completed suicide, especially in the context of disorders of substance use such as alcohol or drug intoxication.

parasympathetic, of or pertaining to the craniosacral division of the autonomic nervous system, consisting of the oculomotor, facial, glossopharyngeal, vagus, and pelvic nerves. The actions of the parasympathetic division are mediated by the release of acetylcholine and primarily involve the protection, conservation, and restoration of body resources. Parasympathetic fibres slow the heart, stimulate peristalsis, promote the secretion of lacrimal, salivary, and digestive glands, induce bile and insulin release, dilate peripheral and visceral blood vessels, constrict the pupils, oesophagus, and bronchioles, and relax sphincters during micturition and defaecation.

parasympathetic nervous system. See **autonomic nervous system.**

parasympatholytic, parasympatholytic drug, an agent antagonizing the effects of parasympathetic nervous system activity, usually an **anticholinergic.**

parasympathomimetic, 1. of or pertaining to a substance producing effects similar to those caused by stimulation of a parasympathetic nerve. **2.** an agent whose effects mimic those resulting from stimulation of parasympathetic nerves, especially the effects produced by acetylcholine.

parasympathomimetic drug, a drug whose effects mimic parasympathetic nervous system activity, usually a **cholinergic.**

parasystole, an independent ectopic rhythm

whose pacemaker cannot be discharged by impulses of the dominant, usually sinus, rhythm because of an area of depressed conduction surrounding the parasystolic focus. In the classic parasystole, the interectopic intervals are exact multiples of a common denominator reflecting the protected status of the parasystolic focus.

parataxic distortion, a defence mechanism in which current interpersonal relationships are perceived and judged according to a mode of reference established by an earlier experience.

parataxic mode, a term introduced by H. S. Sullivan to identify a childhood perception of the physical and social environment as being illogical, disjointed, and inconsistent.

parathion poisoning, a toxic condition caused by the ingestion, inhalation, or absorption through the skin of the highly toxic organophosphorus insecticide parathion. Symptoms include nausea, vomiting, abdominal cramps, confusion, headache, lack of muscular control, convulsions, and dyspnoea.

parathyroid gland, one of several small structures, usually four in number, attached to the dorsal surfaces of the lateral lobes of the thyroid gland. The parathyroid glands secrete parathyroid hormone, which helps maintain the level of blood calcium concentration and ensures normal neuromuscular irritability, blood clotting, and cell membrane permeability.

parathyroid hormone (PH), a hormone secreted by the parathyroid glands that acts to maintain a constant concentration of calcium in the extracellular fluid. The hormone regulates absorption of calcium from the GI tract, mobilization of calcium from the bones, deposition of calcium in the bones, and excretion of calcium in the breast milk, faeces, sweat, and urine.

paratonia. See gegenhalten.

paratrooper fracture, a fracture of the distal tibia and its malleolus, commonly occurring when an individual jumps from an elevated platform and lands feet first on the ground, subjecting the ankles to extreme force.

paratyphoid fever, a bacterial infection, caused by any *Salmonella* species other than *S. typhi,* characterized by symptoms resembling typhoid fever, although somewhat milder.

paraurethral duct, one of two ducts that drain the bulbourethral glands into the vestibule of the vagina. Also called **Skene's duct.**

paravaccinia virus, a member of a subgroup of pox viruses that can infect humans through direct contact with infected livestock. It is related to the smallpox virus and is the cause of pseudocowpox.

paraxial, pertaining to an organ or other

structure located near the axis of the body.

paregoric, a camphorated tincture of opium formerly used in the treatment of diarrhoea and as an analgesic.

parenchyma, the tissue of an organ as distinguished from supporting or connective tissue.

parenchymal cell, any cell that is a functional element of an organ, such as a hepatocyte.

parenchymatous neuritis, any inflammation affecting the substance, axons, or myelin of the nerve.

parent, a mother or father; one who bears offspring.   **parental,** *adj.*

parental generation (P1), the initial cross between two varieties in a genetic sequence; the parents of any individual, organism, or plant belonging to an F1 generation.

parental grief, the behavioural reaction that characterize the grieving process and result in the resolution of the loss of a child from expected or unexpected death. Parental grieving begins with the discovery of the diagnosis of a life-threatening condition. The immediate reaction is shock and disbelief, followed by acute grief at the anticipation of losing the child. Periods of depression, anger, hope, fear, and anxiety alternate during induction therapy, remission, and maintenance of the disease as parents learn to accept and cope with the situation. In sudden, unexpected death, parents are denied the advantages of anticipatory grief and, because of the lack of time to prepare, usually have extreme feelings of guilt and remorse.

parental role conflict, the response by some parents of role confusion and conflict in response to crisis. Defining characteristics include an expression of concerns or feelings of inadequacy to provide for the child's physical and emotional needs during hospitalization or in the home; a demonstrated disruption in caretaking routines; an expression of concerns about changes in parental role, family functioning, family communication, and family health; expressions of concern about perceived loss of control over decisions relating to the child and reluctance to participate in normal caretaking activities; and voiced or demonstrated feelings of guilt, anger, fear, anxiety, and frustrations about the effect of the child's illness on the family process.

parent-child relationship. See **maternal-child attachment.**

parentcraft education, classes for pregnant women and their partners aiming to prepare them for parenthood. Topics covered may include preparation for childbirth, breast feeding, basic infant care and the emotional and practical changes that will occur when the baby has been born.

parent education, any educational experience geared toward the thoughtful conveyance of information enabling the parent to provide quality childrearing.

parent ego state, a part of the self with messages that sound like one's own parents, containing advice and value messages that emphasize what one "ought to" or "should not" do.

parenteral, not in or through the digestive system. Pertaining to substances administered by a route that bypasses the GI tract, such as a drug given by injection. **parenterally,** adv.

parenteral absorption, the taking up of substances within the body by structures other than the digestive tract.

parenteral fluids. See **administration of parenteral fluids.**

parenteral hyperalimentation. See **total parenteral nutrition.**

parenteral nutrition, the administration of nutrients by a route other than through the alimentary canal, such as subcutaneously, intravenously, intramuscularly, or intradermally. The parenteral fluids usually consist of physiological saline with glucose, amino acids, electrolytes, vitamins, and medications.

parent figure, 1. a parent or a substitute parent or guardian who cares for a child, providing the physical, social, and emotional requirements necessary for normal growth and development. **2.** a person who symbolically represents an ideal parent, having those attributes that one conceptualizes as necessary for forming the perfect parent-child relationship.

parent image, a conscious and unconscious concept that a child forms concerning the roles and characteristics of the personality of the mother and father.

parenting, altered, changes in the ability of nurturing figures to create an environment that promotes the optimum growth and development of another human being. Defining characteristics include an observed lack of actions that demonstrate attachment to the child, inattentiveness to the needs of the child, inappropriate caretaking behaviour, a history of abuse or abandonment of the child, constant complaints about the sex or the appearance of the child, verbal self-assessment of inadequacy in the parental role, expressed disgust about the bodily functions of the child, failure to keep health care appointments for the child, inconsistent disciplinary practices, slow growth and development in the child, and an observed need on the part of the parent to receive approval from others.

Parents Anonymous, a self-help group for parents who have abused their children or who feel that they are prone to maltreat them.

parepididymis. See **paradidymis.**

paresis, 1. partial paralysis related in some cases to local neuritis. **2.** a late manifestation of neurosyphilis, characterized by generalized paralysis, tremulous incoordination, transient seizures, Argyll Robertson pupils, and progressive dementia caused by degeneration of cortical neurons. **paretic,** adj.

paretic dementia. See **paresis.**

pareunia. See **coitus.**

paries, pl. **parietes,** the wall of an organ or cavity in the body.

parietal, 1. of or pertaining to the outer wall of a cavity or organ. **2.** of or pertaining to the parietal bone of the skull, or the parietal lobe of the brain.

parietal bone, one of a pair of bones that form the sides of the cranium.

parietal lobe, a portion of each cerebral hemisphere that occupies the parts of the lateral and the medial surfaces that are covered by the parietal bone.

parietal lymph node, one of the small oval glands that filter the lymph coursing through the lymphatic vessels in the walls of the thorax or through the lymphatic vessels associated with the larger blood vessels of the abdomen and the pelvis.

parietal pain, a sharp sensation of distress in the parietal pleura, aggravated by respiration and thoracic movements and caused by pneumonia, empyema, pneumothorax, asbestosis, tuberculosis, neoplasm, or the accumulation of fluid resulting from heart, liver, or kidney disease.

parietal peritoneum, the portion of the largest serous membrane in the body that lines the abdominal wall.

parietal pleura. See **parietal peritoneum.**

parietooccipital, of or pertaining to the parietal and the occipital bones or lobes.

parietooccipital sulcus, a groove on each cerebral hemisphere marking the division of the parietal and occipital lobes of the brain.

Parinaud's syndrome {Henri Parinaud, French ophthalmologist, b. 1844}, a term often used to refer to conjunctivitis that is usually unilateral, follicular, and followed by enlargement of the preauricular lymph nodes and tenderness. The syndrome is frequently caused by infection with a species of the microorganism *Leptothrix.* It may also be associated with other infections, such as tularaemia, cat-scratch fever, and lymphogranuloma venereum.

parity, 1. (in obstetrics) the classification of a woman by the number of live-born children and stillbirths she has delivered at more than 28 weeks of gestation. Commonly, parity is noted with the total number of pregnancies and represented by the letter "P" or the word "para." A para 4 (P4) gravida 5 (G5) has had four deliveries after 28 weeks and one abortion or miscarriage before 28 weeks. **2.** (in epidemiology) the classification of a woman by the number of live-born children she has delivered. **3.** (in computer processing) the condition of a set of items, either even or odd in number, used as a means for checking errors, as in the transmission of information between various elements of the same computer.

parkinsonian equivalents {James Parkinson, English physician, b. 1775}, the side effects of antipsychotic drugs that are behaviours characteristic of parkinsonism, including fine tremors, "pill-rolling" movements of the fingers, drooling, and petit pas gait.

parkinsonism {James Parkinson}, a neurological disorder characterized by tremor, muscle rigidity, hypokinesia, a slow shuffling gait, difficulty in chewing, swallowing, and speaking, caused by various lesions in the extrapyramidal motor system. Signs and symptoms of parkinsonism resemble those of idiopathic Parkinson's disease and may develop during or after acute encephalitis and in syphilis, malaria, poliomyelitis, and carbon monoxide poisoning. Parkinsonism frequently occurs in patients treated with antipsychotic drugs.

Parkinson's disease {James Parkinson}, a slowly progressive, degenerative, neurological disorder characterized by resting tremor, pill rolling of the fingers, a masklike facies, shuffling gait, forward flexion of the trunk, and muscle rigidity and weakness. It is usually an idiopathic disease of persons over 60 years of age, though it may occur in younger persons, especially after acute encephalitis or carbon monoxide or metallic poisoning. Typical pathological changes are destruction of neurons in basal ganglia, loss of pigmented cells in the substantia nigra, and depletion of dopamine in the caudate nucleus, putamen, and pallidum. Signs and symptoms of Parkinson's disease, which include drooling, increased appetite, intolerance to heat, oily skin, emotional instability, and defective judgement, are increased by fatigue, excitement, and frustration. Intelligence is rarely impaired. Also called **paralysis agitans.**

paronychia, an infection of the fold of skin at the margin of a nail. Treatment includes hot compresses or soaks, antibiotics, and, possibly, surgical incision and drainage.

paroophoritis, 1. inflammation of the paroophoron. 2. inflammation of the tissues surrounding the ovary.

paroophoron, a small vestigial remnant of the mesonephros, consisting of a few rudimentary tubules lying in the broad ligament between the epoophoron and the uterus. A similar vestigial structure, the aberrant ductule, is found in the male.

parosmia, any dysfunction or perversion concerning the sense of smell.

parotid duct, a tubular canal, about 7 cm long, that extends from the anterior part of the parotid gland to the mouth.

parotid gland, one of the largest pair of salivary glands that lie at the side of the face just below and in front of the external ear. The main part of the gland is superficial, somewhat flattened and quadrilateral, and lies between the ramus of the mandible, the mastoid process, and the sternocleidomastoideus.

parotitis, inflammation or infection of one or both parotid salivary glands. See also **mumps.**

parovarian, pertaining to residual tissues in the area near the uterine tubes and the ovary.

parovarium. See **epoophoron.**

paroxysm, 1. a marked, u´sually episodic increase in symptoms. 2. a convulsion, fit, seizure, or spasm. **paroxysmal,** *adj.*

paroxysmal atrial tachycardia, a period of very rapid heart beats that begins suddenly and ends abruptly.

paroxysmal cold haemoglobinuria (PCH), a rare autoimmune disorder characterized by haemolysis and haematuria, associated with exposure to cold.

paroxysmal haemoglobinuria, the sudden passage of haemoglobin in urine, occurring after local or general exposure to low temperatures, as in paroxysmal cold haemoglobinuria.

paroxysmal labyrinthine vertigo See **Ménière's disease.**

paroxysmal nocturnal dyspnoea (PND), a disorder characterized by sudden attacks of respiratory distress, usually occurring after several hours of sleep in a reclining position, most commonly caused by pulmonary oedema resulting from congestive heart failure. The attacks are often accompanied by coughing, a feeling of suffocation, cold sweat, and tachycardia with a gallop rhythm.

paroxysmal nocturnal haemoglobinuria (PNH), a disorder characterized by intravascular haemolysis and haemoglobinuria. It occurs in irregular episodes of several days' duration, especially at night. The basic defect in the red blood cell is an unusual sensitivity to lysis by complement or a deficiency or absence of acetylcholinesterase. It is characterized by abdominal pain, back pain, and headache. Its course may be complicated by thrombotic episodes and by iron deficiency, caused by excessive loss of haemoglobin.

paroxysmal supraventricular tachycardia, an ectopic rhythm in excess of 100 per minute and usually faster than 170 per minute that begins abruptly with a premature atrial or junctional beat and is supported by an AV nodal reentry mechanism or by an AV reentry mechanism involving an accessory pathway.

parrot fever. See **psittacosis.**

parry fracture. See **Monteggia's fracture.**

pars, a part, such as the pars abdominalis oesophagi.

part, a portion of a larger area, such as the

condylar part of the occipital bone.

parthenogenesis, a type of nonsexual reproduction in which an organism develops from an unfertilized ovum, as in many lower animals. **parthenogenetic, parthenogenic,** *adj.*

partial bypass, a system of blood circulation in which the heart pumps and maintains a portion of the blood flow while the remainder of the circulation depends on mechanical means.

partial cleavage, mitotic division of only part of a fertilized ovum into blastomeres, usually the activated cytoplasmic portion surrounding the nucleus; restricted division.

partial crown, a restoration that replaces surfaces of a tooth.

partially edentulous arch, a dental arch in which one or more but not all natural teeth are missing.

partial pressure, the pressure exerted by any one gas in a mixture of gases or in a liquid, with the pressure directly related to the concentration of that gas to the total pressure of the mixture. The concentration of oxygen in the atmosphere represents approximately 21% of the total atmospheric pressure, calculated at 760 mm Hg under standard conditions. Therefore, the partial pressure of atmospheric oxygen is about 160 mm Hg (760 x 0.21).

partial pressure of carbon dioxide, the portion of total blood gas pressure exerted by carbon dioxide. The normal pressures of carbon dioxide in arterial blood are 35 to 45 mm Hg; in venous blood, 40 to 45 mm Hg.

partial pressure of oxygen, the part of total blood gas pressure exerted by oxygen gas. The normal partial pressure of oxygen in arterial blood is 95 to 100 mm Hg.

partial response, the condition in which the maximum decrease in treated tumour volume is at least 50% but less than 100%.

partial thromboplastin time (PTT), a test for detecting coagulation defects of the intrinsic system by adding activated partial thromboplastin to a sample of test plasma and to a control sample of normal plasma. The time required for the formation of a clot in test plasma is compared with that in the normal plasma. The normal PTT in plasma is 60 to 85 seconds after the addition to the plasma sample of partial thromboplastin reagent and ionized calcium.

particulate, pertaining to a minute discrete particle or fragment of a substance or material.

partograph, a graph depicting the process of labour, used to faciltate detection of dysfunctional labour.

parturition, the process of giving birth.

parulis. See **gumboil.**

PAS, PASA, abbreviation for **paraaminosalicylic acid.**

PASCAL {Blaise Pascal, French scientist, b.

1623}, a higher level computer compiler language, often used to teach programming.

Pascal's principle {Blaise Pascal}, (in physics) a law stating that a confined liquid transmits pressure applied to it from an external source equally in all directions. Pascal's principle provides the basis for all hydraulic devices.

passive, a state in which behaviour is determined by external forces.

passive-aggressive personality, a personality characterized by passivity and aggression in which forceful actions or attitudes are expressed in an indirect, nonviolent manner, such as pouting, obstructionism, procrastination, inefficiency, stubbornness, and forgetfulness.

passive-aggressive personality disorder, a disorder characterized by the indirect expression of resistance to occupational or social demands, resulting in persistent, pervasive ineffectiveness, lack of self-confidence, poor interpersonal relationships, and pessimism that can lead, in severe cases, to major depression, alcoholism, or drug dependence.

passive algolagnia. See **masochism.**

passive anaphylaxis. See **antiserum anaphylaxis.**

passive-dependent personality, a personality characterized by helplessness, indecisiveness, and a tendency to cling to and seek support from others.

passive euthanasia. See **euthanasia.**

passive exercise, repetitive movement of a part of the body as a result of an externally applied force or the voluntary effort of the muscles controlling another part of the body.

passive immunity, a form of acquired immunity resulting from antibodies that are transmitted naturally through the placenta to a fetus or through the colostrum to an infant or artificially by injection of antiserum for treatment or prophylaxis.

passive movement, the moving of parts of the body by an outside force without voluntary action or resistance by the individual.

passive play, play in which a person does not participate actively. For younger children such activity may include watching and listening to others, observing other children or animals, listening to stories, or looking at pictures.

passive recoil, the normal, quiet act of exhalation caused by the rebound effect of elastic tissue of the lungs, aided by the force of surface tension.

passive smoking, the inhalation by nonsmokers of the smoke from other people's cigarettes, pipes, and cigars.

passive stretching, stretching that involves only noncontractile elements, such as ligaments. An example is during isometric exercises in which there is no range of motion of the body part involved.

passive transfer test. See **Prausnitz-Küstner test.**

passive transport, the movement of small molecules across the membrane of a cell by diffusion. Passive transport is essential to various processes of metabolism, such as the intake of digestive products by the cells lining the intestines.

passive tremor, an involuntary trembling occurring when the person is at rest, one of the signs of Parkinson's disease.

paste, a topical semisolid formulation containing a pharmacologically active ingredient in a fatty base, a viscous or mucilaginous base, or a mixture of starch and petroleum.

Pasteurella {Louis Pasteur, French bacteriologist, b. 1822}, a genus of gram-negative bacilli or coccobacilli, including species pathogenic to humans and domestic animals. *Pasteurella* infections may be transmitted to humans by animal bites.

pasteurization {Louis Pasteur}, the process of applying heat, usually to milk or cheese, for a specified period of time for the purpose of killing or retarding the development of pathogenic bacteria. **pasteurize,** *v.*

pasteurized milk {Louis Pasteur}, milk that has been treated by heat to destroy pathogenic bacteria. By law, pasteurization requires a temperature of 72°C for not less than 20 seconds, or to a temperature of 63°C for 30 minutes, followed by immediate cooling.

pastoral counselling, counselling and support carried out by the hospital chaplaincy service.

Patau's syndrome. See **trisomy 13.**

patch, a small spot of surface tissue that differs from the surrounding area in colour or texture or both and is not elevated above it.

patch test, a skin test for identifying allergens, especially those causing contact dermatitis. The suspected substance (food, pollen, animal fur) is applied to an adhesive patch that is placed on the patient's skin. Another patch, with nothing on it, serves as a control.

patella, a flat, triangular bone at the front of the knee joint, having a pointed apex that attaches to the ligamentum patellae.

patellar ligament, the central portion of the common tendon of the quadriceps femoris. Its superficial fibres are continuous over the front of the patella with those of the tendon of the quadriceps femoris.

patellar reflex, a deep tendon reflex, elicited by a sharp tap on the tendon just distal to the patella, normally characterized by contraction of the quadriceps muscle and extension of the leg at the knee.

patellar-tendon bearing prosthesis (PTB), an ankle-foot orthosis (AFO) that provides prolonged stretch to the posterior leg musculature and may create extension force at the knee joint.

patellar-tendon bearing supracondylar socket (PTB/SC), a patellar-tendon bearing prosthesis with supracondylar (above a condyle) and suprapatellar (above the patella) suspension.

patellar-bearing supracondylar/suprapatellar socket (PTBSC/SP), a type of patellar-tendon below the knee (BK) bearing prosthesis with a socket that extends in front, medially, and laterally to accommodate both the patella and femoral condyles. The higher socket increases knee stability and a suspension strap is not required.

patent, the condition of being open and unblocked, such as a patent airway or a patent anus.

patent ductus arteriosus (PDA), an abnormal opening between the pulmonary artery and the aorta caused by failure of the fetal ductus arteriosus to close after birth. The defect, which is seen primarily in premature infants, allows blood from the aorta to flow into the pulmonary artery and to recirculate through the lungs, causing an increased workload on the left side of the heart and increased pulmonary vascular congestion and resistance.

paternal engrossment. See **bonding.**

Paterson-Kelly syndrome {Donald R. Paterson, Welsh physician, b. 1863; Adam B. Kelly, Scottish physician, b. 1865}, a condition of the digestive system associated with iron deficiency anaemia, characterized by the development of oesophageal webs in the upper oesophagus, making swallowing of solids difficult.

Paterson-Parker dosage system {James R. K. Paterson, English radiologist; H. M. Parker, 20th century American-English physicist}, a method of dosage calculation in brachytherapy to ensure a homogenous dose to the target volume.

pathogen, any microorganism capable of producing disease. **pathogenic,** *adj.*

pathogenesia, the source or cause of an illness or abnormal condition.

pathogenicity, pertaining to the ability of a pathogenic agent to produce a disease.

pathogenic occlusion, an occlusal relationship that is capable of producing pathological changes in the teeth, supporting tissues, and other components of the masticatory system.

pathognomonic, (of a sign or symptom) specific to a disease or condition, such as Koplik's spots on the buccal and lingual mucosa, which are indicative of measles.

pathognomonic symptom. See **symptom.**

pathological, pertaining to a condition that is caused by or involves a disease process.

pathological absorption, the taking up by the blood of an excretory or morbid substance.

pathological anatomy, (in applied anatomy) the study of the structure and morphology of the tissues and cells of the body as related to disease.

pathological diagnosis, a diagnosis arrived at by an examination of the substance and function of the tissues of the body, especially of the abnormal developmental changes in the tissues by histological techniques of tissue examination.

pathological fracture. See **neoplastic fracture.**

pathological mitosis, any cell division that is atypical, asymmetrical, or multipolar and results in the unequal number of chromosomes in the nuclei of the daughter cells. It is indicative of malignancy.

pathological myopia, a type of progressive nearsightedness characterized by changes in the fundus of the eye, posterior staphyloma, and deficient corrected acuity.

pathological physiology, 1. the study of the physical and chemical processes involved in the functioning of diseased tissues. **2.** the study of the modification of the normal functioning processes of an organism caused by disease.

pathological triad, the combination of three respiratory disease conditions: bronchospasm, retained secretions, and mucosal oedema.

pathologist, a doctor who specializes in the study of disease, usually in a hospital, school of medicine, or research institute or laboratory. A pathologist usually specializes in autopsy, or in clinical or surgical pathology.

pathology, the study of the characteristics, causes, and effects of disease, as observed in the structure and function of the body. **Cellular pathology** is the study of cellular changes in disease. **Clinical pathology** is the study of disease by the use of laboratory tests and methods. **pathological,** adj.

pathomimicry. See **Munchausen's syndrome.**

pathophysiology, the study of the biological and physical manifestations of disease as they correlate with the underlying abnormalities and physiological disturbances. **pathophysiological,** adj.

pathosis, a disease condition.

pathway, 1. a network of neurons that provides a transmission route for nerve impulses from any part of the body to the spinal cord and the cerebral cortex or from the central nervous system to the muscles and organs. **2.** a chain of chemical reactions that produces various compounds in critical sequence, such as the Embden-Meyerhof pathway.

patient, 1. a person who is ill and in need of medical or nursing attention. **2.** a health care recipient who is ill or hospitalized. **3.** a client in a health care service.

patient advocate, a person who acts on be-half of the patient and expresses the patient's view to the health care team. See also ombudsman.

patient care plan, a plan of care coordinated to include appropriate participation by each member of the health care team.

patient-controlled analgesia (PCA), a drug-delivery system that dispenses a pre-set IV dose of a narcotic analgesic into a patient when the patient pushes a switch on an electric cord.

patient day (P.D.), a unit in a system of accounting used by health care facilities and health care planners. Each day represents a unit of time during which the services of the institution or facility were used by a patient; thus 50 patients in a hospital for 1 day would represent 50 patient days.

patient held notes, a system of medical record keeping in which the patient has access to his medical notes.

patient interview, a systematic interview of a patient, the purpose of which is to obtain information that can be used to develop an individualized plan for care.

patient mix, 1. the distribution of demographic variables in a patient population, often represented by the percentage of a given race, age, sex, or ethnic derivation. **2.** the distribution of indications for admission in a patient population, such as surgical, maternity, or trauma.

patient record, a collection of documents that provides a record of each episode in which a patient visited or sought treatment and received care or a referral for care from a health care facility.

patient representative. See **ombudsman.**

Patient's Charter, a list of rights for patients receiving health care from the NHS. They can expect to be upheld during patient's care. They are published by the government, and endorsed by health authorities and hospital trusts.

pattern logic, (in cardiology) a feature of an intraaortic balloon pump in which the QRS complex is recognized on a width basis.

pattern theory of pain. This theory holds that the intensity of a stimulus evokes a specific pattern, which is interpreted by the brain as pain. This perception is the result of the intensity and frequency of stimulation of a nonspecific end organ. Some authorities believe that bradykinin and histamine, two chemical substances elaborated by the body, cause pain.

patulous, pertaining to something that is open or spread apart.

Paul-Bunnell test {John R. Paul, American physician, b. 1893; Walls W. Bunnell, American physician, b. 1902}, a blood test for heterophil antibodies, used for confirming a diagnosis of infectious mononucleosis.

Paul's tube {Frank T. Paul, English surgeon, b. 1851}, a large-bore glass drainage tube with a projecting rim, used in performing an enterostomy. Also called **Paul-Mixter tube.**

Pautrier microabscess {Lucien M. A. Pautrier, French dermatologist, b. 1876}, an accumulation of intensely staining mononuclear cells in the epidermis, characterizing malignant lymphoma of the skin, especially mycosis fungoides.

Pauwels' fracture {Friedrich Pauwels, 20th century German surgeon}, a fracture of the proximal femoral neck with varying degrees of angulation.

pavor, a reaction to a frightening stimulus characterized by excessive terror. Kinds of pavor are **pavor diurnus** and **pavor nocturnus.**

pavor diurnus, a sleep disorder occurring in children during daytime sleep in which they cry out in alarm and awaken in fear and panic.

pavor nocturnus, a sleep disorder occurring in children during nighttime sleep that causes them to cry out in alarm and awaken in fear and panic.

Payr's clamp {Erwin Payr, German surgeon, b. 1871}, a heavy clamp used in GI surgery.

Pawlick's grip, a method of assessing engagement of the fetal during abdominal palpation, using one hand. It can cause discomfort if not performed carefully.

Pb, symbol for **lead.**

p.c., (in prescriptions) an abbreviation for the Latin phrases *percentum* meaning *'per cent'* and *post cibum* meaning 'after food'.

PBI, abbreviation for **protein-bound iodine.**

PCB, abbreviation for **polychlorinated biphenyls.**

PCH, abbreviation for **paroxysmal cold haemoglobinuria.**

PCO$_2$, symbol for **partial pressure of carbon dioxide. See partial pressure.**

PCP, 1. abbreviation for **phencyclidine hydrochloride. 2.** abbreviation for **Pneumocystis carinii pneumonia.**

Pd, symbol for **palladium.**

PDA, abbreviation for **patent ductus arteriosus.**

peak, the highest blood level of durg reached during a drug administration cycle.

peak concentration, the maximum amount of a substance or force, such as the highest concentration of a drug measured immediately after the drug has been administered.

peak expiratory flow, the maximum flow rate achieved by an individual during forced expiration.

peak flow meter, an instrument used for measuring peak expiratory flow.

peak height velocity, a point in pubescence in which the iempo of growth is the greatest.

peak level, the highest concentration, usually in the blood, that a substance reaches during the time period under consideration, such as the highest blood glucose level attained during a glucose tolerance test.

peak logic, a feature of the intraaortic balloon pump in which any positive waveform may trigger the pump.

pearly penile papules. See **hirsutoid papilloma of the penis.**

pearly tumour. See **cholesteatoma.**

Pearson's product movement correlation {Karl Pearson, English mathematician, b. 1857}, (in statistics) a statistical test of the relationship between two variables measured in interval or ratio scales. Correlations computed fall between +1.00 and -1.00.

peau d'orange, a dimpling of the skin that gives it the appearance of the skin of an orange.

pectin, a gelatinous carbohydrate substance found in fruits and succulent vegetables and used as the setting agent for jams and jellies and as an emulsifier and stabilizer in many foods. It also adds to the diet bulk necessary for proper GI functioning.

pectineus, the most anterior of the five medial femoral muscles. It functions to flex and adduct the thigh and to rotate it medially.

pectoralis major, a large muscle of the upper chest wall that acts on the joint of the shoulder. The pectoralis major serves to flex, adduct, and medially rotate the arm in the shoulder joint.

pectoralis minor, a thin, triangular muscle of the upper chest wall beneath the pectoralis major. It functions to rotate the scapula, to draw it down and forward, and to raise the third, the fourth, and the fifth ribs in forced inspiration.

pectoriloquy, a phenomenon in which voice sounds, including whispers, are transmitted clearly through the pulmonary structures and are clearly audible through a stethoscope. It is often a sign of lung consolidation.

pectus excavatum. See **funnel chest.**

pedagogy, the art and science of teaching children, based on a belief that the purpose of education is the transmittal of knowledge.

pedicle clamp, a locking surgical forceps used for compressing blood vessels or pedicles of tumours during surgery.

pedicle flap operation, a mucogingival surgical procedure for relocating or sliding gingival tissue from a donor site to an isolated defect, usually a tooth surface denuded of attached gingiva.

pediculicide, any of a group of drugs that kill lice.

pediculosia, infestation with bloodsucking lice. **Pediculosis capitis** is infestation of the scalp with lice. **Pediculosis corporis** is infestation of the skin of the body with lice. **Pediculosis palpebrarum** is infestation of the eyelids and eyelashes with lice. **Pediculosis pubis** is infestation of the pubic hair region with lice. Infestation with lice causes intense itching, often resulting in excoriation of the skin and secondary bacterial infection.

Pediculus pubis. See **crab louse.**

pedigree, 1. line of descent; lineage; ancestry. **2.** (in genetics) a chart that shows the genetic makeup of a person's ancestors, used in the mendelian analysis of an inherited characteristic or disease in a particular family.

peduncle, a stemlike connecting part, such as the pineal peduncle or a peduncle graft. **peduncular, pedunculate,** *adj.*

PEEP, abbreviation for **positive end expiratory pressure.**

Peeping Tom. See **voyeur.**

peer, a person deemed an equal for the purpose at hand. It is usually an "age mate," or companion or associate on roughly the same level of age or mental endowment.

peer review, an appraisal by professional co-workers of equal status of the way an individual nurse or other health professional conducts practice, education, or research.

PEG, abbreviation for **percutaneous gastrostomy.**

Pel-Ebstein fever {Pieter K. Pel, Dutch physician, b. 1852; Wilhelm Ebstein, German physician, b. 1836}, a recurrent fever, occurring in cycles of several days or weeks, characteristic of Hodgkin's disease or malignant lymphoma. Also called **Murchison fever.**

Pelger-Huët anomaly {Karel Pelger, Dutch physician, b. 1885; G. J. Huet, Dutch physician, b. 1879}, an inherited disorder characterized by granulocytes with unusually coarse nuclear material and dumbbell-shaped or peanut-shaped nuclei.

pellagra, a disease resulting from a deficiency of niacin or tryptophan or a metabolic defect that interferes with the conversion of the precursor tryptophan to niacin. It is characterized by scaly dermatitis, especially of the skin exposed to the sun, glossitis, inflammation of the mucous membranes, diarrhoea, and mental disturbances, including depression, confusion, disorientation, hallucination, and delirium. Kinds of pellagra are **pellagra sine pellagra** and **typhoid pellagra. pellagrous,** *adj.*

pellagra sine pellagra, a form of pellagra in which the characteristic dermatitis is not present. See **pellagra.**

pelvic, of or pertaining to the pelvis.

pelvic axis, an imaginary curved line that passes through the centres of the various anteroposterior diameters of the pelvis.

pelvic brim, the curved top of the bones of the hip extending from the anterior superior iliac crest in front on one side around and past the sacrum to the crest on the other side. Below the brim is the pelvis.

pelvic classification, 1. a process in which the anatomical and spatial relationships of the bones of the pelvis are evaluated, usually to assess the adequacy of the pelvic structures for vaginal delivery. Caldwell-Moloy's system of classification is the one most commonly used. **2.** one of the types in a classification system of the pelvis.

pelvic diaphragm, the caudal aspect of the body wall, stretched like a hammock across the pelvic cavity and comprising the levator ani and the coccygeus muscles. It holds the abdominal contents, supports the pelvic viscera, and is pierced by the anal canal, the urethra, and the vagina.

pelvic examination, a diagnostic procedure in which the external and internal genitalia are physically examined using inspection, palpation, percussion, and auscultation.

pelvic exenteration, the surgical removal of all reproductive organs and adjacent tissues.

pelvic floor, the soft tissues enclosing the pelvic outlet.

pelvic floor exercises, a regimen of isometric exercises in which a woman executes a series of voluntary contractions of the muscles of her pelvic diaphragm and perineum in order to increase the contractility of her vaginal introitus or to improve her retention of urine. The exercise involves the familiar muscular squeezing action that is required to stop the urinary stream while voiding: that action is performed in an intensive, repetetive, and systematic way throughout each day.

pelvic inferior aperture. See **pelvic outlet.**

pelvic inflammatory disease (PID), any inflammatory condition of the female pelvic organs, especially one caused by bacterial infection. Characteristics of the condition include fever, vaginal discharge, pain in the lower abdomen, offensive uterine bleeding, pain with coitus, and tenderness or pain in the uterus, affected ovary, or uterine tube on bimanual pelvic examination. If an abscess has already developed, a soft, tender, fluid-filled mass may be palpated.

pelvic kidney. See **ptotic kidney.**

pelvic minilaparotomy, a surgical operation in which the lower abdomen is entered through a small, suprapubic incision, performed most often for tubal sterilization but also for diagnosis and treatment of eccyesis, ovarian cyst, endometriosis, and infertility. It may be performed as an alternative to laparoscopy, often on an outpatient basis.

pelvic outlet, the space surrounded by the bones of the lower portion of the true pelvis. In women, the shape and size of the pelvis vary and are of importance in childbirth. The shapes are classified by the length of the diameters as compared with each other and by the thickness of the bones.

pelvic pain, pain in the pelvis, as occurs in appendicitis, oophoritis, and endometritis. The character and onset of pelvic pain and any factors that alleviate or aggravate it are significant in making a diagnosis.

pelvic pole, the end of the axis at which the

breech of the fetus is located.

pelvic rotation, one of the five major kinematic determinants of gait, involving the alternate rotation of the pelvis to the right and the left of the central axis of the body. The usual pelvic rotation occurring at each hip joint in most healthy individuals is approximately 4 degrees to each side of the central axis. Pelvic rotation occurs during the stance phase of gait and involves a medial to lateral circular motion.

pelvic tilt, one of the five major kinematic determinants of gait that lowers the pelvis on the side of the swinging lower limb during the walking cycle. Through the action of the hip joint the pelvis tilts laterally downward, adducting the lower limb in the stance phase of gait and abducting the opposite extremity in the swing phase of gait. The knee joint of the non-weight-bearing limb flexes during its swing phase to allow the pelvic tilt, which helps minimize the vertical displacement of the centre of gravity of the body, thus conserving energy during walking.

pelvifemoral, of or pertaining to the structures of the hip joint, especially the muscles and the area around the bony pelvis and the head of the femur that make up the pelvic girdle.

pelvifemoral muscular dystrophy. See **Leyden-Moebius muscular dystrophy.**

pelvimeter, a device for measuring the diameter and capacity of the pelvis.

pelvimetry, the act or process of determining the dimensions of the bony birth canal. Kinds of pelvimetry are **clinical pelvimetry** and **x-ray pelvimetry.**

pelvis, *pl.* **pelves,** the lower portion of the trunk of the body, composed of four bones, the two innominate bones laterally and ventrally and the sacrum and coccyx posteriorly. It is divided into the greater or false pelvis and the lesser or true pelvis by an oblique plane passing through the sacrum and the pubic symphysis. The greater pelvis is the expanded portion of the cavity situated cranially and ventral to the pelvic brim. The lesser pelvis is situated distal to the pelvic brim, and its bony walls are more complete than those of the greater pelvis. The inlet and outlet of the pelvis have three important diameters, anteroposterior, oblique, and transverse. **pelvic,** *adj.*

pemoline, a central nervous system stimulant prescribed in the treatment of hyperkinesia in children.

pemphigoid, a bullous disease resembling pemphigus, distinguished by thicker walled bullae arising from erythematous macules or urticarial bases. Oral lesions are uncommon.

pemphigus, an uncommon, serious disease of the skin and mucous membranes, characterized by thin-walled bullae arising from apparently normal skin or mucous membrane. The bullae rupture easily, leaving raw patches. The person loses weight, becomes weak, and is subject to major infections.

pemphigus neonatorum, neonatal impetigo.

pendular knee jerk, an abnormal response to the patellar reflex test in which elicitation of the deep tendon reflex of the knee results in the lower leg oscillating like a pendulum instead of returning immediately to the resting position.

pendular nystagmus, an undulating involuntary movement of the eyeball.

pendulous, hanging loose or lacking proper support.

penetrance, (in genetics) a variable factor that modifies basic patterns of inheritance. It is the regularity with which an inherited trait is manifest in the person who carries the gene. **penetrant,** *adj.*

penicillamine (D-penicillamine), a chelating agent. It is prescribed to bind with and remove metals from the blood in the treatment of heavy metal (especially lead) poisoning, in cystinuria, and in Wilson's disease. It is also prescribed as a palliative in the treatment of and rheumatoid arthritis when other medications have failed.

penicillin, any one of a group of bacterial antibiotics derived from cultures of species of the fungus *Penicillium* or produced semisynthetically. Penicillins administered orally or parenterally for the treatment of bacterial infections exert their antimicrobial action by inhibiting the biosynthesis of bacterial cell wall mucopeptides during active multiplication of the organisms.

penicillin G. See **benzylpenicillin sodium.**

penicillin V. See **phenoxymethylpenicillin.**

penicilliosis, pulmonary infection caused by fungi of the genus *Penicillium.*

Penicillium, a genus of fungi, some species of which have been tentatively linked to disease in humans. Penicillin G is obtained from *Penicillium chrysogenum* and *P. notatum.*

penile cancer, a rare malignancy of the penis occurring in uncircumcised men and associated with genital herpesvirus infection and poor personal hygiene. Leukoplakia or the flat-topped papules of balanitis xerotica obliterans may be premalignant lesions, and the velvety, red, painful papules of Queyrat's erythroplasia are penile squamous cell carcinoma in situ. Cancer of the penis usually presents as a local mass or a bleeding ulcer and metastasizes early in its course.

penis, the external reproductive organ of a man, homologous with the clitoris of a woman. It is attached with ligaments to the front and sides of the pubic arch and is composed of three cylindrical masses of cavernous tissue covered with skin. The corpora cavernosa penis surround a median mass called the corpus spongiosum penis, which contains the greater part of the urethra.

penis envy, a concept of female envy of the

male penis, but generally a female wish for male attributes, position, and advantages. It is believed by some psychiatrists to be a significant factor in female personality development.

penniform, of or pertaining to the shape of a feather, especially the patterns of muscular fasciculi that correlate with the range of motion and the power of muscles.

pentaerythritol tetranitrate, a coronary vasodilator used for the relief of angina pectoris.

pentamidine isethionate, an antiprotozoal drug given by injection or inhalation in the treatment of and prophylaxis pneumonia caused by *Pneumoncystis carinii,* particularly in patients who have AIDS. It is also used in the treatment of leishmaniasis.

pentaploid. See **polyploid.**

pentazocine hydrochloride, an opiate analgesic used for the relief of moderate to severe pain.

pentazocine lactate. See **pentazocine hydrochloride.**

pentose, a monosaccharide made of carbohydrate molecules, each containing five carbon atoms. It is produced by the body and is elevated after the ingestion of certain fruits, such as plums and cherries, and in certain rare diseases.

pentosuria, a rare condition in which pentose is found in the urine. Essential or idiopathic pentosuria is caused by a genetically transmitted error of metabolism.

penumbra, 1. (in radiography) a region of sharpness around the edges of an image due to the finite size of the x-ray tube focus. **2.** (in radiotherapy) a region of low dose outside the defined radiation field due to the finite size of the x-ray focus or source.

Peplau, Hildegard E., one of the pioneers in nursing theory development and a proponent in the 1950s of the concept that nursing is an interpersonal process. Peplau wrote that the nurse-patient relationship occurs in phases during which the nurse functions as a resource person, a counsellor, and a surrogate. The four phases of the process were listed as orientation, identification, exploitation, and resolution.

Pepper syndrome {William Pepper, American physician, b. 1874}, a neuroblastoma of the adrenal glands that usually metastasizes to the liver.

pep pills, *slang.* amphetamines.

pepsin, an enzyme secreted in the stomach that catalyses the hydrolysis of protein. Preparations of pepsin obtained from pork and beef stomachs are sometimes used as digestive aids.

pepsinogen, a zymogenic substance secreted by pyloric and gastric chief cells and converted to the enzyme pepsin in an acidic environment, as in the presence of hydrochloric acid produced in the stomach.

peptic, of or pertaining to digestion or to the enzymes and secretions essential to digestion.

peptic ulcer, a sharply circumscribed loss of the mucous membrane of the stomach or duodenum or of any other part of the GI system exposed to gastric juices containing acid and pepsin. Peptic ulcers may be acute or chronic. Acute lesions are almost always multiple and superficial. They may be totally asymptomatic and usually heal without scarring or other sequelae. Chronic ulcers are true ulcers: They are deep, single, persistent, and symptomatic; the muscular coat of the wall of the organ does not regenerate; a scar forms, marking the site, and the mucosa may heal completely. Peptic ulcers are caused by a combination of poorly understood factors, including excessive secretion of gastric acid, inadequate protection of the mucous membrane, stress, heredity, and the taking of certain drugs, including the corticosteroids, certain antihypertensives, and antiinflammatory medications. Characteristically, ulcers cause a gnawing pain in the epigastrium that does not radiate to the back, is not aggravated by a change in position, and has a temporal pattern that mimics the diurnal rhythm of gastric acidity.

peptide, a molecular chain compound composed of two or more amino acids joined by peptide bonds. See also **amino acid, polypeptide, protein.**

peptone, a derived protein, which may be produced by hydrolysis of a native protein with an acid or enzyme.

peracephalus, *pl.* **peracephali,** a fetus or individual with a malformed head.

perceived severity, (in health belief model) a person's perception of the seriousness of the consequences of contracting a disease.

perceived susceptibility, (in health belief model) a person's perception of the likelihood of contracting a disease.

percentage depth dose, (in radiotherapy) the amount of radiation delivered at a specified depth in skin tissue, usually expressed as a percentage of the maximum dose.

percent solution, a relationship of a solute to a solvent, expressed in terms of weight of solute per weight of solution. An example of a true percent solution is 5 g of glucose dissolved in 95 g of water, forming 100 g of solution.

percent systole, an amount of time of each heartbeat that is devoted to the ejection of blood from the ventricle.

percept, the mental impression of an object that is perceived through the use of the senses.

perception, 1. the conscious recognition and interpretation of sensory stimuli through unconscious associations, especially memory. **2.** the end result or product of the act of perceiving. Kinds of perception include

depth perception, extrasensory perception, facial perception, and **stereognostic perception. perceptive, perceptual,** *adj.*

perceptivity, the ability to receive sense impressions; perceptiveness.

perceptual constancy, in Gestalt psychology, the phenomenon in which an object is seen in the same way under varying circumstances.

perceptual defect, any of a broad group of disorders or dysfunctions of the central nervous system that interfere with the conscious mental recognition of sensory stimuli. Such conditions are caused by lesions at specific sites in the cerebral cortex that may result from any illness or trauma affecting the brain at any age or stage of development.

perceptual deprivation, the absence of or decrease in meaningful groupings of stimuli, which may result from a constant background noise or constant inadequate illumination.

perceptual monotony, a mental state characterized by a lack of variety in the normal pattern of everyday stimuli.

perceptual-motor, pertaining to the interaction of the various channels of perception, including visual, auditory, tactual, and kinaesthetic channels with motor activity.

perceptual-motor match, the process of comparing and collating the input data received through the motor system and through perception.

perchloromethane. See **carbon tetrachloride.**

percolation, 1. the act of filtering any liquid through a porous medium. **2.** (in pharmacology) the removal of the soluble parts of a crude drug by passing a liquid solvent through it.

percussion, a technique in physical examination used to evaluate the size, borders, and consistency of some of the internal organs and to discover the presence and evaluate the amount of fluid in a cavity of the body. **Immediate** or **direct percussion** refers to percussion performed by striking the fingers directly on the body surface; **indirect, mediate,** or **finger percussion** involves striking a finger of one hand on a finger of the other hand as it is placed over the organ. **percuss,** *v.,* **percussable,** *adj.*

percussor, a small, hammerlike diagnostic tool having a rubber head that is used to tap the body lightly in percussion. Also called **plexor.**

percutaneous, performed through the skin, such as a biopsy or the aspiration of fluid from a space below the skin using a needle, catheter, and syringe or the instillation of a fluid in a cavity or space by similar means.

percutaneous absorption, the process of absorption through the skin from topical application.

percutaneous catheter placement, (in arteriography) the technique in which an intracatheter is introduced through the skin into an artery and placed at the site or structure to be studied.

percutaneous endoscopic gastrostomy, a method of placing a gastrostomy tube. An endoscope is passed into the stomach, a small incision made, a guidewire inserted through it and taken up out of the mouth by the endoscope. The PEG tube is passed over the guidewire down into the stomach and partly back out of the incision.

percutaneous nephrolithotomy, a uroradiological procedure performed to extract stones from within the kidney or proximal ureter by percutaneous surgery after the stones have been visualized radiographically.

percutaneous nephroscope, a thin fiberoptics probe that can be inserted into the kidney through an incision in the skin. The device is equipped with a tool that can be used to grasp and remove small stones.

percutaneous transhepatic cholangiography (PCT). See **cholangiography.**

percutaneous transluminal coronary angioplasty (PTCA), a technique in the treatment of atherosclerotic coronary heart disease and angina pectoris in which some plaques in the arteries of the heart are flattened against the arterial walls, resulting in improved circulation. The procedure involves threading a catheter through the vessel to the atherosclerotic plaque and inflating and deflating a small balloon at the tip of the catheter several times, then removing the catheter. The procedure is performed under x-ray or ultrasonic visualization.

Perez reflex {Bernard Perez, French physician, b. 1836}, the normal response of an infant to cry, flex the limbs, and elevate the head and pelvis when supported in a prone position with a finger pressed along the spine from the sacrum to the neck.

perfluorocarbons, a group of chemicals somewhat capable of performing the function of haemoglobin in red blood cells by transporting oxygen through the circulatory system. They can be used for certain blood substitute purposes, regardless of the blood type of the patient.

perforate, 1. to pierce, punch, puncture, or otherwise make a hole. **2.** riddled with small holes. **3.** (of the anus) having a normal opening; not imperforate. **perforation,** *n.*

perforating fracture, an open fracture caused by a projectile, making a small surface wound.

perforation of the uterus, an accidental puncture of the uterus, as may occur with a curette or by an intrauterine contraceptive device.

perfusion, 1. the passage of a fluid through a specific organ or an area of the body. **2.** a therapeutic measure whereby a drug intended for an isolated part of the body is introduced via the bloodstream.

perfusion lung scan, (in radionuclide imaging) an imaging technique to evaluate the perfusion of the lungs using radio-labelled albumin particles injected intravenously and a gamma camera. Usually preceded by a **ventilation lung scan.**

perfusion rate, the rate of blood flow through the capillaries per unit mass of tissue, expressed in ml/minute per 100 g.

perfusion scan. See **perfusion lung scan.**

per gene, a segment of nucleic acid that is associated with circadian rhythms of some animal species. A similar DNA sequence occurs in human genes, but it is not known if it affects human circadian rhythms.

perianal abscess, a focal, purulent, subcutaneous infection in the region of the anus. Treatment includes hot soaks, antibiotics, and, possibly, incision and drainage.

periapical, of or pertaining to the tissues around the apex of a tooth, including the periodontal membrane and the alveolar bone.

periapical abscess, an infection around the root of a tooth, usually a result of spread from dental caries.

periapical cyst. See **radicular cyst.**

periapical fibroma, a mass of benign connective tissue that may form at the apex of a tooth with normal pulp.

periapical infection, infection surrounding the root of a tooth, often accompanied by toothache.

periarteritis, an inflammatory condition of the outer coat of one or more arteries and the tissue surrounding the vessel. Kinds of periarteritis are **periarteritis nodosa** and **syphilitic periarteritis.**

periarteritis gummosa. See **syphilitic periarteritis.**

periarteritis nodosa, a progressive, polymorphic disease of the connective tissue that is characterized by numerous large and palpable or visible nodules in clusters along segments of middle-sized arteries, particularly near points of bifurcation. This process causes occlusion of the vessel, resulting in regional ischaemia, haemorrhage, necrosis, and pain. The early signs of the disease include tachycardia, fever, weight loss, and pain in the viscera.

pericardial artery, one of several small vessels branching from the thoracic aorta, supplying the dorsal surface of the pericardium.

pericardial tamponade. See **cardiac tamponade.**

pericardiocentesis, a procedure for drawing fluid in the pericardial space between the serous membranes by surgical puncture and aspiration of the pericardial sac.

pericarditis, an inflammation of the pericardium associated with trauma, malignant neoplastic disease, infection, uraemia, myocardial infarction, collagen disease, or idiopathic causes. Two stages are observed. The first stage is characterized by fever, substernal chest pain that radiates to the shoulder or neck, dyspnoea, and a dry, nonproductive cough. On examination a rapid and forcible pulse, a pericardial friction rub, and a muffled heartbeat over the apex are noted. The patient becomes increasingly anxious, tired, and orthopnoeic. During the second stage, a serofibrinous effusion develops within the pericardium, restricting cardiac activity; the heart sounds become muffled, weak, and distant on auscultation. A bulge is visible on the chest over the precordial area. If the effusion is caused by bacterial infection, a high fever, sweat, chills, and prostration also occur.

pericardium, *pl.* **pericardia,** a fibroserous sac that surrounds the heart and the roots of the great vessels. It consists of the serous pericardium and the fibrous pericardium. Between the layers is the pericardial space containing a few drops of pericardial fluid, which lubricates opposing surfaces of the space and allows the heart to move easily during contraction. The fibrous pericardium, which constitutes the outermost sac and is composed of tough, white fibrous tissue lined by the parietal layer of the serous pericardium, fits loosely around the heart and attaches to large blood vessels emerging from the top of the heart but not to the heart itself. pericardial, *adj.*

pericholangitis, an inflammatory condition of the tissues surrounding the bile ducts in the liver. Pericholangitis is a complication of ulcerative colitis and is characterized by a recurrent fever, chills, jaundice, and, possibly, portal hypertension.

pericoronitis, an inflammation of the gingival flap (gum tissue) around the crown of a tooth, usually associated with the eruption of a third molar.

peridural anaesthesia. See **epidural anaesthesia.**

perifolliculitis, inflammation of the tissue surrounding a hair follicle. Compare **folliculitis.**

perikaryon, the cytoplasm of a cell body exclusive of the nucleus and any processes, specifically the cell body of a neuron. **perikaryontic,** *adj.*

perilymph, the clear fluid separating the osseous labyrinth from the membranous labyrinth in the internal ear. Compare **endolymph.**

perimetrium the serous membrane enveloping the uterus.

perinatal, around the time of birth.

perinatal asphyxia. See **asphyxia neonatorum.**

perinatal death, 1. the death of a fetus weighing more than 1000 g at 28 or more weeks of gestation. **2.** the death of an infant between birth and the end of the neonatal period.

perinatal mortality rate, the number of stillbirths and deaths in the first week of life per 1000 total births.

perinatal period, a period extending approximately from the twenty-eighth week of gestation to the twenty-eighth day after birth.

perineal care, a cleansing procedure prescribed for cleansing the perineum after various obstetric and gynaecological procedures. Sterile or clean perineal care may be prescribed.

perineometer, a vaginal pressure gauge used to asess the progress of muscle strength.

perineorrhaphy, a surgical procedure in which an incision, tear, or defect in the perineum is repaired by suturing.

perineotomy, a surgical incision into the perineum.

perineum, the part of the body situated dorsal to the pubic arch and the arcuate ligaments, ventral to the tip of the coccyx, and lateral to the inferior rami of the pubis and the ischium and the sacrotuberous ligaments. The perineum supports and surrounds the distal portions of the urogenital and GI tracts of the body. **perineal,** *adj.*

perinodal fibres, the atrial fibres surrounding the sinoatrial node.

period, *nontechnical.* menses.

periodic, (of an event or phenomenon) recurring at regular or irregular intervals. **periodicity,** *n.*

periodic apnoea of the newborn, a normal condition in the full-term newborn infant characterized by an irregular pattern of rapid breathing followed by a brief period of apnoea, usually associated with rapid eye movement (REM) sleep.

periodic breathing. See **Cheyne-Stokes respiration.**

periodic deep inspiration, (in respiratory therapy) periodic deep forced inspiration of compressed gas or air in controlled ventilation.

periodic hyperinflation, a normal phenomenon of an unconscious sighing or deep breathing. Because of the natural need for periodic hyperinflation of the lungs, an artificial sigh is often programmed into the mechanism of mechanical ventilators.

periodontal, of or pertaining to the area around a tooth, such as the peridontium.

periodontal cyst, an epithelium-lined sac that contains fluid, most often occurring at the apex of a pulp-involved tooth. Periodontal cysts that occur lateral to a tooth root are less common.

periodontal disease, disease of the tissues around a tooth, such as an inflammation of the periodontal membrane or periodontal ligament.

periodontal ligament (PDL), the fibrous tissue that attaches the teeth to the alveoli, composed of many bundles of collagenous tissue arranged in groups between which is loose connective tissue interwoven with blood vessels, lymph vessels, and nerves. It invests and supports the teeth.

periodontics, a branch of dentistry concerned with the diagnosis, treatment, and prevention of diseases of the periodontium. Also called **periodontia. periodontic, periodontal,** *adj.*

periodontist, a dentist who specializes in periodontics.

periodontitis, inflammation of the periodontium, which includes the periodontal ligament, the gingiva, and the alveolar bone.

periodontoclasia, the loosening of permanent teeth.

periodontosis, a rare disease that affects young people, especially women, and is characterized by idiopathic destruction of the periodontium.

periorbita, the periosteum of the orbit of the eye. It is continuous with the dura mater and the sheath of the optic nerve.

periorbital, pertaining to the area surrounding the socket of the eye.

periosteum, a fibrous vascular membrane covering the bones, except at their extremities. It consists of an outer layer of collagenous tissue containing a few fat cells and an inner layer of fine elastic fibres. Periosteum is permeated with the nerves and blood vessels that innervate and nourish underlying bone. The membrane is thick and markedly vascular over young bones but thinner and less vascular in late life.

periostitis, inflammation of the periosteum. The condition is caused by chronic or acute infection or trauma and is characterized by tenderness and swelling of the bone affected, pain, fever, and chills.

peripheral, of or pertaining to the outside, surface, or surrounding area of an organ or other structure.

peripheral acrocyanosis of the newborn, a normal, transient condition of the newborn, characterized by pale cyanotic discolouration of the hands and feet, especially the fingers and toes.

peripheral arteriovenography, a radiographic technique to visualize the peripheral arties or veins following the introduction of a radiopaque contrast medium into selected blood vessels.

peripheral device, any hardware device aside from the central processing unit, such as a printer, CRT, or drive.

peripheral embolic phenomena, the clinical signs and symptoms of an embolus in a peripheral vessel.

peripheral glioma. See **schwannoma.**

peripheral nervous system, the motor and sensory nerves and ganglia outside the brain and spinal cord. The system consists of 12 pairs of cranial nerves, 31 pairs of spinal nerves, and their various branches in body organs. Sensory, or afferent, peripheral nerves transmitting information to the central nervous system and motor, or efferent, peripheral nerves carrying impulses from the brain usually travel together but separate at the cord level into a posterior sensory root and an anterior motor root. Fibres innervating the body wall are designated somatic; those supplying internal organs are termed visceral. Nerves in the sympathetic division cause peripheral vasoconstriction, cardiac acceleration, coronary artery dilatation, bronchodilatation, and inhibition of peristalsis. Parasympathetic nerves cause peripheral vasodilatation, cardiac inhibition, and bronchoconstriction, and stimulate peristalsis.

peripheral neuropathy, any functional or organic disorder of the peripheral nervous system. A kind of peripheral neuropathy is paraesthesia.

peripheral odontogenic fibroma, a fibrous connective tissue tumour associated with the gingival margin and believed to originate from the periodontium.

peripheral plasma cell myeloma. See **plasmacytoma.**

peripheral polyneuritis, peripheral polyneuropathy. See **multiple peripheral neuritis.**

peripheral resistance, a resistance to the flow of blood that is determined by the tone of the vascular musculature and the diameter of the blood vessels.

peripheral vascular disease, any abnormal condition that affects the blood vessels outside the heart and the lymphatic vessels. Different kinds and degrees of peripheral vascular disease are characterized by a variety of signs and symptoms, such as numbness, pain, pallor, elevated blood pressure, and impaired arterial pulsations. Various causative factors include obesity, cigarette smoking, stress, sedentary occupations, and numerous metabolic disorders. Some kinds of peripheral vascular disease are **arteriosclerosis** and **atherosclerosis.**

peripheral vision, a capacity to see objects that reflect light waves falling on areas of the retina distant from the macula.

peristalsis, the coordinated, rhythmic, serial contraction of smooth muscle that forces food through the digestive tract, bile through the bile duct, and urine through the ureters.

peristomal, pertaining to the area of skin surrounding a stoma, or surgically created opening in the abdominal wall.

peritoneal cavity, the potential space between the parietal and the visceral layers of the peritoneum.

peritoneal dialysis, a dialysis procedure performed to correct an imbalance of fluid or of electrolytes in the blood or to remove toxins, drugs, or other wastes normally excreted by the kidney. The peritoneum is used as a diffusible membrane. Under local anaesthesia, a many-eyed catheter is sutured in place and is connected to the inflow and outflow tubing with a "Y" connector. The dialysate is introduced through the catheter into the peritoneal cavity. The dialysate remains in the peritoneal cavity; by means of osmosis, diffusion, and filtration, the needed electrolytes pass to the bloodstream via the vascular peritoneum to the blood vessels of the abdominal cavity, and the waste products pass from the blood vessels through the vascular peritoneum into the dialysate. During outflow, the dialysate is allowed to drain from the peritoneal cavity by gravity.

peritoneal dialysis solution, a solution of electrolytes and other substances that is introduced into the peritoneum to remove toxic substances from the body.

peritoneal fluid, a naturally produced fluid in the abdominal cavity that lubricates surfaces, thereby preventing friction between the peritoneal membrane and internal organs.

peritoneoscope. See **laparoscope.**

peritoneum, an extensive serous membrane that covers the entire abdominal wall of the body and is reflected over the contained viscera. It is divided into the parietal peritoneum and the visceral peritoneum. In men, the peritoneum is a closed membranous sac. The free surface of the peritoneum is smooth mesothelium, lubricated by serous fluid that permits the viscera to glide easily against the abdominal wall and against one another. The mesentery of the peritoneum fans out from the main membrane to suspend the small intestine. Other parts of the peritoneum are the transverse mesocolon, the greater omentum, and the lesser omentum. **peritoneal,** *adj.*

peritonitis, an inflammation of the peritoneum produced by bacteria or irritating substances introduced into the abdominal cavity by a penetrating wound or perforation of an organ in the GI tract or the reproductive tract. Peritonitis is caused most commonly by rupture of the vermiform appendix but also occurs after perforations of intestinal diverticula, peptic ulcers, gangrenous gallbladders, gangrenous obstructions of the small bowel, or incarcerated hernias, as well as ruptures of the spleen, liver, ovarian cyst, or uterine tube, especially in ectopic pregnancy. Characteristic signs and symptoms of peritonitis include abdominal distention, rigidity and pain, rebound tenderness, decreased or absent bowel sounds, nausea, vomiting, and tachycardia. The patient has chills and fever, rapid and shallow breathing, is anxious, dehydrated, unable to defaecate, and may vomit faecal material.

Leukocytosis, an electrolyte imbalance, and hypovolaemia are usually present, and shock and heart failure may ensue.

peritonsillar abscess, an infection of tissue between the tonsil and pharynx, usually after acute follicular tonsillitis. The symptoms include dysphagia, pain radiating to the ear, and fever. Redness and swelling of the tonsil and adjacent soft palate are present.

periungual, of or pertaining to the area around the fingernails or the toenails.

perivascular goitre, an enlargement of the thyroid gland surrounding a large blood vessel.

perivitelline, surrounding the vitellus or yolk mass.

perivitelline space, the space between the ovum and the zona pellucida of mammals into which the polar bodies are released at the time of maturation.

perleche. See **cheilosis.**

permanent dentition, the eruption of the 32 permanent teeth, beginning with the appearance of the first permanent molars at about 6 years of age. The process is completed by 12 or 13 years of age except for the four wisdom teeth, which usually do not erupt until 18 to 25 years, or later.

permanent tooth, one of the set of 32 teeth that appear during and after childhood and usually last until old age. In each jaw they include four incisors, two canines, four premolars, and six molars. They replace the 20 deciduous teeth of infancy. The permanent teeth start to develop in the ninth week of fetal life with the thickening of the epithelium along the line of the future jaw. They erupt first in the lower jaw; the first molars in about the sixth year; the two central incisors about the seventh year; the two lateral incisors about the eighth year; the first premolars about the ninth year; the second premolars about the tenth year; the canines between the eleventh and the twelfth years; the second molars between the twelfth and the thirteenth years; the third molars between the seventeenth and the twenty-fifth years.

permeable, a condition of being pervious so that fluids and certain other substances can pass through, such as a permeable membrane.

permethrin, a topical paraciticide used for the treatment of pediculosis and scabies.

pernicious anaemia, a progressive, megaloblastic, macrocytic anaemia, affecting mainly older people, that results from a lack of intrinsic factor essential for the absorption of cyanocobalamin. The maturation of red blood cells in bone marrow becomes disordered, the osterior and lateral columns of the spinal cord deteriorate, and the white blood cell count is reduced. Extreme weakness, numbness and tingling in the extremities, fever, pallor, anorexia, and loss of weight may occur.

pernio. See **chilblain.**

perobrachius, a fetus or individual with deformed arms.

perochirus, a fetus or individual with malformed hands.

perocormus. See **perosomus.**

perodactylus, a fetus or an individual with a deformity of the fingers or the toes, especially the absence of one or more digits.

perodactyly, a congenital anomaly characterized by a deformity of the digits, primarily the complete or partial absence of one or more of the fingers or toes.

peromelia, a congenital anomaly characterized by the malformation of one or more of the limbs. Also called **peromely. peromelus,** *n.*

peroneal, of or pertaining to the outer part of the leg, over the fibula and the peroneal nerve.

peroneal muscular atrophy, an abnormal condition characterized by the symmetrical weakening or atrophy of the foot and the ankle muscles and by hammertoes. Affected individuals may have high plantar arches and an awkward gait, caused by weak ankle muscles.

peroneus brevis, the smaller of the two lateral muscles of the leg, lying under the peroneus longus. It pronates and plantar flexes the foot.

peroneus longus, the more superficial of the two lateral muscles of the leg. The muscle pronates and plantar flexes the foot.

peronia, a congenital malformation or developmental anomaly.

peropus, a fetus or individual with malformed feet, often in association with some defect of the legs.

perosomus, a fetus or individual whose body, especially the trunk, is severely malformed.

perosplanchnia, a congenital anomaly characterized by the malformation of the viscera.

peroxide. See **hydrogen peroxide.**

perphenazine, a dopamine antagonist used in the treatment of psychotic disorders and in the control of severe nausea and vomiting in adults.

PERRLA, abbreviation for *pupils equal, round, react to light, accommodation.* In the process of performing an assessment of the eyes, the size and shape of the pupils, their reaction to light, and their ability to accommodate are evaluated. If all findings are normal, the acronym is noted in the account of the physical examination.

per se, by itself, or of itself.

perseveration, the involuntary and pathological persistence of an idea or response.

persistent cloaca, a congenital anomaly in which the intestinal, urinary, and reproductive ducts open into a common cavity resulting from the failure of the urorectal septum to form during prenatal development. Also called **congenital cloaca.**

persona, *pl.* **personae,** (in analytical psychology) the personality façade or role that a person assumes and presents to the outer world to satisfy the demands of the environment or society or as an expression of some intrapsychic conflict.

personal and social history, (in a health history) an account of the personal and social details of a person's life that serve to identify the person. Place of birth, religion, race, marital status, number of children, occupational history, and place of residence are the usual components of this part of the history.

personal construct theory, an approach to psychology originated by George Kelly in the mid 1950s. It studies the ways in which individuals construe themselves, significant others and their environment. These 'constructs' can be studied and tested by the individual alone or with a therapist in order to understand internal processes, structures and events as well as relationships.

personality, 1. the composite of the behavioural traits and attitudinal characteristics by which one is recognized as an individual. **2.** the pattern of behaviour each person evolves, both consciously and unconsciously, as a means of adapting to a particular environment and its cultural, ethnic, national, and provincial standards.

personality disorder, any of a large group of mental disorders characterized by rigid, inflexible, and maladaptive behaviour patterns that impair a person's ability to function in society by severely limiting adaptive potential. Some kinds of personality disorders are **antisocial personality disorder, histrionic personality disorder, paranoid personality disorder, passive-aggressive personality disorder,** and **schizoid personality disorder.**

personality test, any of a variety of standardized tests used in the evaluation or assessment of various facets of personality structure, emotional status, and behavioural traits.

personal orientation, 1. a continually evolving process in which a person determines and evaluates the relationships that appear to exist between the person and other people. **2.** the assessment derived by a person regarding those relationships.

personal set, the sensory apparatus, beliefs, and patterned operations that a professional brings to the relationship with a patient.

personal space, the area surrounding an individual that is perceived as private by the individual, who may regard a movement into the space by another person as intrusive. Personal space boundaries vary somewhat in different cultures, but in Western cultures it is generally regarded as a distance of 1 m around the individual.

personal unconscious, (in analytical psychology) the thoughts, ideas, emotions, and other mental phenomena acquired and repressed during one's lifetime.

personal zone, an individual protective zone in which the boundaries may contract or expand according to contextual characteristics between distances of about 30cm to 1 metre.

person year, a statistical measure, representing one person at risk of developing a disease during a period of 1 year.

perspiration, 1. the act or process of perspiring; the excretion of fluid by the sweat glands through pores in the skin. **2.** the fluid excreted by the sweat glands. It consists of water containing sodium chloride, phosphate, urea, ammonia, and other waste products. Perspiration serves as a mechanism for excretion and for regulating body temperature. Kinds of perspiration are **insensible perspiration** and **sensible perspiration.**

Perthes' disease {Georg C. Perthes, German surgeon, b. 1869}, osteochondrosis of the head of the femur in children, characterized initially by epiphyseal necrosis or degeneration followed by regeneration or recalcification.

pertussis, an acute, highly contagious respiratory disease, popularly called "whooping cough", characterized by paroxysmal coughing that ends in a loud whooping inspiration. It occurs primarily in infants and in children less than 4 years of age who have not been immunized. The causative organism, *Bordetella pertussis,* is a small, nonmotile, gram-negative coccobacillus. A similar organism, *B. parapertussis,* causes a less severe form of the disease called parapertussis.

pertussis immune globulin, a passive immunizing agent prescribed for immunization against whooping cough.

pertussis vaccine, a killed vaccine used for active immunization against whooping cough when the administration of the combined diphtheria, pertussis, and tetanus vaccine is contraindicated.

pervasive developmental disorder, any of certain disorders of infancy and childhood that are characterized by severe impairment of relatedness and behavioural aberrations previously identified as childhood psychoses. The group of disorders includes infantile autism, childhood schizophrenia, and symbiotic psychosis.

perversion, 1. any deviation from what is considered normal or natural. **2.** the act of causing a change from what is normal or natural. **3.** *informal.* (in psychiatry) any of a number of sexual practices that deviate from what is considered normal adult behavior.

pervert, 1. *informal.* a person whose sexual pleasure is derived from stimuli almost universally regarded as unnatural, such as a fetishist or sadomasochist; a paraphiliac. **2.** one whose sexual behaviour deviates from a social or statistical norm but is not necessarily pathological.

pes, *pl.* **pedes,** the foot or a footlike structure.

pes cavus, a deformity of the foot characterized by an excessively high arch with hyperextension of the toes at the metatarsophalangeal joints, flexion at the interphalangeal joints, and shortening of the Achilles tendon. The condition may be present at birth or appear later because of contractures or an imbalance of the muscles of the foot, as in neuromuscular diseases such as Friedreich's ataxia or peroneal muscular atrophy.

pes planus, an abnormal but relatively common condition characterized by the flattening out of the arch of the foot.

pessary, 1. a solid dose form with a soluble or easily melted base incorporating medication and administered vaginally for local or occasionally, systemic effect. **2.** a device inserted in the vagina to treat uterine prolapse, uterine retroversion, or cervical incompetence. It is employed in the treatment of women whose advanced age or poor general condition precludes procedures required for surgical repair. Pessaries are also used in younger women in evaluating symptomatic uterine retroversion. A **doughnut pessary** is a permanently inflated flexible rubber doughnut that is inserted to support the uterus by blocking the canal of the vagina. An **inflatable pessary** is a collapsible rubber doughnut to which is attached a flexible stem containing a rubber valve. The pessary is inserted collapsed, inflated with a bulb similar to that of a sphygmomanometer, and deflated for removal. A **Bee cell pessary** is a soft rubber cube; in each face of the cube is a conical depression that acts as a suction cup when the pessary is in the vagina. A **diaphragm pessary** is a contraceptive diaphragm used for uterovaginal support. A **stem pessary** is a slim curved rod that is fitted into the cervical canal for uterine positioning.

pessimism, the inclination to anticipate the worst possible results from any action or situation or to emphasize unfavorable conditions, even when progress or gain might reasonably be expected. **pessimist,** *n.*

pesticide poisoning, a toxic condition caused by the ingestion or inhalation of a substance used for the eradication of pests. Kinds of pesticide poisoning include **malathion poisoning** and **parathion poisoning.**

pestis. See **bubonic plague.**

PET, abbreviation for **positron emission tomography.**

petaling, a process of smoothing the raw or ragged edges of a plaster cast to prevent skin irritation.

petechiae, *sing.* **petechia,** tiny purple or red spots that appear on the skin as a result of minute haemorrhages within the dermal or submucosal layers. **petechial,** *adj.*

petechial fever, any febrile illness accompanied by small petechiae on the skin, as seen in the late stage of typhoid fever.

pethidine, an opiate analgesic used to treat moderate to severe pain and as preoperative medication to relieve pain and allay anxiety. It is often used to help alleviate labour pain.

petit mal seizure, an epileptic seizure characterized by a sudden, momentary loss of consciousness occasionally accompanied by minor myoclonus of the neck or upper extremities, slight symmetric twitching of the face, or a loss of muscle tone. The seizures usually occur many times a day without a warning aura. The patient experiencing a typical seizure has a vacant facial expression and ceases all voluntary motor activity; with the rapid return of consciousness, the patient may resume conversation at the point of interruption without realizing what occurred.

petit pas gait, a manner of walking with short, mincing steps and shuffling with loss of associated movements. It is seen in cases of parkinsonism as well as in patients with diffuse cerebral disease resulting from multiple small infarcts.

Petren's gait, a hesitant form of walking in which a patient takes a few steps, halts, and then continues to take a few more steps. In some cases, the patient must be encouraged to begin the next brief period of walking. The condition is seen in elderly persons and those with parietal disease.

petrification, the process of becoming calcified or stonelike.

pétrissage, a technique in massage in which the skin is gently lifted and squeezed. Pétrissage promotes circulation and relaxes the muscles.

petrolatum, a purified mixture of semisolid hydrocarbons obtained from petroleum and commonly used as an ointment base or skin emollient.

petroleum gauze, absorbent gauze permeated with white petrolatum.

petroleum distillate poisoning, a toxic condition caused by the ingestion or inhalation of a petroleum distillate, such as fuel oil, lubricating oil, and various solvents. Nausea, vomiting, chest pain, dizziness, and severe depression of the central nervous system characterize the condition. Severe or fatal pneumonitis may occur if the substance is aspirated.

petrosphenoidal fissure, a fissure on the floor of the cranial fossa between the posterior edge of the great wing of the sphenoid bone and the petrous part of the temporal bone.

Peutz-Jeghers syndrome, an inherited disorder, transmitted as an autosomal dominant trait, characterized by multiple intestinal polyps, and abnormal mucocutaneous pigmentation, usually over the lips and buccal mucosa.

Peyer's patches. See **intestinal tonsil.**

peyote, 1. a cactus from which a hallucinogenic drug, mescaline, is derived. 2. mescaline.

Peyronie's disease {Francois de la Peyronie, French physician, b. 1678}, a disease of unknown cause resulting in fibrous induration of the corpora cavernosa of the penis. The chief symptom of Peyronie's disease is painful erection.

PGI2, abbreviation for **prostacyclin.**

pH, abbreviation for **potential hydrogen,** a scale representing the relative acidity (or alkalinity) of a solution, in which a value 7.0 is neutral, below 7.0 is acid, and above 7.0 is alkaline. The numeric pH value is equal to the negative log of the hydrogen ion concentration expressed in moles per litre.

Ph1c, symbol for **Philadelphia chromosome.**

PHA, abbreviation for **phytohaemagglutinin.**

phacomalacia, an abnormal condition of the eye in which the lens of the eye becomes soft because of the presence of a soft cataract.

phacomatosis. See **phakomatosis.**

phaeochromocytoma, *pl.* **phaeochromocytomas, phaeochromocytomata,** a vascular tumour of chromaffin tissue of the adrenal medulla or sympathetic paraganglia, characterized by hypersecretion of adrenaline and noradrenaline, causing persistent or intermittent hypertension. Typical signs include headache, palpitation, sweating, nervousness, hyperglycaemia, nausea, vomiting, and syncope. There may be weight loss, myocarditis, cardiac arrhythmia, and heart failure. The tumour occurs most frequently in young people, and only a small percentage of the lesions are malignant.

phage. See **bacteriophage.**

phage typing, the identification of bacteria by testing their vulnerability to bacterial viruses.

phagocyte, a cell that is able to surround, engulf, and digest microorganisms and cellular debris. **Fixed phagocytes,** which do not circulate, include the fixed macrophages and the cells of the reticuloendothelial system. **Free phagocytes,** which circulate in the bloodstream, include the leukocytes and the free macrophages. **phagocytic,** *adj.*

phagocytosis, the process by which certain cells engulf and dispose of microorganisms and cell debris.

phakomatosis, *pl.* **phakomatoses,** (in ophthalmology) any of several hereditary syndromes characterized by benign tumourlike nodules of the eye, skin, and brain. The four disorders designated phakomatoses are neurofibromatosis (Recklinghausen's disease), tuberous sclerosis (Bourneville's disease), encephalotrigeminal angiomatosis (Sturge-Weber syndrome), and cerebroretinal angiomatosis (von Hippel-Lindau disease). Also spelled **phacomatosis.**

phalanx, *pl.* **phalanges,** any one of the 14 tapering bones composing the fingers of each hand and the toes of each foot. They are arranged in three rows at the distal end of the metacarpus and the metatarsus. The fingers each have three phalanges; the thumb has two. The toes each have three phalanges; the great toe has two.

phallic stage, (in psychoanalysis) the period in psychosexual development occurring between 3 and 6 years of age when emerging awareness and self-manipulation of the genitals are the predominant source of pleasurable experience.

phalloidine, a poison present in the mushroom *Amanita phalloides.* Ingestion of phalloidine results in bloody diarrhoea, vomiting, severe abdominal pain, kidney failure, and liver damage. Also spelled **phalloidin.**

phallus. See **penis.**

phantom (in radiation dosimetry) a tissue-equivalent device used to mimic the human body for radioation dose meaurements and experimental research.

phantom images, (in computed tomography) false images that appear but are not actually in the focal plane. They are created by the incomplete blurring or fusion of the blurred margins of some structures characteristic of the type of tomographic motion used.

phantom limb syndrome, a phenomenon common after amputation of a limb in which sensation or discomfort is experienced in the missing limb.

phantom tumour, a swelling resembling a tumour, usually caused by muscle contraction or gaseous distention of the intestines.

pharmaceutical, 1. of or pertaining to pharmacy or drugs. 2. a drug.

pharmaceutical chemistry, the science dealing with the composition and preparation of chemical compounds used in medical diagnoses and therapies.

pharmacist, a specialist in formulating and dispensing medications.

pharmacodynamics, the study of how a drug acts on a living organism, including the pharmacological response observed relative to the concentration of the drug at an active site in the organism.

pharmacogenetics, the study of the effects that the genetic characteristics of a group or individual have on the response of the group or the individual to certain drugs.

pharmacokinetics, (in pharmacology) the study of the fate of drugs within the body, including the routes and mechanisms of absorption and excretion, the rate at which a drug's action begins and the duration of the effect, the biotransformation of the substance in the body, and the effects and routes of excretion of the metabolites of the drug.

pharmacological agent, any oral, par-enteral, or topical substance used to alleviate symptoms and treat or control a disease process or aid recovery from an injury.

pharmacologist, a specialist in the science of pharmacology.

pharmacology, the study of the properties, uses, and actions of drugs.

pharmacopoeia, 1. a compendium containing descriptions, recipes, strengths, standards of purity, and dosage forms for selected drugs. **2.** the total of all authorized drugs available within the jurisdiction of a given geographical or political area.

pharmacy, 1. the study of preparing and dispensing drugs. **2.** a place for preparing and dispensing drugs.

pharyngeal aponeurosis, a sheet of connective tissue just beneath the mucosa of the pharynx.

pharyngeal bursa, a blind sac at the base of the pharyngeal tonsil.

pharyngeal reflex. See **gag reflex.**

pharyngeal tonsil, one of two masses of lymphatic tissue situated on the posterior wall of the nasopharynx behind the posterior nares.

pharyngitis, inflammation or infection of the pharynx, usually causing symptoms of a sore throat. Some causes of pharyngitis are diphtheria, herpes simplex virus, infectious mononucleosis, and streptococcal infection.

pharyngoconjunctival fever, an adenovirus infection characterized by fever, sore throat, and conjunctivitis. Contaminated water in lakes and swimming pools is a common source of infection.

pharynx, the throat, a tubular structure that extends from the base of the skull to the oesophagus and is situated just in front of the cervical vertebrae. The pharynx serves as a passageway for the respiratory and digestive tracts and changes shape to allow the formation of various vowel sounds. The pharynx is composed of muscle, is lined with mucous membrane, and is divided into the nasopharynx, the oropharynx, and the laryngopharynx. It contains the openings of the right and the left auditory tubes, the openings of the two posterior nares, the fauces, the opening into the larynx, and the opening into the oesophagus.

phase, in a periodic function, such as rotational or sinusoidal motion, the position relative to a particular part of the cycle.

phase 0, (in cardiology) the upstroke of the action potential.

phase 1, (in cardiology) the initial rapid repolarization phase of the action potential.

phase 2, (in cardiology) the plateau of the action potential.

phase 3, (in cardiology) the terminal rapid repolarization phase of the action potential.

phase 3 aberration, (in cardiology) a ventricular aberration resulting from the arrival of the impulse in the ventricular fascicle during phase 3 of its action potential.

phase 4, (in cardiology) the period of electric diastole and the last of the five phases of cardiac action potential.

phase 4 aberration, (in cardiology) a ventricular aberration resulting from the arrival of the impulse in a spontaneously depolarizing ventricular fascicle late in diastole.

phase of maximum slope, the time of rapid cervical dilatation and rapid fetal descent in the active phase of labour.

phase one study, a clinical trial to assess the risk that might come from administering a new treatment modality. A phase two study evaluates the clinical effectiveness of the new modality, whereas a phase three study compares its effectiveness with the best existing treatment.

phases of crisis, the occurrence of a significant stressor event, onset of disequilibrium, rise in tension levels, decrease in levels of functioning, and resolution with equilibrium reestablished.

phasic, 1. pertaining to a process proceeding in stages or phases. **2.** pertaining to a type of afferent or sensory nerve receptor of the proprioceptive system that responds to rate versus length changes in a muscle spindle.

phencyclidine hydrochloride (PCP), a piperidine derivative with marked hallucinogenic properties, used recreationally.

phenelzine sulphate, a monoamine oxidase inhibitor (MAOI) used in the treatment of depression resistant to less toxic treatments.

phenformin, phenformin hydrochloride, an oral hypoglycaemic.

phenic acid. See **carbolic acid.**

pheniramine maleate, an antihistamine prescribed in the treatment of a variety of hypersensitivity reactions, including rhinitis, skin rash, and pruritus.

phenobarbitone, a barbiturate anticonvulsant and sedative-hypnotic prescribed in the treatment of a variety of seizure disorders and, rarely, as a long-acting sedative.

phenobarbital-phenytoin serum levels, the concentration of phenobarbital and phenytoin in the serum, monitored to maintain concentrations sufficient to control seizures but not high enough to cause toxic reactions.

phenocopy, a phenotypic trait or condition that is induced by environmental factors but closely resembles a phenotype usually produced by a specific genotype. The trait is neither inherited nor transmitted to offspring. Phenocopies may present problems in genetic screening and genetic counselling so that all exogenous factors must be ruled out before any congenital trait or defect is labelled hereditary.

phenol, 1. a highly poisonous, caustic, crystalline chemical derived from coal tar or plant tar or manufactured synthetically and used as a disinfectant and sclerosant. **2.** Any of a large number and variety of chemical products closely related in structure to the alcohols and containing a hydroxyl group attached to a benzene ring.

phenol block, an injection of hydroxybenzene (phenol) into individual nerves, anaesthetizing a selective block of those nerves. The technique is sometimes used to control spasticity in specific muscle groups or to block transmission of nerve impulses in conditions such as trigeminal neuralgia.

phenol camphor, an oily mixture of camphor and phenol, used as an antiseptic and toothache remedy.

phenol coefficient, a measure of the disinfectant activity of a given chemical in relation to carbolic acid.

phenolphthalein, 1. a laxative that acts by stimulating the motor activity of the lower intestinal tract. **2.** an indicator used to determine whether acid is present in aqueous solutions.

phenol poisoning, corrosive poisoning caused by the ingestion of compounds containing phenol, such as carbolic acid, creosote, cresol, guaiacol, and naphthol. Characteristic of phenol poisoning are burns of the mucous membranes, weakness, pallor, pulmonary oedema, convulsion, and respiratory, circulatory, cardiac, and renal failure.

phenolsulfonphthalein, a dye used for testing the excretory capacity of the kidney tubules.

phenomenon, a sign that is often associated with a specific illness or condition and is, therefore, diagnostically important.

phenothiazine derivatives, any of a group of drugs that have a three ring structure in which two benzene rings are linked by a nitrogen and a sulphur. They represent the largest group of antipsychotic compounds in clinical medicine. Of the many phenothiazines and their congeners that are used as adjuncts to general anaesthesia, antiemetics, major tranquillizers (anti-psychotic agents), and antihistamines.

phenotype, 1. the complete observable characteristics of an organism or group, including anatomical, physiological, biochemical, and behavioural traits, as determined by the interaction of both genetic makeup and environmental factors. **2.** a group of organisms that resemble each other in appearance. **phenotypic,** *adj.*

phenoxybenzamine hydrochloride, an antihypertensive used in the control of hypertension and sweating in phaeochromocytoma.

phenoxymethylpenicillin (penicillin V), an antibiotic used in the treatment of susceptible infections.

phentermine, a sympathomimetic amine used as an anorectic agent. It is used to decrease the appetite in the short-term treatment of obesity.

phentolamine mesylate, an antiadrenergic used in the management of hypertensive crises associated with phaeochromocytoma before and during surgery, and as an adjunct to papaverine in the intracavernosal treatment of impotence.

phenylacetic acid, a metabolite of phenylalanine excreted in urine in conjugation with glutamine.

phenylalanine (Phe), an essential amino acid necessary for the normal growth and development of infants and children and for normal protein metabolism throughout life.

phenylalaninaemia, the presence of phenylalanine in the blood.

phenylbutazone, a nonsteroidal antiinflammatory agent used in the treatment of ankylosing spondylitis when other therapy is unsuitable.

phenyl carbinol. See **benzyl alcohol.**

phenylephrine hydrochloride, an alpha-adrenergic agent prescribed to maintain blood pressure and used locally as a nasal or ophthalmic vasoconstrictor.

phenylethyl alcohol, a colourless, fragrant liquid with a burning taste, used as a bacteriostatic agent and preservative in medicinal solutions. Also called **benzyl carbonol.**

phenylic acid, phenylic alcohol. See **carbolic acid.**

phenylketonuria (PKU), abnormal presence of phenylketone and other metabolites of phenylalanine in the urine, characteristic of an inborn metabolic disorder caused by the absence or a deficiency of phenylalanine hydroxylase, the enzyme responsible for the conversion of the amino acid phenylalanine into tyrosine. Accumulation of phenylalanine is toxic to brain tissue. Untreated individuals have very fair hair, eczema, a mousy odour of the urine and skin, and progressive mental deficiency. **phenylketonuric,** *adj.*

phenyl methanol. See **benzyl alcohol.**

phenylpropanolamine hydrochloride, a sympathomimetic amine with vasoconstrictor action used to relieve nasal congestion and related cold symptoms.

phenylpyruvic acid, a product of the metabolism of phenylalanine. The presence of phenylpyruvic acid in the urine is indicative of phenylketonuria.

phenylpyruvic amentia. See **phenylketonuria.**

phenytoin, a drug used as an anticonvulsant and as an antiarrhythmic agent, particularly in digitalis-induced arrhythmias.

pheresis. See **apheresis.**

pheromone, a hormonal substance secreted by an organism that elicits a particular response from another individual of the same species, but usually of the opposite sex.

Philadelphia chromosome (Ph1c), a translocation of the long arm of chromosome 22, often seen in the abnormal myeloblasts, erythroblasts, and megakaryoblasts of patients who have chronic myelocytic leukaemia.

philtrum, the vertical groove in the centre of the upper lip.

phimosis, tightness of the prepuce of the penis that prevents the retraction of the foreskin over the glans. The condition is usually congenital but may be the result of infection.

phimosis vaginalis, congenital narrowness or closure of the vaginal opening.

phi phenomenon, a sensation of apparent motion that is caused by lights that flash on and off at a certain frequency.

phlebitis. See **thrombophlebitis.**

phlebogram, a graphic representation of the venous pulse, obtained by phlebograph.

phlebograph, a device for producing a graphic record of the venous pulse.

phlebography, the technique of preparing a graphic record of the venous pulse by means of a phlebograph.

phlebostatic axis, the approximate location of the right atrium, found by drawing an imaginary line from the fourth intercostal space at the right side of the sternum to an intersection with the midaxillary line.

phlebothrombosis, an abnormal venous condition in which a clot forms within a vein, usually caused by haemostasis, hypercoagulability, or occlusion. In contrast to thrombophlebitis, the wall of the vein is not inflamed.

phlebotomus fever, an acute, mild infection, caused by one of five distinct arboviruses transmitted to humans by the bite of an infected sandfly, characterized by rapidly developing fever, headache, eye pain, conjunctivitis, myalgia, and, occasionally, a macular or urticarial rash.

phlebotomy, the incision of a vein for the letting of blood, as in collecting blood from a donor. Phlebotomy is the chief treatment for polycythaemia vera and may be performed every 6 months, or more frequently if required.

phlegm, thick mucus secreted by the tissues lining the respiratory passages.

phlegmasia alba dolens, thrombophlebitis of the femoral vein, resulting in oedema of the leg and pain. It may occur after childbirth or after a severe febrile illness.

phlegmasia cerulea dolens, a severe form of thrombosis of a deep vein, usually the femoral vein.

phlegmonous gastritis, a rare but severe form of gastritis, involving the connective tissue layer of the stomach wall.

phlyctenular keratoconjunctivitis, an inflammatory condition of the cornea, characterized by tiny, ulcerating nodules, seen most often in children as a response to allergens found in tuberculin, gonococci, *Candida albicans,* or various parasites.

phobia, an anxiety disorder characterized by an obsessive, irrational, and intense fear of a specific object, such as an animal or dirt, of an activity, such as meeting strangers or leaving the familiar setting of the home, or of a physical situation, such as heights and open or closed spaces. Typical manifestations of phobia include faintness, fatigue, palpitations, perspiration, nausea, tremor, and panic. The fear, which is out of proportion to reality, often results from some early painful or unpleasant experience involving the particular object or situation. Some kinds of phobias are **agoraphobia, algophobia, claustrophobia, erythrophobia, laliophobia, mysophobia, nyctophobia, photophobia, xenophobia,** and **zoophobia. -phobic,** *adj.*

phobic, a person who exhibits or is afflicted with a phobia.

phobic disorder, phobic neurosis, phobic reaction. See **phobia.**

phobic state, a condition characterized by extreme anxiety resulting from the excessive, irrational fear of a particular object, situation, or activity. See also **phobia.**

phocomelia, a developmental anomaly characterized by the absence of the upper portion of one or more of the limbs so that the feet or hands or both are attached to the trunk of the body by short, irregularly shaped stumps, resembling the fins of a seal. **phocomelic,** *adj.*

phocomelic dwarf, a dwarf in whom the long bones of any or all of the extremities are abnormally short.

phocomelus, an individual who has phocomelia.

phonation, the production of speech sounds through the vibration of the vocal folds of the larynx.

phonic, of or pertaining to voice, sounds, or speech.

phonocardiogram, a graphic recording obtained from a phonocardiograph.

phonocardiograph, an electroacoustic device that produces graphic heart sound recordings, used in the diagnosis and monitoring of heart disorders. This instrument produces phonocardiograms by using a system of microphones placed on the chest near the base of the heart and another positioned on the chest over the apex of the heart. **phonocardiographic,** *adj.*

phonology, the study of speech sounds, particularly the principles governing the way speech sounds are used in a given language.

phonophoresis, an ultrasound therapeutic

technique in which the high-frequency sound waves are used to force topical medicines into subcutaneous tissues.

phosphatase, an enzyme that acts as a catalyst in chemical reactions involving phosphorus.

phosphate, a salt of phosphoric acid. Phosphates are extremely important in living cells, particularly in the storage and use of energy and the transmission of genetic information.

phosphatide, a phosphatidic acid from which the choline or colamine portion has been removed. It may occur as an intermediate in the biosynthesis of triglycerides and phospholipids.

phosphoglycerate kinase, an enzyme that catalyzes the reversible transfer of a phosphate group from adenosine triphosphate to D-3-phosphoglycerate, forming D-1,3-diphosphoglycerate.

phospholipid, one of a class of compounds, widely distributed in living cells, containing phosphoric acid, fatty acids, and a nitrogenous base. Two kinds of phospholipids are **lecithin** and **sphingomyelin.**

phosphomevalonate kinase, an enzyme that catalyses the transfer of a phosphate group from adenosine triphosphate to produce adenosine diphosphate and 5-pyrophosphomevalonate.

phosphoric acid, a clear, colourless, odourless liquid that is irritating to the skin and eyes and moderately toxic if ingested.

phosphorus (P), a nonmetallic chemical element occurring extensively in nature as a component of phosphate rock. Its atomic number is 15; its atomic weight is 30.975. Phosphorus is essential for the metabolism of protein, calcium, and glucose. A nutritional deficiency of phosphorus can cause weight loss, anaemia, and abnormal growth.

phosphorus poisoning, a toxic condition caused by the ingestion of white or yellow phosphorus, sometimes found in rat poisons, certain fertilizers, and fireworks. Intoxication is characterized initially by nausea, throat and stomach pain, vomiting, diarrhoea, and an odour of garlic on the breath.

photoallergic, exhibiting a delayed hypersensitivity reaction after exposure to light.

photoallergic contact dermatitis, a papulovesicular, eczematous, or exudative skin reaction occurring 24 to 48 hours after exposure to light in a previously sensitized person. The sensitizing substance concentrates in the skin and requires chemical alteration by light to become an active antigen.

photochemotherapy, a kind of chemotherapy in which the effect of the administered drug is enhanced by exposing the patient to light, such as the treatment of psoriasis with oral methoxsalen followed by exposure to ultraviolet light.

photodynamic therapy, a treatment for cancer which involves administering a photosensitive drug to the patient. The drug is then activated in the tumour by shining a laser light directly on to the site, causing a cytotoxic effect.

photoelectric absorption, the process of x-ray interaction with matter in which the incident x-ray photon is completely absorbed; responsible for the differential absorption of x-rays within the body to produce a radiographic image.

photometer, an instrument that measures light intensity.

photomultiplier, a device used in many radiation detection applications that converts low levels of light into electric pulses.

photon, the smallest quantity of electromagnetic energy. It has no mass and no charge but travels at the speed of light. Photons may occur in the form of x-rays, gamma rays, or a quantum of light.

photophobia, **1.** abnormal sensitivity to light, especially by the eyes. The condition is prevalent in albinism and various diseases of the conjunctiva and cornea and may be a symptom of such disorders as measles, psittacosis, encephalitis, Rocky Mountain spotted fever, and Reiter's syndrome. **2.** (in psychiatry) a morbid fear of light with an irrational need to avoid light places. **photophobic,** *adj.*

photopic vision, daylight vision, which depends primarily on the function of the retinal cone cells.

photoprotective, protective against the potential adverse effects of ultraviolet light.

photosensitive, increased reactivity of skin to sunlight caused by a disorder, such as albinism or porphyria, or more frequently resulting from the use of certain drugs. Relatively brief exposure to sunlight or to an ultraviolet lamp may cause oedema, papules, urticaria, or acute burns in individuals with endogenous or acquired photosensitivity.

photosensitivity, any abnormal response to exposure to light, specifically, a skin reaction requiring the presence of a sensitizing agent and exposure to sunlight or its equivalent.

photosynthesis, a process by which green plants containing chlorophyll synthesize chemical substances, chiefly carbohydrates, from atmospheric carbon dioxide and water, using light for energy and liberating oxygen in the process.

phototherapy, the treatment of disorders by the use of light, especially ultraviolet light. Ultraviolet light may be employed in the therapy of acne, decubiti and other indolent ulcers, psoriasis, and hyperbilirubinaemia. **phototherapeutic,** *adj.*

phototherapy in the newborn, a treatment for hyperbilirubinaemia and jaundice in the newborn that involves the exposure of an infant's bare skin to intense fluorescent light. The blue range of light accelerates the excretion of bilirubin in the skin, decomposing it by photooxidation.

phototoxic, characterized by a rapidly developing, nonimmunological reaction of the skin when it is exposed to a photosensitizing substance and light.

phototoxic contact dermatitis, a rapidly appearing, sunburnlike response of areas of skin that have been exposed to the sun after contact with a photosensitizing substance. Hyperpigmentation may follow the acute reaction. Among known photosensitizing materials are coal tar derivatives, oil of bergamot, and many plants containing furocoumarin, such as cowslip, buttercup, and yarrow.

pH paper. See **nitrazine paper.**

phrenic, 1. of or pertaining to the diaphragm. **2.** of or pertaining to the mind.

phrenic nerve, one of a pair of muscular branches of the cervical plexus, arising from the fourth cervical nerve. It contains about one half as many sensory as motor fibres and is generally known as the motor nerve to the diaphragm, although the lower thoracic nerves also help to innervate the diaphragm.

Phthirus, a genus of bloodsucking lice that includes the species *Phthirus pubis,* the pubic louse, or crab.

phychologist, a person who specializes in the study of algae.

phycology, the branch of science that is concerned with algae.

phycomycosis, a fungal infection caused by a species of the order Phycomycetes.

phylloquinone. See **vitamin K1.**

phylogenesis. See **phylogeny.**

phylogenetic, 1. of, relating to, or acquired during phylogeny. **2.** based on a natural evolutionary relationship, as a system of classification. Also **phylogenic.**

phylogeny, the development of the structure of a particular race or species as it evolved from simpler forms of life.

physiatrist, a doctor who tests the physical functioning of a patient and supervises the patient's rehabilitation program.

physical activity level (PAL), a ratio of daily energy expenditure to Basal Metabolic Rate (BMR). Values range from 1. 4 (person with light work energy expenditure and nonactive leisure pursuits) to 1.9 (energy demanding work and active leisure pursuits).

physical abuse, one or more episodes of aggressive behaviour, usually resulting in physical injury with possible damage to internal organs, sense organs, the central nervous system, or the musculoskeletal system of another person.

physical allergy, an allergic response to physical factors, as cold, heat, light, or trauma. Usually, specific antibodies are found in people having physical allergies. Common characteristics include pruritus, urticaria, and angioedema.

physical assessment, the part of the health assessment representing a synthesis of the information obtained in a physical examination.

physical chemistry, the natural science dealing with the relationship between chemical and physical properties of matter.

physical diagnosis, the diagnostic process accomplished by the study of the physical manifestations of health and illness revealed in the physical examination, as guided by the patient's complete history and supported by various laboratory tests.

physical examination, an investigation of the body to determine its state of health, using any or all of the techniques of inspection, palpation, percussion, auscultation, and smell.

physical fitness, the ability to carry out daily tasks with alertness and vigour, without undue fatigue, and with enough energy reserve to meet emergencies or to enjoy leisure time pursuits.

physical science, the study of the laws and properties of nonliving matter. Some kinds of physical science are **chemistry, geology,** and **physics.**

physician, a health professional who has earned a the qualifications M.B. B.S. (or M.B. B.Chir) after a course of undergraduate study at an approved university or medical school, and three years postgraduate study at an approved teaching hospital. Satisfactory completion of examinations, and postgraduate specialization in medicine (as opposed to surgery) is required. In the United Kingdom, a physician will be expected to go on to take the MRCP (Membership of the Royal College of Physicians) examination before specializing in a specific branch of medicine.

physics, the study of the laws and properties of matter and energy, particularly as related to motion and force.

physiological chemistry. See **biochemistry.**

physiological contracture, a temporary condition in which muscles may contract and shorten for a considerable period of time. Drugs, extremes of temperature, and local accumulation of lactic acid are causes.

physiological dead space. See **dead space.**

physiological dwarf. See **primordial dwarf.**

physiological flexion, an excessive amount of flexor tone that is normally present at birth because of the existing level of central nervous system maturation and fetal positioning in the uterus.

physiological hypertrophy, a temporary increase in the size of an organ or part because of normal physiologic functions, as occurs in the walls of the uterus and in the breasts during pregnancy.

physiological motivation, a bodily need,

such as food or water, that initiates behaviour directed toward satisfying the particular need.

physiological occlusion, 1. a closure of the teeth that complements and enhances the functions of the masticatory system. 2. a closure of the teeth that produces no pathologic effects on the stomatognathic system. 3. an acceptable occlusion in a healthy gnathic system.

physiological psychology, the study of the interrelationship of physiological and psychological processes, especially the effects of a change from normal to abnormal.

physiological relaxation, a method of easing tension in veraous muscle groups based on the physiological principle of reciprocal relaxation.

physiological third heart sound, a low-pitched extra heart sound heard early in diastole in a healthy child or young adult. The same sound, heard in an older person who has heart disease, is an abnormal finding called a ventricular gallop.

physiology, 1. the study of the processes and function of the human body. 2. the study of the physical and chemical processes involved in the functioning of living organisms and their component parts. Kinds of physiology are **comparative physiology, developmental physiology, hominal physiology,** and **pathological physiology.**

physiotherapist, a member of The Chartered Institute of Physiotherapists, a person who is trained and qualified to undertake the examination, testing, and treatment of physically disabled or handicapped people and people physically debilitated through injury or illness, employing the use of special exercise, application of heat or cold, use of sonar waves, and other techniques.

physiotherapy, the treatment of disorders with physical agents and methods, such as massage, manipulation, therapeutic exercises, cold, heat (including shortwave, microwave, and ultrasonic diathermy), hydrotherapy, electric stimulation, and light to assist in rehabilitating patients and in restoring normal function after an illness or injury.

physostigmine, an anticholinesterase used as an eyedrop in the treatment of some forms of glaucoma. It has also been used to reverse the toxic effects of anticholinergic poisons.

phytanic acid storage disease, a rare genetic disorder of lipid metabolism in which there are accumulations of phytanic acid in the plasma and tissues. The condition is characterized by ataxia, peripheral neuropathy, retinitis pigmentosa, and abnormalities of the bone and skin.

phytohaemagglutinin (PHA), a haemagglutinin that is derived from a plant, specifically the lectin obtained from the red kidney bean.

phytomenadione, a yellow viscous, oil-soluble vitamin, occurring naturally and produced synthetically. it is used in deficiency states and to counteract the effects of overdose with coumarin anticoagulents.

phytolectin, See **phytohaemagglutinin.**

pia mater, the innermost of the three meninges covering the brain and the spinal cord. It is closely applied to both structures and carries a rich supply of blood vessels, which nourish the nervous tissue. The cranial pia mater covers the surface of the brain and dips deeply into the fissures and the sulci of the cerebral hemispheres. The spinal pia mater is thicker, firmer, and less vascular than the cranial pia mater.

pian. See **yaws.**

pica, a craving to eat substances that are not foods, such as dirt, clay, chalk, glue, ice, starch, or hair. The appetite disorder may occur with some nutritional deficiency states, with pregnancy, and in some forms of mental illness.

picking up, a form of massage in which the tissues are compressed against underlying bone, lifted, squeezed, and released.

Pick's disease {Arnold Pick, Czechoslovakian neurologist, b. 1851}, a form of presenile dementia occurring in middle age. This disorder affects mainly the frontal and temporal lobes of the brain and characteristically produces neurotic behaviour, slow disintegration of intellect, personality, and emotions, and degeneration of cognitive abilities.

pickwickian syndrome, an abnormal condition characterized by obesity, decreased pulmonary function, somnolence, and polycythaemia.

picornavirus, a member of a group of small RNA viruses that are ether-resistant. These viruses cause poliomyelitis, herpangina, and aseptic meningitis, encephalomyocarditis, and foot-and-mouth disease.

picrotoxin, a central nervous system stimulant and potent convulsant obtained from the seeds of Anamirta cocculus, formerly used as an antidote for acute barbiturate poisoning.

PID, abbreviation for **pelvic inflammatory disease.**

PIE, abbreviation for *pulmonary infiltrate with eosinophilia,* a hypersensitivity reaction, characterized by infiltration of alveoli with eosinophils and large mononuclear cells, oedema, and inflammation of the lungs. Simple pulmonary eosinophilia, in which patchy, migratory infiltrates cause minimal symptoms, is a self-limited reaction that is elicited by helminthic infections and by certain drugs. A more prolonged illness, characterized by fever, night sweats, cough, dyspnoea, weight loss, and more severe tissue reaction, occurs in certain drug allergies and bacterial, fungal, and parasitic infections.

piebald, having patches of white hair or skin because of an absence of melanocytes in those nonpigmented areas. It is a hereditary condition.

Piedmont fracture, an oblique fracture of the distal radius, with fragments of bone pulled into the ulna.

Pierre Robin's syndrome {Pierre Robin, French histologist, b. 1867}, a complex of congenital anomalies including a small mandible, cleft lip, cleft palate, other craniofacial abnormalities, and defects of the eyes and ears, including glaucoma. Intelligence is usually normal.

piezoelectric effect, 1. the generation of a voltage across a solid when a mechanical stress is applied. **2.** the dimensional change resulting from the application of a voltage.

pigeon breast, a congenital structural defect characterized by a prominent anterior projection of the xiphoid and the lower part of the sternum and by a lengthening of the costal cartilages. It may cause cardio-respiratory complications. **pigeon-breasted,** *adj.*

pigeon breeder's lung, a respiratory disorder caused by acquired hypersensitivity to antigens in bird droppings.

pigeon-toed. See **metatarsus varus.**

piggyback port, a special coupling for the primary IV tubing that allows a supplementary, or piggyback, solution to run into the IV system.

pigment, 1. any organic colouring material produced in the body, such as melanin. **2.** any coloured, paintlike, medicinal preparation applied to the skin surface. **pigmentary, pigmented,** *adj.*, **pigmentation,** *n.*

pigmentary retinopathy, a disorder of the retina characterized by deposits of pigment and increasing loss of vision.

pigmented villonodular synovitis, a disease of the joints characterized by fingerlike proliferative growths of synovial tissue, with haemosiderin deposition within the synovial tissue.

pilar cyst, an epidermoid cyst of the scalp. It originates from the middle portion of the epithelium of a hair follicle.

piles. See **haemorrhoid.**

pill, 1. *informal.* any oral solid dose form, especially the oral contraceptive. **2.** round, solid oral dose form made by rolling a small ball of a semi-solid pill mass containing active ingredients, bulking and binding agents and allowing to dry. Now superseded by the compressed tablet.

pillion fracture, a T-shaped fracture of the distal femur with displacement of the condyles posterior to the femoral shaft, caused by a severe blow to the knee.

piloerection. See **pilomotor reflex.**

pilomotor reflex, erection of the hairs of the skin in response to a chilly environment, emotional stimulus, or irritation of the skin.

pilonidal cyst, a hairy cyst that often develops in the sacral region of the skin. Pilonidal cysts may sometimes be recognized at birth by a depression, sometimes a hairy dimple, in the midline of the back, sacrococcygeal area.

pilonidal fistula, an abnormal channel containing a tuft of hair, situated most frequently over or close to the tip of the coccyx but also occurring in other regions of the body.

pilosebaceous, of or pertaining to a hair follicle and its oil gland.

pilot view. See **scanogram.**

pilus, *pl.* **pili, 1.** a hair or hairlike structure. **2.** (in microbiology) a fine, filamentous appendage found on certain bacteria and similar to flagellum except that it is shorter, straighter, and found in greater quantities in the organism.

pi-mesons, negatively charged nuclear particles which may be used in external beam radiotherapy.

pimozide, an oral neuroleptic agent used for the treatment of psychoses, mania and hypomania, and the suppression of motor and phonic tics associated with Tourette's syndrome.

pimple, a small papule, pustule, or furuncle.

pin, 1. (in orthopaedics) to secure and immobilize fragments of bone with a nail. **2.** See nail, def. 2. **3.** (in dentistry) a small metal rod or peg, used as a support in rebuilding a tooth.

pin and tube fixed orthodontic appliance, an orthodontic appliance for correcting and improving malocclusion. It employs a labial arch with vertical posts that insert into tubes attached to bands on the teeth.

pinch, a compression or squeezing of the end of the thumb in opposition to the end of one or more of the fingers.

pinch grip. See **tip pinch.**

pinch meter, a type of dynamometer that measures the strength of a finger pinch.

Pindborg tumour. See **calcifying epithelial odontogenic tumour.**

pindolol, a beta-adrenergic blocker with sympathomimetic activity. It is prescribed in the treatment of hypertension and angina pectoris.

pineal body, a small, somewhat flattened, cone-shaped structure, suspended by a stalk in the epithalamus. It consists of glial cells and pinealocytes and apparently elaborates the hormone melatonin.

pineal gland, a cone-shaped structure in the brain, situated between the superior colliculi, the pulvinar, and the splenium of the corpus callosum. Its precise function has not been established. It may secrete the hormone melatonin, which appears to inhibit the secretion of luteinizing hormone.

pineal hyperplasia syndrome, an abnormal condition caused by overgrowth of the pineal gland. It is characterized by severe insulin resistance, dry skin, thick nails, hirsutism, early dentition, and sexual precocity.

pinealoma, *pl.* **pinealomas, pinealomata,** a rare neoplasm of the pineal body in the brain, characterized by hydrocephalus, pupillary changes, gait disturbances, headache, nausea, and vomiting.

pineal tumour, a neoplasm of the pineal body.

pine tar, a topical antieczematic and rubefacient. It is a common ingredient in creams, soaps, and lotions used in the treatment of chronic skin conditions, such as eczema or psoriasis.

pinhole radiograph, a method to measure the size of the focus of an x-ray tube using a lead sheet with a pinhole aligned to the central ray.

pinhole retention, retention developed by drilling one or more holes, 2 to 3 mm in depth, in suitable areas of a cavity preparation to supplement resistance and retention form.

pinhole test, a test performed in examining a person who has diminished visual acuity to distinguish a refractive error from organic disease. Several pinholes are punched in a card; the patient selects one and looks through it with one eye at a time, without wearing glasses. If visual acuity is improved, the defect is refractive; if not, it is organic.

Pin-Index Safety System (PISS), a system for identifying connectors for certain small cylinders of medical gases that have flush valve outlets. The identifying code consists of a combination of two holes in the face of the valve into which connecting pins for a particular type of gas must fit in perfect alignment.

pink disease. See **acrodynia.**

pinkeye. See **conjunctivitis.**

Pinkus' disease. See **lichen nitidus.**

pinna. See **auricle.**

pinocytic, pertaining to a pinocyte, particularly its ability to absorb liquids by phagocytosis in cellular metabolic processes.

pinocytosis, the process by which extracellular fluid is taken into a cell. The cell membrane develops a saccular indentation filled with extracellular fluid, then closes around it, forming a vesicle or a vacuole of fluid within the cell.

pinta, an infection of the skin caused by *Treponema carateum,* a common organism in South and Central America. The bacterium gains entry into the body through a break in the skin. The primary lesion is a slowly enlarging papule with regional lymph node enlargement, followed in 1 to 12 months by a generalized red to slate-blue macular rash, a barbiturate anticonvulsant and sedative-hypnotic prescribed in the treatment of a

variety of seizure disorders and, rarely, as a long-acting sedative.

pin track infection, an abnormal condition associated with skeletal traction and characterized by infection of superficial, deeper, or soft tissues or by osteomyelitis. These infections may develop at skeletal traction pin sites.

pinworm. See *Enterobius vermicularis.*

PIO$_2$, the partial pressure of inspired oxygen.

pions. See **pi-mesons.**

piperazine oestrone sulphate, an oestrogen prescribed in the treatment of menopausal symptoms.

piperocaine hydrochloride, a local anaesthetic for the induction of spinal or caudal anaesthesia.

pipette, 1. a calibrated, transparent open-ended tube of glass or plastic used for measuring or transferring small quantities of a liquid or gas. 2. using a pipette to dispense liquid.

piriform aperture, the anterior nasal opening in the skull.

piriformis, a flat, pyramidal muscle lying almost parallel with the posterior margin of the gluteus medius. It functions to rotate the thigh laterally and to abduct and to help extend it.

Pirquet's test, a tuberculin skin test that consists of scratching the tuberculin material onto the skin.

pisiform bone, a small, spheroidal carpal bone in the proximal row of carpal bones. It articulates with the triangular bone and is attached to the flexor retinaculum, the flexor carpi ulnaris, and the abductor digiti minimi.

PISS, abbreviation for Pin-Index Safety System.

pistol-shot sound, a sharp, slapping sound heard by auscultation over the femoral pulse of a patient with aortic incompetence. It is caused by a large-volume pulse with a sharp rise in pressure.

pit and fissure cavity, a cavity that starts in tiny faults in tooth enamel, usually on occlusal surfaces of molars and premolars.

pitch, the quality of a tone or sound dependent on the relative rapidity of the vibrations by which it is produced.

pitting, 1. small, punctate indentations in fingernails or toenails, often a result of psoriasis. 2. an indentation that remains for a short time after pressing oedematous skin with a finger. 3. small, depressed scars in the skin or other organ of the body. 4. the removal by the spleen of material from within erythrocytes without damage to the cells.

pituicyte, a cell of the neurohypophysis.

pituitary adamantinoma. See **craniopharyngioma.**

pituitary cachexia. See **postpubertal panhypopituitarism.**

pituitary dwarf, a dwarf whose retarded development is caused by a deficiency of growth hormone resulting from hypofunction of the anterior lobe of the pituitary. The body is properly proportioned, with no facial or skeletal deformities, and there is normal mental and sexual development.

pituitary gland, the small gland attached to the hypothalamus and couched in the sphenoid bone, supplying numerous hormones that govern many vital processes. It is divided into an anterior adenohypophysis and a smaller posterior neurohypophysis. The adenohypophysis secretes growth hormone (somatotropin), thyrotropic hormone, adrenocorticotropic hormone (ACTH), two gonadotropic hormones, follicle stimulating hormone (FSH), luteinizing hormone (LH), and prolactin, the hormone that promotes milk secretion. The neurohypophysis stores two hormones, oxytocin and vasopressin.

pituitary nanism, a type of dwarfism associated with hypophyseal infantilism.

pituitary snuff lung, a type of hypersensitivity pneumonitis that sometimes occurs among takers of pituitary snuff. The antigens to which the hypersensitivity reaction occurs are found in serum proteins of cows and pigs and in pituitary tissue. Symptoms of the acute form of the disease include chills, cough, fever, dyspnoea, anorexia, nausea, and vomiting.

pituitary stalk, a structure that connects the pituitary gland with the hypothalamus.

pit viper, any one of a family of venomous snakes found in the Western Hemisphere and Asia, characterized by a heat-sensitive pit between the eye and nostril on each side of the head and hollow, perforated fangs that are usually folded back in the roof of the mouth.

pityriasis alba, a common idiopathic dermatosis characterized by round or oval, finely scaling patches of hypopigmentation, usually on the cheeks.

pityriasis rosea, a self-limited skin disease in which a slightly scaling, pink, macular rash spreads over the trunk and other unexposed areas of the body. A characteristic feature is the **herald patch,** a larger, more scaly lesion that precedes the diffuse rash by several days. The smaller lesions tend to line up with the long axis parallel to normal lines of cleavage of the skin. Mild itching is the only symptom.

Pityrosporum. See *Malassezia.*

pivot joint, a synovial joint in which movement is limited to rotation. The proximal radioulnar articulation is a pivot joint.

pivot transfer, the movement of a person from one site to another, such as from a bed to a wheelchair, when there is a loss of control of one side of the body. The person is helped to a position on the strong side of the body with both feet on the floor, heels behind the knees and knees lower than the hips. The person stands with the weight on the strong leg and pivots on it, and lowers the body into the wheelchair.

pixel, abbreviation for *picture element,* the smallest discrete part of a digital image display.

pKa, the negative logarithm of the ionization constant of an acid that is half dissociated, used as a measure of the strength of an acid.

PK test, abbreviation for **Prausnitz-Küstner test.**

PKU, abbreviation for **phenylketonuria.**

placebo, an inactive substance, such as saline, distilled water, or sugar, or a less than effective dose of a harmless substance, as a water-soluble vitamin prescribed as if it were an effective dose of a needed medication. Placebos are prescribed for patients who cannot be given the medication they request or who, in the judgment of the health care provider, do not need that medication.

placebo effect, a physical or emotional change occurring after a substance is taken or administered that is not the result of any special property of the substance. The change may be beneficial, reflecting the expectations of the patient.

placenta, a highly vascular fetal organ through which the fetus absorbs oxygen, nutrients, and other substances and excretes carbon dioxide and other wastes. It begins to form on approximately the eighth day of gestation when the blastocyst touches the wall of the uterus and adheres to it. At term the normal placenta weighs one seventh to one fifth of the weight of the infant. The maternal surface is lobulated and divided into cotyledons. It has a dark red, rough, liverlike appearance. The fetal surface is smooth and shiny, covered with the fetal membranes, marked by the large white blood vessels beneath the membranes that fan out from the centrally inserted umbilical cord. The time between delivery of the infant and the expulsion of the placenta is the third and last stage of labour.

placenta abruptio. See **abruptio placentae.**

placenta accreta, a placenta that invades the uterine muscle, making it abnormally adherent.

placental hormone, one of the several hormones produced by the placenta, including human placental lactogen, chorionic gonadotropin, oestrogen, progesterone, and a thyrotrophin-like hormone.

placental infarct, a localized ischaemic, hard area on the fetal or maternal side of the placenta.

placental insufficiency, an abnormal condition of pregnancy, manifested clinically by retardation of the rate of fetal and uterine growth.

placenta praevia an abnormally sited placenta, occupying the lower part of the uterus, either completely or partially covering the cervical os. Type I encroaches on the lower segment; Type II reaches to, but does not cover, the os; Type III covers the internal os when it is closed, but not when it is dilated; Type IV completely covers the os.

Plafon fracture, a fracture that involves the buttress portion of the malleolus of a bone.

plagiocephaly, a congenital malformation of the skull in which premature or irregular closure of the coronal or lambdoidal sutures results in asymmetric growth of the head, giving it a twisted, lopsided appearance. **plagiocephalic, plagiocephalous,** *adj.*

plague, an infectious disease transmitted by the bite of a flea from a rodent infected with the bacillus *Yersinia pestis.* Plague is primarily an infectious disease of rats: the rat fleas feed on humans only when their preferred rodent hosts, usually rats, have been killed by the plague in a rat epizootic. Kinds of plague include **bubonic plague, pneumonic plague,** and **septicemic plague.**

plague vaccine, a vaccine containing killed plague bacilli. It is used for active immunization against plague after probable exposure or as protection for travellers in endemic areas, such as Southeast Asia.

planar xanthoma, a yellow or orange flat macule or slightly raised papule containing foam cells and occurring in clusters in localized areas, such as the eyelids, or widely distributed over the body.

Planck's constant, {Max Planck, German physicist, b. 1858}, a fundamental physical constant that relates the energy of radiation to its frequency. It is equal to 6.63×10^{-34} joule-seconds.

plane, 1. a flat surface determined by three points in space. **2.** an extension of a longitudinal section through an axis, such as the coronal, the horizontal, and the sagittal planes used to identify the position of various parts of the body in the study of anatomy. **3.** the act of paring or of rubbing away. **4.** a superficial incision in the wall of a cavity or between tissue layers, especially in plastic surgery. **planar,** *adj.*

planes of anaesthesia. See **Guedel's signs.**

planigraphic principle, a rule of tomography in which the fulcrum or axis of rotation is raised or lowered to alter the level of the focal plane but the tabletop height remains constant.

planned change, (in psychotherapy) an alteration of the status quo by means of a carefully formulated programme that follows four steps: unfreezing the present level, establishing a change relationship, moving to a new level, and freezing at the new level.

planned parenthood, a philosophical framework central to the development of contraceptive methods, contraceptive counselling, and family planning programmes and clinics. Advocates hold that it is the right of each woman to decide when to conceive and bear children and that contraceptive and gynaecological care and information should be available to her to help her become or avoid becoming pregnant.

planning, (in four step nursing process) a category of nursing behaviour in which a strategy is designed for the achievement of the goals of care for an individual patient, as established in the nursing assessment. Planning includes developing and modifying a care plan for the patient, cooperating with other health professionals, and recording relevant information.

plantago seed, a bulk-forming laxative derived from *Plantago psyllium* seeds. It is used in the treatment of constipation and nonspecific diarrhoea.

plantar, of or pertaining to the sole of the foot.

plantar aponeurosis, the tough fascia surrounding the muscles of the soles of the feet.

plantaris, one of three superficial muscles at the back of the leg, between the soleus and the gastrocnemius. It flexes the foot and the leg.

plantar neuroma, a neuroma of the sole of the foot.

plantar reflex, the normal response, elicited by firmly stroking the outer surface of the sole from heel to toes, characterized by flexion of the toes. Compare **Babinski's reflex.**

plantar wart, a painful verrucous lesion on the sole of the foot, primarily at points of pressure, as over the metatarsal heads and the heel. Caused by the common wart virus, it appears as a soft, central core and is surrounded by a firm, hyperkeratotic ring resembling a callus.

plantigrade, of, pertaining to, or characterizing the human gait; walking on the sole of the foot with the heel touching the ground.

plaque, 1. a flat, often raised, patch on the skin or any other organ of the body. **2.** a patch of atherosclerosis. **3.** a thin film on the teeth made up of mucin and colloidal material found in saliva and often secondarily invaded by bacteria.

plasma, the watery, colourless, fluid portion of the lymph and the blood in which the leukocytes, erythrocytes, and platelets are suspended. It contains no cells and is made up of water, electrolytes, proteins, glucose, fats, bilirubin, and gases. It is essential for carrying the cellular elements of the blood through the circulation, transporting nutrients, maintaining the acid-base balance of the body, and transporting wastes from the tissues.

plasma cell, a lymphoid or lymphocyte-like cell found in the bone marrow, connective tissue, and, sometimes, the blood. Plasma cells are involved in the immune mechanism.

plasma cell leukaemia, an unusual neoplasm of blood-forming tissues in which the predominant cells in peripheral blood are plasmacytes. The disease may develop in the course of multiple myeloma or arise independently.

plasma cell myeloma. See **multiple myeloma.**

plasmacytoma, *pl.* **plasmacytomas, plasmacytomata,** a focal neoplasm containing plasma cells. It may develop in the bone marrow, as in multiple myeloma, or outside the bone marrow, as in certain tumours of the viscera.

plasma expander, a substance, usually a high molecular weight dextran, that is administered intravenously to increase the oncotic pressure of a patient.

plasma fibrinogen, normally 2-4g/litre (200-400mg/100ml); increased during pregnancy. Intrauterine foetal death can cause abrupt fall below 1g/litre, causing haemorrhage. See **fibrindex.**

plasma membrane. See **cell membrane.**

plasmapheresis, the removal of plasma from withdrawn blood by centrifugation, the reconstitution of the cellular elements in an isotonic solution, and the reinfusion of this solution into the donor.

plasma protein, any one of the various proteins, including albumin, fibrinogen, prothrombin, and the gamma globulins, which constitute about 6% to 7% of the blood plasma in the body.

plasma renin activity, the action of the enzyme renin, measured in plasma to aid in the diagnosis of adrenal disease associated with hypertension.

plasma thromboplastin antecedent. See **factor XI.**

plasma thromboplastin component deficiency. See **haemophilia.**

plasma volume, the total volume of plasma in the body, elevated in diseases of the liver and spleen and in vitamin C deficiency, lowered in Addison's disease, dehydration, and shock.

plasmid, (in bacteriology) any type of intracellular inclusion considered to have a genetic function, especially a molecule of DNA separate from the bacterial chromosome that determines traits not essential for the viability of the organism but that in some way changes the organism's ability to adapt.

plasmidotrophoblast. See **syncytiotrophoblast.**

plasmin. See **fibrinolysin.**

plasminogen. See **fibrinogen.**

Plasmodium, a genus of protozoa several species of which cause malaria, transmitted to humans by the bite of an infected *Anopheles* mosquito. *Plasmodium falciparum* causes falciparum malaria, the most severe form of the disease; *P. malariae* causes quartan malaria; *P. ovale* causes mild tertian malaria with oval red blood cells; and *P. vivax* causes common tertian malaria.

plasmosome, the true nucleolus of a cell as distinguished from the karyosomes in the nucleus. Also spelled **plasmasome.**

plaster, 1. any composition of a liquid and a powder that hardens when it dries, used in shaping a cast to support a fractured bone as it heals, such as plaster of paris. **2.** a home remedy consisting of a semisolid mixture applied to a part of the body as a counterirritant or for other therapeutic reasons, such as a mustard plaster.

plaster saw, a saw used to cut through a plaster cast.

plastering, the act of encasing a body part in plaster.

plastering tape, an adhesive or resin-impregnated tape used for shaping lightweight casts.

plastic surgery, the alteration, replacement, or restoration of visible portions of the body, performed to correct a structural or cosmetic defect. In performing corrective plastic surgery, the surgeon may use tissue from the patient or from another person or an inert material that is nonirritating, has a consistency appropriate to the use, and is able to hold its shape and form indefinitely. See also specific procedures.

plate, 1. a flat structure or layer, such as a thin layer of bone or the frontal plate between the sides of the ethmoid cartilage and the sphenoid bone in the fetus. **2.** a single partitioning unit of a chromatographic system.

platelet, the smallest of the cells in the blood. Platelets are disc-shaped and contain no haemoglobin. They are essential for the coagulation of blood.

plateletpheresis, the removal of platelets from withdrawn blood, the remainder of the blood being reinfused into the donor.

platinized gold foil, a thin sheet rolled or hammered from platinum sandwiched between two sheets of gold, used for making portions of dental restorations requiring greater hardness than that obtained by using other materials, such as copper amalgam.

platinum (Pt), a silvery-white, soft metallic element. Its atomic number is 78; its atomic weight is 195.09. Platinum is used in dentistry.

platinum foil, a very thin sheet of rolled pure platinum that has a high fusing point, making it an ideal matrix in various soldering procedures for fabricating orthodontic appliances and dentures.

Platyhelminthes, a phylum of parasitic flatworms that includes the Cestoda subclass of tapeworms and Trematoda class of flukes.

platypelloid pelvis, a simple, flat pelvis (incidence 5%). The anteroposterior diameter is short, and the sacrosciatic notch is narrow.

platysma, one of a pair of wide muscles at the side of the neck. It serves to draw down the lower lip and the corner of the mouth.

When the platysma fully contracts, the skin over the clavicle is drawn toward the mandible, increasing the diameter of the neck.

play, any spontaneous or organized activity that provides enjoyment, entertainment, amusement, or diversion. It is essential in childhood for the development of a normal personality and as a means for developing physically, intellectually, and socially. Play provides an outlet for releasing tension and stress. Kinds of play include **active play, associative play, cooperative play, dramatic play, parallel play, passive play, skill play,** and **solitary play.** See also **play therapy.**

play therapy, a form of psychotherapy in which a child plays in a protected and structured environment with games and toys provided by a therapist, who observes the behaviour, affect, and conversation of the child to gain insight into thoughts, feelings, and fantasies.

pleasure principle, (in psychoanalysis) the need for immediate gratification of instinctual drives.

pledget, a small, flat compress made of cotton gauze, or a tuft of cotton wool, lint, or a similar synthetic material, used to wipe the skin, absorb drainage, or clean a small surface.

pleiotropic gene, a gene that produces a complex of unrelated phenotypic effects.

pleiotropy, (in genetics) the production by a single gene of a multiple, different, and apparently unrelated manifestation of a particular disorder, such as the cluster of symptoms in Marfan's syndrome, aortic aneurysm, dislocation of the optic lens, skeletal deformities, and arachnodactyly, any or all of which may be present.

plessimeter. See **pleximeter.**

plethora, a term applied to the beefy red colouration of a newborn. The "boiled lobster" hue of the infant's skin is caused by an unusually high proportion of erythrocytes per volume of blood. **plethoric,** *adj.*

plethysmogram, a tracing produced by a plethysmograph.

plethysmograph, an instrument for measuring and recording changes in the sizes and volumes of extremities and organs by measuring changes in their blood volumes. **plethysmographic,** *adj.*, **plethysmography,** *n.*

pleura, *pl.* **pleurae,** a delicate serous membrane enclosing the lung, composed of a single layer of flattened mesothelial cells resting on a delicate membrane of connective tissue. The pleura divides into the visceral pleura, which covers the lung, dipping into the fissures between the lobes, and the parietal pleura, which lines the chest wall, covers the diaphragm, and reflects over the structures in the mediastinum. **pleural,** *adj.*

pleural cavity, the cavity within the thorax that contains the lungs. Between the ribs and the lungs are the visceral and parietal pleurae.

pleural effusion, an abnormal accumulation of fluid in the interstitial and air spaces of the lungs, characterized by fever, chest pain, dyspnoea, and nonproductive cough. The fluid involved is an exudate or a transudate from inflamed pleural surfaces.

pleural space, the potential space between the visceral and parietal layers of the pleurae. The space contains a small amount of fluid that acts as a lubricant, allowing the pleurae to slide smoothly over each other as the lungs expand and contract with respiration.

pleurisy, inflammation of the parietal pleura of the lungs, characterized by dyspnoea and stabbing pain, leading to restriction of ordinary breathing with spasm of the chest on the affected side. A friction rub may be heard on auscultation. Common causes of pleurisy include bronchial carcinoma, lung or chest wall abscess, pneumonia, pulmonary infarction, and tuberculosis.

pleurodynia, acute inflammation of the intercostal muscles and the muscular attachment of the diaphragm to the chest wall. It is characterized by sudden severe pain and tenderness, fever, headache, and anorexia. These symptoms are aggravated by movement and respiration.

pleuropericardial rub, an abnormal coarse friction sound heard on auscultation of the lungs during late inspiration and early expiration. It is caused by the visceral and parietal pleural surfaces rubbing against each other.

pleuroperitoneal cavity. See **splanchnocoele.**

pleuropneumonia, 1. a combination of pleurisy and pneumonia. **2.** an infection of cattle resulting in inflammation of both the pleura and lungs, caused by microorganisms of the Mycoplasma group.

pleuropneumonia-like organism (PPLO), a group of filterable organisms of the genus *Mycoplasma* similar to *M. mycoides,* the cause of pleuropneumonia in cattle.

pleurothotonos, an involuntary, severe, prolonged contraction of the muscles of one side of the body, resulting in an acute arch to that side. **pleurothotonic,** *adj.*

plexiform neuroma, a neoplasm composed of twisted bundles of nerves.

pleximeter, a mediating device, such as a percussor or finger, used to receive light taps in percussion.

plexor. See **percussor.**

plexus, *pl.* **plexuses,** a network of intersecting nerves and blood vessels or of lymphatic vessels.

plica, *pl.* **plicae,** a fold of tissue within the body, as the plicae transversales of the rectum and the plicae circulares of the small intestine. **plical,** *adj.*

plica circularis. See **circular fold.**

plicae transversales recti, semilunar, transverse folds in the rectum that support the weight of faeces.

plicamycin, an cytotoxic agent used primarily in the treatment of hypercalcaemia associated with cancer. Also called **mithramycin.**

plica semilunaris, the semilunar fold of the conjunctiva that extends laterally from the lacrimal caruncle.

plication, any operation that involves folding, shortening, or decreasing the size of a muscle or hollow organ, such as the stomach, by taking in tucks.

plica umbilicalis lateralis. See **lateral umbilical fold.**

plica umbilicalis mediana. See **middle umbilical fold.**

Plimmer's bodies {Henry G. Plimmer, English biologist, b. 1856}, small, round, encapsulated bodies found in cancers once thought to be the causative parasites.

ploidy, the status of a cell nucleus in regard to the number of complete chromosome sets it contains.

plug, a mass of tissue cells, mucus, or other matter that blocks a normal opening or passage of the body, such as a cervical plug.

Plummer's disease {Henry S. Plummer, American physician, b. 1874}, goitre characterized by a hyperfunctioning nodule or adenoma and thyrotoxicosis.

Plummer-Vinson syndrome {Henry S. Plummer; Porter P. Vinson, American physician, b. 1890}, a rare disorder associated with severe and chronic iron deficiency anaemia, characterized by dysphagia caused by oesophageal webs at the level of the cricoid cartilage.

plunging goitre. See **diving goitre.**

pluricentric blastoma. See **blastoma.**

pluripolar mitosis. See **multipolar mitosis.**

plutonium (Pu), a synthetic transuranic metallic element. Its atomic number is 94; its atomic weight is 242.

Pm, symbol for **promethium.**

PMT, abbreviation for **premenstrual tension.**

PND, abbreviation for **paroxysmal nocturnal dyspnoea.**

pneumatic condenser, (in dentistry) a pneumatic device to deliver a compacting force to restorative material used in filling tooth cavities.

pneumatic heart driver, a mechanical device that regulates compressed air delivery to an artificial heart, controlling heart rate, percent systole, and delay in systole.

pneumatocele, a thin-walled cavity in the lung parenchyma caused by partial airway obstruction.

pneumobelt, a corset with an inflatable bladder that fits over the abdominal area and is connected to a ventilator that delivers positive pressure at an adjustable rate. It is used to assist in the respiratory rehabilitation of patients with high cervical injuries.

pneumococcal, of or pertaining to bacteria of the genus *Pneumococcus.*

pneumococcal vaccine, an active immunizing agent containing antigens of the 14 types of *Pneumococcus* associated with 80% of the cases of pneumococcal pneumonia. It is prescribed for people over 2 years of age who are at high risk of developing severe pneumococcal pneumonia (e.g. those who have had a splenectomy).

pneumococcus, *pl.* **pneumococci,** a grampositive diplococcal bacterium of the species *Diplococcus pneumoniae,* the most common cause of bacterial pneumonia.

pneumoconiosis, any disease of the lung caused by chronic inhalation of dust, usually mineral dusts of occupational or environmental origin. Some kinds of pneumoconioses are **anthracosis, asbestosis, silicosis.**

pneumoconstriction, a dimple of collapsed lung tissue that results from mechanical stimulation of an exposed portion of the lung. It is produced by local reflex muscular closure of alveolar ducts and alveoli.

pneumocystosis, infection with the parasite *Pneumocystis carinii,* usually seen in infants or debilitated or immunosuppressed people and characterized by fever, cough, tachypnoea, and, frequently, cyanosis.

pneumoderma. See **subcutaneous emphysema.**

pneumoencephalography. See **encephalography.**

pneumogastric nerve. See **vagus nerve.**

pneumograph, a device that records breathing movements by means of an inflated coil around the chest.

pneumomediastinum, the presence of air or gas in the mediastinal tissues. The condition may result from bronchitis, acute asthma, pertussis, cystic fibrosis, or bronchial rupture from cough or trauma.

pneumonectomy, the surgical removal of all or part of a lung.

pneumonia, an acute inflammation of the lungs, usually caused by inhaled pneumococci of the species *Diplococcus pneumoniae.* The alveoli and bronchioles of the lungs become plugged with a fibrous exudate. Pneumonia may be caused by other bacteria, as well as by viruses, rickettsiae, and fungi, but in 85% of the cases, pneumococcus infection is the cause. Characteristic of pneumonia are severe chills, a high fever (which may reach 40-41°C), headache, cough, and chest pain. Inflammation of the lower lobe of the right lung may produce a pain suggesting appendicitis. An effusion of red blood cells into the alveolar spaces, resulting from histolytic damage by the microorganism, causes a rust-coloured sputum that may be a diagnostic sign of pneumococcal infection. As the disease progresses, sputum may become thicker and more purulent, and the person may experience painful attacks of coughing. Respiration usually becomes more difficult, painful, shallow, and rapid. The pulse increases in rapidity, often measuring 120 or more beats a minute. Other signs may include profuse sweating and cyanosis. GI disorders and an outbreak of herpes simplex about the face may also occur. In children, pneumonia may be accompanied by convulsion. As the alveoli become filled with exudate, the affected area of a lobe becomes increasingly firm and consolidated. A distinctive kind of rale is heard on auscultation. Kinds of pneumonia are **aspiration pneumonia, bronchopneumonia, eosinophilic pneumonia, interstitial pneumonia, lobar pneumonia, mycoplasma pneumonia,** and **viral pneumonia.**

pneumonic plague, a highly virulent and rapidly fatal form of plague characterized by bronchopneumonia. There are two forms: **Primary pneumonic plague** results from involvement of the lungs in the course of bubonic plague; **secondary pneumonic plague** results from the inhalation of infected particles of sputum from a person having pneumonic plague.

pneumonitis, *pl.* **pneumonitides,** inflammation of the lung. Pneumonitis may be caused by a virus or may be a hypersensitivity reaction to chemicals or organic dusts, such as bacteria, bird droppings, or moulds. It is usually an interstitial, granulomatous, fibrosing inflammation of the lung, especially of the bronchioles and alveoli. Dry cough is a common symptom. A kind of pneumonitis is **humidifier lung.**

pneumoperitoneum, the presence of air or gas within the peritoneal cavity of the abdomen. It may be spontaneous, as from rupture of a hollow gas-containing organ, or induced for diagnostic or therapeutic purposes.

pneumotachometer, a small cylindrical device that measures the change in pressure from the exhausting air of an artificial ventricle.

pneumothorax, a collection of air or gas in the pleural space causing the lung to collapse. Pneumothorax may be the result of an open chest wound that permits the entrance of air, the rupture of an emphysematous vesicle on the surface of the lung, or a severe bout of coughing, or it may occur spontaneously without apparent cause. The onset of pneumothorax is accompanied by a sudden, sharp chest pain, followed by difficult, rapid breathing, cessation of normal chest movements on the affected side, tachycardia, a weak pulse, hypotension, diaphoresis, an elevated temperature, pallor, dizziness, and anxiety.

Po, symbol for **polonium.**

PO₂, symbol for *partial pressure of oxygen.* See **partial pressure.**

podalic, pertaining to the feet.

podiatrist, a health professional trained to diagnose and treat diseases and other disorders of the feet. Also known as a chiropodist.

podiatry, the study of minor disorders of the feet and the practice of treating these disorders.

podophyllotoxin, a cytotoxic substance derived from the roots of *Podophyllum peltatum,* a common plant species known as mayapple, or American mandrake. A paint preparation of podophyllotoxin is used in the treatment of condyloma acuminatum and other types of warts.

podophyllum, the dried rhizome and roots of *Podophyllum peltatum,* from which a caustic resin is derived for use in removing certain warts.

poikilocytosis, an abnormal degree of variation in the shape of the erythrocytes in the blood.

poikiloderma atrophicans vasculare, an abnormal skin condition characterized by hyperpigmentation or hypopigmentation, telangiectasia, and atrophy of the epidermis.

poikiloderma of Civatte, a common benign, progressive dermatitis characterized by erythematous patches on the face and neck that become dry and scaly. As the condition progresses, pigment is deposited around the hair follicles extending down the lateral aspects of the neck.

poikilothermic. See **cold blooded.**

point behaviour, the orientation of body parts in a certain direction within a quantum of space.

point forceps, a dental instrument used in filling root canals. It holds the filling cones during their placement.

point lesion, a disruption of single chemical bonds caused by effects of ionizing radiation on a macromolecule.

point of maximum impulse (PMI), the place in the fifth intercostal space of the thorax, just medial to the left midclavicular line, where the apex beat of the heart is observed.

poise {Jean L. M. Poiseuille, French physiologist, b. 1799}, a unit of liquid or gas (fluid) viscosity expressed in terms of $gm \times cm^{-1} \times sec^{-1}$.

poison, any substance that impairs health or destroys life when ingested, inhaled, or absorbed by the body in relatively small amounts. **poisonous,** *adj.*

poisoning, 1. the act of administering a toxic substance. 2. the condition or physical state produced by the ingestion, injection, inhalation, or exposure of a poisonous substance. Kinds of poisoning include **creosote poi-**

soning, food poisoning, heavy metals poisoning, petroleum distillate poisoning, and salicylate poisoning.

poisoning, potential for, the risk of accidental exposure to or ingestion of drugs or dangerous products in doses sufficient to cause poisoning. The risk factors may be internal (individual) or external (environmental). Internal risk factors include reduced vision, lack of safety or drug education, lack of proper precautions, and cognitive or emotional difficulties. External risk factors include medicines or dangerous products stored in unlocked cabinets; availability of illicit drugs contaminated by poisonous additives; flaking paint or plaster in the presence of young children; chemical contamination of food and water; unprotected contact with heavy metals, chemicals, paint, or lacquer; presence of poisonous vegetation; and presence of atmospheric pollutants.

poisoning treatment, the symptomatic and supportive care given to a patient who has been exposed to or who has ingested a toxic drug, commercial chemical, or other dangerous substance. In the case of oral poisoning, a primary effort should be directed toward recovery of the toxic substance before it can be absorbed into the body tissues. If vomiting does not occur spontaneously, it should be induced after first identifying the poison, if possible. If the poison is a petroleum distillate, such as kerosene, or a caustic or corrosive substance, vomiting should not be induced.

poison ivy, any of several species of climbing vine of the genus *Rhus,* characterized by shiny, three-pointed leaves. It causes severe allergic contact dermatitis in many people. Localized vesicular eruption with itching and burning results.

poisons information centre, one of a number of specialist centres throughout the United Kingdom, that provide 24 hour information and advice on all aspects of poisoning.

poker spine. See **bamboo spine.**

polar, pertaining to molecules that are hydrophilic, or "water-loving." Polar substances tend to dissolve in polar solvents.

polar body, one of the small cells produced during the two meiotic divisions in the maturation process of female gametes, or ova. It is nonfunctional and incapable of being fertilized.

polarity, 1. the existence or manifestation of opposing qualities, tendencies, or emotions, such as pleasure and pain, love and hate, strength and weakness, dependence and independence, masculinity and femininity. **2.** (in midwifery/obstetrics) the co-ordination between the upper and lower uterine segments, described as balanced and harmonious in labour; the upper uterine segment is active and contracts and retracts, while the lower segment is passive. **3.** (in physics) the distinction between a negative and a positive electric charge.

polarity therapy, a technique of massage based on the theory that the body has positive and negative energy patterns that must be balanced to establish physical harmony.

polarization, the concentration within a population or group of members' interests, beliefs, and allegiances around two conflicting positions.

polarographic oxygen analyser, an electrochemical device used to analyse the proportion of oxygen molecules in respiratory care systems. The oxygen is measured in terms of an electron current produced after it acquires electrons from a negative electrode in a hydroxide bath.

pole, 1. (in biology) an end of an imaginary axis drawn through the symmetrically arranged parts of a cell, organ, ovum, or nucleus. **2.** (in anatomy) the point on a nerve cell at which a dendrite originates. **polar,** *adj.*

pol gene, a segment of a retrovirus, such as the human T cell leukaemia virus (HTLV), that encodes its reverse transcriptase enzyme.

policy, a principle or guideline that governs an activity and that employees or members of an institution or organization are expected to follow.

polio. See **poliomyelitis.**

polioencephalitis, an inflammation of the grey matter of the brain caused by infection of the brain by a poliovirus.

polioencephalomyelitis, inflammation of the grey matter of the brain and the spinal cord, caused by infection by a poliovirus.

poliomyelitis, an infectious disease caused by one of the three polioviruses. Asymptomatic, mild, and paralytic forms of the disease occur. It is transmitted from person to person through faecal contamination or oropharyngeal secretions. Asymptomatic infection has no clinical features, but it confers immunity. Abortive poliomyelitis lasts only a few hours and is characterized by minor illness with fever, malaise, headache, nausea, vomiting, and slight abdominal discomfort. Nonparalytic poliomyelitis is longer lasting and is marked by meningeal irritation with pain and stiffness in the back and by all the signs of abortive poliomyelitis. Paralytic poliomyelitis begins as abortive poliomyelitis. The symptoms abate, and for several days the person seems well. Malaise, headache, and fever recur; pain, weakness, and paralysis develop. The peak of paralysis is reached within the first week. In spinal poliomyelitis, viral replication occurs in the anterior horn cells of the spine causing inflammation, swelling, and, if severe, destruction of the neurons. The large proximal muscles of the limbs are most often affected. Bulbar poliomyelitis results from viral multiplication in the brainstem. Bulbar and spinal poliomyelitis often occur together.

poliomyelitis vaccine, vaccines prepared from poliovirus to confer immunity to it. The live oral (Sabin) form of vaccine, is recommended for all individuals who have no specific contraindications. The inactivated (Salk) poliovirus vaccine is recommended for individuals who are immunodeficient. It is given subcutaneously.

poliosis, depigmentation of the hair on the scalp, eyebrows, eyelashes, moustache, beard, or body. The condition may be inherited and generalized or acquired and localized in patches. Acquired localized poliosis often occurs in alopecia areata.

poliovirus, the causative organism of poliomyelitis. There are three serologically distinct types of this very small RNA virus. Infection or immunization with one type does not protect against the others.

poliovirus vaccine. See **poliomyelitis vaccine.**

polishing, a tendency of patients with right temporal lobe lesions to deny dysphoric affect and minimize socially disapproved behaviour while exaggerating other qualities.

pollakiuria, an abnormal condition characterized by unduly frequent passage of urine.

pollen coryza, acute seasonal rhinitis caused by exposure to an allergenic.

pollinosis. See **hay fever.**

pollutant, an unwanted substance that occurs in the environment, usually with health-threatening effects. Pollutants may exist in the atmosphere as gases or fine particles that may be irritating to the lungs, eyes, and skin, as dissolved or suspended substances in drinking water, and as carcinogens or mutagens in foods or beverages.

polonium (Po), a radioactive element that is one of the disintegration products of uranium. Its atomic number is 84; its atomic weight is approximately 210.

polus, *pl.* **poli,** either of the opposite ends of any axis; the official anatomical designation for the extremity of an organ. See also **pole.**

polar, *adj.*

polyacrylamide, a polymer of acrylamide and usually some crosslinking derivative.

polyaesthesia, a sensory disorder involving the sense of touch in which a stimulus to one area of the skin is felt at other sites in addition to the one stimulated.

polyamine, any compound that contains two or moreamine groups, such as spermidine and spermine, which are normally occurring tissue constituents in humans.

polyanionic, pertaining to multiple negative electric charges.

polyarteritis, an abnormal inflammatory condition of several arteries.

polyarteritis nodosa, a severe and poorly understood collagen vascular disease in which there is widespread inflammation and necrosis of small and medium-sized arteries and ischaemia of the tissues they serve. It is characterized by fever, abdominal pain, weight loss, neuropathy, and, if the kidneys are affected, hypertension, oedema, and uraemia. Some symptoms may mimic GI or cardiac disorders.

polyarthritis, an inflammation that involves more than one joint. The inflammation may migrate from one joint to another, or there may be simultaneous involvement of two or more joints.

polychlorinated biphenyls (PCBs), a group of more than 30 isomers and compounds used in plastics, insulation, and flame retardants and varying in physical form from oily liquids to crystals and resins. All are potentially toxic and carcinogenic.

polychromasia. See **polychromatophilia.**

polychromatic, a light of many colours or wavelengths. The term is usually applied to white light although it may also refer to a defined portion of the spectrum.

polychromatophil, any cell that may be stained by several different dyes.

polychromatophilia, an abnormal tendency of a cell, particularly an erythrocyte, to be dyed by a variety of laboratory stains.

polyclonal, 1. of, pertaining to, or designating a group of identical cells or organisms derived from several identical cells. **2.** of, pertaining to, or designating several groups of identical cells or organisms (clones) derived from a single cell.

polyclonal gammopathy. See **gammopathy.**

polycystic, characterized by the presence of many cysts.

polycystic kidney disease (PKD), an abnormal condition in which the kidneys are enlarged and contain many cysts. There are three forms of the disease. **Childhood polycystic disease (CPD)** is uncommon and may be differentiated from adult or congenital polycystic disease by genetic, morphological, and clinical facets. Death usually occurs within a few years as the result of portal hypertension and liver and kidney failure. A portacaval shunt may prolong life into the twenties. **Adult polycystic disease (APD)** may be unilateral, bilateral, acquired, or congenital. The condition is characterized by flank pain and high blood pressure. Kidney failure eventually develops, progressing to uraemia and death. **Congenital polycystic disease (CPD)** is a rare congenital aplasia of the kidney involving all or only a small segment of one or both kidneys. Severe bilateral aplasia results in death shortly after birth.

polycystic ovary syndrome, an abnormal condition characterized by anovulation, amenorrhoea, hirsutism, and infertility. It is caused by an endocrine imbalance with increased levels of testosterone, oestrogen, and luteinizing hormone (LH) and decreased secretion of follicle stimulating hormone (FSH). Numerous follicular cysts, 2 to 6 mm in diameter, may develop. The affected ovary commonly doubles in size and is invested by a smooth, pearly-white capsule.

polycythaemia, an abnormal increase in the number of erythrocytes in the blood. It may be secondary to pulmonary disease or heart disease or to prolonged exposure to high altitudes.

polydactyly, a congenital anomaly characterized by the presence of more than the normal number of fingers or toes. The condition is usually inherited.

polydipsia, excessive thirst characteristic of several different conditions, including diabetes mellitus in which an excessive concentration of glucose in the blood osmotically increases the excretion of fluid via increased urination, which leads to hypovolaemia and thirst.

polyelectrolyte, a substance with many charged or potentially charged groups.

polygene, any of a group of nonallelic genes that individually exert a small effect but together interact in a cumulative manner to produce a particular characteristic within an individual, usually of a quantitative nature, such as size, weight, or skin pigmentation. **polygenic,** *adj.*

polygenic inheritance. See **multifactorial inheritance.**

polyglucosan, a large molecule consisting of many anhydrous polysaccharides.

polyhybrid, (in genetics) pertaining to or describing an individual, organism, or strain that is heterozygous for more than three specific traits.

polyhybrid cross, (in genetics) the mating of two individuals, organisms, or strains that have different gene pairs that determine more than three specific traits.

polyhydramnios. See **hydramnios.**

polyleptic, describing any disease or condition marked by numerous remissions and exacerbations.

polyleptic fever, a fever occurring paroxysmally, such as smallpox and relapsing fever.

polymer, a compound formed by combining or linking a number of monomers, or small molecules. A polymer may be composed of a variety of different monomers or from many units of the same monomer.

polymicrogyria. See **microgyria.**

polymorphism, 1. the state or quality of existing or occurring in several different forms. **2.** the state or quality of appearing in different forms at different stages of development. Kinds of polymorphism are **balanced polymorphism** and **genetic polymorphism.** **polymorphic,** *adj.*

polymorphocytic leukaemia, a neoplasm of blood-forming tissues in which mature, segmented granulocytes are predominant.

polymorphonuclear, having a nucleus with a number of lobules or segments connected by a fine thread.

polymorphonuclear cell (PMN), a leukocyte with a multilobed nucleus, as a neutrophil.

polymorphonuclear leukocyte, a white blood cell containing a segmented lobular nucleus; an eosinophil, basophil, or neutrophil.

polymorphous, occurring in many varying forms, possibly changing in structure or appearance at different stages.

polymorphous light eruption, a common, recurrent, superficial vascular reaction to sunlight or ultraviolet light in susceptible individuals. Within 1 to 4 days after exposure to the light, small, erythematous papules and vesicles appear on otherwise normal skin, then disappear within 2 weeks.

polymyalgia rheumatica, a chronic, episodic, inflammatory disease of the large arteries that usually develops in people over 60 years of age. Polymyalgia rheumatica primarily affects the muscles, and it is characterized by pain and stiffness of the back, shoulder, or neck, usually becoming more severe on rising in the morning. There may also be a cranial headache, as in cranial arteritis, which affects the temporal and occipital arteries, causing a severe, throbbing headache.

polymyositis, inflammation of many muscles, usually accompanied by deformity, edema, insomnia, pain, sweating, and tension.

polymyxin B sulphate, an antibiotic used topically for infections caused by microorganisms sensitive to this drug.

polyneuritic psychosis. See **Korsakoff's psychosis.**

polyopia, a defect of sight in which one object is perceived as many images; multiple vision. The condition can occur in one or both eyes.

polyp, a small tumourlike growth that projects from a mucous membrane surface.

polypeptide, a chain of amino acids joined by peptide bonds. A polypeptide has a larger molecular weight than a peptide but a smaller molecular weight than a protein.

polyphagia, eating to the point of gluttony.

polypharmacy, a term applied to the use of a number of different drugs by a patient who may have one or several health problems.

polyploid, 1. of or pertaining to an individual, organism, strain, or cell that has more than the two complete sets of chromosomes normal for the somatic cell. The multiple of the haploid number characteristic of the species is denoted by the appropriate prefix, as in triploid, tetraploid, pentaploid, and so on. **2.** such an individual, organism, strain, or cell. Also **polyploidic.**

polyploid adenocarcinoma. See **papillary adenocarcinoma.**

polyploidy, the state or condition of having more than two complete sets of chromosomes.

polyposis, an abnormal condition characterized by the presence of numerous polyps on a part.

polyradiculitis, inflammation of many nerve roots, as found in Guillain-Barré syndrome.

polyribosome. See **polysome.**

polysaccharide, a carbohydrate that contains three or more molecules of simple carbohydrates. Examples of polysaccharides include dextrins, starches, glycogens, and pentose.

polysome, (in genetics) a group of ribosomes joined together by a molecule of messenger RNA containing the genetic code.

polysomy, the presence of a chromosome in at least triplicate in an otherwise diploid somatic cell as the result of chromosomal nondisjunction during meiotic division in the maturation of gametes. The chromosome may be duplicated three times (trisomy), four times (tetrasomy), or more times.

polytene chromosome, an excessively large type of chromosome consisting of bundles of unseparated chromonemata filaments. See also **giant chromosome.**

polythiazide, a diuretic and antihypertensive prescribed in the treatment of hypertension and oedema.

polyunsaturated fatty acid. See **unsaturated fatty acid.**

polyuria, the excretion of an abnormally large quantity of urine. Some causes of polyuria are diabetes insipidus, diabetes mellitus, diuretics, excessive fluid intake, hypercalcaemia.

polyvalent antiserum. See **antiserum.**

polyvinyl chloride (PVC), a common synthetic thermoplastic material that releases hydrochloric acid when burned and that may contain carcinogenic vinyl chloride molecules as a contaminant.

POM, abbreviation for **prescription only medicine.**

POMP, abbreviation for a combination drug regimen used in the treatment of cancer, containing three antineoplastics, Purinethol (mercaptopurine), Oncovin (vincristine sulphate), methotrexate, and prednisolone (a glucocorticoid).

Pompe's disease {J. C. Pompe, 20th century Dutch physician}, a form of muscle glycogen storage disease in which there is a generalized accumulation of glycogen, resulting from a deficiency of acid maltase (alpha-1, 4-glucosidase). Children with Pompe's disease appear mentally deficient and hypotonic, seldom living beyond 20 years of age. In adults muscle weakness is progressive, but the disease is not fatal.

pompholyx. See **dyshidrosis.**

ponos. See **kala-azar.**

pons, *pl.* **pontes, 1.** any slip of tissue connecting two parts of a structure or an organ of the body. **2.** a prominence on the ventral surface of the brainstem, between the medulla oblongata and the cerebral peduncles of the midbrain. The pons consists of white matter and a few nuclei and is divided into a ventral portion and a dorsal portion. The dorsal portion comprises the tegmentum, which contains the nucleus of the abducens nerve, the nucleus of the facial nerve, the motor nucleus of the trigeminal nerve, the sensory nuclei of the trigeminal nerve, the nucleus of the cochlear division of the eighth nerve, the superior olive, and the nuclei of the vestibular division of the eighth nerve.

Pontiac fever. See **Legionnaires' disease.**

pontic, the suspended member of a fixed partial denture, such as an artificial tooth, usually occupying the space previously occupied by the natural tooth crown.

pontine centre. See **apneustic centre.**

pooled plasma, a liquid component of whole blood, collected and pooled to prepare various plasma products or to use directly as a plasma expander when whole blood is unavailable or is contraindicated.

poorly differentiated lymphocytic malignant lymphoma, a lymphoid neoplasm containing many cells resembling lymphoblasts that have a fine nuclear structure and one or more nucleoli.

popliteal artery, a continuation of the femoral artery, extending from the opening in the abductor magnus, passing through the popliteal fossa at the knee, dividing into eight branches, and supplying various muscles of the thigh, leg, and foot.

popliteal node, a node in one of the groups of lymph glands in the leg.

popliteal pulse, the pulse of the popliteal artery, palpated behind the knee of a person lying prone with the knee flexed.

population, 1. (in genetics) an interbreeding group of individuals, organisms, or plants characterized by genetic continuity through several generations. **2.** a group of individuals collectively occupying a particular geographic locale. **3.** any group that is distinguished by a particular trait or situation. **4.** any group measured for some variable characteristic from which samples may be taken for statistical purposes.

population at risk, a group of people who share a characteristic that causes each member to be vulnerable to a particular event, such as nonimmunized children who are exposed to poliovirus.

population genetics, a branch of genetics that applies mendelian inheritance to groups and studies the frequency of alleles and genotypes in breeding populations.

porcine graft, a temporary biological heterograft made from the skin of a pig.

pork tapeworm. See *Taenia solium.*

pork tapeworm infection, an infection of

the intestine or other tissues, caused by adult and larval forms of the tapeworm *Taenia solium*. The pork tapeworm is unique in that it can use humans as both intermediate hosts for larvae and definitive hosts for the adult worm. Humans are usually infected with the adult worm after eating contaminated, undercooked pork.

porphobilinogen, a chromogen substance that is an intermediate in the biosynthesis of haem and porphyrins. It appears in the urine of persons with porphyria.

porphyria, a group of inherited disorders in which there is abnormally increased production of substances called porphyrins. Two major classifications of porphyria are **erythropoietic porphyria,** characterized by the production of large quantities of porphyrins in the blood-forming tissue of the bone marrow, and **hepatic porphyria,** in which large amounts of porphyrins are produced in the liver. Clinical signs common to both classifcations of porphyria are photosensitivity, abdominal pain, and neuropathy.

porphyrin, any iron- or magnesium-free pyrrole derivative occurring in many plant and animal tissues.

portacaval shunt, a shunt created surgically to increase the flow of blood from the portal circulation by carrying it into the vena cava.

portal fissure, a fissure on the visceral surface of the liver along which the portal vein, the hepatic artery, and the hepatic ducts pass.

portal hypertension, an increased venous pressure in the portal circulation caused by compression or by occlusion in the portal or hepatic vascular system. It results in splenomegaly, large collateral veins, ascites, and, in severe cases, systemic hypertension and oesophageal varices.

portal of entry, the route by which an infectious agent enters the body.

portal system, the network of veins that drains the blood from the abdominal portion of the digestive tract, the spleen, the pancreas, and the gallbladder and conveys blood from these viscera to the liver.

portal systemic encephalopathy. See **hepatic coma.**

portal vein, a vein that ramifies like an artery in the liver and ends in capillary-like sinusoids that convey the blood to the inferior vena cava through the hepatic veins. The tributaries of the portal vein are the lienal vein, the superior mesenteric vein, the coronary vein, the pyloric vein, the cystic vein, and the paraumbilical vein.

Porter-Silber reaction {Curt C. Porter, American biochemist, b. 1914; Robert H. Silber, American biochemist, b. 1915}, a reaction, visible as a change in colour to yellow, that indicates the amount of adrenal steroids (the 17-hydroxycorticosteroids) excreted per day in the urine. The test is used to evaluate adrenocortical function.

portoenterostomy, a procedure to correct biliary atresis in which the jejunum is anastomosed by a Roux-en-Y loop to the portal fissure region to establish bile flow from the bile ducts to the intestine.

port-wine stain. See **naevus flammeus.**

position, 1. any one of many postures of the body, such as the anatomical position, or lateral recumbent position. See specific positions. **2.** (in obstetrics) the relationship of an arbitrarily chosen fetal reference point, such as the occiput, sacrum, chin, or scapula, on the presenting part of the fetus, with respect to its location in the maternal pelvis.

position of the fetus, the relationship of the part of the fetus that presents in the pelvis to four quadrants of the maternal pelvis identified by initial L(left), R(right), A(anterior) and P(posterior).

positional behaviour, the orientation of the body regions to claim a quantum of space. Positional behaviour involves four body regions: head and neck, upper torso, pelvis and thighs, and lower legs and feet.

positive, 1. (of a laboratory test) indicating that a substance or a reaction is present. **2.** (of a sign) indicating on physical examination that a finding is present, often meaning that there is pathological change. **3.** (of a substance) tending to carry or carrying a positive chemical charge.

positive end expiratory pressure (PEEP), (in respiratory therapy) ventilation controlled by a flow of air delivered in cycles of constant pressure through the respiratory cycle. PEEP is used for the relief of respiratory distress secondary to prematurity, pancreatitis, shock, pulmonary edema, trauma, surgery, or other conditions in which spontaneous respiratory efforts are inadequate and arterial levels of oxygen are deficient.

positive euthanasia. See **euthanasia.**

positive feedback, (in physiology) an increase in function in response to a stimulus; for example, micturition increases once the flow of urine has started.

positive identification, the unconscious modelling of one's personality on that of another who is admired and esteemed.

positive pressure, 1. a greater than ambient atmospheric pressure. **2.** (in respiratory therapy) any technique in which compressed air or gas or air is delivered to the respiratory passages at greater than ambient pressure.

positive pressure breathing unit. See **IPPV unit.**

positive relationship, (in research) a direct relationship between two variables; as one increases, the other can be expected to increase.

positive signs of pregnancy, three unmistakable signs of pregnancy: fetal heart tones, heard on auscultation; fetus visible on ultrasound scan; and fetal parts, felt on palpation.

positron, a positively charged electron emitted from certain neutron-deficient radioactive nuclei.

positron emission tomography (PET), a computerized radionuclide imaging technique that employs radioactive substances to examine the metabolic activity of various body structures. In PET studies the patient either inhales or is injected with a biochemical, such as glucose, carrying a radioactive substance that emits positively charged particles, or positrons, that combine with negatively charged electrons normally found in the cells of the body. When the positrons combine with these electrons, gamma rays are emitted. The electronic circuitry and computers of the PET device detect the gamma rays and convert them into color-coded images that indicate the intensity of the metabolic activity of the organ involved.

Posner-Schlossman syndrome. See glaucomatocyclitic crisis.

postcommissurotomy syndrome, a condition of unknown cause occurring within the first few weeks after cardiac valvular surgery, characterized by intermittent episodes of pain and fever, which may last weeks or months and then resolve spontaneously.

postconcussion syndrome, a condition after head trauma, characterized by dizziness, poor concentration, headache, hypersensitivity, and anxiety.

posterior, **1.** of or pertaining to or situated in the back part of a structure, as of the dorsal surface of the human body. **2.** the back part of something. **3.** toward the back.

posterior Achilles bursitis, a painful heel condition caused by inflammation of the bursa between the Achilles tendon and the calcaneus. It is commonly associated with Haglund's deformity.

posterior asynclitism. See asynclitism.

posterior atlantoaxial ligament, one of five ligaments connecting the atlas to the axis. Compare anterior atlantoaxial ligament.

posterior atlantooccipital membrane, one of a pair of thin, broad fibrous sheets that form part of the atlanto-occipital joint between the atlas and the occipital bone. Compare anterior atlantooccipital membrane.

posterior auricular artery, one of a pair of small branches from the external carotid arteries, dividing into auricular and occipital branches and supplying parts of the ear, scalp, and other structures in the head.

posterior common ligament. See posterior longitudinal ligament.

posterior costotransverse ligament, one of the five ligaments of each costotransverse joint, comprised of a fibrous band passing from the neck of each rib to the base of the vertebra above.

posterior fontanelle, a small triangular area between the occipital and parietal bones at the junction of the sagittal and lambdoidal sutures.

posterior fossa, a depression on the posterior surface of the humerus, above the trochlea, that lodges the olecranon of the ulna when the elbow is extended.

posterior longitudinal ligament, a thick, strong ligament attached to the dorsal surfaces of the vertebral bodies, extending from the occipital bone to the coccyx.

posterior mediastinal node, a node in one of three groups of thoracic visceral nodes, connected to the part of the lymphatic system that serves the esophagus, pericardium, diaphragm, and convex surface of the liver.

posterior mediastinum, the irregularly shaped caudal portion of the mediastinum, parallel with the vertebral column.

posterior nares, a pair of posterior openings in the nasal cavity that connect the nasal cavity with the nasopharynx and allow the inhalation and the exhalation of air.

posterior neuropore, the opening at the caudal end of the embryonic neural tube.

posterior palatal seal area, the area of soft tissues along the junction of the hard and soft palates on which displacement, within the physiologic tolerance of the tissues, can be applied by a denture to aid its retention.

posterior pituitary, posterior pituitary gland. See neurohypophysis.

posterior tibial artery, one of the divisions of the popliteal artery, starting at the distal border of the popliteus muscle, passing behind the tibia, dividing into eight branches, and supplying various muscles of the lower leg, foot, and toes.

posterior tibialis pulse, the pulse of the posterior tibialis artery palpated on the medial aspect of the ankle, just posterior to the prominence of the ankle bone.

posterior tooth, any of the maxillary and mandibular premolars and molars of the permanent dentition, or of prostheses.

posterior vein of left ventricle, one of the five tributaries of the coronary sinus that drains blood from the capillary bed of the myocardium.

posterolateral thoracotomy, a chest surgery technique in which an incision is made in the submammary fold, below the tip of the scapula.

postgastrectomy care, nursing care after the removal of all or part of the stomach. Drainage of the nasogastric tube normally changes from bright red to dark in the first 24 hours. When bowel sounds reappear and a small amount of water given is retained, the nasogastric tube is removed. Small, bland meals are offered hourly as tolerated. An increase in temperature or dyspnoea indicates a leakage of oral fluids around the anastomosis. The diet is changed slowly to a regular diet, with five or six dry small feedings daily. Fluids are given hourly between meals. The most common complication of gastrectomy is the dumping syndrome, with fullness and discomfort, including vertigo, sweating, palpitation, and nausea occurring 5 to 30 minutes after eating, as food enters the small bowel.

posthepatic cirrhosis. See **cirrhosis.**

postictal, of or pertaining to the period following a convulsion. **posticus,** *n.*

postinfectious, occurring after an infection.

postinfectious encephalitis. See **encephalitis.**

postinfectious glomerulonephritis, the acute form of glomerulonephritis, which may follow 1 to 6 weeks after a streptococcal infection, most often in childhood. Characteristics of the disease are haematuria, oliguria, oedema, and proteinuria, especially in the form of granular casts.

postmastectomy exercises, exercises essential to the prevention of shortening of the muscles and contracture of the joints following mastectomy. The woman is asked to flex and extend the fingers of the affected arm and to pronate and supinate the forearm immediately on return to her room after recovery from anaesthesia and surgery. On the first postoperative day she is asked to squeeze a rubber ball in her hand. Brushing her teeth and hair are encouraged as effective exercises.

postmature, **1.** overly developed or matured. **2.** of or pertaining to a postmature infant. **postmaturity,** *n.*

postmature infant, an infant, born after the end of the forty-second week of gestation, bearing the physical signs of placental insufficiency. Characteristically, the baby has dry, peeling skin, long fingernails and toenails, and folds of skin on the thighs and, sometimes, on the arms and buttocks. Hypoglycaemia and hypokalaemia are common. Postmature infants often look as if they have lost weight in utero.

postmenopausal, of or pertaining to the period of life after the menopause.

postmortem, **1.** after death. **2.** *informal.* postmortem examination.

postmyocardial infarction syndrome, a condition that may occur days or weeks after an acute myocardial infarction. It is characterized by fever, pericarditis with a friction rub, pleurisy, pleural effusion, and joint pain. It tends to recur and often provokes severe anxiety, depression, and fear that it is another heart attack.

postnasal drip, a drop-by-drop discharge of nasal mucus into the posterior pharynx, often accompanied by a feeling of obstruction, an unpleasant taste, and fetid breath, caused by rhinitis, chronic sinusitis, or hypersecretion by the nasopharyngeal mucosa.

postnatal period, the period of not less than 10 and not more than 28 days after the end of labour, during which the attendance of a

midwife is mandatory under the UKCC Rules.

postnecrotic cirrhosis, a nodular form of cirrhosis that may follow hepatitis or other inflammation of the liver.

postoperative, of or pertaining to the period of time after surgery. It begins with the patient's emergence from anaesthesia and continues through the time required for the acute effects of the anaesthetic or surgical procedures to abate.

postoperative atelectasis, a form of atelectasis in which collapse of lung tissue is caused by the depressant effects of anaesthetic drugs. Deep breathing and coughing are encouraged at frequent intervals postoperatively to prevent this condition.

postoperative care, the management of a patient after surgery. On the patient's discharge from the operating theatre, the surgical drapes, ground plate, and restraints are removed and a sterile dressing is applied to the incision. The patency and connections of all drainage tubes and the flow rate of parenteral infusions are checked. The patient's cleanliness and dryness are given attention, and the gown is changed, avoiding exposing the individual. Four people transfer the patient slowly and cautiously to a recovery room bed, maintaining body alignment and protecting the limbs. When indicated, an oral or nasal airway is inserted or a previously inserted endotracheal tube is suctioned; respiration may be supported with a pulmonator or intermittent positive pressure breathing (IPPB); if respiration remains impaired, the anaesthetist is notified. The blood pressure, pulse, and respirations are initially reported to the anaesthetist and are then checked every 15 minutes or as ordered. At similar intervals, the level of consciousness, reflexes, and movements of extremities are observed, and the incision, drainage tubes, and intravenous infusion site are inspected. Nothing is given orally; medication, blood or blood components, oxygen, and IPPB are administered as ordered, and fluid intake and output are measured.

postoperative cholangiography. See **operative cholangiography.**

postpartum, after childbirth.

postpartum care care of the mother and her newborn baby during the **postnatal period.**

postpartum depression, a condition that occurs in women after childbirth, typically from 3 days to 6 weeks post partum. It is characterized by symptoms that range from mild "postpartum blues" to an intense, suicidal, depressive psychosis.

postperfusion syndrome, a cytomegalovirus (CMV) infection, occurring between 2 and 4 weeks after the transfusion of fresh blood containing CMV. It is characterized by prolonged fever, hepatitis, rash, atypical lymphocytosis, and, occasionally, jaundice.

postpericardiotomy syndrome, a condition that sometimes occurs days or weeks after pericardiotomy, characterized by symptoms of pericarditis, often without any fever. It appears to be an autoimmune response to damaged muscle cells of the myocardium and pericardium.

postpill amenorrhoea, failure of normal menstrual cycles to resume after discontinuation of oral contraception.

postpolycythaemic myeloid metaplasia, a common late development in polycythaemia vera, characterized by anaemia caused by sclerosis of the bone marrow. The production of red blood cells then occurs only in extramedullary tissue, such as the liver and spleen.

postprandial, after a meal.

postpubertal panhypopituitarism, insufficiency of pituitary hormones, caused by postpartum pituitary necrosis resulting from thrombosis of the circulation of the gland during or after delivery. The disorder, characterized initially by weakness, lethargy, failure to lactate, amenorrhoea, loss of libido, and intolerance to cold, leads to loss of axillary and pubic hair, bradycardia, hypotension, premature wrinkling of the skin, and atrophy of the thyroid and adrenal glands.

postpuberty, a period of approximately 1 to 2 years after puberty during which skeletal growth slows and the physiologic functions of the reproductive years are established. **postpuberal, postpubertal, postpubescent,** *adj.*

postrenal anuria, cessation of urine production caused by obstruction in the ureters.

postresection filling. See **retrograde filling.**

postsynaptic, 1. situated after a synapse. **2.** occurring after a synapse has been crossed.

postsynaptic element, any neurological structure, such as a neuron, situated distal to a synapse.

postterm infant. See **postmature infant.**

posttrauma response, a sustained painful response to unexpected extraordinary life events. Defining characteristics include reexperience of the traumatic event (flashbacks, intrusive thoughts, repetitive dreams or nightmares, talking excessively about the event), emotional numbness, and an altered life-style with self-destructive behaviour and difficulty with interpersonal relationships.

posttraumatic amnesia, a period of amnesia between a brain injury resulting in memory loss and the point at which the functions concerned with memory are restored.

posttraumatic stress disorder, an anxiety disorder characterized by an acute emotional response to a traumatic event or situation involving severe environmental stress, such as a natural disaster, serious accident, military combat or physical torture. Symptoms of the condition include recurrent, intrusive recollections or nightmares, diminished responsiveness to the external world, hyperalertness or an exaggerated startle response, sleep disturbances, irritability, memory impairment, difficulty in concentrating, depression, anxiety, headaches, and vertigo.

postural albuminuria. See **orthostatic proteinuria.**

postural background movements, the spontaneous body adjustments, requiring vestibular and proprioceptive integration, that maintain the center of gravity, keep the head and body in alignment, and stabilize body parts.

postural drainage, the use of positioning to drain secretions from specific segments of the bronchi and the lungs into the trachea. Coughing normally expels secretions from the trachea. Positions are selected that promote drainage from the affected parts of the lungs. Pillows and raised sections of the hospital bed are used to support or elevate parts of the body. The procedure is begun with the patient level, and the head is gradually lowered to a full Trendelenburg position. Inhalation through the nose and exhalation through the mouth is encouraged. Simultaneously the nurse may use cupping and vibration over the affected area of the lungs to dislodge and mobilize secretions. The person is then helped to a position conducive to coughing and is asked to breathe deeply at least three times and to cough at least twice.

postural hypotension. See **orthostatic hypotension.**

postural proteinuria. See **orthostatic proteinuria.**

postural vertigo. See **cupulolithiasis.**

posture, the position of the body with respect to the surrounding space. A posture is determined and maintained by coordination of the various muscles that move the limbs, by proprioception, and by the sense of balance.

potassium (K), an alkali metal element, the seventh most abundant element in the earth's crust. Its atomic number is 19; its atomic weight is 39.1. Potassium salts are necessary to the life of all plants and animals. Potassium in the body constitutes the predominant intracellular cation, helping to regulate neuromuscular excitability and muscle contraction.

potassium chloride (KCl), an electrolyte replenisher prescribed in the treatment of hypokalaemia resulting from a variety of causes and in treating digitalis intoxication.

potassium hydroxide (KOH), a white, soluble, highly caustic compound. Occasionally used in solution as an escharotic for bites of rabid animals, KOH has many laboratory uses as an alkalinizing agent, including the preparation of clinical specimens for examination for fungi under the microscope.

potassium indoxyl sulphate. See **indican.**

potassium iodide, an iodine salt that has been used in the prevention and treatment of iodine deficiency, as an adjunct to antithyroid agents in the preoperative management of hyperthyroidism, to block the uptake of radioactive iodine into the thyroid gland, and as an expectorant.

potassium penicillin V. See **phenoxymethylpenicillin.**

potassium-sparing diuretic. See **diuretic.**

potency, (in embryology) the range of developmental possibilities of which an embryonic cell or part is capable, regardless of whether the stimulus for growth or differentiation is natural, artificial, or experimental.

potential, an expression of the energy involved in transfering a unit of electric charge. The gradient or slope of a potential causes the charge to move.

potential abnormality of glucose tolerance, a classification that includes persons who have never had abnormal glucose tolerance but who have an increased risk of diabetes or impaired glucose tolerance. Factors associated with an increased risk of insulin-dependent diabetes mellitus (IDDM) include circulating islet cell antibodies, being a monozygotic twin or sibling of an IDDM patient, and being the offspring of an IDDM patient.

potential diabetes. See **potential abnormality of glucose tolerance.**

potential difference, the difference in electric potential between two points.

potential trauma, (in dentistry) a change in tissue that may occur because of existing malocclusion or dental disharmony.

potentiate, to increase the strength or degree of activity of something.

potentiation, a synergistic action in which the effect of two drugs given simultaneously is greater than the effect of the drugs given separately.

potentiometer, a voltage measuring device.

Potter-Bucky grid {Hollis E. Potter, American radiologist, b. 1880; Gustav Bucky, American radiologist, b. 1880}, (in radiography) a type of moving secondary radiation grid using a single lateral movement. See also **grid.**

Pott's disease. See **tuberculous spondylitis.**

Pott's fracture {Percival Pott, English physician, b. 1714}, a fracture of the fibula near the ankle, often accompanied by a break of the malleolus of the tibia or rupture of the internal lateral ligament.

potty chair, a small chair that has an open seat over a removable pot, used for the toilet training of young children.

pouch of Douglas, {James Douglas, Scottish anatatomist, b. 1675} a rectouterine pouch or recess formed by a fold of the peritoneum that extends between the rectum and the uterus.

poultice, a soft, moist, pulp spread between layers of gauze or cloth and applied hot to a surface to provide heat or counterirritation.

povidone-iodine, an antiseptic used for disinfection of wounds, as a preoperative surgical scrub, for vaginal infections, and for antiseptic treatment of burns.

powdered gold, a fine granulation of pure gold, produced by atomizing the molten metal or by chemical precipitation. It is used in some dental restorations, such as prepared tooth cavities.

powerlessness, a lack of control over a current health-related situation or problem and the client's perceived knowledge that any action by him or herself will not affect the outcome of the particular situation.

power of attorney, a document authorizing one person to take legal actions in behalf of another, who acts as an agent for the grantor.

power stroke, a working stroke with a dental scaling instrument, used for splitting or dislodging calculus from the surface of a tooth or tooth root.

pox, 1. any of several vesicular or pustular exanthematous diseases. **2.** the pitlike scars of smallpox. **3.** *archaic.* syphilis.

poxvirus, a member of a family of viruses that includes the organisms that cause molluscum contagiosum, smallpox, and vaccinia.

PPD, abbreviation for **purified protein derivative,** the material used in testing for tuberculin sensitivity.

PPLO, abbreviation for **pleuropneumonia-like organism.** See **Mycoplasma.**

ppm, abbreviation for **parts per million.**

PPV, abbreviation for **positive pressure ventilation.** See **positive pressure,** def. 2.

Pr, symbol for **praseodymium.**

practical anatomy. See **applied anatomy.**

practice models, the different patterns in delivery of health care services by means of which health care is made available to diverse groups of people in different settings.

practice nurse, a qualified nurse working in the community and based in a general practice. Their main responsibilities include screening of at-risk groups implementing immunization programmes monitoring the health of the chronically sick and teaching self-care.

practice setting, the context or environment within which nursing care is given.

practice theory, (in nursing research) a theory that describes, explains, and prescribes nursing practice in general. It serves as the basis for specific items in the curriculum of nursing education and for the development of theories in the administration of nursing and nursing education.

practising, the second subphase of the separation-individuation phase in Mahler's system of preoedipal development, when the child is able to move away from the mother and return to her.

practitioner, a person qualified to practice in a special professional field, such as a nurse practitioner.

Prader-Willi syndrome {A. Prader, 20th century Swiss physician; H. Willi}, a metabolic condition characterized by congenital hypotonia, hyperphagia, obesity, and mental retardation. The syndrome is associated with a less than normal secretion of gonadotropic hormones by the pituitary gland.

praevia. See **placenta praevia.**

pragmatic, pertaining to a belief that ideas are valuable only in terms of their consequences.

pralidoxime chloride, a cholinesterase reactivator used as an antidote after organophosphate poisoning or overdosage with cholinesterase inhibitors.

pramoxine hydrochloride, a local anaesthetic for the relief of pain and itching associated with dermatoses, anogenital pruritus, haemorrhoids, anal fissure, and minor burns.

pranayama, rhythmic control of breathing (yoga breath), frequently employed by practitioners of other disciplines, in particular hypnotherapists.

prandial, pertaining to a meal. The term is used in relation to timing, such as postprandial or preprandial. **prandiality** *n.*

praseodymium (Pr), a rare earth metallic element. Its atomic number is 59; its atomic weight is 140.91.

Prausnitz-Küstner (PK) test {Otto C. W. Prausnitz, Polish bacteriologist, b. 1876; Heinz Küstner, Polish gynecologist, b. 1897}, a skin test in which an allergic response is transferred to a nonallergic person who acts as a surrogate to permit identification of the allergen. The test is only performed when skin sensitivity testing cannot be performed directly on the allergic patient.

praxic skills, the skills used in planning and executing motor acts in response to internal or external stimuli. Some individuals may exprience profound difficulty in motor planning (e.g. when given a familiar object being unable to demonstrate its normal use) as a result of development problems or acquired disorders.

prazosin hydrochloride, an alpha-adrenoceptor blocker sued as an antihypertensive in the treatment of hypertension, in congestive heart disease, and in benign protastic hypertrophy.

preagonal ascites, a rapid accumulation of fluid within the peritoneal cavity, representing the transudation of serum from the circulatory system.

preanaesthetic medication. See **premedication.**

preaortic node, a node in one of the three sets of lumbar lymph nodes that serve various abdominal viscera supplied by the coeliac, superior mesenteric, and inferior mesenteric arteries.

precancerous dermatitis. See **intraepidermal carcinoma.**

preceptorship, the position of teacher or instructor.

precession, a comparatively slow gyration of the axis of a spinning body, so as to trace out a cone, caused by the application of a torque.

precipitate, 1. to cause a substance to separate or to settle out of solution. 2. a substance that has separated from or settled out of a solution. 3. occurring hastily or unexpectedly.

precipitate delivery, childbirth that occurs with such speed or in such a situation that the usual preparations cannot be made.

precipitating factor, an element that causes or contributes to the occurrence of a disorder.

precipitin, an antibody that causes formation of an insoluble complex when combined with a specific soluble antigen.

precision rest, a rigid denture support consisting of two tightly fitting parts, the insert of which rests firmly against the gingival portion of the device.

precocious, pertaining to the early, often premature, development of physical or mental qualities.

precocious dentition, the abnormal acceleration of the eruption of the deciduous or permanent teeth, usually associated with an endocrine imbalance, such as excess pituitary growth hormone or hyperthyroidism.

precognition, the foreknowledge of events.

preconscious, 1. before the development of self-consciousness and self-awareness. 2. (in psychiatry) the mental function in which thoughts, ideas, emotions, or memories not in immediate awareness can be brought into the consciousness without encountering any intrapsychic resistance or repression. 3. the mental phenomena capable of being recalled, although not present in the conscious mind.

precordial, of or pertaining to the precordium, which forms the region over the heart and the lower part of the thorax.

precordial movement, any motion of the anterior wall of the thorax localized in the area over the heart. Kinds of precordial movements include **apical impulse, left ventricular thrust,** and **right ventricular thrust.**

precordial thump, a cardiopulmonary resuscitation (CPR) technique used to restore circulation in cardiac arrest. The person performing precordial thumping raises a clenched fist 20 to 30 cm (8 to 12 inches) above the precordium of the patient; the fist is then brought down quickly in a single blow.

precursor, a prognostic characteristic or feature of a patient's health data, such as an x-ray or laboratory finding, that is associated with a higher or lower risk of death than the average.

predeciduous dentition, the epithelial structures found in the mouth of the infant preceding the eruption of the deciduous teeth.

prediabetes. See **potential abnormality of glucose tolerance, previous abnormality of glucose tolerance.**

predicate, (in neurolinguistic programming) the part of a sentence that tells something about the subject. It can refer to direct sensory experience or can be neutral.

predictive hypothesis, (in research) a hypothesis that predicts the nature of a relationship among the variables to be studied.

predictive validity, validity of a test or a measurement tool that is established by demonstrating its ability to predict the results of an analysis of the same data using another test instrument or measurement tool.

predictor variable. See **independent variable.**

predisposing factor, any conditioning factor that influences both the type and amount of resources that the individual can elicit to cope with stress. It may be biological, psychological, or sociocultural in nature.

prednisolone, a glucocorticoid used as an antiinflammatory and immunosuppressant.

prednisone, a glucocorticoid used as an antiinflammatory and immunosuppressant.

pre-eclampsia, now commonly called pregnancy induced hypertension; a syndrome pecular to pregnancy characterized by three signs: raised blood pressure (a rise of 15-20 mmHg above the woman's normal diastolic blood oressure); nondependent oedema; amd proteinuria. The precursor to eclampsia.

pre-excitation, activation of part of the ventricular myocardium earlier than would be expected if the activating impulses travelled only down the normal routes or had experienced a normal delay within the AV node. The degree of preexcitation is determined by how fast the impulse traverses the atrial tissue and the accessory pathway or the AV node.

preferential anosmia, the inability to smell certain odours. The condition is often caused by psychologic factors concerning either a particular smell or the situation in which the smell occurs.

prefix, a portion of a word, usually derived from Latin or Greek, occurring at the beginning of a compound word. In this dictionary, prefixes are called "combining forms." In the words *antiseptic, epidermis, hypoglycaemia, periosteum,* and *semipermeable, anti-, epi-, hypo-, peri-,* and *semi-* are prefixes.

preformation, an early theory in embryology in which the organism is contained in

minute and complete form within the germ cell and after fertilization grows from microscopic to normal size.

preformed water, the water that is contained in foods.

prefrontal lobotomy, a surgical procedure in which connecting fibres between the prefrontal lobes of the brain and the thalamus are severed. After surgery, patients were often apathetic, docile, and lacking social graces. If only the white fibres are severed, the procedure is called a prefrontal leucotomy.

pregnancy, the gestational process, comprising the growth and development within a woman of a new individual from conception through the embryonic and fetal periods to birth. Pregnancy lasts approximately 265 days from the day of fertilization, but it is clinically considered to last 280 days (40 weeks or 9 months and 7 days) from the first day of the last menstrual period.

pregnancy gingivitis, an enlargement or hyperplasia of the gingivae caused by hormonal imbalance during pregnancy.

pregnancy rate, (in statistics) the ratio of pregnancies per 100 woman-years, calculated as the product of the number of pregnancies in the women observed multiplied by 1200 (months) divided by the product of the number of women observed multiplied by the number of months observed. For example, if 50 women used one contraceptive method for 12 months and 5 of them became pregnant, the pregnancy rate would be 10 per 100 woman-years.

pregnanoediol, a crystalline, biologically inactive compound found in the urine of women during pregnancy or the secretory phase of the menstrual cycle.

prehension, the use of the hands and fingers to grasp or pick up objects.

preinvasive carcinoma. See **carcinoma in situ.**

preload, the initial stretch of myocardial fibre at end diastole. The ventricular end diastolic pressure and volume reflect this parameter.

premalignant fibroepithelioma, an elevated Caucasian-flesh-coloured sessile neoplasm formed of interlacing ribbons of epithelial cells on a hyperplastic mesodermal stroma. The tumour occurs most often on the lower trunk of older people.

premature, 1. not fully developed or mature. **2.** occurring before the appropriate or usual time. **prematurity,** *n.*

premature atrial contraction, a cardiac arrhythmia characterized by an atrial beat occurring before the expected excitation, indicated electrocardiographically as an early P wave. The arrhythmia may be the result of atrial enlargement or ischaemia, or may be caused by stress, caffeine, or nicotine.

premature contraction, any contraction of

either the ventricle or atrium that occurs early with respect to the dominant rhythm.

premature ejaculation, uncontrollable, untimely ejaculation of semen often caused by anxiety during sexual intercourse.

premature impulse, any impulse that occurs early with respect to a dominant rhythm.

premature infant. See **preterm infant.**

premature labour. See **preterm labour.**

premature rupture of membranes, the spontaneous rupture of the amniotic membranes before the onset of labour.

premature ventricular contraction (PVC), a cardiac arrhythmia characterized by a ventricular beat preceding the expected electric impulse, shown on the electrocardiogram as an early, wide QRS complex without a preceding related P wave. They may be caused by stress, acidosis, electrolyte imbalance, hypoxaemia, hypercapnia, ventricular enlargement, or a toxic reaction to drugs.

premedication, 1. any sedative, tranquillizer, hypnotic, or anticholinergic medication administered before anaesthesia. The choice of drug depends on such variables as the patient's age and physical condition and the specific operative procedure. 2. the administration of such medications. **premedicate,** *v.*

premenopausal, of or pertaining to the time of life preceding the menopause.

premenstrual syndrome (PMS). See **premenstrual tension.**

premenstrual tension (PMT) a syndrome of nervous tension, irritability, weight gain, oedema, headache, mastalgia, dysphoria, and lack of coordination occurring during the last few days of the menstrual cycle before the onset of menstruation.

premolar, one of eight bicuspid teeth, four in each dental arch, located lateral to and posterior to the canine teeth. The premolars appear during childhood and remain until old age. They are smaller and shorter than the canine teeth.

premonition, a sense of an impending event without prior knowledge of it.

premonitory, an early symptom or sign of a disease. The term is commonly used to describe minor symptoms that precede a major health problem.

premorbid personality, a personality characterized by early signs or symptoms of a mental disorder. The specific defects may indicate whether the condition will progress toward schizophrenia, a bipolar disorder, or another type of condition.

prenatal, prior to birth; occurring or existing before birth, referring to both the care of the woman during pregnancy and the growth and development of the fetus.

prenatal development, the entire process of growth, maturation, differentiation, and development that occurs between conception and birth.

prenatal diagnosis, any of various diagnostic techniques to determine if a developing fetus in the uterus is affected with a genetic disorder or other abnormality. Such procedures include **amniocentesis, fetoscopy,** maternal blood tests and **ultrasound** scanning.

prenatal surgery, any surgical procedure that is performed on a fetus. The technique has been used to correct hydrocephalus and obstructions of the urinary tract.

preoccupation, a state of being self-absorbed or engrossed in one's own thoughts to a degree that hinders effective contact with or relationship to external reality.

preoperational thought phase, a Piagetian phase of child development, during the period of 2 to 7 years of age, when the child focuses on the use of language as a tool to meet his or her needs.

preoperative, of or pertaining to the period of time preceding a surgical procedure. Commonly, the preoperative period begins with the first preparation of the patient for surgery, as when, 12 hours before scheduled procedure, fluids or food by mouth is forbidden. It ends with the induction of surgical anaesthesia in the operating suite.

preoperative care, the preparation and management of a patient before surgery. The patient's nutritional and hygienic state, medical and surgical history, allergies, current medication, physical handicaps, signs of infection, and elimination habits are noted and recorded. The patient's understanding of the operative, preoperative, and postoperative procedures, the patient's ability to verbalize anxieties, and the family's knowledge of the planned surgery are ascertained. The signed informed consent statement, the doctor's preoperative orders, and the patient's identification bands are checked. Blood pressure, temperature, pulse, and respiration are recorded, and any abnormalities are reported to the surgeon. The surgeon is also informed if the electrocardiogram, chest x-ray study, or laboratory studies show any abnormalities. On completion of the patient's blood typing, the number of matched blood units required to be held for a possible blood transfusion is determined.

PREP, abbreviation for Post Registration Education and Practice. Proposals put forward by the UKCC to ensure that nurses undergo regular training to update their skills in order to remain on the register of practising nurses. The proposals are designed so as to promote higher standards of patient care across the range of nursing practice.

preparatory prosthesis, a temporary artificial limb that is fitted to the stump soon after amputation. It permits ambulation and biomechanical adaptation during the first several weeks after surgery.

prepared cavity, a tooth cavity that has been prepared to receive and retain a restoration.

prepatellar bursa, a bursa between the tendon of the quadriceps and the lower part of the femur continuous with the cavity of the knee joint.

preprandial, before a meal.

prepubertal panhypopituitarism, insufficiency of pituitary hormones, caused by damage to the gland usually associated with a suprasellar cyst or craniopharyngioma, occurring in childhood. The disorder is characterized by dwarfism with normal body proportions, subnormal sexual development, impaired thyroid and adrenal function, and yellow, wrinkled skin.

prepuberty, the period immediately preceding puberty, lasting approximately 2 years and characterized by preliminary physical changes, such as accelerated growth and appearance of secondary sex characteristics, that lead to sexual maturity. **prepuberal, prepubertal,** *adj.*

prepubescence, the state of being prepubertal. **prepubescent,** *adj.*

prepuce, a fold of skin that forms a retractable cover, such as the foreskin of the penis or the fold around the clitoris. **prepucial, preputial,** *adj.*

prerenal anuria, cessation of urine production caused by the blood pressure in the kidney being too low to maintain glomerular filtration pressure.

presbycardia, an abnormal cardiac condition, especially affecting elderly individuals and associated with heart failure in the presence of other complications, such as heart disease, fever, anaemia, mild hyperthyroidism, and excess fluid administration. Presbycardia may be associated with decreased elasticity of the musculature of the heart and with mild fibrotic changes of the heart valves, but the basis for these changes and the associated pigmentation of the heart is not known.

presbycusis, the normal loss of hearing acuity, speech intelligibility, auditory threshold, and pitch associated with ageing.

presbyopia, farsightedness resulting from a loss of elasticity of the lens of the eye. The condition commonly develops with advancing age. **presbyopic,** *adj.*

preschizophrenic state, a period before psychosis is evident when the patient deviates from normal behaviour but does not demonstrate psychotic symptoms.

prescribe, 1. to write an order for a drug, treatment, or procedure. **2.** to recommend or encourage a course of action.

prescription, an order for medication, therapy, or a therapeutic device given by a properly authorized person to a person properly authorized to dispense or perform the order. A prescription is usually in written form and includes the name and address of the patient, the date, the name of the medication prescribed (inscription), the dosage, directions to the pharmacist or other dispenser (subscription), directions to the patient that must appear on the label, the prescriber's signature, and, in some instances, an identifying number.

prescription only medicine (POM), a drug that can be dispensed to the public only with a prescription.

prescriptive intervention mode, a therapeutic situation in which the health professional tells the patient explicitly how to solve a problem, so that less collaboration between professional and patient is needed.

prescriptive theory, a theory that is comprised of a description of a specific activity, a statement of the goal of the activity, and an analysis of the elements of the activity that, together, constitute a prescription for reaching the goal.

presenile dementia. See **Alzheimer's disease.**

presentation. See **fetal presentation.**

present health, (in a health history) a chronological, succinct account of any recent changes in the health of the patient and of the circumstances or symptoms that prompted the person to seek health care.

presenting part, the part of the fetus that lies in the lower pole of the uterus.

presenting symptom. See **symptom.**

preservation, the involuntary, persistent repetition of the same verbal response or motor activity regardless of the stimulus or its duration.

presomite embryo, an embryo in any stage of development before the appearance of the first pair of somites, which, in humans, usually occurs around 19 to 21 days after fertilization of the ovum.

pressor, describing a substance that tends to cause a rise in blood pressure.

pressure, a force, or stress, applied to a surface by a fluid or an object, usually measured in units of mass per unit of area, as pounds per square inch.

pressure acupuncture, a system of acupuncture involving the application of pressure, as by the tip of a finger, to certain specified points of the body. See also **acupuncture.**

pressure area care, the management and prevention of pressure sores that occur most frequently on the sacrum, elbows, heels, outer ankles, inner knees, hips, shoulder blades and ear rims of immobilized patients, especially those who are obese, elderly or suffering from infections, injuries or a poor nutritional state. Pressure sores may be prevented by repositioning the immobile patient every 2 hours, keeping the skin dry and inspecting pressure areas every 4 to 6 hours for signs of redness. Assessment of risk can be identified using the Norton or Waterlow Scale.

pressure bandage, a bandage applied to stop bleeding, prevent oedema, or provide support for varicose veins.

pressure dressing, a dressing firmly applied to exert pressure, usually on a wound for haemostasis.

pressure point, 1. a point over an artery where the pulse may be felt. Pressure on the point may be helpful in stopping the flow of blood from a wound distal to the point. **2.** a site that is extremely sensitive to pressure, such as the phrenic pressure point along the phrenic nerve between the sternocleidomastoid and the scalenus anticus on the right side.

pressure sore, an inflammation, sore or ulcer in the skin over a bony prominence. It results from ischaemic hypoxia of the tissues because of prolonged pressure on the part.

pressure support ventilation (PSV), the support of spontaneous breathing with a specific amount of positive airway pressure. The patient controls the inspiratory gas flow and the inspiratory and expiratory frequencies.

pressure ventilator, a ventilator in which gas delivery is limited by a predetermined pressure.

presumptive signs, manifestations that indicate a pregnancy although they are not necessarily positive. Presumptive signs may include cessation of menses and morning sickness.

preswing stance stage, one of the five stages in the stance phase of walking or gait, involving a brief, transitional period of double limb support during which one leg of the body is rapidly relieved of body-bearing weight and prepared for the swing forward.

presymptomatic disease, an early stage of disease when physiological changes have begun although no signs or symptoms are observed.

presynaptic, 1. situated near or before a synapse. **2.** occurring before a synapse is crossed.

presynaptic element, any neurological structure, such as a neuron, situated proximal to a synapse.

presystolic, of or pertaining to the period preceding a systole.

preterm infant. any neonate, regardless of birth weight, born before 37 weeks of gestation. Predisposing factors associated with prematurity include multiple pregnancy, toxaemia, chronic disease, acute infection, sensitization to blood incompatibility, and any severe trauma that may interfere with normal fetal development. In most instances the cause is unknown. The premature infant usually appears small and scrawny, with a large head in relation to body size, and weighs less than 2500 g. The skin is bright pink, smooth, shiny, and translucent with the underlying vessels clearly visible. The arms and legs are extended, not flexed, as in the full-term infant. There is little subcutaneous fat, sparse hair, few creases on the soles and palms, and poorly developed ear cartilage. In boys, the scrotum has few rugae and the testes may be undescended; in girls, the labia gape and the clitoris is prominent.

preterm labour, labour that occurs earlier in pregnancy than normal, before the thirty-seventh week of gestation.

pretibial, of or pertaining to the area of the leg in front of the tibia.

pretibial fever, an acute infection caused by *Leptospira autumnalis,* characterized by headache, chills, fever, enlarged spleen, myalgia, low white blood cell count, and a rash on the anterior surface of the legs.

pretrial discovery. See **discovery.**

prevalence, (in epidemiology) the number of all new and old cases of a disease or occurrences of an event during a particular period of time.

prevention, (in nursing care) any action directed toward preventing illness and promoting health to avoid the need for primary, secondary, or tertiary health care.

preventive, tending to slow, stop, or interrupt the course of an illness or to decrease the incidence of a disease.

preventive care, a pattern of nursing and medical care that focuses on the prevention of disease and health maintenance and includes early diagnosis of disease, discovery and identification of people at risk of developing specific problems, counselling, and other intervention to avert a health problem.

preventive health care. See **preventive care.**

preventive psychiatry, the use of theoretical knowledge and skills to plan and implement programmes designed to achieve primary, secondary, and tertiary prevention.

preventive treatment, a procedure, measure, substance, or programme designed to prevent a disease from occurring or a mild disorder from becoming more severe. Various diseases are prevented by immunizations with vaccines, antiseptic measures, regular exercise, a prudent diet, adequate rest, and screening programs for the detection of preclinical signs of disorders.

previllous embryo, an embryo of a placental mammal at any stage before the development of the chorionic villi, which, in humans, begin to form between the first and second months after fertilization of the ovum.

previous abnormality of glucose tolerance, a classification that includes persons who previously had diabetic hyperglycaemia or impaired glucose tolerance but whose fasting plasma glucose levels have returned to normal. Previously called latent diabetes, prediabetes.

previtamin. See **provitamin.**

prevocational evaluation, an evaluation of the abilities and limitations of a patient undergoing rehabilitation from a disabling disorder. The goal is to find eventual employment in a sheltered workshop or in the general community.

priapism, an abnormal condition of prolonged or constant penile erection, often painful and seldom associated with sexual arousal. It may result from urinary calculi or a lesion within the penis or the central nervous system.

priapitis, inflammation of the penis.

priapus. See **penis.**

prickle cell layer. See **stratum spinosum.**

prickly heat. See **miliaria.**

prilocaine hydrochloride, a local anaesthetic agent of the amide family, used for nerve block, epidural, topical, spinal, and regional anaesthesia.

prima facie rights, rights on the surface, or face, that may be overridden by stronger conflicting rights or by other values.

primal therapy, a form of psychotherapy developed by Arthur Janov that focuses on repressed pain of infancy or childhood. The goal is for the patient to surrender his or her neurotic defenses and "become real."

primaquine phosphate, an antimalarial prescribed in the treatment of malaria.

primary, 1. first in order of time, place, development, or importance. **2.** not derived from any other source or cause, specifically the original condition or set of symptoms in disease processes, as a primary infection or a primary tumor. **3.** (in chemistry) noting the first and most simple compound in a related series, formed by the substitution of one of two or more atoms or of a group in a molecule.

primary afferent fibre, a sensory nerve fibre that transmits impulses from the intrafusal fibres of the muscle spindle to the central nervous system during muscle contraction.

primary amenorrhoea. See **amenorrhoea.**

primary amputation, amputation performed after severe trauma, after the patient has recovered from shock, and before infection has set in.

primary amyloidosis. See **amyloidosis.**

primary apnoea, a self-limited condition characterized by an absence of respiration. It may follow a blow to the head and is common immediately after birth in the newborn who breathes spontaneously when the carbon dioxide in the circulation reaches a certain level. Reflexes are present, and the heart is beating, but the skin colour may be pale or blue and muscle tone is diminished.

primary atelectasis, failure of the lungs to expand fully at birth, most commonly seen in premature infants or those narcotized by maternal anaesthesia. The infant is usually cared for in an incubator in which the temperature and humidity may be closely monitored.

primary atypical pneumonia. See **mycoplasma pneumonia.**

primary biliary cirrhosis, a chronic inflammatory condition of the liver. It is characterized by generalized pruritus, enlargement and hardening of the liver, weight loss, and diarrhoea with pale, bulky stools. Petechiae, epistaxis, or haemorrhage resulting from hypoprothrombinaemia may also be evident. Jaundice, dark urine, pale stools, and cutaneous xanthosis may occur in the later stages of this disease.

primary bronchus, one of the two main air passages that branch from the trachea and convey air to the lungs as part of the respiratory system. The right primary bronchus is about 2.5 cm long, wider and shorter than the left primary bronchus, and enters the right lung nearly opposite the fifth thoracic vertebra. The left primary bronchus is about 5 cm long, passes under the aortic arch, and courses ventral to the oesophagus, the thoracic duct, and the descending aorta before dividing into bronchi for the superior and the anterior lobes of the lung.

primary carcinoma, a neoplasm at its site of origin.

primary care, care given to people in the community at the first point of contact with either the doctor, practice nurse, health visitor or district nurse. This leads to a decision regarding a course of action to resolve the health problem.

primary constriction. See **centromere.**

primary cutaneous melanoma, a primary melanoma on the skin.

primary degenerative dementia. See **senile psychosis.**

primary dental caries, dental caries developing in the enamel of a tooth that was previously unaffected.

primary dentition. See **deciduous tooth.**

primary fissure, a fissure that marks the division of the anterior and posterior lobes of the cerebellum.

primary gain, a benefit, primarily relief from emotional conflict and freedom from anxiety, attained through the use of a defence mechanism or other psychological process.

primary health care, a basic level of health care that includes programmes directed at the promotion of health, early diagnosis of disease or disability, and prevention of disease. Primary health care is provided within the community to people living within a particular geographical area. In any episode of illness, it is the first patient contact with the health care system.

primary health care team, the team is usually made up of doctors, practice nurses, health visitors, district nurses and also physiotherapists. They may be based at one health care centre or general practice.

primary host. See **definitive host.**

primary hypertension. See **essential hypertension.**

primary nurse, a nurse who is responsible for the planning, implementation, and evaluation of the nursing care of one or more clients 24 hours a day for the duration of the hospital stay.

primary nursing, a system for the distribution of nursing care in which care of one patient is managed for the entire 24-hour day by one nurse who directs and coordinates nurses and other personnel, schedules all tests, procedures, and daily activities for that patient, and cares for that patient personally when on duty. In an acute care situation, the primary care nurse might be responsible for only one patient; in an intermediate care situation, the primary care nurse might be responsible for three or more patients.

primary organizer, the part of the dorsal lip of the blastopore that is self-differentiating and induces the formation of the neural plate that gives rise to the main axis of the embryo.

primary physician, 1. the physician who usually takes care of a patient; the physician who first sees a patient for the care of a given health problem. 2. a general practitioner.

primary prevention, a programme of activities directed toward improvement of the general well-being while also involving specific protection for selected diseases, such as immunization against polio.

primary processes, unconscious thought processes seen in dreams and which, in psychoanalytical theory, originate from early per-verbal and non-rational stages of development; e.g. the though disorder of an acutely psychotic person is hypothesized to be the product of primary process thinking.See also secondary process.

primary proximal renal tubular acidosis. See **proximal renal tubular acidosis.**

primary relationships, relationships with intimates, close friends, and family.

primary sensation, a feeling or impression that results directly from a particular stimulus.

primary sequestrum, a piece of dead bone that completely separates from sound bone during the process of necrosis. Compare **secondary sequestrum.**

primary shock, a state of physical collapse comparable to fainting. It may be the result of slight pain, such as that produced by venipuncture, or may be caused by fright. Primary shock is usually mild, self-limited, and of short duration.

primary tooth. See **deciduous tooth.**

primary triad, in Beck's theory of depression, the three major cognitive patterns that force the individual to view self, environment, and future in a negativistic manner.

primary tuberculosis, the childhood form of tuberculosis, most commonly occurring in the lungs, the posterior pharynx, or, rarely, the skin. Infants lack resistance to the disease, being easily infected and especially vulnerable to rapid and extensive spread of the infection through their bodies.

prime mover, a muscle that acts directly to produce a desired movement amid other muscles acting simultaneously to produce indirectly the same movement. Most movements of the body require the combined action of numerous muscles.

primidone, an anticonvulsant prescribed in the treatment of seizure disorders. It is largely converted to phenobarbitone after absorption.

primigravida, a woman pregnant for the first time. **primigravid,** *adj.*

primipara, *pl.* **primiparae,** a woman who has given birth to one viable infant.

primitive, 1. undeveloped; undifferentiated; rudimentary; showing little or no evolution. 2. embryonic; formed early in the course of development; existing in an early or simple form.

primitive fold. See **primitive ridge.**

primitive groove, a furrow in the posterior region of the embryonic disc that indicates the cephalocaudal axis resulting from the active involution of cells forming the primitive streak.

primitive gut. See **archenteron.**

primitive line. See **primitive streak.**

primitive node, a knoblike accumulation of cells at the cephalic end of the primitive streak in the early stages of embryonic development in humans and the higher animals.

primitive pit, a minute indentation at the anterior end of the primitive groove in the early developing embryo.

primitive reflex, any reflex normal in an infant or fetus. Its presence in an adult usually indicates serious neurological disease. Some kinds of primitive reflexes are **grasp reflex, Moro reflex,** and **sucking reflex.**

primitive ridge, a ridge that bounds the primitive groove in the early stages of embryonic development.

primitive streak, a dense area on the central posterior region of the embryonic disc, formed by the morphogenetic movement of a rapidly proliferating mass of cells that spreads between the ectoderm and endoderm, giving rise to the mesodermal layer.

primordial, 1. characteristic of the most undeveloped or primitive state, specifically those cells or tissues that are formed in the early stages of embryonic development. 2. first or original; primitive.

primordial cyst, an odontogenic cyst which develops where a tooth has failed to calcify and which mainly involve the mandibular angle. They are often multilocalar and may expand into soft tissues, envelop unerupted teeth or displace teeth. It appears radiographically as a light area in the affected jaw.

primordial dwarf, a person of extremely short stature who is otherwise perfectly formed, with the usual proportions of body parts and normal mental and sexual development.

primordial germ cell, any of the large spheric diploid cells that are formed in the early stages of embryonic development and are precursors of the oogonia and spermatogonia.

primordial image, (in analytical psychology) the archetype or original parent, representing the source of all life.

primordium, *pl.* **primordia,** the first recognizable stage in the embryonic development and differentiation of a particular organ, tissue, or structure.

principal cell. See **chief cell.**

principle, 1. a general truth or settled rule of action. **2.** a prime source or element from which anything proceeds. **3.** a law on which others are founded or from which others are derived.

PR interval, that part of the electric cardiac cycle shown on the electrocardiogram as beginning with the P wave and ending with the onset of the ventricular complex (which may not be an R wave). The PR interval is a measure of AV conduction time.

printout, a printed copy of information produced by a computer's printer.

Prinzmetal's angina {Myron Prinzmetal, American cardiologist, b. 1908}, an atypical form of angina that occurs at rest rather than with effort and is associated with gross ST elevation in the electrocardiogram that disappears when the pain subsides.

priority, actions established in order of importance or urgency to the welfare or purposes of the organization, patient, or other person at a given time.

privacy, a culturally specific concept defining the degree of one's personal responsibility to others in regulating behaviour that is regarded as intrusive. Some privacy-regulating mechanisms are physical barriers, such as closed doors, and interpersonal types, such as lowered voices.

PRL, abbreviation for **prolactin.**

p.r.n., (in prescriptions) abbreviation for *pro re nata,* a Latin phrase meaning "as needed." The times of administration are determined by the needs of the patient.

Pro, abbreviation for **proline.**

proaccelerin. See **factor V.**

proband. See **propositus.**

probenecid, a uricosuric and adjunct to antibiotics. It is used in the treatment of gout to prolong the activity of penicillin or cephalosporins in some infections, such as gonorrhoea, by reducing their renal excretion.

problem, any health care condition that requires diagnostic, therapeutic, or educational action. An active problem requires immediate action whereas an inactive problem is one of the past. A subjective problem is one reported by the patient whereas one noted by an observer is regarded as an objective problem.

problem-solving approach to patient-centered care, (in nursing) a conceptual framework that incorporates the overt physical needs of a patient with covert psychological, emotional, and social needs. It provides a model for caring for the whole person as an individual, not as an example of a disease or a medical diagnosis. Nursing is defined within this model as a problem-solving process. The patient is viewed as a person who is in an impaired state, less than usually able to perform self-care activities.

probucol, an lipid lowering agent used in the treatment of hyperlipidaemia in patients who have not responded to diet or other therapies.

procainamide hydrochloride, an antiarrhythmic agent prescribed in the treatment of a variety of cardiac arrhythmias, including premature ventricular contractions, ventricular tachycardia, and atrial fibrillation.

procaine hydrochloride, a local anaesthetic of the ester family. Procaine is administered for local anaesthesia by infiltration and injection and for caudal, epidural, and other regional anaesthetic procedures. It is not used for topical anaesthesia.

procaine penicillin, a long acting, depot form of penicillin. It is most commonly used in the treatment of primary syphilis.

procarbazine hydrochloride, a cytotoxic drug used in the treatment of a variety of malignant diseases, especially Hodgkin's disease and other lymphomas.

procaryon. See **prokaryon.**

procaryosis. See **prokaryosis.**

Procaryotae, (in bacteriology) a kingdom of plants that includes all microorganisms in which the nucleoplasm has no basic protein and is not surrounded by a nuclear membrane. The kingdom has two divisions, Cyanobacteria, which includes the blue-green bacteria, and Bacteria.

procaryote. See **prokaryote.**

procerus, one of three muscles of the nose. The procerus functions to draw down the eyebrows and wrinkle the nose.

process, 1. a series of related events that follow in sequence from a particular state or condition to a conclusion or resolution. **2.** a natural growth that projects from a bone or other part. **3.** to put through a particular series of interdependent steps, as in preparing a chemical compound.

processor. 1. (in radiography) See **automatic film processor. 2.** (in computing) See **central processing unit.**

process schizophrenia, a form of schizophrenia caused by organic changes in the brain rather than by environmental influences. The onset of the disease is usually gradual.

processus vaginalis peritonei, a diverticulum of the peritoneal membrane that during embryonic development extends through the inguinal canal. In males it descends into the scrotum to form the processus vaginalis testis; in females it is usually completely obliterated.

prochlorperazine, a phenothiazine antipsychotic and antiemetic used in the treatment of psychotic disorders and for the control of nausea and vomiting.

prochlorperazine maleate, prochlorperazine mesylate. See **prochlorperazine.**

prochromosome. See **karyosome.**

procidentia, the prolapse of an organ. The term is usually applied to a prolapsed uterus.

procoagulant, a precursor or other agent that mediates the coagulation of blood. Examples include fibrinogen and prothrombin.

proconvertin. See **factor VII.**

procreation, the entire reproductive process of producing offspring.   **procreate,** v.

proctitis, inflammation of the rectum and anus caused by infection, trauma, drugs, allergy, or radiation injury. Acute or chronic, it is accompanied by rectal discomfort and the repeated urge to pass faeces with the inability to do so. Pus, blood, or mucus may be present in the stools, and tenesmus may be present. Also called **rectitis.**

proctocele. See **rectocele.**

proctocolectomy, a surgical procedure in which the anus, rectum, and colon are removed. The procedure is a common treatment for severe, intractable ulcerative colitis.

proctodeum, *pl.* **proctodea,** an invagination of the ectoderm, behind the urorectal septum of the developing embryo, that forms the anus and anal canal when the cloacal membrane ruptures. Also spelled **proctodaeum** (*pl.* **proctodaea**). **proctodeal, proctodaeal,** *adj.*

proctologist, a doctor who specializes in proctology.

proctology the branch of medicine concerned with treating disorders of the colon, rectum, and anus.

proctoscope, an instrument used to examine the rectum and the distal portion of the colon. It consists of a light mounted on a tube or speculum.

proctoscopy, the examination of the rectum with an endoscope inserted through the anus.

procyclidine hydrochloride, an anticholinergic prescribed in the treatment of parkinsonism, and to relieve the extrapyramidal side effects of other medications.

prodrome, 1. an early sign of a developing condition or disease. **2.** the earliest phase of a developing condition or disease. **prodromal,** *adj.*

prodrug, an inactive or partially active drug that is metabolically changed in the body to an active drug.

productive cough, a sudden, noisy expulsion of air from the lungs that effectively removes sputum from the respiratory tract and helps clear the air passages, permitting oxygen to reach the alveoli. Coughing is stimulated by irritation or by inflammation of the respiratory tract caused most frequently by infection. Deep breathing, with contraction of the diaphragm and intercostal muscles and forceful exhalation, promotes productive coughing in patients with respiratory infections.

professional liability, a legal concept describing the obligation of a professional person to pay a patient or client for damages caused by the professional's act of omission, commission, or negligence.

professional organization, an organization, whose members share a professional status, created to deal with issues of concern to the professional group or groups involved. Examples of professional organizations are the **British Medical Association** and the **Royal College of Nursing.**

profibrinolysin. See **fibrinogen.**

progenitive, capable of producing offspring; reproductive.

progenitor, 1. a parent or ancestor. **2.** one who or anything that originates or precedes; precursor.

progeny, 1. offspring; an individual or organism resulting from a particular mating. **2.** the descendants of a known or common ancestor.

progeria, an abnormal congenital condition characterized by premature ageing and the appearance in childhood of grey hair and wrinkled skin and by small stature, absence of pubic and facial hair, and the posture and habitus of an aged person. Death usually occurs before 20 years of age.

progestational, of or pertaining to a drug with effects similar to those of progesterone, the hormone produced by the corpus luteum and adrenal cortex during the luteal phase of the menstrual cycle that prepares the uterus for reception of the fertilized ovum.

progestational phase. See **secretory phase.**

progesterone, a natural progestational hormone prescribed in the treatment of various menstrual disorders, infertility associated with luteal phase dysfunction, and repeated spontaneous abortion.

progestin 1. progesterone. **2.** any of a group of hormones, natural or synthetic, secreted by the corpus luteum, placenta, or adrenal cortex that have a progesterone-like effect on the uterus.

progestogen, any natural or synthetic progestational hormone.

proglottid, a sexual segment of an adult tapeworm, containing both male and female reproductive organs.

prognathism, an abnormal facial configuration in which one or both jaws project forward. It is considered real or imaginary, depending on anatomical and developmental factors involved. **prognathic,** *adj.*

prognosis, a prediction of the probable outcome of a disease based on the condition of the person and the usual course of the disease as observed in similar situations.

program, a sequence of instructions, written in computer programming language, that controls the functions of a computer.

program documentation. See **documentation.**

programmer, a person skilled in writing or coding computer programs.

programming language. See **language.**

progression, a carcinogenic process whereby some cells altered by initiators undergo a second genetic mutation that allows them to grow uncontrollably without the stimulus of promoters. They progress to fully malignant cells.

progressive, describing the course of a disease or condition in which the characteristic signs and symptoms become more prominent and severe, such as progressive muscular atrophy.

progressive assistive exercise, an exercise designed to progressively improve the strength of a muscle group by gradually increasing resistance against contractions with the assistance of a therapist.

progressive myonecrosis. See **myonecrosis.**

progressive relaxation, a technique for combating tension and anxiety by systematically tensing and relaxing muscle groups.

progressive resistance exercise, a method of increasing the strength of a weak or injured muscle by gradually increasing the resistance against which the muscle works, as by using graduated weights over a period of time.

progressive spinal muscular atrophy of infants. See **Werdnig-Hoffmann disease.**

progressive subcortical encephalopathy. See **Schilder's disease.**

progressive systemic sclerosis (PSS), the most common form of scleroderma.

progress notes, (in the patient record) notes made by a nurse and doctor that describe the patient's condition and the treatments given or planned. Progress notes may follow the problem-oriented medical record format. The doctor's progress notes usually focus on the medical or therapeutic aspects of the patient's condition and care; the nurse's progress notes, although recording the medical conditions of the patient, usually focus on the objectives stated in the nursing care plan.

Project 2000, a new system of nurse education in the UK. It is a diploma level of education lasting three years. The focus is on health rather than illness, and is a theory and practice programme where students are encouraged to observe, assess and evaluate

projectile vomiting, expulsive vomiting that is extremely forceful.

projection, 1. a protuberance; anything that thrusts or juts outward. 2. the act of perceiving an idea or thought as an objective reality 3. (in psychology) an unconscious defense mechanism by which an individual attributes his or her own unacceptable traits, ideas, or impulses to another.

projection reconstruction imaging, the techniques used in NMR imaging to obtain a cross-sectional image of an object. Such an image is computer reconstructed from a series of NMR profiles.

projective test, a kind of diagnostic, psychological, or personality test that uses unstructured or ambiguous stimuli, such as inkblots, a series of pictures, abstract patterns, or incomplete sentences, to elicit responses that reflect a projection of various aspects of the individual's personality.

prokaryocyte, a cell without a true nucleus and with nuclear material scattered throughout the cytoplasm.

prokaryon, 1. nuclear elements that are not bound by a membrane but are spread throughout the cytoplasm. 2. an organism containing such unbound nuclear elements. Also spelled **procaryon.**

prokaryosis, the condition of not containing a true nucleus surrounded by a nuclear membrane. Also spelled **procaryosis.**

prokaryote, an organism that does not contain a true nucleus surrounded by a nuclear membrane, characteristic of lower forms, such as bacteria, viruses, and blue-green bacteria. Division occurs through simple fission. Also spelled **procaryote. prokaryotic,** *adj.*

prolactin (PRL), a hormone produced and secreted into the bloodstream by the anterior pituitary. Prolactin, acting with oestrogen, progesterone, thyroxine, insulin, growth hormone, glucocorticoids, and human placental lactogen, stimulates the development and growth of the mammary glands. After parturition, prolactin together with glucocorticoids is essential for the initiation and maintenance of milk production.

prolapse, the falling, sinking, or sliding of an organ from its normal position or location in the body, such as a prolapsed uterus.

prolapsed cord, an umbilical cord that protrudes beside or ahead of the presenting part of the fetus.

proliferation, the reproduction or multiplication of similar forms. The term is usually applied to increases of cells or cysts.

proliferative phase, the phase of the menstrual cycle after menstruation. Under the influence of follicle stimulating hormone from the pituitary, the ovary produces increasing amounts of oestrogen, causing the lining of the uterus to become dense and richly vascular.

proline (Pro), a nonessential amino acid found in many proteins of the body, particularly collagen.

promethazine hydrochloride, promethazine theoclate, phenothiazine antiemetics, antihistamines, and sedatives. They are used in the treatment of motion sickness, nausea, rhinitis, itching, and skin rash.

promethium (Pm), a radioactive, rare earth, metallic element. Its atomic number is 61; its atomic weight is 145.

promontory of the sacrum, the superior projecting part of the sacrum at its junction with the L5 vertebra.

promoter, 1. (in molecular genetics) a DNA sequence that initiates RNA transcription of the genetic code. **2.** a cocarcinogenic factor that encourages cells altered by initiators to reproduce at a faster than normal rate, increasing the probability of malignant transformation. Examples include DDT, phenobarbital, and some chemicals in cigarette smoke.

promyelocyte, a large mononuclear blood cell not normally present in the circulating blood. It is intermediate in development between a myeloblast and a myelocyte and is indicative of leukaemia.

pronation, 1. assumption of a prone position, one in which the ventral surface of the body faces downward. **2.** (of the arm) the rotation of the forearm so that the palm of the hand faces downward and backward. **3.** (of the foot) the lowering of the medial edge of the foot by turning it outward and abduction movements in the tarsal and metatarsal joints. **pronate,** v.

pronator reflex, a reflex elicited by holding the patient's hand vertically and tapping the distal end of the radius or ulna, resulting in pronation of the forearm.

pronator teres, a superficial muscle of the forearm, arising from a humeral and an ulnar head. It functions to pronate the hand.

prone, 1. having a tendency or inclination. **2.** (of the body) being in horizontal position when lying face downward. Compare **supine.**

proneness profile, a screening process that evaluates the probability of developmental problems occurring in the early years of a child's life. Several of the variables in the proneness profile that appear to be significant in selecting the infants who are at risk are the perinatal health status of the mother and infant, especially complications of pregnancy, delivery, the neonatal period, and the puerperium; characteristics of the mother; characteristics of the infant, including alertness, activity pattern, and responsiveness; and the behaviours of the infant and care giver as they interact.

prone-on-elbows, a body position in which the person rests the upper part of the body on the elbows while lying face down. The position is used as an initial rehabilitation exercise in training a person with a cerebellar dysfunction to achieve ambulation. From prone-on-elbows the person can practice weight shifting through the hips to a quadruped position without the risk of falling from a standing position.

pronephric duct, one of the paired ducts that connect the tubules of each of the pronephros with the cloaca in the early developing vertebrate embryo.

pronephric tubule, any of the segmentally arranged excretory units of the pronephros in the early developing vertebrate embryo.

pronephros, *pl.* **pronephroi,** the primordial excretory organ in the developing vertebrate embryo.

pronucleus, *pl.* **pronuclei,** the nucleus of the ovum or the spermatozoon after fertilization but before the fusion of the chromosomes to form the nucleus of the zygote.

propantheline bromide, an anticholinergic used to relieve smooth muscle spasm in the urinary or GI tract.

properidin system. See **alternative pathway of complement activation.**

prophase, the first of four stages of nuclear division in mitosis and in each of the two divisions of meiosis.

prophylactic, 1. preventing the spread of disease. **2.** an agent that prevents the spread of disease. **prophylactically,** adv.

prophylactic odontotomy, (in dentistry) mechanical modification of occlusal pits and fissures, and the restoration of non-carious pits and fissures to prevent dental caries.

prophylactic treatment. See **preventive treatment.**

prophylaxis, prevention of or protection against disease, often involving the use of a biologic, chemical, or mechanical agent to destroy or prevent the entry of infectious organisms.

Propionibacterium, a genus of nonmotile, anaerobic, gram-positive bacteria found on the skin of humans, in the intestinal tract of humans and animals, and in dairy products. P. acnes is common in acne pustules (formerly called Corynebacterium acnes).

propionicacidaemia, a rare inherited metabolic defect caused by the failure of the body to metabolize the amino acids threonine, isoleucine, and methionone, characterized by lethargy and mental and physical retardation. Acidosis occurs as a result of the accumulation of propionic acid in the body. **propionicacidaemic,** adj.

propionic fermentation, the production of propionic acid by the action of certain bacteria on sugars or lactic acid.

proportional gas detector, a device for measuring alpha and beta forms of radioactivity.

proportional mortality, a statistical method of relating the number of deaths from a particular condition to all deaths within the same population group for the same time period.

proposition, 1. a statement of a truth to be demonstrated or an operation to be performed. 2. to bring forward or offer for consideration, acceptance, or adoption.

propositus, a person from whom a genealogical lineage is traced, as is done to discover the pattern of inheritance of a familial disease or a physical trait.

propranolol hydrochloride, a beta-adrenergic blocking agent used in the treatment of angina pectoris, cardiac arrhythmias, hypertension and anxiety.

proprietary, 1. of or pertaining to an institution or other organization that is operated for profit. 2. of or pertaining to a product, such as a drug or device, that is made for profit.

proprietary medicine, any pharmaceutical preparation or medicinal substance that is protected from commercial competition because its ingredients or method of manufacture is kept secret or is protected by trademark or copyright.

proprioception, sensation pertaining to stimuli originating from within the body regarding spatial position and muscular activity or to the sensory receptors that they activate.

proprioceptive neuromuscular facilitation (PNF), an activity, such as a therapeutic technique, that helps initiate a proprioceptive response in a person.

proprioceptive reflex, any reflex initiated by stimulation of proprioceptive receptors, such as the increase in respiratory rate and volume induced by impulses arising from muscles and joints during exercise.

proprioceptor, any sensory nerve ending, such as those located in muscles, tendons, joints, and the vestibular apparatus, that responds to stimuli originating from within the body regarding movement and spatial position.

proptosis, bulging, protrusion, or forward displacement of a body organ or area.

propylformic acid. See **butyric acid.**

propylthiouracil, an inhibitor of thyroid hormone biosynthesis. It is used in the treatment of hyperthyroidism, thyrotoxic crisis, and preparation for thyroidectomy.

proscribe, to forbid. **proscriptive,** *adj.*

prosencephalon, the portion of the brain that includes the diencephalon and the telencephalon. **prosencephalic,** *adj.*

prosopalgia. See **trigeminal neuralgia.**

prosopopilary virilism, a heavy growth of facial hair.

prosoposternodidymus, a fetal monster consisting of conjoined twins united laterally from the head through the sternum.

prosopothoracopagus, conjoined symmetric twins who are united laterally in the frontal plane from the thorax through most of the head region.

prospective medicine, the early identification of pathological or potentially pathological processes and the prescription of intervention to stop the processes.

prospective study, a study designed to determine the relationship between a condition and a characteristic shared by some members of a group. A prospective study may involve many variables or only two; it may seek to demonstrate a relationship that is an association or one that is causal.

prostacyclin (PGI), a prostaglandin. It is a biologically active product of arachidonic acid metabolism in human vascular walls, and is a potent inhibitor of platelet aggregation.

prostaglandin (PG), one of several potent, endogenous, hormone-like unsaturated fatty acids that act in exceedingly low concentrations on local target organs. They are produced in small amounts and have a large array of significant effects. Some of the therapeutic uses for the prostaglandins are termination of pregnancy and the protection of gastric mucosa from ulceration by NSAIDs.

prostanoic acid, a 20-carbon aliphatic acid that is the basic framework for prostaglandin molecules, which differ according to the location of hydroxyl and keto substitutions at various positions along the molecule.

prostate, a gland in men that surrounds the neck of the bladder and the urethra and elaborates a secretion that liquefies coagulated semen. It is a firm structure about the size of a chestnut, composed of muscular and glandular tissue. The ejaculatory ducts pass obliquely through the posterior part of the gland. The prostatic secretion consists of alkaline phosphatase, citric acid, and various proteolytic enzymes.

prostatectomy, surgical removal of a portion of the prostate gland, as performed for benign prostatic hypertrophy, or the total excision of the gland, as performed for malignancy. Kinds of approaches include transurethral, the most common, in which a resectoscope is inserted and through it shavings of prostatic tissue are cut off at the bladder opening with a loop, suprapubic, and retropubic. The perineal approach is used for biopsy when early cancer is suspected or for the removal of calculi.

prostatic, pertaining to the prostate gland.

prostatic catheter, a catheter that is approximately 16 inches long and has an angled tip.

It is used in male catheterization to pass an enlarged prostate gland obstructing the urethra.

prostatic ductule, any one of 12 to 20 tiny excretory tubes that convey the alkaline secretion of the prostate gland and open into the floor of the prostatic portion of the urethra.

prostatic hypertrophy. See **prostatomegaly.**

prostatic utricle, the portion of the urethra in men that forms a cul-de-sac about 6 mm long behind the middle lobe of the prostate. It is homologous with the uterus in women.

prostatitis, acute or chronic inflammation of the prostate gland, usually the result of infection. The patient complains of burning, frequency, and urgency.

prostatomegaly, the hypertrophy or enlargement of the prostate gland.

prosthesis, *pl.* **prostheses, 1.** an artificial replacement for a missing part of the body, such as an artificial limb or total joint replacement. **2.** a device designed and applied to improve function, such as a hearing aid.

prosthetic restoration. See **restoration.**

prosthetist, a person who fabricates and fits artificial limbs and similar devices prescribed by a doctor.

prosthodontics, a branch of dentistry devoted to the construction of artificial appliances that replace missing teeth or restore parts of the face.

prostration, a condition of extreme exhaustion and inability to exert oneself further, as in heat prostration or nervous prostration.prostatic

protactinium (Pa), a radioactive element. Its atomic number is 91; its atomic weight is 231.

protamine sulphate, a heparin antagonist derived from fish sperm. It is used to diminish or reverse the anticoagulant effect of heparin, particularly in cases of heparin overdosage.

protamine zinc insulin suspension, a long-acting insulin injection, containing a suspension of insulin complexed with zinc chloride and protamine, that is absorbed slowly at a steady rate.

protanopia, a form of colour blindness in which the person is unable to distinguish shades of red.

protease, an enzyme that is a catalyst in the breakdown of protein.

protective, describing an individual who guards another from danger or injury and provides a safe environment.

protective mechanisms, alterations in, a disruption in the mechanisms that maintain physical integrity through the haematopoietic and immune systems. Defining characteristics include an abnormal blood profile, an abnormal coagulation profile, a delayed hypersensitivity skin reaction, signs and symptoms of infection, bleeding, anaemia or immune deficiency, extremes of age, stress, inadequate nutrition and alcohol, and presence of drugs and treatments.

protein, any of a large group of naturally occurring, complex, organic nitrogenous compounds. Each is composed of large combinations of amino acids containing the elements carbon, hydrogen, nitrogen, oxygen, usually sulphur, and occasionally phosphorus, iron, iodine, or other essential constituents of living cells. Twenty-two amino acids have been identified as vital for proper growth, development, and maintenance of health. The body can synthesize 14 of these amino acids, called nonessential, whereas the remaining eight must be obtained from dietary sources and are termed essential. Protein is the major source of building material for muscles, blood, skin, hair, nails, and the internal organs. It is necessary for the formation of hormones, enzymes, and antibodies and as a source of heat and energy, and it functions as an essential element in proper elimination of waste materials. Excessive intake of protein may in some conditions result in fluid imbalance.

protein-bound iodine (PBI), iodine that is firmly bound to protein in serum, the measurement of which indirectly indicates the concentration of circulating thyroxine (T).

calorie malnutrition. See **energy protein malnutrition.**

protein kinase, a protein that catalyses the transfer of a phosphate group from adenosine triphosphate to produce a phosphoprotein.

protein metabolism, the processes whereby protein foodstuffs are used by the body to make tissue proteins, together with the processes of breakdown of tissue proteins in the production of energy. Food proteins are first broken down into amino acids, then absorbed into the bloodstream, and finally used in body cells to form new proteins. Amino acids in excess of the body's needs may be converted by liver enzymes into keto acids and urea.

proteinuria, the presence in the urine of abnormally large quantities of protein, usually albumin. Persistent proteinuria is usually a sign of renal disease or renal complications of another disease. However, proteinuria can result from heavy exercise or fever.

proteolipid, a type of lipoprotein in which lipid material forms more than one half of the molecule. It is insoluble in water and occurs primarily in the brain.

proteolysis, a process in which water added to the peptide bonds of proteins breaks down the protein molecule. Numerous enzymes may catalyse this process.

proteolytic, of or pertaining to any substance that promotes the breakdown of protein.

Proteus, a genus of motile, gram-negative bacilli often associated with nosocomial infections, normally found in faeces, water, and soil. *Proteus* may cause urinary tract infections, pyelonephritis, wound infections, diarrhoea, bacteraemia, and endotoxic shock.

Proteus morgani, a species of bacteria associated with infectious diarrhoea in infants.

Proteus vulgaris, a species of bacteria that is a frequent cause of urinary tract infections. The bacteria are found in faeces, water, and soil.

prothrombin, a plasma protein that is the precursor to thrombin. It forms thrombin, the first step in blood clotting, when exposed to thromboplastin and calcium. It is synthesized in the liver if adequate vitamin K is present.

prothrombin and proconvertin test, differs from the prothrombin time in that is more sensitive to factor VIII, factor X and prothrombin deficiencies.

prothrombin consumption test, when blood clots, normally 0-30% of the original plasma prothrombin remains (usually <10%). More than 30% indicates a clotting defect.

prothrombin time (PT), a one stage test for detecting certain plasma coagulation defects caused by a deficiency of factors V, VII, or X. Thromboplastin and calcium are added to a sample of the patient's plasma and, simultaneously, to a sample from a normal control. The length of time required for clot formation in both samples is observed.

protocol, a written plan specifying the procedures to be followed in giving a particular examination, in conducting research, or in providing care for a particular condition. See also **standing orders.**

proton, a positively charged particle that is a fundamental component of the nucleus of all atoms. The number of protons in the nucleus of an atom equals the atomic number of the element.

proton density, a measure of proton concentration, or the number of atom nuclei per given volume. It is one of the major determinants of magnetic resonance signal strength in hydrogen imaging.

protopathic, pertaining to the somatic sensations of fast localized pain, slow poorly localized pain, and temperature.

protoplasm, the living substance of a cell, usually composed of myriad molecules of water, minerals, and organic compounds.

protoplast, 1. (in biology) the protoplasm of a cell without its containing membrane. **2.** a first entity or an original. **protoplastic,** *adj.*

protoporphyria, increased levels of protoporphyrin in the blood and faeces.

protoporphyrin, a kind of porphyrin that combines with iron and protein to form a variety of important organic molecules, including catalase, haemoglobin, and myoglobin.

protostoma. See **blastopore.**

prototaxic mode, a stage in infancy, according to Sullivan, characterized by a lack of differentiation between the self and the environment.

protozoa, *sing.* **protozoon,** single-celled microorganisms of the class Protozoa, the lowest form of animal life. Protozoa are more complex than bacteria, forming a self-contained unit with organelles that carry on such functions as locomotion, nutrition, excretion, respiration, and attachment to other objects or organisms. Approximately 30 protozoa are pathogenic to humans. **protozoal, protozoan,** *adj.*

protozoal infection, any disease caused by single-celled organisms of the class Protozoa. Some kinds of protozoal infections are **amoebic dysentery, kala-azar, malaria,** and **trichomonas vaginitis.**

protracted dose, (in radiotherapy) a low amount of radiation delivered continuously over a relatively long period of time.

protriptyline hydrochloride, a tricyclic antidepressant used in the treatment of depression marked by withdrawal and anergy.

protrusio bulbi. See **exophthalmia.**

protrusion, a state or condition of being forward or projecting.

protrusive incisal guide angle, (in dentistry) the inclination of the incisal guide in the sagittal plane.

proud flesh, excessive granulation tissue.

provider, a hospital, clinic, or health care professional, or group of health care professionals, who provide a service to patients.

provirus, a stage of viral replication in which the viral genetic information has been integrated into the genome of the host cell.

provitamin, a precursor of a vitamin; a substance found in certain foods that in the body may be converted into a vitamin. Also called **previtamin.**

provocative diagnosis, a diagnosis in which the identity and cause of an illness are discovered by inducing an episode of the condition.

proxemics, the study of spatial distances between people and its effect on interpersonal behaviour, especially in relation to density of population, placement of people within an area, and the opportunity for privacy.

proximal, nearer to a point of reference, usually the trunk of the body, than other parts of the body. Proximal interphalangeal joints are those closest to the hand.

proximal cavity, a cavity that occurs on the mesial or distal surface of a tooth.

proximal contour, the shape or form of the medial or the distal surface of a tooth.

proximal dental caries, decay that may occur in the mesial or distal surface of a tooth.

proximal radioulnar articulation, the pivot joint between the circumference of the head of the radius and the ring formed by the radial notch of the ulna and the annular ligament. The joint allows the rotary movements of the head of the radius in pronation and supination.

proximal renal tubular acidosis (proximal RTA), an abnormal condition characterized by excessive acid accumulation and bicarbonate excretion. It is caused by the defective reabsorption of bicarbonate in the proximal tubules of the kidney and the resulting flow of excessive bicarbonate into the distal tubules, which normally secrete hydrogen ions. In **primary proximal RTA** the defective reabsorption of bicarbonate is the sole causative factor. **In secondary proximal RTA** the reabsorptive defect is one of several causative factors and may result from tubular cell damage produced by various disorders, such as Fanconi's syndrome.

proximate cause, a legal concept of cause and effect relationships in determining, for example, whether an injury would have resulted from a particular cause.

proximity principle, a rule that when two or more objects are close to each other they may be seen as a perceptual unit.

proxymetacaine hydrochloride, a rapid-acting, topical anaesthetic of the amide family used as a surface anaesthetic prior to ophthalmical procedures.

prurigo, any of a group of chronic inflammatory conditions of the skin characterized by severe itching and multiple, dome-shaped, small papules capped by tiny vesicles. Later (as a result of repeated scratching), crusting and lichenification may occur. Some causes of prurigo are allergies, drugs, endocrine abnormalities, malignancies, and parasites. A mild form of the disease is called **prurigo mitis,** and a more severe form, **prurigo agria** or **prurigo ferox. pruriginous,** *adj.*

pruritus, the symptom of itching, an uncomfortable sensation leading to the urge to scratch. Scratching often results in secondary infection. Some causes of pruritus are allergy, infection, jaundice, lymphoma, and skin irritation. **pruritic,** *adj.*

pruritus ani, a common chronic condition of itching of the skin around the anus. Some causes are candidal infection, contact dermatitis, external haemorrhoids, pinworms, psoriasis, and psychogenic illness.

pruritus vulvae, itching of the external genitalia of a female. The condition may become chronic and result in lichenification, atrophy, and occasionally malignancy. Some causes of pruritus vulvae are contact dermatitis, lichen sclerosus et atrophicus, psychogenic pruritus, trichomoniasis, and vaginal candidiasis.

Prussian blue, a chemical reagent used on microsopic preparations. It demonstrates the presence of copper by developing a bright blue colour.

psammoma, *pl.* **psammomas, psammomata,** a neoplasm containing small calcified granules (psammoma bodies) that occurs in the meninges, choroid plexus, pineal body, and ovaries.

psammoma body, a round, layered mass of calcareous material occurring in benign and malignant epithelial and connective tissue neoplasms and in some chronically inflamed tissue.

pseudaesthesia, a sensation experienced without an external stimulus or a sensation that does not correspond to the causative stimulus, such as phantom limb pain.

pseudoallele, (in genetics) one of two or more closely linked genes on a chromosome that appear to function as a single member of an allelic pair but occupy distinct, nearly corresponding loci on homologous chromosomes. **pseudoallelic,** *adj.,* **pseudoallelism,** *n.*

pseudoanorexia, a condition in which an individual eats secretly while claiming a lack of appetite and inability to eat. Also called **false anorexia.**

pseudochylous ascites, the abnormal accumulation in the peritoneal cavity of a milky fluid that resembles chyle.

pseudocyesis, a condition in which a woman believes she is pregnant when she is not - a spurious pregnancy.

pseudocyst, a space or cavity containing gas or liquid but without a lining membrane. Pseudocysts commonly occur after pancreatitis when digestive juices break through the normal ducts of the pancreas and collect in spaces lined by fibroblasts and surfaces of adjacent organs.

pseudodementia, a depressive condition of elderly patients that is characterized by impaired cognitive funtioning.

pseudoephedrine hydrochloride, a sympathomimetic that acts as a vasoconstrictor and bronchodilator. It is used for the relief of nasal and eustachian tube congestion.

pseudogene, (in molecular genetics) a sequence of nucleotides that resembles a gene and may be derived from one but lacks a genetic function.

pseudoglottis. See **neoglottis.**

pseudogout. See **chondrocalcinosis.**

pseudohermaphroditism, a condition in which a person exhibits the somatic characteristics of both sexes though possessing the physical characteristics of either males (testes) or females (ovaries). Also called **intersex.**

pseudohypertrophic muscular dystrophy. See **Duchenne's muscular dystrophy.**

pseudojaundice, a yellow discoloration of the skin that is not caused by hyperbilirubinaemia. The excessive ingestion of carotene results in a form of pseudojaundice.

pseudomembranous colitis, a severe form of colitis, sometimes caused by an overgrowth of opportunistic organisms. It tends to occur in debilitated individuals who have been taking broad-spectrum antibiotics.

pseudomembranous enterocolitis. See **necrotizing enterocolitis.**

pseudomembranous stomatitis, a severe inflammation of the mouth that produces a membranelike exudate. The inflammation may be caused by a variety of bacteria or by chemical irritants.

pseudomonad, a bacterium of the genus *Pseudomonas.*

Pseudomonas, a genus of gram-negative bacteria that includes several free-living species of soil and water and some opportunistic pathogens, such as *Pseudomonas aeruginosa,* isolated from wounds, burns, and infections of the urinary tract. Pseudomonads are notable for their fluorescent pigments and their resistance to disinfectants and antibiotics.

pseudomutuality, (in psychotherapy) an atmosphere maintained by family members in which there is surface harmony and a high degree of agreement with one another, but in which the atmosphere of agreement covers deep and destructive interpersonal conflicts.

pseudoneurotic schizophrenia. See **latent schizophrenia.**

pseudopsychopathic schizophrenia. See **latent schizophrenia.**

pseudorubella. See **roseola infantum.**

pseudosclerema. See **adiponecrosis subcutanea neonatorum.**

pseudotumour, a false tumour. One kind of pseudotumour is **pseudotumour cerebri.**

pseudotumour cerebri, a condition characterized by increased intracranial pressure, headache, vomiting, and papilloedema without neurological signs, except, occasionally, palsy of the sixth cranial nerve.

pseudoxanthoma elasticum. See **Groünblad-Strandberg syndrome.**

psia, abbreviation for **pounds per square inch, absolute.**

psig, abbreviation for **pounds per square inch, gauge.**

psilocybin, a psychedelic drug and an active ingredient of various Mexican hallucinogenic mushrooms of the genus *Psilocybe mexicana.* It can produce altered states of mood and consciousness and has no acceptable medical use.

psittacosis, an infectious illness caused by the bacterium *Chlamydia psittaci,* characterized by respiratory, pneumonia-like symptoms and transmitted to humans by infected birds, especially parrots. The clinical manifestations of the disease are extremely variable and resemble a great number of infectious diseases, but fever, cough, anorexia, and severe headache are almost always present.

psoas major, a long muscle originating from the transverse processes of the lumbar vertebrae and the fibrocartilages and sides of the vertebral bodies of the lower thoracic vertebrae and the lumbar vertebrae. It acts to flex and laterally rotate the thigh and to flex and laterally bend the spine.

psoas minor, a long, slender muscle of the pelvis, ventral to the psoas major. It functions to flex the spine.

psoralen-type photosynthesizer, any one of the chemical compounds that contain photosensitizing psoralen and that react on exposure to ultraviolet light to increase the melanin in the skin. Naturally occurring psoralen photosynthesizers, such as 5- and 8-methoxypsoralen, are found in buttercups, carrot greens, celery, clover, dill, figs, limes, parsley, and meadow grass. Some psoralentype photosynthesizers produced as pharmaceutical drugs are used to enhance skin pigmentation or tanning in the treatment of skin diseases, such as psoriasis and vitiligo.

psoriasis, a common, chronic, inheritable skin disorder, characterized by circumscribed red patches covered by thick, dry, silvery, adherent scales that are the result of excessive development of epithelial cells. Exacerbations and remissions are typical. Lesions may be anywhere on the body but are more common on extensor surfaces, bony prominences, scalp, ears, genitalia, and the perianal area. An arthritis, particularly of distal small joints, may accompany the skin disease. Subcategories of psoriasis include **guttate psoriasis** and **pustular psoriasis. psoriatic,** *adj.*

psoriatic arthritis, a form of rheumatoid arthritis associated with psoriatic lesions of the skin and nails, particularly at the distal interphalangeal joints of the fingers and toes.

PSS, abbreviation for **progressive systemic sclerosis.**

PSV, abbreviation for **pressure support ventilation.**

psychasthenia. See **obsessive-compulsive disorder.**

psyche, 1. the aspect of one's mental faculty that encompasses the conscious and unconscious processes. **2.** the vital mental or spiritual entity of the individual as opposed to the body or soma. **3.** (in psychoanalysis) the total components of the id, ego, and superego, including all conscious and unconscious aspects. Compare **soma.**

psychedelic, 1. of or describing a mental state characterized by altered sensory perception and hallucination, accompanied by euphoria or fear, usually caused by the deliberate ingestion of drugs or other substances known to produce this effect. **2.** of or describing any drug or substance that causes this state, such as mescaline or psilocybin.

psychiatric assessment, a diagnostic procedure for determining the mental status of a person.

psychiatric disorder. See **mental disorder.**

psychiatric emergency service, a hospital service that provides immediate initial evaluation and treatment to acutely disturbed mental patients on a 24-hour-a-day basis.

psychiatric hospital, a health care facility providing inpatient and outpatient therapeutic services to clients with behavioural or emotional illnesses.

psychiatric inpatient unit, a hospital ward or similar area used for the treatment of inpatients who require psychiatric care.

psychiatric nurse, a qualified nurse has specialized in the study of the care of patients with a mental disorder and of maintaining mental health, thereby gaining the RN(M) qualification or its equivalent.

psychiatric nursing, the branch of nursing concerned with the prevention and cure of mental disorders and their sequelae. Also called **mental health nursing.**

psychiatric social worker. See **psychotherapist, approved social worker.**

psychiatry, the branch of medical science that deals with the causes, treatment, and prevention of mental, emotional, and behavioural disorders. Some kinds of psychiatry are **community psychiatry, descriptive psychiatry, forensic psychiatry,** and **orthopsychiatry. psychiatric,** *adj.*

psychic energy, body energy that is used for psychological tasks such as thinking, perceiving, and remembering. See also **libido.**

psychic infection, the spread of neurotic or psychic effects or influences on others on a small scale, as in folie a deux, or on a large scale, as in the dance and witch manias of the Middle Ages.

psychic suicide, the termination of one's own life without the use of physical means or agents, as by an older person who becomes sufficiently depressed to lose "the will to live."

psychic trauma, an emotional shock or injury or a distressful situation that produces a lasting impression, especially on the subconscious mind. Common causes of psychic trauma are abuse or neglect in childhood, rape, and loss of a loved one.

psychoanalysis, a branch of psychiatry founded by Sigmund Freud devoted to the study of the psychology of human development and behaviour. From its systematized method for investigating the processes of the mind evolved a system of psychotherapy based on the concepts of a dynamic unconscious, using such techniques as free association, dream interpretation, and the analysis of defence mechanisms, especially resistance and transference. Through these devic-

es, emotions and behaviour are traced to the influence of repressed instinctual drives in the unconscious.

psychoanalyst, a psychotherapist, usually a psychiatrist, who has had special training in psychoanalysis and who applies the techniques of psychoanalytical theory.to disinfectants and antibiotics.

psychoanalytical, 1. of or pertaining to psychoanalysis. **2.** using the techniques or principles of psychoanalysis.

psychobiological resilience, a concept that proposes a recurrent human need to weather periods of stress and change throughout life. The ability to weather each period of disruption and reintegration successfully leaves the person better able to deal with the next change.

psychobiology, 1. the study of personality development and functioning in terms of the interaction of the body and the mind. **2.** a school of psychiatric thought introduced by Adolf Meyer that stresses total life experience, including biological, emotional, and sociocultural factors in assessing the psychological makeup or mental status of an individual. Mental disorders are interpreted as dynamic adaptive reactions of the individual to stress or conflict, with little or no emphasis placed on unconscious factors. See **also distributive analysis and synthesis.**

psychocatharsis. See **catharsis.**

psychodrama, a form of group therapy, originated by J. L. Moreno, in which people act out their emotional problems through dramatization and role playing.

psychodynamics, the study of the processes that are hypothesized to constitute mental activity. See **psychoanalysis.**

psychogenesis, 1. the development of the mind or of a mental function or process. **2.** the development or production of a physical symptom or disease from mental or psychological origins rather than organic factors. **3.** the development of emotional states, either normal or abnormal, from the interaction of conscious and unconscious psychological forces.

psychogenic, 1. originating within the mind. **2.** referring to any physical symptom, disease process, or emotional state that is of psychological rather than physical origin. Also **psychogenetic.**

psychogenic pain disorder, a disorder characterized by persistent and severe pain for which there is no apparent organic cause. The condition is often accompanied by other sensory or motor dysfunction, such as paraesthesia or muscle spasm.

psychokinesia, 1. impulsive, maniacal behaviour resulting from deficient or defective inhibitions. **2.** (in parapsychology) psychokinesis.

psychokinesis, the alleged direct influence

of the mind or will on matter that would result in the production of motion in objects without the intervention of the physical senses or a physical force.

psychokinetics, the study of psychokinesis.

psychological test, any of a group of standardized tests designed to measure or ascertain such characteristics of an individual as intellectual capacity, motivation, perception, role behaviour, values, level of anxiety or depression, coping mechanisms, and general personality integration.

psychologist, a person who specializes in the study of the structure and function of the brain and related mental processes of animals and humans. A clinical psychologist is one who is qualified by graduate degree in psychology and training in clinical psychology and who provides testing and counselling services to patients with mental and emotional disorders.

psychology, 1. the study of behaviour and of the functions and processes of the mind, especially as related to the social and physical environment. 2. a profession that involves the practical applications of knowledge, skills, and techniques in the understanding of, prevention of, or solution to individual or social problems, especially in regard to the interaction between the individual and the physical and social environment. 3. the mental, motivational, and behavioural characteristics and attitudes of an individual or group of individuals. Kinds of psychology include **analytical psychology, animal psychology, behaviourism, clinical psychology, cognitive psychology, experimental psychology, humanistic psychology,** and **social psychology. psychological,** *adj.,* **psychologically,** adv.

psychometrics, the development, administration, or interpretation of psychological and intelligence tests.

psychomotor, pertaining to or causing voluntary movements usually associated with neural activity.

psychomotor development, the progressive attainment by the child of skills that involve both mental and muscular activity, such as the ability of the infant to turn over, sit, or crawl at will and of the toddler to walk, talk, control bladder and bowel functions, and begin solving cognitive problems.

psychomotor domain, the area of observable performance of skills that require some degree of neuromuscular coordination.

psychomotor learning, the acquisition of ability to perform motor skills.

psychomotor retardation, a slowing of motor activity related to a state of severe depression.

psychomotor seizure, a temporary impairment of consciousness, often associated with temporal lobe disease and characterized by psychological symptoms, loss of judgment, automatic behaviour, and abnormal acts. No apparent convulsions occur, but there may be loss of consciousness or amnesia for the episode. During the seizure the individual may appear drowsy, intoxicated, or violent; asocial acts or crimes may be committed, but normal activities, such as driving a car, typing, or eating, may continue at an automatic level.

psychoneuroimmunology, a discipline that studies the relationships between psychological states and the immune response.

psychoneurosis. See **neurosis.**

psychoneurotic. See **neurotic.**

psychoneurotic disorder. See **neurotic disorder.**

psychopath, a person who has an antisocial personality disorder.

psychopathia. See **psychopathy.**

psychopathia sexualis, a mental disease characterized by sexual perversion.

psychopathic, of or pertaining to antisocial behaviour. Also **sociopathic.**

psychopathic personality. See **antisocial personality.**

psychopathologist, one who specializes in the study and treatment of mental disorders. **psychopathology,** *n.*

psychopathology, 1. the study of the causes, processes, and manifestations of mental disorders. 2. the behavioural manifestation of any mental disorder.

psychopathy, any disease of the mind, congenital or acquired.

psychopharmacology, the scientific study of the effects of drugs on behaviour and normal and abnormal mental functions.

psychophysical preparation for childbirth, a programme that prepares women for giving birth by teaching them the physiology of the process, exercises to improve muscle tone and physical stamina, and various techniques of breathing and relaxation to promote control and comfort during labour and delivery. Methods of psychophysical preparation for childbirth include **Bradley method, Lamaze method,** and **Read method.**

psychophysics, the branch of psychology concerned with the relationships between physical stimuli and sensory responses.

psychophysiological, 1. of or pertaining to psychophysiology. 2. having physical symptoms resulting from psychogenic origins; psychosomatic.

psychophysiological disorder, any of a large group of mental disorders characterized by the dysfunction of an organ or organ system controlled by the autonomic nervous system, such as a peptic ulcer, which may be caused or aggravated by emotional factors.

psychophysiology, 1. the study of physiology as it relates to various aspects of psychological or behavioural function. 2. the study of mental activity by physical examination and observation.

psychoprophylaxis, a method of preparation for labour, in order to control pain and its perception, by the use of breathing patterns and methods to disassociate from pain.

psychosexual, of or pertaining to the psychological and emotional aspects of sex. **psychosexuality,** n.

psychosexual development, (in psychoanalysis) the emergence of the personality through a series of stages from infancy to adulthood, each stage relatively fixed in time and characterized by a dominant mode of achieving libidinal pleasure through the interaction of the person's biological drives and the restraints of the environment. Resolution of the conflicts encountered at each of the stages theoretically leads to a balanced, heterosexual adjustment and normal development.

psychosexual disorder, any condition characterized by abnormal sexual attitudes, desires, or activities resulting from psychological rather than organic causes.

psychosexual dysfunction, any of a large group of sexual maladjustments or disorders caused by an emotional or psychological problem.

psychosis, pl. **psychoses,** any major mental disorder of organic or emotional origin characterized by extreme derangement or disorganization of the personality, often accompanied by severe depression, agitation, regressive behaviour, illusions, delusions, and hallucinations that so greatly impair perception, thinking, emotional response, and personal orientation that the individual loses touch with reality, is incapable of functioning normally in society, and usually requires hospitalization. Kinds of psychoses include **affective psychosis, alcoholic psychosis, schizophrenia,** and **senile psychosis.**

psychosocial, pertaining to a combination of psychological and social factors.

psychosocial assessment, an evaluation of a person's mental health, social status, and functional capacity within the community. The person's physical status, appearance, and modes of behaviour are observed for factors that may indicate or contribute to emotional distress or mental illness. Posture, facial expressions, manner of dress, speech and thought patterns, degree of motor activity, and level of consciousness are noted. The person is questioned concerning patterns of daily living, including work schedule and social and leisure activities. Pertinent background data include a history of any previous psychiatric problems, the person's response to and methods of coping with stress, relationships, cultural orientation, and any significant life changes, such as serious illnesses, unemployment or change of employment, change of residence, marriage, divorce, or death of a loved one.

psychosocial development, (in child devel-

opment) a description devised by Erik Erikson of the normal serial development of trust, autonomy, identity, and intimacy; the development begins in infancy and progresses as the infantile ego interacts with the environment. For the child to reach a new stage, the preceding one must be fully realized.

psychosomatic, 1. of or pertaining to psychosomatic medicine. 2. relating to, characterized by, or resulting from the interaction of the mind or psyche and the body. 3. the expression of an emotional conflict through physical symptoms.

psychosomatic approach, the interdisciplinary or holistic study of physical and mental disease from a biological, psychosocial, and sociocultural point of view.

psychosomatic illness. See **psychophysiological disorder.**

psychosomatic medicine, the branch of medicine concerned with the interrelationships between mental and emotional reactions and somatic processes, in particular the manner in which intrapsychic conflicts influence physical symptoms.

psychosomatic reaction. See **psychophysiological disorder.**

psychosomatics. See **psychosomatic medicine.**

psychosomatogenic, pertaining to factors that cause or lead to the development of psychophysiological coping measures as learned responses to stressors.

psychosurgery, surgical interruption of certain nerve pathways in the brain, performed to treat selected cases of chronic, unremitting anxiety, agitation, or obsessional neuroses when the condition is severe and when alternative treatments, such as psychotherapy, drugs, and electric shock treatment, have proved ineffective.

psychosynthesis, a form of psychotherapy that focuses on three levels of the unconscious—lower, middle, and higher unconscious. The goal is the recreation or integration of the personality.

psychotherapeutics, the treatment of psychological disorders by means of psychotherapy.

psychotherapist, one who practices psychotherapy, including psychiatrists, psychologists, psychiatric nurses, psychiatric social workers, and persons trained in counselling.

psychotherapy, any of a large number of related methods of treating mental and emotional disorders by psychologic techniques rather than by physical means. Some of the aims of psychotherapy are to change maladaptive behavioural patterns, improve interpersonal relationships, resolve inner conflicts that cause personal distress, modify inaccurate assumptions about the self and the environment, and foster a definite sense of self-identity to promote individual growth leading to a more meaningful and fulfilling existence. Kinds of psychotherapy are **behaviour therapy, group therapy, humanistic existential therapy, interpersonal therapy,** and **psychoanalysis.**

psychotic, 1. of or pertaining to psychosis. **2.** a person exhibiting the characteristics of a psychosis.

psychotic disorder. See **psychosis.**

psychotic insight, a stage in the development of a psychosis that follows an initial experience of confusion, bizarreness, and apprehension. At this point, an insight is reached that enables the patient to interpret the external world in terms of a delusional system of thinking. The factors that had previously been confusing become a part of the systematized pattern of the delusion, which, although irrational to an observer, is perceived by the patient as the attainment of exceptionally lucid thinking.

psychotic reaction. See **psychosis.**

psychotomimetic, a drug or other substance whose effects mimic the symptoms of psychosis, such as hallucinations.

psychotropic, exerting an effect on the mind or modifying mental activity.

psychotropic drugs, drugs that affect the mental functions, behaviour, or experience of a person using them.

psyllium seed. See **plantago seed.**

Pt, symbol for **platinum.**

PT, abbreviation for **prothrombin time.**

PTB, abbreviation for **patellar-tendon bearing (prosthesis).**

PTCA, abbreviation for **percutaneous transluminal coronary angioplasty.**

pteroylglutamic acid. See **folic acid.**

pterygium, a thick, triangular bit of pale tissue that extends medially from the nasal border of the cornea to the inner canthus of the eye.

pterygoideus lateralis, one of the four muscles of mastication. It functions to open the jaws, protrude the mandible, and move the mandible from side to side.

pterygoideus medialis, one of the four muscles of mastication. It acts to close the jaws.

pterygoid plexus, one of a pair of extensive networks of veins between the temporalis and the pterygoideus lateralis, extending between surrounding structures in the infratemporal fossa.

pterygomaxillary notch, a fissure at the junction of the maxilla and the pterygoid process of the sphenoid bone.

ptomaine, an imprecise term introduced in the nineteenth century to identify a group of nitrogenous substances found in putrefied proteins.

ptosis, an abnormal condition of one or both upper eyelids in which the eyelid droops because of a congenital or acquired weakness of the levator muscle or paralysis of the third cranial nerve.

ptotic kidney, a kidney that is abnormally situated in the pelvis, usually over the sacral promontory behind the peritoneum.

PTT. See **partial thromboplastin time.**

ptyalin, a starch-digesting enzyme present in saliva.

ptyalism, excessive salivation, as sometimes occurs in the early months of pregnancy. It is also a clinical sign of mercury poisoning.

Pu, symbol for **plutonium.**

pubarche, the onset of puberty, marked by the beginning of the development of secondary sexual characteristics.

puberty, the period of life at which the ability to reproduce begins.

puberulic acid, an antibiotic isolated from the mold *Penicillium puberulum* that prevents the replication of gram-positive bacteria.

pubic bone. See **pubis.**

pubic region, the most inferior part of the abdomen in the lower zone between the right and left inguinal regions and below the umbilical region.

pubic symphysis, the slightly movable interpubic joint of the pelvis, consisting of two pubic bones separated by a disc of fibrocartilage and connected by two ligaments.

pubis, *pl.* **pubes,** one of a pair of pubic bones that, with the ischium and the ilium, form the hip bone and join the pubic bone from the opposite side at the pubic symphysis. The internal surface of the pubis is smooth; it forms part of the anterior wall of the pelvis.

public health, a field of medicine that deals with the physical and mental health of the community, particularly in such areas as water supply, waste disposal, air pollution, and food safety.

publish or perish, *informal.* a practice followed in many academic institutions in which a contract for employment is renewed at the same or higher rank only if a candidate has demonstrated scholarship and professional status by having had work published in a book or in a reputable professional journal.

pubococcygeus, part of the levator ani muscle.

pubococcygeus exercises. See **pelvic floor exercises.**

pudendal. See **pudendum.**

pudendal block, a form of regional anaesthetic block administered to relieve the discomfort of the expulsive second stage of labour. Pudendal block anaesthetizes the perineum, vulva, clitoris, labia majora, and the perirectal area without affecting the muscular contractions of the uterus. When the block is properly administered, the risk is minimal.

pudendal canal. See **Alcock's canal.**

pudendal nerve, one of the branches of the pudendal plexus that arises from the second, third, and fourth sacral nerves, passes between the piriformis and coccygeus, and leaves the pelvis through the greater sciatic foramen.

pudendal plexus, a network of motor and sensory nerves formed by the anterior branches of the second, the third, and all of the fourth sacral nerves.

pudendum, *pl.* **pudenda,** the external genitalia, especially of women. In a woman it comprises the mons veneris, the labia majora, the labia minora, the vestibule of the vagina, and the vestibular glands. In a man it comprises the penis, scrotum, and testes. **pudendal,** *adj.*

puericulture, the rearing and training of children. **puericulturist,** *n.*

puerile, of or pertaining to children or childhood; juvenile. **puerility,** *n.*

puerperal, of or pertaining to the puerperium.

puerperal mania, a rare, acute mood disorder that sometimes occurs in women after childbirth, characterized by a severe manic reaction.

puerperal sepsis, an infection of the genital tract following childbirth.

puerperium, the time after childbirth, lasting 6 to 8 weeks, during which the anatomical and physiological changes brought about by pregnancy resolve, and a woman adjusts to the new or expanded responsibilities of motherhood and nonpregnant life.

Pulex, a genus of fleas some species of which transmit arthropod-borne infections, such as plague and epidemic typhus.

pulmonary, of or pertaining to the lungs or the respiratory system. Also **pulmonic.**

pulmonary acid aspiration syndrome. See **Mendelson's syndrome.**

pulmonary alveolus, one of the numerous terminal air sacs in the lungs in which oxygen and carbon monoxide are exchanged.

pulmonary anthrax. See **woolsorter's disease.**

pulmonary arteriolar resistance (PAR), pressure loss per unit of blood flow from the pulmonary artery to a pulmonary vein.

pulmonary atrium, any of the spaces at the end of an alveolar duct into which alveoli open.

pulmonary carcinosis. See **alveolar cell carcinoma.**

pulmonary compliance, a measure of the elasticity or expansibility of the lungs.

pulmonary disease, an abnormal condition of the respiratory system, characterized by cough, chest pain, dyspnoea, haemoptysis, sputum production, stridor, and wheezing. Less common symptoms may be anxiety, arm and shoulder pain, tenderness in the calf of the leg, erythema nodosum, swelling of the face, headache, hoarseness, pain in the joints, and somnolence. Pulmonary diseases are either obstructive or restrictive. Obstruc-

tive respiratory diseases are the result of an obstacle in the airway that impedes the flow of air, especially during expiration. Obstructive diseases are characterized by reduced expiratory flow rates and increased total lung capacities. Restrictive respiratory diseases are caused by conditions that limit lung expansion by an actual reduction of the volume of inspired air, such as fibrothorax, a neuromuscular disorder, kyphosis, scoliosis, spondylitis, or surgical removal of lung tissue. Characteristic features of restrictive respiratory diseases are decreased forced vital capacity and total lung capacity, with increased work of breathing and inefficient exchange of gases.

pulmonary oedema, the accumulation of extravascular fluid in lung tissues and alveoli, caused most commonly by congestive heart failure and also occurring in barbiturate and opiate poisoning, diffuse infections, haemorrhagic pancreatitis, renal failure, and after a stroke, skull fracture, near drowning, the inhalation of irritating gases, and the rapid administration of whole blood, plasma, serum albumin, or intravenous fluids. In congestive heart disease serous fluid is pushed back through the pulmonary capillaries into alveoli and quickly enters bronchioles and bronchi. The patient with pulmonary oedema breathes rapidly and shallowly with difficulty, is usually restless, apprehensive, hoarse, pale, or cyanotic, and may cough up frothy, pink sputum. The peripheral and neck veins are usually engorged; the blood pressure and heart rate are increased; and the pulse may be full and pounding or weak and thready. There may be oedema of the extremities, rales in the lungs, respiratory acidosis, and profuse diaphoresis.

pulmonary embolism (PE), the blockage of a pulmonary artery by foreign matter such as fat, air, tumour tissue, or a thrombus that usually arises from a peripheral vein. Predisposing factors include an alteration of blood constituents with increased coagulation, damage to blood vessel walls, and stagnation or immobilization, especially when associated with childbirth, congestive heart failure, polycythaemia vera, or surgery. Pulmonary embolism is difficult to distinguish from myocardial infarction and pneumonia. It is characterized by dyspnoea, sudden chest pain, shock, and cyanosis.

pulmonary emphysema, a chronic obstructive disease of the lungs, marked by an overdistention of the alveoli.

pulmonary function laboratory, an area of a hospital or other health facility used for examination and evaluation of patients' respiratory functions, using electromechanical and other devices.

pulmonary function test (PFT), a procedure for determining the capacity of the lungs to exchange oxygen and carbon dioxide efficiently. There are two general kinds of respiratory function tests. One measures ventilation, or the ability of the bellows action of the chest and lungs to move gas in and out of alveoli; the other kind measures the diffusion of gas across the alveolar capillary membrane and the perfusion of the lungs by blood. Efficient gas exchange in the lungs requires a balanced ventilation-perfusion ratio, with areas receiving ventilation well perfused and areas receiving blood flow capable of ventilation.

pulmonary hypertension, a condition of abnormally high pressure within the pulmonary circulation.

pulmonary infiltrate with eosinophilia. See **PIE.**

pulmonary stenosis, an abnormal cardiac condition, generally characterized by concentric hypertrophy of the right ventricle with relatively little increase in diastolic volume. When the ventricular septum is intact, this condition may be caused by valvular stenosis, by infundibular stenosis, or by both; it produces a pressure difference during systole between the right ventricular cavity and the pulmonary artery.

pulmonary sulcus tumour, a destructive, invasive neoplasm that develops at the apex of the lung and infiltrates the ribs, vertebrae, and the brachial plexus.

pulmonary surfactant, a surfactant agent found in the lungs that functions to reduce the surface tension of the fluid on the surface of the cells of the lower respiratory system, enhancing the elasticity of the alveoli and bronchioles and thus the exchange of gases in the lungs.

pulmonary trunk, the short, wide vessel that conveys venous blood from the right ventricle of the heart to the lungs.

pulmonary tuberculosis. See **tuberculosis.**

pulmonary valve, a cardiac structure composed of three semilunar cusps that close during each heartbeat to prevent blood from flowing back into the right ventricle from the pulmonary artery. The cusps are separated by sinuses that resemble tiny buckets when they are closed and filled with blood. These flaps grow from the lining of the pulmonary artery.

pulmonary vascular resistance (PVR), the resistance in the pulmonary vascular bed against which the right ventricle must eject blood.

pulmonary vein, one of a pair of large vessels that return oxygenated blood from each lung to the left atrium of the heart. The right pulmonary veins pass dorsal to the right atrium and the superior vena cava. The left pulmonary veins pass ventral to the descending thoracic aorta.

pulmonary wedge pressure (PWP), the pressure produced by an inflated latex balloon against a pulmonary artery, as part of a procedure used in the diagnosis of congestive heart failure, myocardial infarction, and other conditions. A balloon-tipped catheter is inserted through a subclavian, jugular, or femoral vein to the vena cava and on through the right atrium and ventricle to the pulmonary artery.

pulmonary Wegener's granulomatosis, a rare, fatal disease of young or middle-aged men, characterized by granulomatous lesions of the respiratory tract, focal necrotizing arteritis, and, finally, widespread inflammation of body organs.

pulmonic. See **pulmonary.**

pulmonic stenosis. See **pulmonary stenosis.**

pulp, any soft, spongy tissue, such as that contained within the spleen, the pulp chamber of the tooth, or the distal phalanges of the fingers and the toes. **pulpy,** *adj.*

pulp canal, the space occupied by the pulp in the radicular portion of the tooth.

pulp cavity, the space in a tooth bounded by the dentin and containing the dental pulp. It is divided into the pulp chamber and the pulp or root canal.

pulpitis, infection or inflammation of the dental pulp.

pulpless tooth, a tooth in which the dental pulp is necrotic or has been removed.

pulp stone. See **denticle.**

pulsatile, pertaining to an activity characterized by a rhythmic pulsation.

pulsatile assist device (PAD), a flexible valveless balloon conduit contained within a rigid plastic cylinder that is inserted into the arterial circulation to provide pulsatile cardiopulmonary bypass perfusion.

pulse, 1. a rhythmic beating or vibrating movement. 2. a brief electromagnetic wave. 3. the regular, recurrent expansion and contraction of an artery produced by waves of pressure caused by the ejection of blood from the left ventricle of the heart as it contracts. The phenomenon is easily detected on superficial arteries, such as the radial and carotid arteries, and corresponds to each beat of the heart. The normal number of pulse beats per minute in the average adult varies from 60 to 80, with fluctuations occurring with exercise, injury, illness, and emotional reactions.

pulse deficit, a condition that exists when the radial pulse is less than the ventricular rate as auscultated at the apex or seen on the electrocardiogram. The condition indicates a lack of peripheral perfusion for some of the heart contractions.

pulse height analyser, a device that accepts or rejects electronic pulses according to their amplitude or energy.

pulseless disease. See **Takayasu's arteritis.**

pulse NMR, NMR techniques that use radiofrequency pulses and Fourier transformation of the NMR signal.

pulse point, any one of the sites on the surface of the body where arterial pulsations can be easily palpated. The most commonly used pulse point is over the radial artery at the wrist. Other pulse points are over the temporal artery in front of the ear, over the common carotid artery at the lower level of the thyroid cartilage, and over the facial artery at the lower margin of the jaw.

pulse pressure, the difference between the systolic and diastolic pressures, normally 30 to 40 mm Hg.

pulsus alternans, a pulse characterized by a regular alternation of weak and strong beats without changes in the length of the cycle.

pulsus paradoxus, an abnormal decrease in systolic pressure and pulse wave amplitude during inspiration.

pulvule, a proprietary capsule containing a dose of a drug in powder form.

pump, 1. an apparatus used to move fluids or gases by suction or by positive pressure, such as an infusion pump or stomach pump. **2.** a physiological mechanism by which a substance is moved, usually by active transport across a cell membrane, such as a sodium pump. **3.** to move a liquid or gas by suction or positive pressure.

pump bump, inflammation of the retrocalcaneal bursa as a result of shoe pressure.

pump lung. See **congestive atelectasis.**

punch biopsy, the removal of living tissue for microscopic examination, usually bone marrow from the sternum, by means of a punch.

punch forceps, a surgical instrument used to cut out a disc of dense or resistant tissue, such as bone and cartilage. The ends of the blades of the punch forceps are perforated to grip the involved tissue.

punctum lacrimale, *pl.* **puncta lacrimalia,** a tiny aperture in the margin of each eyelid that opens into the lacrimal duct. The puncta release tears that travel through the lacrimal ducts to the conjunctiva.

puncture wound, a traumatic injury caused by the penetration of the skin by a narrow object, such as a knife, nail, or slender fragment of metal, wood, glass, or other material.

Punnett square {Reginald C. Punnett, 20th century English geneticist}, a checkerboard, graphlike diagram, used in charting genetic ratios, that shows all of the possible combinations of male and female gametes when one or more pairs of independent alleles are crossed.

pupil, a circular opening in the iris of the eye, located slightly to the nasal side of the centre of the iris. The pupil lies behind the anterior chamber of the eye and the cornea and in front of the lens. Its diameter changes with contraction and relaxation of the muscular fibres of the iris as the eye responds to changes in light, emotional states, and other kinds of stimulation. The pupil is the window of the eye through which light passes to the lens and the retina. **pupillary,** *adj.*

pupillary reflex. See **accommodation reflex, light reflex.**

pupillary skin reflex. See **ciliospinal reflex.**

purgation. See **catharsis.**

purgative, a strong medication usually administered by mouth to promote evacuation of the bowel.

purge, 1. to evacuate the bowels, as with a cathartic. **2.** a cathartic. **3.** to make free of an unwanted substance. **purgative,** *n., adj.*

purified protein derivative (PPD), a dried form of tuberculin used in testing for past or present infection with tubercle bacilli. This product is introduced into the skin during such tests.

purine, any one of a large group of nitrogenous compounds, produced as end products in the digestion of proteins in the diet, or synthesized in the body. Purines are also present in many medications and other substances, including caffeine, theophylline, and various diuretics, muscle relaxants, and myocardial stimulants.

Purkinje cells {Johannes E. Purkinje, Polish physiologist, b. 1787}, large neurons that provide the only output from the cerebellar cortex after the cortex processes sensory and motor impulses from the rest of the nervous system.

Purkinje's fibres, myocardial fibres that are a continuation of the bundle of His and extend into the muscle walls of the ventricles.

Purkinje's network, a complex network of muscle fibres that spread through the right and the left ventricles of the heart and carry the impulses that contract those chambers almost simultaneously.

purposeful activity, activity that depends on consciously planned and directed involvement of the person.

purpura, any of several bleeding disorders characterized by haemorrhage into the tissues, particularly beneath the skin or mucous membranes, producing ecchymoses or petechiae. The two major kinds of purpura are **thrombocytopenic purpura** and **nonthrombocytopenic purpura. purpuric,** *adj.*

pursed-lip breathing, respiration characterized by deep inspirations followed by prolonged expirations through pursed lips.

purulent, producing or containing pus.

pus, a creamy, viscous, pale yellow or yellow-green fluid exudate that is the result of liquefaction necrosis. Its main constituent is an abundance of polymorphonuclear leukocytes. Bacterial infection is its most common cause.

pustular psoriasis, a severe form of psoriasis consisting of bright red patches and sterile pustules all over the body. Crops of lesions lasting 4 to 7 days occur every few days in cycles over weeks or months. Recurrences are inevitable. Fever, leukocytosis, and hypoalbuminaemia are associated.

pustule, a small, circumscribed elevation of the skin containing fluid that is usually purulent. **pustular,** *adj.*

putrefaction, the decay of enzymes, especially proteins, that produces foul-smelling compounds, such as ammonia, hydrogen sulphide, and mercaptans. **putrefactive,** *adj.*

putrefy, to decay, with the production of foul-smelling substances, especially putrescine and mercaptans associated with the decomposition of animal tissues and proteins.

putrescine, a foul-smelling, toxic ptomaine produced by the decomposition of the amino acid ornithine during the decay of animal tissues, bacillus cultures, and faecal bacteria.

putromaine, any toxin produced by the decay of food within a living body.

P value, (in research) the statistical probability attached to the occurrence of a given finding by chance alone in comparison with the known distribution of possible findings, considering the kinds of data, the technique of analysis, and the number of observations.

PVB. See **VBP.**

PVC, **1.** abbreviation for **polyvinyl chloride. 2.** abbreviation for **premature ventricular contraction.**

PVR, abbreviation for **pulmonary vascular resistance.**

P wave, the component of the cardiac cycle shown on an electrocardiogram as an inverted U-shaped curve that follows the end of the T wave and precedes the spike of the QRS complex. It represents atrial depolarization.

P' wave (P prime wave), a P wave that is generated from other than the sinus node; an ectopic P wave.

PWP, abbreviation for **pulmonary wedge pressure.**

pyelitis, *obsolete.* an inflammation of the pelvis of the kidney. See **pyelonephritis.**

pyelography. See **intravenous pyelography.**

pyelolithotomy, a surgical procedure in which renal calculi are removed from the pelvis of the ureter.

pyelonephritis, a diffuse pyogenic infection of the pelvis and parenchyma of the kidney. **Acute pyelonephritis** is usually the result of an infection that ascends from the lower urinary tract to the kidney. **Chronic pyelonephritis** develops slowly after bacterial infection of the kidney and may progress to renal failure. Most cases are associated with some form of obstruction, such as a stone or a stricture of the ureter.

pygmalianism, a psychosexual abnormality in which the individual directs erotic fantasies toward an object that he has created.

pygmy, an extremely small person whose bodily parts are proportioned accordingly; a primordial dwarf.

pygoamorphus, asymmetric, conjoined twins in which the parasitic member is represented by an undifferentiated amorphous mass attached to the autosite in the sacral region.

pygodidymus, **1.** a malformed fetus that has a double pelvis and hips. **2.** conjoined twins that are fused in the cephalothoracic region but separated at the pelvis.

pygomelus, a malformed fetus that has an extra limb or limbs attached to the buttock.

pygopagus, conjoined twins consisting of two fully formed or nearly formed fetuses that are united in the sacral region so that they are back to back.

pyknic, describing a body structure characterized by short, round limbs, a full face, a short neck, stockiness, and a tendency toward obesity.

pylon, an artificial lower limb, often a narrow vertical support consisting of a socket with wooden side-supports and a rubber-clad peg end. It may be used as a temporary prosthesis.

pyloric orifice, the opening of the stomach into the duodenum lying to the right of the middle line at the level of the cranial border of the first lumbar vertebra.

pyloric spasm. See **pylorospasm.**

pyloric sphincter, a thickened muscular ring in the stomach, separating the pylorus from the duodenum.

pyloric stenosis, a narrowing of the pyloric sphincter at the outlet of the stomach, causing an obstruction that blocks the flow of food into the small intestine.

pyloric ulcer. See **peptic ulcer.**

pyloromyotomy, the incision of the longitudinal and circular muscle of the pylorus, which leaves the mucosa intact but separates the incised muscle fibres.

pyloroplasty, a surgical procedure performed to relieve pyloric stenosis.

pylorospasm, a spasm of the pyloric sphincter of the stomach, as occurs in pyloric stenosis.

pylorus, *pl.* **pylori, pyloruses,** a tubular portion of the stomach that angles to the right from the body of the stomach toward the duodenum. **pyloric,** *adj.*

pyoderma, any purulent skin disease, such as impetigo.

pyogenic, pus-producing.

pyogenic granuloma, a small, nonmalignant mass of excessive granulation tissue, usually found at the site of an injury. Most often a dull red colour, it contains numerous capillaries, bleeds easily, and is very tender; it may be attached by a narrow stalk.

pyorrhoea, **1.** a discharge of pus. **2.** a purulent inflammation of the tissues surrounding the teeth. **pyorrhoeal,** *adj.*

pyosalpinx, an accumulation of pus in a uterine tube.

pyramidal, of or pertaining to the shape of a pyramid.

pyramidalis, one of a pair of anterolateral muscles of the abdomen, contained in the lower end of the sheath of the rectus abdominis. It functions to tense the linea alba.

pyramidal tract, a pathway composed of groups of nerve fibres in the white matter of the spinal cord through which motor impulses are conducted to the anterior horn cells from the opposite side of the brain. These descending fibres regulate the voluntary and reflex activity of the muscles through the anterior horn cells.

pyrantel embonate, an anthelmintic used in the treatment of infestation by roundworms, threadworms or hookworms.

pyrazinamide, an antitubercular drug used in the combination therapy in the treatment of tuberculosis.

pyrexia. See **fever.**

pyridostigmine bromide, an anticholinesterase used in the treatment of myasthenia gravis.

pyridoxal phosphate, an enzyme in the body that acts with pyridoxamine phosphate and transaminase to catalyse the reversible transfer of an amino group from an alpha-amino acid to an alpha-keto acid, especially alpha-ketoglutaric acid.

pyridoxamine phosphate, an enzyme that participates with pyridoxal phosphate and transaminase in the reversible transfer of anamino group from an alpha-amino acid to an alpha-keto acid.

pyridoxine, a water-soluble, white, crystalline vitamin that is part of the B complex group, derived from pyridine, and converted in the body to pyridoxal and pyridoxamine for synthesis. It functions as a coenzyme essential for the synthesis of amino acids, the conversion of tryptophan to niacin, the breakdown of glycogen to glucose 1-phosphate, the production of antibodies, the formation of haem in haemoglobin, the formation of hormones important in brain function, the proper absorption of vitamin B12, the production of hydrochloric acid and magnesium, and the maintenance of the balance of sodium and potassium, which regulates body fluids and the functioning of the nervous and musculoskeletal systems.

pyridoxine hydrochloride. See **pyridoxine.**

pyrimethamine, an antimalarial prescribed in the treatment of malaria (in combination with dapsone or sulphadoxine), and toxoplasmosis.

pyrimethamine and sulphadoxine (Fansidar), a fixed-combination antimalarial preparation used for prophylaxis and treatment of malaria.

pyrimidine, an organic compound of heterocyclic nitrogen found in nucleic acids and in many drugs, including the antiviral drugs acyclovir and ribavirin, and the cytotoxic antimetabolite 5-fluorouracil.

pyrogen, any substance or agent that tends to cause a rise in body temperature, such as some bacterial toxins. **pyrogenic,** *adj.*

pyrolagnia, sexual stimulation or gratification from watching or setting fires.

pyromania, an impulse neurosis characterized by an uncontrollable urge to set fires. The condition is found predominantly in men and is usually associated with alcohol intoxication, chronic personal frustrations, resentment of authority figures, or some other psychological disturbance or psychosexual dysfunction.

pyromaniac, 1. a person with or displaying characteristics of pyromania. **2.** of, pertaining to, or exhibiting pyromania. **pyromaniacal,** *adj.*

pyrosis. See **heartburn.**

pyrrole, a heterocyclic substance occurring naturally in many compounds in the body. Haem and porphyrin are pyrrole derivatives.

pyruvate kinase, an enzyme essential for anaerobic glycolysis in red blood cells. It catalyses the transfer of a phosphate group from adenosine triphosphate to produce adenosine diphosphate.

pyruvate kinase deficiency, a congenital haemolytic disorder transmitted as an autosomal recessive trait. The homozygous condition is characterized by severe chronic haemolysis.

pyruvic acid, a compound formed as an end product of glycolysis, the anaerobic stage of glucose metabolism. Exposed to oxygen and acetylcoenzyme A at the entrance to the Krebs citric acid cycle, the compound is changed to citric acid.

pyuria, the presence of white blood cells in the urine, usually a sign of an infection of the urinary tract. Pyuria occurs most often in cystitis, pyelonephritis, urethritis, and tuberculosis of the kidney. See also **bacteriuria.**

Q, 1. symbol for blood volume. **2.** symbol for quantity.

Q, symbol for **rate of blood flow.**

Q angle, the angle of incidence of the quadriceps muscle relative to the patella. The Q angle determines the tracking of the patella through the trochlea of the femur. As the angle increases, the chance of patellar compression problems increases.

QAP, abbreviation for **quality assurance program.**

q.d., (in prescriptions) abbreviation for *quaque die /de*, a Latin phrase meaning "every day."

Q fever, an acute febrile illness, usually respiratory, caused by the rickettsia, *Coxiella burnetii (Rickettsia burnetii).* The disease is spread through contact with infected domestic animals, either by inhaling the rickettsiae from their hides, drinking their contaminated milk, or being bitten by a tick harboring the organism.

q.h., (in prescriptions) abbreviation for *quaque hora,* a Latin phrase meaning "every hour."

q.2h., (in prescriptions) abbreviation for *quaque secunda hora,* a Latin phrase meaning "every 2 hours."

q.3h., (in prescriptions) abbreviation for *quaque tertia hora,* a Latin phrase meaning "every 3 hours."

q.4h., (in prescriptions) abbreviation for *quaque quarta hora,* a Latin phrase meaning "every 4 hours."

q.6h., (in prescriptions) abbreviation for *quaque sex hora,* a Latin phrase meaning "every 6 hours."

q.8h., (in prescriptions) abbreviation for *quaque octa hora,* a Latin phrase meaning "every 8 hours."

q.i.d., (in prescriptions) abbreviation for *quater in die,* a Latin phrase meaning "four times a day."

QRS complex, the components of the ventricular electric events of the cardiac cycle shown on an electrocardiogram as a sharp, angular complex normally less than 0.1 seconds in duration, reflecting the time it takes for the ventricular myocardium to depolarize.

q.s., (in prescriptions) abbreviation for *quantum sufficit,* a Latin phrase meaning "quantity required."

Q's test. See **Queckenstedt's test.**

QT interval, the portion on an electrocardiogram from the beginning of the QRS complex to the end of the T wave, reflecting the length of the refractory period of the heart. An excessively long QT interval is known to cause the life-threatening ventricular tachycardia known as torsades des pointes.

quadratus labii superioris. See **zygomaticus minor.**

quadriceps femoris, the great extensor muscle of the anterior thigh, composed of the rectus femoris, the vastus lateralis, the vastus medialis, and the vastus intermedius. The muscle functions to extend the leg.

quadriceps reflex. See **patellar reflex.**

quadrigeminal, 1. in four parts. **2.** a fourfold increase in size or frequency.

quadrigeminal pulse, a pulse in which a pause occurs after every fourth beat.

quadrilateral socket, a four-sided prosthetic socket design for persons with above the knee amputations. The posterior brim is designed to fit directly beneath the ischial tuberosity so that the person literally sits on it.

quadriplegia, an abnormal condition characterized by paralysis of the arms, the legs, and the trunk of the body below the level of an associated injury to the spinal cord. This disorder may be caused by spinal cord injury, especially in the area of the fifth to the seventh vertebrae. Automobile accidents and sporting mishaps are common causes.

quadruped, 1. any four-footed animal. **2.** a human whose body weight is supported by both arms as well as both legs. See also prone-on-elbows.

quadruplet, any one of four offspring born of the same gestation period during a single pregnancy.

quale, *pl.* **qualia 1.** the quality of a particular thing. **2.** a quality considered as an independent entity. **3.** (in psychology) a feeling, sensation, or other conscious process that has its unique, particular quality regardless of its external meaning or frame of reference.

qualified, pertaining to a health professional or health facility that is formally recognized by an appropriate agency or organization as meeting certain standards of professional competence.

qualitative, of or pertaining to the quality, value, or nature of something.

qualitative melanin test, a test for detecting melanin in the urine of patients with malignant melanomas.

qualitative test, a test that determines the presence or absence of a substance.

quality, (in radiotherapy) specification of the penetrating ability of a beam of x-rays where greater penetrating ability characterizes a beam as "harder," whereas less energy results in a beam being described as "softer."

quality assessment measures, formal, systematic, organizational evaluation of overall patterns or programs of care, including clinical, consumer, and systems evaluation.

quality assurance, (in health care) any evaluation of services provided and the results achieved as compared with accepted standards.

assurance program, a system of review of selected hospital medical records by medical staff members, performed for the purposes of evaluating the quality and effectiveness of medical care in relation to accepted standards.

quality factor, (in radiotherapy) evaluation of the biologic damage that radiation can produce. In the field of radiation protection, biologically equivalent doses are set equal to one another by multiplying the actual absorbed dose by a number called the quality factor.

quantitative inheritance. See **multifactorial inheritance.**

quantitative test, a test that determines the amount of a substance per unit volume or unit weight.

quantum mechanics. See **quantum theory.**

quantum theory, (in physics) a theory dealing with the interaction of matter and electromagnetic radiation, particularly at the atomic and subatomic levels, according to which radiation consists of small units of energy called quanta.

quarantine, 1. isolation of people with communicable disease or of those exposed to communicable disease during the contagious period in an attempt to prevent spread of the illness. **2.** the practice of detaining travellers or vessels coming from places of epidemic disease, originally for 40 days, for the purpose of inspection or disinfection.

quartan, recurring on the fourth day, or at about 72-hour intervals.

quartan malaria, a form of malaria, caused by the protozoan *Plasmodium malariae,* characterized by febrile paroxysms that occur every 72 hours.

quarternary ammonium derivative, a substance whose chemical structure has four carbon groups attached to a nitrogen atom. It is usually a strong base, highly water soluble but relatively insoluble in lipids.

quartz silicosis. See **silicosis.**

Queckenstedt's test, {Hans H. G. Queckenstedt, German physician, b. 1876}, a test for an obstruction in the spinal canal in which the jugular veins on each side of the neck are compressed alternately. Normally, occlusion of the veins of the neck causes an immediate rise in spinal fluid pressure; if the vertebral canal is blocked, no rise occurs.

quellung reaction, the swelling of the cap-

sule of a bacterium, seen in the laboratory when the organism is exposed to specific antisera. This phenomenon is used to identify the genera, species, or subspecies of the bacteria causing a disease.

Quengle cast, a two-section, hinged orthopaedic cast for immobilizing the lower extremities from the foot or ankle to below the knee and the upper thigh to a level just above the knee. The two parts of the cast are connected by special hinges at knee level.

quercetin, a yellow, crystalline, flavonoid pigment found in oak bark, the juice of lemons, asparagus, and other plants. It is used to reduce abnormal capillary fragility.

querulous paranoia, a form of paranoia characterized by extreme discontent and habitual complaining, usually about imagined slights by others.

quick connect , a plastic or similar connecting device that is attached to or implanted in a patient who will be joined to an electromechanical or other apparatus.

quickening, the first feeling by a pregnant woman of movement of her baby in utero, usually occurring between 16 and 20 weeks of gestation.

Quick's test {Armand J. Quick, American physician, b. 1894}, **1.** a test for jaundice. The patient is given an oral dose of sodium benzoate, which is conjugated in the liver with glycine to form hippuric acid. The amount of hippuric acid excreted in the urine is inversely proportional to the degree of liver damage. **2.** a test for haemophilia. A solution of thromboplastin is added to oxalated blood plasma and calcium chloride. The amount of time required for formation of a firm clot is inversely proportional to the amount of prothrombin in the plasma.

quinacrine hydrochloride, an anthelmintic and an antimalarial. It is prescribed in the treatment of giardiasis and cestodiasis and in the treatment and suppression of malaria.

Quincke's pulse, {Heinrich I. Quincke, German physician, b. 1842}, an abnormal alternate blanching and reddening of the skin that may be observed in several ways, as by pressing the front edge of the fingernail and watching the blood in the nail bed recede and return.

quinethazone, a diuretic and antihypertensive prescribed in the treatment of hypertension and oedema.

quinidine, an antiarrhythmic agent used as a bisulfate, gluconate, polygalacturonate, or sulfate. It is prescribed in the treatment of atrial flutter, atrial fibrillation, premature ventricular contractions, and tachycardias.

quinidine gluconate. See **quinidine.**

quinine, a white, bitter crystalline alkaloid, made from cinchona bark, used in antimalarial medications.

quinine dihydrochloride, an antimalarial.

quinine sulfate, an antimalarial with antipyretic, analgesic, and muscle relaxant activity. It is prescribed in the treatment of malaria, particularly malaria caused by *Plasmodium falciparum,* and nocturnal leg cramps.

quinolone, any of a class of antibiotics that act by interrupting the replication of DNA molecules in bacteria.

quinsy. See **peritonsillar abscess.**

quintan, recurring on the fifth day, or at about 96-hour intervals. See also trench fever.

quintana fever. See **trench fever.**

quintuplet, any one of five offspring born of the same gestation period during a single pregnancy.

quotid. See **q.d.**

Q wave, the component of the cardiac cycle shown on an electrocardiogram as a short abrupt downward line from the end of the tail of the P wave before the sudden sharp ascent of the R wave. It represents the first part of the QRS complex.rocardiogram from the(-KSbeginning of the QRS complex to the end of the T wave)

-racetam, a suffix for piracetam-type nootrope substances.

-renone, a suffix for spironolactone-type aldosterone antagonists.

R, 1. abbreviation for **metabolic respiratory quotient. 2.** abbreviation for **resolution. 3.** abbreviation for **respiratory exchange ratio.**

R factor, an episome in bacteria that is responsible for drug resistance. It is transmissible to progeny and other bacterial cells by conjugation. The portion of the episome involved in replication and transmission is called **resistance transfer factor.**

R wave. See **QRS complex.**

r-loop, (in molecular genetics) a distinctive loop formation seen under an electron microscope. It is composed of a single helical strand of DNA, wound with a hybrid strand containing another single strand of DNA with a strand of RNA.

R-on-T phenomenon, an arrhythmia characterized by premature ventricular contraction that occurs on or before completion of the T wave of the previous beat.

R-R interval, the interval from the peak of one QRS complex to the peak of the next, as shown on an electrocardiogram.

RCP, abbreviation for **Royal College of Physicians.**

RCS, abbreviation for **Royal College of Surgeons.**

r.t.c., abbreviation for **return to clinic,** noted on the chart, usually followed by a date on which a subsequent appointment has been made for the patient.

Ra, symbol for **radium.**

RA latex test, abbreviation for **rheumatoid arthritis latex test.** See **latex fixation test.**

rabbit fever. See **tularaemia.**

rabies, an acute and usually fatal viral disease of the central nervous system of animals. It is transmitted from animals to people by infected blood, tissue or, most commonly, saliva. The reservoir of the virus is primarily wild animals, including skunks, bats, foxes, dogs, raccoons and cats. After introduction into the human body, often by a bite of an infected animal, the virus travels along nerve pathways to the brain, and later to other organs. An incubation period ranges from 10 days to 1 year, and is followed by a prodromal period characterized by fever, malaise, headache, paraesthesia and myalgia. After several days, severe encephalitis, delirium, agonizingly painful muscular spasms, seizures, paralysis, coma and death ensue.

rabies immunoglobulin (RIG), a preparation of immunoglobulins obtained from the plasma of donors immunized against rabies and containing specific antibodies to the rabies virus. It is used in the passive immunization of persons suspected of exposure to rabies.

rabies vaccine (DEV), a sterile suspension of killed rabies virus used for active immunization and postexposure prophylaxis against rabies.

race, a vague, unscientific term for a group of genetically related people who share certain physical characteristics.

racemic, pertaining to a compound made up of levorotatory isomers, rendering it optically inactive under polarized light.

racemose, resembling a bunch of grapes. The term is used to describe a structure in which many branches terminate in nodular, cyst-like forms, such as pulmonary alveoli.

racemose aneurysm, a pronounced dilatation of lengthened and tortuous blood vessels, some of which may be distended up to 20 times their normal size.

rachiopagus, conjoined symmetrical twins that are united back-to-back along the spinal column.

rachischisis, a congenital fissure of one or more vertebrae.

rachischisis totalis. See **complete rachischisis.**

rachitic, 1. of, or pertaining to, rickets. **2.** resembling or suggesting the condition of a person afflicted with rickets.

rachitic dwarf, a person whose retarded growth is caused by rickets.

rachitis, 1. rickets. **2.** an inflammatory disease of the vertebral column.

racial immunity, a form of natural immunity shared by most of the members of a genetically related population.

racial unconscious. See **collective unconscious.**

rackets, (in psychology) feelings or behaviours used to cover other feelings.

rad, abbreviation for **radiation absorbed dose;** it is the basic unit of absorbed dose of ionizing radiation. One rad is equivalent to 0.01 Gy.

radarkymography, a radar (radio detection and ranging) technique for showing the size and outline of the heart, using a radar tracking device and a fluoroscopic screen to display images produced by electrical impulses passed over the chest surface.

Radford nomogram, a mathematical chart device used in respiratory therapy to estimate combined tidal volumes and rates for mechanical ventilation. It is based on the three parameters of body weight, sex and respiratory rate.

radial artery, an artery in the forearm, starting at the bifurcation of the brachial artery and passing in 12 branches to the forearm, wrist and hand.

radial keratotomy, a surgical procedure in which a series of tiny, shallow incisions are made on the cornea, causing it to bulge slightly to correct for near-sightedness.

radial nerve, the largest branch of the brachial plexus, arising on each side as a continuation of the posterior cord. It supplies the skin of the arm and forearm as well as their extensor muscles.

radial nerve palsy, a compression or entrapment neuropathy involving the radial nerve. Symptoms of muscle weakness and sensory loss are due to compression of the radial nerve against the humerus.

radial notch of ulna, the narrow, lateral depression in the coronoid process of the ulna that receives the head of the radius.

radial pulse, the pulse of the radial artery palpated at the wrist over the radius. The radial pulse is the one most often taken, because of the ease with which it is palpated.

radial recurrent artery, a branch of the radial artery. It arises just distal to the elbow, ascends between the branches of the radial nerve, and supplies several muscles of the arm and the elbow.

radial reflex, a normal reflex elicited by tapping over the distal radius, with the response being flexion of the forearm.

radiant energy, the energy emitted by electromagnetic radiation, such as radio waves, visible light, x-rays and gamma rays.

radiate, to diverge or spread from a common point.

radiate ligament, a ligament that connects the head of a rib with a vertebra and an associated intervertebral disk.

radiation, 1. the emission of energy, rays or waves. **2.** (in medicine) the use of a form of ionizing radiation for the diagnosis or treatment of disease.

radiation caries, tooth decay which characteristically affects the cervical areas and encircles the tooth. It is caused by ionizing radiation of the oral and maxillary tissues, which may damage the salivary glands and reduce the normal flow of saliva.

radiation detector, a device for converting radiant energy to an observable form, used for detecting the presence and sometimes the amount of radiation, such as a Geiger-Mller tube or scintillation counter.

Effects Research Foundation (RERF), an organization that studies the long-term effects of survivers of atomic bombings of Hiroshima and Nagasaki during World War II. The RERF is successor to the Atomic Bomb Casualty Commission.

radiation exposure, a measure of the ionization produced in air by x-rays or gamma rays. It is the sum of the electrical charges on all ions of one sign that are produced when all electrons liberated by photons in a volume of air are completely stopped, divided by the mass of air in the volume element. The SI unit of exposure is joules per kilogram of air; the special unit is the roentgen (R), and 1 R is equal to 2.58×10^{-4} coulombs per kilogram.

radiation oncologist. See **radiotherapist.**

radiation oncology, the treatment of cancer using radiation.

radiation sensitivity, a measure of the response of tissue to ionizing radiation.

radiation sickness. See **acute radiation exposure.**

radiation syndrome. See **acute radiation exposure.**

radiation therapy. See **radiotherapy.**

radical, 1. a group of atoms that act together and form a component of a compound. The group tends to remain bound together when a chemical reaction removes it from a compound and attaches it to another. A radical does not exist freely in nature. **2.** pertaining to drastic therapy, such as the surgical removal of an organ, limb or other part of the body.

radical dissection, the surgical removal of tissue in an extensive area surrounding the operative site. Most often it is performed to identify and excise all tissue that may be malignant, so as to decrease the chance of recurrence.

radical mastectomy, the surgical removal of an entire breast, pectoral muscles, axillary lymph nodes and all fat, fascia and adjacent tissues. It is performed for the treatment of breast cancer. Chemotherapy and radiotherapy may continue after surgery. The woman is told never to allow blood to be drawn from the affected arm; intravenous injection is also to be avoided in that arm.

radical neck dissection, dissection and removal of all lymph nodes and removable tissues under the skin of the neck, performed to prevent the spread of malignant tumours of the head and neck that have a reasonable chance of being controlled.

radical therapy, 1. a treatment intended to cure, not palliate. **2.** a definitive, extreme treatment; not conservative, such as radical mastectomy rather than simple or partial mastectomy.

radical vulvectomy. See **vulvectomy.**

radicular retainer, a type of retainer that lies within the body of a tooth, usually in the root portion, such as a dowel crown.

radicular retention, retention developed by placing metal projections into the root canals of pulpless teeth.

radioactive, unstable atomic nucleus which disintegrates spontaneously, usually with the emission of charged particles.

radioactive contamination, the undesirable addition of radioactive material to the body or part of the environment, such as clothing or equipment. Beta radiation contamination of healthcare personnel is only possible through ingestion, inhalation or absorption of the source, as when the skin is contaminated with a beta emitter contained in an absorbable chemical form. Instruments, drapes, surgical gloves and clothing that come in contact with serous fluids, blood and urine of patients containing beta or gamma radiation emitters may be contaminated.

radioactive decay, the spontaneous disintegration of an unstable nucleus, for example by alpha decay or beta minus decay.

radioactive element, an element subject to spontaneous degeneration of its nucleus accompanied by the emission of alpha particles, beta particles or gamma rays. All elements with atomic numbers greater than 83 are radioactive.

radioactive half-life. See **half-life.**

radioactive iodine (RAI). See **iodine.**

radioactive iodine excretion test. See **thyroid function test.**

radioactive iodine uptake (RAIU). See **thyroid function test.**

radioactivity, the emission of corpuscular or electromagnetic radiations as a consequence of nuclear disintegration.

radioallergosorbent test (RAST), a test in which a radioimmunoassay is used to identify and quantify IgE in serum that has been mixed with any of 45 known allergens. If an atopic allergy to a substance exists, an antigen-antibody reaction occurs with characteristic conjugation and clumping.

radiobiology, the branch of the natural sciences dealing with the effects of radiation on biological systems. **radiobiological,** *adj.*

radiocarpal articulation, the condyloid joint at the wrist that connects the radius and distal surface of an articular disk with the scaphoid, the lunate, and the triangular bones. The joint involves four ligaments and allows all movements but rotation.

radiochemistry, the branch of chemistry that deals with the properties and behaviour of radioactive materials and the use of radionuclides in the study of chemical and biologic problems.

radiocurable, the susceptibility of tumour cells to destruction by ionizing radiation.

radiofrequency (rf), that portion of the electromagnetic spectrum with frequencies lower than about 10^{10} Hz.

radiograph, an x-ray image.

radiographer, a healthcare professional qualified to direct ionizing radiations physically (IRR, 1988). Competence to practise is assessed by the College of Radiographers (UK) and the Council of Professions Supplementary to Medicine (UK), following 3 years of study for the award of either the Diploma of the College of Radiographers (DCR) or Bachelor of Science in Radiography. The qualification may be in either **diagnostic radiography** or **therapeutic radiography.**

radiographic magnification. See **magnification.**

radiography, the use of ionizing radiation to produce images of the anatomy, and often function, of the body's organs. **radiographic,** *adj.*

radioimmunoassay (RIA), a technique in radiology used to determine the concentration of an antigen, antibody or other protein in the serum.

radioimmunosorbent assay test, a test that uses serum immunoglobulin E to detect allergies to various substances, such as certain cosmetics, animal fur, dust and grasses.

radioiodine. See **iodine.**

radioisotope, a radioactive isotope of an element, used for therapeutic and diagnostic purposes.

radioisotope scan. See **radionuclide imaging.**

radiological anatomy, (in applied anatomy) the study of structure and morphology of tissues and organs of the body, based on their x-ray visualization.

radiologist, a medical practitioner further qualified in radiology, who interprets diagnostic images and clinically directs medical exposures for examination purposes.

radiology, the branch of medicine concerned with the diagnosis of disease using methods of imaging, such as **radiography, computerized tomography, ultrasound, radionuclide imaging** and **magnetic resonance imaging.** **radiological,** *adj.*

radiolucency, a characteristic of materials of low atomic number that attenuate very few of the x-ray photons passing through, resulting in a high intensity of x-rays reaching the image-recording medium. On a radiograph, radiolucent materials appear dark; for example, air-filled lungs. **radiolucent,** *adj.*

radionecrosis, tissue death caused by radiation.

radionuclide, 1. an isotope (or nuclide) that undergoes radioactive decay. **2.** any of the radioactive isotopes of cobalt, iodine, phosphorus, strontium and other elements, used in nuclear medicine for the treatment of tumours and cancers, and for nuclear imaging of internal parts of the body.

radionuclide imaging, a method of imaging the functional anatomy of the body, following administration of a radiopharmaceutical, by detection of the precise site and intensity of the radioactivity emitted using a gamma camera.

radionuclide organ imaging. See **radionuclide imaging.**

radiopaque, a material of relatively high atomic number that attenuates the majority of x-ray photons passing through, resulting in a low intensity of x-rays reaching the recording medium. On a radiograph, radiopaque materials appear white; for example, bone. **radiopacity,** *n.*

radiopaque contrast medium, a chemical substance of relatively high atomic number, which attenuates most of the x-ray photons passing through; for example, barium sulphate used in radiographic examinations of the GI tract, and iodine compounds used intravenously.

radiopaque dye. See **radiopaque contrast medium.**

radiopharmaceutical, a selected drug labelled with a radionuclide. It is used in radionuclide imaging and targets the organ or site of interest to allow detection of the emitted gamma rays by a gamma camera.

radiopharmacy, a facility for the preparation and dispensing of radioactive drugs, as well as the storage of radioactive materials, inventory records and prescriptions of radioactive substances.

radioresistance, the relative resistance of cells, tissues, organs, organisms, chemical compounds or any others substances, to the effects of radiation.

radioresistant, unchanged by, or protected against, damage by radioactive emissions such as x-rays, alpha particles or gamma rays.

radiosensitive, capable of being changed by, or reacting to, radioactive emissions such as x-rays, alpha particles or gamma rays.

radiosensitivity, the relative susceptibility of cells, tissues, organs, organisms or any other living substances to the effects of radiation. Cells of self-renewing systems, such as those in the crypts of the intestine, are the most radiosensitive. Cells that divide regularly but mature between divisions, such as spermatogonia and spermatocytes, are next in radiosusceptibility. Long-lived cells that usually do not undergo mitosis unless there is a suitable stimulus include the less radiosensitive cells of the liver, kidney and thyroid. Least sensitive are fixed postmitotic cells that have lost the ability to divide, such as neurons.

radiosensitizers, drugs that enhance the killing effect of radiation on cells. If radiosensitizers can be selectively introduced into the cells of a tumour while being absent from the surrounding normal tissue, the effect of tumour irradiation will be increased.

radiotherapist, a medical practitioner further qualified in radiotherapy for the clinical detection of medical exposures for treatment purposes.

radiotherapy, the branch of medicine concerned with the use of ionizing radiations such as x-rays, gamma rays, electrons, neutrons and protons, for the treatment of disease, primarily malignancy. The volume to be irradiated is precisely defined so as to deliver maximum radiation dose to the target volume and minimal dose to surrounding normal tissues.

radioulnar articulation, the articulation of the radius and ulna, consisting of a proximal articulation, a distal articulation and three sets of ligaments.

radium (Ra), a radioactive metallic element of the alkaline earth group. Its atomic number is 88. Four radium isotopes occur naturally and have different atomic weights 223, 224, 226 and 228.

radium insertion, the introduction of metallic radium (Ra) into a body area, such as the uterus or cervix, for the treatment of cancer.

radius, *pl.* **radii,** one of the bones of the forearm, lying parallel to the ulna. Its proximal end is small and forms a part of the elbow joint. The distal end is large and forms a part of the wrist joint.

radix. See **root.**

radon (Rn), a radioactive, inert, gaseous, non-metallic element. Its atomic number is 86 and its atomic weight is 222.

radon daughters, electrically charged ions that are decay products of radon gas. Radon daughters are regarded as a potential health hazard because they tend to adhere to surfaces, such as alveoli of the lungs, where they can cause ionizing radiation damage. Radon is released by rocks, soil and groundwater.

radon seed, a small, sealed tube of glass or gold containing radon, and visible radiographically, for insertion into body tissues in the treatment of malignancies.

RAI, abbreviation for **radioactive iodine.**

RAIU, abbreviation for **radioactive iodine uptake.**

rale, a common abnormal respiratory sound heard on auscultation of the chest during inspiration, characterized by discontinuous bubbling noises. Fine rales have a crackling sound produced by air entering distal bronchioles or alveoli that contain serous secretions, as in congestive heart failure, pneumonia or early tuberculosis. Coarse rales originate in the larger bronchi or trachea and have a lower pitch. Kinds of rales are **sibilant rale** and **sonorous rale.** Compare **rhonchus, wheeze.**

Ramsay Hunt's syndrome {James Ramsay Hunt, American neurologist, b. 1874}, a neurological condition resulting from invasion of the seventh nerve ganglia and the geniculate ganglion by varicella zoster virus. It is characterized by severe ear pain, facial nerve paralysis, vertigo, hearing loss and often mild, generalized encephalitis.

ramus, *pl.* **rami,** a small, branch-like structure extending from a larger one or dividing into two or more parts, such as a branch of a nerve or artery, or one of the rami of the pubis.   **ramification,** *n.* **ramify,** *v.*

random genetic drift.   See **genetic drift.**

random selection,   a method of choosing subjects for a research study in which all members of a particular group have an equal chance of being selected.

random voided specimen,   a voided urine specimen obtained at any point during a 24-hour period.

range of motion exercise,   any body action involving the muscles, joints and natural directional movements, such as abduction, extension, flexion, pronation and rotation.

ranitidine,   a histamine H2 receptor antagonist used in the treatment of duodenal and gastric ulcers and gastric hypersecretory conditions.

Rankine scale {William J. M. Rankine, Scottish physicist, b. 1820}, an absolute temperature scale calculated in degrees Fahrenheit. Absolute zero on the Rankine scale is -460° F, equivalent to -273° C.

ranula, *pl.* **ranulae,**   a large mucocele in the floor of the mouth, usually caused by obstruction of the ducts of sublingual salivary glands and less commonly by obstruction of the ducts of submandibular salivary glands.

Ranvier's nodes,   constrictions in the medullary substance of a nerve fibre at more or less regular intervals.

rape,   a sexual assault, homosexual or heterosexual involving unlawful sexual intercourse. Rape is a crime of violence, or a crime committed under the threat of violence, and its victims are treated for medical and psychological trauma.

rape counselling,   counselling by a trained person provided to a victim of rape.

rape-trauma syndrome,   the forced, violent sexual penetration against the victim's will and consent. The trauma syndrome includes an acute phase of disorganization and a longer phase of reorganization in the victim's life. Defining characteristics are divided into three subcomponents: **rape trauma, compound reaction** and **silent reaction. Rape trauma** in the acute phase includes emotional reactions of anger, guilt and embarrassment, fear of physical violence and death, humiliation, wish for revenge and multiple physical complaints. The long-term phase includes changes in the usual patterns of daily life, nightmares and phobias, and a need for support from friends and family. The **compound reaction** includes all of the defining characteristics of rape trauma, reliance on alcohol or drugs, or the recurrence of symptoms of previous conditions. The **silent reaction** sometimes occurs in place of the rape trauma or compound reaction. Defining characteristics are an abrupt change in the victim's usual sexual relationships, an increase in nightmares, an increasing anxiety during the interview about the rape incident, a marked change in sexual behaviour, denial of the rape or refusal to discuss it, and the sudden development of phobic reactions.

raphe, a line of union of the halves of various symmetrical parts; for example, the abdominal raphe of the linea alba, or the raphe penis which appears as a narrow, dark streak on the inferior surface of the penis. Also spelt **rhaphe.**

rapid eye movement.   See **sleep.**

rapport,   a sense of mutuality and understanding; harmony, accord, confidence and respect, underlying a relationship between two persons. This is an essential bond between a therapist and patient in psychotherapy.

rapprochement,   (in psychology) the third subphase of the separation-individuation phase of Mahler's system of preoedipal development. This stage is characterized by the rediscovery of mother after the initial separation of the practising subphase.

raptus, 1. a state of intense emotional or mental excitement, often characterized by uncontrollable activity or behaviour resulting from an irresistible impulse; ecstasy; rapture. **2.** any sudden or violent seizure or attack.

raptus haemorrhagicus,   a sudden, massive haemorrhage.

raptus maniacus,   a sudden violent attack of mania.

raptus melancholicus,   an attack of extreme agitation or frenzy that occurs during the course of depression.

raptus nervorum,   a sudden, violent attack of nervousness that may be marked by cramps.

rare earth element,   a metallic element with an atomic number that ranges from 57 up to, and including, 71. These closely related substances are classified in three groups: cerium metals, terbium metals and yttrium metals.

rare earth screen,   See **intensifying screen.**

RAS,   abbreviation for **reticular activating system.**

rash, a skin eruption. Kinds of rashes·include **butterfly rash, nappy rash, drug rash** and **heat rash.**

Rashkind procedure {William J. Rashkind, American physician, b. 1922}, the enlargement of an opening in the cardiac septum between the right and left atria. It is performed to relieve congestive heart failure in newborns with certain congenital heart defects, by improving the oxygenation of the blood.

Rasmussen's aneurysm {Fritz W. Rasmussen, Danish physician, b. 1922}, a localized dilatation of a blood vessel in a tuberculous cavity that causes haemorrhage when it ruptures.

RAST. See **radioallergosorbent test.**

rat typhus. See **murine typhus.**

rat-bite fever, either of two distinct infections transmitted to humans by the bite of a rat or mouse, characterized by fever, headache, malaise, nausea, vomiting and rash. Rat-bite fever resulting from infection caused by *Streptobacillus moniliformis* is also known as **Haverhill fever;** infection caused by *Spirillum minus* is also called **sodoku.**

rate, a numeric ratio, often used in the compilation of data concerning the prevalence and incidence of events. The number of actual occurrences appears as the numerator, and the number of possible occurrences appears as the denominator. Standard rates are stated in conventional units of population, such as neonatal mortality per 1000 or maternal mortality per 100,000.

rate-pressure product, the heart rate multiplied by the systolic blood pressure. It is a clinical indicator of myocardial oxygen demand.

Rathke's pouch, a depression that forms in the roof of the mouth of an embryo around the fourth week of gestation. The walls of the diverticulum develop into the anterior lobe of the pituitary gland.

Rathke's pouch tumour. See **craniopharyngioma.**

ratio, the relationship of one quantity to one or more other quantities, expressed as a proportion of one to the others and written either as a fraction (8/3) or linearly (8:3).

ratio solution, the relationship of a solute to a solvent, expressed as a proportion, such as 1:100 or parts per thousand.

rational, 1. of, or pertaining to, a measure, method or procedure based on reason. **2.** of, or pertaining to, a therapeutic method based on an understanding of the cause and mechanisms of a specific disease and the potential effects of drugs or procedures used in treating the disorder. **3.** sane; capable of normal reasoning or behaviour.

rational emotive therapy (RET), a form of psychotherapy, originated by Albert Ellis. It emphasizes a reorganization of one's cognitive and emotional functions, a redefinition of one's problems, and a change in one's attitudes to develop more effective and suitable patterns of behaviour.

rational treatment. See **treatment.**

rationale, a system of reasoning or a statement of the reasons used in explaining data or phenomena.

rationalization, a process of constructing plausible reasons to explain and justify one's behaviour.

rattle, an abnormal sound heard by auscultation of the lungs in some forms of pulmonary disease. It consists of a coarse vibration caused by the movement of moisture and separation of the walls of small air passages during respiration.

rattlesnake, a poisonous pit viper with a series of loosely connected, horny segments at the end of the tail that make a noise like a rattle when shaken. Rattlesnakes have a haematoxin in their venom. See **snakebite.**

rauwolfia {Leonhard Rauwolf, 16th century German botanist}, the dried roots of *Rauwolfia serpentina*, formerly used as a source of extracts and alkaloids, such as reserpine, with hypotensive and tranquillizing activity.

rauwolfia alkaloid, any one of more than 20 alkaloids derived from the root of the climbing shrub *Rauwolfia serpentina*, indigenous to India and the surrounding area. It was formerly used as an antipsychotic agent and in the treatment of hypertension.

rauwolfia serpentina. See **Rauwolfia.**

raw data, (in magnetic resonance imaging) the information obtained by radio reception of the MR signal as stored by a computer. Specific computer manipulation of these data is required to construct an image from it.

ray, a beam of radiation, such as heat or light, moving away from a source.

Raynaud's phenomenon (Maurice Raynaud, French physician, b. 1834}, intermittent attacks of ischaemia of the body extremities, especially the fingers, toes, ears and nose, caused by exposure to cold or emotional stimuli. The attacks are characterized by severe blanching of the extremities, followed by cyanosis and then redness; they are usually accompanied by numbness, tingling, burning and often pain. The condition is called **Raynaud's disease** when there is a history of symptoms for at least 2 years with no progression of symptoms and no evidence of an underlying cause.

Raynaud's sign. See **acrocyanosis.**

Rb, symbol for **rubidium.**

RBC, abbreviation for **red blood cell.** See **erythrocyte.**

RBE, abbreviation for **relative biological effectiveness.**

RCM, abbreviation for **Royal College of Midwives.**

RCN, abbreviation for **Royal College of Nursing.**

RD, abbreviation for **registered dietician.**

RDS, abbreviation for **respiratory distress syndrome.** See **respiratory distress syndrome of the newborn.**

Re, symbol for **rhenium.**

reabsorption, the process of something being absorbed again, such as the removal of calcium from the bone back into the blood.

reacher, a pair of extended tongs that can be used by persons with upper extremity disabilities to grasp objects on shelves and similar areas beyond their usual range.

reaction, a response in opposition to a substance, treatment or other stimulus, such as an antigen-antibody reaction in immunology, a hypersensitivity reaction in allergy or an adverse reaction in pharmacology. **react,** *v.,* **reactive,** *adj.*

reaction formation, a defence mechanism in which a person avoids anxiety through overt behaviour and attitudes that are the opposite of repressed impulses and drives, serving to conceal those unacceptable feelings.

reactive decision, (in psychology) a decision made by an individual in response to the influence or goals of others.

reactive depression, an emotional disorder characterized by an acute feeling of despondency, sadness and depressive dysphoria, which varies in intensity and duration. See **situational depression.**

reactive schizophrenia, a form of schizophrenia caused by environmental factors rather than organic changes in the brain. The onset of disease is usually rapid; symptoms are of brief duration, and the affected individual appears well immediately before and after the schizophrenic episode.

reactor, 1. (in psychology) a family therapist who lets a family in therapy take the lead and then follows in that direction. **2.** (in radiology) a cubicle in which radioisotopes are artificially produced.

reading, (in molecular genetics) the linear process in which the genetic information contained in a nucleotide sequence is decoded, as in the translation of the messenger RNA directives for the sequence of amino acids in a polypeptide.

readthrough, (in molecular genetics) transcription of RNA beyond the normal termination sequence in the DNA template, caused by the occasional failure of RNA polymerase to respond to the end-point signal.

reagent, a chemical substance known to react in a specific way. A reagent is used to detect or synthesize another substance in a chemical reaction.

reagin, 1. an antibody associated with human atopy, such as asthma and hay fever. In antigen-antibody reactions it triggers the release of histamine and other mediators that cause atopic symptoms. **2.** a non-specific, non-treponemal antibody-like substance found in the serum of individuals with syphilis. **reaginic,** *adj.*

reagin-mediated disorder, a hypersensitivity reaction, such as hay fever or an allergic response to an insect sting, produced by reaginic antibodies (IgE immunoglobulins). It causes degranulation and the release of histamine, bradykinin, serotonin and other vasoactive amines. An initial sensitizing dose of the antigen induces the formation of specific IgE antibodies, and their attachment to mast cells and basophils results in hypersensitivity to a subsequent challenging dose of the antigen. Abundance of mast cells in the skin, nose and lungs makes those areas susceptible to IgE-mediated reactions.

reaginic antibody, an IgE immunoglobulin that is elevated in hypersensitive individuals.

real time, an application of computerized equipment that allows data to be processed with relation to ongoing external events, so that the operators can make immediate diagnostic or other decisions based on the current data output.

real-time scanning, the scanning or imaging of an entire object, or a cross-sectional slice of the object, at a single moment. To produce such a "snapshot" image, scanning data must be recorded quickly over a very short time rather than by accumulation over a longer period.

reality, that which is thought to exist.

reality orientation, techniques used to orientate individuals suffering from organic confusional states. Awareness of the temporal, environmental and personal dimensions is fostered through use of this technique.

reality principle, an awareness of the demands of the environment and the need for an adjustment of behaviour to meet those demands. It is expressed primarily by the renunciation of immediate gratification of instinctual pleasures to obtain long-term and future goals.

reality testing, a process of evaluating the physical and social aspects of one's environment so as to differentiate between external reality and any inner imaginative world, and to behave in a manner that exhibits an awareness of accepted norms and customs.

reality therapy, a form of psychotherapy in which the aims are to help define and assess basic values within the framework of a current situation, and to evaluate the person's present behaviour and future plans in relation to those values.

reamer, 1. a tool with a straight or spiral cutting edge, used in a rotating motion to enlarge a hole or clear an opening. **2.** (in dentistry) an instrument with a tapered and loosely spiralled metal shaft, used for enlarging and cleaning root canals.

reapproximate, to rejoin tissues separated by surgery or trauma so that their anatomical relationship is restored. **reapproximation,** *n.*

reasonable care, the degree of skill and knowledge used by a competent health practitioner in treating and caring for the sick and injured.

rebase, a process of refitting a denture by replacing its base material without changing the occlusal relationships of the teeth.

rebirthing, a form of psychotherapy that focuses on the breath and breathing apparatus. The goal of treatment is to overcome the trauma of the hypothesized birth-damaged breathing apparatus so that the person is able to use the breath as a supportive and creative part of life.

rebound, 1. recovery from illness. **2.** a sudden contraction of muscle after a period of relaxation, often seen in conditions in which inhibitory reflexes are lost.

rebound congestion, swelling and congestion of the nasal mucosa that follows the vasodilator effects of decongestant medications.

rebound tenderness, a sign of inflammation of the peritoneum in which pain is elicited by the sudden release of a hand pressing on the abdomen.

rebreathing, breathing into a closed system. Exhaled gas mixes with the gas in the closed system, and some of this mixture is then reinhaled. Rebreathing may result in progressively decreasing concentrations of oxygen and progressively increasing concentrations of carbon dioxide.

rebreathing bag, (in anaesthesia) a flexible bag attached to a mask. It may function as a reservoir for anaesthetic gases during surgery, or for oxygen during resuscitation. It may be squeezed to pump the gas or air into the lungs.

recalcification time, the time taken for a fibrin clot to appear after the addition of calcium to plasma, normally 90-125 seconds; it is increased in haemophilia and other clotting disorders.

recannulate, to make a new opening through an organ or tissue, such as opening a passage through an occluded blood vessel.

recapitulation theory, the theory, formulated by German naturalist Ernst Heinrich Haeckel, that an organism during the course of embryonic development passes through stages that resemble the structural form of several ancestral types of the species as it evolved from a lower to a higher form of life. It is summarized by the statement "Ontogeny recapitulates phylogeny".

receiver, (in communication theory) the person or persons to whom a message is sent.

reception deprivation, an inability to receive stimuli properly because of damage to tissue receptors, resulting in partial or total loss of sensation.

receptive aphasia, a form of speech disorder marked by impaired comprehension of language. This term has now been replaced by more precise descriptions of various communication disorders.

receptor, 1. a chemical structure on the surface of a cell that combines with an antigen to produce a discrete immunological component. **2.** a sensory nerve ending that responds to various kinds of stimulation. **3.** a specific cellular protein that must first bind a hormone before cellular response can be elicited.

receptor theory of drug action, the concept that certain drugs produce their effects by acting at some specific receptor site within the cell or on its membrane.

recess, a small, hollow cavity, such as the epitympanic recess in the tympanic cavity of the inner ear, or the retrocaecal recess extending as a small pocket behind the caecum.

recessive, of, pertaining to or describing a gene, the effect of which is masked or hidden if there is a dominant gene at the same locus.

recessive gene, the member of a pair of genes that lacks the ability to express itself in the presence of its more dominant allele; it is expressed only in the homozygous state.

recessive trait, a genetically determined characteristic expressed only when present in the homozygotic state.

reciprocal, a type of body movement that aids in communication, such as body language that indicates affiliation between people.

reciprocal gene. See **complementary gene.**

reciprocal inhibition, a theory in behaviour therapy, according to which, if an anxiety-producing stimulus occurs simultaneously with a response that diminishes anxiety, the stimulus may cause less anxiety; for example, deep chest or abdominal breathing and relaxation of the deep muscles appear to diminish anxiety and pain in childbirth.

reciprocal translocation, the mutual exchange of genetic material between two non-homologous chromosomes.

Recklinghausen's canal {Friedrich D. von Recklinghausen, German pathologist, b. 1833}, the small lymph space in the connective tissues of the body.

Recklinghausen's disease. See **neurofibromatosis.**

Recklinghausen's tumour {Friedrich Recklinghausen}, a benign tumour derived from smooth muscle containing connective tissue and epithelial elements. It occurs in the wall of the oviduct or posterior uterine wall.

reclining, leaning backwards. **recline,** *v.*

recombinant, 1. the cell or organism that results from recombination of genes within the DNA molecule, regardless of whether naturally or artificially induced. **2.** of, or pertaining to, such an organism or cell.

recombinant DNA, a DNA molecule in which rearrangement of the genes has been artificially induced. Enzymes are used to break isolated DNA molecules into fragments that are then rearranged in the desired sequence. Portions of DNA material from another organism of the same or a different species may also be introduced into the molecule.

recombination, 1. (in genetics) the formation of new combinations and arrangements of genes within the chromosome, as a result of independent assortment of unlinked genes, crossing over of linked genes, or intracistronic crossing over of nucleotides. See also **recombinant DNA. 2.** a method of measuring radiation by ionometric techniques in which it is necessary to collect the liberated charges to arrive at a value of total charge per unit mass of air. Recombination of ions will lower the value collected.

recon, (in molecular genetics) the smallest genetic unit that is capable of recombination, thought to be a triplet of nucleotides.

reconstitution, the continuous repair of tissue damage.

reconstruction time, (in computed tomography) the period between the end of a scan and the appearance of an image.

record, a written form of communication that permanently documents information relevant to the care of a patient.

recovery room (RR), an area adjoining the operating room to which patients are taken post-surgery, while still under anaesthesia, before being returned to their rooms. Vital signs and adequacy of ventilation are carefully observed as the patient recovers conciousness.

recreational therapy, a form of adjunctive psychotherapy in which games or other group activities are used as a means of modifying maladaptive behaviour, awakening social interests, or improving the ability to communicate in depressed, withdrawn people.

recrudescence, a return of symptoms of a disease during a period of recovery.

recrudescent hepatitis, a form of acute viral hepatitis marked by a relapse during the period of recovery.

recrudescent typhus. See **Brill-Zinsser disease.**

rectal anaesthesia general anaesthesia achieved by the insertion, injection or infusion of an anaesthetic agent into the rectum; this procedure is rarely performed, because of the unpredictability of absorption of the drug into the blood.

rectal cancer. See **colorectal cancer.**

rectal instillation of medication, the instillation of a medicated suppository, cream or gel into the rectum. Some conditions treated by this method are constipation, pruritus ani and haemorrhoids. Occasionally, a drug may be given in a medicated enema.

rectal reflex, the normal response (defaecation) to the presence of an accumulation of faeces in the rectum.

rectal tube, a flexible tube inserted into the rectum to assist in the relief of flatus.

rectifier, an electrical device that converts alternating current (AC) to direct current (DC).

rectitis. See **proctitis.**

rectocele, a protrusion of the rectum and posterior wall of the vagina into the vagina. The condition occurs where the muscles of the vagina and pelvic floor have been weakened by childbearing, old age or surgery.

rectosigmoid, a portion of anatomy that includes the lower portion of the sigmoid and upper portion of the rectum.

rectouterine excavation, rectouterine pouch. See **pouch of Douglas.**

rectovaginal ligament, one of the four main uterine support ligaments. It helps to hold the uterus in position by maintaining traction on the cervix.

rectum, *pl.* **rectums, recta,** the portion of the large intestine, about 12 cm long, continuous with the descending sigmoid colon, just proximal to the anal canal. It follows the sacrococcygeal curve, and ends in the anal canal. **rectal,** *adj.*

rectus abdominis, one of a pair of anterolateral muscles of the abdomen, extending the whole length of the ventral aspect of the abdomen. It functions to flex the vertebral column, tense the anterior abdominal wall, and assist in compressing the abdominal contents.

rectus femoris, a fusiform muscle of the anterior thigh, one of the four parts of the quadriceps femoris. It functions to flex the leg.

rectus muscle, a muscle of the body that has a relatively straight form. Some rectus muscles are **rectus abdominis, rectus capitis anterior** and **rectus capitis lateralis.**

recumbent, lying down or leaning backwards. See also **reclining. recumbency,** *n.*

recuperate, to recover one's health and strength.

recurrent bandage, a bandage that is wrapped several times around itself, usually applied to the head or an amputated stump.

recurrent fever. See **relapsing fever.**

recurvatum, backward thrust of the knee, caused by weakness of the quadriceps or a joint disorder.

red blindness. See **protanopia.**

red blood cell count, a count of the erythrocytes in a specimen of whole blood, commonly made with an electronic counting device. The normal concentrations of red blood cells in the whole blood of males are 4.6 to 6.2 million/mm^3; in females, the concentrations are 4.2 to 5.4 million/mm^3.

red blood cell. See **erythrocyte.**

red bug. See **chigger.**

red cell mass, the total volume of all the circulating red cells, normally 30ml/kg for males and 27ml/kg for females. It is increased in polycythaemia.

red cell indexes, a series of relationships that characterize the red cell population in terms of size, haemoglobin content and haemoglobin concentration. The indexes are useful in making differential diagnoses of several kinds of anaemia.

red cell. See **erythrocyte.**

red cell mass, the total volume of all circulating red cells, normally 30 ml/kg for males and 27 ml/kg for females. It is increased in polycythaemia.

red corpuscle. See **erythrocyte.**

Red Cross. See **British Red Cross, International Red Cross Society.**

red fever. See **dengue fever.**

red hepatization. See **hepatization.**

red infarct, a pathological change that occurs in brain tissue that has been rendered ischaemic by lack of blood. Diapedesis of red blood cells occurs into the parenchyma of the brain, producing only infiltration of erythrocytes.

red marrow, the red vascular substance that consists of connective tissue and blood vessels containing primitive blood cells, macrophages, megakaryocytes and fat cells. It is found in the cavities of many bones, including the flat and short bones, the bodies of vertebrae, sternum, ribs and the articulating ends of long bones.

red tide. See **shellfish poisoning.**

redon, the smallest unit of the DNA molecule capable of recombination; it may be as small as one deoxyribonucleotide pair.

redox, an abbreviation for **reduction-oxidation (reaction).**

reduce, 1. (in surgery) the restoration of a part to its original position after displacement, as in the reduction of a fractured bone by bringing ends or fragments back into alignment. 2. to decrease the amount, size, extent or number of something, as of body weight.

reduction, 1. also called **hydrogenation.** The addition of hydrogen to a substance. 2. the removal of oxygen from a substance. 3. the decrease in the valence of the electronegative part of a compound. 4. the addition of one or more electrons to a molecule or atom of a substance. 5. the correction of a fracture, hernia or luxation. 6. the reduction of data, as in converting interval data to an ordinal or nominal scale of measurement.

reduction diet, a diet that is low in calories, used for reduction of body weight. The diet must supply fewer calories than the individual expends each day, while supplying all the essential nutrients for maintaining health. A diet of this type may provide 1200 calories per day from the basic food groups.

reduction division. See **meiosis.**

reductionism, an approach that tries to explain a form of behaviour or an event in terms of a specific category of phenomena, such as biological, psychological or cultural, negating the possibility of an interrelation of causal phenomena.

Reed-Sternberg cell {Dorothy M. Reed, American pathologist, b. 1874; Karl Sternberg, Austrian pathologist, b. 1872}, one of a number of large, abnormal, multinucleated reticuloendothelial cells in the lymphatic system in Hodgkin's disease. The number and proportion of cells are the basis for the histopathological classification of Hodgkin's disease.

reefer, cigarette containing an illicit drug, usually cannabis. Reefers containing measured amounts of diamorphine are sometimes used in the treatment of injecting opiate addicts, to try and reduce their desire to inject.

reentry, (in cardiology) the reactivation of myocardial tissue for the second or subsequent time by the same impulse. Reentry is one of the most common arrhythmogenic mechanisms.

journal, a professional or literary journal in which articles or papers are selected for publication by a panel of referees who are experts in the field.

reference electrode, an electrode that has an established potential and is used as a reference against which other potentials may be measured.

reference group, a group with which a person identifies or wishes to belong.

reference nutrient intake (RNI), this applies to protein, vitamins and minerals. The value is set at 2 standard deviations above the mean (EAR), and is sufficient for 97% of people in a group.

referential idea. See **idea of reference.**

referential index deletions, a neurolinguistic programming term that pertains to the omission of the specific person being discussed.

referral, a process whereby a patient or the patient's family is introduced to further health resources following the initial contact with a member of the health care team.

referred pain, pain felt at a site different from that of an injured or diseased organ or part of the body. In disease of the gallbladder, pain may be felt in the right shoulder or scapular region.

referred sensation, a feeling or impression that occurs at a site other than at which the stimulus is initiated.

refined birth rate, the ratio of total births to the total female population, considered during a period of 1 year.

reflecting, a communication technique in which the listener picks up the feeling tone of the patient's message and repeats it back to the patient. It encourages the patient to continue with clarifying comments.

reflection, 1. (in cardiology) a form of reentry in which, after encountering delay in one fibre, an impulse enters a parallel fibre and returns retrogradely to its source. 2. (in ultrasonography) the re-entry of acoustic energy where there is a discontinuity in the characteristic acoustic impedance along the propagation path.

reflective layer, (in radiography) a thin layer of magnesium oxide or titanium oxide between the phosphor and the base of an intensifying screen. Its function is to intercept and redirect isotropically emitted light from the phosphor to the x-ray film.

reflective practice, the process by which individuals reflect on their actions and outcomes achieved and learn from these experiences to refine and develop practice.

reflex, 1. a backward or return flow of energy or image, as a reflection. **2.** a reflected action, particularly an involuntary action or movement.

reflex action, the involuntary functioning or movement of any organ or part of the body in response to a particular stimulus.

reflex apnoea, involuntary cessation of respiration caused by irritating, noxious vapours or gases.

reflex bladder. See **spastic bladder.**

reflex dyspepsia, an abnormal condition characterized by impaired digestion associated with disease of an organ not directly involved with digestion.

reflex hammer, a small hammer with a flexible handle, used to elicit a reflex.

reflex inhibiting pattern (RIP), a conscious set of neuromuscular actions directed towards inhibition of a natural reflex, as in suppressing a sneeze.

reflex sensation. See **referred sensation.**

reflexology, a system of treating certain disorders by massaging the soles of the feet, using principles similar to those of acupuncture.

reflux, an abnormal backward or return flow of a fluid. Kinds of reflux include **gastroesophageal reflux, hepatojugular reflux** and **vesicoureteral reflux.**

reflux oesophagitis, oesophageal irritation and inflammation that results from reflux of the stomach contents into the oesophagus.

refracting medium. See **medium.**

refraction, 1. the change of direction of energy as it passes from one medium to another of different density. **2.** an examination to determine and correct refractive errors of the eye. **3.** (in ultrasonography) the phenomenon of bending wave fronts as the acoustic energy propagates from the medium of one acoustic velocity to a second medium of differing acoustic velocity.

refractive error, a defect in the ability of the lens of the eye to focus an image accurately, as occurs in near-sightedness and far-sightedness.

refractive index, a numerical expression of the refractive power of a medium, as compared with that of air, which has a refractive index value of 1. It is related to the number, charge and mass of vibrating particles in the material through which light passes.

refractometer, an instrument for measuring the refractive index of a substance and used primarily for measuring the refractivity of solutions.

refractoriness, the property of excitable tissue that determines how closely together two action potentials can occur.

refractory, pertaining to a disorder that is resistant to treatment.

refractory period, the interval after excitation of a neuron or contraction of a muscle, during which repolarization of the cell membrane occurs.

reframing, changing the viewpoint in relation to which a situation is experienced, and placing it in a different frame that fits the "facts" of a concrete situation equally well, thereby changing its entire meaning.

Refsum's syndrome {Sigvald Refsum, Norwegian physician, b. 1907}, a rare, hereditary disorder of lipid metabolism in which phytanic acid cannot be broken down. The syndrome is characterized by ataxia, abnormalities of the bones and skin, peripheral neuropathy and retinitis pigmentosa.

regimen, a strictly regulated therapeutic programme, such as a diet or exercise schedule.

region of interest (ROI), (in positron emission tomography) an area that circumscribes a desired anatomical location. Image processing systems permit drawing of ROIs on images.

region of recombination, the first stage of amplitude of an electrical signal in a gas-filled radiation detector, when the voltage is very low. No electrons are attracted to the central electrode, and ion pairs produced in the chamber will recombine.

regional, of, or pertaining to, a geographic area; for example, a regional medical facility or a part of the body, such as regional anaesthesia.

regional anatomy, the study of structural relationships within the organs and parts of the body. Kinds of regional anatomy are **surface anatomy** and **cross-sectional anatomy.**

regional anaesthesia, anaesthesia of an area of the body by injecting a local anaesthetic to block a group of sensory nerve fibres. Kinds of regional anaesthesia include **brachial plexus anaesthesia, caudal anaesthesia, epidural anaesthesia, intercostal anaesthesia, paracervical block, pudendal block** and **spinal anaesthesia.**

regional control, the control of cancer in sites that represent the first stages of spread from the local origin.

regional enteritis. See **Crohn's disease.**

regional health services, a geographical region designated under the National Health Planning and Resources Department Act of 1974 covering such factors as population and health resources for the effective planning and development of health services to meet local needs.

regional hyperthermia, the elevation of

temperature over an extended volume of tissue.

register, (in computed tomography) a device in the central processing unit (CPU) that stores information for future use.

registered general nurse (RGN), the title given to a nurse who has undergone a course of study in the care of adults, and who has passed an examination qualifying him or her for entry to the register of Nurses. This qualification was replaced in 1992 by the generic Registered Nurse (RN), but existing RGNs are entitled to continue to use this abbreviation.

registered mental nurse (RMN), the title given to a nurse who has undergone a course of study in the care of people with mental health disorders, and who has passed an examination qualifying him or her for entry to the national professional register of nurses maintained in the Central Council for Nurses, Midwives and Health Visitors (in the UK). This qualification was replaced in 1992 by the generic Registered Nurse (RN), but existing RMNs are entitled to continue to use the abbreviation of their original qualification.

registered nurse (RN), a professional nurse who has undertaken a course of study at a Board approved college of nursing, and has passed assessments to demonstrate competency to the required national standard so as to qualify for the Register of Nurses. A registered nurse will have specialised in the care of adults, or children, or those with mental health problems or with learning disabilities. A registered nurse may use the initials RN after his or her signature.

registered nurse for the mentally handicapped (RNMH), the title given to a nurse who has undergone a course of study in the care of people with learning disabilities, and who has passed an examination qualifying him or her for entry to the national professional register of nurses maintained by the Central Council for Nurses, Midwives and Health Visitors (in the UK). This qualification was replaced in 1992 by the generic Registered Nurse (RN), but existing RNMHs are entitled to continue to use the abbreviation of their original qualification.

registered nursing home, an institution devoted to providing care for an individual over a prolonged period of time.

registered sick children's nurse (RSCN), the title given to a nurse who has undergone a course of study in the care of children, and who has passed an examination qualifying him or her for entry to the Register of Nurses. This qualification was replaced in 1992 by the generic Registered Nurse (R), but existing RSCNs are entitled to continue to use this abbreviation.

registrar, 1. a doctor who is training in a medical speciality. **2.** an administrative officer whose responsibility is to maintain the records of an institution.

registry, (in epidemiology) a listing service for incidence data pertaining to the occurrence of specific diseases or disorders, such as a tumour registry.

regression, 1. a retreat or backward movement in conditions, signs or symptoms. **2.** a return to an earlier, more primitive form of behaviour. **3.** a tendency in physical development to become more typical of the population than of the parents. **regress,** *v.*

regulative cleavage. See **indeterminate cleavage.**

regulative development, a type of embryonic development in which the fertilized ovum undergoes indeterminate cleavage, producing blastomeres that have similar developmental potencies and are each capable of giving rise to a single embryo. Determination of the particular organs and parts of the embryo occurs during later stages of development and is influenced by inductors and intercellular interactions.

regulator gene, (in molecular genetics) a genetic unit that regulates or suppresses the activity of one or more structural genes.

regulatory sequence, (in molecular genetics) a series of DNA nucleotides that regulate the expression of a gene.

regurgitation, 1. the return of swallowed food into the mouth. **2.** the backward flow of blood through a defective heart valve, named according to the affected valve, as in **aortic regurgitation.**

rehabilitation, the restoration of an individual or a part to normal or near-normal function after a disabling disease, injury, addiction or incarceration. **rehabilitate,** *v.*

rehabilitation centre, a facility that provides therapy and training for rehabilitation. The centre may offer occupational therapy, physical therapy, vocational training and special training, such as speech therapy.

Reid's base line {Robert W. Reid, Scottish anatomist, b. 1851}, the base line of the skull. It is a hypothetic line extending from the infraorbital point to the superior border of the external auditory meatus.

Reifenstein's syndrome {Edward C. Reifenstein, Jr., American physician, b. 1908}, male hypogonadism of unknown origin, marked by azoospermia, undescended testes, gynaecomastia, testosterone deficiency and elevated gonadotrophin titres.

reinforcement, (in psychology) a process in which a response is strengthened by an event which is important to the organism; for example, food, water, pain pleasure. **Positive reinforcement** is the presentation of an event as a consequence of an operant (behaviour), increasing the probability of the operant's recurrence. **Negative reinforcement** refers to a procedure whereby removal of an aversive stimulus follows the emission of a response and results in an increase in the rate of responding.

reinforcement-extinction, a process of socialization in which one learns to engage in certain behaviours (reinforcement) or avoid certain behaviours (extinction).

reinforcer, (in psychology) a consequence that increases the probability that a behaviour will recur.

Reiter's syndrome {Hans Reiter, German physician, b. 1862}, an arthritic disorder of adult males, believed to result from a myxovirus or *Mycoplasma* infection. The syndrome most often affects the ankles, feet and sacroiliac joints, and is usually associated with conjunctivitis and urethritis. Lesions that become superficial ulcers may form on the palms and soles. Arthritis usually persists after conjunctivitis and urethritis subside, but may become episodic.

reject analysis, (in radiology) the study of repeated radiographs to determine the cause for their being discarded.

rejection, 1. (in medicine) an immunological response to organisms or substances that the system recognizes as foreign, including grafts or transplants. **2.** (in psychiatry) the act of excluding or denying affection to another person.

rejunctive, (in psychology) a relationship in therapy characterized by moves towards trustworthy relatedness.

relapse, 1. to re-exhibit the symptoms of a disease from which a patient appears to have recovered. **2.** the recurrence of a disease after apparent recovery.

relapsing fever, any one of several acute infectious diseases, marked by recurrent febrile episodes, caused by various strains of the spirochaete *Borrelia*. The disease is transmitted by both lice and ticks, and is often seen during wars and famines. The first episode usually starts with a sudden high fever 40°C (104°F), accompanied by chills, headache, neuromuscular pains and nausea. A rash may appear over the trunk and extremities, and jaundice is common during the later stages. Each attack lasts 2 or 3 days and culminates in a crisis of high fever, profuse sweating and a rise in heart and respiratory rate. This is followed by an abrupt drop in temperature and a return to normal blood pressure. People typically relapse after 7 to 10 days of normal temperature, and eventually recover completely.

relapsing polychondritis, a rare disease of unknown cause, resulting in inflammation and destruction of cartilage with replacement by fibrous tissue. Autoimmunity may be involved in this condition. Most commonly the ears and noses of middle-aged people are affected, with episodes of tender swelling often accompanied by fever, arthralgia and episcleritis.

relation searching, (in nursing research) a study design used to discover and describe relationships between and among variables.

relationship therapy, a therapy based on a totality of patient-therapist relationship, encouraging the growth of self in the patient.

relative biological effectiveness (RBE), (in radiotherapy) a measure of the cell-killing ability of a particular radiation compared with a reference radiation. RBE represents the ratio of cells killed with the test radiation over that of 250 keV radiation.

relative centrifugal force (RCF), a method of comparing the force generated by various centrifuges, based on the speeds of rotation and distance from the centre of rotation.

relative growth, the comparison of various increases in the size of similar organisms, tissues or structures, at different time intervals.

relative humidity, the amount of moisture in the air, compared with the maximum the air could contain at the same temperature.

relative refractory period. See **refractory period.**

relative risk, an assessment of the degree or incidence of adverse effects that may be expected in the presence of a particular factor or event, compared with the expected adverse effects in the absence of the factor or event.

relative value unit, a comparable service measure used by hospitals to permit comparison of the amounts of resources required to perform various services within a single department or between departments.

relaxation, 1. reduction of tension, as when a muscle relaxes between contractions. **2.** lessening of pain. **3.** (in magnetic resonance imaging) the return of excited nuclei to their normal unexcited state by the release of energy.

relaxation oven, (in xeroradiography) a part of the xerographic plate conditioner system used to eliminate ghost images. The plate is heated in the oven so that any residual electrostatic charge on the surface will be removed.

relaxation response, a protective mechanism against stress. It brings about decreased heart rate, lower metabolism and decreased respiratory rate. It is the physiological opposite of the "fight or flight" or stress response.

relaxation therapy, a kind of treatment which teaches patients to perform breathing and relaxation exercises and concentrate on a pleasant situation when a noxious stimulus is applied.

relaxation time, (in radiotherapy) the characteristic time required by a sample of atoms, whose nuclei have first been aligned along a static magnetic field and then excited to a higher energy (MRI) state by a radiofrequency signal, to return to a lower energy equilibrium state.

release therapy, a type of paediatric psycho-therapy used to treat children with stress and anxiety related to a specific, recent event.

releasing hormone (RH), one of several peptides produced by the hypothalamus and secreted directly into the anterior pituitary via a connecting vein. Each of the releasing hormones stimulates the pituitary to secrete a specific hormone; thus, corticotrophic releasing hormone stimulates the pituitary to secrete adrenocorticotrophic hormone.

releasing stimulus, (in psychology) an action or behaviour by one individual that serves as a cue to trigger a response in others. An example is yawning by one person, which results in yawning by others in the group.

reliability, (in research) the extent to which a test measurement or a device produces the same results with different investigators, observers or administration of the test over time.

relief area, the portion of tissue surface under a prosthesis, on which pressures are reduced or eliminated.

relieving factor, an agent that alleviates a symptom.

religiosity, a psychiatric symptom characterized by the demonstration of excessive or affected piety.

reline, the resurfacing of the tissue side of a denture with new base material.

REM, abbreviation for **rapid eye movement.**

rem, abbreviation for **roentgen equivalent man.** A dose of ionizing radiation that produces in humans the same effect as one roentgen of x-radiation or gamma radiation.

REM rebound, the occurrence of greater than normal REM activity following cessation of a drug that suppresses REM time.

remasking, (in digital fluoroscopy) the production of one or more additional mask images, where the first is inadequate due to patient motion, noise or other factors.

remedial activity, purposeful activity forming part of a therapeutic programme designed to overcome functional deficits caused by illness or trauma.

reminiscence, the recollection of past personal experiences and significant events.

reminiscence therapy, individuals are encouraged to enter into reflective and expressive discussion, following the triggering of past events by the introduction of artefacts from those times. The reminiscence engaged in allows those involved to share previous experiences which can strengthen role identity and social interaction.

remission, the partial or complete disappearance of the clinical and subjective characteristics of a chronic or malignant disease. Remission may be spontaneous or the result of therapy.

remittent fever, diurnal variations of an elevated temperature. There are exacerbations and remissions, but temperature does not return to normal.

remnant radiation, the measurable radiation that passes through an object, capable of producing an image on radiographic film.

remote afterloading, a brachytherapy technique in which applicators are positioned in the patient and verified using dummy sources. They are subsequently connected to a radioactive source safe, from which sources may be driven remotely into the applicators. This technique allows the applicators to be optimally positioned while the medical team receive no radiation dose. See **manual afterloading.**

remotivation, the use of special techniques that stimulate patient motivation to learn and interact.

remotivation group, a treatment group organized with the purpose of stimulating the interest, awareness and communication of withdrawn and institutionalized mental patients.

removable lingual arch, an orthodontic arch wire designed to fit the lingual surface of teeth and aid orthodontic movement of the dentition involved.

removable orthodontic appliance, a device placed inside the mouth to correct or alleviate malocclusion. It is designed to be removed or replaced by the patient.

removable rigid dressing, a dressing similar to a cast, used to encase the stump of an amputated limb. It is usually applied to permit the fitting of a temporary prosthesis so that ambulation can begin soon after surgery.

renal, of, or pertaining to, the kidney.

renal adenocarcinoma. See **renal cell carcinoma.**

renal angiography, a radiographic technique for visualizing the renal artery and associated blood vessels, following introduction of a radiopaque contrast medium.

renal anuria, cessation of urine production, caused by intrinsic renal disease.

renal artery, one of a pair of large, visceral branches of the abdominal aorta that supply the kidneys, suprarenal glands and ureters.

renal biopsy, the removal of kidney tissue for microscopic examination. It is conducted to establish the diagnosis of a renal disorder and to aid in determining the stage of disease, appropriate therapy and prognosis. An open biopsy involves an incision, permits better visualization of the kidney and carries a lower risk of haemorrhage; a closed or percutaneous biopsy is performed by aspirating a specimen of tissue with a needle; it requires a shorter period of recovery, and is less likely to cause infection.

renal calculus, a concretion occurring in the kidney.

renal calyx, the first unit in the system of

ducts in the kidney, carrying urine from the renal pyramid of the cortex to the renal pelvis for excretion through the ureters. There are two divisions: The minor calyx, with several others, drains into a larger major calyx, which in turn joins other major calyces to form the renal pelvis.

renal cell carcinoma, a malignant neoplasm of the kidney, composed predominantly of large cells with clear cytoplasm that originate in tubular epithelium. The tumour may develop in any part of the kidney, becoming a large mass that may grow into the tributaries of the renal vein. Haematuria and pain are usually present.

renal colic, sharp, severe pain in the lower back over the kidney, radiating forward into the groin. Renal colic usually accompanies forcible dilatation of a ureter, followed by spasm as a stone is lodged or passed through it.

renal corpuscle. See **malpighian corpuscle.**

renal cortex, the soft, granular, outer layer of the kidney, containing approximately **1.** 25 million renal tubules which remove body wastes in the form of urine.

renal diet, a diet prescribed in chronic renal failure and designed to control the intake of protein, potassium, sodium, phosphorus and fluids, depending on individual conditions. Carbohydrates and fats are the principal sources of energy. Protein is limited, and the allowed amount is determined by the patient's condition.

renal dwarf, a dwarf whose retarded growth is caused by renal failure.

renal failure, inability of the kidneys to excrete waste, concentrate urine and conserve electrolytes. The condition may be acute or chronic. **Acute renal failure** is characterized by oliguria and rapid accumulation of nitrogenous wastes in the blood. It is caused by haemorrhage, trauma, burn, toxic injury to the kidney, acute pyelonephritis or glomerulonephritis, or lower urinary tract obstruction. **Chronic renal failure** may result from other diseases. The early signs include sluggishness, fatigue and mental dullness. Later, anuria, convulsions, GI bleeding, malnutrition and various neuropathies may occur. The skin may turn yellow-brown and become covered with uraemic frost. Congestive heart failure and hypertension are frequent complications, resulting from hypervolaemia.

renal hypertension, hypertension resulting from kidney disease, including chronic glomerulonephritis, chronic pyelonephritis, renal carcinoma and renal calculi. Analgesic abuse and certain drug reactions may also result in renal hypertension. Untreated renal hypertension is likely to lead to kidney damage and cardiovascular disease.

renal nanism, dwarfism associated with infantile renal osteodystrophy.

renal osteodystrophy, a condition resulting from chronic renal failure. It is characterized by uneven bone growth and demineralization.

renal papilla. See **papilla.**

renal rickets, a condition characterized by rachitic changes in the skeleton. It is caused by chronic nephritis.

renal scan, a radionuclide image of the kidneys, obtained with a gamma camera following intravenous administration of a radiopharmaceutical.

renal tubular acidosis (RTA), an abnormal condition associated with persistent dehydration, metabolic acidosis, hypokalaemia, hyperchloraemia and nephrocalcinosis. It is caused by the inability of the kidneys to conserve bicarbonate and acidify the urine adequately. Prolonged RTA can cause hypercalciuria and formation of kidney stones. Some common signs and symptoms of RTA, especially in children, may include anorexia, vomiting, constipation, retarded growth, polyuria, nephrocalcinosis and rickets. In children and adults, RTA can also cause urinary tract infections and pyelonephritis.

Rendu-Osler-Weber syndrome. See **Osler-Weber-Rendu syndrome.**

renin, a proteolytic enzyme produced by and stored in the juxtaglomerular apparatus that surrounds each arteriole as it enters a glomerulus. The enzyme affects blood pressure by catalysing the change of angiotensinogen to angiotensin. Compare **rennin.**

renin test. See **plasma renin activity.**

rennin, a milk-curdling enzyme that occurs in the gastric juices of infants. It is also present in the rennet produced in the stomach of calves and other ruminants. It is an endopeptidase that converts casein to paracasein.

renography, a radionuclide imaging technique for assessing kidney function, following intravenous administration of a radiopharmaceutical.

renovascular hypertension. See **portal hypertension.**

reovirus, any one of three ubiquitous, double-stranded RNA viruses found in the respiratory and alimentary tracts in healthy and ill individuals. Reoviruses have been implicated in some cases of upper respiratory tract disease and infantile gastroenteritis.

repetition compulsion, an unconscious need to revert to and repeat earlier situations, patterns of behaviour and acts, so as to experience previously felt emotions or relationships.

repetition maximum, the maximum weight or resistance against which muscles can be worked either through one lift, the 1 repetition maxium (1 RM), or 10 lifts, the 10 repetition maximum (10 RM).

replacement, substitution of a missing part or substance with a similar structure or substance, such as the replacement of an amputated limb with a prosthesis or replacement of lost blood with donor blood.

replication, 1. a process of duplicating, reproducing or copying; literally, a folding back of a part to form a duplicate. **2.** (in research) the exact repetition of an experiment performed to confirm the initial findings. **3.** (in genetics) the duplication of the polynucleotide strands of DNA or the synthesis of DNA. **replicate,** *v*.

replicator, (in genetics) the segment of the DNA molecule that initiates and controls replication of the polynucleotide strands.

replicon, (in genetics) a replication unit; the segment of the DNA molecule undergoing replication.

repolarization, (in cardiology) the process by which the cell is restored to its resting potential. It encompases the effective and relative refractory periods, and is measured by the QT interval.

report, (in nursing) the transfer of information from the nurses on one shift to the nurses on the following shift. Report is given systematically at the time of change of shift.

representative group, a group of individuals whose members represent the various sectors of a community.

repression, 1. the act of restraining, inhibiting, or suppressing. **2.** (in psychoanalysis) an unconscious defence mechanism whereby unacceptable thoughts, feelings, ideas, impulses or memories, especially those concerning some traumatic past event, are pushed from the consciousness because of their painful guilt association or disagreeable content and are submerged in the unconscious, where they remain dormant but operant and dynamic. **repress,** *v*, **repressive,** *adj*.

repressive-inspirational approach, a psychotherapeutic approach used in some groups to encourage focus on positive feelings and group strengths.

repressor, (in molecular genetics) a protein produced by the regulator gene. It binds to a sequence of nucleotides in the operator gene, which regulates the structural gene.

repressor gene. See **regulator gene.**

reproduction, 1. the process by which animals and plants give rise to offspring; procreation; the sum total of cellular and genetic phenomena involved in the transmission of organic life from one organism to successive generations similar to the parents, so that perpetuation and continuity of the species is maintained. Kinds of reproduction include **asexual reproduction, cytogenic reproduction, sexual reproduction, somatic reproduction** and **unisexual reproduction. 2.** the creation of a similar structure, situation or phenomenon; duplication;

replication. **3.** (in psychology) the recalling of a former idea, impression or something previously learned. **reproductive,** *adj*.

reproductive system, the male and female gonads, associated ducts and glands, and the external genitalia that function in the procreation of offspring. In women, these include the ovaries, uterine tubes, uterus, vagina, clitoris and vulva. In men, these include the testes, epididymis, vas deferens, seminal vesicles, ejaculatory duct, prostate and penis.

repulsion, 1. the act of repelling, disjoining. **2.** a force that separates two bodies or things. **3.** (in genetics) the situation in linked inheritance in which the alleles of two or more mutant genes are located on homologous chromosomes so that each chromosome of the pair carries one or more mutant and wild-type genes, which are located close enough to be inherited together.

required arch length, the sum of the mesiodistal widths of all natural teeth in a dental arch.

RES, abbreviation for **reticuloendothelial system.**

research, the diligent enquiry or examination of data, reports and observations in a search for facts or principles.

research instrument, a testing device for measuring a given phenomenon, such as a paper and pencil test, a questionnaire, an interview, or a set of guidelines for observation.

research measurement, an evaluation of the quantity or incidence of a given variable as obtained by using a research instrument.

resect, to remove tissue from the body by surgery.

resection, the cutting out of a significant portion of an organ or structure. Resection of an organ may be partial or complete. A kind of resection is a **wedge resection.**

reserpine, an antihypertensive used in the treatment of high blood pressure and certain neuropsychiatric disorders.

reserve, an alkaloid formerly used in the treatment of high blood pressure and certain neuropsychiatric disorders.

reserve cell carcinoma. See **oat cell carcinoma.**

reservoir, a chamber or receptacle for holding or storing a fluid.

reservoir bag, a component of an anaesthesia apparatus in which gas accumulates, forming a reserve supply of gas for use when the quantity of flow is inadequate.

reservoir host, a non-human host that serves as a means of sustaining an infectious organism as a potential source of human infection. Wild monkeys are reservoir hosts for the yellow fever virus.

reservoir of infection, a continuous source of infectious disease. People, animals and plants may be reservoirs of infection.

resident bacteria, bacteria living in a specific area of the body.

residential care centre, a centre that provides custodial care to people who, because of physical, mental or emotional disorders, are not able to live independently.

residual, pertaining to the portion of something that remains after an activity that removes the bulk of the substance.

residual cyst, an odontogenic cyst that develops or remains in the jaw after removal of a tooth.

residual dental caries, any decayed material left in a prepared tooth cavity.

residual ridge, the portion of dental ridge that remains after the alveolar process has disappeared following tooth extraction.

residual urine, urine that remains in the bladder after urination.

residual volume, the volume of gas in the lungs at the end of a maximum expiration.

residue schizophrenia, a form of schizophrenia in which there is a history of at least one psychotic schizophrenic episode. Objective signs of the illness persist, and are marked by social withdrawal, eccentric behaviour, illogical thinking and inappropriate emotional reactions.

resistance, **1.** an opposition to a force, such as the resistance offered by the constriction of peripheral vessels to the blood flow in the circulatory system. **2.** the frictional force that opposes the flow of an electrical charge, as measured in ohms. **3.** (in respiratory therapy) the process of acting against a force placed on it, pertaining to thoracic resistance, tissue resistance and airway resistance.

resistance form, the shape given to a prepared tooth cavity so as to impart strength and durability to the restoration and remaining tooth structure.

resistance to flow, (in respiratory therapy) the pressure differential required to produce a unit flow change.

resistance transfer factor. See **R factor.**

resistance vessels, the blood vessels, including small arteries, arterioles and metarterioles, that form the major portion of the total peripheral resistance to blood flow.

resistive magnet, a simple electromagnet in which electricity passing through coils of wire produces a magnetic field.

resocialization, the reintegration of a patient into family and community life after critical or long-term hospitalization.

resolution, **1.** the ability of an imaging process to distinguish adjacent structures in the object. **2.** the state of having made a firm determination or decision on a course of action. **3.** the ability of a chromatographic system to separate two adjacent peaks.

resolving power, the ability to separate closely migrating substances, as in electrophoresis.

resonance, **1.** an echo or other sound produced by percussion of an organ or cavity of the body during a physical examination. **2.** the process of energy absorption by an object that is tuned to absorb energy of a specific frequency. Other frequencies do not affect the object. An example is the effect of vibration of a tuning fork, causing other tuning forks of the same frequency to vibrate. **resonant,** *adj.*

resorcinated camphor, a mixture of camphor and resorcinol, used for the treatment of pediculosis and itching.

resorcinol, an antiseptic substance and keratolytic agent used in the treatment of acne, other dermatoses and anorectal disorders.

resorcinol test. See **Boas' test.**

resorption, **1.** the loss of substance or bone by physiological or pathological means. **2.** the cementoclastic and dentinoclastic action that may occur on a tooth root.

respiration, the process of molecular exchange of oxygen and carbon dioxide within the body's tissues, from the lungs to cellular oxidation processes. Some kinds of respiration are **Biot's respiration, Cheyne-Stokes respiration** and **Kussmaul's respiration.**

respirator, an apparatus used to modify air for inspiration, improve pulmonary ventilation, or to give artificial ventilation.

respiratory, of, or pertaining, to respiration.

respiratory acidosis, an abnormal condition characterized by increased arterial PCO_2, excess carbonic acid and increased plasma hydrogen ion concentration. It is caused by reduced alveolar ventilation or suppression of respiratory reflexes with narcotics, sedatives, hypnotics or anaesthetics. The hypoventilation associated with this condition inhibits the excretion of carbon dioxide, which consequently combines with water in the body to produce excessive carbonic acid and thus reduces blood pH. Some common signs and symptoms of respiratory acidosis are headache, dyspnoea, fine tremors, tachycardia, hypertension and vasodilatation. Ineffective treatment of acute respiratory acidosis can lead to coma and death.

respiratory alkalosis, an abnormal condition characterized by decreased PCO_2, decreased hydrogen ion concentration and increased blood pH. It is caused by pulmonary and non-pulmonary problems. Some pulmonary causes are acute asthma, pulmonary vascular disease and pneumonia. Non-pulmonary causes include aspirin toxicity, anxiety, fever, metabolic acidosis, inflammation of the central nervous system, gram-negative septicaemia and hepatic failure. Hyperventilation associated with respiratory alkalosis usually stems from extreme anxiety. Deep and rapid breathing at rates as high as 40 respirations per minute is a major sign of respiratory alkalosis. Other symptoms are light-headedness, dizziness, peripheral paraesthesia, spasms of the hands and feet, muscle weakness, tetany and cardiac arrhythmia. Confirming diagnosis is often based on PCO_2 levels below 35 mm Hg, but the measurement of blood pH is critical in differentiating between metabolic acidosis and respiratory alkalosis.

respiratory arrest, the cessation of breathing.

respiratory assessment, an evaluation of the condition and function of a person's respiratory system. Signs of confusion, anxiety, restlessness, flaring nostrils, cyanotic lips, gums, earlobes or nails, clubbing of extremities, fever, anorexia and a tendency to sit upright, are noted if present. The person's breathing is closely observed for evidence of slow, rapid, irregular, shallow or Cheyne-Stokes respiration, hyperventilation, a long expiratory phase or periods of apnoea, and for retractions in the suprasternal, supra-clavicular, substernal or intercostal areas during breathing. Percussion is performed to evaluate resonance, hyper-resonance, tympany and dull or flat sounds. Rales, rhonchi, wheezing, friction rubs, transmission of spoken words through the chest wall and decreased or absent breath sounds are detected by auscultation. Background information pertinent to the evaluation includes allergies, recent exposure to infection, immunizations, exposure to environmental irritants, previous respiratory disorders and operations, pre-existing chronic conditions, currently taken medications, smoking habits and family history.

respiratory bronchiole. See **bronchiole.**

respiratory burn, tissue damage to the respiratory system resulting from inhalation of a hot gas or burning particles, as may occur in a fire or explosion.

respiratory centre, a group of nerve cells in the pons and medulla of the brain that control the rhythm of breathing in response to changes in levels of oxygen and carbon dioxide in the blood and cerebrospinal fluid. Changes in the concentration of oxygen and carbon dioxide or hydrogen ion levels in the arterial circulation and cerebrospinal fluid activate central and peripheral chemoreceptors; these send impulses to the respiratory centre, increasing or decreasing the breathing rate.

respiratory component (αPCO_2), the acid component of an acid-base control system that is modified by the respiratory status.

respiratory cycle, an inspiration followed by an expiration.

respiratory distress syndrome of the newborn (RDS), an acute lung disease of the newborn, characterized by airless alveoli, inelastic lungs, more than 60 respirations a minute, nasal flaring, intercostal and subcostal retractions, grunting on expiration and peripheral oedema. It is caused by a deficiency of pulmonary surfactant, resulting in overdistended alveoli and, at times, hyaline membrane formation, alveolar haemorrhage, severe right-to-left shunting of blood, increased pulmonary resistance, decreased cardiac output and severe hypoxaemia.

respiratory exchange ratio (R), the ratio of net expiration of carbon dioxide to the concurrent net inspiration of oxygen, expressed by the formula VCO_2/VO_2.

respiratory failure, the inability of the cardiac and pulmonary systems to maintain an adequate exchange of oxygen and carbon dioxide in the lungs. Respiratory failure may be hypoxaemic or ventilatory. Hypoxaemic failure is characterized by hyperventilation and occurs in diseases that affect the alveoli or interstitial tissues of the lobes of lungs, such as alveolar oedema, emphysema, fungal infections, leukaemia, lobar pneumonia, lung carcinoma, various pneumoconioses, pulmonary eosinophilia, sarcoidosis or tuberculosis. Ventilatory failure, characterized by increased arterial tension of carbon dioxide, occurs in acute conditions in which retained pulmonary secretions cause increased airway resistance and decreased lung compliance, as in bronchitis and emphysema.

respiratory medicine, the branch of medicine that deals with the treatment, maintenance or improvement of the ventilatory function of the respiratory tract.

respiratory muscles, the muscles that produce volume changes of the thorax during breathing. The inspiratory muscles include the hemidiaphragms, external intercostals, scaleni, sternomastoids, trapezius, pectoralis major, pectoralis minor, subclavius, latissimus dorsi, serratus anterior and the muscles that extend the back. The expiratory muscles are the internal intercostals, abdominals and the muscles that flex the back.

respiratory quotient (RQ), the body's total exchange of oxygen for carbon dioxide, expressed as the ratio of the volume of carbon dioxide produced to the volume of oxygen consumed per unit of time.

respiratory rate, the normal rate of breathing at rest, about 14 inspirations per minute. The rate may be more rapid in fever, acute pulmonary infection, diffuse pulmonary fibrosis, gas gangrene, left ventricular failure, thyrotoxicosis, and in states of tension. Slower breathing rates may result from head injury, coma or narcotic overdose.

respiratory rhythm, a regular oscillating cycle of inspiration and expiration, controlled by neuronal impulses transmitted between the muscles of inspiration in the chest and respiratory centres in the brain.

respiratory syncytial virus (RSV, RS virus), a member of a subgroup of myxoviruses that in tissue culture causes formation of giant cells or syncytia. It is a common cause of epidemics of acute bronchiolitis, bronchopneumonia, the common cold in young children, and sporadic acute bronchitis and mild upper respiratory tract infections in adults. Symptoms of infection with this virus include fever, cough and severe malaise.

respiratory system. See **respiratory tract.**

respiratory tract, the complex of organs and structures that performs the pulmonary ventilation of the body as well as the exchange of oxygen and carbon dioxide between ambient air and blood circulating through the lungs. It also warms the air passing into the body and assists in the speech function by providing air for the larynx and vocal cords.

respiratory tract infection, any infectious disease of the upper or lower respiratory tract. Upper respiratory tract infections include the common cold, laryngitis, pharyngitis, rhinitis, sinusitis and tonsillitis. Lower respiratory tract infections include bronchitis, bronchiolitis, pneumonia and tracheitis.

respiratory zone, the terminal air units where gas exchange actually occurs, usually below the seventeenth division of bronchi.

respite care, 1. short-term health services to the dependent older adult, either at home or in an institutional setting. **2.** the provision of temporary care for a patient who requires specialized or intensive care or supervision that is normally provided by his or her family at home.

respite time, relief time from responsibilities for the care of a patient.

respondent conditioning. See **classical conditioning.**

responder, a tumour that shrinks in volume by at least 50% as a result of chemotherapy, radiation or other treatment.

response, (in psychology) an event that follows a stimulus. Patterns of responses may be studied in order to find associative and causal relationships.

response time, 1. the period between the input of information into a computer and the response or output. **2.** the period between the application of a stimulus and the response of a cell or cells.

rest, an extension from a prosthesis that affords vertical support for a dental restoration.

rest angle. See **occlusal rest angle.**

rest area, a surface prepared on a tooth or fixed restoration into which the rest fits, providing support for a removable partial denture.

rest joint position, the position of a joint where the joint surfaces are relatively incongruent and the support structures are relatively lax. The position is used extensively in passive mobilization procedures.

rest seat. See **rest area.**

resting cell, a cell that is not undergoing division. See **interphase.**

resting jaw relationship, (in dentistry) the postural relation of the mandible to the maxillae when the patient is resting comfortably in the upright position.

resting membrane potential, the transmembrane voltage that exists when the heart muscle is at rest.

resting metabolic expenditure (RME), the basal metabolic rate (BMR) with an additional allowance, usually 10% for the energy needed for eating, digestion, respiration and minimal physical activity. RME is preferred to BMR for the critically ill patient.

resting tremor. See **passive tremor.**

restitution, the spontaneous turning of the fetal head to the right or left after it has extended through the vulva.

restless legs syndrome, a benign condition of unknown origin, characterized by an irritating sensation of uneasiness, tiredness and itching deep within the muscles of the leg, especially the lower part of the limb, accompanied by twitching and sometimes pain. The only relief is walking or moving the legs.

restoration, any tooth filling, inlay, crown, partial or complete denture, or prosthesis that restores or replaces lost tooth structure, teeth or oral tissues.

restoration contour, the profile of the surfaces of teeth that have been restored.

restoration of cusps, a reduction and inclusion of tooth cusps within a tooth cavity preparation and their restoration to functional occlusion with an artificial dental material.

restraint, any one of numerous devices used in aiding the immobilization of patients, especially children in traction.

restriction endonuclease, (in molecular genetics) an enzyme that cleaves DNA at a specific site. Each of the many different endonucleases acts at a species-specific cleavage site.

restriction fragment, a fragment of viral or cellular nucleic acid produced by cleavage of the DNA molecule by specific endonucleases.

restriction fragment length polymorphism (RFLP), a marker for a DNA segment of a chromosome associated with a hereditary disease. RFLPs are used in the detection of sequence variations in human genomic DNA segments.

restrictive disease, a respiratory disorder characterized by restriction of expansion of the lungs or chest wall, resulting in diminished lung volumes and capacities.

resuscitation, the process of sustaining the vital functions of a person in respiratory or cardiac failure while reviving him or her, using techniques of artificial respiration and cardiac massage, correcting acid-base imbalance and treating the cause of failure. **resuscitate,** *v.*

resuscitator, an apparatus for pumping air into the lungs. It consists of a mask snugly applied over the mouth and nose, a reservoir for air and a manually or electrically powered pump.

RET, abbreviation for **rational emotive therapy.**

retained placenta, the retention of all or part of the placenta in the uterus after birth.

retainer, 1. the part of a dental prosthesis that connects an abutment tooth with the suspended portion of a bridge. **2.** an appliance for maintaining teeth and jaw positions gained by orthodontic procedures. **3.** the portion of a fixed prosthesis that attaches a pontic to the abutment teeth. **4.** any clasp, attachment or device for fixing or stabilizing a dental prosthesis.

retaining orthodontic appliance, an orthodontic device for holding the teeth in place, following orthodontic tooth movement, until the occlusion is stabilized.

retarded, (of physical, intellectual, social or emotional development) abnormally slow. **retard,** *v.*, **retardation,** *n.*

retarded dentition, the abnormal delay of eruption of deciduous or permanent teeth, resulting from malnutrition, malposition of the teeth, a hereditary factor or a metabolic imbalance, such as hypothyroidism.

retarded depression, the depressive phase of bipolar disorder.

retarded ejaculation, the inability of a male to ejaculate after having achieved an erection. This often accompanies the ageing process.

retch, a staining but ineffective attempt to vomit, hence there is no expulsion of stomach contents.

rete, a network, especially of arteries or veins. **retial,** *adj.*

rete peg. See epithelial peg.

retention, 1. a resistance to movement or displacement. **2.** the ability of the digestive system to hold food and fluid. **3.** the inability to urinate or defaecate. **4.** the ability of the mind to remember information acquired from reading, observation or other processes. **5.** the inherent property of a dental restoration to maintain its position without displacement under axial stress. **6.** a characteristic of proper tooth cavity preparation in which provision is made for preventing vertical displacement of the cavity filling. **7.** a period of treatment during which an individual wears an appliance to maintain teeth in positions to which they have been moved by orthodontic procedures. **retain,** *v.*

retention form, the provision made in a prepared tooth cavity to prevent displacement of the restoration.

retention groove, a depression formed by the opposing vertical constrictions in the preparation of a tooth, which improves the retention of a restoration.

retention of urine, an abnormal, involuntary accumulation of urine in the bladder as a result of a loss of muscle tone in the bladder, neurological dysfunction or damage to the bladder, obstruction of the urethra or administration of a narcotic analgesic.

retention pin, a frictional grip of a small metal projection that extends from a dental metal casting into the dentine of a tooth, to improve the retention of a tooth restoration.

retention time (ta), 1. (in chromatography) the amount of elapsed time, from injection of a sample into the chromatographic system to the recording of peak (band) maximum of the component in the chromatogram. **2.** the length of time that a compound is retained on a chromatography column.

reticular, (of a tissue or surface) having a net-like pattern or structure of veins.

reticular activating system (RAS), a functional system in the brain essential for wakefulness, attention, concentration and introspection. A network of nerve fibres in the thalamus, hypothalamus, brainstem and cerebral cortex contribute to the system.

reticular formation, a small, thick cluster of neurons, nestled within the brainstem, that controls breathing, heartbeat, blood pressure, level of consciousness and other vital functions of the body. The reticular formation constantly monitors the state of the body through connections with the sensory and motor tracts.

reticulin, an albuminoid substance found in the connective fibres of reticular tissue.

reticulocyte, an immature erythrocyte characterized by a mesh-like pattern of threads and particles at the former site of the nucleus.

reticulocyte count, a count of the number of reticulocytes in a whole blood specimen, used in determining bone marrow activity. The reticulocyte count is lowered in haemolytic diseases and elevated after haemorrhage or during recovery from anaemia.

reticulocytopenia, a decrease below the normal range of 0.5% to 1.5% in the number of reticulocytes in a blood sample.

reticulocytosis, an increase in the number of reticulocytes in the circulating blood.

reticuloendothelial cells, cells lining vascular and lymph vessels, capable of phagocytosing bacteria, viruses and colloidal particles, or forming immune bodies against foreign particles.

reticuloendothelial system (RES), a functional system of the body involved primarily in defence against infection and disposal of the products of breakdown of cells. It is made up of macrophages, Kupffer cells of the liver, and reticulum cells of the lungs, bone marrow, spleen and lymph nodes. Disorders of this system include **eosinophilic granuloma, Gaucher's disease, Hand-Schüller-Christian syndrome** and **Niemann-Pick disease.**

reticuloendotheliosis, an abnormal condition characterized by increased growth and proliferation of the cells of the reticuloendothelial system. See **reticuloendothelial system.**

reticulogranular, pertaining to a cloudy appearance of the lungs, on the chest radiograph of a patient with respiratory distress syndrome.

reticulosarcoma. See **undifferentiated malignant lymphoma.**

reticulum cell sarcoma. See **histiocytic malignant lymphoma.**

retina, a 10-layered, delicate nervous tissue membrane of the eye, continuous with the optic nerve. It receives images of external objects and transmits visual impulses through the optic nerve to the brain. The retina is soft, semitransparent, and contains rhodopsin which gives it a purple tint. The retina becomes clouded and opaque if exposed to direct sunlight. The outer surface of the retina is in contact with the choroid; the inner surface with the vitreous body.

retinaculum, pl. **retinacula, 1.** a structure that retains an organ or tissue. **2.** an instrument for retracting tissues during surgery.

retinaculum extensorum manus, the thick band of antebrachial fascia that wraps the tendons of extensor muscles of the forearm at the distal ends of the radius and ulna.

retinaculum flexorum manus, the thick, fibrous band of antebrachial fascia that wraps the carpal canal surrounding the tendons of flexor muscles of the forearm at the distal ends of the radius and ulna.

retinal, 1. an aldehyde precursor of vitamin A produced by the enzymatic dehydration of retinol. **2.** pertaining to the retina.

retinal detachment, a separation of the retina from the choroid in the back of the eye. It usually results from a hole in the retina that allows the vitreous humor to leak between the choroid and retina. Severe trauma to the eye, such as a contusion or penetrating wound, may be the proximate cause. However, in the great majority of cases retinal detachment is the result of internal changes in the vitreous chamber associated with ageing or, less frequently, inflammation of the interior of the eye. In most cases, retinal detachment develops slowly. The first symptom is often the sudden appearance of a large number of spots floating loosely and suspended in front of the affected eye. The person may also notice a curious sensation of flashing lights as the eye is moved. Because the retina does not contain sensory nerves that relay sensations of pain, the condition is painless. Detachment usually be-

gins at the thin peripheral edge of the retina and extends gradually beneath the thicker, more central areas. The person perceives a shadow that begins laterally and grows in size, slowly encroaching on central vision. If the process of detachment is not halted, total blindness of the eye ultimately results. The condition does not resolve spontaneously.

retinene, either of the two carotenoid pigments found in the rods of the retina; they are precursors of vitamin A and are activated by light. See also **retinal, retinol.**

retinoblastoma, pl. **retinoblastomas, retinoblastomata,** a congenital, hereditary neoplasm developing from retinal germ cells. Characteristic signs are diminished vision, strabismus, retinal detachment and an abnormal pupillary reflex. The rapidly growing tumour may invade the brain and metastasize to distant sites.

angiomatosis. See **cerebroretinal angiomatosis.**

retinodialysis, a separation or tear in the retina in its anterior part, in the area of the ora serrata, just behind the ciliary body.

retinol, the cis-trans form of vitamin A, found in the retinas of mammals. Also called **vitamin A1.**

retinopathy, a non-inflammatory eye disorder resulting from changes in the retinal blood vessels.

retraction, 1. the displacement of tissues to expose a part or structure of the body. **2.** a distal movement of the teeth. **3.** a distal or retrusive position of the teeth, dental arch or jaw.

retraction of the chest, the visible sinking-in of the soft tissues of the chest between and around the firmer tissue of the cartilaginous and bony ribs, as occurs with increased inspiratory effort.

retractor, an instrument for holding back the edges of tissues and organs to maintain exposure of the underlying anatomic parts, particularly during surgery, such as an army retractor or a double-ended Richardson retractor.

retroaortic node, a node in one of three sets of lumbar lymph nodes that serve various structures in the abdomen and pelvis.

retroclusion, a method of controlling haemorrhage from an artery by compressing it between tissues on either side. A needle is inserted through the tissues above the bleeding vessel, then turned around and down so that it also passes through the tissues beneath the artery.

retroflexion, an abnormal position of an organ in which the organ is tilted back acutely, folded over on itself.

retroflexion, a position of the uterus in which the body of the uterus is bent backwards on itself, at the isthmus of the cervix and the lower uterine segment.

retroflexion of the uterus, a condition in

which the body of the uterus is bent backwards at an angle with the cervix, the position of which remains unchanged.

retrognathism, a facial abnormality in which one or both jaws, usually the mandible, are posterior to their normal facial positions.

retrograde, 1. moving backwards; moving in the opposite direction to that which is considered normal. **2.** degenerating; reverting to an earlier state or worse condition. **3.** catabolic.

retrograde amnesia, the loss of memory for events occurring shortly before an event that precipitates amnesia.

retrograde cystography, a radiographic technique for visualizing the urinary bladder, following administration of a radiopaque contrast medium via a catheter into the bladder. **retrograde cystogram,** n.

retrograde cystoscopy. See **cystoscopy.**

retrograde infantilism. See **acromegalic eunuchoidism.**

retrograde infection, an infection that spreads along a tubule or duct against the flow of secretions or excretions, as in the urinary and lymphatic systems.

retrograde menstruation, a backflow of menstrual discharge through the uterine cavity and uterine tubes into the peritoneal cavity.

retrograde pyelography, a radiographic technique for visualizing the ureters and kidneys, following administration of a radiopaque contrast medium via a ureteric catheter.

retrograde root filling, a filling placed in the apical portion of a tooth root to seal the apical portion of the root canal.

retrograde urography. See **retrograde pyelography.**

retrograde Wenckebach, a progressively lengthening conduction of impulses from the ventricles or AV junction to the atria until an impulse fails to reach the atria.

retrogression, a return to a less complex state, condition or behavioural adaptation; degeneration; deterioration.

retrolental fibroplasia, a formation of fibrous tissue behind the lens of the eye, resulting in blindness. The disorder is caused by administration of excessive concentrations of oxygen to premature infants.

retromolar pad, a mass of soft tissue, usually pear-shaped, that marks the distal termination of the mandibular residual ridge.

retromylohyoid space, the part of the alveolingual sulcus that is distal to the distal end of the mylohyoid ridge.

retroperitoneal, of, or pertaining to, organs closely attached to the abdominal wall and partly covered by peritoneum, rather than suspended by that membrane.

retroperitoneal fibrosis, a chronic inflammatory process, usually of unknown cause, in which fibrous tissue surrounds the large blood vessels in the lower lumbar area. Symptoms include low-back and abdominal pain, weakness, weight loss, fever and, with urinary tract involvement, frequency of urination, haematuria, polyuria or anuria.

retroperitoneal lymph node dissection, surgical removal of lymph nodes behind the peritoneum. It is usually performed in an attempt to eliminate sites of lymphoma or metastases from malignancies originating in pelvic organs or genitalia.

retropharyngeal abscess, a collection of pus in the tissues behind the pharynx, accompanied by difficulty in swallowing, fever and pain. Occasionally, the airway becomes obstructed.

retroplacental, behind the placenta.

retrospective nursing audit. See **nursing audit.**

retrospective study, a study in which a search is made for a relationship between one (usually current) phenomenon or condition and another that occurred in the past.

retrouterine, behind the uterus.

retroversion, a common condition in which an organ is tipped backwards, usually without flexion or other distortion. Uterine retroversion is measured as first-, second- or third-degree, depending on the angle of tilt with respect to the vagina.

retroverted gravid uterus, a pregnant uterus that is tilted backwards. This usually reverts to anteflexion as the uterus grows. If it persists, incarceration of the retroverted gravid uterus occurs, causing retention of urine.

retrovirus, any of a family of RNA viruses containing reverse transcriptase in the virion. During replication, the viral DNA becomes integrated into the DNA of the host cell. Retroviruses are enveloped and assemble their capsids in the cytoplasm of the host cell. The HTLV-III/LAV, which causes AIDS, is a retrovirus.

retrusion. See **retroversion.**

revascularization, the restoration, by surgical means, of blood flow to an organ or tissue that is being replaced, as in bypass surgery.

reverberation, the phenomenon of multiple reflections within a closed system.

Reverdin's needle {Albert Reverdin, Swiss surgeon, b. 1881}, a surgical needle with an eye that can be opened and closed with a slide.

reversal film, (in radiography) a reverse-tone duplicate of an x-ray image, showing black changed to white and white to black. It is produced by exposing single-emulsion film through a standard x-ray film.

reverse anaphylaxis. See **inverse anaphylaxis.**

reverse Barton's fracture {John R. Barton, American surgeon, b. 1794}, a fracture of the volar articular surface of the radius with associated displacement of the carpal bones and radius.

reverse bevel. See **contra bevel.**

reverse curve, (in dentistry) a convex curve of occlusion, as viewed in the frontal plane.

reverse isolation, isolation procedures designed to protect a patient from infectious organisms that might be carried by staff, other patients or visitors, and on air droplets, equipment or materials. Handwashing, gowning, gloving, sterilization or disinfection of materials brought into the area, and other details of housekeeping, vary with the reason for isolation and the usual practices of the hospital.

reverse transcriptase (RT), an enzyme present in the virion of retroviruses. Reverse transcriptase occurs in leukoviruses and RNA tumour viruses of eukaryotic cells.

reverse Trendelenburg, a position in which the lower extremities are lower than the body and head.

reversed coarctation. See **Takayasu's arteritis.**

reversed phase, a chromatographic mode in which the mobile phase is more polar than the stationary phase.

reversible brain syndrome, any of a group of acute brain disorders characterized by a disruption of cognition. The disorder is related to a variety of biological stressors; recovery is possible.

review of systems (ROS), (in a health history) a system-by-system review of the body functions. The ROS is started during the initial interview with the patient and completed during physical examination, as physical findings prompt further questions.

Reye's syndrome {Ralph D. K. Reye, 20th century Australian pathologist}, a combination of acute encephalopathy and fatty infiltration of internal organs that may follow acute viral infections. This syndrome has been associated with influenza B, chickenpox (varicella), the enteroviruses and the Epstein-Barr virus. It usually affects people under 18 years of age, characteristically causing an exanthematous rash, vomiting and confusion about 1 week after the onset of a viral illness. In the late stage, there may be extreme disorientation followed by coma, seizures and respiratory arrest.

RF, abbreviation for **rheumatoid factor.**

Rf, symbol for a ratio used in paper chromatography and thin-layer chromatography. It represents the distance from the origin to the centre of the separated zone, divided by the distance from the origin to the solvent front.

rf, abbreviation for **radiofrequency.**

RF test. See **latex fixation test.**

Rh, symbol for **rhodium.**

Rh factor, an antigenic substance present in the erythrocytes of 85% of people. A person having the factor is Rh positive (Rh+); a person lacking the factor is Rh negative (Rh–). If an Rh– person receives Rh+ blood, haemolysis and anaemia occur. Rh+ infants may be exposed to antibodies to the factor produced in the Rh– mother's blood, resulting in red cell destruction and erythroblastosis fetalis. Transfusion, blood typing and cross-matching depend on Rh+ and ABO classification. The Rh factor was first isolated and identified in the blood of a species of the rhesus (Rh) monkey.

Rh incompatibility, (in haematology) a lack of compatibility between two groups of blood cells that are antigenically different, because of the presence of the Rh factor in one group and its absence in the other.

Rh negative. See **Rh factor.**

Rh positive. See **Rh factor.**

rhabdomyoma, *pl.* **rhabdomyomas, rhabdomyomata,** a tumour of striated muscle that may occur in the uterus, vagina, pharynx or tongue, or in the heart as congenital neoplastic nodules.

rhabdomyosarcoma, *pl.* **rhabdomyosarcomas, rhabdomyosarcomata,** a highly malignant tumour, derived from primitive striated muscle cells. It occurs most frequently in the head and neck, but is also found in the genitourinary tract, extremities, body wall and retroperitoneum. In some cases, the onset is associated with trauma. The initial symptoms depend on the site and indicate local tissue or organ destruction, such as dysphagia, vaginal bleeding, haematuria or obstruction of the flow of urine.

rhabdovirus, a member of a family of viruses that includes the organism causing rabies.

rhagades, cracks or fissures in skin that has lost its elasticity, especially common around the mouth.

rhaphe. See **raphe.**

rhenium (Re), a hard, brittle metallic element. Its atomic number is 75 and its atomic weight is 186.2. Rhenium has a high melting point and is used in thermometers for measuring high temperatures.

Rhesus factor. See **Rh factor.**

rheumatic, of, or pertaining to, rheumatism.

rheumatic aortitis, an inflammatory condition of the aorta, occurring in rheumatic fever and characterized by disseminated focal lesions that may progressively form patches of fibrosis.

rheumatic arteritis, a complication of rheumatic fever characterized by generalized inflammation of arteries and arterioles. Fibrin, mixed with cellular debris, may invade, thicken and stiffen the vessel wall; the vessel may be surrounded by haemorrhage and exudate.

rheumatic chorea. See **Sydenham's chorea.**

rheumatic fever, an inflammatory disease that may develop as a delayed reaction to inadequately treated Group A beta-haemolytic streptococcal infection of the upper respiratory tract. Its onset is usually sudden, often occurring between 1 to 5 symptom-free weeks following recovery from a sore throat or scarlet fever. Early symptoms usually include fever, joint pains, nose bleeds, abdominal pain and vomiting. The major manifestations of this disease include migratory polyarthritis affecting numerous joints, and carditis which causes palpitations, chest pain and, in severe cases, symptoms of cardiac failure. Sydenham's chorea, which may develop, is usually the sole, late sign of rheumatic fever; it may manifest initially as an increased awkwardness and an associated tendency to drop objects. As the chorea progresses, irregular body movements may become extensive, occasionally involving the tongue and facial muscles, resulting in incapacitation of the affected individual.

rheumatic heart disease, damage to heart muscle and heart valves caused by episodes of rheumatic fever. When a susceptible person acquires a group A beta-haemolytic streptococcal infection, an autoimmune reaction may occur in heart tissue, resulting in permanent deformities of heart valves or chordae tendineae. Involvement of the heart may be evident during acute rheumatic fever, or may be discovered long after the acute disease has subsided. Rheumatic heart disease is characterized by heart murmurs resulting from stenosis or insufficiency of the valves, and compensatory alterations in the size of heart chambers and the thickness of their walls. Abnormalities of pulse rate and rhythm, heart block and congestive heart failure are also common. Death is usually the result of heart failure or bacterial endocarditis.

rheumatism *non-technical*, **1.** any of a large number of inflammatory conditions of the bursae, joints, ligaments or muscles, characterized by pain, limitation of movement and structural degeneration of single or multiple parts of the musculoskeletal system. **2.** the syndrome of pain, limitation of movement and structural degeneration of elements in the musculoskeletal system, as may occur in gout, rheumatoid arthritis, systemic lupus erythematosus, ankylosing spondylitis and other diseases. **rheumatic, rheumatoid,** *adj.*

rheumatoid arthritis, a chronic, destructive, sometimes deforming collagen disease that has an autoimmune component. Rheumatoid arthritis is characterized by symmetrical inflammation of the synovium and increased synovial exudate, leading to synovial thickening and swelling of the joint. The course of the disease is variable but is most frequently marked by remissions and exacerbations. **Still's disease** is a kind of rheumatoid arthritis that affects children and young people.

rheumatoid coronary arteritis, an abnormal condition characterized by a thickening of the tunica intima of the coronary arteries, which may produce coronary insufficiency. Rheumatoid coronary arteritis is a collagen disease that affects the connective tissue by inflammation and fibrinoid degeneration.

rheumatoid factor (RF), antiglobulin antibodies often found in the serum of patients with a clinical diagnosis of rheumatoid arthritis. RF may also be found in widely divergent diseases such as tuberculosis, parasitic infections, leukaemia and connective tissue disorders.

rheumatologist, a specialist in rheumatology.

rheumatology, the study of disorders characterized by inflammation, degeneration or metabolic derangement of connective tissue and related structures of the body.

rhinencephalon, *pl.* **rhinencephala,** a portion of each cerebral hemisphere that contains the limbic system, which is associated with the emotions. **rhinencephalic,** *adj.*

rhinitis, inflammation of the mucous membranes of the nose, usually accompanied by mucosal swelling and a nasal discharge. Rhinitis may be acute, allergic, atrophic or vasomotor.

rhinopathy, any disease or malformation of the nose.

rhinophycomycosis, an infection of the nasal and paranasal sinuses caused by the phycomycete *Entomophthora coronata*. The infection often spreads to surrounding tissues, including the eye and brain.

rhinophyma, a form of rosacea in which there is sebaceous hyperplasia, redness, prominent vascularity, swelling and distortion of the skin of the nose.

rhinoplasty, a procedure in plastic surgery in which the structure of the nose is changed. Bone or cartilage may be removed, tissue grafted from another part of the body, or synthetic material implanted to alter the shape. The procedure is most frequently performed for cosmetic reasons.

rhinorrhoea, 1. the free discharge of a thin nasal mucus. **2.** the flow of cerebrospinal fluid from the nose after a head injury.

rhinoscope, an instrument for examining the nasal passages, through the anterior nares or the nasopharynx.

rhinoscopy, an examination of the nasal passages to inspect the mucosa and detect inflammation, deformities or asymmetry, as in deviation of the septum. The nasal passages may be examined anteriorly, by introducing a speculum into the anterior nares, or posteriorly, by introducing a rhinoscope through the nasopharynx. **rhinoscopic,** *adj.*

rhinosporidiosis, an infection caused by the fungus *Rhinosporidium seeberi*, characterized by fleshy red polyps on mucous membranes of the nose, conjunctiva, nasopharynx and soft palate. The disease may be acquired by swimming or bathing in infected water.

rhinotomy, a surgical procedure in which an incision is made along one side of the nose. It is performed to drain accumulated pus from an abscess or a sinus infection.

rhinovirus, any of about 100 serologically distinct, small RNA viruses that cause about 40% of acute respiratory illnesses. Infection is characterized by dry, scratchy throat, nasal congestion, malaise and headache. Fever is minimal. Nasal discharge lasts 2 or 3 days, and there is usually complete recovery.

rhizomelic, pertaining to the hip and shoulder joints.

rhizotomy, the surgical resection of the dorsal root of a spinal nerve, performed to relieve pain.

Rho immunoglobulin. See **anti-D (Rho) immunoglobulin.**

rhodium (Rh), a greyish-white metallic element. Its atomic number is 45 and its atomic weight is 102.91.

rhodopsin, the purple pigmented compound in the rods of the retina. It is formed by a protein, opsin, and a derivative of vitamin A, retinal. Rhodopsin gives the outer segments of the rods a purple colour and adapts the eye to low-density light. The compound breaks down when struck by light, and this chemical change triggers the conduction of nerve impulses.

rhomboid glossitis. See **median rhomboid glossitis.**

rhomboideus major, a muscle of the upper back, below and parallel to the rhomboideus minor. It functions to draw the scapula towards the vertebral column while supporting it and drawing it slightly upwards.

rhomboideus minor, a muscle of the upper back, above and parallel to the rhomboideus major. It acts to draw the scapula towards the vertebral column while supporting the scapula and drawing it slightly upwards.

rhonchi, *sing.* **rhonchus,** abnormal sounds heard on auscultation of a respiratory airway obstructed by thick secretions, muscular spasm, neoplasm or external pressure. Sibilant rhonchi are high-pitched and are heard in the small bronchi, as in asthma. Sonorous rhonchi are low-pitched and are heard in the large bronchi, as in tracheobronchitis. Dry rales are called rhonchi.

rhotacism, a speech disorder characterized by a defective pronunciation of words containing the sound /r/, the excessive use of the sound /r/, or the substitution of another sound for /r/. Compare **lallation, lambdacism.**

rhus dermatitis, a skin rash resulting from contact with a plant of the genus *Rhus*, such as poison ivy. See also **contact dermatitis.**

rhythm, the relationship of one impulse to neighbouring impulses, as measured in time, movement or regularity of action.

rhythm method. See **natural family planning method.**

rhytidoplasty, a procedure in reconstructive plastic surgery, in which the skin of the face is tightened, wrinkles are removed and the skin is made to appear firm and smooth.

rhytidosis, wrinkling, especially of the cornea. Also spelt rhitidosis.

Ri, symbol for inhibitory receptor molecule.

RIA. See **radioimmunoassay.**

rib, one of the 12 pairs of elastic arches of bone, forming a large part of the thoracic skeleton. The first seven ribs on each side are called true ribs because they articulate directly with the sternum and vertebrae. The remaining five ribs are called false ribs; the first three attaching ventrally to ribs above; the last two ribs are free at their ventral extremities and are called **floating ribs.**

rib fracture, a break in a bone of the thoracic skeleton, caused by a blow, a crushing injury or violent coughing or sneezing. The ribs most commonly broken are the fourth to eighth; if the bone is splintered or the fracture displaced, sharp fragments may pierce the lung, causing haemothorax or pneumothorax. The patient with a fractured rib suffers pain, especially on inspiration, and usually breathes rapidly and shallowly. The site of the break is generally very tender to the touch, and the crackling of bone fragments rubbing together may be heard on auscultation. Breath sounds may be absent, decreased or accompanied by rales and rhonchi.

rib shaking, a procedure in physiotherapy, involving constant downward pressure with an intermittent shaking motion of the hands on the rib cage over the area being drained. It is performed with the flat part of the palm of the hand over the lung segment being drained.

rib vibration, a procedure in physiotherapy similar to rib shaking, but performed with a downward vibrating pressure with the flat part of the palm during exhalations.

ribavirin, See **tribavirin.**

riboflavin, a yellow crystalline, water-soluble pigment, one of the heat-stable components of the B vitamin complex. It combines with specific flavoproteins, and functions as a coenzyme in the oxidative processes of carbohydrates, fats and proteins. Deficiency of riboflavin produces cheilosis; local inflammation; desquamation; encrustation; glossitis; photophobia; corneal opacities; proliferation of corneal vessels; seborrhoeic dermatitis around the nose, mouth, forehead, ears and scrotum; trembling; sluggishness; dizziness; oedema; inability to urinate; and vaginal itching. There is no known toxicity of riboflavin.

ribonucleic acid (RNA), a nucleic acid, found in both the nucleus and cytoplasm of cells. It transmits genetic instructions from the nucleus to the cytoplasm. In the cytoplasm, RNA functions in the assembly of proteins.

ribose, a 5-carbon pentose sugar that occurs as a component of ribonucleic acid.

ribosome, a cytoplasmic organelle composed of ribonucleic acid and protein that functions in the synthesis of protein. Ribosomes interact with messenger RNA and transfer RNA to join together amino acid units into a polypeptide chain according to the sequence determined by the genetic code.

Richet's aneurysm. See **fusiform aneurysm.**

rickets, a condition caused by the deficiency of vitamin D, calcium and usually phosphorus. It is seen primarily in infancy and childhood, and is characterized by abnormal bone formation. Symptoms include soft, pliable bones causing deformities such as bowlegs and knock-knees, nodular enlargements on the ends and sides of the bones, muscle pain, enlarged skull, chest deformities, spinal curvature, enlargement of the liver and spleen, profuse sweating and general tenderness of the body when touched. Kinds of rickets include **adult rickets, coeliac rickets, renal rickets** and **vitamin D-resistant rickets.**

rickettsia, pl. **rickettsiae** {Howard T. Ricketts, American pathologist, b. 1871}, any organism of the genus *Rickettsia*. Rickettsiae are small, round or rod-shaped specialized bacteria that live as virus-like intracellular parasites in lice, fleas, ticks and mites. They are transmitted to humans by bites of these insects. The various species are distinguished on the basis of similarities in the diseases they cause: the spotted fever group includes Rocky Mountain spotted fever, rickettsialpox and others; the typhus group includes epidemic typhus, scrub typhus and murine typhus; and a miscellaneous group includes Q fever and trench fever. **rickettsial,** adj.

rickettsialpox {Howard T. Ricketts}, a mild, acute infectious disease caused by *Rickettsia akari* and transmitted from mice to humans through mites. It is characterized by an asymptomatic, crusted primary lesion, chills, fever, headache, malaise, myalgia and a rash resembling chickenpox. Approximately 1 week after the onset of symptoms, small, discrete, maculopapular lesions appear on any part of the body.

rickettsiosis, pl. **rickettsioses** {Howard T. Ricketts}, any of a group of infectious diseases caused by micro-organisms of the genus *Rickettsia*. Kinds of rickettsioses include a spotted fever group (**boutonneuse fever, rickettsialpox, Rocky Mountain**

spotted fever), a typhus group (**epidemic typhus, murine typhus, scrub typhus**) and a miscellaneous group (**Q fever, trench fever**).

rider's bone, a bony deposit that sometimes develops in horseback riders on the inner side of the lower end of the tendon of the adductor muscle of the thigh.

ridge, a projection or projecting structure, such as the gastrocnemial ridge on the posterior surface of the femur, giving attachment to the gastrocnemius muscle.

Riedel's struma, Riedel's thyroiditis. See **fibrous thyroiditis.**

Rieder's cell leukaemia {Hermann Rieder, German physician, b. 1858}, a malignant neoplasm of blood-forming tissues, characterized by the presence in blood of large numbers of atypical myeloblasts with immature cytoplasm and relatively mature, lobulated, indented nuclei.

rifampicin, an antibacterial used in the treatment of tuberculosis, in meningococcal prophylaxis and as an antileprotic.

Rift Valley fever, an arbovirus infection of Egypt and east Africa, spread by mosquitoes or by handling infected sheep and cattle. It is characterized by abrupt fever, chills, headache and generalized aches, followed by epigastric pain, anorexia, loss of the sense of taste and photophobia.

RIG, abbreviation for **rabies immune globulin.**

Riga-Fede disease {Antonio Riga, Italian physician, b. 1832; Francesco Fede, Italian pediatrician, b. 1832}, an ulceration of the lingual frenum in some infants, caused by abrasion of the frenum by natal or neonatal teeth.

right atrial catheter, an indwelling intravenous catheter, inserted centrally or peripherally and threaded into the superior vena cava and right atrium.

right atrioventricular valve. See **tricuspid valve.**

right brachiocephalic vein, a vessel, about 2.5 cm long, starting in the root of the neck at the junction of the internal jugular and subclavian veins on the right side, and descending vertically from behind the sternal end of the clavicle to join the left brachiocephalic vein and form the superior vena cava.

right bundle branch block, an abnormal cardiac condition characterized by an impaired electrical signal associated with the bundle of fibres that transmit impulses from the bundle of His to the right ventricle. A right bundle branch block is often associated with right ventricular hypertrophy, especially in persons under 40 years of age. In older individuals, a right bundle branch block is commonly caused by coronary artery disease.

right common carotid artery, the shorter of

the two common carotid arteries, springing from the brachiocephalic trunk, passing obliquely from the level of the sternoclavicular articulation to the cranial border of the thyroid cartilage, and dividing into the right carotid arteries.

right coronary artery, one of a pair of branches of the ascending aorta, arising in the right posterior aortic sinus. It passes along the right side of the coronary sulcus, divides into the right interventricular artery and a large marginal branch, and supplies both ventricles, the right atrium and sinoatrial node.

right coronary vein. See **small cardiac vein.**

right hepatic duct, the duct that drains bile from the right lobe of the liver into the common bile duct.

right interventricular artery. See **dorsal interventricular artery.**

right lymphatic duct, a vessel that conveys lymph from the right upper quadrant of the body into the blood-stream in the neck, at the junction of the right internal jugular and the right subclavian veins.

right pulmonary artery, the longer and slightly larger of the two arteries conveying venous blood from the heart to the lungs, rising from the pulmonary trunk, bending to the right behind the aorta and dividing into two branches at the root of the right lung.

right subclavian artery, a large artery that arises from the brachiocephalic artery. It has several important branches: the axillary, vertebral thoracic and internal thoracic arteries, and the cervical and costocervical trunks, perfusing the right side of the upper body.

right ventricle, the relatively thin-walled chamber of the heart that pumps blood received from the right atrium into the pulmonary arteries to the lungs for oxygenation. The right ventricle is shorter and rounder than the long, conical, left ventricle. See **heart.**

right-hand rule, a principle of physics, according to which the direction of current flow in a wire is related to the position of the imaginary lines of force of the magnetic field around the wire.

right-handedness, a natural tendency to favour the use of the right hand.

right-heart failure, an abnormal cardiac condition characterized by impairment of the right side of the heart, as well as congestion and elevated pressure in the systemic veins and capillaries. Right-heart failure is usually related to left-heart failure, because both sides of the heart are part of a circuit and whatever affects one side will eventually affect the other. Compare **left-heart failure.**

right-sided failure. See **right-heart failure.**

righting reflex, any reflex that tends to return an animal to its normal body position in space when it has been moved from the normal position, and adjusts head-to-body position or vice versa. The head and trunk are thus kept in alignment.

rigidity, a condition of hardness, stiffness or inflexibility. **rigid,** *adj.*

rigidus, a deformity characterized by limited motion, especially dorsiflexion of the great toe.

rigor, 1. a rigid condition of the tissues of the body, as in rigor mortis. **2.** a violent attack of shivering that may be associated with chills and fever.

rigor mortis, the rigid stiffening of skeletal and cardiac muscle shortly after death.

rima glottidis. See **glottis.**

ring chromosome, a circular chromosome formed by the fusion of the two ends. It is the primary type of chromosome found in bacteria.

ring pad, a pad designed to protect an injured joint. It is cut to fit over the site of injury and cause force on the body part to be transferred to the surrounding area.

Ringer's lactate solution, a fluid and electrolyte replenisher. It is used for correction of fluid and electrolyte depletion.

ringworm. See **tinea.**

Rinne tuning fork test {Heinrich A. Rinne, German otologist, b. 1819}, a method of assessing auditory acuity. It is useful in distinguishing conductive from sensorineural hearing loss. The test is performed with tuning forks of 256, 512 and 1024 cycles; while each ear is tested, the other is masked. The stem of a vibrating fork is alternately placed 0.5 inches from the external auditory meatus of the ear and on the adjacent mastoid bone, until the sound is no longer heard at each of these positions.

Rio Grande fever. See **abortus fever.**

RIP, abbreviation for **reflex inhibiting pattern.**

risk factor, a factor that causes a person or a group of people to be particularly vulnerable to an unwanted, unpleasant or unhealthy event; for example, immunosuppression, which increases the incidence and severity of infection.

risk management, a function of a hospital administration or other health care centre, directed towards the identification, evaluation and correction of potential risks that could lead to injury to patients, staff members or visitors, and in property loss or damage.

risorius, one of the 12 muscles of the mouth. It arises in the fascia over the masseter and inserts into the skin at the corner of the mouth. It acts to retract the angle of the mouth, as in a smile.

Risser cast {Joseph C. Risser, American surgeon, b. 1892}, an orthopaedic device for encasing the entire trunk of the body, extending over the cervical area to the chin. In rare cases, it extends over the hips to the knees.

risus sardonicus, a wry, mask-like grin caused by spasm of the facial muscles, as seen in tetanus.

ritodrine hydrochloride, a beta-sympathomimetic agent used to stop the uterus from contracting in premature labour, and during fetal asphyxia due to hypertonic uterine contractions.

Ritter's disease {Gottfried Ritter von Rittershain, Czechoslovakian paediatrician, b. 1820}, a rare, staphylococcal infection of newborns. It begins with red spots around the mouth and chin, gradually spreading over the entire body and followed by generalized exfoliation. Vesicles and yellow crusts may also be present. Ritter's disease is usually fatal unless treated with antibiotics.

river blindness. See onchocerciasis.

Rivermead perceptual assessment battery, a standardized battery of tests, used selectively or as a whole, and administered by a therapist to provide a comprehensive analysis of an individual's perceptual ability. Developed by Whitting, Lincoln, Bhavnani and Cockburn.

Rivinus' notch {Augustus Q. Rivinus, German anatomist, b. 1652}, a deficiency in the tympanic sulcus of the ear that forms an attachment for the flaccid part of the tympanic membrane and mallear folds.

RMN, abbreviation for registered mental nurse.

RMSF, abbreviation for Rocky Mountain spotted fever.

RN, abbreviation for registered nurse.

Rn, symbol for radon.

RNA, abbreviation for ribonucleic acid.

RNA polymerase, (in molecular genetics) an enzyme that catalyses the assembly of ribonucleoside triphosphates into RNA, with single-stranded DNA serving as the template.

RNA splicing, (in molecular genetics) the process by which base pairs that interrupt the continuity of genetic information in DNA are removed from the precursors of messenger RNA.

RNMH, abbreviation for registered nurse for the mentally handicapped.

robertsonian translocation, the exchange of entire chromosome arms. The break occurs at the centromere, usually between two non-homologous acrocentric chromosomes, to form one large metacentric chromosome and one extremely small chromosome that carries little genetic material; through successive cell divisions this small chromosome may be lost.

rock fever. See brucellosis.

Rocky Mountain spotted fever (RMSF), a serious tick-borne infectious disease occurring throughout the temperate zones of North and South America, caused by *Rickettsia rickettsii* and characterized by chills fever, severe headache, myalgia, mental confusion and rash. Erythematous macules first appear on wrists and ankles, spreading rapidly over the extremities, trunk, face and usually on the palms and soles. Haemorrhagic lesions, constipation and abdominal distention are also common. Care must be taken not to crush ticks, as infection may be acquired through skin abrasions.

rod, 1. a straight cylindric structure. **2.** one of the tiny cylindric elements arranged perpendicular to the surface of the retina. Rods contain the chemical rhodopsin, which adapts the eye to detect low-intensity light and gives the rods a purple colour.

rodent ulcer, a slowly developing serpiginous ulceration of a basal cell carcinoma of the skin.

rodenticide poisoning, a toxic condition caused by the ingestion of a substance intended for the control of rodent populations

roentgen (R) {William K. Roentgen, German physicist, b. 1845}, the quantity of x- or gamma radiation that creates 1 electrostatic unit of ions in 1 ml of air at 0° C and 760 mm of pressure. In radiotherapy or radio-diagnosis, the roentgen is the unit of exposure.

Rohrer's constants, the constants in an empiric equation for airway resistance. It is expressed as $R = K_1 + K_2 V$, where R is resistance, V is instantaneous volumetric flow rate, K_1 is a constant representing gas viscosity and airway geometry, and K_2 is a constant representing gas density and airway geometry.

Rokitansky's disease. See Budd-Chiari syndrome.

Rolando's fracture {Luigi Rolando, Italian anatomist, b. 1773}, a fracture of the base of the first metacarpal.

role, a socially expected behaviour pattern associated with an individual's function in various social groups. Roles provide a means for social participation and a way to test identities for consensual validation by significant others. The term derives from the word for a character in a play.

role blurring, the tendency for professional roles to overlap and become indistinct.

role change, a situation in which status is retained while role expectations change.

role clarification, gaining the knowledge, information and cues required to perform a role.

role conflict, the presence of contradictory and often competing role expectations.

role overload, a condition in which there is insufficient time for carrying out all of the expected role functions.

role performance, altered, a disruption in the way one perceives one's role performance. Characteristics include a change in self-perception of one's role, denial of the role, a change in others' perception of one's role, conflict in roles, a change in physical capacity to resume one's role, lack of knowledge of role and change in usual patterns of responsibility.

role playing, a psychotherapeutic technique in which a person acts out a real or simulated situation as a means of understanding intrapsychic conflicts.

role playing therapy. See **psychodrama.**

role reversal act, the act of assuming the role of another person to appreciate how the person feels, perceives and behaves in relation to self and others.

role strain, stress associated with expected roles or positions, experienced as frustration. **Role ambiguity** occurs when shared specifications set for an expected role are incomplete or insufficient to inform the involved individual of what is desired and how it is to be done. **Role incongruence** occurs when an individual undergoes role transitions requiring a significant modification in attitudes and values. **Role overqualification** occurs when a role does not require full use of a person's resources.

Rolfing. See **structural integration.**

roll, intrinsic joint movements on an axis parallel to the articulating surface. The axis can remain stationary or move in a plane parallel to the joint surface.

roller bandage, a long, tightly wound strip of material that may vary in width. It is generally applied as a circular bandage.

roller clamp, a device, usually made of plastic, equipped with a small roller that may be rolled counter-clockwise to close off primary intravenous tubing, or clockwise to open it.

rolling effleurage, a circular rubbing stroke used in massage to promote circulation and muscle relaxation, especially on the shoulder and buttocks. It is performed with the hand flat, the palm and closely held fingers acting as a unit.

Romberg sign {Moritz H. Romberg, German physician, b. 1795}, an indication of loss of the sense of position in which the patient loses balance when standing erect, feet together and eyes closed.

rongeur forceps, a kind of biting forceps that is strong and heavy, used for cutting bone.

root, the lowest part of an organ or structure by which something is firmly attached, such as the anatomical root of the tooth.

root amputation. See **apicectomy.**

root canal file, a small metal hand instrument with tightly spiralled blades, used for cleaning and shaping a root canal.

root canal filling, a material placed in the root canal system of a tooth to seal the space previously occupied by the dental pulp.

root canal. See **pulp canal.**

root curettage, debridement and planing of the root surface of a tooth, to remove accretions and induce the development of healthy gingival tissues.

root end cyst. See **radicular cyst.**

root furcation, a pathological condition involving the alveolar bone in the furcation area of a multi-rooted tooth.

root resection. See **apicectomy.**

root retention, a technique that removes the crown of a root canal-treated tooth, but retains enough of the root and gingival attachment to support a removable prosthesis.

root submersion, a root retention in which the tooth structure is reduced below the level of the alveolar crest, and the soft tissue is allowed to heal over it.

rooting reflex, a normal response in newborns when the cheek is touched or stroked along the side of the mouth to turn the head towards the stimulated side and so that sucking can begin.

Rorschach test {Hermann Rorschach, Swiss psychiatrist, b. 1884}, a projective personality assessment test. It consists of 10 pictures of inkblots, five in black and white, three in black and red and two multicoloured, to which the subject responds by telling, in as many interpretations as is desired, what images and emotions each design evokes. The test is designed to assess the degree to which intellectual and emotional factors are integrated in the subject's perception of the environment.

rosacea, a chronic form of acne seen in adults of all ages and associated with telangiectasia, especially of the nose, forehead and cheeks.

rose fever, a common misnomer for seasonal allergic rhinitis caused by pollen, most frequently of grasses, that is airborne at the time roses are in bloom.

rose spots, small erythematous macules occurring on the upper abdomen and anterior thorax and lasting 2 or 3 days, characteristic of typhoid and paratyphoid fever.

Rosenmüller's organ. See **epoophoron.**

Rosenthal's syndrome. See **haemophilia C.**

roseola, any rose-coloured rash.

roseola infantum, a benign, presumably viral, endemic illness of infants and young children, characterized by abrupt, high sustained or spiking fever, mild pharyngitis and lymph node enlargement. Febrile convulsions may occur. After 4 or 5 days the fever suddenly drops to normal, and a faint, pink, maculopapular rash appears on the neck, trunk and thighs. The rash may last a few hours to 2 days.

rostral, beak-shaped. **rostrum,** *n.*

rotameter, a device operated by a needle valve in an anaesthetic gas machine that measures gases by speed of flow, according to their viscosity and density.

rotating tourniquet, one of four constricting devices used in a rotating order to pool blood in the extremities, so as to relieve congestion in the lungs for the treatment of acute pulmonary oedema. Tourniquets are applied to the upper parts of three extremities at one time. Every 15 minutes, in clockwise order, a tourniquet is placed on the nonconstricted extremity, and one tourniquet is removed; as a result of this rotation, the blood vessels of each of the four extremities are constricted for 45 minutes of each hour of the procedure.

rotation, 1. a turning around an axis. 2. one of the four basic kinds of motion allowed by various joints: the rotation of a bone around its central axis, which may lie in a separate bone, as in the pivot formed by the dens of the axis around which the atlas turns. A bone, such as the humerus, may also rotate around its own longitudinal axis, or the axis of rotation may not be quite parallel to the long axis of the rotating bone, as in movement of the radius on the ulna during pronation and supination of the hand. 3. (in obstetrics) the turning of the fetal head to descend through the pelvis.

rotavirus, a double-stranded RNA molecule that appears as a tiny wheel, with a clearly defined outer layer, or rim, and an inner layer of spokes. The organism is a cause of acute gastroenteritis with diarrhoea.

Rotokinetic treatment table, a special bed equipped with an automatic turning device that completely immobilizes patients while rotating them from 90 to 270 degrees around a horizontal axis.

Rotor syndrome, a rare condition of the liver, inherited as an autosomal recessive trait. It is similar to Dubin-Johnson syndrome.

roughage. See dietary fibre.

rouleaux, *sing.* **rouleau,** an aggregation of red cells in what looks like a stack of coins or checkers. The formation may sometimes be caused by abnormal proteins.

round ligament, 1. a curved fibrous band, attached at one end to the fovea of the head of the femur and at the other to the transverse ligament of the acetabulum. 2. a fibrous cord extending from the umbilicus to the anterior part of the liver. 3. in the female, a fibromuscular band that extends from the anterior surface of the uterus through the inguinal canal to the labium majus. The structure is homologous to the spermatic cord in the male.

rounds *informal,* a teaching conference or meeting in which the clinical problems encountered in the practice of nursing, medicine or other service are discussed; for example, **nursing rounds, teaching rounds, walking rounds.**

roundworm, any worm of the class Nematoda, including *Ancylostoma duodenale, Ascaris lumbricoides, Enterobius vermicularis* and *Strongyloides stercoralis.*

route of administration, (of a drug) any one of the ways in which a drug may be administered, such as intramuscularly, intranasally, intravenously, orally, rectally, subcutaneously, sublingually, topically or vaginally.

Rovsing's sign {Nils T. Rovsing, Danish surgeon, b. 1862}, an indication of acute appendicitis in which pressure on the left lower quadrant of the abdomen causes pain in the right lower quadrant.

Royal College of Physicians (RCP), a professional organization of physicians in the UK.

Royal College of Radiologists (RCR), a professional organization of radiologists in the UK.

Royal College of Surgeons (RCS), a professional organization of surgeons in the UK.

Royal Pharmaceutical Society of Great Britain (RPSGB), the professional and disciplinary body for pharmacists practising in the UK. Membership is mandatory for those wishing to practice as pharmacists. The Society has statutory responsibility for enforcing many aspects of legislation concerning medicines and pharmacy.

RPF, abbreviation for **renal plasma flow.**

RQ, abbreviation for **respiratory quotient.**

Rs, symbol for **stimulatory receptor molecule.**

RSCN, abbreviation for **registered sick children's nurse.**

RSV, RS virus, abbreviation for **respiratory syncytial virus.**

RT, abbreviation for **radiotherapy.**

RTA, abbreviation for **road traffic accident.**

Ru, symbol for **ruthenium.**

rubber *informal,* condom.

rubber dam, a thin sheet of latex rubber for isolating one or more teeth during a dental procedure.

rubber dam clamps forceps, (in dentistry) a type of forceps with beaks designed to engage holes in a rubber dam clamp, to facilitate its placement.

rubber-band ligation, a method of treating haemorrhoids by placing a rubber band around the haemorrhoidal portion of the blood vessel, causing it to slough off after a period of time.

rubefacient, 1. a substance or agent that increases the reddish colouration of the skin. 2. increasing the reddish colouration of the skin.

rubella, a contagious viral disease characterized by fever, symptoms of a mild upper respiratory tract infection, lymph node enlargement, arthralgia and a diffuse, fine, red, maculopapular rash. The virus is spread by droplet infection, and the incubation time is from 12 to 23 days. The symptoms usually last only 2 or 3 days, except for arthralgia which may persist longer or recur. One attack confers lifelong immunity. If a woman acquires rubella in the first trimester of pregnancy, fetal anomalies may result, including heart defects, cataracts, deafness and mental retardation. An infant exposed to the virus in utero at any time during gestation may shed the virus for up to 30 months after birth. Complications of postnatal rubella are rare.

rubella embryopathy, any congenital abnormality in an infant caused by maternal rubella in the early stages of pregnancy.

rubella panencephalitis. See **panencephalitis.**

rubella vaccine, a suspension containing live attenuated rubella virus. It is used for active immunization against rubella.

rubeola. See **measles.**

rubescent, reddening.

rubidium (Rb), a soft, metallic element of the alkali metals group. Its atomic number is 37 and its atomic weight is 85.47. Slightly radioactive, it is used in radioisotope scanning.

Rubin's test {Isador C. Rubin, American gynaecologist, b. 1883}, a test performed in the process of evaluating the cause of infertility, by assessing the patency of the uterine tubes. Carbon dioxide gas (CO_2) is introduced into the tubes under pressure through a cannula inserted into the cervix. The CO_2 is passed through from a syringe connected to a manometer at pressures of up to 200 mm Hg. If the tubes are open, the gas enters the abdominal cavity and the recorded pressure falls below 180 mm Hg.

rubivirus, a member of the togavirus family, which includes the rubella virus.

rubor, redness, especially when accompanying inflammation.

rubricyte, a nucleated red blood cell; the marrow stage in the normal development of an erythrocyte.

ructus. See **eructation.**

rudiment, an organ or tissue that is incompletely developed or non-functional. **rudimentary,** *adj.*

Ruffini's corpuscles {Angelo Ruffini, Italian histologist, b. 1864}, a variety of ovalshaped nerve endings in the subcutaneous tissue, located principally at the junction of the corium and subcutaneous tissue.

ruga, *pl.* **rugae,** a ridge or fold, such as the rugae of the stomach, which presents large folds in the mucous membrane of that organ.

rule of bigeminy, (in cardiology) the tendency of a lengthened ventricular cycle to precipitate a ventricular premature beat.

rule of co-occurrence, a mandate that a person will use the same level of lexical and syntactic structure when speaking.

rule of confidentiality, a principle that personal information about others, particularly patients, should not be revealed to persons not authorized to receive such information.

rule of nines, a formula for estimating the amount of body surface covered by burns, by assigning 9% to the head and each arm, twice 9% (18%) to each leg and the anterior and posterior trunk, and 1% to the perineum. This is modified in infants and children because of the different body proportions.

rule of three, (in respiratory therapy) an arterial oxygen tension that is three times the value of inspired oxygen concentration. It is regarded as an empirical guide to a temporarily acceptable minimal oxygenation or expression of clinical observation.

rumination, habitual regurgitation of small amounts of undigested food with little force after every feeding. It is commonly seen in infants, and may be a symptom of overfeeding, eating too fast or swallowing air.

rupture, 1. a tear or break in the continuity or configuration of an organ or body tissue, including those instances where other tissue protrudes through the opening. **2.** to cause a break or tear.

ruptured intervertebral disk. See **herniated disk.**

Russell dwarf {Alexander Russell, 20th century Scottish physician}, a person affected with **Russell's syndrome,** a congenital disorder in which short stature is associated with various anomalies of the head, face and skeleton, with varying degrees of mental retardation.

Russell traction {R. Hamilton Russell, 20th century Australian surgeon}, a unilateral or a bilateral orthopaedic mechanism that combines suspension and traction to immobilize, position and align the lower extremities in the treatment of fractured femurs, hip and knee contractures, and in the treatment of disease processes of the hip and knee.

Russell's bodies {William Russell, Scottish physician, b. 1852}, the mucoprotein inclusions found in globular plasma cells in cancer and inflammations. The bodies contain surface gamma globulins.

Russell's syndrome. See **Russell dwarf.**

ruthenium (Ru), a hard, brittle, metallic element. Its atomic number is 44 and its atomic weight is 101.07.

rutin, a bioflavonoid obtained from buckwheat and used in the treatment of capillary fragility.

RV, abbreviation for **residual volume.**

RVC, abbreviation for **responds to verbal commands.**

S, **1.** symbol for **sulphur.** **2.** symbol for **saturation of haemoglobin.**

s, **1.** abbreviation for **steady state.** **2.** abbreviation for **sinister** (left). **3.** abbreviation for **second.**

S wave, the component of the cardiac cycle shown on an electrocardiogram as a line slanting downwards sharply from the peak of the R wave to the beginning of the upward curve of the T wave. It represents the final phase of the QRS complex.

S's test. See **Sulkowitch's test.**

S-phase, the phase of a cell reproductive cycle in which DNA is synthesized before mitosis.

S-plasty, a technique of plastic surgery in which an S-shaped instead of a straight line incision is made to reduce tension and improve healing in areas where the skin is loose.

s.o.s., (in prescriptions) abbreviation for *si opus sit,* a Latin phrase meaning "if necessary".

S1, the first heart sound in the cardiac cycle occurring with ventricular systole. It is associated with closure of the mitral and tricuspid valves and is synchronous with the apical pulse.

S2, the second heart sound in the cardiac cycle. It is associated with closure of the aortic and pulmonary valves just before ventricular diastole.

S3, the third heart sound in the cardiac cycle. Normally, it is audible only in children and physically active young adults. In older people, it is an abnormal finding and usually indicates myocardial failure.

S4, the fourth heart sound in the cardiac cycle. It occurs late in diastole on contraction of the atria. Rarely heard in normal subjects, it indicates an abnormally increased resistance to ventricular filling.

SA, **1.** abbreviation for **sinoatrial.** **2.** abbreviation for **surface area.**

SA conduction time, the conduction time for an impulse from the sinus node to the atrial musculature, measured from the SA deflection in the SA nodal electrocardiogram to the beginning of the P wave in a bipolar record, or to the beginning of the high right atrial electrogram in a unipolar record.

SA electrogram, a direct electric recording of the SA node.

SA node. See **sinoatrial node.**

Sabin vaccine. See **poliomyelitis vaccine.**

Sabin-Feldman dye test {Albert B. Sabin, American virologist, b. 1906; H. A. Feldman}, a diagnostic test for toxoplasmosis, basd on the presence of specific antibodies that block the uptake of methylene blue dye by the cytoplasm of the *Toxoplasma* organisms.

sac, a pouch or a bag-like organ, such as the abdominal sac of the embryo that develops into the abdominal cavity.

saccade, pertaining to something jerky, broken or abrupt, such as rapid shifts of eye movement or a staccato voice.

saccadic eye movement, an extremely fast voluntary movement of the eyes, allowing the eyes to fix accurately on a still object in the visual field as the person moves or the head turns.

saccharide, any of a large group of carbohydrates, including all sugars and starches. Almost all carbohydrates are saccharides. See also **carbohydrate, sugar.**

saccharin, **1.** a white, crystalline synthetic sweetener, which has a sweeter taste than table sugar (sucrose). **2.** having a sweet taste, especially cloyingly sweet.

Saccharomyces, a genus of yeast fungi, including brewer's and baker's yeast, as well as some pathogenic fungi, that cause diseases such as bronchitis, moniliasis and pharyngitis.

saccharomycosis, **1.** infection with yeast fungi, such as the genera *Candida* or *Cryptococcus.* **2.** *obsolete.* cryptococcosis or European blastomycosis.

saccular, pertaining to a pouch, or shaped like a sac.

saccular aneurysm, a localized dilatation of an artery in which only a small area of the vessel is distended, forming a sac-like swelling or protrusion.

saccule, a small bag or sac, such as the air saccules of the lungs. saccular, *adj.*

sacculus, *pl.* **sacculi,** a little sac or bag, especially the smaller of the two divisions of the membranous labyrinth of the vestibule, which communicates with the cochlear duct through the ductus reuniens in the inner ear. See also **saccule.**

Sachs' disease. See **Tay-Sachs disease.**

sacral, of or pertaining to the sacrum.

sacral foramen, one of several openings between the fused segments of the sacral vertebrae in the sacrum through which the sacral nerves pass.

sacral node, a node in one of the seven groups of parietal lymph nodes of the abdomen and the pelvis, situated within the sacrum.

sacral plexus, a network of motor and sensory nerves formed by the lumbosacral trunk from the fourth and fifth lumbar, and by the first, second and third sacral nerves. They converge towards the caudal portion of the greater sciatic foramen and unite to become a large, flattened band, most of which continues into the thigh as the sciatic nerve.

sacral vertebra, one of the five segments of the vertebral column that fuse in the adult to form the sacrum. The ventral border of the first sacral vertebra projects into the pelvis. The bodies of the other sacral vertebrae are smaller than that of the first and are flattened and curved ventrally, forming the convex, anterior surface of the sacrum.

sacroiliac, pertaining to the part of the skeletal system that includes the sacrum and the ilium bones of the pelvis.

sacroiliac articulation, an immovable joint in the pelvis formed by the articulation of each side of the sacrum with an iliac bone.

sacrospinalis, a large, fleshy muscle of the back that divides into a lateral iliocostalis column, an intermediate longissimus column and a medial spinalis column.

sacrum, the large, triangular bone at the dorsal part of the pelvis, inserted like a wedge between the two hip bones. The base of the sacrum articulates with the last lumbar vertebra, and its apex articulates with the coccyx. **sacral,** *adj.*

saddle block anaesthesia, a form of regional nerve block that anaesthetizes the parts of the body that would touch a saddle, if the patient was sitting astride one. It is performed by injecting a local anaesthetic into the spinal cavity as the patient sits with the head on the chest, the back curved and the legs down.

saddle joint, a synovial joint in which surfaces of contiguous bones are reciprocally concavoconvex. A saddle joint permits no axial rotation but allows flexion, extension, adduction and abduction.

sadism {Donatien A. F. de Sade, French Marquis, b. 1740}, **1.** abnormal pleasure derived from inflicting physical or psychological pain or abuse on others; cruelty. **2.** (in psychiatry) a psychosexual disorder characterized by the infliction of physical or psychological pain or humiliation on another person, either a consenting or non-consenting partner, to achieve sexual excitement or gratification. Kinds of sadism are **anal sadism** and **oral sadism.** **sadistic,** *adj.*

sadist, a person who is afflicted with or practices sadism.

sadomasochism {Marquis de Sade, b. 1740; Leopold von Sacher-Masoch, Austrian author, b. 1836}, a personality disorder characterized by traits of sadism and masochism.

safe period. See **natural family planning method.**

safety manager, a member of a hospital staff whose activities are related to safety functions, such as fire prevention, environmental safety and disaster planning activities.

sagittal, (in anatomy) of, or pertaining to, a suture or an imaginary line extending from the front to the back in the midline of the body or a part of the body.

sagittal axis, a hypothetical line through the mandibular condyle that serves as an axis for rotation movements of the mandible.

sagittal fontanelle, a soft area located in the sagittal suture, halfway between the anterior and posterior fontanelles. It may be found in some normal newborns and in some newborns with Down's syndrome.

sagittal plane, the anterioposterior plane or the section parallel to the median plane of the body.

sagittal suture, the serrated connection between the two parietal bones of the skull, coursing down the midline from the coronal suture to the upper part of the lambdoidal suture.

SaH, SAH, abbreviation for **subarachnoid haemorrhage.**

salicylate, any of several widely prescribed drugs derived from salicylic acid. Salicylates exert analgesic, antipyretic and anti-inflammatory actions. The most important is acetylsalicylic acid, or aspirin. Sodium salicylate has also been used systemically, and it exerts similar effects. Methyl salicylate is the active ingredient in many rubefacient preparations. Another salicylate, salicylic acid, is too irritating to be used systemically and is used topically as a keratolytic agent, for removing warts and treating other hyperkeratotic and fungal skin conditions.

salicylate poisoning, a toxic condition caused by the ingestion of salicylate, most often in aspirin or oil of wintergreen. Intoxication is characterized by rapid breathing, vomiting, headache, irritability, ketosis, hypoglycaemia and, in severe cases, convulsions and respiratory failure.

salicylazosuphpyridine. See **sulphasalazine.**

salicylic acid. See **salicylate.**

salicylism, a syndrome of salicylate toxicity.

saline infusion, the therapeutic introduction of a physiological salt solution into a vein.

saline irrigation, the washing out of a body cavity or wound with a stream of salt solution, usually an isotonic aqueous solution of sodium chloride.

saline laxative, one of a large group of laxatives administered to achieve prompt, complete evacuation of the bowel. A watery semi-fluid evacuation usually occurs within 3 to 4 hours.

saline solution, a solution containing sodium chloride. Depending on the use, it may be hypotonic, isotonic or hypertonic with body fluids.

saliva, the clear, viscous fluid secreted by the salivary and mucous glands in the mouth. Saliva contains water, mucin, organic salts and the digestive enzyme ptyalin. It serves to moisten the oral cavity, initiate the digestion of starches, and aid in the chewing and swallowing of food.

salivary, of, or pertaining to, saliva or the formation of saliva.

salivary duct, any one of the ducts through which saliva passes. Kinds of salivary ducts are **Bartholin's duct, duct of Rivinus, parotid duct,** and **submandibular duct.**

salivary fistula, an abnormal communication from a salivary gland or duct to an opening in the mouth or on the skin of the face or neck.

salivary gland, one of the three pairs of glands that pour their secretions into the mouth, thus aiding the digestive process. The salivary glands are the parotid, the submandibular, and the sublingual glands. They are racemose structures consisting of numerous lobes subdivided into smaller lobules connected by dense areolar tissue, vessels, and ducts.

salivary gland cancer, a malignant disease of a salivary gland, occurring most frequently in the parotid gland. About 75% of tumours that develop in the salivary glands are benign, characteristically slow-growing, painless, mobile masses that are cystic or rubbery in consistency. The most common malignant neoplasms are mucoepidermoid, adenoid cystic, solid and squamous cell carcinomas.

salivation, the process of saliva secretion by the salivary glands.

Salk vaccine. See **poliomyelitis vaccine.**

salmon calcitonin. See **calcitonin.**

Salmonella {Daniel E. Salmon, American pathologist, b. 1850}, a genus of motile, gram-negative, rod-shaped bacteria that includes species causing typhoid fever, paratyphoid fever and some forms of gastroenteritis.

salmonellosis {Daniel E. Salmon}, a form of gastroenteritis, caused by ingestion of food contaminated with a species of *Salmonella*, characterized by an incubation period of 6 to 48 hours followed by sudden, colicky abdominal pain, fever and bloody, watery diarrhoea. Nausea and vomiting are common, and abdominal signs may resemble acute appendicitis or cholecystitis. Symptoms usually last from 2 to 5 days, but diarrhoea and fever may persist for up to 2 weeks. Dehydration may occur.

salol camphor, a clear, oily mixture of two parts of camphor and three parts of phenyl salicylate, used as a local antiseptic.

Salonica fever. See **trench fever.**

salpingectomy, surgical removal of one or both uterine tubes, performed to remove a cyst or tumour, excise an abscess, or, if both tubes are removed, as a sterilization procedure.

salpingitis, an inflammation or infection of the uterine tube.

salpingo-oophorectomy, the surgical removal of a uterine tube and an ovary.

salpingography. See **hysterosalpingography.**

salpingostomy, the formation of an artificial opening in a uterine tube, performed to restore patency in a tube whose fimbriated opening has been closed by infection or chronic inflammation, or drain an abscess or an accumulation of fluid. A prosthesis may be inserted to maintain the patency of the uterine tube and direct the route of the ova to assist fertilization.

salpinx, *pl.* **salpinges,** a tube, such as *salpinx auditiva* or *salpinx uterina*. **salpingian,** *adj.*

salt, 1. a compound formed by the chemical reaction of an acid and a base. Salts are usually composed of a metal and a nonmetal, and may behave chemically as metals or non-metals. **2.** sodium chloride (common table salt). **3.** a substance, such as magnesium sulfate (Epsom salt), used as a purgative.

salt cake, sodium sulfate anhydrous; a technical grade of sodium sulfate used in detergents, dyes, soaps and other industrial products.

salt depletion, the loss of salt from the body through excessive elimination of body fluids by perspiration, diarrhoea, vomiting or urination, without corresponding replacement.

salt-free diet. See **low-sodium diet.**

saltation, (in genetics) a mutation causing a significant difference in appearance between parent and offspring, or an abrupt variation in the characteristics of the species. **saltatorial, saltatoric, saltatory,** *adj.*

saltatory conduction, impulse transmission that skips from node to node.

saltatory evolution, the appearance of a sudden, abrupt change within a species, caused by mutation; the progression of a species by sudden major changes rather than by the gradual accumulation of minor changes.

Salter fracture. See **epiphyseal fracture.**

salvage therapy, therapy administered to sites at which previous therapies have failed and the disease has recurred.

salve. See **ointment.**

samarium (Sm) {Colonel Samarski, 19th century Russian mine official}, a rare earth, metallic element. Its atomic number is 62 and its atomic weight is 150.35.

San Joaquin fever, the primary stage of coccidioidomycosis.

sand bath, the application of warm, dry sand

or damp sand to the body.

sand flea. See **chigoe.**

sand tumour. See **psammoma.**

sandfly fever. See **phlebotomus fever.**

Sandhoff's disease, a variant of Tay-Sachs disease that includes defects in the enzymes haexosaminidase A and B. It is characterized by a progressively more rapid course and is found in the general population, as opposed to the restricted incidence of Tay-Sachs disease.

sanguineous, pertaining to blood.

sanitary landfill, a solid waste disposal site, usually a swamp area, ravine or canyon where the waste is compacted by heavy machines and covered with earth.

SaO$_2$, symbol for the percent of *saturation of arterial blood*.

saphenous nerve, the largest and longest branch of the femoral nerve, supplying the skin of the medial side of the leg.

saphenous vein. See **great saphenous vein.**

saponified, pertaining to a substance chemically hydrolysed into soaps or acid salts and glycerol by heating with an alkali.

saponin, a soapy material found in some plants, especially soapwort (Bouncing Bet) and certain lilies. It has been used in pharmaceutical formulations as a wetting agent.

saprophyte, an organism that lives on dead organic matter. **saprophytic,** *adj.*

saralasin, a competitive antagonist of angiotensin. It is administered by intravenous injection to assess the role of the renin-angiotensin system in the maintenance of blood pressure.

sarcoidosis, a chronic disorder of unknown origin characterized by the formation of tubercles of non-necrotizing epithelioid tissue. Common sites are the lungs, spleen, liver, skin, mucous membranes and lacrimal and salivary glands, usually with involvement of the lymph glands. The lesions usually disappear over a period of months or years but progress to widespread granulomatous inflammation and fibrosis.

sarcoidosis cordis, a form of sarcoidosis in which granulomatous lesions develop in the myocardium. In severe cases the myocardium may be infiltrated by several tumours and cardiac failure may follow.

sarcoma, *pl.* **sarcomas, sarcomata,** a malignant neoplasm of the soft tissues arising in fibrous, fatty, muscular, synovial, vascular or neural tissue, usually presenting initially as a painless swelling. The tumour, composed of closely packed cells in a fibrillar or homogeneous matrix, tends to be vascular and highly invasive. Trauma probably does not play a role in the cause, but sarcomas may arise in burn or radiation scars. See **specific sarcomas.**

sarcoma botryoides, a tumour derived from primitive striated muscle cells, occurring most frequently in young children. It is char-

acterized by a painful, oedematous, polypoid, grape-like mass in the upper vagina, uterine cervix or neck of the urinary bladder.

sarcomagenesis, the process of initiating and promoting the development of a sarcoma. **sarcomagenetic,** *adj.*

sarcomere, the smallest functional unit of a myofibril. Sarcomeres occur as repeating units along the length of a myofibril, occupying the region between Z disks of the myofibril.

sarcoplasmic reticulum, a network of tubules and sacs in skeletal muscles that plays an important role in muscle contraction and relaxation by releasing and storing calcium ions.

Sarcoptes scabiei, the genus of itch mite that causes scabies.

sartorius, the longest muscle in the body, extending from the pelvis to the calf of the leg. It acts to flex the thigh and rotate it laterally and to flex the leg and rotate it medially.

satiety, the satisfied feeling of being full after eating.

saturated, 1. having absorbed or dissolved the maximum amount of a given substance, such as a solution in which no more of the solute can be dissolved. **2.** an organic compound that contains the maximum number of hydrogen atoms so that only single valence bonds exist in the carbon chain.

saturated calomel electrode (SCE), a reference electrode commonly used in polarography.

saturated fatty acid, any of a number of glyceryl esters of certain organic acids in which all the atoms are joined by single-valence bonds. These fats are chiefly of animal origin and include beef, lamb, pork, veal, whole-milk products, butter, most cheeses and a few plant fats such as cocoa butter, coconut oil and palm oil.

saturated hydrocarbon. See **saturated.**

saturated solution, a solution in which the solvent contains the maximum amount of solute it can take up.

saturation-dependent drugs, drugs that act diffusely on tissues rather than at specific receptor sites.

satyriasis, excessive or uncontrollable sexual desire in the male.

sauna bath, a bath in which hot vapour is used to induce sweating, followed by rubbing of the body, and finishing with a cold shower.

Sayre's jacket {Lewis A. Sayre, American surgeon, b. 1820}, a cast applied for support and immobilization in the treatment of certain abnormalities of the spinal column.

Sb, symbol for **antimony.**

SBE, 1. abbreviation for **self-breast examination. 2.** abbreviation for **subacute bacterial endocarditis.**

Sc, symbol for **scandium.**

sc, abbreviation for *sine correctione*, a Latin phrase meaning "without correction".

scab. See **eschar.**

scabicide, any one of a group of drugs that destroy the mite Sarcoptes scabiei, for example, lindane. These drugs are applied topically in a lotion or cream-based preparation. All are potentially toxic and irritating to the skin.

scabies, a contagious disease caused by *Sarcoptes scabiei*, the itch mite. It is characterized by intense itching of the skin and excoriation from scratching. The mite, transmitted by close contact with infected humans or domestic animals, burrows into outer layers of the skin where the female lays eggs. Two to 4 months after the first infection, sensitization to the mites and their products begins, resulting in a pruritic papular rash. Secondary bacterial infection may occur.

scalded skin syndrome. See **toxic epidermal necrolysis.**

scale, 1. a small, thin flake of keratinized epithelium. **2.** to remove encrusted material from the surface of a tooth.

scalp, the skin covering the head, not including the face and ears.

scalp medication, 1. a cream, ointment, lotion or shampoo used to treat dermatological conditions of the scalp. **2.** the application of a medication to the scalp.

scalp vein needle, a thin-gauge needle designed for use on the veins of the scalp or other small veins, especially in children.

scamping speech, abnormal speech in which consonants or whole syllables are left out of words because of the person's inability to shape the sounds.

scandium (Sc), a grayish metallic element. Its atomic number is 21 and its atomic weight is 44.956.

scanning, a method of imaging where an area, organ or system of the body is studied and an image recorded and displayed. Methods include **computerized tomography, radionuclide imaging, magnetic resonance imaging** and **ultrasonography. scan,** *n., v.*

scanning electron microscope (SEM), an instrument that resembles an electron microscope in that a beam of electrons, instead of visible light, is used to scan the surface of a specimen. The image produced is of less magnification than that produced by an electron microscope, but it appears to be three-dimensional and life-like.

scanning electron microscopy, the technique using a scanning electron microscope on an electrically conducting sample.

scanning speech, abnormal speech characterized by a staccato-like articulation in which the words are clipped and broken because the person pauses between syllables.

scanogram, (in computerised tomography) frontal or lateral projection of the area of interest to determine the required levels to be scanned. Also called **scout view, pilot view.**

scapegoating, the projection of blame, hostility or suspicion onto one member of a group by other members to avoid self-confrontation.

scaphocephaly, a congenital malformation of the skull in which premature closure of the sagittal suture results in restricted lateral growth of the head, giving it an abnormally long, narrow appearance with a cephalic index of 75 or less. **scaphocephalic, scaphocephalous,** *adj.*

scaphoid abdomen, an abdomen with a sunken anterior wall.

scaphoid bone, either of two similar bones of the hand and the foot. The scaphoid bone of the hand is slanted at the radial side of the carpus. The scaphoid bone of the foot is located at the medial side of the tarsus between the talus and cuneiform bones.

scapula, one of the pair of large, flat, triangular bones that form the dorsal part of the shoulder girdle.

scapular line, an imaginary vertical line drawn through the inferior angle of the scapula.

scapulohumeral, of, or pertaining to, the structures of muscles and the area around the scapula and humerus that make up the shoulder girdle.

scapulohumeral muscular dystrophy. See **Erb's muscular dystrophy.**

scapulohumeral reflex, a normal response to tapping the vertebral border of the scapula, resulting in adduction of the arm.

scar. See **cicatrix.**

scarification, multiple superficial scratches or incisions in the skin, such as those made for the introduction of a vaccine.

scarify, to make multiple superficial incisions into the skin; to scratch. Vaccination against smallpox is achieved by scarifying the skin under a drop of vaccine.

scarlatina. See **scarlet fever.**

scarlatiniform, resembling the rash of **scarlet fever.**

scarlet fever, an acute contagious disease of childhood caused by an erythrotoxin-producing strain of group A haemolytic *Streptococcus.* The infection is characterized by sore throat, fever, enlarged lymph nodes in the neck, prostration and a diffuse, bright red rash.

scattered radiation, radiation that travels in a direction other than that of its source energy, such as secondary radiaiion and stray radiation.

scattergram, a graph representing the distribution of two variables in a sample population. One variable is plotted on the vertical axis; the second on the horizontal axis. A scattergram demonstrates the degree or tendency to which the variables occur in association with each other.

scattering, (in radiation dosimetry) attenuation of a radiation beam where x-ray photons interact with matter and are deviated from their original direction.

scavenging system. See **gas scavenging system.**

Schedule I, a category of drugs not considered legitimate for medical use, under the Misuse of Drugs Regulations, 1985. Special Home Office authorization is required to supply or possess such agents.

Schedule II, a category of drugs specified in the Misuse of Drugs regulations, 1985, and considered to have a strong potential for abuse or addiction; however, they have legitimate medical use. Among the substances classified as Schedule II are morphine, cocaine, quinalbarbitone, oxycodone, methadone, diamorphine (heroin), amphetamine and glutethimide. They are subject to the fullest and strictest requirements for custody, record keeping and prescription writing under the Regulations.

Schedule III, a category of drugs specified in the Misuse of Drugs Regulations, 1985. They have less potential for abuse or addiction than Schedule II or I drugs. Among the substances classified as Schedule III are most barbiturates, buprenorphine, diethylpropion meprobamate and phentermine. They are subject to special prescription writing requirements, in addition to the requirement of keeping invoices to cover their sale for 2 years.

Schedule IV, a category of drugs specified in the Misuse of Drugs Regulations, 1985. They have less potential for abuse or addiction than those of Schedules I to III. Among the substances classified as Schedule IV are 34 benzodiazepines and pemoline. They are subject to minimal controls beyond those covering other prescription-only medicines.

Schedule V, a category of preparations of drugs appearing in other Schedules of the Misuse of Drugs Regulations, 1985. They are exempted from most of the regulations that normally apply, because of their low strength.

schema, an innate knowledge structure that allows a child to organize in his or her mind ways to behave in the environment.

Scheuermann's disease {Holger W. Scheuermann, Danish surgeon, b. 1877}, an abnormal skeletal condition characterized by a fixed kyphosis that develops at puberty and is caused by wedge-shaped deformities of one or several vertebrae. The cause of the disease is unknown, but it is thought that it may result from infection, inflammatory processes, aseptic necrosis, disk deterioration, mechanical influences,

inadequate circulation during rapid growth, or disturbances of epiphyseal growth resulting from protrusion of the intervertebral disk through deficient or defective cartilaginous plates. The most striking pathological feature of Scheuermann's disease is the presence of wedge-shaped vertebral bodies, seen on radiographic examination, that cause an excessive curvature.

Schick test {Bela Schick, Austrian-American physician, b. 1877}, a skin test to determine immunity to diphtheria, in which diphtheria toxin is injected intradermally. A positive reaction, indicating susceptibility, is marked by redness and swelling at the site of injection.

Schilder's disease {Paul F. Schilder, American neurologist, b. 1886}, a group of progressive, severe, neurological diseases beginning in childhood. All are characterized by demyelination of the white matter of the brain with muscle spasticity, optic neuritis, aphasia, deafness, adrenal insufficiency and dementia. Many of the signs resemble those of multiple sclerosis.

Schiller's test {Walter Schiller, American pathologist, b. 1887}, a procedure for indicating areas of abnormal epithelium in the vagina or on the cervix of the uterus as a guide in selecting biopsy sites for cancer detection. A potassium iodide or aqueous iodine solution is painted on the vaginal walls and cervix under direct visualization. Normal epithelium contains glycogen and stains a deep brown colour; abnormal epithelium, containing no glycogen, will not stain, and non-staining sites may then be included in tissue biopsies.

Schilling test {Robert Schilling, American physician, b.1919}, a diagnostic test for pernicious anaemia. Vitamin B12, tagged with radioactive cobalt, is administered orally, and GI absorption is measured by determining the radioactivity of urine samples collected over a 24-hour period.

Schilling's leukaemia. See **monocytic leukaemia.**

schindylesis, an articulation of certain bones of the skull in which a thin plate of one bone enters a cleft formed by the separation of two layers of another bone.

Schiötz' tonometer {Hjalmar Schötz, Norwegian ophthalmologist, b. 1850}, a tonometer used to measure intraocular pressure by observing the depth of indentation of the cornea made by the weighted plunger on the device after a topical anaesthetic is applied.

schistocyte, a cell fragment of an erythrocyte, a characteristic of haemolysis or cell fragmentation associated with severe burns and intravascular coagulation.

Schistosoma, a genus of blood flukes that may cause urinary, GI or liver disease in humans. It requires freshwater snails as intermediate hosts. *Schistosoma haemato-*

bium, found chiefly in Africa and the Middle East, affects the bladder and pelvic organs, causing painful, frequent urination and haematuria. *S. japonicum,* found in Japan, the Philippines and Eastern Asia, causes GI ulcerations and fibrosis of the liver. *S. mansoni,* found in Africa, the Middle East, Caribbean and tropical America, causes symptoms similar to those caused by S. japonicum.

schistosomiasis, a parasitic infection caused by a species of fluke of the genus *Schistosoma,* transmitted to humans, the definitive host, by contact with fresh water contaminated by human faeces. A single fluke may live in one part of the body, depositing eggs frequently for up to 20 years. The eggs are irritating to mucous membrane, causing it to thicken and become papillomatous. Symptoms depend on the part of the body infected.

schistosomicide, a drug destructive to schistosomes, blood flukes transmitted by snails to human hosts. **schistosomicidal,** *adj.*

schizoaffective disorder, a condition that includes characteristics of schizophrenia and bipolar disorder or other major affective disorders.

schizogenesis, reproduction by fission. **schizogenetic, schizogenic, schizogenous,** *adj.*

schizogony, 1. reproduction by multiple fission. **2.** the asexual reproductive stage of sporozoans, specifically the portion of lifecycle of the malarial parasite that occurs in the erythrocytes or liver cells.

schizoid, 1. characteristic of, or resembling, schizophrenia; schizophrenic. **2.** a person, not necessarily a schizophrenic, who exhibits the traits of a schizoid personality.

schizoid personality, a functioning but maladjusted person whose behaviour is characterized by extreme shyness, oversensitivity, introversion, seclusiveness and avoidance of close interpersonal relationships.

schizoid personality disorder, a condition characterized by a defect in the ability to form social relationships, as shown by emotional coldness and aloofness, withdrawn and seclusive behaviour, and indifference to praise, criticism and the feelings of others. The condition may precede schizophrenia.

schizont, the multinucleated cell stage during the sexual reproductive phase in the lifecycle of a sporozoan, such as the malarial parasite *Plasmodium.* It is produced by the multiple fission of the trophozoite in a cell of the vertebrate host, subsequently segmenting into merozoites.

schizonticide, a substance that destroys schizonts. **schizonticidal,** *adj.*

schizophasia, the disordered, incomprehensible speech characteristic of some forms of schizophrenia.

schizophrene, a person afflicted with schizophrenia.

schizophrenia, any one of a large group of psychotic disorders characterized by gross distortion of reality, disturbances of language and communication, withdrawal from social interaction, and the disorganization and fragmentation of thought, perception and emotional reaction. Characteristics include apathy and confusion; delusions and hallucinations; rambling or stylized patterns of speech, such as evasiveness, incoherence and echolalia; withdrawn, regressive and bizarre behaviour; and emotional lability. No single cause of the disease is known; genetic, biochemical, psychological, interpersonal and sociocultural factors are usually involved. Kinds of schizophrenia include **acute schizophrenia, catatonic schizophrenia, childhood schizophrenia, disorganized schizophrenia, latent schizophrenia, paranoid schizophrenia, process schizophrenia, reactive schizophrenia** and **residual schizophrenia.** Also called **schizophrenic disorder, schizophrenic reaction.**

schizophrenic, 1. of, or pertaining to, schizophrenia. **2.** a person with schizophrenia.

schizophrenic disorder, schizophrenic reaction. See **schizophrenia.**

schizophreniform disorder, a condition exhibiting the same symptoms as schizophrenia but characterized by an acute onset with resolution in 2 weeks to 6 months.

schizophrenogenic, tending to cause or produce schizophrenia.

schizotypal personality disorder, a condition characterized by oddities of thought, perception, speech and behaviour that are not severe enough to meet the clinical criteria for schizophrenia. Symptoms include magical thinking, such as belief in clairvoyance and telepathy; ideas of reference; recurrent illusions, such as sensing the presence of a person not actually present; social isolation; peculiar speech patterns, including words used deviantly; and hypersensitivity to criticism.

Schlatter-Osgood disease, Schlatter's disease. See **Osgood-Schlatter disease.**

Schlemm's canal. See **canal of Schlemm.**

Schneiderian carcinoma, an epithelial malignancy of the nasal mucosa and paranasal sinuses.

Schönlein-Henoch purpura. See **Henoch-Schönlein purpura.**

Schofield equation, an equation used for estimating the Basal Metabolic Rate (BMR) from the weight of older children, adolescents, adults and the elderly.

school phobia, an extreme separation anxiety disorder of children, usually in the elementary grades, characterized by a persistent, irrational fear of going to school or being in a school-like atmosphere. Such children are usually oversensitive, shy, timid, nervous and emotionally immature, and have pervasive feelings of inadequacy. They typically try to cope with their fears by becoming overdependent on others, especially the parents.

Schüffner's dots, coarse pink or red granules seen in the red blood cells of patients with tertiary malaria. They are signs of *Plasmodium vivax* or *P. ovale* and are absent in blood cells of patients infected with other types of malaria.

Schultz-Charlton phenomenon {Werner Schultz, German physician, b. 1878; Willy Charlton, German physician, b. 1889}, a cutaneous reaction to the intradermal injection of scarlatina antiserum in a person with a scarlatiniform rash. The rash blanches.

Schultze mechanism, the delivery of a placenta with the fetal surfaces presenting. It is the most common method of expulsion.

Schwann cells {Friedrich T. Schwann, German anatomist, b. 1810}, cells of ectodermal origin that comprise the neurilemma.

Schwann's sheath. See **neurilemma.**

schwannoma, *pl.* **schwannomas, schwannomata** {Friedrich Schwann}, a benign, solitary, encapsulated tumour arising in the neurilemma (Schwann's sheath) of peripheral, cranial or autonomic nerves.

Schwartz bed. See **hyperextension bed.**

Schwartzman-Sanarelli phenomenon {Gregory Schwartzman, American physician, b. 1896; Guiseppe Sanarelli, Italian physician, b. 1864}, a phenomenon induced experimentally in the investigation of the role of coagulation in renal disease. Animals injected twice with a bacterial endotoxin develop massive disseminated intravascular coagulation with thrombosis of the blood vessels in the kidneys.

sciatic, near the ischium, such as the sciatic nerve or sciatic vein.

sciatic nerve, a long nerve originating in the sacral plexus and extending through the muscles of the thigh, leg and foot, with numerous branches.

sciatica, an inflammation of the sciatic nerve, usually marked by pain and tenderness along the course of the nerve through the thigh and leg. It may result in a wasting of the muscles of the lower leg.

SCID, abbreviation for **severe combined immunodeficiency disease.**

science, a systematic attempt to establish theories to explain observed phenomena, and the knowledge obtained through these efforts. **Pure science** is concerned with the gathering of information solely for the sake of obtaining new knowledge. **Applied science** is the practical application of scientific theory and laws.

scientific method, a systematic, ordered approach to the gathering of data and solving of problems. The basic approach is statement of the problem, followed by statement of a hypothesis. An experimental method is established to help prove or disprove the

hypothesis. The results of the experiment are observed, and conclusions are drawn from the observed results.

scientific rationale, reasoning, based on supporting scientific evidence, to justify the selection of a particular action.

scintigraph, a photographic recording produced by an imaging device showing the distribution and intensity of radioactivity in various tissues and organs following the administration of a radiopharmaceutical.

scintillation detector, 1. a device that relies on the emission of light or ultraviolet radiation from a crystal subjected to ionizing radiation. The light is detected by a photomultiplier tube and converted to an electric signal that can be processed further. **2.** a device used to measure the amount of radioactivity in an area of the body.

scintiscan, a photographic display of the distribution of a radiopharmaceutical within the body.

scirrhous carcinoma, a hard, fibrous, particularly invasive tumour in which the malignant cells occur singly, in small clusters or strands in dense connective tissue. It is the most common form of breast cancer. Also called **carcinoma fibrosum.**

scissors, a sharp instrument composed of two opposing cutting blades, held together by a central pin on which the blades pivot. The most common dissecting scissors are the straight **Mayo,** for cutting sutures; the **Snowden-Pencer,** for deep, delicate tissue; the long, curved **Mayo,** for deep, heavy or tough tissue; the short, curved Metzenbaum, for superficial, delicate tissue; and the long, blunt, curved Metzenbaum, for deep, delicate tissue.

sclera, the tough, inelastic, opaque membrane covering the posterior five sixths of the eyebulb. It maintains the size and form of the bulb and attaches to muscles that move the bulb. Posteriorly, it is pierced by the optic nerve; with the transparent cornea it comprises the outermost of three tunics covering the eyebulb.

sclerema neonatorum, a progressive generalized hardening of the skin and subcutaneous tissue of the newborn. It is usually a fatal condition that occurs as a result of severe cold stress in severely ill premature infants.

sclerodactyly, a musculoskeletal deformity affecting the hands of persons with scleroderma. The fingers are fixed in a semi-flexed position, and the fingertips are pointed and ulcerated.

scleroderma, a relatively rare autoimmune disease affecting the blood vessels and connective tissue. The disease is characterized by fibrous degeneration of the connective tissue of the skin, lungs and internal organs, especially the oesophagus and kidneys. Scleroderma is most common in middle-aged women. The most common initial complaints are changes in the skin of the face and fingers. Raynaud's phenomenon occurs with a gradual hardening of the skin and swelling of the distal extremities. In the early stages, the disease may be confused with rheumatoid arthritis or Raynaud's disease. As the disease progresses, there is deformity of the joints and pain on movement. Skin changes include oedema, then pallor, followed by firming of the skin. Skin finally becomes slightly pigmented and fixed to the underlying tissues. At this stage, the skin of the face is taut, shiny and mask-like, and the patient may have difficulty in chewing and swallowing.

scleroedema, an idiopathic skin disease characterized by non-pitting induration beginning on the face or neck and spreading downwards over the body, sparing the hands and feet. There also may be swelling of the tongue, restriction of the movements of the eyes, and pericardial, pleural and peritoneal effusions.

scleromalacia perforans, a condition of the eyes in which devitalization and sloughing of the sclera occur as a complication of rheumatoid arthritis. The pigmented uvea becomes exposed. Glaucoma, cataract formation and retinal detachment may result.

sclerose, to harden or cause hardening. **sclerotic,** *adj.*

sclerosing haemangioma, a solid, cellular tumour-like nodule of the skin or a mass of histiocytes, thought to arise from a haemangioma by the proliferation of endothelial and connective tissue cells.

sclerosing solution, a liquid containing an irritant that causes inflammation and resulting fibrosis of tissues. It may be used in cauterizing ulcers, arresting haemorrhage and treating haemangiomas.

sclerosis, a condition characterized by hardening of tissue resulting from any of several causes, including inflammation, the deposit of mineral salts and infiltration of connective tissue fibres. **sclerotic,** *adj.*

sclerotomal pain distribution, the referral of pain from pain-sensitive tissues covering the axial skeleton along a sclerotomal segment.

sclerotome, (in embryology) the part of the segmented mesoderm layer in the early developing embryo that originates from the somites and gives rise to the skeletal tissue of the body.

scolex, *pl.* **scoleces,** the head-like segment or organ of an adult tapeworm that has hooks, grooves or suckers by which it attaches itself to the wall of the intestine.

scoliosis, lateral curvature of the spine, a common abnormality of childhood. Causes include congenital malformations of the spine, poliomyelitis, skeletal dysplasias, spastic paralysis and unequal leg length. Unequal heights of hips or shoulders may be a sign of this condition.

scope, the breadth of opportunity to function; range of activity.

scopolamine. See **hyoscine.**

scopophilia, 1. pleasure derived from looking. **2.** voyeurism. **scopophiliac, scopophilic,** *adj., n.*

scopophobia, an anxiety disorder characterized by a morbid fear of being seen or stared at by others. The condition is commonly seen in schizophrenia.

scorbutic pose, the characteristic posture of a child with scurvy, with thighs and legs semiflexed and hips rotated outwards. The child usually lies motionless without voluntary movements of the extremities because of the pain that accompanies any motion. See **scurvy.**

scorbutus. See **scurvy.**

scorpion sting, a painful wound produced by a scorpion, an arachnid with a hollow stinger in its tail. The stings of many species are only slightly toxic, but some, including Centruroides sculpturatus of the southwestern United States, may inflict fatal injury, especially in small children. Initial pain is followed within several hours by numbness, nausea, muscle spasm, dyspnoea and convulsion.

scotoma, a defect of vision in a defined area in one or both eyes. A common prodromal symptom is a shimmering film appearing as an island in the visual field.

scout view, See **scanogram.**

scratch test, a skin test for identifying an allergen, performed by placing a small quantity of a solution containing a suspected allergen on a lightly scratched area of the skin. If a wheal forms within 15 minutes, allergy to the substance is indicated.

screamer's nodule. See **vocal cord nodule.**

screen memory, a consciously tolerable memory that replaces one that is emotionally painful to recall.

screening, 1. a preliminary procedure, such as a test or examination, to detect the most characteristic sign or signs of a disorder that may require further investigation. **2.** the examination of a large sample of a population to detect a specific disease or disorder, such as hypertension.

screw clamp, a device, usually made of plastic, equipped with a screw that can be manipulated to close and open the primary intravenous tubing for regulating the flow of intravenous solution.

Scribner shunt {Belding S. Scribner, American physician, b. 1921}, a type of arteriovenous bypass, used in haemodialysis, consisting of a special tube connection outside the body.

scripting, a technique of family therapy involving the development of new family transactional patterns.

scrotal cancer, an epidermoid malignancy

of the scrotum, characterized initially by a small sore that may ulcerate. The lesion occurs most frequently in elderly men who have been exposed to soot, pitch, crude oil, mineral oils, polycyclic hydrocarbons or arsenic fumes from copper smelting. In the eighteenth century, Sir Percival Pott associated scrotal cancer in chimney sweeps with exposure to soot. It is the first malignancy shown to be caused by an environmental carcinogen.

scrotal raphe, a line of union of the two halves of the scrotum. It is generally more highly pigmented than the surrounding tissue.

scrotal tongue, a non-pathological condition in which the tongue is deeply furrowed and resembles the surface of the scrotum.

scrotum, the pouch of skin containing the testes and parts of the spermatic cords. It is divided on the surface into two lateral portions by a ridge that continues ventrally to the undersurface of the penis and dorsally along the middle line of the perineum to the anus. The two layers of the scrotum are the skin and dartos tunic. The skin is very thin, it has a brownish colour and is usually wrinkled. It is supplied with sebaceous follicles that secrete a substance with a characteristic odour and has thinly scattered, kinky hairs with roots that are visible through the skin. The dartos tunic is composed of a thin layer of unstriated muscular fibres around the base of the scrotum, continuous with the two layers of the superficial fascia of the groin and perineum. The tunic projects an internal septum that divides the pouch into two cavities for the testes, extending between the scrotal ridge and root of the penis. **scrotal,** *adj.*

scrub nurse, a registered nurse or operating room technician who assists surgeons during operations.

scrub room, a special hospital area where surgeons and surgical teams use disposable sterile brushes and bactericidal soaps to wash and scrub their fingernails, hands, and forearms before performing or assisting in surgical operations.

scrub typhus, an acute, febrile disease of Asia, India, northern Australia and the western Pacific islands, caused by several strains of the genus *Rickettsia tsutsugamushi* and transmitted from infected rodents to humans by mites. The clinical course is characterized by a necrotic papule or black eschar at the site of the lesion caused by the bite of the small arachnid. Tender, enlarged regional lymph nodes, fever, severe headache, eye pain, muscle aches and a generalized rash usually occur. In severe cases, the myocardium and central nervous system may be involved.

scrub. See **surgical scrub.**

scrubbed team members, surgeons and physicians, nurses and technicians who are scrubbed for surgical procedures in a sterile environment.

scruple, a measure of weight in the apothecaries' system, equal to 20 grains or 1.296 g.

sculpting, a technique of family therapy involving construction of a live family portrait that depicts family alliances and conflicts.

scultetus bandage {Johann Schultes, German surgeon, b. 1595}, a many-tailed bandage with an attached central piece. The tails are overlapped; the last two tied or pinned act to secure the others. A scultetus bandage may be opened or removed without moving the bandaged part of the body.

scurvy, a condition resulting from lack of ascorbic acid in the diet. It is characterized by weakness, anaemia, oedema, spongy gums, often with ulceration and loosening of teeth, a tendency to mucocutaneous haemorrhage and induration of the leg muscles.

SD, abbreviation for **standard deviation.**

Se, symbol for **selenium.**

sealed source, (in brachytherapy) a radionuclide which is sealed within a metal container to prevent leakage.

sealer cement, a compound used in filling a root canal. It is applied as a plastic that solidifies after insertion and fills depressions in the surface of the canal.

seal limbs. See **phocomelia.**

seasickness. See **motion sickness.**

seasonal affective disorder (SAD), a mood disorder associated with the shorter days and longer nights of autumn and winter. Symptoms include lethargy, depression and work difficulties. The patients also consume excess amounts of carbohydrates. The symptoms recede in the spring. The condition is associated with the effect of light on melatonin secretion, and is treated with exposure to bright light.

seatworm. See *Enterobius vermicularis.*

sea urchin sting, an injury inflicted by any of a variety of sea urchins. The skin is punctured and some species release venom. A venomous sting is characterized by pain, muscular weakness, numbness around the mouth and dyspnoea..

seawater bath, a bath taken in warm seawater or in saline solution.

sebaceous, fatty, oily or greasy, usually referring to the oil-secreting glands of the skin or their secretions.

sebaceous cyst, a misnomer for epidermoid cyst or pilar cyst.

sebaceous gland, one of several small sacculated organs in the dermis. They are located throughout the body in close association with all types of body hair but are especially abundant in the scalp, face, anus, nose, mouth and external ear. Each gland consists of a single duct that emerges from a cluster of oval alveoli. Each alveolus is composed of a transparent basement membrane enclosing epithelial cells. The ducts from most sebaceous glands open into the hair follicles but some open onto the surface of the skin. The sebum secreted by the glands oils hair and surrounding skin helps prevent evaporation of sweat and aids in the retention of body heat.

seborrheic dermatitis, a common, chronic, inflammatory skin disease characterized by dry or moist, greasy scales and yellowish crusts. Common sites are the scalp, eyelids, face, external surfaces of the ears, axillae, breasts, groin and gluteal folds. In acute stages there may be exudate and infection resulting in secondary furunculosis. In some people seborrhoeic dermatitis is associated with paralysis agitans, diabetes mellitus, malabsorption disorders, epilepsy or an allergic reaction to gold or arsenic. Types of seborrhoeic dermatitis include **cradle cap, dandruff** and **seborrhoeic blepharitis.**

seborrhoea, any of several common skin conditions in which there is an overproduction of sebum resulting in excessive oiliness or dry scales. **seborrhoeic,** *adj.*

seborrhoeic blepharitis, a form of seborrhoeic dermatitis in which the eyelids are erythematous and the margins are covered with a granular crust.

seborrhoeic keratosis, a benign, well circumscribed, slightly raised, tan to black, warty lesion of the skin of the face, neck, chest or upper back. The macules are loosely covered with a greasy crust that leaves a raw pulpy base when removed. Itching is common.

sebum, the oily secretion of the sebaceous glands of the skin, composed of keratin, fat and cellular debris. Combined with sweat, sebum forms a moist, oily, acidic film that is mildly antibacterial and antifungal and protects the skin against drying.

Seckel's syndrome. See **bird headed dwarf.**

seclusion, (in psychiatric nursing) the isolation of a patient in a special room to decrease stimuli that might be causing or exacerbating the patient's emotional distress.

second cuneiform bone. See **intermediate cuneiform bone.**

second filial generation. See **F2.**

second intention. See **intention.**

second messenger, a chemical substance inside a cell that carries information along the signal pathway from the internal portion of a membrane-spanning receptor embedded in the cell membrane.

second nerve. See **optic nerve.**

second opinion, a patient privilege of requesting an examination and evaluation of a health condition by a second physician to verify or challenge the diagnosis by a first physician.

second sight. See **senopia.**

second-order change, a change that changes

the system itself.

second-order kinetics, a chemical reaction in which the rate of the reaction is determined by the concentration of two chemical entities involved.

secondary, second in importance or in incidence, or belonging to the second order of sophistication or development, such as a secondary healthcare facility or secondary education.

secondary amenorrhoea. See **amenorrhoea.**

secondary amputation, amputation performed after suppuration has begun following severe trauma.

secondary amyloidosis. See **amyloidosis.**

secondary analysis, the study of a problem using previously compiled data.

secondary apnoea, an abnormal condition in which respiration is absent and will not begin again spontaneously. Secondary apnoea may result from any event that severely impedes the absorption of oxygen into the bloodstream.

secondary areola, a second ring appearing around the areola of the breast during pregnancy that is more pigmented than the areola before pregnancy.

secondary biliary cirrhosis, an abnormal hepatic condition characterized by obstruction of the bile duct with or without infection.

secondary bronchus, a lobar or segmental bronchus.

secondary care, 1. the provision of a specialized medical service by a specialist or hospital on referral by a primary care doctor. **2.** the retardation of an existing illness or other pathological condition.

secondary dementia, dementia resulting from another, concurrent form of psychosis.

secondary dental caries, dental caries developing in a tooth already affected by the condition; often a new cavity forms adjacent to, or beneath, the restorative filling of an old cavity.

secondary dentition. See **permanent dentition.**

secondary diabetes. See other types of diabetes.

secondary fissure, a fissure between the uvula and the pyramid of the cerebellum.

secondary fracture. See **neoplastic fracture.**

secondary gain, an indirect benefit, usually obtained through an illness or debility. Such gains may include monetary and disability benefits, personal attentions, or escape from unpleasant situations and responsibilities.

secondary healthcare, an intermediate level of healthcare that includes diagnosis and treatment, performed in a hospital having specialized equipment and laboratory facilities.

secondary host. See **intermediate host.**

secondary hypertension, elevated blood pressure associated with several primary diseases, such as renal, pulmonary, endocrine, and vascular diseases. See **hypertension.**

secondary hypertrophic osteoarthropathy. See **clubbing.**

secondary infection, an infection by a micro-organism that follows an initial infection by another kind of organism.

secondary memory device, a peripheral computer device outside the internal memory, used for storage of computer programmes and data.

secondary nutrient, a substance that acts as a stimulant to activate the flora of the GI tract to synthesize other nutrients.

secondary occlusal traumatism, occlusal stress that affects previously weakened periodontal structures.

secondary port, a control device for regulating the flow of a primary and a secondary intravenous solution. It consists of a Y-shaped plastic apparatus that attaches to the primary intravenous tubing and allows the primary and secondary intravenous solutions to flow separately or flow simultaneously.

secondary postpartum haemorrhage, haemorrhage occurring later than 24 hours after delivery, until up to 6 weeks after birth. It is most often caused by retained fragments of the placenta, a laceration of the cervix or vagina that was not discovered or was not completely sutured, or by subinvolution of the placental site within the uterus.

secondary prevention, a level of preventive medicine that focuses on early diagnosis, use of referral services, and rapid initiation of treatment to stop the progress of disease processes or a debilitating disorder.

secondary process, a form of thought process, hypothesized in phsychoanalytic theory to develop as the child learns to use language; it is characterized by the use of grammar and logic. See **primary process.**

secondary proximal renal tubular acidosis. See **proximal renal tubular acidosis.**

secondary radiation, radiation produced following the interaction of the primary radiation with matter. It includes **scattered radiation, characteristic radiation, annihilation radiation** and **secondary electrons.**

secondary radiation grid, (in radiography) a device consisting of parallel lead strips placed in front of the x-ray cassette during an exposure, to prevent scattered radiation reaching the x-ray film and degrading the image.

secondary relationships, relationships with those who provide or accept services, or with acquaintances and friends, as distinguished from family members and intimate friends.

secondary sequestrum, a piece of dead bone that partially separates from sound bone during the process of necrosis but may be pushed back into position.

secondary sex characteristic, any of the external physical characteristics of sexual maturity secondary to hormonal stimulation that develops in the maturing individual.

secondary shock, a state of physical collapse and prostration caused by numerous traumatic and pathological conditions. It develops over a period of time after severe tissue damage and may merge with primary shock, accompanied by various signs, such as weakness, restlessness, low body temperature, low blood pressure, cold sweat and reduced urinary output. Blood pressure drops progressively in this state, and death may occur within a relatively short time after onset unless appropriate treatment intervenes. Secondary shock is often associated with heat stroke, crushing injuries, myocardial infarction, poisoning, fulminating infections, burns and other life-threatening conditions. The pathology of this state reflects changes in the capillaries, which become dilated and engorged with blood.

secondary thrombocytosis. See **thrombocytosis.**

secrete, to discharge a substance into a cavity, vessel or organ or onto the surface of the skin, such as a gland.   **secretion,** *n.*

secretin, a digestive hormone produced by certain cells lining the duodenum and jejunum when fatty acids of partially digested food enter the intestine from the stomach. It stimulates the pancreas to produce a fluid high in salts but low in enzymes.

secretin test, a test of pancreatic function after stimulation with a hormone, secretin. The test measures the volume and bicarbonate concentration of pancreatic secretions.

secretory duct, (of a gland) a small duct that has a secretory function and joins with an excretory duct.

secretory phase, the phase of menstrual cycle after the release of an ovum from a mature ovarian follicle. The corpus luteum secretes progesterone, which stimulates the development of the glands and arteries of the endometrium, causing it to become thick and spongy. In a negative feedback response to the increased level of progesterone in the blood, the secretion of LH from the pituitary decreases.

secretory piece, a polypeptide chain attached to an IgA molecule. The secretory piece is necessary for secretion of the immunoglobulin molecule into mucosal spaces.

sectional arch wire, a wire attached to only a few teeth, usually on one side of a dental arch or in the anterior segment of the arch to cause or guide orthodontic tooth movement.

security operations, (in psychology) mechanisms described by Sullivan, such as apathy and selective inattention, that are defences against recognizing or experiencing anxiety.

sedation, an induced state of quiet, calmness or sleep, such as by means of a sedative or hypnotic medication.

sedative, 1. of or pertaining to a substance, procedure or measure that has a calming effect. **2.** an agent that decreases activity, diminishes irritability and allays excitement.

sedative bath, the immersion of the body in water for a prolonged period of time, used especially as a calming procedure for agitated patients.

sedative-hypnotic, a drug that depresses reversibly the activity of the central nervous system. It is used primarily for inducing sleep and allaying anxiety. Barbiturates and many non-barbiturate sedative-hypnotics with diverse chemical and pharmacological properties share the ability to depress the activity of all excitable tissue, but the arousal centre in the brainstem is especially sensitive to their effects. Various sedative-hypnotics are used in the treatment of insomnia, acute convulsive conditions and anxiety states, and also for facilitating the induction of anaesthesia.

sedimentation rate. See **erythrocyte sedimentation rate.**

segmental bronchus, a bronchus branching from a lobar bronchus to a bronchiole.

segmental fracture, a bone break in which several large bone fragments separate from the main body of a fractured bone. The ends of such fragments may pierce the skin, as in an open fracture, or remain contained within the skin, as in a closed fracture.

segmental resection, a surgical procedure in which a part of an organ, gland or other part of the body is excised; for example, segmental resection of part of an ovary performed to diminish the hormonal secretion of the gland by decreasing the amount of secretory tissue in the gland.

segmentation, 1. the repetition of structured parts or the process of dividing into segments or similar parts, such as the formation of somites or metameres. **2.** the division of the zygote into blastomeres; cleavage.

segmentation cavity. See **blastocoele.**

segmentation cell. See **blastomere.**

segmentation method, a technique for filling tooth root canals in which a preselected gutta-percha cone is cut into segments and the tip section is sealed into the apex of a root. The other sections are usually warmed and condensed against the first piece with a plugger.

segmentation nucleus, the nucleus of the zygote resulting from the fusion of the male and female pronuclei in the fertilized ovum. It is the final stage in fertilization.

segmented hyalinizing vasculitis, a chronic, relapsing inflammatory condition of the blood vessels of the lower legs, associated with nodular or purpuric skin lesions that may become ulcerated and leave scars.

segmented neutrophil, a neutrophil with a filament between the lobes of its nucleus.

segregation, (in genetics) a principle stating that the pairs of chromosomes bearing genes derived from both parents are separated during meiosis. Chance alone determines which gene, maternal or paternal, will travel to which gamete.

seizure, a sudden, violent involuntary series of contractions of a group of muscles that may be paroxysmal and episodic, as in a seizure disorder, or transient and acute, for instance after a head concussion. A seizure may be clonic or tonic, focal, unilateral or bilateral.

seizure threshold, the amount of stimulus necessary to produce a convulsive seizure. All humans can have seizures if there is sufficient provocation.

selection, 1. the act or product of choosing. **2.** (in genetics) the process by which various factors or mechanisms determine and modify the reproductive ability of a genotype within a specific population, thus influencing evolutionary change. Kinds of selection are **artificial selection, natural selection** and **sexual selection.**

selective abstraction, a type of cognitive distortion in which focus on one aspect of an event negates all other aspects.

selective angiography, a radiographic technique for visualizing a selected vessel, following introduction of a radiopaque contrast medium via a percutaneous catheter.

selective grinding, any modification of the occlusal forms of teeth, produced by corrective grinding at selected places to improve occlusion and tooth function.

selective inattention, the screening out of unwanted stimuli, particularly the part of a message the listener does not want to hear.

selectivity, the capacity factor ratios of two substances measured under identical chromatographic conditions.

selectivity coefficient, the degree to which an ion-selective electrode (ISE) responds to a particular ion with respect to a reference ion.

selenium (Se), a metalloid element of the sulphur group. Its atomic number is 34 and its atomic weight is 78.96. Selenium occurs as a trace element in foods, and research continues to determine the most effective daily allowances for different age groups.

selenium sulfide, an antifungal and antiseborrhoeic used for the management of dandruff and seborrhoeic dermatitis of the scalp.

self, *pl.* **selves, 1.** the total essence or being of a person; the individual. **2.** those affective, cognitive and spiritual qualities that distinguish one person from another; individuality. **3.** a person's awareness of his or her own being or identity; consciousness; ego.

self-actualization, (in humanistic psychology) the fundamental tendency towards the maximum realization and fulfilment of one's human potential.

self-alien. See **ego-dystonic.**

self-alienation. See **depersonalization.**

self-anaesthesia, the self-administered inhalational anaesthesia in which whiffs of anaesthetic gas are inhaled from a hand-operated breathing device controlled by the patient.

self-breast examination (SBE), a procedure in which a woman examines her breasts and their accessory structures for evidence of change that could indicate a malignant process. This is usually performed 1 week to 10 days after the first day of the menstrual cycle, when the breasts are smallest and cyclic nodularity is least apparent. The techniques are similar to those of the examination of the breast as performed in the health assessment or physical examination.

self-care, 1. the personal and medical care carried out by the patient, usually in collaboration with, and following instruction by, a medical professional. **2.** medical care provided by laypersons to their families, friends and themselves, including identification and evaluation of symptoms, medication and treatment. **3.** personal care accomplished without technical assistance, such as eating, washing, dressing, using the telephone, attending to one's own elimination, appearance and hygiene. The goal of rehabilitation medicine is maximal personal self-care.

self-care deficit, bathing/hygiene, a person's impaired ability to perform or complete personal bathing and hygiene activities. Defining characteristics include an inability to wash the body or parts of the body, an inability to obtain or reach water for bathing, and an inability to regulate water temperature or flow.

self-care deficit, dressing/grooming, a person's impaired ability to perform or complete personal dressing and grooming activities. Defining characteristics include an impaired ability to put on or remove necessary items of clothing, an impaired ability to fasten clothing, obtain or replace articles of clothing and maintain a satisfactory appearance.

self-care deficit, feeding, a person's impaired ability to perform or complete personal feeding activities. The major defining characteristic is an inability to bring food from a receptacle to the mouth.

self-care deficit, toileting, a person's impaired ability to perform or complete personal toileting activities. Defining characteristics include an inability to reach the toilet or commode, sit or rise from the toilet or commode, remove or put on the necessary clothing and perform the usual toilet hygiene.

self-care theory, a model used to provide a conceptual framework for nursing care directed towards self-care by the patient to the greatest degree possible. The model requires an assessment of the patient's capability for self-care and need for care.

self-catheterization, a procedure performed by a patient to empty the bladder and prevent it from becoming overdistended with urine. The patient who cannot empty the bladder completely but can retain urine for 2 to 4 hours at a time can be taught self-catheterization if he or she is willing to learn and has some manual dexterity and the ability to palpate the bladder.

self-concept, the composite of ideas, feelings and attitudes that a person has about his own identity, worth, capabilities and limitations.

self-confrontation, a technique for behaviour modification that depends on a patient's recognition of and dissatisfaction with inconsistencies in his or her own values, beliefs and behaviours, or between his or her own personal system and that of a significant other.

self-conscious, 1. the state of being aware of oneself as an individual entity that experiences, desires and acts. **2.** a heightened awareness of oneself and one's actions as reflected by the observations and reactions of others; socially ill at ease. **self-consciousness,** *n.*

self-destructive behaviour, any behaviour, either direct or indirect, that if uninterrupted, will ultimately lead to the death of the individual.

self-diagnosis, the diagnosis of one's own health problems, usually without direction or assistance from a physician.

self-differentiation, specialization and diversification of a tissue or part resulting solely from intrinsic factors.

self-disclosure, the process by which one person lets his or her inner being, thoughts and emotions be known to another. This is important for psychological growth in individual and group psychotherapy.

self-esteem, chronic low, a long-standing negative self-evaluation and negative feelings about the self or self-capabilities. Defining characteristics include self-negating verbalization, expression of shame or guilt, evaluation of self as unable to deal with events, rejection of positive feedback, exaggeration of negative feedback, hesitation to try new situations, frequent lack of success in the work environment or social life, being over-conforming and dependent on others' opinions, being non-assertive, indecisive and excessively seeking reassurance.

self-esteem, situational low, a negative self-evaluation with feelings towards the self that develop in response to a loss or change in an individual who previously had a positive self-evaluation. Defining characteristics include an episodic occurrence of negative self-appraisal in response to life events, verbalization of negative feelings about the self, such as helplessness or uselessness, self-negating verbalizations, expression of shame or guilt, evaluation of oneself as unable to handle situations or events, and difficulty in making decisions.

self-esteem, the degree of worth and competence one attributes to oneself.

self-esteem disturbance, a negative self-evaluation and negative feelings towards the self or self-capabilities, which may be expressed directly or indirectly. Defining characteristics include self-negating verbalization, expressions of shame or guilt, evaluation of self as unable to deal with events, rationalization or rejection of positive feedback, exaggeration of negative feedback, hesitation to try new situations, denial of problems obvious to others, projection of blame or responsibility for problems on others, rationalization of personal failures, hypersensitivity to slight or criticism and grandiose behaviour.

self-fulfilling prophecy, a principle that states that a belief in or the expectation of a particular resolution is a factor that contributes to its fulfilment.

self-help group, a group of people who meet to improve their health through discussion and special activities. Characteristically, self-help groups are not led by a professional.

self-ideal, a perception of how one should behave, based on personal standards. The standard may be either a carefully constructed image of the kind of person one would like to be, or a number of aspirations one would like to achieve.

self-image, the total concept, idea or mental image that a person has for oneself and his or her role in society; the person one believes oneself to be.

self-imposed guilt, a restrictive type of guilt that the individual is aware of and from which he or she is unable to break free.

self-limited, (of a disease or condition) tending to end without treatment.

self-management approach, a treatment approach in which patients assume responsibility for their behaviour, changing their environment and planning their future.

self-other, a concept that characterizes persons believing that sources of power are within the self, as opposed to those who believe that the source of power is in others.

self-radiolysis, a process in which a compound is damaged by radioactive decay products originating in an atom within the compound.

self-responsibility, a concept of holistic health by which individuals assume responsibility for their own health.

self-retaining catheter, an indwelling urinary catheter that has a double lumen. One channel allows urine to drain from the bladder into a collecting bag; the other channel has a balloon at the bladder end and a diaphragm at the other end. Several centimetres of air or sterile water are injected through the diaphragm to fill the balloon in the bladder and hold the catheter in place.

self-system, the organization of experiences that acts as a protective mechanism against anxiety.

self-theory, a personality theory that uses one's self-concept in integrating the function and organization of the personality.

self-threading pin, a threaded pin screwed into a hole drilled in tooth dentine to improve the retention of a restoration.

self-transcendence, the ability to focus attention on doing something for the sake of others, as opposed to self-actualization in which doing something for oneself is an end goal.

sella turcica, a transverse depression crossing the midline on the superior surface of the body of the sphenoid bone, and containing the pituitary gland.

SEM. See **scanning electron microscope.**

semen, the thick, whitish secretion of the male reproductive organs discharged from the urethra on ejaculation. It contains various constituents, including spermatozoa in their nutrient plasma and secretions of the prostate, seminal vesicles and various other glands. **seminal,** *adj.*

semi-Fowler's position {George R. Fowler}, placement of the patient in an inclined position, with the upper half of the body raised by elevating the head of the bed.

semicircular canal, any of three bony, fluid-filled loops in the osseous labyrinth of the internal ear, associated with the sense of balance.

semicircular duct, one of three ducts that make up the membranous labyrinth of the inner ear.

semicoma. See **coma.**

semiconductor, a solid crystalline substance whose electrical conductivity is intermediate between that of a conductor and an insulator. An **n-type semiconductor** has loosely bound electrons that are relatively free to move inside the material. A **p-type semiconductor** has holes, or positive traps, in which electrons may be bound. The holes may be free to migrate through the material.

semifixed feature space, (in psychology) objects in the environment, such as furniture, that have some degree of mobility.

semilunar bone. See **lunate bone.**

semilunar valve, 1. a valve with half-moon-shaped cusps, such as the aortic valve and the pulmonary valve. **2.** any one of the cusps constituting such a valve.

semimembranosus, one of three posterior femoral muscles. The tendon of insertion forms one of the two medial hamstrings. The functions of the muscle are flexion and medial rotation of the leg and extension of the thigh.

seminal duct, any duct through which semen passes, such as the vas deferens or the ejaculatory duct.

seminal fluid test, any of several tests of semen to detect abnormalities in a male reproductive system and determine fertility. Some common factors considered are seminal fluid liquefaction time, spermatic quantity, morphology, motility, volume and pH.

seminal fluid. See **semen.**

seminal vesicle, either of the paired, sac-like glandular structures that lie behind the urinary bladder in the male and function as part of the reproductive system. The seminal vesicles produce a fluid that is added to the secretion of the testes and other glands, forming the semen.

seminal vesiculitis, inflammation of a seminal vesicle.

seminarcosis. See **twilight sleep.**

semination, the introduction of semen into the female genital tract.

seminiferous, transporting or producing semen, such as the tubules of the testis.

seminoma, *pl.* **seminomas, seminomata,** a malignant tumour of the testis. It is the most common testicular tumour and is believed to arise from the seminiferous epithelium of the mature or maturing testis.

semipermeable membrane, a membrane barrier to the passage of substances above a specific size, but which allows the movement through the membrane of substances below that size.

semirecumbent, a reclining position.

semitendinosus, one of three posterior femoral muscles of the thigh. Its functions are leg flexion and medial rotation, and extension of the thigh.

semustine, a cytotoxic nitrosurea compound used in the treatment of Lewis lung carcinoma, brain tumours, malignant melanoma and Hodgkin's disease. It is not commercially available in the UK.

sender, (in communication theory) the person by whom a message is encoded and sent.

senescent, ageing or growing old. **senescence,** *n.*

Sengstaken-Blakemore tube {Robert W. Sengstaken, American neurosurgeon, b. 1923; Arthur H. Blakemore, American surgeon, b. 1987}, a thick catheter having a triple lumen and two balloons, used to produce pressure to arrest haemorrhage from oesophageal varices. Attached to a tube, one balloon is blown up in the stomach and exerts pressure against the upper orifice. Sim-

ilarly attached, another balloon exerts pressure on the walls of the oesophagus. The third tube is used for withdrawing gastric contents.

senile, pertaining to, or characteristic of, old age or the process of ageing, especially the physical or mental deterioration accompanying ageing. **senescent,** *adj.,* **senility,** *n.*

senile angioma. See **cherry angioma.**

senile cataract, a kind of cataract, associated with ageing, in which a hard opacity forms in the nucleus of the lens of the eye.

senile delirium, disorientation and mental feebleness associated with extreme age. It is characterized by restlessness, insomnia, aimless wandering and, less commonly, hallucination.

senile dementia. See **senile psychosis.**

senile dental caries, tooth decay occurring at an advanced age. Senile dental caries is usually characterized by cavity formation in or around the cementum layer and root surfaces.

senile involution, a pattern of retrograde changes occurring with advancing age and resulting in the progressive shrinking and degeneration of tissues and organs.

senile keratosis. See **actinic keratosis.**

senile nanism, dwarfism associated with progeria.

senile psychosis, an organic mental disorder of the aged, resulting from the generalized atrophy of the brain with no evidence of cerebrovascular disease. Symptoms include loss of memory, impaired judgment, decreased moral and aesthetic values, inability to think abstractly, periods of confusion, confabulation and irritability, all of which may range from mild to severe.

senile wart. See **actinic keratosis.**

senna, the dried leaflets of pods of *Cassia acutifolia,* or *Cassia augustifolia,* or a standardized formula prepared from them, used as a laxative.

senopia, an improvement in the near vision of the elderly, caused by the myopia associated with increasing lenticular nuclear sclerosis.

sensate focus technique, a therapeutic programme for the treatment of erectile dysfunction in males.

sensation, 1. a feeling, impression or awareness of a bodily state or condition that results from the stimulation of a sensory receptor site and transmission of the nerve impulse along an afferent fibre to the brain. Kinds of sensation include **delayed sensation, epigastric sensation, primary sensation, referred sensation** and **subjective sensation. 2.** a feeling or awareness of a mental or emotional state, which may or may not result in response to an external stimulus.

sense, 1. the faculty by which stimuli are perceived and conditions outside and within the body are distinguished and evaluated.

The major senses are sight, hearing, smell, taste, touch and pressure. Other senses include hunger, thirst, pain, temperature, proprioception, spatial, time and visceral sensations. **2.** the ability to feel; a sensation. **3.** the capacity to understand; normal mental ability. **4.** to perceive through a sense organ.

sensible perspiration, loss of fluid from the body through the secretory activity of the sweat glands in a quantity sufficient to be observed.

sensitive volume, (in magnetic resonance imaging) the region of the object from which an MRI signal will be acquired preferentially, because of strong magnetic field inhomogeneity elsewhere.

sensitivity, 1. capacity to feel, transmit or react to a stimulus. **2.** susceptibility to a substance, such as a drug or antigen. **sensitive,** *adj.*

sensitivity test, a laboratory method for testing the effectiveness of antibiotics. It is usually done on organisms known to be potentially resistant to antibiotic therapy in vitro. A report of "resistant" means that the antibiotic is not effective in inhibiting the growth of a pathogen, whereas use of an effective antibiotic results in a "sensitive" report.

sensitization, 1. an acquired reaction in which specific antibodies develop in response to an antigen. This is deliberately caused in immunization by injecting a disease-causing organism that has been altered in such a way that it is no longer infectious yet remains capable of causing the production of antibodies to fight the disease. **2.** a photodynamic method of destroying microorganisms by inserting into a solution substances, such as fluorescing dyes, that absorb visible light and emit energy at wavelengths destructive to the organism. **3.** *nontechnical*, anaphylaxis. **sensitize,** *v.*

sensitized, pertaining to tissues that have been made susceptible to antigenic substances.

sensorimotor phase, the developmental phase of childhood, encompassing the period from birth to 2 years of age, according to piagetian psychology.

sensorimotor therapy, a kind of therapy designed to enhance the integration of reflex phenomena and emergence of voluntary motor behaviours, concerned with posture and locomotion.

sensorineural hearing loss, a form of hearing loss in which sound is conducted through the external and middle ear in a normal way but a defect in the inner ear results in its distortion, making discrimination difficult.

sensorium, (in psychology) the part of the consciousness that includes the special sensory perceptive powers and their central correlation and integration in the brain. A clear sensorium conveys the presence of a reasonably accurate memory together with a correct orientation for time, place, and person.

sensory apraxia. See **ideational apraxia.**

sensory deficit, a defect in the function of one or more of the senses.

sensory discrimination, the ability to distinguish specific characteristics of a sensation, such as one versus two points of pressure on the skin.

sensory integration, the organization of sensory input for use, a perception of the body or environment, an adaptive response, a learning process, or the development of some neural function.

sensory integrative dysfunction, a disorder or irregularity in brain function that makes sensory integration difficult. Many learning disorders stem form sensory integrative dysfunctions.

sensory integrative therapy, therapy that involves sensory stimulation and adaptive responses to it, according to a child's neurological needs. Treatment usually involves full body movements that provide vestibular, proprioceptive and tactile stimulation. The goal is to improve the ability of the brain to process and organize sensations.

sensory nerve, a nerve consisting of afferent fibres that conduct sensory impulses from the periphery of the body to the brian or spinal cord via the dorsal spinal roots. Compare motor nerve.

sensory-based language, the use of nonverbal behaviour in neurolinguistic communication. Examples include puzzled expressions and finger-pointing.

sensory-perceptual overload, a state in which the volume and intensity of various stimuli overcome the ability of the individual to discriminate among the varying stimuli.

sensory/perceptual alterations (visual, auditory, kinaesthetic, gustatory, tactile, olfactory), a change in the amount or patterns of incoming stimuli accompanied by a diminished, exaggerated, distorted or impaired response to such stimuli. Defining characteristics include disorientation, change in the ability to abstract, conceptualize or solve problems, change in behaviour and sensory acuity, restlessness, irritability, inappropriate response to stimuli, lack of concentration, rapid mood changes and exaggerated emotional responses, non-compliance, motor incoordination, hallucination, complaints of fatigue, changes in posture and muscular tension, and inappropriate responses.

sentinel node. See **Virchow's node.**

SEP, abbreviation for somatosensory evoked potential.

separation anxiety, fear and apprehension caused by separation from familiar surroundings and significant persons. The syndrome may occur in an infant when separated from its mother or from its mothering figure, or when it is approached by a stranger.

separation factor. See **selectivity.**

separator, an instrument for wedging teeth apart, used in the examination of proximal tooth surfaces and in finishing proximal restorations.

sepsis, infection, contamination. **septic,** *adj.*

septal defect, an abnormal, usually congenital defect in the wall separating two chambers of the heart. Oxygenated and deoxygenated blood mix, causing a decrease in the amount of oxygen carried in the blood to the peripheral tissues. Kinds of septal defects are **atrial septal defect** and **ventricular septal defect.**

septate, pertaining to a structure divided by a septum.

septic abortion, spontaneous or induced termination of a pregnancy in which the life of the mother may be threatened because of invasion of germs into the endometrium, myometrium and beyond, requiring immediate and intensive care, massive antibiotic therapy, evacuation of the uterus and often emergency hysterectomy, in order to prevent death from overwhelming infection and septic shock.

septicaemia, systemic infection in which pathogens are present in the circulating bloodstream, having spread from an infection in any part of the body. Characteristically, septicaemia causes fever, chill, prostration, pain, headache, nausea or diarrhoea. **septicaemic,** *adj.*

septicaemic plague, a rapidly fatal form of bubonic plague in which septicaemia with meningitis occur before buboes have had time to form.

septic arthritis, an acute form of arthritis. It is characterized by bacterial inflammation of a joint caused by the spread of bacteria through the bloodstream from an infection elsewhere in the body, or by contamination of a joint during trauma or surgery. The joint is stiff, painful, tender, warm and swollen.

septic fever, an elevation of body temperature associated with infection by pathogenic micro-organisms or in response to a toxin secreted by a micro-organism.

septic shock, a form of shock that occurs in septicaemia when endotoxins are released from certain bacteria in the bloodstream. The endotoxins cause decreased vascular resistance, resulting in a drastic fall in blood pressure. Fever, tachycardia, increased respirations and confusion or coma may also occur. Septic shock is usually preceded by signs of severe infection, often of the genitourinary or gastrointestinal system. Kings of septic shock include **toxic shock syndrome** and **bacteraemic shock.**

septostomy, surgical formation of an opening in a septum.

septum, septa, a partition, such as the interauricular septum that separates the atria of the heart.

sequela, *pl.* **sequelae,** any abnormal condition that follows and is the result of a disease, treatment or injury, such as paralysis following poliomyelitis.

sequential imaging, (in radionuclide imaging) a diagnostic procedure in which a series of closely timed images of the rapidly changing distribution of an administered radioactive tracer are used to determine a physiological process or precesses within the body.

sequential line imaging, (in magnetic resonance imaging) techniques in which the image is built up from successive lines through the object.

sequential multiple analysis (SMA), the biochemical examination of various substances in the blood, such as albumin, alkaline phosphatase, bilirubin, calcium, cholesterol and others. A computerized laboratory analyser is used, which produces a printout of measured values of the substances tested.

sequential plane imaging, (in magnetic resonance imaging) a technique in which the image of an object is built up from successive planes in the object.

sequential point imaging, (in magnetic resonance imaging) techniques in which the image is built from successive point positions in the object.

sequester, to detach, separate or isolate, such as a patient sequestered to prevent the spread of an infection.

sequestered antigens theory, a theory of autoimmunity, stressing the relationship between antigen exposure, immunogenic cells and body cells.

sequestered oedema, oedema localized in the tissues surrounding a newly created surgical wound.

sequestrum, *pl.* **sequestra,** a fragment of dead bone that is partially or entirely detached from the surrounding or adjacent healthy bone.

sequestrum forceps, a forceps with small, powerful teeth used for extracting necrotic or sharp fragments of bone from surrounding tissue.

sequoiasis, a type of hypersensitivity pneumonitis common among workers in sawmills where redwood is processed. The antigens are the fungus *Pullalaria pullulans* and species of the genus *Graphium*, found in mouldy redwood sawdust. Characteristics of the acute disease include chills, fever, cough, dyspnoea, anorexia, nausea and vomiting. Symptoms of the chronic disease include productive cough, dyspnoea on exertion, fatigue and weight loss.

Ser, abbreviation for **serine.**

serendipity {Serendip, author Horace Walpole's mythic land of pleasant surprises}, the act of accidental discovery. A number of important medications have evolved through serendipity, such as the discovery of antidepressant activity in a drug originally developed for the treatment of tuberculosis.

serial determination, a laboratory test that is repeated at stated intervals, as in a series of repeated tests for cardiac enzymes in blood samples taken from a patient with suspected myocardial infarction.

serial dilution, a laboratory technique in which a substance, such as blood serum, is decreased in concentration in a series of proportional amounts.

serial extraction, the extraction of selected primary teeth over a period of years. Sometimes it concludes with the removal of the first premolar teeth to relieve crowding of the dental arches during eruption of the lateral incisors, canines and premolars.

serial speech, overlearned speech involving a series of words, such as counting or reciting days of the week.

series, *pl.* **series,** a chain of objects or events arranged in a predictable order, such as the series of stages through which a mature blood cell develops.

serine (Ser), a non-essential amino acid found in many proteins in the body. It is a precursor of the amino acids, glycine and cysteine.

serological diagnosis, a diagnosis that is made through laboratory examination of antigen-antibody reactions in the serum.

serologist, a bacteriologist or medical technologist who prepares or supervises the preparation of sera used to diagnose and treat diseases, and immunize persons against infectious diseases.

serology, the branch of laboratory medicine that studies blood serum for evidence of infection by evaluating antigen-antibody reactions in vitro. **serological,** *adj.*

serosa, any serous membrane, such as the tunica serosa that lines the walls of body cavities and secretes a watery exudate.

serosanguineous, (of a discharge) thin and red; composed of serum and blood. Also **serosanguinous.**

serotonin, a naturally occurring derivative of tryptophan found in platelets and in cells of the brain and intestine. It acts as a potent vasoconstrictor and a neurotransmitter.

serous fluid, a fluid that has the characteristics of serum.

serous membrane, one of the many thin sheets of tissue that line closed cavities of the body, such as the pleura lining the thoracic cavity, the peritoneum lining the abdominal cavity, and the pericardium lining the sac that encloses the heart. Between the visceral layer of serous membrane covering various organs and the parietal layer lining the cavity containing such organs there is a potential space moistened by serous fluid. This fluid reduces the friction of the structures covered by the serous membrane, for example the lungs which move against the thoracic walls in respiration.

serpent ulcer, an ulceration of the skin that heals in one area while extending to another.

Serratia, a genus of motile, gram-negative bacilli capable of causing infection in humans, including bacteraemia, pneumonia and urinary tract infections. *Serratia* organisms are frequently acquired in hospitals.

serratus anterior, a thin muscle of the chest wall extending from the ribs under the arm to the scapula. It acts to rotate the scapula and raise the shoulder, as in full flexion and abduction of the arm.

Sertoli-Leydig cell tumour. See **arrhenoblastoma.**

serum, 1. any serous fluid, especially that moistening the surfaces of serous membranes. 2. any clear, watery fluid that has been separated from its more solid elements, such as the exudate from a blister. 3. the clear, thin and sticky fluid portion of the blood that remains after coagulation. 4. a vaccine or toxoid prepared from the serum of a hyperimmune donor for prophylaxis against a particular infection or poison.

serum albumin, a major protein in blood plasma, important in maintaining the oncotic pressure of the blood.

serum C-reactive protein. See **C-reactive protein.**

serum creatinine level, the concentration of creatinine in the serum, used as a diagnostic sign of possible renal impairment.

serum diagnosis. See **serological diagnosis.**

serum glutamic oxaloacetic transaminase (SGOT), a catalytic enzyme found in various parts of the body, especially the heart, liver and muscle tissue. Increased amounts of the enzyme occur in the serum as a result of myocardial infarction, acute liver disease, the actions of certain drugs, and any disease or condition in which cells are seriously damaged. See also **transaminase.**

serum glutamic pyruvic transaminase (SGPT), a catalytic enzyme normally found in high concentration in the liver. Greater than normal amounts in the serum indicate liver damage.

serum hepatitis. See **hepatitis B.**

serum sickness, an immunological disorder that may occur 2 to 3 weeks after the administration of an antiserum. It is caused by antibody reaction to an antigen in the donor serum, and is characterized by fever, splenomegaly, swollen lymph nodes, skin rash and joint pain.

sesamoid bone, any one of numerous small, round, bony masses embedded in certain tendons that may be subjected to compression and tension. The largest sesamoid bone is the patella, which is embedded in the tendon of the quadriceps femoris at the knee.

sessile, 1. (in biology) attached by a base rather than by a stalk or a peduncle; for instance, a leaf that is attached directly to its stem. 2. permanently connected.

set, a predisposition to behave in a certain way.

setup, 1. an arrangement of teeth on a trial denture base. 2. a laboratory procedure in which teeth are removed from a plaster cast and repositioned in wax. It is used as a diagnostic procedure or to produce a mould for a positioner appliance.

seventh cranial nerve. See **facial nerve.**

Sever's disease. See **calcaneal epiphysitis.**

severe combined immunodeficiency disease (SCID), an abnormal condition characterized by the complete absence or marked deficiency of B cells and T cells, with the consequent lack of humoral immunity and cell-mediated immunity. This disease occurs as an X-linked recessive disorder only in males, and as an autosomal recessive disorder affecting both males and females. It results in a pronounced susceptibility to infection, and is usually fatal. The precise cause of SCID is not known, but research indicates that it may be caused by a cytogenic dysfunction of the embryonic stem cells in differentiating B cells and T cells. Consequently, the affected individual has a very small thymus and little or no protection against infection.

sex, 1. a classification of male or female based on many criteria, among them anatomical and chromosomal characteristics. 2. coitus.

sex chromatin, a densely staining mass within the nucleus of all non-dividing cells of normal mammalian females. It represents the facultative heterochromatin of the inactivated X chromosome.

sex chromosome, a chromosome responsible for the sex determination of offspring; it carries genes that transmit sex-linked traits and conditions. In humans and other mammals there are two distinct sex chromosomes, the X and the Y chromosomes.

sex chromosome mosaic, an individual or organism whose cells contain variant chromosomal numbers involving the X or Y chromosomes. Such variations are found in most of the syndromes associated with sex chromosome aberrations, primarily Turner's syndrome. They may be caused by non-disjunction of the chromosomes during the second meiotic division of gametogenesis, or by some error in chromosome distribution during cell division of the fertilized ovum.

sex factor. See **F factor.**

sex hormones, chemical substances produced in the body, causing specific regulatory effects on the activity of organs of the reproductive system.

sex mosaic. See **sex chromosome mosaic.**

sex role, the expectations held by society regarding types of behaviour that are appropriate or inappropriate for each sex.

sex therapist, a healthcare professional with specialized knowledge, skill and competence in assisting individuals who experience sexual difficulties.

sex therapy, a type of counselling that aids in the resolution of pathological conditions so that a healthy sexuality can be maintained.

sex-controlled. See **sex-influenced.**

sex-influenced, of or pertaining to an autosomal genetic trait or condition, such as patterned baldness or gout, that in one sex is expressed phenotypically in both homozygotes and heterozygotes, whereas in the other sex a phenotypic effect is produced in homozygotes only.

sex-limited, of or pertaining to an autosomal genetic trait or condition expressed phenotypically in only one sex, although the genes for them may be carried by both sexes.

sex-linked, pertaining to genes or to the normal or abnormal characteristics or conditions they transmit. The genes are carried on the sex chromosomes, specifically the X chromosome.

sex-linked disorder, any disease or abnormal condition determined by the sex chromosomes or a defective gene on a sex chromosome. These may involve a deviation in the number of either the X or Y chromosomes, as occurs in Turner's syndrome and Klinefelter's syndrome. Most occurrences are a result of non-disjunction during meiosis.

sex-linked ichthyosis, a congenital skin disorder characterized by large, thick, dry scales that are dark in colou, covering the neck, scalp, ears, face, trunk and flexor surfaces of the body, such as the folds of the arms and back of the knees. It is transmitted by females as an X-linked recessive trait and appears only in males.

sexism, a belief that one sex is superior to the other and that the superior sex has endowments, rights, prerogatives and status greater than those of the inferior sex. sexist, n.

sexual, of or pertaining to sex.

sexual abuse, the sexual mistreatment of another person by fondling, rape or forced participation in unnatural sex acts or other perverted behaviour.

sexual assault, the forcible perpetration of an act of sexual contact on the body of another person, male or female, without his or her consent. Legal criteria vary among different communities.

sexual aversion disorder, a persistent or extreme aversion to or avoidance of all or nearly all genital sexual contact with a partner.

sexual dwarf, an adult dwarf whose genital organs are normally developed.

sexual dysfunction, a state in which a person experiences a change in sexual functions, viewed as unsatisfying, unrewarding, or inadequate. The patient reports a perceived dysfunction, a physical alteration or limitation imposed by disease or treatment, an inability to achieve sexual satisfaction, an alteration in the sexual relationship with the partner, and a change in interest in the self or in others.

sexual fantasy, mental images of an erotic nature that can lead to sexual arousal.

sexual generation, reproduction by the union of male and female gametes.

sexual harassment, an aggressive, sexually motivated act of physical or verbal violation of a person over whom the aggressor has some power. Sexual harassment may be heterosexual or, as is common in prison, homosexual.

sexual history, (in a patient record) the portion of the patient's personal history concerned with sexual function and dysfunction. It may include age at onset of sexual intercourse, the kind and frequency of sexual activity, and the satisfaction derived from it.

sexual intercourse. See **coitus.**

sexual orientation, the clear, persistent desire of a person for affiliation with one sex rather than the other.

sexual psychopath, an individual whose sexual behaviour is openly perverted, antisocial and criminal.

sexual reassignment, a change in the gender identity of a person by legal, surgical, hormonal or social means.

sexual reflex, (in males) a reflex in which tactile or cerebral stimulation results in penile erection, priapism or ejaculation.

sexual response cycle, the four phases of biological sexual response: excitement, plateau, orgasm and resolution.

sexual sadism. See **sadism.**

sexual selection, the theory that mates are chosen according to the attraction or preference for certain characteristics, such as colouration or behaviour patterns, so that eventually only those particular traits appear in succeeding generations.

sexual tasks, specific skills learned in various phases of development in the lifecycle continuum, allowing an adult to function normally in the sexual realm.

sexuality, 1. the sum of the physical, functional and psychological attributes that are expressed by one's gender identity and sexual behaviour, whether or not related to the sex organs or procreation. 2. the genital characteristics that distinguish male from female.

sexuality patterns, altered, an individual's concern regarding his or her sexuality. Defining characteristics include reported difficulties, limitations or changes in sexual behaviours or activities. Related factors include a knowledge or skill deficit about alternative responses to health-related transitions, or altered body functions or structure (illness or medical).

sexually deviant personality, a sexual behaviour that differs significantly from what is considered normal for a society.

sexually transmitted disease (STD), a contagious disease usually acquired by sexual intercourse or genital contact. Historically, the five venereal diseases were gonorrhoea, syphilis, chancroid, granuloma inguinale and lymphogranuloma venereum. Other STDs include scabies, herpes genitalis, anorectal herpes and warts, pediculosis, trichomoniasis, genital candidiasis, molluscum contagiosum, non-specific urethritis, chlamydial infections, cytomegalovirus and AIDS.

SFD, abbreviation for **small for dates.** See **small for gestational age infant.**

SGA, abbreviation for **small for gestational age.** See **small for gestational age infant.**

SGOT, abbreviation for **serum glutamic oxaloacetic transaminase.**

SGPT, abbreviation for **serum glutamic pyruvic transaminase.**

shadow, (in psychology) an archetype that represents the unacceptable aspects and components of behaviour.

shadow cells, red blood cells that have lost their haemoglobin because of exposure to urine.

shadow chart, a copy of the data contained in the permanent patient record, available for use when the information is required but retrieval of the record may be difficult or time-consuming.

shake test, a "foam" test for fetal lung maturity. It is more rapid than determination of the L/S ratio.

shallow breathing, a respiration pattern marked by slow, shallow, and generally ineffective inspirations and expirations. It is usually caused by drugs and indicates depression of the medullary respiratory centres.

shaping, a procedure used for conditioning a person undergoing behaviour therapy to develop new behavioural responses.

shared paranoid disorder, a psychopathological condition characterized by identical manifestations of the same mental disorder, usually ideas, in two closely associated or related persons.

shared services, administrative, clinical or other service functions that are common to two or more hospitals or other healthcare facilities, and are used jointly or cooperatively by them.

Sharpey's fibre {William Sharpey, English

anatomist, b. 1802}, (in dentistry) any one of the many collagenous fibres that blend with the cementum of a tooth.

shaving stroke, a phase of the working stroke of a periodontal curet, used for smoothing or planing a tooth or tooth root surface.

shear, an applied force or pressure exerted against the surface and layers of the skin as tissues slide in opposite but parallel planes.

shearling, a sheepskin placed on a bed to help prevent decubitus ulcers.

sheath, a tubular structure that surrounds an organ or any other part of the body, such as the sheath of the rectus abdominis muscle.

Sheehan's syndrome {Harold L. Sheehan, English pathologist, b. 1900}, a postpartum condition of pituitary necrosis and hypopituitarism after circulatory collapse resulting from uterine haemorrhage.

sheep cell test, a method that mixes human blood cells with the red blood cells of sheep to determine the absence or deficiency of human T-lymphocytes. When mixed with human blood cells, the red blood cells of sheep cluster around the human T-lymphocytes and form characteristic rosettes.

sheet bath, the application of wet sheets to the body, used primarily as an antipyretic procedure.

sheet wadding, stretchable sheets of cotton padding used to cover the skin before a cast is applied. The stretching allows for some extremity oedema without the cast becoming too tight.

shell shock *obsolete,* any of a number of mental disorders, ranging from extreme fear to dementia, resulting from a traumatic reaction to the stress of combat.

shell teeth, a type of dental dysplasia characterized by large pulp chambers, insufficient coronal dentin and usually no roots.

shellfish poisoning, a toxic, neurological condition that results from eating clams, oysters or mussels that have ingested the poisonous protozoa commonly called the "red tide". The characteristic symptoms appear within a few minutes and include nausea, light-headedness, vomiting and tingling or numbness around the mouth, followed by paralysis of the extremities and possibly respiratory paralysis. Saxitoxin, the causative agent, is not destroyed by cooking.

sheltered workshop, a facility or programme, either for outpatients or residents of an institution, that provides vocational experience in a controlled working environment.

shiatsu (acupressure), a type of therapy in which pressure is applied on the acupuncture points for treatments and for giving pain relief. It is unique in that it combines the principles of acupuncture with physical masssage.

shield, (in radiation technology) a device used in radiation protection to reduce exposure to ionizing radiation.

shift, 1. (in nursing) the particular hours of the day during which a nurse is scheduled to work. The evening shift is also called "relief", presumably because nurses originally worked 12-hour shifts and the evening and night shift was thought to be relief for the day nurse. Nurses are said to "work shift" when they work assigned hours. **2.** an abrupt change in an analytical system that continues at the new level.

shift to the left *informal,* a predominance of immature lymphocytes, noted in a differential white blood cell count. The term derives from a graph of blood components in which immature cell frequencies appear on the left side of the graph.

shift to the right, (in haematology) a preponderance of polymorphonuclear neutrophils having three or more lobes, indicating maturity of the cell. It indicates a relative lack of blood-forming activity.

Shigella {Kiyoshi Shiga, Japanese bacteriologist, b. 1870}, a genus of gram-negative pathogenic bacteria that causes gastroenteritis and bacterial dysentery, such as *Shigella dysenteriae.*

shigellosis, an acute bacterial infection of the bowel, characterized by diarrhoea, abdominal pain and fever. It is transmitted by hand-to-mouth contact with the faeces of individuals infected with bacteria of a pathogenic species of the genus *Shigella.* These organisms may be carried in the stools of asymptomatic people for up to several months and may be spread through contact with contaminated objects, food or flies, especially in poor, crowded areas.

shin bone. See **tibia.**

shin splints, a painful condition of the lower leg caused by strain of the long flexor muscle of the toes after strenuous athletic activity, such as running.

shingles. See **herpes zoster.**

Shirodkar's operation, a surgical procedure called a cerclage in which the cervical canal is closed by a purse-string suture embedded in the uterine cervix encircling the canal. It is performed to correct an incompetent cervix that has failed to retain previous pregnancies. If labour begins with the suture in place, the suture is removed promptly or the infant is delivered by caesarean section, before rupture of the uterus occurs.

SHO, abbreviation for **Senior House Officer.**

shock, an abnormal condition of inadequate blood flow to the body's peripheral tissues, with life-threatening cellular dysfunction, hypotension, and oliguria. The condition is usually associated with inadequate cardiac output, changes in peripheral blood flow resistance and distribution, and tissue damage. Causal factors include haemorrhage, vomiting, diarrhoea, inadequate fluid intake or excessive renal loss, resulting in hypovolaemia. The signs and symptoms of different kinds of shock are similar and are related to the condition of hypovolaemia. There is decreased blood flow with a resulting reduction in the delivery of oxygen, nutrients, hormones and electrolytes to the body's tissues and a concomitant decreased removal of metabolic wastes. Pulse and respirations are increased. There may be tachycardia. Blood pressure may decline moderately at first. The patient often shows signs of restlessness and anxiety, an effect related to decreased blood flow to the brain. There may also be weakness, lethargy, pallor and a cool, moist skin. As shock progresses, the body temperature falls, respirations become rapid and shallow, and the pulse pressure (i.e. the difference between systolic and diastolic blood pressures) narrows. Urinary output is reduced. Haemorrhage may be apparent or concealed although other factors, such as vomiting or diarrhoea, may account for the deficiency of body fluids. Kinds of shock include **anaphylactic shock, bacteraemic shock, cardiogenic shock, diabetic shock, electric shock, hypovolaemic shock** and **neurogenic shock**.

shock lung. See **acute respiratory distress syndrome.**

shock trousers, pneumatic trousers designed to counteract hypotension, associated with internal or external bleeding and hypovolemia. Shock trousers may be contraindicated in patients with pulmonary oedema, cardiogenic shock, increased intracranial pressure or eviscerations. The shock trousers are required when the patient loses consciousness, has a decreased or falling blood pressure and shows signs of respiratory distress, such as dyspnoea, rapid breathing, a cough and pink, frothy sputum. The leg pulses may be diminished or absent, and the feet may appear pale, mottled and cold.

short bones, bones that occur in clusters and usually permit movement of the extremities, such as the carpals and tarsals.

short gut syndrome, a congenital disorder in which an infant's intestine is too short or underdeveloped to allow normal food digestion. The child is maintained on parenteral nutrition until the intestine grows or develops further or is replaced by surgical transplant.

short sight. See **myopia.**

short-acting, pertaining to, or characterizing, a therapeutic agent, usually a drug, with a brief period of effectiveness, generally beginning soon after the substance or measure is administered.

short-acting insulin. See **soluble insulin.**

short-arm cast, an orthopaedic cast applied to immobilize the hand or wrist. It is used in treating fractures, for postoperative positioning, and for correction or maintenance of correction of deformities of the hand and wrist.

short-leg cast, an orthopaedic cast used for immobilizing fractures in the lower extremities from the toes to the knee.

short-leg cast with walker, an orthopaedic cast applied to immobilize the lower extremities from the toes to the knee, while allowing the patient to walk by incorporating a rubber walker on the bottom of the cast.

short-PR-normal-QRS syndrome. See **Lown-Ganong-Levine syndrome.**

short-term memory, the definition of this term depends of the theory of memory. It usually refers to recall that is of limited duration.

shotgun therapy *informal,* any treatment that has a wide range of effect and which, therefore, can be expected to correct the abnormal condition even though the particular cause is unknown.

shoulder, the junction of the clavicle and scapula at the point where the arm attaches to the trunk of the body.

shoulder blade. See **scapula.**

shoulder joint, the ball and socket articulation of the humerus with the scapula. The joint includes eight bursae and five ligaments.

shoulder spica cast, an orthopaedic cast applied to immobilize the trunk of the body to the hips, wrist and hand. It is used in the treatment of shoulder dislocations and injuries, or in the positioning and immobilization of the shoulder after surgery.

shoulder subluxation, the separation of the humeral head from the glenoid cavity, resulting in strain on the soft tissues surrounding the joint.

shoulder-hand syndrome, a neuromuscular condition characterized by pain and stiffness in the shoulder and arm, limited joint motion, swelling of the hand, muscle atrophy and decalcification of the underlying bones. The condition occurs most commonly after myocardial infarction but may be associated with other known or unknown causes.

show. See **operculum.**

shreds, glossy filaments of mucus in the urine, indicating inflammation in the urinary tract.

shunt, left to right, a diversion of blood from the left side of the heart to the right, as through a septal defect, or from the systemic to the pulmonary circulation, as from a patent ductus arteriosus.

shunt, 1. to redirect the flow of a body fluid from one cavity or vessel to another. **2.** a tube or device implanted in the body to redirect a body fluid from one cavity or vessel to another.

Shy-Drager syndrome {G. Milton Shy, American neurologist, b. 1919; Glenn A. Drager, American physician, b. 1917}, a rare, progressive neurological disorder characterized by orthostatic hypotension, bladder and bowel incontinence, atrophy of the iris, anhidrosis, tremor, rigidity, incoordination, ataxia and muscle wasting.

SI, abbreviation for **Système International d'Unités,** the French name for the **International System of Units.**

Si, symbol for **silicon.**

SI units, the international units of physical amounts. Examples of these units are the volume of a litre, the length of a metre, or the precise amount of time in a minute. A group of scientists (Comité International des Poids et Mesures) meets regularly to define the units.

SIADH, abbreviation for **syndrome of inappropriate antidiuretic hormone secretion.**

sialadenitis, any inflammation of one or more of the salivary glands.

sialogogue, anything that stimulates the secretion of saliva.

sialography, a radiographic technique for visualizing the parotid or submandibular glands, following introduction of a radiopaque contrast medium into the selected duct. **sialogram,** *n.*, **sialographic,** *adj.*

sialolith, a calculus formed in a salivary gland or duct.

sialolithiasis, a pathological condition in which one or more calculi or stones are formed in a salivary gland.

sialorrhoea, an excessive flow of saliva that may be associated with a variety of conditions, such as acute inflammation of the mouth, mental retardation, mercurialism, pregnancy, teething, alcoholism or malnutrition.

Siamese twins {Chang and Eng, conjoined twins born in Siam (now Thailand) in 1811}, conjoined, equally developed twin fetuses that were produced from the same ovum. The severity of the condition ranges from superficial fusion, as of the umbilical vessels, to that in which the heads or complete torsos are united and several internal organs are shared.

Siberian tick typhus, a mild, acute febrile illness seen in Asia, caused by *Rickettsia siberica,* transmitted by ticks and characterized by a diffuse maculopapular rash, headache, conjunctival inflammation and a small ulcer or eschar at the site of the tick bite.

sibilant rale, an abnormal whistling sound that may emanate from the lungs of an individual with a respiratory disorder or disease. It is caused by the passage of air through a lumen narrowed by the accumulation of mucus or other viscid fluid.

sibling, 1. one of two or more children who have both parents in common; a brother or sister. **2.** of or pertaining to a brother or sister.

sibship, 1. the state of being related by blood. **2.** a group of people descended from a common ancestor who are used as a basis for genetic studies. **3.** brothers and sisters considered as a group.

sick role, a pattern of behaviour in which a person adopts the symptoms of a physical or mental disorder to be cared for, sympathized with and be protected from the demands and stresses of life.

sick sinus syndrome, a complex of syndromes associated with sinus node dysfunction. The condition may result from a variety of cardiac diseases. It is characterized by severe sinus bradycardia alone, sinus bradycardia alternating with tachycardia, or sinus bradycardia with atrioventricular block. The most common symptoms are lethargy, weakness, light-headedness, dizziness and episodes of near syncope to actual loss of consciousness.

sickle cell, an abnormal, crescent-shaped red blood cell containing haemoglobin S, an abnormal form of haemoglobin characteristic of sickle cell anaemia.

sickle cell anaemia, a severe, chronic, incurable, anaemic condition that occurs in people homozygous for haemoglobin S (Hb S). The abnormal haemoglobin results in distortion and fragility of the erythrocytes. Sickle cell anaemia is characterized by crises of joint pain, thrombosis and fever, and by chronic anaemia, with splenomegaly, lethargy and weakness.

sickle cell crisis, an acute, episodic condition that occurs in children with sickle cell anaemia. The crisis may be vasoocclusive, resulting from the aggregation of misshapen erythrocytes, or anaemic, resulting from bone marrow aplasia, increased haemolysis, folate deficiency, or splenic sequestration of erythrocytes. Painful vasoocclusive crisis is the most common of the sickle cell crises. It is usually preceded by an upper respiratory or GI infection without exacerbation of anaemia. The clumps of sickled erythrocytes obstruct blood vessels, resulting in occlusion, ischaemia and infarction of adjacent tissue. Characteristic of this kind of crisis are leukocytosis, acute abdominal pain from visceral hypoxia, painful swelling of the soft tissue of the hands and feet (hand-foot syndrome) and migratory, recurrent or constant joint pain, often so severe that movement of the joint is limited. Persistent headache, dizziness, convulsions, visual or auditory disturbances, facial nerve palsies, coughing, shortness of breath and tachypnoea may occur if the central nervous system or lungs are affected.

sickle cell thalassaemia, a heterozygous blood disorder in which the genes for sickle cell and for thalassaemia are both inherited. A mild form and a severe form may be identified, depending on the degree of suppression of beta-chain synthesis by the thalassaemia gene. The clinical course is relatively mild. When beta-chain synthesis is completely suppressed, as in the severe form, only haemoglobin S appears in the red cells, and the clinical course is generally as severe as in homozygous sickle cell anaemia.

sickle cell trait, the heterozygous form of sickle cell anaemia, characterized by the presence of both haemoglobin S and haemoglobin A in the red blood cells. Anaemia and the other signs of sickle cell anaemia do not occur. People with this trait are informed and counselled regarding the possibility of having an infant with sickle cell disease if both parents have the trait. See **haemoglobin S.**

side effect, any reaction or consequence that results from a medication or therapy. Usually, although not necessarily, the effect is undesirable, and may manifest as nausea, dry mouth, dizziness, blood dyscrasias, blurred vision, discoloured urine or tinnitus.

sideroblastic anaemia, any one of a heterogenous group of chronic haematologic disorders characterized by normocytic or slightly macrocytic anaemia, hypochromic and normochromic red blood cells, and decreased erythropoiesis and haemoglobin synthesis. The red blood cells contain a perinuclear ring of iron-stained granules. The condition may be acquired or hereditary, primary or secondary to another condition or situation.

siderocyte, an abnormal erythrocyte in which there are visible particles of non-haemoglobin iron.

sideropenic dysphagia. See **Plummer-Vinson syndrome.**

siderosis, 1. a variety of pneumoconiosis caused by the inhalation of iron dust or particles. **2.** the introduction of colour in any tissue caused by the presence of excess iron. **3.** an increase in the amounts of iron in the blood.

siderotic granules, inclusion bodies seen in the red blood cells of splenectomy patients and in cases of haemoglobin synthesis and haemolytic anaemia. The granules contain iron.

SIDS, abbreviation for **sudden infant death syndrome.**

sievert (Sv) {R. M. Sievert, 20th century Swedish physicist}, the SI unit of dose equivalent. It is equal to the absorbed dose multiplied by a quality factor, the value of which depends on the biological effect of the specific ionising radiation.

sigh. See **periodic deep inspiration.**

sight, 1. the special sense that enables the shape, size, position and colour of objects to be perceived; the faculty of vision. It is the major function of the eye. **2.** that which is seen.

sigmoid, 1. of, or pertaining to, an S shape. **2.** the sigmoid colon.

sigmoid colon, the portion of the colon that extends from the end of the descending colon in the pelvis to the juncture of the rectum.

sigmoid flexure. See **sigmoid colon.**

sigmoid mesocolon, a fold of peritoneum that connects the sigmoid colon with the pelvic wall.

sigmoid notch, a concavity on the superior surface of the mandibular ramus between the coronoid and condyloid processes.

sigmoidectomy, excision of the sigmoid flexure of the colon, most commonly performed to remove a malignant tumour.

sigmoidoscope, an instrument used to examine the lumen of the sigmoid colon. It consists of a tube and a light, allowing direct visualization of the mucous membrane lining the colon.

sigmoidoscopy, the inspection of the rectum and sigmoid colon by the aid of a sigmoidoscope.

sign, an objective finding as perceived by an examiner, such as a fever, a rash, the whisper heard over the chest in pleural effusion, or the light band of hair seen in children after recovery from kwashiorkor. Many signs accompany symptoms; for instance, erythema and a maculopapular rash are often seen when a patient complains of pruritus.

signal molecule, a hormone, neurotransmitter or other agent that transfers information from one cell or organ to another. Examples include steroid hormones, insulin and growth factors.

signal node. See **Virchow's node.**

signal symptom. See **symptom.**

signal-to-noise ratio (SNR), the number used to describe the relative contribution to a detected signal of the true signal and random superimposed signals or "noise".

significance, 1. (in research) the statistical probability that a given finding is very unlikely to have occurred by chance alone. **2.** the importance of a study in developing a practice or theory, as in nursing practice.

silanization, (in chromatography) the chemical process of converting the SiOH moieties of a stationary form to the ester form.

silent ischaemia, an asymptomatic form of myocardial ischaemia that may result in severe damage (myocardial infarction) or sudden death. Silent ischaemia is most likely to occur during the first six hours after awakening in the morning.

silent mutation, (in molecular genetics) an alteration in a sequence of nucleotides that does not result in an amino acid change.

silhouette sign, an x-ray artefact caused by an infiltrate that obscures the demarcating line between lung segments.

silicate dental cement, a relatively hard,

translucent material used primarily to restore anterior teeth.

silicon (Si), a non-metallic element, second to oxygen as the most abundant of the elements. Its atomic number is 14 and its atomic weight is 28. It occurs in nature as silicon dioxide and in silicates. The silicates are used as detergents, corrosion inhibitors, adhesives and sealants.

silicone, any organic silicon polymer compound used in medicine, such as an adhesive, lubricant or a substitute for rubber, especially in prosthetic devices.

silicone septum, a vascular access device used in intravenous therapy. It consists of a silicone partition that covers the port chamber housed in the metal or plastic body of an implanted infusion port.

silicosis, a lung disorder caused by continued, long-term inhalation of the dust of an inorganic compound, silicon dioxide, which is found in sands, quartzes, flints and a number of other stones. Silicosis is characterized by the development of nodular fibrosis in the lungs. In advanced cases, severe dyspnoea may develop.

silk suture, a braided, fine, black suture material used to close incisions, wounds and cuts in the skin. It is not absorbed by the body.

silo filler's disease, a rare, acute, respiratory condition seen in agricultural workers who have inhaled nitrogen oxide whilst working with fermented fodder in closed, poorly ventilated areas such as silos. Characteristically, symptoms of respiratory distress and pulmonary oedema occur several hours after exposure. Loss of consciousness may occur.

silver (Ag), a whitish precious metal occurring mainly as a sulphide. Its atomic number is 47 and its atomic weight is 107.88. It is used extensively as a component of amalgams of dental fillings and many medications, especially antiseptics and astringents. Silver nitrate is used externally as an antiseptic and astringent, especially in the prevention of ophthalmia neonatorum.

silver cone method, a technique for filling tooth root canals. A prefitted silver cone is sealed into the apex of a root canal, and any remaining canal space is filled with guttapercha or sealer.

Silver dwarf {Henry K. Silver, American pediatrician, b. 1918}, a person who has Silver's syndrome, a congenital disorder in which short stature is associated with lateral asymmetry, various anomalies of the head, face and skeleton, and precocious puberty.

silver nitrate, a caustic, astringent and antiinfective, nowadays mostly used to treat overgranulation of wounds. It is usually applied as a pencil.

silver salts poisoning, a toxic condition caused by the ingestion of silver nitrate, characterized by discolouration of the lips, vomiting, abdominal pain, dizziness and convulsions.

silver sulphadiazine, a topical antimicrobial used to prevent or treat infection in secondand third-degree burns.

Silver's syndrome. See **Silver dwarf.**

silver-fork fracture. See **Colles' fracture.**

Silverman-Anderson score, a system of assessing the degree of respiratory distress.

simethicone, an antifoaming agent used as an antiflatulent.

simian crease, a single crease across the palm from the fusion of proximal and distal palmar creases, seen in congenital disorders such as Down's syndrome.

simian virus 40, a vacuolating virus isolated from the kidney tissue of rhesus monkeys.

similarity principle, a rule that objects similar to one another will become organized into one perceptual unit.

Simmonds' disease. See **postpubertal panhypopituitarism.**

simplate bleeding time test, a blood test for determining how quickly platelets form a plug when exposed to air. Platelet plug formation is the first step in clotting.

simple angioma, a tumour consisting of a network of small vessels or distended capillaries surrounded by connective tissue.

simple cavity, a cavity that involves only one surface of a tooth.

simple fission. See **binary fission.**

simple fracture, an uncomplicated, closed fracture in which the bone does not break the skin.

simple mastectomy, a surgical procedure in which a breast is completely removed and the underlying muscles and adjacent lymph nodes are left intact.

simple phobia, an anxiety disorder characterized by a persistent, irrational fear of specific things, such as animals, dirt, light or darkness.

simple protein, a protein that yields amino acids as the only or chief product on hydrolysis. The class includes albumins, globulins, glutelins, alcohol-soluble proteins, albuminoids, histones and protamines.

simple schizophrenia, a slow, insidiously progressive form of schizophrenia characterized by apathy, withdrawal, lack of initiative, gradual depletion of emotional reactions and an impoverishment in human relationships.

simple sugar, a monosaccharide, such as glucose.

simple tubular gland, one of the many multicellular glands with only one tubeshaped duct, such as various glands within the epithelium of the intestine.

simple vulvectomy. See **vulvectomy.**

Sims' position {James M. Sims, American gynaecologist, b. 1813}, a position in which the patient lies on the left side with the right knee and thigh drawn upwards towards the chest. The chest and abdomen are allowed to fall forward.

simulation, a mode of computer-assisted instruction in which a student receives basic information about a topic and then must interact with the computer to gain deeper understanding of the information and topic.

sinciput, the anterior or upper part of the head.

sinew, the tendon of a muscle, such as the thick, flattened tendon attached to the short head of the biceps brachii.

singer's nodule. See **vocal cord nodule.**

single-emulsion film, film that is coated with light-sensitive emulsion on only one side. Used in radiography to record images in multiformat, such as in **radionuclide imaging, ultrasonography, computerise tomography, laser imaging.**

single monster, a fetus with a single body and head but severely malformed or duplicated parts or organs.

single-blind study, an experiment in which either the subject or the person collecting data does not know whether the subject is in the control group or the experimental group.

single-case experimental design, the comparison of baseline measurements of one or more subjects' behaviours, with repeated measures of the same behaviour following the introduction and withdrawal or reversal of one or more interventions.

single-emulsion film, film that is coated with light-sensitive emulsion on only one side. It is used in radiography to record images in multiformat, as in radionuclide imaging, ultrasound, computerized tomography and laser imaging.

single-parent family, a family consisting of only the mother or father and one or more dependent children.

single-photon emission computed tomography (SPECT), a variation of computed tomography (CT) scanning in which the ray sum is defined by the collimator holes on the gamma-ray detector rotating around the patient. SPECT units usually consist of large crystal gamma cameras mounted on a gantry that permits rotation of the camera around the patient. Multiple detectors are used to reduce the imaging time.

singultus. See **hiccough.**

sinistrality. See **left-handedness.**

sinoatrial (SA) block, a conduction disturbance in the heart during which an impulse formed within the SA node is blocked from depolarizing the atrial myocardium. The condition is indicated on the electrocardiogram by the absence of some P waves. Causes include excessive vagal stimulation, acute infections and atherosclerosis. SA block may also be an adverse reaction to quinidine or digitalis.

sinoatrial (SA) node, a cluster of hundreds of cells located in the right atrial wall of the heart, near the opening of the superior vena cava. It comprises a knot of modified heart muscle that generates impulses that travel swiftly throughout the muscle fibres of both atria, causing them to contract. Specialized pacemaker cells in the node have an intrinsic rhythm that is independent of any stimulation by nerve impulses from the brain and the spinal cord. The sinoatrial node will normally "fire" at a rhythmic rate of 70 to 75 beats per minute. If the node fails to generate an impulse, pacemaker function will shift to another excitable component of the cardiac conduction system, such as the atrioventricular node or Purkinje's fibres.

sinus, a cavity or channel; as a cavity within a bone, a dilated channel for venous blood, or one permitting the escape of pus.

sinus arrhythmia, an irregular heart rhythm caused by interference in the impulses arising from the sinoatrial node.

sinus bradycardia. See **bradycardia.**

sinus node, an area of specialized heart tissue near the entrance of the superior vena cava that generates the cardiac electric impulse and is in turn controlled by the autonomic nervous system.

sinus pacemaker. See **sinus node.**

sinus rhythm, an expected regular cardiac rhythm stimulated by the sinoatrial node.

sinus tachycardia. See **tachycardia.**

sinus venosus defect. See **atrial septal defect.**

sinusitis, an inflammation of one or more paranasal sinuses. It may be a complication of an upper respiratory infection, dental infection, allergy, a change in atmosphere, as in air travel or underwater swimming, or a structural defect of the nose. With swelling of nasal mucous membranes the openings from sinuses to the nose may be obstructed, resulting in an accumulation of sinus secretions, causing pressure, pain, headache, fever and local tenderness. Complications include cavernous sinus thrombosis and spread of infection to bone, brain or meninges.

sinusoid, an anastomosing blood vessel, somewhat larger than a capillary, lined with reticuloendothelial cells.

sireniform fetus. See **sirenomelus.**

sirenomelia, a congenital anomaly in which there is complete fusion of the lower extremities and no feet.

sirenomelus, an infant who has sirenomelia.

siriasis, sunstroke.

Sister Kenny's treatment {Elizabeth Kenny, Australian nurse, b. 1886}, poliomyelitis therapy in which the patient's limbs and back are wrapped in warm, moist woollen cloths, and after the pain subsides the patient is taught to exercise affected muscles, especially by swimming. Equally important is passive movement of affected limbs with simultaneous stimulation at the site of muscle origins, carried out after application of hot packs.

site, 1. location. See also **situs. 2.** a quantum of space occupied and defined by a cluster of people.

site visit, a visit made by designated officials to evaluate or gather information about a department or institution. A site visit is a step in the accreditation of an institution.

situation therapy. See **milieu therapy.**

situational anxiety, a state of apprehension, discomfort and anxiety precipitated by the experience of new or changed situations or events. Situational anxiety is not abnormal and requires no treatment; it usually disappears as the person adjusts to the new experiences.

situational crisis, (in psychiatry) a crisis that arises suddenly in response to an external event or a conflict concerning a specific circumstance.

situational depression, (in psychiatry) an episode of emotional and psychological depression that occurs in response to a specific set of external conditions or circumstances.

situational loss, the loss of a person, thing or quality, resulting from a change in a life situation, including changes related to illness, body image, environment and death.

situational psychosis, (in psychiatry) a psychotic episode that results from a specific set of external circumstances.

situational theory, a leadership theory in which the manager chooses a leadership style to match the particular situation.

situational therapy, (in psychiatry) a kind of psychotherapy in which the milieu is part of the treatment program.

situs, the normal position or location of an organ or part of the body.

sitz bath, a bath in which only the hips and buttocks are immersed in water or saline solution. The procedure is used for patients who have had rectal or perineal surgery.

sixth disease. See **roseola infantum.**

sixth nerve. See **abducens nerve.**

Sjögren's syndrome {Henrik S. C. Sjögren, Swedish ophthalmologist, b. 1899}, an immunological disorder characterized by deficient moisture production of the lacrimal, salivary and other glands, and resulting in abnormal dryness of the mouth, eyes and other mucous membranes. Atrophy of the lacrimal glands can lead to desiccation of the cornea and conjunctiva. When the lungs are affected, the dryness increases susceptibility to pneumonia and other respiratory infections. Treatment includes application of artificial tears.

Sjögren-Larsson syndrome {Torsten Sjögren, Swedish paediatrician, b. 1859; T. Larsson, 20th century Swedish pediatrician}, a congenital condition, inherited as an autosomal recessive trait and characterized by ichthyosis, mental deficiency and spastic paralysis.

skeletal enchondromatosis. See **enchondromatosis.**

skeletal fixation, any method of holding together the fragments of a fractured bone by the attaching of wires, screws, plates or nails.

skeletal muscle. See **striated muscle.**

skeletal system, all of the bones and cartilage of the body that collectively provide the supporting framework for muscles and organs.

skeletal traction, one of the two basic kinds of traction used in orthopaedics for the treatment of fractured bones and the correction of orthopaedic abnormalities. Skeletal traction is applied to the affected structure by a metal pin or wire inserted in the tissue of the structure and attached to traction ropes. Skeletal traction is often used when continuous traction is desired to immobilize, position and align a fractured bone properly during the healing process. Infection of the pin tract is one of the complications that may develop with skeletal traction.

skeleton, the supporting framework for the body, comprising 206 bones that protect delicate structures, provide attachments for muscles, allow body movement, serve as major reservoirs of blood, and produce red blood cells. The skeleton is divided into the axial skeleton, which has 74 bones, the appendicular skeleton with 126 bones and the 6 auditory ossicles. The skeleton is derived from the mesoderm that grows from the primitive streak as skeletal cells multiply, change, migrate into various regions and form the membranous skeleton. Most of the membranous skeleton changes to cartilaginous skeleton in which ossification centres spread to form the bony skeleton. The four types of bones composing the skeleton are the long bones, including the humerus and phalanges of the fingers; the short bones, including the carpals and tarsals; the flat bones, including the frontal bone and parietal bone of the cranium; and the irregular bones, including the vertebrae. **skeletal,** *adj.*

Skene's duct. See **paraurethral duct.**

Skene's glands {Alexander J. C. Skene, American gynaecologist, b. 1838}, the largest of the glands that open into the female urethra.

skew, a deviation from a line or symmetrical pattern, such as data in a research study that do not follow the expected statistical curve of distribution because of the unwitting introduction of another variable.

skill play, a form of play in which a child persistently repeats an action or activity until it has been mastered, such as throwing or catching a ball.

Skillern's fracture {Penn G. Skillern, American surgeon, b. 1882}, an open fracture of the distal radius associated with a greenstick fracture of the distal ulna.

skills training, the teaching of specific verbal and non-verbal behaviours and the practicing of these behaviours by the patient.

skimmed milk, milk from which the fat has been removed. Most of the vitamin A is removed with the cream, although all other nutrients remain.

skin, the tough, supple cutaneous membrane that covers the entire surface of the body. It is the largest organ of the body and is composed of five layers of cells. The deepest layer is the stratum basale. It anchors the more superficial layers to the underlying tissues, and provides new cells to maintain the cells lost by abrasion from the outermost layer. The cells of each layer migrate upwards as they mature. Above the stratum basale lies the stratum spinosum. The cells in this layer are polygonal with tiny spines on their surfaces. As the cells migrate to the next layer, the stratum granulosum, they become flat, lying parallel with the surface of the skin. Over this layer lies a clear, thin band of homogeneous tissue called the stratum lucidum. The outermost layer, the stratum corneum, is composed of scaly, squamous plaques of dead cells that contain keratin. This horny layer is thick over areas of the body subject to abrasion, such as the palms of the hands. The colour of the skin varies according to the amount of melanin in the epidermis. Genetic differences determine the amount of melanin.

skin barrier, an artificial layer of skin, usually made of plastic, applied to skin before the application of tape or ostomy drainage bags. It protects the real skin from chronic irritation.

skin button, a plastic and fabric device that covers the drivelines of an artificial heart at their exit point from the skin. Its purpose is to eliminate the transmission of pumping pressure to the surrounding tissues.

skin cancer, a cutaneous neoplasm caused by ionizing radiation, certain genetic defects or chemical carcinogens, including arsenics, petroleum, tar products and fumes from some molten metals, by overexposure to the sun or other sources of ultraviolet light. Skin cancers, the most common and most curable malignancies, are also the most frequent secondary lesions in patients with cancer in other sites. Risk factors are a fair complexion, xeroderma pigmentosa, vitiligo, senile and seborrhoeic keratitis, Bowen's disease, radiation dermatitis and hereditary basal cell naevus syndrome. The most common skin cancers are basal cell carcinomas and squamous cell carcinomas.

skin graft, a portion of skin implanted to cover areas where skin has been lost through burns or injury or by surgical removal of diseased tissue. To prevent tissue rejection of permanent grafts, the graft is taken from the patient's own body or from the body of an identical twin. Skin from another person or animal can be used as a temporary cover for large burned areas to decrease fluid loss. Various techniques are used including pinch, split-thickness, full-thickness, pedicle and mesh grafts. In pinch grafting, 1-4 inch pieces of skin are placed as small islands on the donor site that they will grow to cover. The split-thickness graft consists of sheets of superficial and some deep layers of skin. The grafts are sutured into place; compression dressings may be applied for firm contact, or the area may be left exposed. A full-thickness graft contains all of the layers of skin and is more durable and effective for weight-bearing and friction-prone areas. In a pedicle graft, a portion remains attached to the donor site whereas the remainder is transferred to the recipient site. Its own blood supply remains intact, and it is not detached until the new blood supply has developed fully. A mesh graft is composed of multiple slices of new skin. A successful new graft of any type is well established in about 72 hours.

skin integrity, impaired, a state in which an individual's skin is adversely altered. Defining characteristics include disruption of the surface of the skin, destruction of cell layers of the skin, and invasion of structures of the body through the skin.

skin integrity, impaired, potential, a state in which an individual's skin is at risk of being adversely altered. Defining characteristics include the environmental (external) or somatic (internal) risk factors that may contribute to the cause of the breakdown of the integument. Among the environmental factors are hypothermia or hyperthermia; presence of an injurious chemical substance; shearing force or pressure, restraint, or laceration; radiation; physical immobilization; presence on the skin of excretions or secretions; and an abnormally high humidity. Somatic factors include reaction to some medications; obesity or emaciation; an abnormal metabolic state; alteration in circulation, sensory function or pigmentation; bony prominences; adverse developmental factors; decrease in normal skin turgor; and psychogenic or immunological abnormalities.

skin prep, a procedure for cleansing the skin with an antiseptic prior to surgery or venipuncture. Skin preps are performed to kill bacteria and pathological organisms and reduce the risk of infection. Various devices are available for this procedure, commonly constructed of plastic filled with a specific antiseptic, and equipped with an applicator. The antiseptic is applied by rubbing the device in a circular motion over the skin.

skin-sparing effect, (in radiotherapy) an effect occurring in megavoltage external beam radiotherapy, where the maximum radiation dose is delivered at a depth below the skin surface.

skin tag. See **cutaneous papilloma.**

skin test, a test to determine the reaction of the body to a substance, by observing the results of injecting the substance intradermally or applying it topically to the skin. Skin tests are used to detect allergens, determine immunity and diagnose disease. Kinds of skin tests include **patch test, Schick test** and **tuberculin test.**

skin traction, one of the two basic types of traction used in orthopaedics for the treatment of fractured bones and correction of orthopaedic abnormalities. Skin traction applies pull to an affected body structure by straps attached to the skin surrounding the structure. Kinds of skin traction are **adhesive skin traction** and **non-adhesive skin traction.**

skinfold calipers, an instrument used to measure the breadth of a fold of skin, usually on the posterior aspect of the upper arm or over the lower ribs of the chest.

Skinner box {Burrhus F. Skinner, American psychologist, b. 1904}, a box-like laboratory apparatus used in operant conditioning in animals, usually containing a lever or other device that when pressed produces reinforcement by either giving a reward, such as food or an escape outlet, or avoiding a punishment, such as an electric shock.

skull, the bony structure of the head, consisting of the cranium and skeleton of the face. The cranium, which contains and protects the brain, consists of eight bones. The skeleton of the face is composed of 14 bones.

slander, any words spoken with malice that are untrue and prejudicial to the reputation, professional practice, commercial trade, office or business of another person.

slant of occlusal plane, (in dentistry) the inclination measured by the angle between the extended occlusal plane and the axisorbital plane.

SLE, abbreviation for systemic lupus erythematosus.

sleep, a state marked by reduced consciousness, diminished activity of the skeletal muscles and depressed metabolism. People normally experience sleep in patterns that follow four observable, progressive stages. During Stage 1, the brainwaves are of the theta type, followed in Stage 2 by the appearance of distinctive sleep spindles; during Stages 3 and 4, the theta waves are replaced by delta waves. These four stages represent three-fourths of a period of typical sleep, and are collectively called **non-rapid eye movement (NREM)** sleep. The remaining time is usually occupied with **rapid eye movement (REM)** sleep; this can be detect-

ed with electrodes placed on the skin around the eyes so that tiny electrical discharges from contractions of the eye muscles are transmitted to the recording equipment. The REM sleep periods, lasting from a few minutes to half an hour, alternate with NREM periods. Dreaming occurs during REM time.

sleep apnoea, a sleep disorder characterized by periods of an absence of attempts to breathe. The person is momentarily unable to move respiratory muscles or maintain airflow through the nose and mouth.

sleep pattern disturbance, a disruption of the hours of sleep, causing discomfort or interference with normal daily activities. Defining characteristics include difficulty in falling asleep, wakening earlier than usual, interruption of night sleep by periods of wakefulness, or not feeling rested after sleep. There may also be changes in behaviour and performance, such as increased irritability, restlessness, disorientation, lack of energy and fatigue.

sleep terror disorder, a condition occurring during stages 3 or 4 of non-rapid eye movement sleep. It is characterized by repeated episodes of abrupt awakening, usually with a panicky scream, accompanied by intense anxiety, confusion, agitation, disorientation, unresponsiveness, marked motor movements and total amnesia concerning the event. The disorder is usually seen in children.

sleeping pill, *informal* a sedative taken for insomnia.

sleeping sickness. See **African trypanosomiasis.**

sleepwalking. See **somnambulism.**

slide clamp, a device, usually constructed of plastic, employed to regulate the flow of intravenous solution. The slide clamp has a graduated opening through which the intravenous tubing passes. Pushing the tube into the narrow end of the opening constricts the tube and reduces the flow rate.

sliding filaments, interdigitated thick and thin filaments of a sarcomere. In muscle contraction, they slide past each other so that the sarcomere becomes shorter although the filament lengths do not change. The action of the sliding filaments contributes to the increased thickness of a muscle in contraction.

sliding transfer, the movement of a person in a sitting position from one site to another, for example, from a bed to a wheelchair, by sliding the person along a transfer board.

sling, a bandage or device used to support an injured part of the body.

sling restraint, a therapeutic device, usually constructed of felt. It is used to assist in the immobilization of patients, especially orthopaedic patients in traction. The sling is placed over the pelvis to reduce pelvic motion with lower extremity traction, or over the abdominal area as counter-traction with Dunlop traction.

slip-on blood pump, a plastic mesh device with an attached squeeze bulb, rubber tubing and pressure gauge, used to help administer large amounts of blood quickly. The plastic mesh slips over the blood bag and applies pressure to the bag when the bulb is squeezed.

slipped disk. See **herniated disk.**

slipped femoral epiphysis, a failure of the femoral epiphyseal plate that tends to occur primarily in overweight adolescents as a result of hormonal changes. Clinical features include hip stiffness and pain. There may also be knee pain and external rotation of the affected leg. The condition is treated by orthopaedic surgery.

slipping rib, a chest pain caused by a loose ligament that allows slippage of one of the lower five ribs. One of the ribs may slip inside or outside an adjacent rib, causing pain or discomfort that may mimic a disorder of the pancreas, gallbladder or other upper abdominal organ.

slit lamp, an instrument used in ophthalmology for examining the conjunctiva, lens, vitreous humor, iris and cornea. A high-intensity beam of light is projected through a narrow slit, and a cross-section of the illuminated part of the eye is examined through a magnifying lens.

slit lamp microscope, a microscope for ophthalmic examination. It permits the viewer to examine the endothelium of the posterior surface of the cornea in a projected band of light that is shaped like a slit.

slough, 1. to shed or cast off dead tissue cells of the endometrium, such as during menstruation. **2.** the tissue that has been shed.

slow diastolic depolarization, the slow loss of negativity that occurs during phase 4 of the action potential in cardiac cells having automaticity.

slow response action potential, (in cardiology) an action potential produced when one of the fast sodium channels is available for depolarization and the fibre is separated only via slower Na^+/Ca^+ channels, producing an action potential with a slow upstroke velocity, low amplitude and consequent slow conduction.

slow virus, a virus that remains dormant in the body after initial infection. Years may elapse before symptoms occur.

slow-twitch (ST) fibre, a muscle fibre that develops less tension more slowly than a fast-twitch fibre. The ST fibre is usually fatigue- resistant and has adequate oxygen and enzyme activity.

slurred speech, abnormal speech in which words are not enunciated clearly or completely but are run together or are partially eliminated. The condition may be caused by weakness of the muscles of articulation, damage to a motor neurone, cerebellar disease, drug usage or carelessness.

Sm, symbol for **samarium.**

SMA, abbreviation for **sequential multiple analysis.**

SMA-6, SMA-12, SMA-18. See **sequential multiple analysis.**

small calorie. See **calorie.**

small cardiac vein, one of the five tributaries of the coronary sinus that drains blood from the myocardium. It conveys blood from the back of the right atrium and the right ventricle; in some individuals, it is joined by the right marginal vein.

small cell carcinoma. See **oat cell carcinoma.**

small for gestational age (SGA) infant, an infant whose weight and size at birth falls below the tenth percentile of appropriate for gestational age infants, whether delivered at term or earlier or later than term. Factors associated with smallness or retardation of intrauterine growth other than genetic influences include any disorder causing short stature, such as dwarfism, malnutrition caused by placental insufficiency, and certain infectious agents, including cytomegalovirus, rubella virus and *Toxoplasma gondii.* Other factors associated with the smallness of an SGA infant include cigarette smoking by the mother during pregnancy, her addiction to alcohol or heroin, and her having received methadone treatment.

small intestine, the longest portion of the digestive tract, extending approximately 7 m from the pylorus of the stomach to the iliocaecal junction. It is divided into the duodenum, jejunum and ileum.

small omentum. See **lesser omentum.**

smallest cardiac vein, one of the tiny vessels that drain deoxygenated blood from the myocardium into the atria. A few of these vessels end in the ventricles.

smallpox, a highly contagious viral disease characterized by fever, prostration and a vesicular, pustular rash. It is caused by one of two species of poxvirus: variola minor (alastrim) or variola major. Because human beings are the only reservoir for the virus, worldwide vaccination with vaccinia, a related poxvirus, has been effective in eradicating smallpox.

smallpox vaccine, a vaccine prepared from dried smallpox virus. It is indicated only for laboratory workers exposed to pox viruses.

smear, a laboratory specimen for microscopic examination prepared by spreading a thin film of tissue on a glass slide. A dye, stain, reagent, diluent or lysing agent may be applied to the specimen.

smegma, a secretion of sebaceous glands, especially the cheesy, foul-smelling secretion often found under the foreskin of the penis and at the base of the labia minora, near the glans clitoris.

smell, 1. the special sense that enables odours to be perceived through the stimulation of the olfactory nerves; olfaction. 2. any odour, pleasant or unpleasant.

Smith fracture {Robert W. Smith, Irish surgeon, b. 1807}, a reverse Colles' fracture of the wrist, involving volar displacement and angulation of a distal bone fragment.

Smith-Petersen nail {Marius N. Smith-Petersen, American surgeon, b. 1886}, a three-flanged stainless steel nail used in orthopaedic surgery to anchor the fractured neck of the femur to its head. It is introduced below the prominence of the greater trochanter and passed through the fractured part into the head of the femur.

smoke inhalation, the inhalation of noxious fumes or irritating particulate matter that may cause severe pulmonary damage. Respiratory burns are difficult to distinguish from simple smoke inhalation. Chemical pneumonitis, asphyxiation and physical trauma to the respiratory passages may occur. Characteristics include irritation of the upper respiratory tract, singed nasal hairs, dyspnoea, hypoxia, dusty gray sputum, rhonchi, rales, restlessness, anxiety, cough and hoarseness. Pulmonary oedema may develop up to 48 hours after exposure.

smooth muscle, one of two kinds of muscle, composed of elongated, spindle-shaped cells in muscles that are not under voluntary control, such as the smooth muscle of the visceral organs. The heart muscle is an exception because it is a striated involuntary muscle. The nucleated cells of smooth muscle are arranged parallel to one another, and also to the long axis of the muscle they form. Smooth muscle fibres are shorter than striated muscle fibres, and have only one nucleus per fibre.

smooth pursuit eye movement, the tracking of the eyes following a slowly moving object at a steady coordinated velocity, rather than in saccades.

smooth surface cavity, a cavity formed by decay that starts on surfaces of teeth without pits, fissures or enamel faults.

smudge cell, a degenerated leukocyte as seen in blood smears from patients with chronic lymphatic leukaemia.

SN, abbreviation for student nurse, used in signing nursing notes.

Sn, symbol for tin.

snail, an invertebrate of the order *Gastropoda*, several species of which are intermediate hosts of the blood flukes that cause schistosomiasis in humans.

snakebite, a wound resulting from penetration of the flesh by the fangs of a snake. Bites by snakes known to be non-venomous are treated as puncture wounds; those produced by an unidentified or poisonous snake require immediate attention.

snare, a device designed for holding a wire noose, used in removing small pedunculated growths. The operator tightens the wire around the peduncle, thus removing the growth.

sneeze, a sudden, forceful, involuntary expulsion of air through the nose and mouth, occurring as a result of irritation to the mucous membranes of the upper respiratory tract; for example, by dust, pollen or viral inflammation.

Snellen chart {Hermann Snellen, Dutch ophthalmologist, b. 1834}, one of several charts used in testing visual acuity. Letters, numbers, or symbols are arranged on the chart in decreasing size from top to bottom.

Snellen test, a test of visual acuity, using a Snellen chart. The tested person stands 20 feet from the chart and reads as many of the symbols as possible, reading each line downwards from the top. A score is assigned in the form of a ratio, comparing the individual's performance to that of a statistically normal performance. A person who can read what the average person can read at 20 feet has 20/20 vision.

snout reflex, an abnormal sign elicited by tapping the nose, resulting in a marked facial grimace. It usually indicates bilateral corticopontine lesions.

Snowden-Pencer scissors. See **scissors.**

SNP, abbreviation for **sodium nitroprusside.**

snuff dipping, the practice of extracting juices from chewing tobacco placed in the mucobuccal fold of the mouth. The practice has been associated with an increased incidence of leukoplakia, tooth and gum diseases and possible oral cancer.

snuffles, a nasal discharge in infancy, characteristic of congenital syphilis.

soap, 1. a compound of fatty acids and an alkali. Soap cleanses because molecules of fat are attracted to molecules of soap in a water solution, and are pulled off the dirty surface into the water. 2. a metallic salt of any salt produced from an acid. Compare **detergent.**

social adjustment rating scale. See **social readjustment rating scale.**

social breakdown syndrome, the progressive deterioration of social and interpersonal skills in long-term psychiatric patients.

social class, a grouping of persons with similar values, interests, income, education and occupations.

social deviance, behaviour that violates social standards, engendering anger, resentment, and a desire for punishment in a significant segment of the society.

social interaction, impaired, an insufficient or excessive quantity or ineffective quality of social exchange. Defining characteristics include verbalized or observed discomfort in social situations; verbalized or observed inability to receive or communicate a satisfying sense of belonging, caring, interest or shared history; observed use of unsuccessful social interaction behaviours; and dysfunctional interaction with peers, family and/or others.

social isolation, a condition in which a feeling of aloneness is experienced, which the patient acknowledges as a negative or threatening state imposed by others. Defining characteristics may be objective or subjective, or both. Objective characteristics include absence of family and friends; absence of a significant personal relationship with another person; the patient's withdrawal and preoccupation with his or her own thoughts and interests; meaningless actions or interests and activities inappropriate to the patient's developmental age; a physical or mental handicap or illness; or unacceptable social behaviour. Subjective characteristics include the verbal expression of feeling different from and rejected by others, the acknowledgment of values unacceptable to the dominant cultural group, absence of a significant purpose in life, inability to meet the expectations of others and the expressed feeling of insecurity in social situations.

social learning theory, a concept that the impulse to behave aggressively is subject to the influence of learning, socialization and experience.

social margin, the sum total of all resources (material, personal and interpersonal) available to assist an individual in coping with stress.

social medicine, an approach to the prevention and treatment of disease, based on the study of human heredity, environment, social structures and cultural values.

social mobility, the process of moving upwards or downwards in the social hierarchy.

social motivation, an incentive or drive resulting from a sociocultural influence that initiates behaviour towards a particular goal.

social network, an interconnected group of cooperating significant others, who may or may not be related, with whom a person interacts.

social network therapy, the gathering together of patient, family and other social contacts into group sessions, for the purpose of problem solving.

social order, the manner in which a society is organized, and the rules and standards required to maintain that organization.

social phobia, an anxiety disorder characterized by an avoidance and a persistent, irrational fear of situations in which the individual may be exposed to scrutiny by others, such as speaking, eating, performing in public, or using public lavatories or transportation.

social psychiatry, a branch of psychiatry based on the study of social influences on the development and course of mental disorders.

social psychology, the study of the effects of group membership on the behaviour, attitudes and beliefs of the individual.

social radical therapy, a form of psychotherapy that attempts to bring about change by merging treatment into a radical political movement, usually one that represents the personal views of the therapist. Its major premise is that all therapy is characterized by numerous social and political value choices.

social readjustment rating scale, a scale of 43 common life events associated with some degree of disruption of an individual's life. The scale was developed by psychologists T. Holmes and R. J. Rahe, who found that a number of serious physical disorders, such as myocardial infarction, peptic ulcer and infections, as well as a variety of psychiatric disorders, were associated with an accumulation of 200 or more points on the rating scale within a period of 1 year. According to the psychologists, the most disruptive event in one's life was the death of a spouse, which warranted 100 points. The lowest rated event was a minor law violation, rated at 11 points.

social sanctions, the measures used by a society to enforce its rules of acceptable behaviour.

social worker, a person with special training in dealing with social, emotional and environmental problems associated with illness or disability. A **medical social worker** is qualified and experienced in counselling patients and their families in the hospital setting. A **psychiatric social worker** may specialize in counselling individuals and families so that they can deal with social, emotional or environmental problems resulting from mental illness.

socialization, 1. the process by which an individual learns to live in accordance with the expectations and standards of a group or society, acquiring the beliefs, habits, values and accepted modes of behaviour primarily through imitation, family interaction and educational systems; the procedure by which society integrates the individual. **2.** (in psychoanalysis) the process of adjustment, beginning in early childhood, by which the individual becomes aware of the need to accommodate inner drives to the demands of external realty.

society, a nation, community or broad group of people who establish particular aims, beliefs or standards of living and conduct.

sociogenic, pertaining to personal or group activities that are motivated by social values and constraints.

sociolinguistics, the study of the relationship between language and the social context in which it occurs.

sociology, the study of group behaviour

within a society.

sociopath. See **psychopath.**

sociopathic personality. See **antisocial personality.**

sociopathic. See **psychopathic.**

socket, the part of a prosthesis into which the stump of the remaining limb fits. Most modern prosthetic sockets are made of plastic materials, which are lighter, odourless and easier to clean than traditional leather sockets.

soda, a compound of sodium, particularly sodium bicarbonate, sodium carbonate or sodium hydroxide.

soda lime (SL), a mixture of sodium and calcium hydroxides used to absorb exhaled carbon dioxide in an anaesthesia rebreathing system.

sodium (Na) {coined by Sir Humphry Davy, English chemist, b. 1778)}, a soft, greyish metal of the alkaline metals group. Its atomic number is 11 and its atomic weight is 22.99. Sodium is one of the most important elements in the body. Sodium ions are involved in acid-base balance, water balance, transmission of nerve impulses and contraction of muscles. Sodium is the chief electrolyte in interstitial fluid, and its interaction with potassium as the main intracellular electrolyte is critical to survival. A decrease in the sodium concentration of the interstitial fluid immediately decreases osmotic pressure, making it hypotonic to intracellular fluid osmotic pressure.

sodium acid glutamate. See **sodium glutamate.**

sodium arsenite poisoning, a toxic condition caused by the ingestion of sodium arsenite, an insecticide and weed-killer. The characteristic symptoms of arsenite poisoning are similar to those of arsenic poisoning.

sodium bicarbonate, an antacid, electrolyte and urinary alkalinizing agent. It is used in the treatment of acidosis and gastric acidity, and to encourage the urinary excretion of weakly acidic drugs such as methotrexate.

sodium chloride, common table salt (NaCl), used in solution as a fluid and electrolyte replenisher, isotonic vehicle and irrigating solution.

sodium chloride and dextrose. See **dextrose and sodium chloride injection.**

sodium etidronate. See **etidronate disodium.**

sodium glutamate, a salt of glutamic acid used to enhance the flavour of foods. It has been used in the treatment of hepatic coma.

sodium hypochlorite solution, an aqueous solution of NaOCl, used as a disinfectant for utensils not harmed by its bleaching action, and occasionally for cleaning sloughy wounds.

sodium iodide, an iodine with uses similar to potassium iodide.

sodium lactate injection, an electrolyte

replenisher that has been used for metabolic acidosis.

sodium nitroprusside (SNP), a vasodilator used primarily in the emergency treatment of hypertensive crises, in heart failure, and for producing hypotension during surgery.

sodium perborate, an oxygen-liberating antiseptic ($NaBO_3.H2O_2.3H_2O$) that may be used in the treatment of necrotizing ulcerative gingivitis and other kinds of gingival inflammation, as well as for bleaching pulpless teeth.

sodium phosphate, a saline laxative, occasionally used to achieve prompt and thorough evacuation of the bowel. It has also been administered with other phosphates, orally or intravenously, for the treatment of hypercalcaemia.

sodium phosphate P32, a myelosuppressive radioactive agent. It is used to treat polycythaemia vera. It has also been used for other malignancies including myelocytic leukaemia, and to diagnose tumours of the eye, brain and skin.

sodium pump, a theoretical mechanism for transporting sodium ions across cell membranes against an opposing concentration gradient. Energy for this transport system is obtained from the hydrolysis of adenosine triphosphate by special enzymes.

sodium salicylate, an analgesic, antipyretic and antirheumatic, sometimes used to relieve pain and fever.

sodium sulphate anhydrous. See **salt cake.**

sodium valproate. See **valproate.**

sodium-calcium edetate, a parenteral chelating agent. It is used in the treatment of poisoning with heavy metals, especially lead.

sodium-restricted diet. See **low-sodium diet.**

sodoku. See **rat-bite fever.**

sodomy, 1. anal intercourse. **2.** intercourse with an animal. **3.** a vague term for "unnatural" sexual intercourse. **sodomite,** *n.*, **sodomize,** *v.*

soft data, health information that is mainly subjective, as provided by the patient and the patient's family, including pain or other sensations, lifestyle habits and family health history.

soft diet, a diet that is soft in texture, low in residue, easily digested and well tolerated. It provides the essential nutrients in the form of liquids and semisolid foods, such as milk, fruit juices, eggs, cheese, custards, tapioca and puddings, strained soups and vegetables.

soft fibroma, a fibroma that contains several cells.

soft neurological sign, a mild or slight neurological abnormality that is difficult to detect or interpret.

soft palate, the structure composed of mucous membrane, muscular fibres and mucous glands, suspended from the posterior border of the hard palate forming the roof of the mouth. When the soft palate rises, as in swallowing and sucking, it separates the nasal cavity and nasopharynx from the posterior part of the oral cavity and oral portion of the pharynx.

soft radiation, (in radiography) low energy ionizing radiation which could be absorbed in the skin and not contribute to the radiographic image. Such radiation is usually selectively removed from the beam by a filter.

sol, a colloidal state in which a solid is suspended in a liquid, such as a soap or starch in water. The fluidity of cytoplasm depends on its sol/gel balance.

solar fever. See **dengue fever, sunstroke.**

solar keratosis. See **actinic keratosis.**

solar plexus, a dense network of nerve fibres and ganglia that surrounds the roots of the coeliac and superior mesenteric arteries at the level of the first lumbar vertebra. It is one of the great autonomic plexuses of the body in which the nerve fibres of the sympathetic system and parasympathetic system combine.

solar radiation, the emission and diffusion of actinic rays from the sun. Overexposure may result in sunburn, keratosis, skin cancer or lesions associated with photosensitivity.

soleus, one of three superficial posterior muscles of the leg. It is a broad flat muscle lying just under the gastrocnemius. The soleus plantar flexes the foot.

solid, 1. a dense body, figure, structure or substance that has length, breadth and thickness, is not a liquid or a gas, contains no significant cavity or hollowness, and has no breaks or openings on its surface. **2.** describing such a body, figure, structure or substance.

solitary coin lesion, a nodule identified on a chest x-ray film by clear normal lung tissue surrounding it. A coin lesion is usually between 1 and 6 cm in size and often malignant.

solitary play, a form of play among a group of children within the same room or area in which each child engages in an independent activity using toys that are different from other children's and showing no interest in joining in or interfering with the play of others.

soluble insulin, a fast-acting insulin used in the treatment of diabetes mellitus when the desired action is prompt, intense, and short-acting. Insulin injection is the only form of insulin suitable for intramuscular and intravenous administration. It is also the only form of insulin suitable for use during a diabetic emergency or during surgery.

solute, a substance dissolved in a solution.

solution, a mixture of one or more substances dissolved in another substance. The molecules of each of the substances disperse homogeneously and do not change chemically. A solution may be a gas, a liquid or a solid.

solvent, 1. any liquid in which another substance can be dissolved. **2.** *informal,* an organic liquid, such as benzene, carbon tetrachloride and other volatile petroleum distillate which, when inhaled, can cause intoxication as well as damage to mucous membranes of the nose and throat and the tissues of the kidney, liver and brain.

soma, *pl.* **somas, somata, 1.** the body as distinguished from the mind or psyche. **2.** the body, excluding germ cells. **3.** the body of a cell. **somatic, somal,** *adj.*

somatic cavity. See **coelom.**

somatic cell, any of the cells of body tissue that have the diploid number of chromosomes as distinguished from germ cells, which contain the haploid number. Compare **germ cell.**

somatic chromosome, any chromosome in a diploid or somatic cell, as contrasted to those in a haploid or gametic cell; an autosome.

somatic delusion, a false notion or belief concerning body image or body function.

somatic therapy, a form of treatment that affects one's physiological functioning.

somatic. See **soma, psychosomatic.**

somatist, a psychotherapist or other health professional who believes that every neurosis and psychosis has an organic cause.

somatization disorder, a disorder characterized by recurrent, multiple, physical complaints and symptoms for which there is no organic cause. The symptoms vary according to the individual and the underlying emotional conflict. Some common symptoms are GI dysfunction, paralysis, temporary blindness, cardiopulmonary distress, painful or irregular menstruation, sexual indifference and pain during intercourse.

somatoform disorder, any of a group of neurotic disorders, characterized by symptoms suggesting physical illness or disease, for which there are no demonstrable organic causes or physiological dysfunctions. Kinds of somatoform disorders are **conversion disorder, hypochondriasis, psychogenic pain disorder** and **somatization disorder.**

somatogenesis, 1. (in embryology) the development of the body from the germ plasm. **2.** the development of a physical disease or of symptoms from an organic patho-physiological cause. **somatogenic, somatogenetic,** *adj.*

somatoliberin. See **growth hormone releasing factor.**

somatomedin. See **growth hormone.**

somatomegaly, a condition in which the body is abnormally large because of an excessive secretion of somatotropin or an inadequate secretion of somatostatin.

somatoplasm, the non-reproductive protoplasmic material of the body cells, as distinguished from the reproductive material of the germ cells.

somatopleure, the tissue layer that forms the body wall of the early developing embryo. **somatopleural,** *adj.*

somatosensory evoked potential (SEP), evoked potential elicited by repeated stimulation of the pain and touch systems. It is the least reliable of the evoked potentials studied as monitors of neurological function during surgery.

somatosplanchnic, of or pertaining to the trunk of the body and visceral organs.

somatostatin, a hormone produced in the hypothalamus that inhibits the release of the growth hormone somatotrophin from the anterior pituitary gland. It also inhibits the release of certain other hormones, including thyrotrophin, adrenocorticotrophic hormone, glucagon, insulin and cholecystokinin, and of some enzymes, including pepsin, renin, secretin and gastrin.

somatotherapy, the treatment of physical disorders, as distinguished from psychotherapy.

somatotropic hormone, somatotropin. See **growth hormone.**

somatotype, 1. body build or physique. **2.** the classification of individuals according to body build based on certain physical characteristics. The primary types are **ectomorph, endomorph and mesomorph.**

somatropin, a synthetic polypeptide growth hormone produced by recombinant DNA technology. It is prescribed for patients who fail to grow because of limited endogenous growth hormone secretion.

somite, any of the paired, segmented masses of mesodermal tissue that form along the length of the neural tube during the early stage of embryonic development in vertebrates.

somite embryo, an embryo in any stage of development between the formation of the first and last pairs of somites, which in humans occurs in the third and fourth weeks after fertilization of the ovum.

somnambulism, 1. a condition occurring during stages 3 or 4 of non-rapid eye movement sleep. It is characterized by complex motor activity, usually culminating in leaving the bed and walking about, with no recall of the episode on awakening. The episodes usually last from several minutes to half an hour or longer. **2.** a hypnotic state in which the person has full possession of the senses but no recollection of the episode.

somnolent, 1. the condition of being sleepy or drowsy. **2.** tending to cause sleepiness. **somnolence,** *n.*

somnolent detachment, (in psychology) a term introduced by Sullivan for a type of security operation in which a person falls asleep when confronted by a highly threatening, anxiety-producing experience.

sonography. See **ultrasonography.**

sonorous rale, a snoring sound that may be produced by the vibration of a mass of thick secretion lodged in a bronchus. This sound is associated with various lung or respiratory disorders.

soot wart. See **scrotal cancer.**

soporific, 1. of or pertaining to a substance, condition or procedure that causes sleep. **2.** a soporific drug.

sorbent, the property of a substance that allows it to interact with another compound, usually to enable it to bind.

sorbic acid, a compound occurring naturally in berries of the mountain ash. Commercial sorbic acid derived from acetaldehyde is used in fungicides, food preservatives, lubricants and plasticizers.

sordes, *pl.* **sordes,** dirt or debris, especially the crusts consisting of food, micro-organisms and epithelial cells that accumulate on teeth and lips during a febrile illness. Sordes gastricae is undigested food and mucus in the stomach.

sore, 1. a wound, ulcer or lesion. **2.** tender or painful.

Sorrin's operation, a surgical technique for treating a periodontal abscess, used especially when the marginal gingiva appears healthy and provides no access to the abscess. A semilunar incision is made below the abscess area in the attached gingiva, leaving the gingival margin undisturbed. The tissue flap produced by the incision is raised, accessing the abscessed area for curettage, after which the wound is sutured.

souffle, a soft murmur heard through a stethoscope. When detected over the uterus in a pregnant woman, it is coincident with the maternal pulse and is caused by blood circulating in the large uterine arteries.

sound, an instrument used to locate the opening of a cavity or canal, test the patency of a canal, ascertain the depth of a cavity, or reveal the contents of a canal or cavity.

source-image receptor distance. See **focus-film distance.**

South African genetic porphyria. See **variegate porphyria.**

South American blastomycosis. See **paracoccidioidomycosis.**

Southern blot test, a gene analysis method used in the identification of specific DNA fragments and the diagnosis of cancers and haemoglobinopathies.

sp. (*pl.* **spp.**), abbreviation for species.

space, an actual or potential cavity of the body, such as the complemental spaces in the pleural cavity that are not occupied by lung tissue, and the lymph spaces occupied by lymph.

space maintainer, a fixed or movable appliance for preserving the space created by the premature loss of one or more teeth.

space obtainer, an appliance for increasing the space between adjoining teeth.

space regainer, a fixed or removable appliance for moving a displaced permanent tooth into its normal position in a dental arch.

Spalding's sign, overlapping of the fetal cranial bones, seen on X-ray, indicating intrauterine death.

Spanish fly. See **cantharis.**

sparganosis, an infection with larvae of the fish tapeworm the pseudogenus *Sparganum*, characterized by painful subcutaneous swellings or swelling and destruction of the eye. It is acquired by ingesting larvae in contaminated water or in inadequately cooked, infected frog flesh.

spasm, 1. an involuntary muscle contraction of sudden onset, such as habit spasms, hiccups, stuttering or a tic. **2.** a convulsion or seizure. **3.** a sudden, transient constriction of a blood vessel, bronchus, oesophagus, pylorus, ureter or other hollow organ.

spasmodic dysphonia, a speech disorder in which phonation is intermittently blocked by spasms of the larynx.

spasmodic torticollis, a form of torticollis characterized by episodes of spasms of the neck muscles. In some cases, severe stress and muscular spasm may be the cause.

spasmogen, any substance that can produce smooth muscle contractions, as in the bronchioles, such as histamine, bradykinin and serotonin.

spastic, of, or pertaining to, spasms or other uncontrolled contractions of the skeletal muscles. **spasticity,** *n.*

spastic aphonia, a condition in which a person is unable to speak because of spasmodic contraction of the abductor muscles of the throat.

spastic bladder, a form of neurogenic bladder caused by a lesion of the spinal cord above the voiding reflex center. It is marked by loss of bladder control and bladder sensation, incontinence and automatic, interrupted, incomplete voiding. It is often caused by trauma, a tumour or multiple sclerosis.

spastic colon. See **irritable bowel syndrome.**

spastic dysphonia. See **spasmodic dysphonia.**

spastic entropion. See **ectropion, entropion.**

spastic hemiplegia, paralysis of one side of the body with increased tendon reflexes and uncontrolled contraction occurring in the affected muscles.

spastic paralysis, an abnormal condition characterized by the involuntary contraction of one or more muscles with associated loss of muscular function. Compare **flaccid paralysis.**

spastic pseudoparalysis. See **Creutzfeldt-Jakob disease.**

spasticity, a form of muscular hypertonicity with increased resistance to stretch. It usually involves the flexors of the arms and extensors of the legs. Moderate spasticity is characterized by movements that require great effort and lack of normal coordination. Slight spasticity may be marked by gross movements that are coordinated, but combined selective movement patterns are incoordinated.

spatial dance, the body shifts or movements used by individuals as they try to adjust the distance between them. See also **spatial zones.**

spatial relationships, 1. orientation in space; the ability to locate objects in the three-dimensional external world using visual or tactile recognition, and make a spatial analysis of the observed information. **2.** the relative locations of various personnel and equipment in an operating room, with particular emphasis on what is sterile, clean or contaminated.

spatial summation. See **summation,** def. 2.

spatial zones, the areas of personal space in which most people interact. Four basic spatial zones are the intimate zone, in which distance between individuals is less than 18 inches; the personal zone, between 18 inches and 4 feet; the social zone, extending between 4 and 12 feet; and the public zone, beyond 12 feet.

SPE, abbreviation for **sucrose polyester.**

Spearman's rho {Charles E. Spearman, English psychologist, b. 1863}, a statistical test for correlation between two rank-ordered scales. It yields a statement of the degree of interdependence of the scores of the two scales.

special care unit, a hospital unit with the necessary specialized equipment and personnel for handling critically ill or injured patients, such as an intensive care unit, burn unit or cardiac care unit.

special gene system, a plasmid, transposon or other genetic fragment that is able to transfer genetic information from one cell to another.

special sense, the sense of sight, smell, taste, touch or hearing.

specialing *informal,* **1.** (in psychiatric nursing) the constant attendance of a professional staff member on a disturbed patient, to protect the patient from harming the self or others and observe the patient's behaviour. **2.** (in nursing) the giving of nursing care only to one person, as when caring for a patient whose needs are so great that a nurse is required at all times.

specialist, a healthcare professional who practises a specialty. A specialist usually has advanced clinical training and may have a postgraduate academic degree.

specialty, a branch of medicine or nursing in

which the professional is specially qualified to practise by having attended an advanced programme of study, having passed an examination given by an organization of specialty members, or having gained experience by extensive practice in the specialty.

specialty care, specialized medical services provided by a medical specialist.

species (Sp), *pl.* **species (sp., spp.),** the category of living things below genus in rank. A species includes individuals of the same genus who are similar in structure and chemical composition and can interbreed.

species immunity, a form of natural immunity shared by all members of a species.

specific absorption rate (SAR), (in hyperthermia treatment) the rate of absorption of heat energy (W) per unit mass of tissue in units of W/kg.

specific activity, 1. (in nuclear medicine) the radioactivity of a radioisotope per unit mass of the element or compound, expressed in disintegrations per second per milligram. **2.** the relative activity per unit mass, expressed as counts per minute per milligram.

specific gravity, the ratio of the density of a substance to the density of another substance accepted as a standard. The usual standard for liquids and solids is water. Thus, a liquid or solid with a specific gravity of 4 is four times as dense as water.

specific immune globulin, a special preparation obtained from human blood that is preselected for its high antibody count against a specific disease, such as varicella zoster immune globulin.

specific rates, statistical rates in which the events in both numerator and denominator are restricted to a specific subgroup of a population.

specific treatment. See **treatment.**

specificity of association, the uniqueness of a relationship between a causal factor and the occurrence of a disease.

specimen, a small sample of something, intended to show the nature of the whole, such as a urine specimen.

SPECT, abbreviation for **single-photon emission computed tomography.**

spectator ions, ions that are not involved in proton transfer in a chemical reaction.

spectinomycin hydrochloride, an antibiotic prescribed in the treatment of gonorrhoea.

spectrometer, an instrument for measuring wavelengths of rays of the spectrum, the deviation of refracted rays, and the angles between faces of a prism. Kinds of spectrometer are **mass spectrometer** and **Mössbauer spectrometer.**

spectrometry, the procedure of measuring wavelengths of light and other electromagnetic waves. **spectrometric,** *adj.*

spectrophotometry, the measurement of colour in a solution by determining the amount of light absorbed in the ultraviolet, infrared or visible spectrum, widely used in clinical chemistry to calculate the concentration of substances in solution. **spectrophotometric,** *adj.*

spectrum, *pl.* **spectra, 1.** a range of phenomena or properties occurring in increasing or decreasing magnitude. Radiant or electromagnetic energy is arranged on the basis of wavelength and frequency. **2.** the range of effectiveness of an antibiotic. A broad-spectrum antibiotic is effective against a wide range of micro-organisms.

speculum, a retractor used to separate the walls of a cavity to make examination possible, such as an ear speculum, an eye speculum or a vaginal speculum.

speech, 1. the utterance of articulate vocal sounds that form words to give expression to one's thoughts or ideas. **2.** communication by means of spoken words. **3.** the faculty of language production, which involves the complex coordination of the muscles and nerves of the organs of articulation. Kinds of dysfunctions include **ataxic speech, explosive speech, mirror speech, scamping speech, scanning speech, slurred speech** and **staccato speech.**

speech audiometry. See **audiometry.**

speech dysfunction, any defect or abnormality of speech, including aphasia, alexia, stammering, stuttering, aphonia and slurring.

speech pathology, 1. the study of abnormalities of speech or the organs of speech. **2.** the diagnosis and treatment of abnormalities of speech as practised by a speech pathologist or a speech therapist.

speech therapist, a person trained in speech pathology, who treats people with disorders affecting normal oral communication.

speech-language pathologist, an individual with professional training in human communication, its development and disorders. The person specializes in the measurement and evaluation of language abilities, auditory processes and speech production, clinical treatment of children and adults with speech, language and hearing disorders, and research methods in the study of communication processes.

speed, 1. the rate of change of position with time. **2.** *slang.* any stimulating drug, such as amphetamine. **3.** a reciprocal of the amount of radiation used to produce an image with various components of an x-ray imaging system, such as screens, film and image intensifiers. A system using little radiation is "fast", whereas one requiring more radiation is "slow". **4.** the amount of exposure of film to light or x-rays needed to produce a desired image.

speed shock, a sudden adverse physiological reaction of a patient to intravenous medications or drugs that are administered too quickly. Some signs of speed shock are a flushed face, headache, a tight feeling in the chest, irregular pulse, loss of consciousness and cardiac arrest.

sperm. See **semen, spermatozoon.**

spermatic cord, a structure extending from the deep inguinal ring in the abdomen to the testis, descending nearly vertically into the scrotum.

spermatic duct. See **vas deferens.**

spermatic fistula, an abnormal passage communicating with a testis or a seminal duct.

spermatid, a male germ cell that arises from a spermatocyte and becomes a mature spermatozoon in the last phase of the continual process of spermatogenesis.

spermatocele, a cystic swelling, either of the epididymis or of rete testis, that contains spermatozoa.

spermatocide. See **spermicide.**

spermatocyte, a male germ cell that arises from a spermatogonium.

spermatocytogenesis. See **spermatogenesis.**

spermatogenesis, the process of development of spermatozoa, including the first stage, called spermatocytogenesis, in which spermatogonia become spermatocytes that develop into spermatids, and the second stage, called spermiogenesis, in which the spermatids become spermatozoa.

spermatogonium, *pl.* **spermatogonia,** a male germ cell that gives rise to a spermatocyte early in spermatogenesis.

spermatozoon, *pl.* **spermatozoa,** a mature male germ cell that develops in the seminiferous tubules of the testes. Resembling a tadpole, it is about 50 μm (1/500 inch) long and has a head with a nucleus, a neck and a tail that provides propulsion. See **spermatogenesis.**

spermicide, a chemical substance that kills spermatozoa. **spermicidal,** *adj.*

spermiogenesis. See **spermatogenesis.**

sphenoid bone, the bone at the base of the skull, anterior to the temporal bones and the basilar part of the occipital bone.

sphenoid fontanelle, an anterolateral fontanelle, usually not palpable.

sphenoidal fissure, a cleft between the great and small wings of the sphenoid bone.

sphenoidal sinus, one of a pair of cavities in the sphenoid bone of the skull, lined with mucous membrane that is continuous with that of the nasal cavity.

sphenomandibular ligament, one of a pair of flat, thin ligaments comprising part of the temporomandibular joint between the mandible of the jaw and temporal bone of the skull.

spherocyte, an abnormal spheric red blood cell that contains more than the normal amount of haemoglobin. **spherocytic,** *adj.*

spherocytic anaemia, a haematological disorder characterized by haemolytic anaemia caused by the presence of red blood cells that are spheric rather than round and biconcave. The cells are fragile and tend to haemolyse in the oxygen-poor peripheral circulatory system. Episodic crises of abdominal pain, fever, jaundice and splenomegaly occur.

spherocytosis, the abnormal presence of spherocytes in the blood.

spheroidea. See **ball-and-socket joint.**

sphincter, a circular band of muscle fibres that constricts a passage or closes a natural opening in the body, such as the external anal sphincter, which closes the anus.

sphincter pupillae, a muscle that expands the iris, narrowing the diameter of the pupil of the eye. It is composed of circular fibres arranged in a narrow band about 1 mm wide, surrounding the margin of the pupil towards the posterior surface of the iris.

sphingolipid, a compound that consists of a lipid and a sphingosine. It is found in high concentrations in the brain and other tissues of the nervous system.

sphingomyelin, any of a group of sphingolipids containing phosphorus. It occurs primarily in the tissue of the nervous system.

sphingomyelin lipidosis, any of a group of diseases characterized by an abnormality in the ability of the body to store sphingolipids. Kinds of sphingomyelin lipidosis include **Gaucher's disease, Niemann-Pick disease** and **Tay-Sachs disease.**

sphingosine, a long-chain unsaturated amino alcohol, a major constituent of sphingolipids and sphingomyelin.

sphygmogram, a pulse tracing produced by a sphygmograph. Sphygmographic abnormalities of rate, rhythm and form may be diagnostically useful in the assessment of cardiovascular function.

sphygmograph, an instrument that records the force of the arterial pulse on a tracing called a sphygmogram. **sphygmographic,** *adj.*

sphygmomanometer, a device for measuring the arterial blood pressure. It consists of an arm or leg cuff with an air bladder connected to a tube and a bulb for pumping air into the bladder, and a gauge for indicating the amount of air pressure being exerted against the artery.

spica bandage, a figure-of-eight bandage in which each turn generally overlaps the next to form a succession of V-like designs. It may be used to give support, apply pressure or hold a dressing in place.

spica cast, an orthopaedic cast applied to immobilize part or all of the trunk of the body and part or all of one or more extremities. Kinds of spica casts are **bilateral long-leg spica cast, one-and-a-half spica cast, shoulder spica cast** and **unilateral long-leg spica cast.**

spicule, a sharp body with a needle-like

point.

spider angioma, a form of telangiectasis characterized by a central, elevated red dot, the size of a pinhead, from which small blood vessels radiate.

spider antivenom. See **black widow spider antivenom.**

spider bite, a puncture wound produced by the bite of a spider, an arachnid related to ticks and mites.

spider naevus. See **spider angioma.**

spikeboard, a device that enables individuals with upper extremity handicaps to stabilize foods when only one hand is available for meal preparation.

spillway, a channel or passageway through which food normally escapes from the occlusal surfaces of teeth during mastication.

spin, 1. the intrinsic angular momentum of an elementary particle or a nucleus of an atom. 2. intrinsic joint movements about an axis perpendicular to the articular surface.

spin density, (in magnetic resonance imaging) a measure of hydrogen concentration. It is a quantity proportional to the number of hydrogen nuclei precessing at the Larmor frequency and contributing to the MRI signal.

spin-lattice relaxation time. See **relaxation time.**

spin-spin relaxation time. See **relaxation time.**

spina, *pl.* **spinae,** 1. the spinal column. 2. a spine or a thorn-like projection, such as the bony projection on the anterior border of the ilium, forming the anterior end of the iliac crest.

spina bifida, congenital neural tube defect characterized by a developmental anomaly in the posterior vertebral arch. Spina bifida that does not involve herniation of the meninges or contents of the spinal canal rarely requires treatment.

spina bifida anterior, incomplete closure along the anterior surface of the vertebral column.

spina bifida cystica, a developmental defect of the central nervous system in which a hernial cyst containing meninges (meningocoele), spinal cord (myelocoele) or both (myelomeningocoele) protrudes through a congenital cleft in the vertebral column. The protruding sac is encased in a layer of skin or a fine membrane that can rupture easily, causing leakage of cerebrospinal fluid and an increased risk of meningeal infection.

spina bifida occulta, defective closure of the laminae of the vertebral column in the lumbosacral region, without hernial protrusion of the spinal cord or meninges. Because the neural tube has closed, there are usually no neurological impairments associated with the defect. However, any abnormal adhesion of the spinal cord to the area of malformation may lead to neuromusucular

disturbances.

spinal, 1. of, or pertaining, to a spine; especially the spinal column. 2. *informal*; spinal anaesthesia, such as saddle block or caudal anaesthesia.

spinal accessory nerve. See **accessory nerve.**

spinal aperture, a large opening formed by the body of a vertebra and its arch.

spinal arachnoid. See **arachnoidea spinalis.**

spinal canal, the cavity within the vertebral column.

spinal caries. See **tuberculous spondylitis.**

spinal column. See **vertebral column.**

spinal cord, a long, nearly cylindrical structure lodged in the vertebral canal and extending from the foramen magnum at the base of the skull to the upper part of the lumbar region. A major component of the central nervous system, the adult cord is approximately 1 cm in diameter with an average length of 42 to 45 cm and a weight of 30 g. The cord conducts sensory and motor impulses to and from the brain, and controls many reflexes. Thirty-one spinal nerves originate from the cord: 8 cervical, 12 thoracic, 5 lumbar, 5 sacral and 1 coccygeal. It has an inner core of grey material consisting mainly of nerve cells and is enclosed by three protective membranes (meninges): the dura mater, arachnoid and pia mater. The cord is an extension of the medulla oblongata of the brain and ends near the third lumbar vertebra.

spinal cord compression, an abnormal and often serious condition resulting from pressure on the spinal cord. The symptoms range from temporary numbness of an extremity to permanent quadriplegia, depending on the cause, severity and location of the pressure. Causes include spinal fracture, vertebral dislocation, tumour, haemorrhage and oedema associated with contusion.

spinal cord injury, any one of the traumatic disruptions of the spinal cord, often associated with extensive musculoskeletal involvement. Common spinal cord injuries are spinal fractures and dislocations, such as those commonly suffered by individuals involved in accidents. Such trauma may cause varying degrees of paraplegia and quadriplegia. Injuries to spinal structures below the first thoracic vertebra may produce paraplegia. Injuries to the spine above the first thoracic vertebra may cause quadriplegia. Injuries that completely transect the spinal cord cause permanent loss of motor and sensory functions activated by neurons below the level of the lesions involved. Spinal cord injuries produce a state of spinal shock, characterized by placid paralysis and complete loss of skin sensation at the time of the injury. Musculoskeletal complications are associated with the neurological involvement of spinal cord injuries.

spinal cord tumour, a neoplasm of the spinal cord of which more than 50% are extramedullary, about 25% are intramedullary, and the rest are extradural. Symptoms usually develop slowly and may progress from unilateral paraesthesia and a dull ache to lancinating pain, weakness in one or both legs, abnormal deep tendon reflexes and, in advanced cases, monoplegia, hemiplegia or paraplegia. Function of the autonomic nervous system is sometimes disturbed, causing areas of dry, cold, bluish pink skin or profuse sweating of the lower extremities.

spinal curvature, any persistent, abnormal deviation of the vertebral column from its normal position, such as **kyphoscoliosis, kyphosis, lordosis** and **scoliosis.**

spinal dysrhaphis. See **spina bifida.**

spinal fasciculi. See **spinal tract.**

spinal fluid. See **cerebrospinal fluid.**

spinal fusion, the fixation of an unstable segment of the spine, accomplished by skeletal traction or immobilization of the patient in a body cast but most frequently by a surgical procedure.

spinal headache, a headache occurring after spinal anaesthesia or lumbar puncture, caused by a loss of cerebrospinal fluid (CSF) from the subarachnoid space. It results in traction of the meninges on the pressure-sensitive intracranial structures. Severe spinal headache may be accompanied by diminished aural and visual acuity. Treatment usually includes keeping the patient flat in bed to relieve the meningeal irritation, encouraging an increased fluid intake to increase the production and volume of cerebrospinal fluid, and administering analgesics to reduce pain.

spinal manipulation, the forced passive flexion, extension and rotation of vertebral segments, carrying the elements of articulation beyond the usual range of movement to the limit of anatomical range.

spinal nerves, the 31 pairs of nerves without special names that are connected to the spinal cord and numbered according to the level of the cord at which they emerge. There are 8 cervical, 12 thoracic, 5 lumbar and 5 sacral pairs and 1 coccygeal pair. The first cervical pair of nerves emerges from the spinal cord in the space between the first cervical vertebra and occipital bone. The rest of the cervical pairs and all the thoracic pairs emerge horizontally through the intervertebral foramen of their respective vertebrae. The lumbar, sacral and coccygeal nerve pairs descend from their points of origin at the lower end of the cord before reaching the intervertebral foramina of their respective vertebrae. Each spinal nerve attaches to the spinal cord by an anterior root and a posterior root. The posterior roots accompany a distended spinal ganglion within the vertebral foramina. Emerging from the cord, each spinal nerve divides into the anterior, posterior and white rami; the anterior and posterior rami serve the voluntary nervous system, and the white rami serve the autonomic nervous system.

spinal puncture. See **lumbar puncture.**

spinal shock, a form of shock associated with acute injury to the spinal cord.

spinal tract, any one of the ascending and descending pathways for motor or sensory nerve impulses, found in the white matter of the spinal cord. Twenty-one different tracts lie within the dorsal, ventral and lateral funiculi of the white substance. Ascending tracts conduct impulses up the spinal cord to the brain; descending tracts conduct impulses down the cord from the brain. Touch, pressure, proprioception, temperature and pain are sensory stimuli transmitted via the spinal tracts. Reflex and voluntary motor activity are regulated by motor nerve stimulation from the brain and brainstem to the motor neurons of the spinal cord.

spindle, 1. the fusiform figure of achromatin in the cell nucleus during the late prophase and metaphase of mitosis. **2.** a type of brainwave, consisting of a short series of changes in electrical potential with a frequency of 14 per second. **3.** any one of the special receptor organs comprising the neurotendinous and neuromuscular spindles distributed throughout the body.

spindle cell carcinoma, a rapidly growing neoplasm composed of fusiform squamous cells. It may be difficult to distinguish from a sarcoma.

spindle cell naevus. See **benign juvenile melanoma.**

spine, the vertebral column, or backbone.

spinocerebellar, of, or pertaining to, the spinal cord and cerebellum.

spinocerebellar disorder, an inherited disorder characterized by a progressive degeneration of the spinal cord and cerebellum, but it may often also involve other parts of the nervous system. These disorders tend to occur within families and can be inherited as dominant or recessive traits. Some kinds of spinocerebellar degeneration are **ataxia telangiectasia, Charcot-Marie-Tooth atrophy, Dejerine-Sottas disease, Friedreich's ataxia, olivopontocerebellar atrophy,** and **Refsum's syndrome.**

spiral fracture, a bone break in which the disruption of bone tissue is spiral, oblique or transverse to the long axis of the fractured bone.

spiral organ of Corti. See **organ of Corti.**

spiral reverse bandage, a spiral bandage that is turned and folded back on itself as necessary to make it fit the contour of the body more securely.

spirillary rat-bite fever, spirillum fever. See **rat-bite fever.**

spirit, 1. any volatile liquid, particularly one that has been distilled. **2.** a volatile substance dissolved in alcohol.

spiritual distress (distress of the human spirit), a disruption in the life principle which pervades a person's entire being and which integrates and transcends biopsychosocial nature. Defining characteristics include stated anger against the deity or questions about the meaning of the suffering being experienced. The client may joke in a macabre fashion, regard the illness as punishment, have nightmares, cry, act in a hostile or apathetic manner, express self-blame or deny all responsibility for the problem, express anger or resentment against religious figures, and cease participation in religious practices.

spirochaete, any bacterium of the genus *Spirochaeta* that is motile and spiral-shaped with flexible filaments. Kinds of spirochaetes include the organisms responsible for leptospirosis, relapsing fever, syphilis and yaws. **spirochaetal,** *adj.*

spirogram, a visual record of respiratory movements made by a spirometer, used in the assessment of pulmonary function and capacity.

spirograph, a device for recording respiratory movements. **spirographic,** *adj.*

spirometer, an instrument that measures and records the volume of inhaled and exhaled air, used to assess pulmonary function. **spirometric,** *adj.*

spirometry, laboratory evaluation of the air capacity of the lungs by means of a spirometer. **spirometric,** *adj.*

spironolactone, an aldosterone antagonist used in the treatment of primary hyperaldosteronism, cirrhosis of the liver accompanied by oedema, nephrotic syndrome, and malignant and cirrhotic ascites.

Spitz naevus. See **benign juvenile melanoma.**

splanchnic, of, or pertaining to, the internal organs; visceral.

splanchnic engorgement, the excessive filling or pooling of blood within the visceral vasculature following the removal of pressure from the abdomen, as in the excision of a large tumour or birth of a child.

splanchnocele, hernial protrusion of any abdominal viscera.

splanchnocoele, a part of the embryonic body cavity, or coelom, that gives rise to the abdominal, pericardial and pleural cavities.

splanchnopleure, a layer of tissue in the early developing embryo, formed by the union of endoderm and splanchnic mesoderm. **splanchnopleural,** *adj.*

spleen, a soft, highly vascular, roughly ovoid organ situated between the stomach and diaphragm in the left hypochondriac region of the body. It is considered part of the lymphatic system, because it contains lymphatic nodules. It is of a dark purple colour and varies in shape in different individuals. Macrophages lining the sinuses of the spleen destroy micro-organisms by phagocytosis. The spleen also produces leukocytes, monocytes, lymphocytes and plasma cells. If the body suffers severe haemorrhage, the spleen can increase the blood volume from 350 ml to 550 ml in less than 60 seconds. **splenic,** *adj.*

spleen scan, an imaging technique for studying the spleen, such as radionuclide imaging or ultrasound.

splenectomy, the surgical excision of the spleen.

splenic flexure syndrome, a recurrent pain and abdominal distention in the left upper quadrant of the abdomen. It is caused by a pocket of gas trapped in the large intestine below the spleen, at the flexure of the transverse and descending colon.

splenic gland. See **pancreaticolienal node.**

splenic vein. See **lienal vein.**

splenius capitis, one of a pair of deep muscles of the back. It acts to rotate, extend and bend the head.

splenius cervicis, one of a pair of deep muscles of the back. The splenius cervicis acts to rotate, bend and extend the head and neck.

splenomedullary leukaemia. See **acute myelocytic leukaemia, chronic myelocytic leukaemia.**

splenomegaly, an abnormal enlargement of the spleen, as is associated with portal hypertension, haemolytic anaemia, Niemann-Pick disease or malaria.

splenomyelogenous leukaemia. See **acute myeloblastic leukaemia, chronic myeloblastic leukaemia.**

splint, 1. an orthopaedic device for immobilization, restraint or support of any part of the body. It may be rigid (made of metal, plaster or wood) or flexible (made of felt or leather). **2.** (in dentistry) a device for anchoring teeth or modifying the bite.

splinter fracture, a comminuted fracture with thin, sharp bone fragments.

splinter haemorrhage, linear bleeding under a fingernail or toenail, resembling a splinter.

splinting, the process of immobilizing, restraining or supporting a body part.

split gene, (in molecular genetics) a genetic unit whose continuity is interrupted.

split personality. See **multiple personality.**

split Russell traction, an orthopaedic mechanism that combines suspension and traction to immobilize, position and align the lower extremities in the treatment of congenital hip dislocation, hip and knee contractures, and in the correction of orthopaedic deformities.

splitting, a primitive defence mechanism which, when overused, represents a developmental arrest.

spondylitis, an inflammation of any of the spinal vertebrae, usually characterized by stiffness and pain. The condition may follow traumatic injury to the spine; it may also be the result of infection or rheumatoid disease.

spondylolisthesis, the partial forward dislocation of one vertebra over the one below it.

spondylosis, a condition of the spine characterized by fixation or stiffness of a vertebral joint.

spondylosyndesis. See **spinal fusion.**

sponge, 1. a resilient, absorbent mass used to absorb fluids, apply medication or cleanse. **2.** *informal,* a folded gauze square used in surgery.

sponge bath, the procedure of washing the patient with a damp washcloth or sponge. It is used when a full bath is not necessary or as a method of reducing body temperature.

sponge gold. See **mat gold.**

spongioblastoma, *pl.* **spongioblastomas, spongioblastomata,** a neoplasm composed of spongioblasts, embryonic epithelial cells that develop around the neural tube and transform into cells of the supporting connective tissue of nerve cells or cells of lining membranes of the ventricles and spinal cord canal. A kind of spongioblastoma is **spongioblastoma unipolare.**

spongioblastoma multiforme. See **glioblastoma multiforme.**

spongioblastoma unipolare, a rare neoplasm composed of approximately parallel spongioblasts. It may occur near the third ventricle, in the pons and brainstem, basal ganglia or the terminal filament of the spinal cord.

spongiocytoma. See **spongioblastoma.**

spontaneous, occurring naturally and without apparent cause, such as spontaneous remission.

spontaneous abortion, expulsion of the products of conception before the twenty-fourth week of gestation.

spontaneous delivery, a vaginal birth without assistance.

spontaneous fracture. See **neoplastic fracture.**

spontaneous generation, the theoretical origin of living organisms from inanimate matter; abiogenesis.

spontaneous PEEP (sPEEP), a spontaneous breathing system with end-expiratory pressure.

spontaneous ventilation, normal unassisted breathing, in which the patient creates the pressure gradient through muscle and chest wall movements that move the air into and out of the lungs.

sporadic, (of a number of events) occurring at scattered, intermittent and apparently random intervals.

spore, 1. a reproductive unit of some genera of fungi or protozoa. **2.** a form assumed by some bacteria; it is resistant to heat, drying, and chemicals. Diseases caused by spore-forming bacteria include anthrax, botulism, gas gangrene and tetanus.

sporicide, any agent effective in destroying spores, such as compounds of chlorine and formaldehyde, and gluteraldehyde.

sporiferous, producing or bearing spores.

spork, a spoon-like food utensil with fork tines, specially designed for persons with upper extremity disabilities.

sporoblast, any cell that gives rise to a sporozoite or spore during the sexual reproductive phase of the lifecycle of a sporozoan, specifically the cells resulting from the multiple fission of the encysted zygote of the malarial parasite *Plasmodium* from which the sporozoites develop.

sporocyst, 1. any structure containing spores or reproductive cells. **2.** a sac-like structure, or oocyst, secreted by the zygote of certain protozoa before sporozoite formation. **3.** the second larval stage in the lifecycle of parasitic flukes.

sporogenesis, 1. the formation of spores. **2.** reproduction by means of spores. **sporogenic,** *adj.*

sporogenous, describing an animal or plant that reproduces by spores.

sporogeny. See **sporogenesis.**

sporogony, reproduction by means of spores, specifically the formation of sporozoites during the sexual stage of the lifecycle of a sporozoan, primarily the malarial parasite *Plasmodium.*

sporont, a mature protozoan parasite in the sexual reproductive stage of its lifecycle.

sporonticide, any substance that destroys sporonts, such as chloroquine and other antimalarial drugs. **sporonticidal,** *adj.*

sporophore, the part of an organism or plant that produces spores.

sporophyte, the asexual, spore-bearing stage in plants that reproduce by alternation of generations.

sporotrichosis, a common, chronic fungal infection caused by the species *Sporothrix schenckii,* usually characterized by skin ulcers and subcutaneous nodules along lymphatic channels. The fungus is found in soil and decaying vegetation, and usually enters the skin by accidental injury.

Sporotrichum, a genus of soil-inhabiting fungi formerly thought to cause sporotrichosis.

Sporozoa, a class of parasite in the phylum Protozoa that is characterized by the absence of any external organs of locomotion. Included in this class are the genera *Toxoplasma* and *Plasmodium.*

sporozoite, any of the cells resulting from the sexual union of spores during the lifecycle of a sporozoan.

sport, 1. an individual or organism that differs drastically from its parents or others of its type because of genetic mutation; a mutant. **2.** a genetic mutation. **3.** See **lusus naturae.**

sports medicine, a branch of medicine that specializes in the prevention and treatment of injuries resulting from training and participation in athletic events. Among the most common sports injuries are shin splints, runner's knee, pulled hamstring muscles, Achilles tendonitis, ankle sprain, tennis elbow, baseball finger, dislocations, muscle cramps and bursitis.

sporulation, 1. a type of reproduction that occurs in lower plants and animals, such as fungi, algae and protozoa. It involves the formation of spores by the spontaneous division of the cell into four or more daughter cells, each of which contains a portion of the original nucleus. **2.** the formation of a refractile body, or resting spore, within certain bacteria that makes the cell resistant to unfavourable environmental conditions.

spot, (in psychotherapy) a small quantum of space that becomes the territorial object and extension of point behaviour.

spot film, a radiograph made instantly during fluoroscopy.

spotted fever. See **Rocky Mountain spotted fever.**

sprain, a traumatic injury to the tendons, muscles, or ligaments around a joint, characterized by pain, swelling and discolouration of the skin over the joint. The duration and severity of the symptoms vary with the extent of damage to the supporting tissues.

sprain fracture, a fracture that results from the separation of a tendon or ligament at the point of insertion, associated with the separation of a bone at the same insertion site.

spreader bar, a metal bar with curved hoop areas for attaching hooks or pins for traction.

spring forceps, a kind of forceps that includes a spring mechanism, used for grasping an artery to arrest or prevent haemorrhage.

spring lancet, a lancet with a spring-triggered blade. It may be used for collecting small specimens of blood for laboratory tests.

sprinter's fracture, a fracture of the anterior superior or anterior inferior spine of the ilium, caused by a fragment of bone forcibly pulled by a violent muscle spasm.

sprue, a chronic disorder resulting from malabsorption of nutrients from the small intestine and characterized by diarrhoea, weakness, weight loss, poor appetite, pallor, muscle cramps, bone pain, ulceration of the mucous membrane lining the digestive tract and a smooth, shiny tongue. It occurs in both tropical and non-tropical forms.

spurious pregnancy. See **pseudocyesis.**

sputum, material coughed up from the lungs and expectorated through the mouth. It contains mucus, cellular debris or micro-organisms, and may also contain blood or pus. The amount, colour and constituents of sputum are important in the diagnosis of many illnesses.

squama, *pl.* **squamae, 1.** a flattened scale from the epidermis. **2.** the thin, expanded part of a bone, especially in the cranial wall.

squamous cell, a flat, scale-like epithelial cell.

squamous cell carcinoma, a slow-growing, malignant tumour of squamous epithelium, frequently found in the lungs and skin. It may also occur in the anus, cervix, larynx, nose, bladder and other sites. The typical skin lesion is a firm, red, horny, painless nodule and is often the result of overexposure to sunlight.

square window, an angle of the wrist between the hypothenar prominence and forearm. It is used as a reference point for estimating the gestational age of a newborn infant.

squeeze dynamometer, a dynamometer for measuring the muscular strength of the grip of the hand.

squeeze-film lubrication, the exudation of fluid from the cartilage of joints, forming a film in the transient area of impending contact.

squint. See **strabismus.**

squinting eye, the abnormal eye in a person with strabismus that cannot be focused with the fixated eye.

Sr, symbol for **strontium.**

ss, abbreviation for **steady state.**

ST, abbreviation for *slow-twitch.* See **slow-twitch fibre.**

ST segment, the component of the cardiac cycle shown on an electrocardiogram as a short, gradual upward curve after the spiked QRS complex, before the ascent of the T wave. It represents the interval between complete depolarization at the end of ventricular contraction and the beginning of repolarization.

St. Louis encephalitis, an arbovirus infection of the brain transmitted from birds to humans by an infected mosquito. It is characterized by headache, malaise, fever, stiff neck, delirium and convulsions. Sequelae may include visual and speech disturbances, difficulty in walking and personality changes. Convalescence may be prolonged, and death may ensue.

stab, a non-segmented neutrophil.

stab form. See **band.**

stabile diabetes. See **non-insulin-dependent diabetes.**

stabilization, 1. the physiological and metabolic process of attaining homeostasis. **2.** the seating of a fixed or removable denture so that it does not tilt or becomes displaced under pressure. **3.** the control of induced stress loads and development of measures to counteract such forces, so that the movement of teeth or a prosthesis does not irritate surrounding tissues.

stable element, a non-radioactive element, one not subject to spontaneous nuclear degeneration. Some kinds of stable elements are calcium, iron, lead, potassium and sodium.

staccato speech, abnormal speech in which the person pauses between words, breaking the rhythm of the phrase or sentence. The condition is sometimes observed in association with multiple sclerosis.

stadium, *pl.* **stadia,** a significant stage in a fever or illness, such as the fastigium of a febrile illness or the prodromal stage of a viral infection.

staff, **1.** people who work towards a common goal and are employed or supervised by someone of higher rank. **2.** a designation by which a staff nurse is distinguished from a head nurse or other nurse. **3.** (in nursing education) the non-professional employees of an institution, such as librarians, technicians, secretaries and clerks.

staff development, (in nursing) a process that assists individual nurses in attaining new skills and knowledge, gaining increasing levels of competence and growing professionally. The process may include programmes such as orientation, practical training and continuing education.

staff of Æsculapius, a staff carried by Æsculapius, the Greek god of medicine. It is used as the traditional symbol of the physician. A single serpent entwines the staff of Æsculapius.

staffing, the process of assigning people to fill the roles designed for an organizational structure through recruitment, selection and placement.

staffing pattern, (in hospital or nursing administration) the number and type of staff assigned to the particular units and departments of a hospital. Staffing patterns vary with the unit, department and shift.

stages of anaesthesia. See **Guedel's signs.**

stages of dying, the five emotional and behavioural stages that often occur after a person first learns of approaching death. The stages, identified and described by Elizabeth Kübler-Ross, are denial and shock, anger, bargaining, depression and acceptance. The stages may occur in sequence or may recur, as the person fluctuates—especially between denial, anger and bargaining.

stagnant anoxia, a condition in which there is inadequate blood flow in the capillaries, causing low tissue oxygen tension and reduced oxygen exchange.

stain, **1.** a pigment, dye or substance used to impart colour to microscopic objects or tissues, so as to facilitate their examination and identification. Kinds of stains include **acid-fast stain, Gram's stain** and **Wright's stain. 2.** to apply pigment to a substance or tissue for examination under a microscope. **3.** an area of discolouration.

stammering, a speech dysfunction characterized by spasmodic pauses, hesitations and faltering utterances, such as mispronunciation or transposition of letters within a word.

stance phase of gait, the first phase of the normal gait cycle that begins with the strike of the heel on the ground and ends with the lift of the toe at the beginning of the swing phase of gait: the brief period in which both feet are on the ground.

standard, **1.** an evaluation that serves as a basis of comparison for evaluating similar phenomena or substances, such as a standard for the preparation of a pharmaceutical substance or a standard for the practice of a profession. **2.** a pharmaceutical preparation or chemical substance of known quantity, ingredients and strength, used to determine the constituents or strength of another preparation. **3.** of known value, strength, quality or ingredients. **4.** agreed criteria used for guidance in the operation of a healthcare or other facility, so as to ensure quality performance. **standardize,** *v.,* **standardization,** *n.*

standard air chamber, a radiation measuring device used by national and international calibration laboratories, to provide exposure calibrations of secondary ionization chambers.

standard bicarbonate, the bicarbonate ion concentration of plasma separated anaerobically from whole blood that has been saturated with oxygen and equilibrated at carbon dioxide pressure of 40 torr at 38° C. It is a measure of the metabolic disturbance of acid-base balance in a sample of blood after any respiratory disturbance present has been corrected.

standard deviation (SD), (in statistics) a mathematic statement of the dispersion of a set of values or scores from the mean. Each sample value is subtracted from the sample mean and squared, and the squares are summed. The square root of the summed squares gives a mathematically standardized value so that sample deviations can be compared.

standard environmental chamber. See **Skinner box.**

standard error, (in statistics) the variability in scores that can be expected if measurements are made on random samples of the same size from the same universe of population, phenomena or observations. The standard error provides a framework within which a determination of the difference between groups may be made.

standardized death rate, the number of deaths per 1000 people of a specified population during 1 year. This rate is adjusted to avoid distortion by the age composition of the population.

standing orders, a written document containing rules, policies, procedures, regulations and orders for the conduct of patient care in various stipulated clinical situations. Standing orders usually name the condition and prescribe the action to be taken in caring for the patient, including the dosage and route of administration for a drug or schedule for the administration of a therapeutic procedure.

stanozolol, an androgenic anabolic steroid used in the treatment of the vascular manifestations of Behet's disease, hereditary angioedema and aplastic anaemia.

stapedectomy, removal of the stapes of the middle ear and insertion of a graft and prosthesis. It is performed for restoration of hearing in the treatment of otosclerosis. The stapes that has become fixed is replaced so that vibrations once again transmit sound waves through the oval window to the fluid of the inner ear.

stapes, one of the three ossicles in the middle ear, resembling a tiny stirrup. It transmits sound vibrations from the incus to the internal ear.

staphylococcal infection, an infection caused by any one of several pathogenic species of Staphylococcus, commonly characterized by the formation of abscesses of the skin or other organs. Staphylococcal infections of the skin include carbuncles, folliculitis, furuncles and hidradenitis suppurativa. Bacteraemia is common and may result in endocarditis, meningitis or osteomyelitis. *Staphylococcal* pneumonia often follows influenza or other viral disease, and may be associated with chronic or debilitating illness. Acute gastroenteritis may result from an enterotoxin produced by certain species of staphylococci in contaminated food.

staphylococcal scalded skin syndrome (SSSS), an abnormal skin condition, characterized by epidermal erythema, peeling and necrosis, giving the skin a scalded appearance. This disorder primarily affects infants 1 to 3 months of age as well as children, but may also affect adults. It is caused by strains of *Staphylococcus aureus,* especially Group II phage types. Individuals contracting the disease may be predisposed to it by deficient immune functions and renal insufficiency. SSSS is more common in the newborn because of undeveloped immunity and renal systems. A prodromal upper respiratory tract infection with concomitant purulent conjunctivitis is commonly associated with SSSS. Epidermal complications develop in the erythemal stage, the exfoliation stage and the desquamation stage. Erythema often spreads around the mouth and other orifices, and may extend over the entire body in wide circles as the skin becomes tender and the superficial layer of the skin sloughs from friction. The exfoliation stage follows the erythema stage by 24 to 48 hours, and is commonly manifested by slight crusting and erosion which may spread from around the orifices to wider skin areas.

Staphylococcus, a genus of non-motile, spheric, gram-positive bacteria. Some species are normally found on the skin and in the throat; certain species cause severe, purulent infections or produce an enterotoxin which may cause nausea, vomiting and diarrhoea. *Staphylococcus aureus* is a species frequently responsible for abscesses, endocarditis, impetigo, osteomyelitis, pneumonia and septicaemia. See also **staphylococcal infection. staphylococcal,** *adj.*

staphylokinase, an enzyme, produced by certain strains of staphylococci, that catalyses the conversion of plasminogen to plasmin in various animal hosts of the micro-organism.

staple, a piece of stainless steel wire used to close certain surgical wounds.

starch, the principal molecule used for the storage of food in plants. Starch is a polysaccharide and is composed of long chains of glucose subunits. In animals, excess glucose is stored as glycogen.

Starling's law of the heart {Ernest H. Starling, English physiologist, b. 1866}, a rule that the force of the heartbeat is determined by the length of the fibres comprising the myocardial walls.

Starr-Edwards prosthesis {A. Starr, 20th century American physician; M. L. Edwards, 20th century American physician}, an artificial cardiac valve. A caged-ball form of device, it obstructs the valve opening and prevents the backward flow of blood.

start codon. See **initiation codon.**

start point, (in molecular genetics) the initial nucleotide transcribed from the DNA template in the formation of messenger RNA.

startle reflex. See **Moro reflex.**

starvation, 1. a condition resulting from the lack of essential nutrients over a long period of time, and characterized by multiple physiological and metabolic dysfunctions. **2.** the act or state of starving or being starved. See also **malnutrition.**

stasis, 1. a disorder in which the normal flow of a fluid through a vessel of the body is slowed or halted. **2.** stillness.

stasis dermatitis, a common result of venous insufficiency of the legs, beginning with ankle oedema and progressing to tan pigmentation, patchy erythema, petechiae and induration. Ultimately, there may be atrophy and fibrosis of the skin and subcutaneous tissue, with ulcerations that are slow to heal. The tan pigment is haemosiderin from blood leaking through capillary walls under elevated venous pressure. The involved skin is very easily irritated or sensitized to topical medications.

stasis ulcer, a necrotic crater-like lesion of the skin of the lower leg, caused by chronic venous congestion. The ulcer is often associated with stasis dermatitis and varicose veins.

static, without motion, at rest, in equilibrium.

static cardiac work, the energy transfer that occurs during the development and maintenance of ventricular pressure immediately before the opening of the aortic valve.

static electricity film fault, a defect in a radiograph or a developed photographic film, which appears as lightning-like streaks. It is caused by too rapid opening of the film packet or transfer of static electricity from the film to the user.

static equilibrium, the ability of an individual to adjust to displacements of his or her centre of gravity while maintaining a constant base of support.

static imaging, (in nuclear medicine) a diagnostic procedure in which a radioactive substance is administered to a patient to visualize an internal organ or body compartment. An image or set of images is made of the fixed or slowly changing distribution of the radioactivity.

station, the location of the presenting part of the fetus in labour, in relation to the level of the ischial spines. If the level is above the ischial spines, this is described as -1 to -5. If it is below, it is described as +1 to +5.

stationary grid, (in radiography) a secondary radiation grid that does not move or oscillate during exposure.

stationary lingual arch, an orthodontic arch wire designed to fit the lingual surface of teeth and soldered to the associated anchor bands.

statistical, a number that describes a property of a set of data or other numbers.

statistics, a mathematical science concerned with measuring, classifying and analysing objective information.

statotonic reflex. See **attitudinal reflex.**

status, 1. a specified state or condition, such as emotional status. **2.** an unremitting state or condition, such as status asthmaticus.

status asthmaticus, an acute, severe and prolonged asthma attack. Hypoxia, cyanosis and unconsciousness may follow.

status dysraphicus. See **dysraphia.**

status epilepticus, a medical emergency characterized by continual attacks of convulsive seizures occurring without intervals of consciousness. Unless convulsions are arrested, irreversible brain damage results. Status epilepticus can be precipitated by the sudden withdrawal of anticonvulsant drugs, inadequate body levels of glucose, brain tumour, head injury, a high fever or poison-

ing.

spongiosus, a condition of toxic and degenerative brain alteration usually associated with dissolution of the brain substance.

STD, abbreviation for **sexually transmitted disease.**

steady state (s, ss), a basic physiological concept implying that the various forces and processes of life are in a state of homeostasis.

stearyl alcohol, a solid substance, prepared by the catalytic hydrogenation of stearic acid. It is used in various ointments.

steatorrhoea, greater than normal amounts of fat in the faeces, characterized by frothy, foul-smelling faecal matter that floats, as in coeliac disease, some malabsorption syndromes and any condition in which fats are poorly absorbed by the small intestine.

Steele-Richardson-Olszewski syndrome {John C. Steele; J. Clifford Richardson; Jerzy Olszewski; 20th century Canadian neurologists}, a rare, progressive, neurological disorder of unknown cause, occurring in middle age and more often in men. It is characterized by paralysis of eye muscles, ataxia, neck and trunk rigidity, pseudobulbar palsy and parkinsonian facies. Dementia and inappropriate emotional responses are also common.

steeple head. See **oxycephaly.**

Stein-Leventhal syndrome. See **polycystic ovary syndrome.**

Steinert's disease. See **myotonic muscular dystrophy.**

stellate, star-shaped or arranged in the pattern of a star.

stellate fracture, a fracture that involves the central point of impact or injury and radiates numerous fissures throughout surrounding bone tissue.

stem cell, a formative cell; a cell whose daughter cells may give rise to other cell types. A **pluripotential stem cell** is one that has the potential to develop into several different types of mature cells, including lymphocytes, granulocytes, thrombocytes and erythrocytes.

stem cell leukaemia, a malignant neoplasm of blood-forming organs in which the predominant neoplastic cell is too immature to classify.

stem cell lymphoma. See **undifferentiated malignant lymphoma.**

stenosis, an abnormal condition characterized by the constriction or narrowing of an opening or passageway in a body structure. Kinds of stenosis include aortic stenosis and pyloric stenosis. **stenotic,** adj.

Stensen's duct. See **parotid duct.**

stent {Charles R. Stent, 19th century English dentist}, **1.** a compound used in making dental impressions and medical moulds. **2.** a mould or device made of stent, used in anchoring skin grafts and for supporting body openings and cavities during grafting, or vessels and tubes of the body during surgical anastomosis.

step reflex. See **dance reflex.**

stepwedge, a device used to put a series of increasing exposures on a radiographic film when exposed by a radiographic beam.

stereognosis, 1. the faculty of perceiving and understanding the form and nature of objects by the sense of touch. **2.** perception by the senses of the solidity of objects. **stereognostic,** *adj.*

stereognostic perception, the ability to recognize objects by the sense of touch.

stereoisomeric specificity, specificity of an enzyme for one form of a DL pair of compounds with an asymmetrical carbon atom.

stereopsis, the quality of visual fusion.

stereoradiography, a technique for producing radiographs that give a three-dimensional view of an internal body structure.

stereoscopic microscope, a microscope that produces three-dimensional images through the use of double eyepieces and double objectives.

stereoscopic parallax. See **binocular parallax.**

stereoscopic radiograph, a composite of two radiographs, made by shifting the position of the x-ray tube a few centimetres between each of two exposures. The result is a three-dimensional presentation of the radiograph when viewed through stereoscopic lenses.

stereotaxic neuroradiography, an x-ray procedure commonly performed during neurosurgery to guide the insertion of a needle into a specific area of the brain.

stereotype, a generalization concerning a form of behaviour, an individual or a group.

stereotypic behaviour, a pattern of body movements that has autistic and symbolic meaning for an individual.

stereotypy, the persistent, inappropriate, mechanical repetition of actions, body postures or speech patterns, usually occurring with a lack of variation in thought processes or ideas. **stereotypical,** *adj.*

sterile, 1. barren; unable to produce children because of a physical abnormality, often the absence of spermatogenesis in a man or blockage of the uterine tubes in a woman. **2.** aseptic. **sterility,** *n.*

sterile field, 1. a specified area considered free of micro-organisms. **2.** an area immediately around a patient that has been prepared for a surgical procedure. The sterile field includes the scrubbed team members and all furniture and fixtures in the area.

sterilization, 1. a process or act that renders a person unable to produce children. **2.** a technique for destroying micro-organisms using heat, water, chemicals or gases. **sterilize,** *v.*

sternal node, a node in one of the three groups of thoracic parietal lymph nodes.

Sternheimer-Malbin stain, a crystal violet and safranin stain, used in urinalysis to provide additional contrast for certain casts and cells.

sternoclavicular articulation, the double gliding joint between the sternum and clavicle.

sternocostal articulation, the gliding articulation of the cartilage of each true rib and the sternum, except for the articulation of the first rib in which the cartilage is directly united with the sternum to form a synchondrosis.

sternohyoideus, one of the four infrahyoid muscles. It acts to depress the hyoid bone.

sternothyroideus, one of the four infrahyoid muscles. It acts to depress the thyroid cartilage.

sternum, the elongated, flattened bone forming the middle portion of the thorax. It supports the clavicles, articulates with the first seven pairs of ribs, and comprises the manubrium, gladiolus (body) and xiphoid process.

sternutation. See **sneeze.**

steroid, any of a large number of hormonal substances with a similar basic chemical structure. They are produced mainly in the adrenal cortex and gonads.

sterol, a large subgroup of steroids containing an OH group at position 3 and a branched aliphatic side chain of eight or more carbon atoms at position 17. Kinds of sterols include **cholesterol and ergosterol.**

stertorous, pertaining to a respiratory effort that is strenuous or struggling; having a snoring sound.

stethomimetic, pertaining to any condition causing or associated with a reduction in chest volume below its normal value.

stethoscope, an instrument, used in auscultation, consisting of two earpieces connected by flexible tubing to a diaphragm, which is placed against the skin of the patient's chest or back to hear heart and lung sounds.

Stevens-Johnson syndrome {Albert M. Stevens, American paediatrician, b. 1884; F. C. Johnson, American physician, b. 1894}, a serious and sometimes fatal inflammatory disease affecting children and young adults. It is characterized by the acute onset of fever, bullae on the skin and ulcers on the mucous membranes of the lips, eyes, mouth, nasal passage and genitalia. Pneumonia, joint pain and prostration are common. Perforation of the cornea may be a complication. The syndrome may be an allergic reaction to certain drugs; it may also follow pregnancy, herpesvirus I infection or other infection.

sthenic fever, high body temperature associated with thirst, dry skin and often delirium.

sticky ends. See **cohesive termini.**

Stieda's fracture {Alfred Steida, German

surgeon, b. 1869}, a fracture of the internal condyle of the femur.

stiff lung. See **congestive atelectasis.**

stigma, *pl.* **stigmata, stigmas, 1.** a moral or physical blemish. **2.** a physical characteristic that serves to identify a disease or condition.

stilboestrol. See **diethylstilboestrol.**

stilet, stilette. See **stylet.**

Still's disease. See **juvenile rheumatoid arthritis.**

stillbirth, a baby who has issued forth from its mother after the 24th week of pregnancy, and did not, at any time after being expelled, breathe or show any signs of life.

stimulant, any agent that increases the rate of activity of a body system.

stimulant laxative, a laxative that acts by promoting the motility of the bowel, especially the longitudinal peristalsis of the colon. Stimulant laxatives include **cascara** and **senna.**

stimulating bath, a bath taken in water in which an aromatic substance, an astringent or a tonic has been added.

stimulus, *pl.* **stimuli,** anything that excites or incites an organism or part to function, become active or respond. **stimulate,** *v.*

stimulus control, a strategy for self-modification that depends on manipulating the antecedents of behaviour to increase goals or behaviours desired by a patient while decreasing those that are undesired.

stimulus duration, the length of time that a stimulus must be applied for the resulting nerve impulse to produce excitation in the receptor tissue. In general, more intense stimuli require shorter excitation times to effect a cellular response.

stimulus generalization, a type of conditioning in which the reaction to one stimulus is reinforced to allow transfer of the reaction to other occurrences.

sting, an injury caused by a sharp, painful penetration of the skin, often accompanied by exposure to an irritating chemical or the venom of an insect or animal. Kinds of stings include bee, jellyfish, scorpion, sea urchin and shellfish stings. See also **stingray, wasp.**

stingray, a flat, long-tailed fish bearing barbed spines on its back that are connected to sacs of venom. Spasm of the skeletal muscles, severe local pain, seizures and dyspnoea may occur if the skin is broken by the spines. See also **sea urchin sting.**

stochastic effect, (in radiobiology) the biological effect of ionizing radiation for which there is a risk of occurrence with any dose, where the probability of occurrence increases with dose; for example, induction of malignancy, genetic mutations.

stocking aid, a device that enables a handicapped person to pull on a pair of stockings. One type consists of a dowel with a cuphook on the end.

stoker's cramp. See **heat cramp.**

Stokes-Adams syndrome. See **Adams-Stokes syndrome.**

stoma, *pl.* **stomas, stomata, 1.** a pore, orifice or opening on a surface. **2.** an artificial opening of an internal organ on the surface of the body, created surgically, as for a colostomy, ileostomy or tracheostomy. **3.** a new opening created surgically between two body structures, as for a gastroenterostomy.

stoma care, the management and support of a patient with a surgical opening created in the bladder, ileum, or colon for the temporary or permanent passage of urine or faeces, necessitated by carcinoma, intestinal obstruction, trauma, or severe ulceration distal to the site of the incision. In most cases the opening is covered with a temporary disposable bag in the operating theatre.

stomach, the major organ of digestion, located in the right upper quadrant of the abdomen and divided into a body and a pylorus. It receives and partially processes food and drink funneled from the mouth through the oesophagus and moves nutritional bulk into the intestines. The stomach is lined with a mucous coat, a submucous coat, a muscular coat and a serous coat, all richly supplied with blood vessels and nerves. It contains fundic, cardiac and pyloric gastric glands.

stomach pump, a pump for withdrawing the contents of the stomach through a tube passed into the stomach through the mouth or nose.

stomadaeum. See **stomodaeum.**

stoma irrigation, a procedure for cleansing, stimulating, and regulating evacuation of an artificially created orifice. Fluids used in irrigation include tap water and saline or medicated solutions. Loop and double-barrel colostomies require a sequential irrigation of the proximal loop, distal loop, and rectum to prevent the accumulation of discharge.

stomal peptic ulcer, a marginal peptic ulcer. See also **peptic ulcer.**

Stoma therapist, a nurse specializing in the care of patients with stomas, providing advise and support in hospital and the community.

stomatitis, any inflammatory condition of the mouth. It may result from infection by bacteria, viruses or fungi, exposure to certain chemicals or drugs, vitamin deficiency, or a systemic inflammatory disease. Kinds of stomatitis include **aphthous stomatitis, pseudomembranous stomatitis, thrush** and **Vincent's infection.**

stomatognathic system, the combination of organs, structures and nerves involved in speech and reception, mastication and deglutition of food. This system consists of the teeth, jaws, masticatory muscles, tongue, lips and surrounding tissues, and the nerves that control these structures.

stomatology, the study of morphology, structure, function and diseases of the oral cavity. **stomatologist,** *n.,* **stomatological,** *adj.*

stomion, the median point of the oral slit when the mouth is closed.

stomodaeum, *pl.* **stomodaeums, stomodaea,** an invagination in the ectoderm located in the foregut of the developing embryo that forms the mouth. Also spelt **stomadaeum.** **stomodaeal, stomadaeal,** *adj.*

stone. See **calculus.**

stool softener. See **fecal softener.**

stool. See **faeces.**

stop needle, a needle with a shoulder flange that stops it from penetrating beyond a certain distance.

stopcock, a valve that controls the flow of fluid or air through a tube.

storage capacity, the amount of data that can be stored on a computer disk or tape, usually expressed in kilobytes or megabytes.

stored-energy foot, a lower-limb prosthesis designed to imitate the spring-like action of a natural foot and leg. A device stores energy when weight is placed on the artificial leg. When the weight is shifted to the other leg, the stored energy is released, returning the prosthesis to its original shape.

storing fermentation, the rapid, gaseous clotting of milk caused by *Clostridium perfringens.*

stork bite. See **telangiectatic naevus.**

STP, *slang.* a psychedelic agent, dimethoxy-4-methylamphetamine (DOM). STP is an abbreviation for **serenity, tranquility and peace.**

STPD, abbreviation for **standard temperature, standard pressure, dry.**

STPD conditions of a volume of gas, the conditions of a volume of gas at 0° C, 760 torr, and containing no water vapour. It should contain a calculable number of moles of a particular gas.

strabismus, an abnormal ophthalmic condition in which the eyes are crossed. There are two kinds of strabismus, paralytic and nonparalytic. Paralytic strabismus results from the inability of the ocular muscles to move the eye because of neurological deficit or muscular dysfunction. The dysfunctional muscle may be identified by watching as the patient attempts to move the eyes to each of the cardinal positions of gaze. Non-paralytic strabismus is a defect in the position of the two eyes in relation to each other, and is an inherited condition. The person cannot use both eyes together, but has to fix with one or the other. The eye that looks straight at a given time is the fixing eye. Some individuals have alternating strabismus, using one eye and then the other; some have monocular strabismus affecting only one eye. Visual acuity decreases with diminished use of an eye and suppression amblyopia may develop. **strabismal, strabismic, strabismical,**

adj.

straight line blood set, a common device composed of plastic components, used for delivering blood infusions. It consists of a plastic tubing, a clamp, a drip chamber and a filter.

straight sinus, one of the six posterior-superior venous channels of the dura mater, draining blood from the brain into the internal jugular vein. It has no valves and is located at the junction of the falx cerebri with the tentorium cerebelli.

straight wire fixed orthodontic appliance, an orthodontic appliance used for correcting and improving malocclusion. It is designed to decrease arch wire adjustments by reorientating arch wire slots.

strain, 1. to exert physical force in a manner that may result in injury, usually muscular. **2.** to separate solids or particles from a liquid with a filter or sieve. **3.** damage, usually muscular, that results from excessive physical effort. **4.** a taxon that is a subgroup of a species. **5.** an emotional state reflecting mental pressure or fatigue.

straitjacket, a coat-like garment of canvas with long sleeves that can be tied behind the wearer's back to prevent movement of the arms. It is used for restraining violent or uncontrollable people.

strangulation, the constriction of a tubular structure of the body, such as the trachea, a segment of bowel or the blood vessels of a limb, that prevents function or impedes circulation. **strangulate,** *v.,* **strangulated,** *adj.*

strap, 1. a band, such as that made of adhesive plaster, used to hold dressings in place or attach one thing to another. **2.** to bind securely.

strapping, the application of overlapping strips of adhesive tape to an extremity or body area, so as to exert pressure and hold a structure in place. It is used in the treatment of strains, sprains, dislocations and certain fractures.

stratiform cartilage. See **fibrocartilage.**

stratiform fibrocartilage, a structure made of fibrocartilage that forms a thin coating of osseous grooves through which tendons of certain muscles glide.

stratum, *pl.* **strata,** a uniformly thick sheet or layer, usually associated with other layers, such as the stratum basale of the epidermis.

stratum basale, 1. also called **basal layer, stratum germinativum.** The deepest of the five layers of the skin, composed of tall cylindric cells. This layer provides new cells by mitotic cell division. **2.** the deepest layers of the uterine decidua, containing uterine gland terminals.

stratum corneum, the horny, outermost layer of the skin, composed of dead cells converted to keratin that flakes away continuously. It is thick on the palms of the hands and soles of the feet but thin over more protected areas.

stratum germinativum. See **stratum basale.**

stratum granulosum, one of the layers of the epidermis situated just below the stratum corneum, except in the palms of the hands and soles of the feet where it lies just under the stratum lucidum.

stratum lucidum, one of the layers of the epidermis, situated just beneath the stratum corneum and present only in the thick skin of the palms of the hands and soles of the feet.

stratum spinosum, one of the layers of the epidermis, composed of several layers of polygonal cells. It lies on top of the stratum basale and beneath the stratum granulosum, and contains tiny fibrils within its cellular cytoplasm.

stratum spongiosum, one of the three layers of the endometrium of the uterus, containing tortuous, dilated uterine glands and a small amount of interglandular tissue.

strawberry gallbladder, a tiny, yellow gallbladder spotted with deposits on the red mucous membrane, characteristic of cholesterolosis.

strawberry haemangioma, strawberry mark. See **capillary haemangioma.**

strawberry tongue, a clinical sign of scarlet fever, characterized by a strawberry-like colouration of the inflamed tongue papillae.

stray light, radiant energy that reaches a photodetector and which consists of wavelengths other than those defined by the filter or monochromator.

stray radiation. See **leakage radiation.**

streak, a line or a stripe, such as the primitive streak at the caudal end of the embryonic disk.

strength, the ability of a muscle to produce or resist a physical force.

strength of association, the degree of relationship between a causal factor and the occurrence of a disease, usually expressed in terms of a relative risk ratio.

strep throat *informal,* an infection of the oral pharynx and tonsils caused by a haemolytic species of *Streptococcus,* usually belonging to group A. The infection is characterized by a sore throat, chills, fever, swollen lymph nodes in the neck and sometimes nausea and vomiting. The symptoms usually begin abruptly a few days after exposure to the organism in airborne droplets, or after direct contact with an infected person.

streptobacillary rat-bite fever. See **Haverhill fever.**

Streptobacillus moniliformis, a species of necklace-shaped bacteria that can cause rat-bite fever in humans.

streptococcal angina, a condition in which

feelings of choking, suffocation and pain occur as a result of streptococcal infection.

streptococcal infection, an infection caused by pathogenic bacteria of one of several species of the genus *Streptococcus* or their toxins. The infections occur in many forms including cellulitis, endocarditis, erysipelas, impetigo, meningitis, pneumonia, scarlet fever, tonsillitis and urinary tract infection.

streptococcal sore throat. See **strep throat.**

Streptococcus, a genus of non-motile, grampositive cocci classified by serological types (Lancefield groups A through T), haemolytic action (alpha, beta, gamma) when grown on blood agar, and reaction to bacterial viruses (phage types 1 to 86). Many species cause disease in humans. *Streptococcus viridans,* a member of the normal flora of the mouth, is the most common cause of bacterial endocarditis, especially when introduced into the bloodstream during dental procedures.

streptokinase, a fibrinolytic activator that enhances the conversion of plasminogen to the fibrinolytic enzyme plasmin. It is used in the emergency treatment of pulmonary and coronary embolism.

streptokinase-streptodornase, two enzymes derived from a strain of *Streptococcus haemolyticus.* They are used in combination for sloughy and necrotic wounds.

streptolysin, a substance produced by various streptococci, liberating haemoglobin from red blood cells.

streptomycin sulphate, an aminoglycoside antibiotic used in the treatment of tuberculosis.

streptozocin, an investigational cytotoxic drug used in the treatment of a variety of neoplasms, especially metastatic islet cell tumours of the pancreas. It is an antibiotic substance from *Streptomyces acromogenes.*

stress, any emotional, physical, social, economic or other factor that requires a response or change, such as dehydration which can cause an increase in body temperature, or the separation from parents which can cause distress to a young child.

stress behaviour, a change from a person's normal behaviour in response to a stressor.

stress fracture, a fracture, especially of one or more of the metatarsal bones, caused by repeated, prolonged or abnormal stress.

stress inoculation, a procedure useful in helping patients to control anxiety by substituting positive coping statements for statements that bring about anxiety.

stress kinesic, a type of behavioural characteristic of personal conversation, such as the use of body shifts or movements. It marks the flow of speech and generally coincides with linguistic stress patterns.

stress management, methods of controlling factors that require a response of change within a person by identifying the stressors, eliminating negative stressors and developing effective coping mechanisms. Examples include progressive relaxation, guided imagery, biofeedback and active problem solving.

stress reaction.   See **general adaptation syndrome, post-traumatic stress disorder.**

stress response syndrome.   See **post-traumatic stress disorder.**

stress test, a test that measures the function of a system of the body when subjected to carefully controlled amounts of stress. The data produced allow the examiner to evaluate the condition of the tested system.

stress ulcer, a gastric or duodenal ulcer that develops in previously unaffected individuals subjected to severe stress, as when severely burned. See also **Curling's ulcer.**

stress-adaptation theory, a concept that stress depletes the reserve capacity of individuals, thereby increasing their vulnerability to health problems.

stressor, anything that causes wear and tear on the body's physical or mental resources.

stretch mark. See **stria.**

stria, *pl.* **striae,** a streak or linear scar that often results from rapidly developing tension in the skin, as seen on the abdomen after pregnancy. Purplish striae are one of the classic findings in hyperadrenocorticism. Also called **stretch mark.**

stria atrophica. See **linea albicantes.**

stria gravidarum, irregular depressions with red to purple colourations that appear in the skin of the abdomen, thighs and buttocks of pregnant women.

striated muscle, muscle tissue, including all the skeletal muscles, that appears microscopically to consist of striped myofibrils. Striated muscles are composed of bundles of parallel, striated fibres under voluntary control; the heart, a striated involuntary muscle, is an exception. Each myofibril comprises thick filaments that consist of molecules of myosin, and thin filaments that consist of actin and two other protein compounds. Muscle contraction occurs when an electrochemical impulse crosses the myoneural junction, causing the thin filaments to shorten.

strict vegetarian, a vegetarian whose diet excludes the use of all foods of animal origin. Such diets may be deficient in many essential nutrients, particularly vitamin B12.

stricture, an abnormal temporary or permanent narrowing of the lumen of a hollow organ, such as the oesophagus, pylorus of the stomach, ureter or urethra, because of inflammation, external pressure or scarring. Treatment varies depending on the cause.

stridor, an abnormal, high-pitched, musical respiratory sound, caused by an obstruction in the trachea or larynx. It is usually heard during inspiration. Stridor may indicate several neoplastic or inflammatory conditions, including glottic oedema, asthma, diphtheria, laryngospasm or papilloma.

string carcinoma, a malignancy of the large intestine, usually of the ascending or transverse colon. On radiological visualization, the intestine appears tied in segments, like a string of large beads.

strip membranes, (in obstetrics) a procedure in which an examiner digitally frees the membranes of the amniotic sac from the wall of the lower segment of the uterus in the small area around the cervical os.

stripping, 1. *non-technical,* a surgical procedure for the removal of the long and short saphenous veins of the legs. **2.** the mechanical removal of a very small amount of enamel from the mesial or distal surfaces of teeth, to alleviate crowding.

stroboscopic illusion.   See **phi phenomenon.**

stroke risk profile, a predictive index using a complex of risk factors that indicate susceptibility of a person to cerebrovascular accident (CVA). Factors include advanced age, hypertension, a history of transient ischaemic attacks, cigarette smoking, heart disorders, associated embolism, family history of CVA, use of oral contraceptives, diabetes mellitus, physical inactivity, obesity, hypercholesteraemia and hyperlipidaemia.

stroke volume, the amount of blood ejected by the ventricle during a ventricle contraction.

stroke volume index, the stroke volume divided by the body surface area.

stroke. See **cerebrovascular accident.**

stroking, a form of massage in which the operator produces unidirectional movements, usually proximal to distal down the length of tissues, and varying the speed to produce the required effect.

stroma, *pl.* **stromata,** the supporting tissue or matrix of an organ as distinguished from its parenchyma.   **stromatic,** *adj.*

Strongyloides, a genus of parasitic intestinal nematode. A species of *Strongyloides*, *S. stercoralis*, causes strongyloidiasis.

strongyloidiasis, infection of the small intestine by the roundworm *Strongyloides stercoralis*. It is acquired when larvae from the soil penetrate intact skin, incidentally causing a pruritic rash. The larvae pass to the lungs via the bloodstream, sometimes causing pneumonia. Larvae then migrate up the air passages to the pharynx, they are swallowed, and develop into adult worms in the small intestine. Bloody diarrhoea and intestinal malabsorption may result. Wearing shoes prevents contagion from contaminated soil.

strontium (Sr), a metallic element. Its atomic number is 38 and its atomic weight is 87.62. Chemically similar to calcium, it is found in bone tissue. Isotopes of strontium are used in radioisotope scanning procedures of bone. Strontium 90, the longest-lived, is the most dangerous constituent of fallout from atomic bomb tests. It can replace some of the calcium in food, become concentrated in teeth and bones, and continue to emit electrons that can cause death in the host. Cows concentrate strontium 90 in their milk.

structural chemistry, the science dealing with the molecular structure of chemical substances.

structural gene, (in molecular genetics) a unit of genetic information that specifies the amino acid sequence of a polypeptide.

structural integration, a technique of deep massage intended to help in body realignment by altering the length and tone of myofascial tissues. The basis of the practice is the belief that misalignment of myofascial tissues may have an overall detrimental effect on a person's energy level, self-image, muscular efficiency, perceptions and general health. Also called **Rolfing.**

structural model, a model of family therapy that views the family as an open system and identifies subsystems within the family that carry out specific family functions.

structure, a part of the body, such as the heart, a bone, gland, cell or limb.

structure-activity relationship (SAR), the relationship between the chemical structure of a drug and its activity.

struma lymphomatosa. See **Hashimoto's disease.**

Stryker wedge frame, an orthopaedic bed that allows the patient to be rotated as required to either the supine or prone position. As with the Foster bed, the Stryker wedge frame is used in the immobilization of patients with an unstable spine, postoperative management of multilevel spinal fusions and management of severe burns. The Stryker wedge frame comes in one size, the only accommodation to different body builds being an adjustable crossbar on the anterior circle of the frame. If the crossbar is properly adapted, the patient is held firmly between the frames without the need for pillows or extra padding.

Stuart-Power factor. See **factor X.**

stump, the part of a limb after amputation that is proximal to the portion amputated.

stump hallucination, the sensation of the continued presence of an amputated limb.

stupor, a state of lethargy and unresponsiveness in which a person seems unaware of the surroundings. Kinds of stupor are **anergic stupor, benign stupor, delusion stupor** and **epileptic stupor.**

Sturge-Weber syndrome {William A. Sturge, English physician, b. 1850; Frederick P. Weber, English physician, b. 1863}, a congenital neurocutaneous disease marked by a port wine-coloured capillary haemangioma over a sensory dermatome of a branch of the trigeminal nerve of the face. The cerebral cortex may atrophy; generalized or focal seizures, angioma of the choroid, secondary glaucoma, optic atrophy and new cutaneous haemangiomas may develop.

stuttering, a speech dysfunction characterized by spasmodic enunciation of words, involving excessive hesitations, stumbling, repetition of the same syllables and prolongation of sounds. The condition may result from cerebellar disease, a neuromuscular defect, or injury of the organs of articulation. However, in most cases the cause is emotional or psychological.

stye, a purulent infection of a meibomian or sebaceous gland of the eyelid, often caused by a staphylococcal organism.

stylet, a thin metal probe for inserting into or passing through a needle, tube or catheter to clean the hollow bore, or for inserting in a soft, flexible catheter to make it shift as the catheter is placed in a vein or passed through an orifice of the body.

stylohyoid ligament, the ligament attached to the tip of the styloid process of the temporal bone and to the lesser cornu of the hyoid bone.

stylohyoideus, one of four suprahyoid muscles, lying anterior and superior to the posterior belly of the digastricus. It serves to draw the hyoid bone up and back.

stylomandibular ligament, one of a pair of specialized bands of cervical fascia, forming an accessory part of the temporomandibular joint. It extends from the styloid process of the temporal bone to the ramus of the mandible between the masseter and pterygoideus muscles, and separates the parotid gland from the submandibular gland.

styptic, 1. a substance used as an astringent, often to control bleeding. A chemical styptic induces blood coagulation. A mechanical styptic is a cotton pledget used as a compress to control bleeding. **2.** acting as an astringent or agent to control bleeding.

subacromial bursa, the bursa separating the acromion and deltoid muscle from the insertion of the supraspinatus muscle and greater tubercle of the humerus.

subacute, 1. less than acute. **2.** of, or pertaining to, a disease or other abnormal condition present in a person who appears to be clinically well.

subacute bacterial endocarditis (SBE), a chronic bacterial infection of the heart valves. It is characterized by a slow, quiet onset with fever, heart murmur, splenomegaly and the development of clumps of abnormal tissue, called vegetations, around an intracardiac prosthesis or on the cusps of a valve. Various species of *Streptococcus* or *Staphylococcus* are commonly the cause of SBE. Dental procedures are associated with infection by *Streptococcus viridans*, surgical procedures with *Streptococcus faecalis*, and self-infection (especially by drug abusers) with *Staphylococcus aureus*.

subacute glomerulonephritis, an uncommon, non-infectious disease of the glomerulus of the kidney, characterized by proteinuria, haematuria, decreased production of urine and oedema. The disease is of unknown cause, it may progress rapidly, and renal failure may occur. Kidney transplantation and dialysis are the only treatments available.

subacute myeloptic neuropathy (SMON), a condition of muscular pain and weakness, usually below the T12 vertebra, painful dysaesthesia of the limbs and, in some cases, optic atrophy.

subacute sclerosing panencephalitis, an uncommon, slow viral infection caused by the measles virus. It is characterized by diffuse inflammation of brain tissue, personality change, seizures, blindness, dementia, fever and death.

subacute thyroiditis. See **de Quervain's thyroiditis.**

subaortic, pertaining to the area of the body below the aorta.

subarachnoid, situated under the arachnoid membrane and above the pia mater.

subarachnoid block anaesthesia, a form of spinal anaesthesia involving the injection of an anaesthetic into the space between the arachnoidea and pia mater.

subarachnoid haemorrhage (SaH, SAH), an intracranial haemorrhage into the cerebrospinal fluid filled space between the arachnoid and pial membranes on the surface of the brain. The haemorrhage may extend into the brain if the force of bleeding from the broken vessel is sudden and severe. The cause may be trauma, rupture of a berry aneurysm, or an arteriovenous anomaly. The first symptom of a subarachnoid haemorrhage is a sudden extremely severe headache that begins in one localized area and then spreads, becoming dull and throbbing. The localized pain results from vascular distortion and injury. The generalized ache is the result of meningeal irritation from blood in the subarachnoid space. Other characteristics of subarachnoid haemorrhage include dizziness, rigidity of the neck, pupillary inequality, vomiting, drowsiness, sweating and chills, stupor and loss of consciousness. There is commonly a brief period of unconsciousness immediately after the rupture; severe haemorrhage may result in continued unconsciousness, coma and death. Delirium and confusion often persist through the first weeks of recovery, and permanent brain damage is common.

subarachnoid space, the space between the arachnoid and pia mater membranes.

subcapital fracture, a fracture of tissue just below the head of a bone that pivots in a ball and socket joint, such as the head of the femur.

subcapsular cataract, a condition marked by opacity or cloudiness beneath the anterior or posterior capsule of the lens of the eye.

subclavian, situated under the clavicle, such as the subclavian vein.

subclavian artery, one of a pair of arteries that vary in origin, course and in the height to which they rise in the neck, but having six similar main branches supplying the vertebral column, spinal cord, ear and brain.

subclavian steal syndrome, a vascular syndrome caused by an occlusion in the subclavian artery proximal to the origin of the vertebral artery. The block results in a reversal of the normal blood pressure gradient in the vertebral artery and decreased blood flow distal to the occlusion. This condition is characterized by episodes of flaccid paralysis of the arm, pain in the mastoid and occipital areas, and a diminished or absent radial pulse on the involved side.

subclavian vein, the continuation of the axillary vein in the upper body, extending from the lateral border of the first rib to the sternal end of the clavicle, where it joins the internal jugular to form the brachiocephalic vein.

subclavius, a short muscle of the chest wall. It acts to draw the shoulder down and forward.

subclinical, of, or pertaining to, a disease or abnormal condition which is so mild that it produces no symptoms.

subclinical diabetes. See **impaired glucose tolerance.**

subconscious, imperfectly or partially conscious. **subconsciousness,** *n*.

subconscious memory, a thought, sensation or feeling that is not immediately available for recall to the conscious mind.

subculture, an ethnic, regional, economic or social group with characteristic patterns of behaviour and ideals that distinguish it from the rest of a culture or society.

subcutaneous, beneath the skin.

subcutaneous emphysema, the presence of free air or gas in the subcutaneous tissues. The air or gas may originate in the rupture of an airway or alveoli and migrate through the subpleural spaces to the mediastinum and neck. The face, neck and chest may appear swollen. Skin tissues can be painful and may produce a "crackling" sound as air moves under them. The patient may experience dyspnoea and appear cyanotic if the air leak is severe. Treatment may require an incision to release the trapped air.

subcutaneous fascia, a continuous layer of connective tissue over the entire body between the skin and deep fascial investment of the specialized structures of the body, such as the muscles. It comprises an outer, normally fatty layer and an inner, thin elastic layer.

subcutaneous fat necrosis. See **adiponecrosis subcutanea neonatorum.**

subcutaneous injection, the introduction of a hypodermic needle into the subcutaneous tissue beneath the skin, usually on the upper arm, thigh or abdomen.

subcutaneous mastectomy, a surgical procedure in which all the breast tissue of one or both breasts is removed leaving the skin, areola and nipple intact. The adjacent lymph nodes and the pectoralis major and pectoralis minor are not removed. It may be performed on women who are at great risk of developing breast cancer.

subcutaneous nodule, a small, solid boss or node beneath the skin; it can be detected by touch.

subcutaneous test. See **intradermal test.**

subcutaneous tunnel, a tunnel under the skin between the exit site of an atrial catheter and the entrance into the vein.

subdural, situated under the dura mater and above the arachnoid membrane.

subdural hygroma, a collection of fluid between the dura mater and arachnoid layers, resulting from a spinal fluid leak through a rupture in the arachnoid tissue.

subendocardial infarction, a myocardial infarction that involves only the innermost layer of the myocardium and, in some cases, portions of the middle layer of tissue, but does not extend to the epicardial region.

subgerminal cavity. See **blastocoele.**

subgingival calculus, a deposit of various mineral salts, such as calcium phosphate and calcium carbonate, which accumulates with organic matter and oral debris on the teeth or within the gingival crevice, the gingival pocket or the periodontal pocket. It is usually darker, more pigmented and denser than supragingival calculus.

subgingival curettage, the debridement of an ulcerated epithelial attachment and subjacent gingival corium to eliminate inflammation and shrink and restore gingival tissue.

subintentional suicide. See **benign suicide.**

subintimal, the area beneath the intima or membrane lining a blood vessel, usually a large artery.

subinvolution, the delayed or incomplete return of the uterus to its pre-pregnant size and shape. This is usually due to retained products of conception.

subjective, 1. pertaining to the essential nature of an object as perceived in the mind rather than to a thing in itself. **2.** existing only in the mind. **3.** that which arises within or is perceived by the individual, as contrasted with something modified by external circumstances or something that may be evaluated by objective standards. **4.** pertaining

to a person who places excessive importance on his own moods, attitudes or opinions; egocentric.

subjective data collection, the process in which data relating to the patient's problem are elicited from the patient. The interviewer encourages a full description of the onset, course and character of the problem, and of any factors that aggravate or ameliorate it.

subjective sensation, a feeling or impression that is not associated with or does not directly result from any external stimulus.

subjects, people, animals or events selected for a study to examine a particular variable or condition, such as the effects of a new medication or therapy.

sublethal gene, a gene whose presence causes abnormalities or impairs the functioning of an organism but does not cause its death.

subleukaemic leukaemia. See **aleukaemic leukaemia.**

sublimate, to refine or divert instinctual impulses and energy from their immediate goal to one that can be expressed in a social, moral or aesthetic manner acceptable to the person and society.

sublimation, 1. a defence mechanism by which an unacceptable instinctive drive is unconsciously diverted to and expressed through a personally approved, socially accepted means. **2.** (in psychoanalysis) the process of diverting certain components of the sex drive to a socially acceptable, nonsexual goal.

subliminal, taking place below the threshold of sensory perception or outside the range of conscious awareness.

sublingual, beneath the tongue.

sublingual administration of a medication, the administration of a drug, such as nitroglycerin, usually in tablet form, by placing it beneath the tongue until the tablet dissolves.

sublingual duct. See **Bartholin's duct, duct of Rivinus.**

sublingual gland, one of a pair of small salivary glands situated under the mucous membrane of the floor of the mouth, beneath the tongue. It is a narrow, almond-shaped structure, and secretes mucus produced by its alveoli.

subluxation, a partial dislocation.

submandibular duct, a duct through which a submandibular gland secretes saliva.

submandibular gland, one of a pair of round, walnut-sized salivary glands in the submandibular triangle. The gland secretes both mucus and a thinner serous fluid, which aid the digestive process.

submaxillary duct. See **submandibular duct.**

submentovertex, a reference point at the base of the skull, used in preparing radiographic projections of the skull and its associated structures.

submetacentric, pertaining to a chromosome in which the centromere is located approximately equidistant between the centre and one end, so that the arms of the chromatids are not equal in length.

submucous, beneath a mucous membrane.

subperiosteal fracture, a fracture in a bone beneath the periosteum that does not disrupt the periosteal covering.

subphrenic, pertaining to the area beneath or under the diaphragm.

subserous fascia, one of three kinds of fascia, lying between the internal layer of deep fascia and the serous membranes lining the body cavities, in much the same manner as the subcutaneous fascia lies between the skin and the deep fascia. It is thin in some areas, such as between the pleura and chest wall, and thick in other areas, where it forms a pad of adipose tissue.

subspecialty, (in nursing) a nurse's particular professional and highly specialized field of practice, such as nursing in dialysis, oncology, neurology or newborn intensive care.

substance, 1. any drug, chemical or biological entity. **2.** any material capable of being self-administered or abused because of its physiological or psychological effects.

substance abuse, the overindulgence in and dependence on a stimulant, depressant or other chemical substance, leading to effects that are detrimental to the individual's physical or mental health, or the welfare of others.

substance P, a polypeptide neurotransmitting substance synthesized by the body. It acts to stimulate vasodilatation and contraction of intestinal and other smooth muscles. It also plays a part in salivary secretion, diuresis and natriuresis, and affects the function of the peripheral and central nervous systems.

substantive epidemiology, the body of knowledge derived from epidemiological studies. For each disease, it includes the natural history of the disorder, patterns of occurrence and risk factors for developing disease.

substantivity, the property of continuing therapeutic action despite removal of the vehicle, as applied to certain shampoos.

substernal goitre, an enlargement of the thyroid gland, a portion of which is located beneath the sternum.

substitution, a mental mechanism, operating unconsciously, by which an unattainable or unacceptable goal, emotion, or object is replaced by one that is more attainable or acceptable.

substrate, a substance acted on and changed by an enzyme in any chemical reaction.

substrate depletion phase, a period during an enzyme assay where the concentration of substrate is falling and the assay is not following zero-order kinetics.

substratum, any underlying layer; a foundation.

subsystem, a smaller component of a large system composed of individuals or dyads. It is formed by generation, gender, interest or function.

subthalamus, a portion of the diencephalon that serves as a correlations centre for optic and vestibular impulses relayed to the globus pallidus. **subthalamic,** *adj.*

subtle, having a low intensity; not severe and having no serious sequelae, such as a mild infection or inflammation.

subungual, under a fingernail or toenail.

subungual haematoma, a collection of blood beneath a nail, usually resulting from trauma.

succinic acid, a compound found in certain hydatid cysts and in lichens, amber and fossils.

succinylcholine chloride, a depolarizing non-muscular blocker, used to reduce muscle skeletal muscle contractions during surgery or mechanical ventilation, and facilitates endotracheal intubation.

succus, *pl.* **succi,** a juice or fluid, usually one secreted by an organ, such as succus prostaticus of the prostate.

succussion splash, the sound elicited by shaking the body of an individual who has free fluid and air or gas in a hollow organ or body cavity. This sound may be present over a normal stomach, but may also be heard with hydropneumothorax, large hiatal hernia, or intestinal or pyloric obstruction.

suck, 1. to draw a liquid or semiliquid into the mouth by creating a partial vacuum through motions of the lips and tongue. **2.** to hold on the tongue and dissolve by the movements of the mouth and action of the saliva. **3.** to draw fluid into the mouth, specifically to draw milk from the breast or nursing bottle.

sucking blisters, the pale, soft pads on the upper and lower lips of a baby that look like blisters but are not. They seem to augment the seal of the lips around the nipple or breast. Some babies are born with them, having sucked on their own fingers, hand or arm before birth.

sucking reflex, involuntary sucking movements of the circumoral area in newborns in response to stimulation. The reflex continues throughout infancy and often occurs without stimulation, such as during sleep.

suckle, 1. to provide nourishment, specifically to breast feed. **2.** to take in as nourishment, especially by feeding from the breast.

suckling, an infant that has not been weaned.

sucrose, sugar derived from sugar cane, sugar beets and sorghum.

sucrose polyester (SPE), an experimental, synthetic, non-absorbable fat. When added to the diet, it reduces plasma cholesterol levels by increasing the excretion of cholesterol in the faeces.

suction, the aspiration of a gas or fluid by reducing air pressure over its surface, usually by mechanical means.

suction curettage, a method of curettage in which a specimen of the endometrium or the products of conception are removed by aspiration.

suction drainage. See **drainage.**

suction lipectomy. See **liposuction.**

sudden infant death syndrome (SIDS), the unexpected and sudden death of an apparently normal and healthy infant that occurs during sleep and with no physical or postmortem evidence of disease. Multiple causes have been proposed, including lack of biotin in the diet, abnormality of the endogenous-opioid system, mechanical suffocation, a defect in respiratory mucosal defence, prolonged apnoea, an unknown virus, anatomical abnormality of the larynx, and immunoglobulin abnormalities. It is seen more often among babies who have recently had a minor illness such as upper respiratory infection. The syndrome is neither contagious nor hereditary, although there is a greater than average risk of its occurrence within the same family, which may indicate the influence of polygenic factors.

sudoriferous duct, a duct leading from a sweat gland to the surface of the skin.

sudoriferous gland, one of about 3 million tiny structures within the dermis that produce sweat. The average quantity of sweat secreted in 24 hours varies from 700 to 900 g. Most of these glands are eccrine glands, producing sweat that carries away sodium chloride, the waste products urea and lactic acid, and the breakdown products from garlic, spices and other substances. Each sudoriferous gland consists of a single tube with a deeply coiled body and a superficial duct.

sudorific, 1. of, or pertaining to, a substance or condition, such as heat or emotional tension, that promotes sweating. **2.** a sudorific agent. Sweat glands are stimulated by cholinergic drugs.

suffocation, potential for, the accentuated risk of accidental suffocation (inadequate air available for inhalation). The risk factors may be internal (individual) or external (environmental). Internal risk factors include reduced olfactory sensation, reduced motor abilities, lack of safety education, lack of safety precautions, cognitive or emotional difficulties, and disease or injury processes. External risk factors include a pillow or a propped bottle placed in an infant's crib, a vehicle warming in a closed garage, children playing with plastic bags or inserting small objects into their mouths or noses, discarded or unused refrigerators or freezers without removed doors, unattended children in bathtubs or pools, household gas leaks, smoking in bed, eating too large mouthfuls of food, use of non-vented fuel-burning heaters, low-strung clothesline, and a pacifier hung around infant's neck.

suffocative goitre, an enlargement of the thyroid gland, causing a sensation of suffocation on pressure.

sugar, any of several water-soluble carbohydrates. The two principal categories of sugars are monosaccharides and disaccharides. A monosaccharide is a single sugar, such as glucose, fructose or galactose. A disaccharide is a double sugar, such as sucrose (table sugar) or lactose.

sugar alcohol, an alcohol produced by the reduction of an aldehyde or ketone of a sugar.

suggestibility, pertaining to a person's susceptibility to having his or her ideas or actions changed by the influence of others.

suggestion, 1. the process by which one thought or idea leads to another, as in the association of ideas. **2.** the use of persuasion, exhortation or another device to implant an idea, thought, attitude or belief in the mind of another, as a means of influencing or altering behaviour or states of mind. **3.** an idea, belief or attitude implanted in the mind of another.

suicidal, of, relating to or tending towards self-destruction.

suicide, 1. the intentional taking of one's own life. **2.** *informal,* the ruin or destruction of one's own interests. **3.** a person who commits or attempts self-destruction.

suicidology, the study of the causes and prevention of suicide. **suicidologist,** *n.*

sulcus, *pl.* **sulci,** a shallow groove, a depression or a furrow on the surface of an organ, such as a sulcus that separates the convolutions of the cerebral hemisphere. **sulcate,** *adj.*

sulcus centralis cerebri. See **fissure of Rolando.**

sulcus pulmonalis, a depression on each side of the vertebral bodies that accommodates the posterior portion of the lung.

sulfacetamide, a topical antibacterial used for the prophylaxis of infection after injury to the cornea, and in the treatment of bacterial conjunctivitis.

sulindac, a non-steroidal anti-inflammatory agent used in the treatment of osteoarthritis, rheumatoid arthritis and ankylosing spondylitis, other musculoskeletal disorders and acute gout.

Sulkowitch's test {Hirsh W. Sulkowitch, American physician, b. 1906}, an examination of the urine for the presence of calcium. It is a reagent containing oxalic acid, ammonium oxalate and glacial acetic acid; when mixed with urine, it causes calcium to precipitate out of the urine.

sulphadiazine, a sulphonamide antibacterial used in the treatment of infection, particularly of the urinary tract.

sulphaemoglobin, a form of haemoglobin containing an irreversibly bound sulphur molecule that prevents normal oxygen binding. It is present in the blood in trace amounts.

sulphaemoglobinaemia, the presence of abnormal sulphur-containing heamoglobin circulating in the blood.

sulphamethizole, a sulphonamide antibacterial used in the treatment of infection, particularly of the urinary tract.

sulphamethoxazole, a sulphonamide antibacterial used in the treatment of various bacterial infections, usually in combination with trimethoprim. See **co-trimoxazole.**

sulphamethoxazole and trimethoprim. See **co-trimoxazole.**

sulphanilic acid, a red-tinged, white crystalline compound used in the synthesis of sulphonamides and as a reagent in tests for phenol, faecal matter in water, albumin, aldehydes and glucose.

sulphasalazine, a sulphonamide with anti-inflammatory activity. It is used in the treatment of ulcerative colitis, Crohn's disease and rheumatoid arthritis.

sulphate, a salt of sulphuric acid. Natural sulphates, such as sodium sulphate, calcium sulphate and potassium sulphate, are plentiful in the body.

sulphathiazole, a sulphonamide antibacterial, occasionally used topically in the treatment of bacterial vaginitis and cervicitis.

sulphatide lipidosis, an inherited lipid metabolism disorder of childhood caused by a deficiency of cerebroside sulphatase enzyme. It results in an accumulation of metachromatic lipids in tissues of the central nervous system, kidney, spleen and other organs, leading to dementia, paralysis and death by the age of 10 years.

sulphinpyrazone, a uricosuric used in the prophylaxis of gout and hyperuricaemia.

sulphiting agents, food preservatives composed of potassium or sodium bisulphite or potassium metabisulphite. Sulphiting agents are used in the processing of beer, wine, baked goods, soup mixes and some imported seafoods, and by restaurants to impart a "fresh" appearance to salad fruits and vegetables. The chemicals can cause a severe allergic reaction in persons hypersensitive to sulphites. The reactions are marked by flushing, faintness, hives, headache, GI distress, breathing difficulty and, in extreme cases, loss of consciousness and death.

sulphobromophthalein, a substance used in its disodium salt form for evaluating liver function.

sulphonamide, one of a large group of synthetic, bacteriostatic drugs that are effective in treating infections caused by many gram-negative and gram-positive micro-organisms. The drugs act by preventing the normal growth, development and multiplication of the bacteria, but do not kill mature organisms. They are bacteriostatic rather than bactericidal.

sulphonates, a class of anticholinesterase compounds used as insecticides.

sulphonylurea, any one of a group of antidiabetic agents that stimulate the pancreatic production of insulin. Hypersensitivity to sulphonamides is a contraindication for using these agents. They are used in the treatment of non-insulin-dependent (type 2) diabetes mellitus. Sulphonylureas include glibenclamide, tolbutamide and gliclazide.

sulphosalicylic acid, a white or faintly pink crystalline substance that is highly water-soluble, used as a reagent in tests for albumin and as an intermediate compound in the manufacture of dyes and surfactants.

sulphur (S), a non-metallic, multivalent, tasteless, odourless chemical element that occurs abundantly in yellow crystalline form or in masses, especially in volcanic areas. Its atomic number is 16 and its atomic weight is 32.06. Sulphur has been used in the treatment of gout, rheumatism and bronchitis, and as a mild laxative. The sulphonamides, or sulpha drugs, are used in the treatment of various bacterial infections.

sulphuric acid, a clear, colourless, oily, highly corrosive liquid that generates great heat when mixed with water. An extremely toxic substance, sulphuric acid causes severe skin burns, blindness on contact with the eyes, serious lung damage if the vapours are inhaled, and death if it is ingested. It was formerly called oil of vitriol.

summation, 1. an accumulative effect or action; a total aggregate; totality. **2.** (in neurology), the accumulation of concentration of a neurotransmitter at a synapse, either by increasing the frequency of nerve impulses in each fibre (temporal summation) or by increasing the number of fibres stimulated (spatial summation), so that the threshold of the postsynaptic neuron is overcome and an impulse is transmitted.

sun bath, exposure of the naked body to the sun.

sundowning, a condition in which elderly patients tend to become confused or disorientated at the end of the day. With less light, they lose visual cues that help them to compensate for their sensory impairments.

sunrise syndrome, a condition of unstable cognitive ability on rising in the morning.

sunstroke, a morbid condition caused by overexposure to the sun and characterized by a high fever, convulsions and coma.

superego, (in Freudian psychoanalysis) that part of the psyche, functioning mostly in the unconscious, that develops when the standards of parents and society are incorporated into the ego. The superego has two parts, the conscience and the ego ideal.

superfecundation, the fertilization of two or

more ova, released during one menstrual cycle, by spermatozoa from the same or different males during separate acts of sexual intercourse.

superfetation, the fertilization of a second ovum after the onset of pregnancy, resulting in the presence of two fetuses of different degrees of maturity developing within the uterus simultaneously.

superficial, 1. of, or pertaining to, the skin or another surface. **2.** not grave or dangerous.

superficial fading infantile haemangioma, a superficial, transient, salmon-coloured patch in the centre of the forehead, face or occiput of many newborns.

superficial implantation, (in embryology) the partial embedding of the blastocyst within the uterine wall, so that the blastocyst, and later the chorionic sac, protrude into the uterine cavity.

superficial inguinal node, a node in one of the two groups of inguinal lymph glands in the upper femoral triangle of the thigh.

superficial reflex, any neural reflex initiated by stimulation of the skin. Kinds of superficial reflexes are **abdominal reflex, anal reflex** and **cremasteric reflex.** Compare **deep tendon reflex.**

superficial sensation, the awareness or perception of feelings in the superficial layers of the skin in response to touch, pressure, temperature and pain.

superficial spreading melanoma, a melanoma that grows outwards, spreading over the surface of the affected organ or tissue, most commonly on the lower legs of women and the torso of men.

superficial temporal artery, an artery at each side of the head that can be easily felt in front of the ear and is often used for taking the pulse. It is the smaller of the two terminal branches of the external carotid.

superficial vein, one of the several veins between the subcutaneous fascia just under the skin.

superinfection, an infection occurring during antimicrobial treatment for another infection.

superior, situated above or oriented towards a higher place, as the head is superior to the torso.

superior aperture of minor pelvis, an opening bounded by the crest and pecten of the pubic bones, the arch-shaped lines of the ilia, and the anterior margin of the base of the sacrum.

superior aperture of thorax, an elliptical opening at the summit of the thorax bounded by the first thoracic vertebra, the first ribs and the upper margin of the sternum.

superior conjunctival fornix, the space in the fold of the conjunctiva, created by the reflection of the conjunctiva covering the eyeball and the lining of the upper lid.

superior costotransverse ligament, one of five ligaments associated with each costotransverse joint, except that of the first rib. It passes from the neck of each rib to the transverse process of the vertebra immediately above.

superior gastric node, a node in one of two sets of gastric lymph glands, accompanying the left gastric artery.

superior haemorrhagic polioencephalitis. See **Wernicke's encephalopathy.**

superior mediastinum, the cranial portion of the mediastinum in the middle of the thorax, containing the trachea, oesophagus, the aortic arch, and the origins of the sternohyoidei and sternothyroidei.

superior mesenteric artery, a visceral branch of the abdominal aorta, arising caudal to the coeliac artery, dividing into five branches, and supplying most of the small intestine and parts of the colon.

superior mesenteric node, a node in one of the three groups of visceral lymph nodes that serve the viscera of the abdomen and pelvis.

superior mesenteric vein, a tributary of the portal vein that drains blood from the small intestine, caecum and the ascending and transverse colons. See also **portal vein.**

superior profunda artery. See **deep brachial artery.**

superior radioulnar joint. See **proximal radioulnar articulation.**

superior sagittal sinus, one of the six venous channels in the posterior of the dura mater, draining blood from the brain into the internal jugular vein.

superior subscapular nerve, one of two small nerves on opposite sides of the body that supply the superior part of the subscapularis.

superior thyroid artery, one of a pair of arteries in the neck, usually rising from the external carotid artery, that supplies the thyroid gland and several muscles in the head.

superior ulnar collateral artery, a long, slender division of the brachial artery, arising just distal to the middle of the arm, descending to the elbow, and anastomosing with the posterior ulnar recurrent and inferior ulnar collateral arteries.

superior vena cava, the second largest vein of the body, returning deoxygenated blood from the upper half of the body to the right atrium. It is formed by the junction of the two brachiocephalic veins at the level of the first intercostal space behind the sternum on the right side. The section of the superior vena cava closest to the heart comprises about one-half of the length of the vessel and is within the pericardial sac, covered by the serous pericardium.

supernatant, the clear upper portion of any mixture after it has been centrifuged.

supernormal conduction, (in cardiology) conduction that occurs when a block is expected.

supernormal excitability, the ability of the myocardium to respond to a stimulus that would be ineffective earlier or later in the cardiac cycle.

supernormal period, a period at the end of phase 3 of the cardiac cycle when activation can be initiated with less stimulus than is required at maximal repolarization.

supernumerary nipples, an excessive number of nipples which are usually not associated with underlying glandular tissue. They may vary in size from small pink dots to that of normal nipples.

superoxide, a common reactive form of oxygen. It is formed when molecular oxygen gains a single electron. Superoxide radicals can attack susceptible biological targets, including lipids, proteins and nucleic acids.

superoxide dismutase (SOD), an enzyme composed of metal-containing proteins, that converts superoxide radicals into less toxic agents. It is the main enzymatic mechanism for clearing superoxide radicals from the body.

supervision, (in psychology) a process whereby a therapist is helped to become a more effective clinician through the direction of a supervisor who provides theoretical knowledge and therapeutic techniques.

supinate, pertaining to a supine position or turning the palm upwards.

supination, 1. one of the types of rotation allowed by certain skeletal joints, such as the elbow and wrist joints, which enable the palm of the hand to turn up. **2.** the position of lying on the back. **supinate,** *v.*

supinator longus. See **brachioradialis.**

supine, lying horizontally on the back.

supine hypotensive syndrome, a fall in blood pressure that occurs when a pregnant woman is lying on her back. It is caused by impaired venous return that results from pressure of the gravid uterus on the vena cava.

supplemental inheritance, the acquisition or expression of a genetic trait or condition from the presence of two independent pairs of non-allelic genes that interact in such a way that one gene supplements the action of the other.

supplementary gene, one of two pairs of non-allelic genes that interact in such a way that one pair needs the presence of the other to be expressed, whereas the second pair can produce an effect independent of the first.

support, 1. to sustain, hold up or maintain in a desired position or condition, as in physically supporting the abdominal muscles with a scultetus binder or emotionally supporting a patient under stress. **2.** the assistance given to this end, such as physical support, emotional support or life support.

supporting area, any of the areas of maxil-

lary or mandibular edentulous ridges that are considered best suited to bear the forces of mastication with functioning dentures.

supportive psychotherapy, a form of psychotherapy that concentrates on creating an effective means of communication with an emotionally disturbed person, rather than trying to produce psychological insight into the underlying conflicts.

supportive treatment. See **treatment.**

suppository, an easily melted, cone-shaped, medicated mass for insertion into the rectum. Theobroma oil, glycerinated gelatin and high molecular weight-polyethylene glycols are common suppository bases.

suppressant, an agent that suppresses or diminishes a physical or mental activity, such as a medication that reduces hyperkinetic behaviour.

suppression, (in psychoanalysis) the conscious inhibition or effort to conceal unacceptable or painful thoughts, desires, impulses, feelings or acts.

suppression amblyopia, a partial loss of vision, usually in one eye, caused by cortical suppression of central vision to avoid diplopia. It commonly occurs in strabismus where the eye deviates and does not fixate.

suppressor gene, (in molecular genetics) a genetic unit that is able to reverse the effect of a specific kind of mutation in other genes.

suppressor mutation, (in molecular genetics) a mutation that restores, partially or completely, a function lost by a primary mutation occurring in a different genetic site.

suppressor T cell. See **T cell.**

suppurate, to produce purulent matter. **suppuration,** *n.,* **suppurative,** *adj.*

supraclavicular, the area of the body above the clavicle, or collar bone.

supraclavicular nerve, one of a pair of cutaneous branches of the cervical plexus, arising from the third and fourth cervical nerves, mostly from the fourth nerve.

supracondylar fracture, a fracture involving the area between the condyles of the humerus or femur.

supragingival calculus, a deposit composed of various mineral salts, such as calcium phosphate and calcium carbonate, which accumulates with organic matter and oral debris on the teeth occlusal or coronal to the gingival crest.

suprainfection, a secondary infection usually caused by an opportunistic pathogen, such as a fungal infection after the antibiotic treatment of another infection.

suprapubic, located above the symphysis pubis.

suprarenal, situated above the kidney, such as the suprarenal gland.

suprascapular nerve, one of a pair of branches from the cords of the brachial plexus.

suprasellar cyst. See **craniopharyngioma.**

supraspinal ligament, the ligament that connects the apices of the spinous processes from the seventh cervical vertebra to the sacrum. Between the spinous processes it is continuous with the interspinal ligaments.

suprasternal, pertaining to the area above the sternum, adjacent to the neck.

supraventricular tachycardia , an impulse that originates above the ventricles but cannot be clearly identified as arising from the SA node, atria or AV node.

suramin sodium, an antitrypanosomal drug with some antineoplastic activity. It is not available commercially in the UK.

surface anaesthesia. See **topical anaesthesia.**

surface anatomy, the study of the structural relationships of the external features of the body to the internal organs and parts.

surface area (SA), the total area exposed to the outside environment. The surface area of an object increases with the square of the object's linear dimensions; volume increases as the cube of the object's linear dimensions.

surface biopsy, the removal of living tissue for microscopic examination, by scraping the surface of a lesion.

surface tension, the tendency of the surface of a liquid to minimize the area of its surface by contracting. This property causes liquids to rise in a capillary tube, affects the exchange of gases in the pulmonary alveoli; it also alters the ability of various liquids to wet another surface.

surface therapy, a form of radiotherapy administered by placing one or more radioactive sources on or near an area of body surface.

surface thermometer, a device that detects and indicates the temperature of the surface of any part of the body.

surfactant, 1. an agent, such as soap or detergent, dissolved in water to reduce its surface tension or tension at the interface between the water and another liquid. **2.** certain lipoproteins that reduce the surface tension of pulmonary fluids, allowing the exchange of gases in the alveoli of the lungs and contributing to the elasticity of pulmonary tissue.

surfer's nodules, nodules on the skin of the knees, ankles, feet or toes of a surfer caused by repeated contact of the skin with an abrasive, sandy surfboard.

surgery, a branch of medicine concerned with diseases and trauma requiring operative procedures. **surgical,** *adj.*

surgery assistant (SA), a medical professional trained to assist during surgery and in the preoperative and postoperative periods, under the supervision of a surgeon.

surgical abdomen. See **acute abdomen.**

surgical anaesthesia, the third stage of general anaesthesia.

surgical anatomy, (in applied anatomy) the study of the structure and morphology of tissues and organs of the body as they relate to surgery.

surgical diathermy. See **electrocoagulation.**

surgical microscope. See **operating microscope.**

surgical pathology, the study of tissue specimens obtained during surgery. The surgical pathologist often examines specimens during surgery to determine how the operation should be modified or completed. Various techniques are used. The appearance of the specimen is first noted; slices of tissue are then prepared and examined microscopically.

surgical scrub, 1. a bactericidal soap or solution used by surgeons and surgical nurses before performing or assisting in surgery. **2.** the act of washing the fingernails, hands and forearms with a bactericidal soap or solution before a surgical procedure.

surgical sectioning, an oral surgery procedure for dividing a tooth to facilitate its removal.

surgical spirit, a skin disinfectant, containing industrial methylated spirit, water, methyl salicylate, diethyl pthalate and castor oil. Surgical spirit may cause skin dryness. It is only for external use, and is flammable.

surgical suite, a group of one or more operating rooms and adjunct facilities, such as sterile storage area, scrub room and recovery room.

surgical treatment. See **treatment.**

surrogate, 1. a substitute; a person or thing that replaces another. **2.** (in psychoanalysis) a substitute parental figure, a symbolic image or representation of another, as may occur in a dream.

surveillance, supervising or observing a patient or a health condition.

surveyed height of contour, a line, scribed or marked on a cast, that designates the greatest convexity relative to a selected path of denture placement and removal.

survival curve, a curve obtained by plotting the number or percentage of organisms surviving at different intervals against doses of radiation.

survivor, a term sometimes used interchangeably with 'victim'. It usually implies that the victim has adapted to his or her changed circumstances by managing to regain a sense of well-being, health and control of his or her own life. See **victimology.**

susceptibility, the condition of being more than normally vulnerable to a disease or disorder. **susceptible,** *adj.*

suspension, 1. a liquid in which small particles of a solid are dispersed, but not dissolved, and in which the dispersal is maintained by stirring or shaking the mixture. **2.**

a treatment, used primarily in spinal disorders, consisting of suspending the patient by the chin and shoulders. **3.** a temporary cessation of pain or a vital process.

suspension sling, a sling usually made of muslin or lightweight canvas and employed primarily to provide support. An example is a common triangular sling.

suspensory ligament of the lens. See **zonula ciliaris.**

sustenance, 1. the act or process of supporting or maintaining life or health. **2.** the food or nutrients essential for maintaining life.

sutura, *pl.* **suturae,** an immovable, fibrous joint in which certain bones of the skull are connected by a thin layer of fibrous tissue.

sutura dentata, an immovable fibrous joint; it is one kind of true suture in which tooth-like processes interlock along the margins of connecting bones of the skull.

sutura limbosa, an immovable fibrous joint; it is one kind of true suture in which beveled and serrated edges of certain connecting bones of the skull overlap and interlock.

sutura plana, a fibrous joint; it is one kind of false suture in which rough, contiguous edges of certain bones of the skull, such as the maxillae, form a connection.

sutura serrata, an immovable fibrous joint; it is one kind of true suture in which connecting bones interlock along serrated edges that resemble fine-toothed saws.

sutura squamosa, an immovable fibrous joint; it is one kind of false suture in which overlapping, bevelled edges unite certain bones of the skull.

suture, 1. a border or a joint, as between the bones of the cranium. **2.** to stitch together cut or torn edges of tissue with suture material. **3.** a surgical stitch taken to repair an incision, tear or wound. **4.** material used for surgical stitches, such as absorbable or non-absorbable silk, catgut, wire or synthetic material.

suture forceps. See **needle holder.**

Sv, abbreviation for **sievert.**

SV40, abbreviation for **simian virus 40.**

SvO$_2$, symbol for the percent of saturation of mixed venous blood.

swab, a stick or clamp for holding absorbent gauze or cotton, used for washing, cleansing, or drying a body surface, for collecting a specimen for laboratory examinations, or for applying a topical medication.

swallowing, impaired, a decreased ability to pass fluids and/or solids voluntarily from the mouth to the stomach. Defining characteristics include observed evidence of difficulty in swallowing, such as stasis of food in the oral cavity, coughing, choking and evidence of aspiration.

swamp fever. See **leptospirosis, malaria.**

swan neck deformity, 1. an abnormal condition of the finger characterized by flexion of the distal interphalangeal joint and hyper-

extension of the proximal interphalangeal joint. The condition is most often seen in rheumatoid arthritis. **2.** a structural abnormality of the kidney tubules associated with rickets. The kidney tubule connecting the glomerulus with the convoluted portion of the tubule is narrowed into a configuration referred to as "swan" neck.

Swan-Ganz catheter {Harold J. C. Swan, American physician, b. 1922; William Ganz, American cardiologist, b. 1919}, a long, thin cardiac catheter with a tiny balloon at its tip.

sweat bath, a bath given to induce sweating.

sweat duct, any one of the tiny tubules conveying sweat to the surface of the skin from sweat glands throughout the body. Each sweat duct is the most superficial part of a coiled tube that forms the body of each sweat gland, and opens onto the surface through a funnel-shaped opening. The sweat ducts in the armpits and groin are larger than in other parts of the body.

sweat gland. See **sudoriferous gland.**

sweat test, a method for evaluating sodium and chloride excretion from the sweat glands; this is often the first test performed in the diagnosis of cystic fibrosis. The sweat glands are stimulated with a drug, such as pilocarpine, and the perspiration produced is analysed. The eccrine glands of patients with cystic fibrosis produce sodium and chloride concentrations that are three to six times those of the normal.

sweat. See **perspiration.**

sweating. See **diaphoresis.**

Sweet localization method, a radiographic technique for locating a foreign body in the eye, by making two x-ray films of the eye with the patient's head immobilized. A small metal ball and a cone are placed at precise distances from the centre of the cornea as register marks, while lateral and perpendicular x-ray views of the eye are made. A three-dimensional view of the eye is constructed from the two x-ray films, and location of the foreign body in the eye is plotted from the intersection of lines through the ball and cone.

Swift's disease. See **acrodynia.**

swimmer's ear *informal,* otitis externa resulting from infection transmitted in the water of a swimming pool.

swimmer's itch, an allergic dermatitis caused by sensitivity to schistosome cercarias that die under the skin, leading to erythema, urticaria and a papular rash lasting 1 or 2 days.

swimming pool conjunctivitis. See **pharyngoconjunctival fever.**

swing phase of gait, one of the two phases in the rhythmic process of walking. The swing phase of gait follows the stance phase and is divided into the initial swing stage, midswing stage and terminal swing stage.

swinging ventricular tachycardia, tachycardia in which the polarity of the wide QRS complexes swings between positive and negative.

sycosis barbae, an inflammation of hair follicles of skin that has been shaved.

Sydenham's chorea, a form of chorea associated with rheumatic fever, usually occurring during childhood. The cause is a streptococcal infection of the vascular and perivascular tissues of the brain. The choreic movements increase over the first 2 weeks, when they reach a plateau, and then diminish.

sylvatic plague, an endemic disease of wild rodents caused by *Yersinia pestis*, transmissable to humans by the bite of an infected flea. It is found in every continent except Australia.

symbiosis, 1. (in biology) a mode of living characterized by close association between organisms of different species, usually in a mutually beneficial relationship. **2.** (in psychiatry) a state in which two mentally disturbed people are emotionally dependent on each other. **3.** pathological inability of a child to separate from its mother emotionally and, sometimes, physically. **symbiotic,** *adj.*

symbiotic phase, in Mahler's system of preoedipal development, the stage between 1 and 5 months when the infant participates in a "symbiotic orbit" with the mother. All parts of the mother, including voice, gestures, clothing and space in which she moves, are joined with the infant.

symbol, 1. an image, object, action or other stimulus that represents something else by reason of conscious association, convention or other relationship. **2.** an object, mode of behaviour or feeling that disguises a repressed emotional conflict through an unconscious association rather than through an objective relationship, as in dreams and neuroses.

symbolism, 1. the representation or evocation of one idea, action or object by the use of another, as in systems of writing, poetic language or dream metaphor. **2.** (in psychiatry) an unconscious mental mechanism characteristic of all human thinking, in which a mental image stands for but disguises some other object, person or thought.

symelus. See **symmelus.**

symmelia, a fetal anomaly characterized by the fusion of the lower limbs with or without feet. Kinds of symmelia are **apodial symmelia, dipodial symmelia, monopodial symmelia** and **tripodial symmelia.**

symmelus, a malformed fetus characterized by symmelia.

Symmer's disease. See **giant follicular lymphoma.**

symmetric tonic neck reflex, a normal response in infants to assume the crawl position by extending the arms and bending the knees when the head and neck are extended.

symmetrical, (of the body or parts of the body) equal in size or shape; very similar in relative placement or arrangement about an axis. **symmetry,** *n.*

symmetrical lipomatosis. See **nodular circumscribed lipomatosis.**

sympathectomy, a surgical interruption of part of the sympathetic nerve pathways, performed for the relief of chronic pain in vascular diseases, such as arteriosclerosis, claudication, Buerger's disease and Raynaud's phenomenon. The sheath around an artery carries the sympathetic nerve fibres that control constriction of the vessel. Removal of the sheath causes the vessel to relax and expand, and allows more blood to pass through it.

sympathetic amine, a drug that produces effects resembling those manifested by stimulation of the sympathetic nervous system.

sympathetic nervous system. See **autonomic nervous system.**

sympathetic ophthalmia, a granulomatous inflammation of the uveal tract of both eyes, occurring after injury to the uveal tract of one eye.

sympathetic trunk, one of a pair of chains of ganglia extending along the side of the vertebral column from the base of the skull to the coccyx. Each trunk is part of the sympathetic nervous system and consists of a series of ganglia connected by cords that contain various types of fibres. Each sympathetic trunk distributes branches with postganglionic fibres to the autonomic plexuses, cranial nerves, individual organs, nerves accompanying arteries and spinal nerves.

sympathizing eye, (in sympathetic ophthalmia) the uninfected eye that becomes infected by lymphatic or blood-borne metastasis of a micro-organism.

sympatholytic, sympatholytic agent. See **antiadrenergic.**

sympathomimetic, denoting a pharmacological agent that mimics the effects of stimulation of organs and structures by the sympathetic nervous system, by occupying adrenergic receptor sites and acting as an agonist or increasing the release of the neurotransmitter norepinephrine at postganglionic nerve endings. Various sympathomimetic agents are used as decongestants of nasal and ocular mucosa, bronchodilators in the treatment of asthma, bronchitis, bronchiectasis and emphysema, and vasopressors and cardiac stimulants in the treatment of acute hypotension and shock.

sympathomimetic amine, any one of a group of amine compounds with pharmacological actions similar to noradrenaline, the neurotransmitter in post-ganglionic sympathetic nerves.

sympathomimetic bronchodilator, a medication that reduces bronchial muscle spasm. This is an action that mimics that of the sympathetic nervous system in producing smooth muscle relaxation. Most agents in this category are beta-adrenergic agonists; for example, salbutamol.

sympathy, 1. an expressed interest or concern regarding the problems, emotions, or states of mind of another. **2.** the relation that exists between the mind and body causing the one to be affected by the other. **3.** mental contagion or influence exerted by one individual or group on another, and the effects produced, such as the spread of panic, uncontrollable laughter or yawning. **4.** the physiological or pathological relationship between two organs, systems or parts of the body. **sympathetic,** *adj.,* **sympathize,** *v.*

symphalangia, 1. a condition, usually inherited, characterized by ankylosis of the fingers or toes. **2.** a congenital anomaly in which webbing of the fingers or toes occurs in varying degrees.

symphocephalus, twin fetuses joined at the head. The term is often used as a general designation for fetuses with varying degrees of the anomaly.

symphyseal angle, (in dentistry) the angle of the chin, which may be protruding, straight or receding, according to type.

symphysic teratism, a congenital anomaly in which there is a fusion of normally separated parts or organs, such as a horseshoe kidney.

symphysis, *pl.* **symphyses, 1.** a line of union, especially a cartilaginous joint in which adjacent bony surfaces are firmly united by fibrocartilage. **2.** *informal,* symphysis pubis. **symphysic,** *adj.*

symphysis pubis. See **pubic symphysis.**

sympodia, a congenital developmental anomaly characterized by fusion of the lower extremities.

symptom, a subjective indication of a disease or a change in condition as perceived by the patient. Several symptoms are accompanied by objective signs, such as pruritus. Some symptoms may be confirmed objectively, such as numbness of a body part confirmed by absence of response to a pin prick. **Primary symptoms** are symptoms that are intrinsically associated with a disease process. **Secondary symptoms** are a consequence of a disease process.

symptom neurosis, psychological disorders in which dysfunctional coping mechanisms appear as clinical symptoms that represent direct manifestations of anxiety.

symptom-bearer, (in psychology) a family member frequently seen as the patient who is functioning poorly because family dynamics interfere with functioning at a higher level.

symptomatic nanism, dwarfism associated with defects in bone growth, tooth formation and sexual development.

symptomatic oesophageal peristalsis, a condition in which peristaltic progression in the body of the oesophagus is normal but contractions in the distal oesophagus are of increased amplitude and duration.

symptomatic treatment. See **treatment.**

symptothermal method of family planning, a natural method of family planning that incorporates the ovulation and basal body temperature methods of family planning.

sympus, a malformed fetus in which the lower extremities are completely fused or rotated and the pelvis and genitalia are defective. Kinds of sympuses are **sirenomelus, sympus dipus** and **sympus monopus.**

sympus apus. See **sirenomelus.**

sympus dipus, a malformed fetus in which the lower extremities are fused and both feet are formed.

sympus monopus, a malformed fetus in which the lower extremities are fused and one foot is formed.

synadelphus, *pl.* **synadelphi,** a conjoined twin fetal monster with a single head and trunk and eight limbs.

synapse, 1. the region surrounding the point of contact between two neurons or between a neuron and an effector organ, across which nerve impulses are transmitted through the action of a neurotransmitter, such as acetylcholine or norepinephrine. Synapses are polarized so that nerve impulses normally travel in only one direction; they are also subject to fatigue, oxygen deficiency, anaesthetics and other chemical agents. Types of synapses include **axoaxonic synapse, axodendritic synapse, axodendrosomatic synapse, axosomatic synapse** and **dendrodendritic synapse. 2.** to form a synapse or connection between neurons. **3.** (in genetics) to form a synaptic fusion between homologous chromosomes during meiosis. **synaptic,** *adj.*

synapsis, *pl.* **synapses,** the pairing of homologous chromosomes during the early meiotic prophase stage in gametogenesis to form double or bivalent chromosomes.

synaptic cleft, the microscopic, extracellular space at the synapse that separates the membrane of terminal nerve endings of a presynaptic neuron and the membrane of a postsynaptic cell.

synaptic junction, the membranes of both the presynaptic neuron and the postsynaptic receptor cell, together with the synaptic cleft.

synaptic transmission, the passage of a neural impulse across a synapse from one nerve fibre to another, by means of a neurotransmitter.

synarthrosis. See **fibrous joint.**

syncephalus, a conjoined twin monster having a single head and two bodies.

syncheilia, a congenital anomaly in which

there is complete or partial fusion of the lips; atresia of the mouth.

synchondrosis, *pl.* **synchondroses,** a cartilaginous joint between two immovable bones, such as the pubic symphysis.

synchorial, pertaining to multiple fetuses that share a common placenta, as in monozygosity.

synchronized intermittent mandatory ventilation (SIMV), periodic assisted mechanical breaths occurring at preset intervals when the patient makes an inspiratory effort that is sensed by the ventilator. Spontaneous breathing by the patient occurs between the assisted mechanical breaths.

synclitism, 1. (in obstetrics) a condition in which the sagittal suture of the fetal head is in line with the transverse diameter of the inlet, equidistant from the maternal symphysis pubis and sacrum. **2.** (in haematology) the normal condition in which the nucleus and the cytoplasm of the blood cells mature simultaneously and at the same rate.

syncopal attack, any episode of unconsciousness or fainting, especially one associated with fear or pain. Many individuals suffer such attacks during violent coughing spells because of associated rapid changes in arterial blood pressure.

syncope, a brief lapse in consciousness caused by transient cerebral hypoxia. It is usually preceded by a sensation of light-headedness, and may often be prevented by lying down or sitting with the head between the knees.

syncretic thinking, a stage in the development of the cognitive thought processes of the child. During this phase, thought is based purely on what is perceived and experienced. The child is incapable of making deductions or generalizations. In Piaget's classification, this stage occurs between 2 and 7 years of age. **syncresis,** *n.*

syncytial, pertaining to a syncytium.

syncytial virus, a virus that induces the formation of syncytia, particularly in cell cultures. Syncytial viruses are members of the spumavirinae subfamily of retroviridae.

syncytiotrophoblast, the outer syncytial layer of the trophoblast of the early mammalian embryo that erodes the uterine wall during implantation and gives rise to the villi of the placenta. **syncytiotrophoblastic,** *adj.*

syncytium, *pl.* **syncytia,** a group of cells in which the protoplasm of one cell is continuous with that of adjoining cells.

syndactylus, a person with webbed fingers or toes.

syndactyly, a congenital anomaly characterized by the fusion of the fingers or toes. **syndactyl, syndactylous,** *adj.*

syndesmosis, a fibrous articulation in which two bones are connected by interosseous ligaments, such as the anterior and posterior ligaments in the tibiofibular articulation. Compare **gomphosis, sutura.**

syndrome, a complex of signs and symptoms resulting from a common cause, or appearing in combination to present a clinical picture of a disease or inherited abnormality. See also specific syndromes.

syndrome of inappropriate antidiuretic hormone secretion (SIADH), an abnormal condition characterized by the excessive release of antidiuretic hormone (ADH) that upsets the fluid and electrolytic balances of the body. It results from various malfunctions, such as the inability of the body to produce and secrete dilute urine, water retention, increased extracellular fluid volume and hyponatraemia. SIADH develops in association with diseases that affect the osmoreceptors of the hypothalamus. Oat cell carcinoma of the lung is the most common cause. Common signs and symptoms of SIADH are weight gain despite anorexia, vomiting, nausea, muscle weakness and irritability. In some patients, SIADH may produce coma and convulsions. Most of the free water associated with this syndrome is intracellular; associated oedema is rare unless excess water volume exceeds 4 mOsm.

synechia, *pl.* **synechiae,** an adhesion, especially of the iris to the cornea or lens of the eye. It may develop from glaucoma, cataracts, uveitis or keratitis, or as a complication of surgery or trauma to the eye. Synechiae prevent or impede flow of aqueous fluid between the anterior and posterior chambers of the eye, and may lead rapidly to blindness.

syneresis, the drawing together or coagulation of particles of a gel with separation from the medium in which the particles were suspended, as occurs in blood clot retraction.

synergism. See **synergy.**

synergist, an organ, agent or substance that augments the activity of another organ, agent or substance.

synergistic agent, a substance that augments or adds to the activity of another substance or agent.

synergistic muscles, groups of muscles that contract together to accomplish the same body movement.

synergy, 1. the process in which two organs, substances or agents work simultaneously to enhance the function and effect of one another. **2.** the coordinated action of a set of muscles that work together to produce a specific movement. **3.** a combined action of different parts of the autonomic nervous system, as in the sympathetic and parasympathetic innervation of secreting cells of the salivary glands. **4.** the interaction of two or more drugs to produce a certain effect. **synergistic, synergic,** *adj.*

syngeneic, 1. (in genetics) denoting an individual or cell type that has the same genotype as another individual or cell. **2.** (in transplantation biology) denoting tissues that are antigenically similar. Also **isogeneic.**

synophthalmia. See **cyclopia.**

synostotic joint, a joint in which bones are joined to bones and there is no movement between them, as in the bones of the adult sacrum or skull.

synotia, a congenital malformation characterized by the union or approximation of the ears in front of the neck, often accompanied by the absence or defective development of the lower jaw.

synotus, a fetus with synotia.

synovectomy, the excision of a synovial membrane of a joint.

synovia, a transparent, viscous fluid, resembling the white of an egg, secreted by synovial membranes and acting as a lubricant for many joints, bursae and tendons. It contains mucin, albumin, fat and mineral salts. **synovial,** *adj.*

synovial bursa, one of the many closed sacs filled with synovial fluid in the connective tissue between the muscles, tendons, ligaments and bones.

synovial chondroma, a rare cartilaginous growth developing in the connective tissue below the synovial membrane of the joints, tendon sheaths, or bursa.

synovial crypt, a pouch in the synovial membrane of a joint.

synovial fluid. See **synovia.**

synovial joint, a freely movable joint in which contiguous bony surfaces are covered by articular cartilage and connected by ligaments lined with synovial membrane. Kinds of synovial joints are **ball and socket joint, condyloid joint, gliding joint, hinge joint, pivot joint, saddle joint** and **uniaxial joint.**

synovial membrane, the inner layer of an articular capsule surrounding a freely movable joint. The synovial membrane is loosely attached to the external fibrous capsule. It secretes into the joint a thick fluid that normally lubricates the joint, but it may accumulate in painful amounts when the joint is injured.

synovial sarcoma, a malignant tumour, composed of synovioblasts, that begins as a soft swelling. It often has metastasized through the bloodstream to the lung, before it is discovered.

synovial sheath, any one of the membranous sacs that enclose a tendon of a muscle and facilitate the gliding of a tendon through a fibrous or bony tunnel, such as that under the flexor retinaculum of the wrist.

synovial tendon sheath, one of the many membranous sacs enclosing various tendons that glide through fibrous and bony tunnels in the body, such as those under the flexor retinaculum of the wrist. One layer of the

synovial sheath lines the tunnel; the other covers the tendon.

synovitis, an inflammatory condition of the synovial membrane of a joint, as a result of an aseptic wound or a traumatic injury, such as a sprain or severe strain. The knee is most commonly affected. Fluid accumulates around the capsule, the joint is swollen, tender and painful, and motion is restricted.

syntax, a property of language involving structural cues for the arrangement of words as elements in a phrase, clause or sentence.

syntaxic mode, the ability to perceive whole, logical, coherent pictures as they occur in reality, according to the Sullivan theory of psychology.

synteny, (in genetics) the presence on the same chromosome of two or more genes that may or may not be transmitted as a linkage group but appear to be able to undergo independent assortment during meiosis.

synthesis, a level of cognitive learning in which the individual puts together the elements of previous learning levels to create a unified whole.

synthetic, of, or pertaining to, a substance produced by an artificial rather than a natural process or material.

synthetic chemistry, the science dealing with the formation of chemical compounds from simpler substances.

synthetic oleovitamin D. See **viosterol.**

Syntometrine, an oxytocic drug containing 0.5 mg of ergometrine and 5 units of Syntocinon in 1 ml, commonly given to shorten the third stage of labour.

syntrophoblast. See **syncytiotrophoblast.**

syphilis, a sexually transmitted disease caused by the spirochaete, *Treponema pallidum,* characterized by distinct stages of effects over a period of years. Any organ system may become involved. The spirochaete is able to pass through the human placenta, resulting in congenital syphilis.

syphilitic aortitis, an inflammatory condition of the aorta, occurring in tertiary syphilis and characterized by diffuse dilatation with grey, wheal-like plaques containing calcium on the inner coat and scars and wrinkles on the outer coat. The middle layer of the vascular wall is usually infiltrated with plasma cells and contains fragments of damaged elastic tissue and many newly formed blood vessels. There may be damage to the aortic valves, narrowing of the mouths of the coronary arteries, and formation of thrombi. Cerebral embolism may result. Signs of syphilitic aortitis are substernal pain, dyspnoea, bounding pulse and high systolic blood pressure.

syphilitic meningoencephalitis. See **general paresis.**

syphilitic periarteritis, an inflammatory condition of the outer coat of one or more arteries occurring in tertiary syphilis and characterized by soft gummatous perivascular lesions infiltrated with lymphocytes and plasma cells.

syringe, a device for withdrawing, injecting or instilling fluids. A syringe for the injection of medication usually consists of a calibrated glass or plastic cylindric barrel having a close-fitting plunger at one end and a small opening at the other to which the head of a hollow-bore needle is fitted. Medication of the desired amount may be pulled up into the barrel by suction, as the plunger is withdrawn and injected by pushing the plunger back into the barrel, thus forcing the liquid out through the needle. Kinds of syringe include Asepto syringe, **bulb syringe, hypodermic syringe, Luer-Lok syringe** and **tuberculin syringe.**

syringomyelocele, a hernial protrusion of the spinal cord through a congenital defect in the vertebral column, in which the cerebrospinal fluid within the central cavities of the cord is greatly increased so that the cord tissue forms a thin-walled sac that lies close to the membrane of the cavity.

system, 1. a collection or assemblage of parts that, unified, make a whole. Physiological systems, such as the cardiovascular or reproductive systems, are made up of structures specifically able to engage in processes that are essential to a vital function in the body. **2.** a set of computer programmes and hardware that work together for some specific purpose.

systematic error, a non-random statistical error that affects the mean of a population of data, and defines the bias between the means of two populations.

systematic heating, the elevation of temperature of the whole body.

systematic tabulation, (in research) mechanical or manual techniques for recording and classifying data for statistical analysis.

system documentation. See **documentation.**

systemic, of, or pertaining to, the whole body rather than a localized area or regional portion of the body.

systematic desensitization, a technique used in behaviour therapy for eliminating maladaptive anxiety associated with phobias. The procedure involves the construction by the person of a hierarchy of anxiety-producing stimuli, and the general presentation of these stimuli until they no longer elicit the initial response of fear.

systemic lupus erythematosus (SLE), a chronic inflammatory disease affecting many systems of the body. The pathophysiology of SLE includes severe vasculitis, renal involvement and lesions of the skin and nervous system. The primary cause of the disease has not been determined; viral infection or dysfunction of the immune system have been suggested. Adverse reaction to certain drugs may also cause a lupus-like syndrome. SLE affects women four times more frequently than men. The initial manifestation is often arthritis. An erythematous rash over the nose and malar eminences, weakness, fatigue and weight loss are also frequently seen early in the disease. In addition, there may be photosensitivity, fever, skin lesions on the neck, and alopecia where the skin lesions extend beyond the hairline. The skin lesions may spread to the mucous membranes and other tissues of the body. They do not ulcerate but cause degeneration of the affected tissues. Depending on the organs involved, the patient may also have glomerulonephritis, pleuritis, pericarditis, peritonitis, neuritis or anaemia. Renal failure and severe neurological abnormalities are among the most serious manifestations of the disease.

systemic oxygen consumption, the amount of oxygen consumed by the tissues of the body, as measured during a period of 60 seconds.

systemic remedy, a medicinal substance given orally, parenterally or rectally, to be absorbed into the circulation for treatment of a health problem. Medication administered systemically may have various local effects, but the intent is to treat the whole body.

systemic vascular resistance (SVR), the resistance against which the left ventricle must eject to force out its stroke volume with each beat. As the peripheral vessels constrict, the SVR increases.

systemic vein, one of a number of veins that drain deoxygenated blood from most of the body. Systemic veins arise in tiny plexuses that receive blood from the billions of capillaries lacing the body tissues and converge into trunks that increase in size as they pass towards the heart. They are larger and more numerous than the arteries, have thinner walls, and collapse when they are empty. Kinds of systemic veins are identified according to location, such as deep veins, superficial veins and venous sinuses.

system of care, a framework within which healthcare is provided, comprising: healthcare professionals; recipients, consumers, or patients; energy resources or dynamics; organizational and political contexts or frameworks; and processes or procedures.

system overload, an inability to cope with messages and expectations from a number of sources within a given time limit.

systems design, the art or technique of analysing a problem, modifying it for processing or solution by data processing equipment, and determining the best means and equipment by which a solution can be reached. **systems designer,** *n.*

systole, the contraction of the heart, driving blood into the aorta and pulmonary arteries. The occurrence of systole is indicated by the first heart sound heard on auscultation, the palpable apex beat and peripheral pulse.

systolic click, an extra sound that has a click-like quality heard in mid- or late systole. It is believed to originate from the abnormal motion of the mitral valve. The most frequent cause of systolic clicks is prolapse of a mitral valve leaflet.

systolic ejection period, the amount of time spent in systole per minute.

systolic gradient, the difference in pressure in the left atrium and left ventricle during systole.

systolic murmur, cardiac murmur occurring during systole. Systolic murmurs are generally less significant than diastolic murmurs, and occur in many people who have no evidence of heart disease.

systolic pressure, blood pressure measured during the period of ventricular contraction (systole). In blood pressure readings, it is normally the higher of the two measurements.

24-hour clock system, a method of designating time by using the numerical sequence from 00 to 23 for the hours and the numbers 00 to 59 for the minutes, in a daily cycle beginning with 0000 (midnight) and ending with 2359 (1 minute before the following midnight).

T, 1. symbol for **temperature. 2.** abbreviation for **tumour. See cancer staging.**

T bandage, a bandage in the shape of the letter T. It is used for the perineum and sometimes for the head.

T cell, a small circulating lymphocyte, produced in the bone marrow, that matures in the thymus or as a result of exposure to thymosin secreted by the thymus. T cells, which live for years, have several functions but primarily mediate cellular immune responses, such as graft rejection and delayed hypersensitivity. One kind of T cell, the **helper cell,** affects the production of antibodies by B cells; the **suppressor T cell** suppresses B cell activity.

t.d.s., (in prescriptions) abbreviation for the Latin phrase 'ter die sumendus, a, um' meaning "three times a day".

T fracture, an intercondylar fracture in which the fracture lines are T-shaped.

T lymphocyte. See lymphocyte, T cell.

t test, a statistical test used to determine whether there are differences between two means or between a target value and a calculated mean.

T tube, 1. a tubular device in the shape of a T, inserted through the skin into a cavity or a wound and used for drainage. **2.** an apparatus used to connect a source of humidified oxygen to the endotracheal tube so that a spirometer can be attached for evaluation of tidal volume and appropriate removal of the endotracheal tube.

T tube cholangiography, a type of biliary tract radiographic examination in which a water-soluble iodinated contrast medium is injected into the bile duct through an indwelling T tube.

T tubule system, a system of invaginations along the surface of myocardial cell membranes, providing an extension of the membrane into the cells. The system is believed to be a method of storing calcium ions, for the movement of substrates into the cells and the removal of metabolic end-products from the cells.

T wave, the component of the cardiac cycle shown on an electrocardiogram as a short, inverted, U-shaped curve following the ST segment.

t.i.d., (in prescriptions) abbreviation for ter in die, a Latin phrase meaning "three times a day".

t.n.t.c., abbreviation for too numerous to count, usually applied to organisms or cells viewed on a slide under a microscope.

T1, T2. See relaxation time.

T3, symbol for **triiodothyronine.**

T4, symbol for **thyroxine.**

TA, abbreviation for **transactional analysis.**

Ta, symbol for **tantalum.**

tabes dorsalis, an abnormal condition characterized by the slow degeneration of all or part of the body, and the progressive loss of peripheral reflexes. This disease involves the posterior columns and posterior roots of the spinal cord, and destroys the large joint of affected limbs in some individuals. It is often accompanied by incontinence, impotence and severe flashing pains in the abdomen and the extremities.

tablet, a small, solid dosage form of a medication. It may be of almost any size, shape, weight and colour. Most tablets are intended to be swallowed whole, but some may be dissolved in the mouth, chewed or dissolved in liquid before swallowing; some may be placed in a body cavity.

taboo, something that is forbidden by a society as unacceptable or improper. Incest is a taboo common to many societies.

tabula rasa, a term used to describe a child's mind at birth as a receptive "blank slate".

tache noire, a local ulcerous lesion marking the point of infection in certain rickettsial diseases, such as African tick typhus and scrub typhus.

tachycardia, an abnormal condition in which the myocardium contracts regularly but at a rate greater than 100 beats per minute. The heart rate normally accelerates in response to fever, exercise or nervous excitement. Pathological tachycardia accompanies anoxia, as caused by anaemia, congestive heart failure, haemorrhage or shock. Tachycardia acts to increase the amount of oxygen delivered to the cells of the body by increasing the amount of blood circulated through the vessels.

tachykinin. See substance P.

tachyphylaxis, 1. (in pharmacology) a phenomenon in which the repeated administration of some drugs results in a marked decrease in effectiveness. **2.** (in immunology) rapidly developing immunity to a toxin because of previous exposure, such as from previous injection of small amounts of the toxin.

tachypnoea, an abnormally rapid rate of breathing, such as seen with hyperpyrexia. See also **respiratory rate.**

tactile, of, or pertaining to, the sense of touch.

tactile anaesthesia, the absence or lack of the sense of touch in the fingers, possibly as a result of injury or disease. This condition may cause the patient to incur severe burns, serious cuts, contusions or abrasions.

tactile corpuscle, any one of many small, oval end-organs associated with the sense of touch, widely distributed throughout the body in peripheral areas; for example, the skin of the lips, mucous membrane of the tongue, palpebral conjunctivae and the skin of mammary papillae.

tactile corpuscle of Meissner. See **Wagner-Meissner corpuscle.**

tactile defensiveness, a sensory integrative dysfunction characterized by tactile sensations that cause excessive emotional reactions, hyperactivity or other behaviour problems.

tactile fremitus, a tremulous vibration of the chest wall during respiration, palpable on physical examination.

tactile image, a mental concept of an object as perceived through the sense of touch.

Taenia, a genus of large, parasitic, intestinal flatworm, having an armed scolex and a series of segments in a chain. Taeniae are among the most common parasites infecting humans; they include *Taenia saginata,* the beef tapeworm, and *T. solium,* the pork tapeworm.

Taenia saginata, a species of tapeworm that inhabits the tissues of cattle during its larval stage and infects the intestine of humans in its adult form.

Taenia solium, a species of tapeworm that most commonly inhabits the tissues of pigs during its larval stage and infects the intestine of humans in its adult form.

taeniasis, an infection with a tapeworm of the genus *Taenia.*

TAF, abbreviation for **tumour angiogenesis factor.**

TAG, a contraction for **3,4,6-tri-O-acetyl-D-glucal.**

taijin kyofu, a culturally patterned fear of meeting people, observed in some areas of Japan.

tail fold, a curved ridge formed at the caudal end of the early developing embryo.

tail of Spence, the upper outer tail of breast tissue that extends into the axilla.

tailor's bottom. See **weaver's bottom.**

tailor's bunion. See **bunionette.**

Takayasu's arteritis {Michishige Takayasu, Japanese physician, b. 1871}, a disorder characterized by progressive occlusion of the innominate and left subclavian and left common carotid arteries above their origin in the aortic arch. Signs of the disorder are absence of a pulse in both arms and in the carotid arteries, transient paraplegia, transient blindness and atrophy of facial muscles.

talipes, a deformity of the foot, usually congenital, in which the foot is twisted and relatively fixed in an abnormal position. Talipes refers to deformities that involve the foot and ankle. Kinds of talipes include talipes calcaneovalgus, talipes calcaneovarus and talipes equinovarus.

talipes calcaneovalgus. See **clubfoot.**

talipes cavus. See **pes cavus.**

talipes equinovarus. See **clubfoot.**

talus, *pl.* **tali,** the second largest tarsal bone. It supports the tibia, rests on the calcaneus, and articulates with the malleoli and navicular bones.

Tamm-Horsfall protein (THP), a mucoprotein found in the matrix of renal tubular casts. THP is secreted in the loop of Henle.

tamoxifen, a non-steroidal oestrogen receptor antagonist used in the palliative treatment of advanced breast cancer in postmenopausal women whose tumours are oestrogen-dependent. It is also used as an adjuvant to the surgical treatment of breast cancer, and in the treatment of anovulatory female infertility.

tampon, a pack of cotton, sponge or other material for checking bleeding or absorbing secretions in cavities or canals, or for holding displaced organs in position.

tamponade, stoppage of the flow of blood to an organ or a part of the body by pressure, or by the compression of a part by accumulation of fluid, as in cardiac tamponade.

tangentiality, an association disturbance characterized by a tendency to digress from an original topic of conversation.

tangible elements, objects that can be seen or touched, as distinguished from emotions, knowledge or abstractions.

Tangier disease, a rare familial deficiency of high-density lipoproteins, characterized by low blood cholesterol and an abnormal orange or yellow discolouration of the tonsils and pharynx.

tannin, any of a group of astringent substances obtained from plants. Tannic acid, a mixture of tannins, is used in the treatment of burns.

tanning, a process in which the pigmentation of skin deepens as a result of exposure to ultraviolet light. Skin cells containing melanin darken immediately.

tantalum (Ta), a silvery metallic element. Its atomic number is 73 and its atomic weight is 180.95. Relatively inert chemically, tantalum is used in prosthetic devices such as skull plates and wire sutures.

tantrum, a sudden outburst or violent display of rage, frustration and bad temper, usually occurring in a maladjusted child and certain emotionally disturbed persons.

tapering arch, a dental arch that converges from the molars to the central incisors, to such a degree that lines passing through the central grooves of the molars and premolars intersect within 2.5 cm anterior to the central incisors.

tapeworm, a parasitic, intestinal worm belonging to the class Cestoda and having a scolex and a ribbon-shaped body composed of segments in a chain. Humans usually acquire tapeworms by eating the undercooked meat of intermediate hosts contaminated by the cysticerus or larval form of the tapeworm. Kinds of tapeworm include *Diphyllobothrium latum, Taenia saginata* and *Taenia solium.*

tapeworm infection, an intestinal infection by one of several species of parasitic worms, caused by eating raw or undercooked meat infested with tapeworm or its larvae. Tapeworms live as larvae in one or more vertebrate intermediate hosts, and grow to adulthood in the intestine of humans. Symptoms of intestinal infection with adult worms are usually mild or absent, but diarrhoea, epigastric pain and weight loss may occur.

tapotement, a type of massage in which the body is tapped in a rhythmic manner with the tips of fingers or sides of hands, using short, rapid, repetitive movements.

tardive dyskinesia, an abnormal condition characterized by involuntary, repetitious movements of the muscles of the face, limbs and trunk. This disorder most commonly affects older people who have been treated for extended periods with phenothiazine drugs to alleviate the symptoms of parkinsonism.

tardy peroneal nerve palsy, a type of mononeuropathy in which the peroneal nerve is excessively compressed where it crosses the head of the fibula. Such compression may occur when an individual falls asleep with the legs crossed.

tardy ulnar nerve palsy, an abnormal condition characterized by atrophy of the first dorsal interosseous muscle and difficulty in the performance of fine manipulations. It may be caused by injury of the ulnar nerve at the elbow, and commonly affects individuals with a shallow ulnar groove or those who persistently rest their weight on their elbows. Signs and symptoms of this disorder may include numbness of the small finger, the contiguous half of the proximal and middle phalanges of the ring finger, and the ulnar border of the hand.

target, (in radiography) area or anode of an x-ray tube which is bombarded by electrons and emits x-rays.

target cell, 1. also called **leptocyte.** An abnormal red blood cell which, when stained and examined under a microscope, is characterized by a densely stained centre surrounded by a pale unstained ring circled by a dark, irregular band. **2.** any cell having a specific receptor that reacts with a specific hormone, antigen, antibody, antibiotic, sensitized T cell or other substance.

target organ, 1. (in radionuclide imaging) an organ intended to receive the greatest concentration of a diagnostic radioactive tracer. **2.** (in endocrinology) an organ most affected by a specific hormone.

target symptoms, symptoms of an illness that are most likely to respond to a specific treatment, such as a particular psychopharmacological drug.

target volume, (in radiotherapy) the volume of tissue intended to receive the prescribed dose of radiation. It includes the known tumour volume plus a margin of normal tissue to allow for microscopic invasion.

tarnishing, a tendency by left foci temporal lobe epilepsy patients to make a harsh assessment of themselves by emphasizing negative qualities in their self-descriptions.

tarsal, of, or pertaining to, the tarsus, or ankle bone.

tarsal bone, any one of seven bones comprising the tarsus of the foot, consisting of the talus, calcaneus, cuboid, navicular and the three cuneiforms.

tarsal gland, one of numerous modified sebaceous glands on the inner surfaces of the eyelids.

tarsal tunnel syndrome, an abnormal condition and a kind of mononeuropathy, characterized by pain and numbness in the sole of the foot. This disorder may be caused by fractures of the ankle that compress the posterior tibial nerve.

tarsometatarsal, of, or pertaining to, the metatarsal bones and tarsus of the foot.

tarsus, *pl.* **tarsi, 1.** the area of articulation between the foot and the leg. **2.** also known as **tarsal plate.** any one of the plates of cartilage, about 2.5 cm long, forming the eyelids. One tarsal plate shapes each eyelid. The superior tarsal plates form the upper eyelids. The inferior tarsal plates form the lower eyelids.

tart, abbreviation for **tartrate carboxylate anion.**

tartar, 1. a hard, gritty deposit composed of organic matter, phosphates and carbonates, collecting on the teeth and gums. **2.** any of several compounds containing tartrate, the salt of tartaric acid.

tartaric acid, a colourless or white powder found in various plants and prepared commercially from maleic anhydride and hydrogen peroxide. It is used in baking powder, certain beverages and in tartar emetic.

task analysis, the analysis of the components (tasks) involved in an activity. This may include the identification of the physical, interactive and psychological skills necessary for that task.

task functions, behaviours that focus on, or direct activities towards, movements with work or labour overtones.

task group, a group in which structured verbal or non-verbal exercises are used to help a person gain emotional, physical and other personal awareness.

task-oriented behaviour, actions involving a person's cognitive abilities in an attempt to solve problems and gratify the person's needs in order to reduce or avoid distress.

taste, the sense of perceiving different flavours in soluble substances that contact the tongue and trigger nerve impulses to special taste centres in the cortex and thalamus of the brain. The four basic traditional tastes are sweet, salty, sour and bitter. The front of the tongue is most sensitive to salty and sweet substances; the sides of the tongue are most sensitive to sour substances; and the back of the tongue is most sensitive to bitter substances. The middle of the tongue produces virtually no taste sensation. The sense of taste is intricately linked with the sense of smell.

taste bud, any one of many peripheral taste organs distributed over the tongue and the roof of the mouth. Each taste bud rests in a spheric pocket which extends through the epithelium. Gustatory cells and supporting cells form each bud, which has a surface opening and an opening in the basement membrane.

tattoo, a permanent colouration of the skin by the introduction of foreign pigment. A tattoo may occur accidentally when a piece of graphite from a broken pencil point is embedded in the skin. **tattoo,** v.

tautomer, any of several compounds related through a dynamic equilibrium between isomers. The classic example is the enol-keto tautomer, in which molecules of a compound can exist in two forms at the same time, depending on the position of a hydrogen atom next to a carbonyl group.

taxonomy, a system for classifying organisms on the basis of natural relationships and assigning them appropriate names. **taxonomic,** adj.

Tay's spot. See **cherry-red spot.**

Tay-Sachs disease {Warren Tay, English ophthalmologist, b. 1843; Bernard Sachs, American neurologist, b. 1858}, an inherited, neurodegenerative disorder of lipid metabolism, caused by a deficiency of the enzyme hexosaminidase A. It results in the accumulation of sphingolipids in the brain. The condition, which is transmitted as an autosomal recessive trait, occurs predominantly in families of Eastern European Jewish origin, specifically the Ashkenazic Jews, and is characterized by progressive mental and physical deficiency and early death.

Taylor brace {Charles F. Taylor, American surgeon, b. 1827}, a padded steel brace used to support the spine.

TB, abbreviation for **tuberculosis.**

TBI, abbreviation for **total body irradiation.**

Tb, symbol for **terbium.**

TBT, abbreviation for **tracheobronchial tree.**

TBW, abbreviation for **total body water.**

TBZ, abbreviation for **tetrabenazine, an anaesthetic adjuvant.**

Tc, symbol for **technetium.**

TD, abbreviation for **toxic dose.**

TDCR, abbreviation for **Teachers' Diploma of the College of Radiographers.**

TD₅₀. See **median toxic dose.**

tDNA, abbreviation for **transfer DNA.**

Te, symbol for **tellurium.**

tea. See **cannabis.**

teacher's nodule. See **vocal cord nodule.**

Teachers' Diploma of the College of Radiographers (TDCR), post-higher diploma and post-teaching certificate qualification awarded by the College of Radiographers (UK).

teaching hospital, a hospital with accredited educational and training programmes in medical, nursing or professions supplementary to medicine.

team nursing, a decentralized system in which the care of a patient is distributed among the members of a team.

tear duct, any duct that carries tears, including the lacrimal ducts, nasolacrimal ducts and the excretory ducts of the lacrimal glands.

teardrop fracture, an avulsion fracture of one of the short bones, such as a vertebra, causing a tear-shaped disruption of bone tissue.

tearing, watering of the eye, usually caused by excessive tear production due to strong emotion, infection or mechanical irritation by a foreign body. If the normal amount of fluid tears is produced but not drained into the lacrimal punctum at the nasal border of the eye, tearing will occur.

tebutate, a contraction for tertiary butyl acetate.

technetium (Tc), a radioactive metallic element. Its atomic number is 43 and its atomic weight is 99. Isotopes of technetium are used in radioisotope scanning procedures of internal organs. Formerly called **masurium.**

technetium 99, the radionuclide most commonly used to image the body in radionuclide imaging scans. It has a half-life of six hours, and is a pure gamma ray emitter.

technique, the method and details followed in performing a procedure, such as those used in conducting a laboratory test, a physical examination, a psychiatric interview, a surgical operation or any process requiring certain skills or an ordered sequence of actions.

teenager. See **adolescent.**

teether, an object, such as a teething ring, on which an infant can bite or chew during the teething process.

teething, the physiological process of eruption of deciduous teeth through the gums. It normally begins between the sixth and eighth months of life, and occurs periodically until the complete set of 20 teeth has appeared at about 30 months. Discomfort and inflammation result from the pressure exerted against the periodontal tissue as the crown of the tooth breaks through the membranes. General signs of teething include excessive drooling, biting on hard objects, irritability, difficulty in sleeping and refusal of food. **teethe,** *v.*

teething ring, a circular device, usually made of plastic or rubber, on which an infant may chew or bite during the teething process.

TEIB, abbreviation for **triethylene immunobenzoquinone.**

telangiectasia, permanent dilatation of groups of superficial capillaries and venules. Common causes are actinic damage, atrophy-producing dermatoses, rosacea, elevated oestrogen levels and collagen vascular diseases.

telangiectatic epulis, a benign red tumour of the gingiva, containing prominent blood vessels. Low-grade or chronic irritation is usually associated, and the lesion is easily traumatized.

telangiectatic fibroma. See **angiofibroma.**

telangiectatic glioma, a tumour composed of glial cells and a network of blood vessels, which give the mass a vivid pink appearance.

telangiectatic granuloma. See **pyogenic granuloma.**

telangiectatic lipoma. See **angiolipoma.**

telangiectatic naevus, a common skin condition of neonates, characterized by flat, deep-pink localized areas of capillary dilatation that occur predominantly on the back of the neck, lower occiput, upper eyelids, upper lip and bridge of the nose.

telangiectatic sarcoma, a malignant tumour of mesodermal cells with an unusually rich vascular network.

telegraphic speech, a type of language dysfunction commonly experienced by persons with organic brain syndrome and some forms of aphasia. It is characterized by replies that are relevant but carry a minimum amount of information.

telepathist, 1. a person who believes in telepathy. **2.** a person who claims to have telepathic powers.

telepathy, the alleged communication of thought from one person to another, by means other than the physical senses. **telepathic,** *adj.*, **telepathize,** *v.*

telereceptive, pertaining to the exteroceptors of hearing, sight and smell that detect stimuli distant from the body.

teletherapy, radiotherapy administered by a machine positioned at some distance from the patient.

tellurium (Te), an element exhibiting metallic and non-metallic chemical properties. Its atomic number is 52 and its atomic weight is 127.60.

telocentric, pertaining to a chromosome in which the centromere is located at the end, so that the chromatids appear as straight filaments.

telogen. See **hair.**

telophase, the final of the four stages of nuclear division in mitosis and in each of the two divisions in meiosis.

temazepam, a hypnotic benzodiazepine used for the relief of transient and intermittent insomnia.

temper tantrum. See **tantrum.**

temperate phage, a bacteriophage whose genome is incorporated into the host bacterium.

temperature, 1. a relative measure of sensible heat or cold. **2.** (in physiology) a measure of sensible heat associated with the metabolism of the human body, normally maintained at a constant level of $37°$ C ($98.6°$ F). **3.** informal, a fever.

template, (in genetics) the strand of DNA that acts as a mould for the synthesis of messenger RNA.

temporal arteritis, a progressive inflammatory disorder of cranial blood vessels, principally the temporal artery. Symptoms are intractable headache, difficulty in chewing, weakness, rheumatic pains and loss of vision if the central retinal artery becomes occluded.

temporal artery, any one of three arteries on each side of the head: superficial temporal artery, middle temporal artery and deep temporal artery.

temporal bone, one of a pair of large bones forming part of the lower cranium and containing various cavities and recesses associated with the ear, such as the tympanic cavity and auditory tube.

temporal bone fracture, a break of the temporal bone of the skull, sometimes characterized by bleeding from the ear.

temporal lobe, the lateral region of the cerebrum, below the lateral fissure.

temporal lobe epilepsy. See **psychomotor seizure.**

temporal muscle. See **temporalis.**

temporal subtraction, the subtraction of two or more digitized x-ray images that were acquired at different times. The subtraction process eliminates information in the image that was static.

temporal summation. See **summation,** def. 2.

temporalis, one of the four muscles of mastication. It is a broad radiating muscle that arises from the whole of the temporal fossa and from the surface of the temporal fascia. The temporalis acts to close the jaws and retract the mandible.

temporary filling, a mixture of gutta-percha, zinc oxide, white wax and colouring, used for temporarily sealing dressings in tooth cavities.

temporary tooth. See **deciduous tooth.**

temporomandibular joint, one of two joints connecting the mandible of the jaw to the temporal bone of the skull. It is a combined hinge and gliding joint, formed by the anterior parts of the mandibular fossae of the temporal bone, articular tubercles, condyles of the mandible and five ligaments.

temporomandibular joint pain dysfunction syndrome (TMJ), an abnormal condition characterized by facial pain and mandibular dysfunction, apparently caused by a defective or dislocated temporomandibular joint. Some common indications of this syndrome are clicking of the joint when the jaws move, limitation of jaw movement, subluxation and temporomandibular dislocation.

temporoparietalis, one of a pair of broad, thin muscles of the scalp, which fan out over the temporal fascia. It acts in combination with the occipitofrontalis to wrinkle the forehead, widen the eyes and raise the ears.

TEN, abbreviation for **toxic epidermal necrolysis.**

tenacious, pertaining to secretions that are sticky or adhesive or otherwise tend to hold together, such as mucus and sputum.

tenaculum, *pl.* **tenacula,** a clip or clamp with long handles used to grasp, immobilize and hold an organ or a piece of tissue. Kinds of tenacula include the **abdominal tenaculum,** which has long arms and small hooks, the **forceps tenaculum,** which has long hooks and is used in gynaecological surgery, and the **uterine** or **cervical tenaculum,** which has short hooks or open, eye-shaped clamps used to hold the cervix.

tendinitis, an inflammatory condition of a tendon, usually resulting from strain. Also spelt **tendonitis.**

tendinous cords. See **chordae tendineae.**

tendo calcaneus. See **Achilles tendon.**

tendon, one of many white, glistening fibrous bands of tissue that attach muscle to bone. Except at points of attachment, tendons are sheathed in delicate fibroelastic connective tissue. Tendons are extremely strong and flexible, inelastic, and occur in various lengths and thicknesses. **tendinous,** *adj.*

tendon of Achilles. See **Achilles tendon.**

tendon reflex. See **deep tendon reflex.**

tendonitis. See **tendinitis.**

tenesmus, persistent, ineffectual spasms of the rectum or bladder, accompanied by the desire to empty the bowel or bladder.

tennis elbow. See **lateral humeral epicondylitis.**

tenofibril. See **tonofibril.**

Tenon's capsule. See **fascia bulbi.**

tenosynovitis, inflammation of a tendon sheath caused by calcium deposits, repeated strain or trauma, high levels of blood cholesterol, rheumatoid arthritis, gout or gonorrhoea.

tenotomy, the total or partial severing of a tendon, performed to correct a muscle imbalance, such as in the correction of strabismus of the eye or in clubfoot.

TENS, abbreviation for **transcutaneous electric nerve stimulation.**

tension, 1. the act of pulling or straining until taut. **2.** the condition of being taut, tense or under pressure. **3.** a state or condition resulting from the psychological and physiological reaction to a stressful situation, characterized physically by a general increase in muscle tonus, heart rate, respiration rate and alertness, and psychologically by feelings of strain, uneasiness, irritability and anxiety.

tension headache, pain that affects the occipital region of the body as a result of overwork or emotional strain. It tenses the body and inhibits rest and relaxation.

tensor, any one of the muscles of the body that tenses a structure, such as the tensor fasciae latae of the thigh.

tensor fasciae latae, one of the 10 muscles of the gluteal region. It functions to flex the thigh and rotate it slightly medially.

tent, 1. a transparent cover, usually of plastic, supported over the upper part of a patient by a frame. Used in the treatment of respiratory conditions, it provides a controlled environment into which steam, oxygen, vapourised medication or droplets of cool water may be sprayed, such as an oxygen tent. **2.** a cone made of various materials inserted into a cavity or orifice of the body to dilate its opening, such as a laminaria tent. **3.** a pack placed in a wound to hold it open so as to ensure that healing progresses from the base of the wound upwards to the skin.

tenth nerve. See **vagus nerve.**

tenth-value layer (TVL), the thickness of material required to attenuate a beam of radiation to one-tenth of its original intensity.

tentorial herniation, the protrusion of brain tissue into the tentorial notch, caused by increased intracranial pressure resulting from oedema, haemorrhage or tumour. Characteristic signs are severe headache, fever, flushing, sweating, abnormal pupillary reflex, drowsiness, hypotension and loss of consciousness.

tentorium, *pl.* **tentoria,** any part of the body

that resembles a tent, such as the tentorium of hypophysis that covers the hypophyseal fossa.

tentorium cerebelli, one of the three extensions of the dura mater that separates the cerebellum from the occipital lobe of the cerebrum.

tepid, moderately warm to the touch.

teramorphous, of the nature, or characteristic, of a monster.

teras, *pl.* **terata,** a severely deformed fetus. **teratic,** *adj.*

teratism, any congenital or developmental anomaly produced by inherited or environmental factors, or by a combination of the two; any condition in which a severely malformed fetus is produced. Kinds of teratism include **atresic teratism, ceasmic teratism, ectopic teratism, ectrogenic teratism, hypergenetic teratism** and **symphysic teratism.**

teratogen, any substance, agent or process that interferes with normal prenatal development, causing the formation of one or more developmental abnormalities in the fetus. Teratogens act directly on the developing organism, or indirectly, affecting supplemental structures such as the placenta or some maternal system. The period of highest vulnerability in the developing embryo is from about the third through the twelfth week of gestation, when differentiation of the major organs and systems occurs. **teratogenic,** *adj.*

teratogenesis, the development of physical defects in the embryo. **teratogenetic,** *adj.*

teratogenic agent. See **teratogen.**

teratogeny. See **teratogenesis.**

teratoid, of, or pertaining to, abnormal physical development.

teratoid tumour. See **dermoid cyst.**

teratologist, a specialist in the science of teratology.

teratology, the study of the causes and effects of congenital malformations and developmental abnormalities. **teratological,** *adj.*

teratoma, *pl.* **teratomas, teratomata,** a tumour composed of different kinds of tissue, none of which normally occur together or at the site of the tumour.

teratosis. See **teratism.**

terbium (Tr), a rare earth metallic element. Its atomic number is 65 and its atomic weight is 158.294.

terbutaline sulphate, a beta-adrenergic stimulant used as a bronchodilator in the treatment of asthma, bronchitis and emphysema, and as a uterine relaxant to treat premature labour.

teres, *pl.* **teretes,** a long, cylindrical muscle, such as the teres minor or teres major. **teres,** *adj.*

teres major, a thick, flat muscle of the shoulder. It functions to adduct, extend and rotate the arm medially.

teres minor, a cylindrical, elongated muscle of the shoulder. It functions to rotate the arm laterally, adduct the arm weakly, and draw the humerus towards the glenoid fossa of the scapula, strengthening the shoulder joint.

terfenadine, a non-sedating histamine H1-receptor antagonist, used to relieve symptoms of seasonal allergic rhinitis and other allergic conditions.

term, a pregnancy that reaches 37 weeks, until 42 completed weeks.

terminal, 1. (of a structure or process) near or approaching its end, such as a terminal bronchiole or a terminal disease. **2.** an input/output (I/O) device that has a two-way communication capability with a computer. **terminate,** *v.,* **terminus,** *n.*

terminal bronchiole. See **bronchiole.**

terminal disinfection, the process of cleaning equipment and airing of a room after the release of a patient who has been treated for an infectious disease.

terminal drop, a rapid decline in cognitive function and coping ability that occurs 1 to 5 years before death.

terminal nerve, a small nerve originating in the cerebral hemisphere in the region of the olfactory trigone, classified by most anatomists as part of the olfactory, or first cranial, nerve.

terminal stance, one of the five stages in the stance phase of a walking gait, directly associated with the continuation of single limb support or the period during which the body moves forward on the supporting foot.

terminal sulcus of right atrium, a shallow channel on the external surface of the right atrium between the superior and inferior venae cavae.

termination codon, (in molecular genetics) a unit in the genetic code that specifies the end of the sequence of amino acids in a polypeptide.

termination phase, the last stage of a therapeutic relationship when attained goals are evaluated and outcomes achieved.

termination sequence, (in molecular genetics) a DNA segment at the end of a unit that is transcribed to messenger RNA from the DNA template.

territorial, a type of body movement that aids in communication. A territorial will frame an interaction and define an individual's "territory".

territoriality, an emotional attachment to, and defence of, certain areas related to one's existence.

tertian, occurring every 48 hours or 3 days, including the first day of occurrence, such as vivax or tertian malaria in which fever occurs every third day.

tertian malaria, a form of malaria, caused by the protozoan *Plasmodium vivax* or *Plasmodium ovale*. It is characterized by febrile paroxysms that occur every 48 hours. Vivax malaria, caused by *Plasmodium vivax,* is the most common form of malaria, and although rarely fatal, it is the most difficult form to cure and relapses are common. **Ovale malaria,** caused by *Plasmodium ovale,* is usually milder and causes only a few short attacks.

tertiary, third in frequency or in order of use.

tertiary healthcare, a specialized, highly technical level of healthcare that includes diagnosis and treatment of disease and disability in sophisticated, large research and teaching hospitals. It offers a highly centralized care to the population of a large region, and sometimes at national and international level.

tertiary prevention, a level of preventive medicine that deals with the rehabilitation and return of a patient to a status of maximum usefulness with a minimum risk of recurrence of a physical or mental disorder.

tesla {Nikola Tesla, American engineer, b. 1856}, a unit of magnetic flux density, defined by the International System of Units as 1 weber per square metre, the equivalent of 1 volt/second per square metre.

test, 1. an examination or trial intended to establish a principle or determine a value. **2.** a chemical reaction or reagent that has clinical significance. **3.** to detect, identify or conduct a trial.

test method, a method chosen for experimental testing or study by means of method evaluation.

test tube, a tube made of transparent material having one open end. It is used in many common laboratory functions.

testcross, 1. (in genetics) the cross of a dominant phenotype with a recessive phenotype, to determine either the degree of genetic linkage or whether the dominant phenotype is homozygous or heterozygous. **2.** the subject undergoing such a test.

testes determining factor (TDF), a Y-chromosome gene believed to determine male sexual development.

testicle. See **testis.**

testicular, of or pertaining to the testicle.

testicular artery, one of a pair of long, slender branches of the abdominal aorta, arising caudal to the renal arteries and supplying the testis.

testicular cancer, a malignant neoplastic disease of the testis. An undescended testicle is often involved. In many cases the tumour is detected after an injury, but trauma is not considered a causative factor. Patients with early testicular cancer are often asymptomatic, and metastases may be seeded in lymph nodes, the lungs and liver before the primary lesion is palpable. In the later stages there may be pulmonary symptoms, ureteral obstruction, gynaecomastia and an abdominal mass.

testicular duct. See **vas deferens.**

testicular feminization. See **feminization.**

testicular self-examination (TSE), a recommended procedure for detecting tumours or other abnormalities in the male testes. Each testicle is examined with both hands, placing the fingers under the testicle while the thumbs are placed on top. The testicle is then rolled gently between the thumbs and fingers.

testicular vein, one of a pair of veins that emerge from convoluted venous plexuses, forming the greater mass of the spermatic cords.

testis, one of the pair of male gonads that produce semen. The adult testes are suspended in the scrotum by the spermatic cords. Each testis is a laterally compressed oval body about 4 cm long and 2.5 cm wide, and weighs about 12 g. The convoluted epididymis lying on the posterior border of the testis is about 20 feet long and connects with the vas deferens through which spermatozoa pass during ejaculation. Each testis consists of several hundred conical lobules containing the tiny coiled seminiferous tubules in which spermatozoa develop.

testosterone, a naturally occurring anabolic acid androgenic hormone, used for androgen deficiency, female breast cancer and for stimulation of growth, weight gain and red blood cell production.

testosterone derivative. See **anabolic steroid.**

testosterone enanthate, testosterone isocaproate, testosterone phenylpropionate, testosterone propionate, esters of testosterone given intramuscularly as components of depot injections. See **testosterone; anabolic steroid.**

testosterone undecanoate, an ester of testosterone given orally. See **testosterone; anabolic steroid.**

tetanus, an acute, potentially fatal infection of the central nervous system caused by an exotoxin, tetanospasmin, elaborated by an anaerobic bacillus, *Clostridium tetani.* The toxin is a neurotoxin and is one of the most lethal poisons known. *C. tetani* infects only wounds that contain dead tissue. The bacillus is a common resident of the superficial layers of the soil and a normal inhabitant of the intestinal tracts of cows and horses. The bacillus may enter the body through a puncture wound, abrasion, laceration or burn. The infection occurs in two clinical forms: (a) with an abrupt onset, high mortality and a short incubation period (3 to 21 days); (b) with less severe symptoms, a lower mortality and a longer incubation period (4 to 5 weeks). The disease is characterized by irritability, headache, fever and painful spasms of the muscles resulting in lockjaw, risus sardonicus, opisthotonos and laryngeal spasm; eventually, every muscle of the body is in tonic spasm. The motor nerves transmit the impulses from the infected central nervous system to the muscles. There is no lesion; even at autopsy no organic lesion is seen, and the cerebrospinal fluid is clear and normal.

tetanus antiserum, a tetanus immune serum of animal origin, that neutralizes exotoxins in tetanus infection. It has been used for short-term immunization against tetanus after possible exposure to the organism, and for tetanus treatment. However, allergic reactions to it are frequent and it has largely been superseded by tetanus immunoglobulin.

tetanus immunoglobulin, an injectable antibody preparation derived from the blood of immune humans. It is effective and much safer than tetanus antitoxin. It is used for short-term immunization against tetanus after possible exposure to the organism, and for tetanus treatment.

tetanus toxoid, an active immunizing agent prepared from detoxified tetanus toxin that produces an antigenic response in the body, conferring permanent immunity to tetanus infection. It is used for active immunization against tetanus.

tetany, a condition characterized by cramps, convulsions, twitching of the muscles and sharp flexion of the wrist and ankle joints. Tetany is a manifestation of an abnormality in calcium metabolism which can occur in association with vitamin D deficiency, hypoparathyroidism, alkalosis or ingestion of alkaline salts. Kinds of tetany are **duration tetany, grass tetany, hyperventilation tetany** and **lactation tetany.**

tetrachlormethane. See **carbon tetrachloride.**

tetracycline, a broad spectrum antibiotic used for the treatment of many bacterial and rickettsial infections, and as a sclerosing agent in the treatment of pleural effusions.

tetrad, (in genetics) a group of four chromatids of a synapsed pair of homologous chromosomes during the first meiotic prophase stage of gametogenesis. **tetradic,** *adj.*

tetrahydrocannabinol (THC). See **delta-9-tetrahydrocannabinol.**

tetraiodothyronine. See **thyroxine.**

tetramer, something that is composed of four parts, such as a protein composed of four polypeptide subunits.

tetraploid (4n), 1. also tetraploidic. Of, or pertaining to, an individual, organism, strain or cell that has four complete sets of chromosomes. **2.** such an individual, organism, strain or cell.

tetraploidy, the state or condition of having four complete sets of chromosomes.

TGF, abbreviation for **transforming growth factor.**

Th, symbol for **thorium.**

thalamus, *pl.* **thalami,** one of a pair of large oval organs forming most of the lateral walls of the third ventricle of the brain and part of the diencephalon. It relays sensory impulses to the cerebral cortex. It is composed mainly of gray substance and translates impulses from appropriate receptors into crude sensations of pain, temperature and touch. It also participates in associating sensory impulses with pleasant and unpleasant feelings, in the arousal mechanisms of the body, and in the mechanisms that produce complex reflex movements. **thalamic,** *adj.*

thalassaemia, haemolytic anaemia characterized by microcytic, hypochromic and short-lived red blood cells caused by deficient haemoglobin synthesis. It is genetically transmitted disease, occurring in two forms: (a) **thalassaemia major (Cooley's anaemia),** the homozygous form, is evident in infancy and is recognized by anaemia, fever, failure to thrive and splenomegaly; it is confirmed by characteristic changes in the red blood cells on microscopic examination. The spleen may become so enlarged that respiratory excursion is impeded, and the abdominal organs are crowded. Headache, abdominal pain, fatigue and anorexia often occur. (b) **Thalassaemia minor,** the heterozygous form, is characterized only by a mild anaemia and minimal red blood cell changes. Thalassaemia minima is a form that lacks clinical symptoms, although patients show haematological evidence of the disease.

thalidomide, a sedative-hypnotic with immunosuppressive activity. It has been withdrawn from general use because of its potential for teratogenic effects, particularly phocomelia, when taken during pregnancy. It is sometimes used for the treatment of leprosy, Behcet's syndrome and other conditions where its immunosuppressant activity is useful.

thallium (Tl), a soft, bluish-white metallic element that exhibits some non-metallic chemical properties. Its atomic number is 81 and its atomic weight is 204.37. Many of its compounds are highly toxic.

thallium poisoning, a toxic condition caused by the ingestion, or absorption through the skin, of thallium salts, especially thallium sulphate. Characteristic of the condition are abdominal pain, vomiting, bloody diarrhoea, tremor, delirium and alopecia.

thanatology, the study of death and dying. **thanatologist.**

thanatophoric dwarf, an infant with severe micromelia, the limbs usually extending straight out from the trunk, an extremely narrow chest and flattened vertebral bodies with wide intervertebral spaces.

THC, abbreviation for **tetrahydro-**

cannabinol.

theca, *pl.* **thecae,** a sheath or capsule, such as the theca cordis or pericardium.

theca cell tumour, an uncommon, benign, fibroid tumour of the ovary, composed of theca cells and usually containing granulosa (follicular) cells.

thecocellulare xanthomatodes, thecoma. See **theca cell tumour.**

thenar, 1. the ball of the thumb. **2.** of, or pertaining to, the thumb side of the palm.

theobromine, a substance (methylxanthine) that is related chemically to caffeine and theophylline; it differs from them by the number and distribution of methyl groups. Theobromine occurs naturally in cocoa, cola nuts and tea. It acts as a diuretic, vasodilator, cardiac stimulant and smooth muscle relaxant.

theophylline, a xanthine bronchodilator used to relax the smooth muscle of the bronchial passages in the treatment of asthma, bronchitis and emphysema.

theorem, 1. a proposition to be proved by a chain of reasoning and analysis. **2.** a rule expressed by symbols or formulae.

theoretic plate number (N), a number defining the efficiency of a chromatographic column.

theory, an abstract statement formulated to predict, explain or describe the relationships among concepts, constructs or events.

theotherapy, a therapeutic approach to the prevention, diagnosis and treatment of disease and dysfunction based on religious or spiritual beliefs.

therapeutic, 1. beneficial. **2.** pertaining to a treatment.

therapeutic abortion, 1. a termination of pregnancy performed in accordance with the Abortion Act of 1967 (UK), amended in 1990. **2.** informal, any legal induced abortion.

therapeutic communication, (in psychiatric nursing) a process in which the nurse consciously influences a patient, or helps the patient to a better understanding through verbal or non-verbal communication.

therapeutic community, (in mental health) a treatment facility in which the entire milieu is part of the treatment. The physical environment, other patients, staff and policies of the facility influence the function of the individual.

therapeutic equivalent, a drug that has essentially the same effect in the treatment of a disease or condition as one or more other drugs.

therapeutic exercise, any exercise planned and performed to attain a specific physical benefit, such as maintenance of the range of motion, strengthening of weakened muscles, increased flexibility of a joint or improved cardiovascular and respiratory function.

therapeutic gain, the ratio of the biological effect of a therapy on a tumour, compared with the effect on surrounding normal tissue.

therapeutic index, the difference between the minimum therapeutic and minimum toxic concentrations of a drug.

therapeutic radiography. See **radiotherapy.**

therapeutic radiopharmaceutical, a radioactive drug administered to a patient to deliver radiation to body tissues internally, such as iodine 131 which is used to ablate thyroid tissue in hyperthyroid patients.

therapeutic temperature, (in hyperthermia treatment) temperatures between 42° and 45° C (107° and 113° F).

therapist, a person with special skills, obtained through education and experience, in one or more areas of healthcare.

therapy, the treatment of any disease or a pathological condition, such as inhalation therapy which administers various medicines to patients suffering from diseases of the respiratory tract.

thermal, of, or pertaining to, the production, application or maintenance of heat. Also thermic.

thermal burn, tissue injury, usually of the skin, caused by exposure to extreme heat.

thermal dilution, a method of cardiac output determination. A bolus of solution of known volume and temperature is added to the bloodstream; the resultant cooling of blood temperature is detected by a thermister previously placed in the pulmonary artery with a catheter.

thermal field size, the area over which therapeutic heating is likely to be produced.

thermic fever. See **heat hyperpyrexia.**

thermistor, a kind of thermometer for measuring minute changes in temperature.

thermocautery, the use of a needle or wire heated by direct flame, a heated hydrocarbon vapour or an electric current, for the destruction of tissue.

thermocouple, a temperature-measuring device that relies on the production of a temperature-dependent voltage at the junction of two dissimilar metals.

thermodilution, a cardiac output testing method in which a small amount of a cold liquid, such as a saline solution, is injected into the bloodstream. Cardiac output is calculated as a function of the flow rate of the saline solution, multiplied by a factor derived from the temperature differences.

thermogenesis, production of heat, especially by the cells of the body. **thermogenetic,** *adj.*

thermography, a technique for sensing and recording on film hot and cold areas of the body, by means of an infrared detector that reacts to blood flow. **thermographic,** *adj.*

thermolabile, easily destroyed or altered by heat.

thermoluminescent dosimetry, a method of measuring the ionizing radiation to which a person is exposed, using a device that stores the radiant energy and releases it later as ultraviolet or visible light.

thermometer, an instrument for measuring temperature. It usually consists of a sealed glass tube, marked in degrees of Celsius or Fahrenheit, containing liquid such as mercury or alcohol. The liquid rises or falls as it expands or contracts according to changes in temperature. Some kinds of thermometers are clinical thermometer, digital thermometer and electronic thermometer.

thermoneutral environment, 1. an environment that keeps body temperature at an optimal point at which the least amount of oxygen is consumed for metabolism. **2.** an environment that enables a neonate to maintain a body temperature of 36.5° C (97.7° F) with a minimal requirement of energy and oxygen.

thermoregulation, ineffective, the state in which an individual's temperature fluctuates between hypothermia and hyperthermia. The critical characteristic is the fluctuation in body temperature above or below the normal range.

thermoregulation, the control of heat production and heat loss, specifically the maintenance of body temperature through physiological mechanisms.

thermostable, unaffected by or resistant to change by an increase in temperature.

thermostat, a device for the automatic control of a heating or cooling system. **thermostatic,** *adj.*

thermotaxis, 1. the normal adjustment and regulation of body temperature. **2.** the movement of an organism in response to heat, either towards the stimulus (positive thermotaxis) or away from the stimulus (negative thermotaxis).

thermotherapeutic penetration, the depth to which heating to therapeutic temperatures is likely to extend.

thermotherapy, the treatment of disease by the application of heat. Thermotherapy may be administered as dry heat with heat lamps, diathermy machines, electric pads, hot water bottles, as moist heat with warm compresses, or by immersion in warm water. **thermotherapeutic,** *adj.*

thermotropism. See **thermotaxis.**

theta wave, one of the several types of brain waves, characterized by a relatively low frequency of 4 to 7 Hz and a low amplitude of 10 µV. Theta waves are the "drowsy waves" of the temporal lobes of the brain.

thiabendazole, an anthelmintic used in the treatment of a variety of worm infestations, including hookworms, roundworms, threadworms and strongyloidiasis.

thiamine, a water-soluble, crystalline compound of the B complex vitamin group, es-

sential for normal metabolism and for the health of the cardiovascular and nervous systems. Thiamine combines with pyruvic acid to form a coenzyme necessary for the breakdown of carbohydrates into glucose. A deficiency of thiamine affects chiefly the nervous system, circulation and GI tract. Symptoms include irritability, emotional disturbances, loss of appetite, multiple neuritis, increased pulse rate, dyspnoea, reduced intestinal motility and heart irregularities. Severe deficiency causes beriberi. Also spelt thiamin.

thiazide diuretic. See **diuretic.**

thigh, the section of the lower limb between the hip and knee.

thigh bone. See **femur.**

thinking, 1. the cognitive process of forming mental images or concepts. **2.** the process of cognitive problem solving through the sorting, organizing and classification of facts. Kinds of thinking include abstract thinking, concrete thinking and syncretic thinking.

thioctic acid, a pyruvate oxidation factor found in liver and yeast, used in bacterial culture media.

thioester, an important group of biological chemicals formed by the hydrosulphides and carboxylic acids and identified by an ester bond involving the -SH radical. Examples include the coenzyme A thioesters.

thioguanine, a cytotoxic antimetabolite used in the treatment of a variety of malignant diseases, especially the acute leukaemias.

thiopentone sodium, a potent short-acting barbiturate, used as a general anaesthetic for surgical procedures that are expected to require 15 minutes or less, as an induction agent for other general anaesthetics, as a hypnotic component in balanced anaesthesia, and as an adjunct to regional anaesthesia.

thioridazine hydrochloride, a phenothiazine antipsychotic used in the treatment of severe childhood behavioural disorders, geriatric mental disorders, psychoses and mania.

thiotepa, a cytotoxic alkylating agent, most often used as an intracavity instillation in the treatment of bladder cancer or malignant effusions.

thiothixene, any one of a group of thioxanthene antipsychotics used in the treatment of acute agitation and mild to severe psychotic disorders.

thiourea derivative, one of a group of antithyroid drugs used in the treatment of hyperthyroidism. Thiourea drugs act by inhibiting the synthesis of thyroid hormone.

thioxanthene derivative, any one of a group of antipsychotic drugs, each of which is similar to the phenothiazenes in its indication, action and adverse effects. They include flupenthixol.

third cranial nerve. See **oculomotor nerve.**

third cuneiform bone. See **lateral cuneiform bone.**

third ventriculostomy, a surgical procedure for draining cerebrospinal fluid into the cisterna chiasmatis of the subarachnoid space in hydrocephalus, usually in the newborn.

thirst, a perceived desire for water or other fluid. The sensation of thirst is usually referred to the mouth and throat.

Thiry-Vella fistula {Ludwig Thiry, Austrian physiologist, b. 1817; Luigi Vella, Italian physiologist, b. 1825}, an artificial passage from the abdominal surface of an experimental animal to an isolated intestinal loop, created surgically for the study of intestinal secretions.

Thomas' splint {Hugh Owen Thomas, English surgeon, b. 1834}, **1.** a rigid splint constructed of steel bars that are curved to fit the involved limb and held in place by a cast or a rigid bandage. **2.** A rigid metal splint that extends from a ring at the hip to beyond the foot.

Thompson scattering. See **scattering.**

Thomsen's disease. See **myotonia congenita.**

thoracentesis. See **thoracocentesis.**

thoracic, of, or pertaining to, the thorax.

thoracic actinomycocis. See **actinomycosis.**

thoracic aorta, the large upper portion of the descending aorta, starting at the caudal border of the fourth thoracic vertebra, dividing into seven branches and supplying many parts of the body, such as the heart, ribs, chest muscles and stomach.

thoracic duct, the common trunk of all lymphatic vessels in the body, except those on the right side of the head, neck and thorax, right upper limb, right lung, right side of the heart and the diaphragmatic surface of the liver. The thoracic duct contains various valves, including two at this orifice that prevent venous blood from flowing into the lymphatic system.

thoracic fistula, an abnormal opening in the chest wall that ends blindly or communicates with the thoracic cavity.

thoracic medicine, the branch of medicine concerned with the diagnosis and treatment of disorders of the structures and organs of the chest, especially the lungs.

thoracic nerves, the 12 spinal nerves on each side of the thorax, including 11 intercostal nerves and one subcostal nerve. They are distributed mainly to the walls of the thorax and abdomen. The first two intercostal nerves innervate the upper limb and thorax; the next four supply only the thorax; and the lower five supply the walls of the thorax and abdomen.

thoracic outlet syndrome, an abnormal condition and a type of mononeuropathy characterized by paraesthesia of the fingers. It may be caused by a nerve root compression by a cervical disk or carpal tunnel syndrome.

thoracic parietal node, one of the lymph glands in the thorax, associated with various lymphatic vessels and divided into sternal nodes, intercostal nodes and diaphragmatic nodes.

thoracic vertebra, one of the 12 bony segments of the spinal column of the upper back, designated T1 to T12. T1 is just below the seventh cervical vertebra (C7) and T12 is just above the first lumbar vertebra (L1). The thoracic portion of the spine is flexible and has a concave ventral curvature.

thoracic visceral node, a node in the three groups of lymph nodes connected to the part of the lymphatic system that serves certain structures within the thorax, such as the thymus, pericardium, oesophagus, trachea, lungs and bronchi.

thoracocentesis, the surgical perforation of the chest wall and pleural space with a needle. It is performed for the aspiration of fluid for diagnostic or therapeutic purposes or the removal of a specimen for biopsy.

thoracodorsal nerve, a branch of the brachial plexus, usually arising between the two subscapular nerves. It courses along the posterior wall of the axilla and terminates in branches that supply the latissimus dorsi.

thoracolumbar fascia, a non-contractile structure that functions in a manner similar to a ligament in the lumbar area. It extends from the iliac crest and sacrum to the thoracic cage and envelops the paravertebral musculature.

thoracostomy, an incision made into the chest wall to provide an opening for the purpose of drainage.

thoracotomy, a surgical opening into the thoracic cavity.

Thoraeus filters, combinations of metals, usually tin, copper and aluminum, used to modify the quality of orthovoltage x-ray beams to improve the penetrating ability.

thorax, *pl.* **thoraces, thoraxes,** the cage of bone and cartilage containing the principal organs of respiration and circulation, and covering part of the abdominal organs. It is formed ventrally by the sternum and costal cartilages, and dorsally by the 12 thoracic vertebrae and dorsal parts of the 12 ribs.

thorium (Th), a heavy, greyish, radioactive, metallic element. Its atomic number is 90 and its atomic weight is 232.04. Thorium is used in radiographic procedures and radiation therapy.

thought broadcasting, a symptom of psychosis in which the patient believes that his or her thoughts are "broadcast" beyond the head so that other persons can hear them.

thought insertion, a belief by some mentally ill patients that thoughts of other persons can be inserted into their own minds.

thought processes, altered, a state in which an individual experiences disruption in cognitive operations and activities. Characteristics include distraction; egocentrism; abnormal cognitive function; abnormal interpretations of the environment; decreased ability to grasp ideas; impaired ability to reason, solve problems, calculate, conceptualize or make decisions; disorientation; inappropriate social behaviour; altered sleep patterns; delusions or hallucinations; and attention to environmental cues which is either more or less acute than might normally be expected.

thought transference. See **telepathy.**

Thr, abbreviation for **threonine.**

threadworm infection. See **strongyloidiasis.**

threadworm. See *Enterobius vermicularis.*

thready pulse, an abnormal pulse that is weak and often fairly rapid; the artery does not feel full, and the rate may be difficult to count.

threatened abortion, a condition in pregnancy before the twenty-fourth week of gestation characterized by uterine bleeding and cramping sufficient to suggest that miscarriage may result.

three-day fever. See **phlebotomus fever.**

three-day measles. See **rubella.**

threonine (Thr), an essential amino acid required for the proper growth of infants and maintenance of nitrogen balance in adults. See also **amino acid, protein.**

threshold, the point at which a stimulus is great enough to produce an effect; for example, a pain threshold is the point at which a person becomes aware of pain.

threshold limit values, the maximum concentration of a chemical to which workers can be exposed for a fixed period, such as 8 hours per day, without developing a physical impairment.

thrill, a fine vibration, felt by an examiner's hand on the body of a patient over the site of an aneurysm or on the precordium, indicating the presence of an organic murmur.

throat. See **pharynx.**

throb, a deep, pulsating kind of discomfort or pain. **throbbing,** *adj., n.*

thrombapheresis. See **plateletpheresis.**

thrombasthenia, a rare haemorrhagic disease characterized by a defect in platelet mediated haemostasis. It is caused by an abnormality in the membrane surface of the platelet. The platelets do not aggregate, a clot does not form and haemorrhage ensues, often from the mucous membrane.

thrombectomy, the removal of a thrombus from a blood vessel, performed as emergency surgery to restore circulation to the affected part.

thrombin, an enzyme formed in plasma during the clotting process from prothrombin, calcium and thromboplastin.

thrombin clotting time, a test for detecting inhibitors to the clotting process which is normally 10-15 seconds. It is prolonged in DIC, liver disease and heparin therapy.

thromboangiitis obliterans, an occlusive vascular condition, usually of a leg or a foot, in which the small and medium-sized arteries become inflamed and thrombotic. Early signs of the condition are burning, numbness and tingling of the foot or leg distal to the lesion. Phlebitis and gangrene may develop as the disease progresses. Pulsation in the limb below the damaged blood vessels is often absent.

thrombocytapheresis. See **plateletapheresis.**

thrombocyte. See **platelet.**

thrombocytopathy, any disorder of the blood coagulation mechanism caused by an abnormality or dysfunction of platelets. Kinds of thrombocytopathies include thrombocytopenia and thrombocytosis. **thrombocytopathic,** *adj.*

thrombocytopenia, an abnormal haematological condition in which the number of platelets is reduced, usually by destruction of erythroid tissue in bone marrow associated with certain neoplastic diseases or an immune response to a drug. There may be decreased production of platelets, decreased survival of platelets, increased consumption of platelets and splenomegaly. Thrombocytopenia is the most common cause of bleeding disorders.

thrombocytopenic purpura, a bleeding disorder characterized by a marked decrease in the number of platelets, resulting in multiple bruises, petechiae and haemorrhage into the tissues. It may occur secondary to a number of causes, including infection and drug sensitivity and toxicity. It is considered to be a manifestation of an autoimmune response.

thrombocytosis, an abnormal increase in the number of platelets in the blood. **Benign thrombocytosis,** or **secondary thrombocytosis,** is asymptomatic and usually occurs after splenectomy, inflammatory disease, haemolytic anaemia, haemorrhage or iron deficiency, as a response to exercise or after treatment with vincristine. **Essential thrombocythaemia** is characterized by episodes of spontaneous bleeding alternating with thrombotic episodes.

thromboembolism, a condition in which a blood vessel is blocked by an embolus carried in the bloodstream from the site of clot formation. The area supplied by an obstructed artery may tingle and become cold, numb and cyanotic. An embolus in the lungs causes a sudden, sharp thoracic or upper abdominal pain, dyspnoea, a violent cough, fever and haemoptysis. Obstruction of the pulmonary artery or one of its branches may be rapidly fatal.

thrombolytic, pertaining to the dissolution

of blood clots.

thrombophlebitis, inflammation of a vein, often accompanied by formation of a clot. It occurs most commonly as a result of trauma to the vessel wall, hypercoagulability of blood, infection, chemical irritation, postoperative venous stasis, prolonged sitting, standing or immobilization, or a long period of intravenous catheterization. Thrombophlebitis of a superficial vein is generally evident; the vessel feels hard and thready or cord-like, and is extremely sensitive to pressure; the surrounding area may be erythematous and warm to the touch, and the entire limb may be pale, cold and swollen. Deep vein thrombophlebitis is characterized by aching or cramping pain, especially in the calf when the patient walks or dorsiflexes the foot (Homan's sign).

thrombophlebitis migrans. See **migratory thrombophlebitis.**

thrombophlebitis purulenta, an inflammation of a vein associated with the formation of a soft purulent thrombus that infiltrates the wall of the vessel.

thromboplastin, a complex substance that initiates the clotting process by converting prothrombin to thrombin in the presence of calcium ion.

thrombosis, *pl.* **thromboses,** an abnormal vascular condition in which thrombus develops within a blood vessel of the body. See also **blood clotting.**

thrombotest, an alternative to the prothrombin ratio for monitoring anticoagulant therapy, using fingerprick blood (thus avoiding venepuncture), normally 100%. The therapeutic level is 10-20%.

thrombotic thrombocytopenic purpura (TTP), a disorder characterized by thrombocytopenia, haemolytic anaemia and neurological abnormalities. It is accompanied by a generalized purpura together with deposition of microthrombi within the capillaries and smaller arterioles.

thrombus, *pl.* **thrombi,** an aggregation of platelets, fibrin, clotting factors and the cellular elements of blood attached to the interior wall of a vein or artery, sometimes occluding the lumen of the vessel. Kinds of thrombi include **agonal thrombus, hyaline thrombus, laminated thrombus, marasmic thrombus, parasitic thrombus** and **white thrombus.**

through transmission, (in ultrasonography) the process of imaging by transmitting the sound field through a specimen and picking up the transmitted energy on a far surface or a receiving transducer.

thrush, candidiasis of the tissues of the mouth.

thulium (Tm), a rare earth metallic element. Its atomic number is 69 and its atomic weight is 168.93.

thumb, the first and shortest digit of the hand, classified by some anatomists as one of the fingers because its metacarpal bone ossifies in the same manner as those of the phalanges. Other anatomists classify the thumb separately, regarding it as composed of one metacarpal bone and only two phalanges.

thumb forceps, a surgical instrument used to grasp soft tissue, especially while suturing.

thumbsucking, the habit of sucking the thumb for oral gratification. It is normal in infants and young children as a pleasure-seeking or comforting device, especially when the child is hungry or tired. The habit reaches its peak when the child is between 18 and 20 months of age, and it normally disappears as the child develops and matures.

thymic, of, or pertaining to, the thymus gland.

thymic hypoplasia, thymic parathyroid aplasia. See **DiGeorge's syndrome.**

thymol, a synthetic or natural thyme oil, used as an antibacterial and antifungal. It is an ingredient in some over-the-counter mouthwashes, gargles and cold preparations.

thymoma, *pl.* **thymomas, thymomata,** a usually benign tumour of the thymus gland that may be associated with myasthenia gravis or an immune deficiency disorder.

thymosin, 1. a naturally occurring immunological hormone secreted by the thymus gland. It is present in greatest amounts in young children and decreases in amount throughout life. **2.** an investigational drug derived from bovine thymus extracts and used as an immunomodulator.

thymus, *pl.* **thymuses, thymi,** a single unpaired gland located in the mediastinum. It extends superiorly into the neck to the lower edge of the thyroid gland and inferiorly as far as the fourth costal cartilage. The thymus is the primary central gland of the lymphatic system. T cells of the cell-mediated immune response develop in this gland before migrating to the lymph nodes and spleen. The gland consists of two lateral lobes closely bound by connective tissue, which also encloses the entire organ in a capsule. Compare **spleen.**

thyrocalcitonin. See **calcitonin.**

thyrocervical trunk, one of a pair of short, thick arterial branches, arising from the first portion of the subclavian arteries, close to the medial border of the scalenus anterior. It supplies numerous muscles and bones in the head, neck and back.

thyroid acropathy, swelling of subcutaneous tissue of the extremities and clubbing of the digits, occurring rarely in patients with thyroid disease and usually associated with pretibial myxoedema or exophthalmos.

thyroid cancer, a tumour of the thyroid gland. The first sign of cancer may be an increase in size of the thyroid gland, a palpable nodule, hoarseness, dysphagia, dyspnoea or pain on pressure. Diagnostic measures include x-ray examination, transillumination of the gland, radioisotope scanning, needle biopsy and ultrasound examination. More than half of thyroid malignancies are papillary carcinomas, about one-third are follicular carcinomas, and the rest consist of rapidly growing invasive anaplastic carcinomas, medullary carcinomas that secrete calcitonin, and metastatic lesions from primary tumours in the breast, kidneys or lungs.

thyroid cartilage, the largest cartilage of the larynx, consisting of two laminae fused together at an acute angle in the middle line of the neck to form the Adam's apple. Compare **cricoid.**

thyroid dermoid cyst, a tumour derived from embryonal tissues, believed to have developed in the thyroid gland or thyrolingual duct.

thyroid function test, any of several laboratory tests performed to evaluate the function of the thyroid gland. Thyroid function tests include protein-bound iodine, butanol-extractable iodine, T3, T4, free thyroxine index, thyroxin-binding globulin, thyroid stimulating hormone, long-acting thyroid stimulator, radioactive iodine uptake and radioactive iodine excretion.

thyroid gland, a highly vascular organ at the front of the neck, usually weighing about 30 g, consisting of bilateral lobes connected in the middle by a narrow isthmus. The thyroid gland secretes the hormone thyroxin directly into the blood and is part of the endocrine system of ductless glands. It is essential to normal body growth in infancy and childhood. Its removal greatly reduces the oxidative processes of the body, producing a lower metabolic rate that is characteristic of hypothyroidism.

thyroid hormone, an iodine-containing compound secreted by the thyroid gland, predominantly as thyroxine (T4) and in smaller amounts as four times more potent triiodothyronine (T3). These hormones increase the rate of metabolism, affect body temperature, regulate protein, fat and carbohydrate catabolism in all cells, maintain growth hormone secretion, skeletal maturation, cardiac rate, force and output, promote CNS development, stimulate the synthesis of many enzymes, and are necessary for muscle tone and vigour. Derivatives of thyronine, T4 and T3, are synthesized in the thyroid gland by a complex process involving the uptake, oxidation and incorporation of iodide and production of thyroglobulin, the form in which the hormones are apparently stored in thyroid follicular colloid.

thyroid releasing hormone. See **thyrotrophin releasing hormone.**

thyroid stimulating hormone (TSH), a substance, secreted by the anterior lobe of the pituitary gland, that controls the release of thyroid hormone. It is necessary for the growth and function of the thyroid gland, and its secretion is regulated by thyrotrophin releasing factor elaborated in the median eminence of the hypothalamus.

thyroid storm, a crisis in uncontrolled hyperthyroidism, caused by the release into the bloodstream of increased amounts of thyroid hormones. The storm may occur spontaneously, or it may be precipitated by infection, stress or a thyroidectomy performed on a patient who is inadequately prepared with antithyroid drugs. Characteristic signs are fever that may reach 41° C (106° F), a rapid pulse, acute respiratory distress, apprehension, restlessness, irritability and prostration. The patient may become delirious, lapse into a coma and die of heart failure.

thyroid. See **thyroid gland, thyroid hormone.**

thyroidectomy, the surgical removal of the thyroid gland, performed for colloid goitre, tumours or hyperthyroidism that does not respond to iodine therapy and antithyroid drugs. The whole of the gland, except for 5-10%, is removed; regrowth usually begins shortly after surgery, and thyroid function may return to normal. For cancer of the thyroid, the entire gland is removed along with surrounding structures from neck to collarbone, in a radical neck dissection.

thyroiditis, inflammation of the thyroid gland. Acute thyroiditis, caused by staphylococcal, streptococcal or other infections, is characterized by suppuration and abscess formation and may progress to subacute diffuse disease of the gland. Subacute thyroiditis is marked by fever, weakness, sore throat and a painfully enlarged gland that contains granulomas composed of colloid masses surrounded by giant cells and mononuclear cells. Chronic lymphocytic thyroiditis (Hashimoto's disease), characterized by lymphocyte and plasma cell infiltration of the gland and diffuse enlargement, seems to be transmitted as a dominant trait and may be associated with various autoimmune disorders. Another chronic form of thyroiditis is Riedel's struma, a rare progressive fibrosis usually of one lobe of the gland, but sometimes involving both lobes, the trachea and surrounding muscles, nerves and blood vessels. Radiation thyroiditis occasionally occurs 7 to 10 days after treatment of hyperthyroidism with radioactive iodine [131]I.

thyronine. See **thyroid hormone.**

thyrotoxicosis. See **Graves' disease.**

thyrotrophin, See **thyroid stimulating hormone.**

thyrotrophin releasing hormone, a substance elaborated in the median eminence of the hypothalamus; it stimulates the release of thyrotrophin (thyroid stimulating hormone) from the anterior pituitary gland.

thyroxine (T4), a hormone of the thyroid gland, derived from tyrosine, that influences metabolic rate.

thyroxine-binding globulin, a plasma protein that binds with and transports thyroxine in the blood.

TI, abbreviation for *therapeutic index.*

Ti, symbol for **titanium.**

TIA, abbreviation for **transient ischaemic attack.**

tibia, the second longest bone of the skeleton, located at the medial side of the leg. It articulates with the fibula laterally, the talus distally and the femur proximally, forming part of the knee joint.

tibial torsion, a lateral or medial twisting rotation of the tibia on its longitudinal axis.

tibialis anterior, one of the anterior crural muscles of the leg, situated on the lateral side of the tibia. It dorsiflexes and supinates the foot.

tic douloureux. See **trigeminal neuralgia.**

tic. See **mimic spasm.**

ticarcillin, an injectable penicillin antibiotic used in the treatment of serious bacterial infections.

tick bite, a puncture wound produced by the toothed beak of a bloodsucking tick which is a small, tough-skinned arachnid. Ticks transmit several diseases to humans, and a few species carry a neurotoxin in their saliva that may cause ascending paralysis beginning in the legs. Nervousness, loss of appetite, tingling and headache may occur, followed by muscle pain and, in extreme cases, respiratory failure.

tick fever. See **relapsing fever.**

tick paralysis, a rare, progressive, reversible disorder caused by several species of ticks that release a neurotoxin that causes weakness, incoordination and paralysis. The tick must feed on the host for several days before the symptoms appear.

tidal drainage. See **drainage.**

tidal volume (TV), the amount of air inhaled and exhaled during normal ventilation. Inspiratory reserve volume, expiratory reserve volume and tidal volume make up vital capacity.

tide, a variation, increase or decrease, in the concentration of a particular component of body fluids, such as acid tide, fat tide. **tidal,** *adj.*

tidemark, a transitional zone, appearing as a wavy line, that marks the junction between calcified and uncalcified cartilage.

Tietze's syndrome, 1. a disorder characterized by non-suppurative swellings of one or more costal cartilages causing pain that may radiate to the neck, shoulder or arm, and mimic the pain of coronary artery disease.

2. albinism, except for normal eye pigment, accompanied by deaf mutism and hypoplasia of the eyebrows.

timed collection, the collection of a specimen, such as a urine or stool sample, for a specific period of time.

timolol maleate, a beta-adrenergic receptor blocking agent. It is used in eyedrops for reducing intraocular pressure in chronic open-angle, aphakic and secondary glaucoma. It is also used orally in the treatment of hypertension, to prevent myocardial infarction after a previous infarct, and in the prophylaxis of migraine.

tin (Sn), a whitish metallic element. Its atomic number is 50 and its atomic weight is 118.69. Tin oxide is used in dentistry as a polishing agent for teeth and in some restorative procedures.

tincture, a substance in a solution that is diluted with alcohol.

tine test, a tuberculin skin test in which a small disposable disk with multiple tines bearing tuberculin antigen is used to puncture the skin. Induration around the puncture site indicates previous exposure or active disease, requiring further testing.

tinea, a group of fungal skin diseases caused by dermatophytes of several kinds, characterized by itching, scaling and sometimes painful lesions. Tinea is a general term that refers to infections of various causes, which are seen on several sites; the specific type is usually designated by a modifying term.

tinea capitis, a contagious fungal disease characterized by circular bald patches ranging between 1 to 6 cm in diameter, with slight erythema, scaling and crusting. Also called **ringworm.**

tinea corporis, a superficial fungal infection of the non-hairy skin of the body, most prevalent in hot, humid climates and usually caused by species of *Trichophyton* or *Microsporum.*

tinea cruris, a superficial fungal infection of the groin, caused by species of *Trichophyton* or *Epidermophyton floccosum.* It is most common in the tropics and among males.

tinea pedis, a chronic superficial fungal infection of the foot, affecting especially the skin between the toes and the skin of the soles. It is common worldwide and is usually caused by *Trichophyton mentagrophytes, T. rubrum* and *Epidermophyton floccosum.*

tinea unguium, a superficial fungal infection of the nails, caused by various species of *Trichophyton* and occasionally by *Candida albicans.* It is more common on the toes than the fingers, and can cause complete crumbling and destruction of the nails.

tinea versicolor, a fungous infection of the skin characterized by finely desquamating, pale tan patches on the upper trunk and upper arms that may itch and fail to tan, caused by *Malassezia furfur.* The fungus fluoresces under Wood's light and may be easily identified in scrapings viewed under a microscope.

Tinel's sign {Jules Tinel, French neurosurgeon, b. 1879}, an indication of irritability of a nerve, resulting in a distal tingling sensation on percussion of a damaged nerve.

tingling, a prickly sensation in the skin or a part of the body, accompanied by diminished sensitivity to stimulation of the sensory nerves. It is felt as the area is numbed by local anaesthetic, or by exposure to the cold, or as it numbs from pressure on a nerve.

tinnitus, tinkling or ringing heard in one or both ears. It may be a sign of acoustic trauma, Ménière's disease, otosclerosis, presbycusis, or an accumulation of cerumen impinging on the eardrum or occluding the external auditory canal.

tinted denture base, a denture base that simulates the colouring of natural oral tissue.

tip pinch, a grasp in which the tip of the thumb is pressed against any or each of the tips of the other fingers.

tip seal, the closure of an ampoule accomplished by melting a bead of glass at the neck of the ampule.

tissue, a collection of similar cells that act together in the performance of a particular function.

tissue activator. See **fibrinokinase.**

tissue dextrin. See **glycogen.**

tissue fixation, a process in which a tissue specimen is placed in a fluid that preserves the cells as nearly as is possible in their natural state.

tissue fixative, a fluid that preserves cells in their natural state, so that they may be identified and examined.

tissue integrity, impaired, damage to mucous membrane, corneal, integumentary or subcutaneous tissue. The major characteristic is damaged or destroyed tissue. Related factors are altered circulation, nutritional deficit or excess, knowledge deficit and impaired physical mobility.

tissue kinase. See **fibrinokinase.**

tissue perfusion, altered (renal, cerebral, cardiopulmonary, gastrointestinal, peripheral), a state in which an individual experiences a decrease in nutrition and oxygenation at cellular level, due to a deficit in capillary blood supply. Characteristics include coldness of the affected extremity, paleness on elevation of the extremity, diminished arterial pulses, and changes in the arterial blood pressure when measured in the affected extremity. Claudication, gangrene, brittle nails, slowly healing ulcers or wounds, shiny skin and absence of hair are also commonly seen.

tissue plasminogen activator (TPA), a clot-dissolving substance produced naturally by cells in the walls of blood vessels. TPA activates plasminogen to dissolve clots, and has been used therapeutically to remove blood clots that block coronary arteries.

tissue response, any reaction or change in living cellular tissue when it is acted on by disease, toxin or other external stimulus. Some kinds of tissue responses are **immune response, inflammation and necrosis.**

tissue typing, a systematized series of tests to evaluate the intraspecies compatibility of tissues of a donor and a recipient prior to transplantation.

tissue-base relationship, (in dentistry) the relationship of the base of a removable prosthesis to subjacent structures.

titanium (Ti), a greyish, brittle metallic element. Its atomic number is 22 and its atomic weight is 47.9. An alloy of titanium is used in the manufacture of orthopaedic prostheses.

titre, 1. a measurement of concentration of a substance in a solution. **2.** the quantity of a substance required to produce a reaction with another substance. **3.** the smallest amount of a certain substance that indicates the presence of a colon bacillus under standard conditions. **4.** the highest dilution of a serum that causes clumping of bacteria.

titubation, unsteady posture characterized by a staggering or stumbling gait and a swaying head or trunk while sitting. It may be a manifestation of cerebellar disease.

Tl, symbol for **thallium.**

TLC, abbreviation for **total lung capacity.**

TLI, abbreviation for **total lymphoid irradiation.**

Tm, symbol for **thulium.**

TMJ, abbreviation for **temporomandibular joint.**

TMP/SMX, abbreviation for **trimethoprim/ sulphamethoxazole.** See **co-trimoxazole.**

TNM, a system for staging malignant disease.

toadstool poisoning, a toxic condition caused by ingestion of certain varieties of poisonous mushrooms.

tobacco, a plant whose leaves are dried and used for smoking and chewing, and in snuff.

tobacco withdrawal syndrome, a change in mood or performance associated with the cessation or reduction in exposure to nicotine. Symptoms may range from lack of concentration to anxiety and temper outbursts.

TOBEC, abbreviation for total body electrical conductivity.

tobramycin sulphate, an aminoglycoside antibiotic used in the treatment of external ocular infection and serious systemic bacterial infections.

Tobruk plaster, a plaster cast splint with tapes for skin traction coming through openings in the plaster and connected with Thomas' splint. It covers and immobilizes the leg from foot to groin.

tocainide hydrochloride, an oral, lignocaine-type antiarrhythmic drug, used for the suppression of symptomatic ventricular arrhythmias.

tocodynamometer, an electronic device for monitoring and recording uterine contractions in labour. It consists of a pressure transducer applied to the fundus of the uterus by means of a belt, which is connected to a machine that records the contractions on graph paper. Also spelt **tokodynamometer.**

tocolytic drug, any drug used to suppress premature labour.

tocopherol. See **vitamin E.**

tocotransducer, an electronic device used to measure uterine contractions.

toddler, a child between 12 and 36 months of age. During this period of development, the child acquires a sense of autonomy and independence through the mastery of various specialized tasks, such as control of bodily functions, refinement of motor and language skills, and acquisition of socially acceptable behaviour.

toe, any one of the digits of the feet.

toeing in. See **metatarsus varus.**

toeing out. See **metatarsus valgus.**

toenail, one of the ungual structures covering the terminal phalanges of the toes.

togaviruses, a family of arboviruses that includes the organisms causing encephalitis, dengue, yellow fever and rubella.

toilet training, the process of teaching a child to control the functions of the bladder and bowel. Training often begins between 18 and 24 months of age, when voluntary control of the anal and urethral sphincters is achieved by most children. Night time bladder control may not be achieved until the child is 4 or 5 years of age or older.

tokodynamometer. See **tocodynamometer.**

tolazamide, an oral sulphonylurea anti-diabetic used in the treatment of non-insulin-dependent diabetes mellitus.

tolbutamide, an oral sulphonylurea anti-diabetic used in the treatment of non-insulin-dependent diabetes mellitus.

tolerance, the ability to endure hardship, pain or ordinarily injurious substances, such as drugs, without apparent physiological or psychological injury. A kind of tolerance is work tolerance.

tolerance dose, (in radiobiology) the maximum radiation dose that can be absorbed by a specific organ or tissue without causing long-term damage.

tolmetin sodium, a non-steroidal anti-inflammatory agent used in the treatment of rheumatoid arthritis, juvenile rheumatoid arthritis, osteoarthritis and other musculoskeletal disorders.

tolnaftate, an antifungal used in the treatment of superficial fungal infections of the skin, including tinea pedis, tinea cruris and tinea versicolor.

tomographic DSA, the visualization of blood vessels in the body in three dimensions.

tomography, an x-ray technique that produces a film representing a detailed cross-section of tissue structure at a predetermined depth. It is a valuable diagnostic tool for the discovery and identification of space-occupying lesions, as might be found in the brain, liver, pancreas and gallbladder.

tone. See **tonus.**

tongue, the principal organ of the sense of taste that also assists in the mastication and deglutition of food. It is located in the floor of the mouth within the curve of the mandible. Its root is connected to the hyoid bone posteriorly by the hypoglossi and genioglossi muscles. The use of the tongue as an organ of speech is not anatomical but a secondary acquired characteristic.

tongue-thrust swallow, an immature form of swallowing in which the tongue is projected forward instead of being retracted during the act of swallowing. It may result in forward displacement of the maxilla, with consequent malocclusion of teeth.

tongue-tie. See **ankyloglossia.**

tonic, pertaining to a type of afferent or sensory nerve receptor that responds to length changes placed on the non-contractile portion of a muscle spindle. It may be triggered by a mechanical external force such as positioning, or an internal stretch caused by intrafusal muscle contraction.

tonic labyrinthine reflex, a normal postural reflex in animals, abnormally accentuated in decerebrate humans. It is characterized by extension of all four limbs when the head is positioned in space at an angle above the horizontal in quadrupeds or in the neutral, erect position in humans.

tonic neck reflex, a normal response in newborns to extend the arm and leg on the side of the body to which the head is quickly turned while the infant is supine, and to flex the limbs of the opposite side.

tonicity, the quality of possessing tone, or tonus.

tonification, to build up energy, especially for individuals that are weak and exhausted, and for those suffering from chronic illnesses.

tonofibril, a bundle of fine filaments found in the cytoplasm of epithelial cells. The individual strands, or **tonofilaments,** spread throughout the cytoplasm and extend into the intercellular bridge to converge at the desmosome. In keratinizing epithelium, the strands are the main precursor of keratin.

tonometer, an instrument used in measuring tension or pressure, especially intraocular pressure.

tonometry, the measuring of intraocular pressure by determining the resistance of the eyeball to indentation by an applied force. The air-puff tonometer, which does not touch the eye, records deflections of the cornea from a puff of pressurized air. The Schiötz impression and applanation tonometers record the pressure required to indent or flatten the corneal surface.

tonsil, a small rounded mass of tissue, especially lymphoid tissue, such as that comprising the palatine tonsils in the oropharynx.

tonsillectomy, the surgical excision of the palatine tonsils, performed to prevent recurrent streptococcal tonsillitis. Tonsillectomy is often combined with adenoidectomy.

tonsillitis, an infection or inflammation of a tonsil. Acute tonsillitis, frequently caused by streptococcus infection, is characterized by severe sore throat, fever, headache, malaise, difficulty in swallowing, earache and enlarged, tender lymph nodes in the neck. Acute tonsillitis may accompany scarlet fever.

tonus, 1. the normal state of balanced tension in the tissues of the body, especially the muscles. Partial contraction or alternate contraction and relaxation of neighbouring fibres of a group of muscles hold the organ or part of the body in a neutral, functional position without fatigue. **2.** the state of tissues of the body being strong and fit.

tooth, *pl.* **teeth,** one of numerous dental structures that develop in the jaws as part of the digestive system and are used to cut, grind and process food in the mouth for ingestion. Each tooth consists of a crown which projects above the gum; two to four roots embedded in the alveolus; and a neck which stretches between the crown and root. Each tooth also contains a cavity filled with pulp, richly supplied with blood vessels and nerves that enter the cavity through a small aperture at the base of each root. The solid portion of the tooth consists of dentine, enamel and a thin layer of bone on the surface of the root. The dentine comprises the bulk of the tooth. Enamel covers the exposed portion of the crown. Two sets of teeth appear at different periods of life: the 20 deciduous teeth appear during infancy; the 32 permanent teeth appear during childhood and early adulthood.

tooth alignment, the arrangement of teeth in relation to their supporting bone or alveolar process, adjacent teeth and opposing dentitions.

tooth form, the identifying curves, lines, angles and contours of a tooth that differentiate it from other teeth.

tooth fulcrum, axis of movement of a tooth subjected to lateral forces, considered to be at the middle third of the portion of the tooth root embedded in the alveolus.

tooth germ, a primitive cell in the embryo that is the precursor of a tooth.

tooth inclination, the angle of slope of a tooth or teeth from the vertical plane, such as mesially, distally, lingually, buccally or labially inclined.

tooth-borne, describing a dental prosthesis or part of a prosthesis that depends entirely on abutment teeth for support.

tooth-borne base, a denture base restoring an edentulous area that has abutment teeth at each end for support.

toothbrush, an implement with bristles fixed to a head at the end of a handle, used for brushing and cleaning the teeth and gingivae and massaging the gingival tissues. It is the most effective implement for removing bacterial plaque.

tophaceous, pertaining to the presence of tophi.

tophus, *pl.* **tophi,** a calculus containing sodium urate deposits; it develops in periarticular fibrous tissue, typically in patients with gout.

topical, 1. of, or pertaining to, the surface of a part of the body. **2.** of, or pertaining to, a drug or treatment applied topically.

topical anaesthesia, surface analgesia produced by application of a topical anaesthetic in the form of a solution, gel or ointment to the skin, mucous membrane or cornea.

topognosis, the ability to recognize tactile stimuli.

topographic, figurative use of a word pertaining to a Freudian conceptualization of the layers of human consciousness.

topographic disorientation, a form of disorientation based on Freud's topographic model of the mental apparatus. It consists of conscious, preconscious and unconscious sytems for interpreting perceptions of the outside world and internal perceptions.

TORCH, an abbreviation for toxoplasmosis, other, rubella virus, cytomegalovirus and herpes simplex viruses; they are a group of agents that can infect the fetus or newborn infant, causing a constellation of morbid effects called the TORCH syndrome.

TORCH syndrome, infection of the fetus or newborn by one of the TORCH agents. The outcome of a pregnancy complicated by a TORCH agent may be abortion or stillbirth, intrauterine growth retardation or premature delivery. At delivery and during the first days after birth, an infant infected with any one of the organisms may demonstrate various clinical manifestations such as fever, lethargy, poor feeding, petechiae on the skin, purpura, pneumonia, hepatosplenomegaly, jaundice, haemolytic and other anaemias, encephalitis, microcephaly, hydrocephalus, intracranial calcifications, hearing deficits, chorioretinitis and microphthalmia.

Torkildsen's procedure. See **ventriculocisternostomy.**

torque, 1. a twisting force produced by contraction of the medial femoral muscles that tend to rotate the thigh medially. **2.** (in dentistry) a force applied to a tooth to rotate it on a mesiodistal or buccolingual axis. **3.** a rotary force applied to a denture base.

torr {Evangelista Torricelli, Italian physicist, b. 1608}, a unit of pressure equal to 1333.22 dynes/cm², or 1.33322 millibars. One torr is the pressure required to support a column of mercury 1 mm high when the mercury is of standard density and subjected to standard acceleration.

torsades de pointes, a type of ventricular tachycardia with a spiral-like appearance ("twisting of the points") and complexes that at first look positive and then negative on electrocardiography. It is precipitated by a long Q-T interval, which is often drug-induced but may also be the result of hypokalaemia or profound bradycardia.

torsion, 1. the process of twisting in a positive (clockwise) or negative (counter-clockwise) direction. **2.** the state of being turned. **3.** (in dentistry) the twisting of a tooth on its long axis.

torsion dystonia. See **dystonia musculorum deformans.**

torsion fracture, a spiral fracture, usually caused by a torsion injury.

torsion of the testis, the axial rotation of the spermatic cord that cuts off blood supply to the testicle, epididymis and other structures. Complete ischaemia for 6 hours may result in gangrene of the testis. Partial loss of circulation may result in atrophy.

torsion spasm. See **dystonia musculorum deformans.**

torticollis, an abnormal condition in which the head is inclined to one side as a result of contraction of the muscles on that side of the neck. It may be congenital or acquired.

Torula histolytica. See *Cryptococcus neoformans.*

torulopsosis, an infection with the yeast *Torulopsis glabrata,* a normal inhabitant of the oropharynx, GI tract and skin. It causes disease in severely debilitated patients or those with impaired immune function.

torulosis. See **cryptococcosis.**

torus fracture. See **lead pipe fracture.**

total anomalous venous return, a rare congenital cardiac anomaly in which the pulmonary veins attach directly to the right atrium or to various veins draining into the right atrium, rather than directing flow to the left atrium. Clinical manifestations include cyanosis, pulmonary congestion and heart failure.

total body electrical conductivity (TOB-EC), a method of measuring body composition by the differences in electrical conductivity of fat, bone and muscle. It is used in clinical studies of weight control in which physicians want to determine whether weight loss is due to fat, water or other tissues.

total body irradiation (TBI), a technique in external beam radiotherapy, to expose the whole body to a uniform prescribed dose of radiation. It may be used to induce immunosuppression and treat certain lymphomas, and is followed by a bone marrow transplant.

total body water (TBW), the amount of water contained within the body, including intracellular and extracellular water plus water in the GI and urinary tracts.

total cleavage, mitotic division of the fertilized ovum into blastomeres.

total iron, the total iron concentration in the blood. The normal concentrations in serum are 50 to 150 µg/dl.

total joint replacement, a surgical procedure for the treatment of severe arthritis and other disorders, in which the normal articulating surfaces are replaced by metal and plastic prostheses. The operation most commonly involves replacement of the hip joint with a metallic femur head and a plastic-coated metal acetabulum.

total lung capacity (TLC), the volume of gas in the lungs at the end of a maximum inspiration. It equals vital capacity plus residual capacity.

total lymphoid irradiation (TLI). See **total body irradiation.**

total macroglobulins, the heavy serum macroglobulins that are elevated in various diseases, such as cancer and infections.

total nitrogen, the nitrogen content of faeces, measured to detect various disorders such as pancreatic insufficiency and impaired protein digestion. The normal amount in a 24-hour faecal specimen is 10% of intake, or 1-2 g.

total parenteral nutrition (TPN), administration of a nutritionally adequate hypertonic solution consisting of glucose, protein hydrolysates, minerals and vitamins, through an indwelling catheter into the superior vena cava. The procedure is used in prolonged coma, severe uncontrolled malabsorption, extensive burns, GI fistulas and other conditions in which feeding by mouth cannot provide adequate amounts of essential nutrients.

total peripheral resistance, the maximum degree of resistance to blood flow caused by constriction of systemic blood vessels.

total renal blood flow (TRBF), the total volume of blood that flows into the renal arteries. The average TRBF in a normal adult is 1200 ml per minute.

touch, 1. the ability to feel objects and distinguish their various characteristics; the tactile sense. **2.** the ability to perceive pressure when it is exerted on the skin or body mucosa. **3.** to palpate or examine with the hand, such as digital examination of the abdomen, rectum or vagina.

touch deprivation, a lack of tactile stimulation, especially in early infancy, which if continued for a sufficient length of time may lead to serious developmental and emotional disturbances, such as stunted growth, personality disorders and social regression. See also **hospitalism.**

Tourette's syndrome. See **Gilles de la Tourette's syndrome.**

tourniquet, a device used in controlling haemorrhage, consisting of a wide constricting band applied to the limb proximal to the site of bleeding. The use of a tourniquet is a drastic measure and should be employed only if the haemorrhage is life-threatening and other safer measures have proved ineffective.

tourniquet infusion method, a technique of intra-arterial regional chemotherapy used in the treatment of osteogenic sarcoma. The technique uses one or two external tourniquets, depending on the location of the tumour, which slow or interrupt the blood flow to a limb temporarily while a cytotoxic drug, such as adriamycin, is infused into the area.

tourniquet test, a test of capillary fragility in which a blood pressure cuff is applied for 5 minutes to a person's arm, and is inflated to a pressure halfway between the diastolic and systolic blood pressure. The number of petechiae within a circumscribed area of the skin may be counted.

tower head, tower skull. See **oxycephaly.**

toxaemia, the presence of bacterial toxins in the bloodstream. **toxaemic,** *adj.*

toxic, 1. of, or pertaining to, a poison. **2.** (of a disease or condition) severe and progressive.

toxic amblyopia, partial loss of vision because of retro-optic bulbar neuritis, caused by poisoning with quinine, lead, wood alcohol, nicotine, arsenic or other poisons.

toxic dementia, dementia resulting from excessive use of, or exposure to, a poisonous substance.

toxic dose (TD), (in toxicology) the amount of a substance that may be expected to produce a toxic effect.

toxic epidermal necrolysis (TEN), a rare skin disease, characterized by epidermal erythema, superficial necrosis and skin erosions. This condition makes the skin appear scalded, often leaving scars. TEN may result from toxic or hypersensitive reactions. It is commonly associated with drug reactions, and has also been associated with airborne toxins such as carbon monoxide. TEN may also indicate an immune response, or may be associated with severe physiological stress. Early signs of the condition include inflammation of the mucous membranes, fever, malaise, a burning sensation in the conjunctivae and pervasive tenderness of the skin. The first phase of TEN is manifested by diffuse erythema. The second phase involves vesiculation and blistering. The third phase is marked by extensive epidermal necrolysis and desquamation. As the disease progresses, large flaccid bullae develop and rupture, exposing wide areas of denuded skin. Tissue fluids and electrolytes are consequently lost, resulting in extensive systemic complications such as pulmonary oedema, bronchopneumonia, GI and oesophageal haemorrhage, sepsis, shock, renal failure and disseminated intravascular coagulation. These extreme conditions contribute to the high mortality associated with TEN.

toxic gastritis. See **corrosive gastritis.**

toxic goitre, enlargement of the thyroid gland associated with exophthalmia and systemic disease.

toxic haemoglobinuria. See **haemoglobinuria.**

toxic nodular goitre, an enlarged thyroid gland characterized by numerous discrete nodules and hypersecretion of thyroid hormones. Typical signs of thyrotoxicosis are usually present, such as nervousness, tremor, weakness, fatigue, weight loss and irritability, but exophthalmia is rare; anorexia is more common than hyperphagia, and cardiac arrhythmia or congestive heart failure may be a predominant manifestation.

toxic psychosis, psychosis that results from the effects of chemicals or drugs, including those produced by the body itself.

toxic shock syndrome (TSS), a severe, acute disease caused by infection with strains of *Staphylococcus aureus,* phage group I, that produces a unique toxin, enterotoxin F. It is most common in menstruating women using high-absorbency tampons, but has also been seen in newborn infants, children and men. The onset of the syndrome is characterized by sudden high fever, headache, sore throat with swelling of the mucous membranes, diarrhoea, nausea and erythroderma. Acute renal failure, abnormal liver function, confusion and refractory hypotension usually follow, and death may ensue.

toxicity, 1. the degree to which something is poisonous. **2.** a condition that results from exposure to a toxin or toxic amounts of a substance which, given in smaller amounts, does not cause adverse effects.

toxicokinetics, the passage through the body system of a toxic agent or its metabolites, usually in an action similar to that of pharmacokinetics.

toxicologist, a specialist in toxicology.

toxicology, the scientific study of poisons, their detection, effects and methods of treatment of the conditions they produce. **toxicological,** *adj.*

toxin, a poison, usually one produced by, or occurring in, a plant or micro-organism.

toxocariasis, infection with the larvae of

Toxocara canis, the common roundworm of dogs and cats. Ingestion of viable eggs, commonly found in soil, leads to the spread of tiny larvae throughout the body and results in respiratory symptoms, enlarged liver, skin rashes, eosinophilia and delayed ocular lesions. Children who eat dirt are particularly subject to this disease.

toxoid, a microbial toxin that has been treated with chemicals or heat so as to decrease its toxic effect, but which retains its antigenic power. It is given to produce immunity by stimulating the creation of antibodies which will react with the original toxin.

Toxoplasma, a genus of protozoa with only one known species, *Toxoplasma gondii;* it is an intracellular parasite of cats and other hosts that causes toxoplasmosis in humans.

toxoplasmosis, a common infection with the protozoan intracellular parasite *Toxoplasma gondii.* The congenital form is characterized by liver and brain involvement with cerebral calcification, convulsions, blindness, microcephaly or hydrocephaly and mental retardation. The acquired form is characterized by rash, lymphadenopathy, fever, malaise, CNS disorders, myocarditis and pneumonitis.

TPA, abbreviation for **tissue plasminogen activator.**

TPAL. See **parity.**

TPN, abbreviation for **total parenteral nutrition.**

trabecula carnea, any one of the irregular bands and bundles of muscle that project from the inner surfaces of the ventricles, except in the arterial cone of the right ventricle.

trabecula septomarginalis. See **moderator band.**

trabeculae, (in ophthalmology) the portion of the eye in front of the canal of Schlemm and within the angle created by the iris and cornea.

trabeculectomy, the surgical removal of a section of corneosclerial tissue to increase the outflow of aqueous humour in patients with severe glaucoma.

trabeculotomy, a surgical opening in an orbital trabecula to increase the outflow of aqueous humour.

trace element, an element essential to nutrition or physiological processes, found in such minute quantities that analysis yields a presence of virtually zero amounts.

trace gas, a gas or vapour that escapes into the atmosphere during an anaesthetic procedure.

tracer, 1. see radioisotope scan. A radioactive isotope, used in radionuclide imaging, to allow a biological process to be seen. Kinds of tracers include radioactive iodine (^{131}I) and radioactive carbon(^{14}C). **2.** a device that records graphically the outline or

movements of an object or part of the body. **3.** a dissecting instrument used to isolate vessels and nerves.   **trace,** *v.*

tracer depot method, (in nuclear medicine) a technique used to determine local skin or muscle blood flow, based on the rate at which a radioactive tracer deposited in a tissue is removed by diffusion into the capillaries and washed out by the local blood supply.

trachea, an almost cylindrical tube in the neck, composed of cartilage and membrane. It extends from the larynx at the level of the sixth cervical vertebra to the fifth thoracic vertebra, where it divides into two bronchi. The trachea conveys air to the lungs.   **tracheal,** *adj.*

tracheal breath sound, a normal breath sound heard in auscultation of the trachea. Inspiration and expiration are equally loud, the expiratory sound being heard during the greater part of expiration, whereas the inspiratory sound stops abruptly at the height of inspiration.

tracheitis, any inflammatory condition of the trachea. It may be acute or chronic, resulting from infection, allergy or physical irritation.

trachelodynia. See **cervicodynia.**

tracheobronchial tree (TBT), an anatomical complex that includes the trachea, bronchi and bronchial tubes. It conveys air to and from the lungs.

tracheobronchitis, inflammation of the trachea and bronchi; it is a common form of respiratory infection.

tracheobronchomegaly, an abnormally large upper airway, in which the trachea may be as wide as the spinal column.

tracheoesophageal fistula, a congenital malformation in which there is an abnormal tube-like passage between the trachea and oesophagus.

tracheoesophageal shunt, a surgical procedure enabling a patient who has had a laryngectomy to speak, by constructing a passageway between the trachea and oesophagus. The operation results in an ability to produce oesophageal speech with normal respiration as a source of air, without the need to belch to produce voice sounds.

tracheomalacia, an eroding of the trachea, usually caused by excessive pressure from a cuffed endotracheal tube.

tracheostomy, an opening through the neck into the trachea, through which an indwelling tube may be inserted. After tracheostomy, the patient's chest is auscultated for breath sounds indicative of pulmonary congestion; mucous membranes and fingertips are observed for cyanosis; and humidified oxygen is given via tent or directly into the tracheostomy tube. The patient is reassured that the tube is open and that air can pass through it. The tube is suctioned frequently to keep it free from tracheobronchial secretions using a suction catheter attached to a Y-connector. The patient is taught to cough so as to move secretions out of the bronchi. If the procedure is performed as an emergency, the tracheostomy is closed once normal breathing is restored. If the tracheostomy is permanent, as with a laryngectomy, the patient is taught self-care.

tracheotomy, an incision made into the trachea through the neck below the larynx, performed to gain access to the airway below a blockage with a foreign body, tumour or oedema of the glottis. The opening may be made as an emergency measure at an accident site.

trachoma, a chronic infectious disease of the eye caused by the bacterium *Chlamydia trachomatis*. It is characterized initially by inflammation, pain, photophobia and lacrimation. If untreated, follicles form on the upper eyelids and grow larger until the granulations invade the cornea, eventually causing blindness.

tracing, a graphic record of a physical event, such as an electrocardiograph tracing made by pens on a moving sheet of paper while recording the electric impulses of heart muscle contractions.

tract, 1. an elongate group of tissues and structures that function together as a pathway, such as the digestive tract or respiratory tract. **2.** (in neurology) the neuronal axons that are grouped together to form a pathway.

traction, 1. (in orthopaedics) the process of putting a limb, bone or group of muscles under tension by means of weights and pulleys, to align or immobilize the part or relieve pressure on it. **2.** the process of pulling a part of the body along, through or out of its socket or cavity, such as axis traction with obstetric forceps in delivering an infant. Kinds of traction include **Bryant's traction, Buck's extension traction, Russell traction, skeletal traction,** and **skin traction.**

traction frame, an orthopaedic apparatus that supports the pulleys, ropes and weights by which traction is applied to various parts of the body or various parts of the body are suspended. The main components of a traction frame are metal uprights that attach to the bed and support an overhead metal bar.

traction response, the response to traction applied to the spine. Alterations of certain signs and symptoms of a musculoskeletal disorder may be revealed by traction tests.

trademark, a word, symbol or device assigned to a product by its manufacturer and registered as a part of its identity.

tragus, *pl.* **tragi,** a projection of the cartilage of the auricle at the opening of the external auditory meatus.

trained reflex. See **conditioned response.**

training effect, a rehabilitation training effect for heart patients, that can be measured by changes in cardiac function.

trait, 1. a characteristic mode of behaviour or any mannerism or physical feature that distinguishes one individual or culture from another. **2.** any characteristic quality or condition that is genetically determined and inherited as a specific genotype.

trance, 1. a sleep-like state characterized by complete or partial suspension of consciousness and loss or diminution of motor activity. **2.** a dazed or bewildered condition; stupor. **3.** a state of detachment from one's immediate surroundings. Kinds of trances are **alcoholic trance, death trance, hypnotic trance, hysteric trance** and **induced trance.**

tranquillizer, a drug prescribed to calm anxious or agitated people, ideally without decreasing their consciousness. Major tranquillizers are generally used in the treatment of psychoses. Minor tranquillizers are used for the treatment of anxiety, irritability, tension or neurosis. Tranquillizers tend to induce drowsiness and have the potential for causing physical and psychological dependence.

transactional analysis (TA), a form of psychotherapy based on a theory that three different, coherent, organized egos exist throughout life, simultaneously in every person, representing the child, the adult and the parent. Interactions between people are transactions, originating from a person in one of the ego states, received by another person who may be in a complementary or a crossed ego state.

transaminase, an enzyme that catalyses the transfer of an amino group from an alpha-amino acid to an alpha-keto acid, with pyridoxal phosphate and pyridoxamine phosphate acting as coenzymes.

transcellular water, the portion of extracellular water enclosed by an epithelial membrane, whose volume and composition is determined by the cellular activity of that membrane.

transcendence, the rising above one's previously perceived limits or restrictions.

transcondylar fracture, a fracture that occurs transversally and distal to the epicondyles of any one of the long bones.

transconfiguration, 1. (in genetics) the presence of the dominant allele of one pair of genes and recessive allele of another pair on the same chromosome. **2.** the presence of at least one mutant gene and one wild-type gene of a pair of pseudoalleles on each chromosome of a homologous pair.

transcortical apraxia. See **ideomotor apraxia.**

transcortin, a diglobulin protein that binds a majority of cortisol in the plasma.

transcriptase, an enzyme that induces transcription.

transcription, (in molecular genetics) the process by which RNA is formed from a DNA template in the process of manufacturing a protein.

transcultural nursing, a field of nursing in which the nurse transcends ethnocentricity and practises nursing in other cultural environments.

transcutaneous, pertaining to a procedure that is performed through the skin.

transcutaneous electric nerve stimulation (TENS), a method of pain control by the application of electric impulses to the nerve endings through electrodes placed on the skin. The electric impulses generated are similar to those of the body, but different enough to block transmission of pain signals to the brain.

transcutaneous nerve stimulation. See transcutaneous electric nerve stimulation.

transcutaneous oxygen/carbon dioxide monitoring, a method of measuring the oxygen or carbon dioxide in the blood, by attaching electrodes to the skin. Oxygen is commonly measured through an oximeter, which contains heating coils to raise the skin temperature and increase blood flow at the surface. Transcutaneous carbon dioxide electrodes are similar to blood gas electrodes.

transdermal delivery system, a method of applying a drug to unbroken skin. The drug is absorbed continuously through the skin and enters the system.

transducer, 1. a device activated by some type of received energy that is then converted to a signal suitable for transmission, usually over electric circuits. 2. a device used in ultrasound to convert electric signals into sound waves and vice versa.

transduction, (in molecular genetics) a method of genetic recombination by which DNA is transferred from one cell to another by a viral vector.

transect, to sever or cut across, as in preparing a cross-section of tissue.

transfection, (in molecular genetics) the process by which a cell is infected with DNA or RNA isolated from a virus or a viral vector.

transfer DNA (tDNA), (in molecular genetics) DNA transferred from its original source and present in transformed cells.

transfer factor, a leukocyte extract that transfers delayed hypersensitivity from one person to another.

transfer factor of lungs. See diffusing capacity.

transfer RNA (tRNA), (in molecular genetics) a kind of RNA that transfers the genetic code from messenger RNA for the production of a specific amino acid. There are at least 20 different kinds of tRNA, each of which is able to combine covalently with a specific amino acid.

transferase, any of a group of enzymes that catalyses the transfer of a chemical group or radical, such as the phosphate, methyl, amine or keto groups, from one molecule to another.

transference, 1. the shifting of symptoms from one part of the body to another, as occurs in conversion disorder. 2. (in psychiatry) an unconscious defence mechanism whereby feelings and attitudes originally associated with important people and events in one's early life are attributed to others in current interpersonal situations. 3. (in psychoanalysis and psychotherapy) the feelings of a patient for the analyst to whom the patient has attributed or assigned the qualities, attitudes and feelings of a person or persons significant in his or her emotional development, usually a figure from childhood.

transferrin, a trace protein present in the blood; it is essential in the transport of iron.

transformation, (in molecular genetics) the process in which exogenous genes are integrated into chromosomes in a form that is recognized by the replicative and transcriptional apparatus of the host cell.

transforming growth factor (TGF), a protein or group of proteins produced by the cells of a tumour that, when inoculated into a normal cell culture, causes a disorderly and abnormal increase in the number of cells in the culture.

transfusion, the introduction into the bloodstream of whole blood or blood components, such as plasma, platelets or packed red cells. Whole blood may be infused into the recipient directly from a donor matched for the ABO blood group and antigenic subgroups, but more frequently the donor's blood is collected and stored by a blood bank.

transfusion reaction, a systemic response by the body to the administration of blood incompatible with that of the recipient. The causes include red cell incompatibility, allergic sensitivity to leukocytes, platelets or plasma protein components of the transfused blood, or to the potassium or citrate preservative in the banked blood. Fever is the most common transfusion reaction; urticaria is a relatively common allergic response. Asthma, vascular collapse and renal failure occur less commonly. A haemolytic reaction from red cell incompatibility is serious and must be diagnosed and treated promptly. Symptoms develop shortly after beginning the transfusion, before 50 ml have been given, and include a throbbing headache, sudden, deep and severe lumbar pain, precordial pain, dyspnoea and restlessness. Objective signs include ruddy facial flushing followed by cyanosis and distended neck veins, rapid, thready pulse, diaphoresis and cold, clammy skin. Profound shock may occur within 1 hour.

transient, pertaining to a condition that is temporary, such as transient ischaemic attack.

transient ischaemic attack (TIA), an episode of cerebrovascular insufficiency, usually associated with a partial occlusion of an artery by an atherosclerotic plaque or embolism. Disturbance of normal vision in one or in both eyes, dizziness, weakness, dysphasia, numbness or unconsciousness may occur. The attack is usually brief, lasting a few minutes; rarely, symptoms continue for several hours.

transillumination, 1. the passage of light through a solid or liquid substance. 2. the passage of light through body tissues for the purpose of examining a structure interposed between the observer and the light source.

transition, the last phase of the first stage of labour.

transitional cell carcinoma, a malignant, usually papillary tumour derived from transitional stratified epithelium, occurring most frequently in the bladder, ureter, urethra or renal pelvis. The majority of tumours in the collecting system of the kidney are of this kind.

transitional dentition. See **mixed dentition.**

transitional object, an object used by a child to provide comfort and security while he or she is away from a secure base, such as mother or home.

transitory mania, a mood disorder characterized by the sudden onset of manic reactions that are of short duration, usually lasting from 1 hour to a few days.

translation, (in molecular genetics) the process in which the genetic information carried by nucleotides in messenger RNA directs the amino acid sequence in the synthesis of a specific polypeptide.

translocation, (in genetics) the rearrangement of genetic material within the same chromosome, or the transfer of a segment of one chromosome to another non-homologous one. Kinds of translocations are **balanced translocation, reciprocal translocation** and **robertsonian translocation.**

transmission, the transfer or conveyance of something, or a condition, such as a neural impulse, infectious or genetic disease or a hereditary trait, from one person or place to another.   **transmissible,** *adj.*

transmission electron microscopy. See **electron microscopy.**

transmission scanning electron microscope, an instrument that transmits a highly magnified, well-resolved, three-dimensional image on a television screen, thus combining the advantages of the electron and scanning electron microscopes.

transmission scanning electron microscopy (TSEM), a technique using a transmission scanning electron microscope, in which the atomic number of the portion of the sample being scanned is determined and used to modulate a beam of electrons in a cathode-ray tube and in the beam scanning the sample.

transmitter substance. See **neurotransmitter.**

transmural, pertaining to the entire thickness of the wall of an organ, such as a transmural myocardial infarction.

transmural infarction, the death of myocardial tissue that extends from the endocardium to the epicardium as a result of a myocardial infarction.

transneuronal degeneration, degeneration of irreparably damaged nerve cells that may progress proximally or distally to involve neurons more than one synapse removed.

transplacental, across or through the placenta, specifically in reference to the exchange of nutrients, waste products and other material between the developing fetus and mother.

transplant, 1. to transfer an organ or tissue from one person to another, or from one body part to another, so as to replace a diseased structure, restore function or change appearance. Skin and kidneys are the most frequently transplanted structures; others include cartilage, bone, corneal tissue, portions of blood vessels and tendons, hearts and livers. Preferred donors are identical twins or persons having the same blood type and immunological characteristics. 2. any tissue or organ that is transplanted. 3. of, or pertaining to, a tissue or organ that is transplanted, a recipient of a donated tissue or organ, or a phenomenon associated with the procedure.

transposable element, (in molecular genetics) a DNA fragment or segment that can move or be moved from one site in the genome to another.

transposase, (in molecular genetics) an enzyme involved in the movement of a DNA fragment or segment from one site in the genome to another.

transposition, 1. an abnormality occurring during embryonic development in which a part of the body normally on the left is found on the right, or vice versa. 2. the shifting of genetic material from one chromosome to another at some point in the reproductive process.   **transpose,** *v.*

transposition of the great arteries, a developmental abnormality of the heart, in which the roots of the aorta and pulmonary artery do not bear their normal relationship to each other. There are several varieties of transposition of the great arteries. This abnormality is always associated with other structural abnormalities of the heart.

transposition of the great vessels. See **transposition of the great arteries.**

transposon, a gene or group of genes that are mobile and, like plasmids, act to transfer genetic instructions from one place to another. Transposons travel saddled on bacteriophages from one virus to another.

transpulmonary pressure, the difference between alveolar and intrapleural pressure, or the pressure acting across the lung from the intrapleural space to the alveoli.

transseptal fibre, (in dentistry) any one of the many fibres of the gingival fibre system that extends horizontally from the supra-alveolar cementum of a tooth, through the interdental attached gingiva above the septum of the alveolar bone, to the cementum of an adjacent tooth.

transsexual, a person whose gender identity is opposite his or her biological sex.

transtentorial herniation, a bulge of brain tissue out of the cranium through the tentorial notch, caused by increased intracranial pressure.

transudate, a fluid passed through a membrane or squeezed through a tissue or into the space between the cells of a tissue.

transudation, 1. the passage of a substance through a membrane as a result of a difference in hydrostatic pressure. **2.** the passage of a fluid through a membrane with nearly all the solutes of the fluid remaining in solution or suspension.

transudative ascites, an abnormal accumulation in the peritoneal cavity of a fluid that characteristically contains scant amounts of protein and cells.

transurethral resection (TUR), a surgical procedure through the urethra, as in transurethral prostatectomy.

transverse, at right angles to the long axis of any common part, such as the planes that cut the long axis of the body into upper and lower portions, and are at right angles to the sagittal and frontal planes.

transverse colon, the segment of colon that extends from the end of ascending colon at the hepatic flexure on the right side, across the mid-abdomen, to the beginning of the descending colon at the splenic flexure on the left side.

transverse fissure, a fissure dividing the dorsal surface of the diencephalon and the ventral surface of the cerebral hemisphere.

transverse fracture, a fracture that occurs at right angles to the longitudinal axis of the bone involved.

transverse lie, abnormal presentation of a fetus in which the long axis of the fetus is across the long axis of the mother's body.

transverse ligament of the atlas, a thick, strong ligament stretched across the ring of the atlas, holding the dens against the anterior arch.

transverse mesocolon, a broad fold of the peritoneum connecting the transverse colon to the dorsal wall of the abdomen.

transverse palatine suture, the line of junction between the processes of maxilla and horizontal portions of the palatine bones that form the hard palate.

transverse plane, any one of the planes that cut across the body perpendicular to the sagittal and frontal planes, dividing the body into caudal and cranial portions.

transverse relaxation time. See **relaxation time.**

transverse sinus, one of a pair of large venous channels in the posterior superior group of sinuses serving the dura mater.

transversus abdominis, one of a pair of transverse abdominal muscles that are the anterolateral muscles of the abdomen, lying immediately under the obliquus internus abdominis. It serves to constrict the abdomen and, by compressing the contents, to assist in micturition, defaecation, emesis, parturition and forced expiration.

transvestism, a tendency to achieve psychic and sexual relief by dressing in the clothing of the opposite sex.

tranylcypromine sulphate, a monoamine oxidase inhibitor antidepressant. It is used in the treatment of severe reactive or endogenous depression which has been unresponsive to less toxic treatments.

trapezium, *pl.* **trapeziums, trapezia,** a carpal bone in the distal row of carpal bones. The trapezium articulates with the scaphoid proximally, the first metacarpal distally, and the trapezoideum and second metacarpal medially.

trapezius, a large, flat, triangular muscle of the shoulder and upper back. It acts to rotate the scapula, raise the shoulder and abduct and flex the arm.

trapezoid bone, the smallest carpal bone, located in the distal row of carpal bones between the trapezium and capitate.

trapezoidal arch, a dental arch that has slightly less convergence than that of a tapering arch.

trauma, potential for, the accentuated risk of accidental tissue injury, such as a wound, burn or fracture. The risk factors may be internal (individual) or external (environmental). Internal risk factors include weakness, poor vision, balancing difficulties, reduced temperature or tactile sensation, reduced muscle or eye-hand coordination, lack of safety education, precautions or equipment, cognitive or emotional difficulties and history of previous trauma. External risk factors include slippery floors, stairs or passages, a bath without anti-slip equipment, unsteady chairs or ladders, defective electrical wires or appliances, obstructed paths, potential igniting gas leaks, unscreened fires or heaters, inadequately stored combustibles or corrosives, contact with intense cold or heat (including very hot water), overexposure to sun, sunlamps or radiotherapy, and exposure to dangerous machinery.

trauma, 1. physical injury caused by violent or disruptive action, or by the introduction into the body of a toxic substance. **2.** psychological injury resulting from a severe emotional shock. **traumatic,** *adj.,* **traumatize,** *v.*

traumatic anaesthesia, a total lack of normal sensation in a part of the body, resulting from injury, destruction of nerves or interruption of nerve pathways.

traumatic delirium, delirium following severe head injury, characterized by alertness and consciousness with disorientation, confabulation and amnesia apparent. See also **delirium.**

traumatic fever, an elevation in body temperature secondary to mechanic trauma, particularly a crushing injury. The increased body temperature may help provide resistance to subsequent infection, and increased wound temperature may accelerate local healing.

traumatic myositis, inflammation of the muscles resulting from a wound or other trauma.

traumatic neuroma, a tangled mass of nerve elements and fibrous tissue produced by the proliferation of Schwann cells and fibroblasts after severe injury to a nerve. A kind of traumatic neuroma is amputation neuroma.

traumatic occlusion, a closure of teeth that injures the teeth, periodontal tissues, residual ridge and other oral structures.

traumatopathy, a pathological condition resulting from a wound or injury. **traumatopathic,** *adj.*

traumatophilia, a psychological state in which the individual derives unconscious pleasure from injuries and surgical operations. **traumatophiliac,** *n.,* **traumatophilic,** *adj.*

traumatopnoea, partial asphyxia with collapse of the patient, caused by a penetrating thoracic wound permitting air to enter the pleural space and compress the lungs.

traumatopyra, an elevated temperature resulting from a wound or injury.

traumatropism, the tendency of damaged tissue to attract micro-organisms and promote their growth, frequently causing infections after injuries, especially burns.

travail, 1. physical or mental exertion, especially when distressful. **2.** (in obstetrics) the effort of labour and childbirth.

traveller's diarrhoea, any of several diarrhoeal disorders commonly seen in people visiting foreign parts of the world. Some strains of *Escherichia coli,* which produce a powerful exotoxin, are the common cause. Other causative organisms include *Giardia lamblia* and species of *Salmonella* and *Shigella.* Symptoms include abdominal cramps, nausea, vomiting, slight fever and watery stools.

TRBF, abbreviation for **total renal blood flow.**

Treacher Collins' syndrome, an inherited disorder characterized by mandibulofacial dysostosis.

treatment, 1. the care and management of a patient to combat, ameliorate or prevent a disease, disorder or injury. **2.** a method of combating, ameliorating or preventing a disease, disorder or injury. Active or curative treatment is designed to cure; palliative treatment is directed to relieve pain and distress; prophylactic treatment prevents a disease or disorder; causal treatment focuses on the cause of a disorder. Treatment may be pharmacological, using drugs; surgical, involving operative procedures; or supportive, building the patient's strength.

treatment room, a room in a hospital or health centre, in which various treatments or procedures requiring special equipment are performed, such as removing sutures.

treatment simulator, (in radiotherapy) diagnostic x-ray unit isocentrically mounted on a gantry to simulate the movements and other parameters of a radiotherapy megavoltage unit. Used to perform localisation and verification techniques.

Trechona, a genus of spiders, family *Dipluridae,* the bite of which is toxic and irritating to humans.

tree, (in anatomy) an anatomic structure with branches that spread out like those of a tree, such as the bronchial tree.

trematode, any species of flatworm of the class *Trematoda,* some of which are parasitic to humans, infecting the liver, lungs and intestines. Kinds of trematodes include the organisms causing **clonorchiasis, fascioliasis, paragonimiasis** and **schistosomiasis.**

tremor, rhythmic, purposeless, quivering movements resulting from the involuntary alternating contraction and relaxation of opposing groups of skeletal muscles. Tremors occur in some elderly individuals, in certain families, and in patients with various neurodegenerative disorders. Kinds of tremors are continuous tremor and intention tremor.

tremulous, pertaining to tremors or involuntary muscular contractions.

trench fever, a self-limited infection, caused by *Rochalimaea quintana,* a rickettsial organism transmitted by body lice. It is characterized by weakness, fever, rash and pain in the legs.

trench mouth. See **acute necrotizing gingivitis.**

Trendelenburg gait {Friederich Trendelenburg, German surgeon, b. 1844}, an abnormal gait associated with a weakness of the gluteus medius. It is characterized by a drop of the pelvis on the unaffected side of the body at the moment of heelstrike on the affected side.

Trendelenburg's operation, the ligation of varicose veins whose valves are ineffective, performed to remove weakened portions of veins and pockets in which thrombi might lodge. The saphenous vein is ligated at the groin, where it joins the femoral vein. A wire device, called a stripper, is threaded through the lumen of the vein from groin to ankle; the wire and vein are then pulled from the groin incision.

Trendelenburg's position, a position in which the head is low and the body and legs are on an inclined plane. It is sometimes used in pelvic surgery to displace the abdominal organs upwards, out of the pelvis, or to increase blood flow to the brain in hypotension and shock.

Trendelenburg's test, a simple test for incompetent valves in a person with varicose veins. The individual lies down and elevates the leg to empty the vein, then stands, and the vein is observed as it fills. If the valves are incompetent, the vein fills from above; if the valves are normal, they do not allow backflow of blood, and the vein fills from below.

trephine, a circular, saw-like instrument used in removing pieces of bone or tissue, usually from the skull. Also called **trepan.**

Treponema, a genus of spirochaetes, including some that are pathogenic to humans, such as the organisms causing bejel, pinta, syphilis and yaws.

Treponema pallidum, an actively motile, slender spirochaetal organism that causes syphilis.

treponematosis, *pl.* **treponematoses,** any disease caused by spirochaetes of the genus *Treponema.* All these infections are effectively treated with penicillin. Kinds of treponematoses are **bejel, pinta, syphilis** and **yaws.**

tretinoin, a keratolytic used in the topical treatment of acne vulgaris.

TRF, abbreviation for **thyrotrophin releasing factor.** See **thyrotrophin releasing hormone.**

triad, pertaining to a combination of three, such as two parents and a child.

triage, 1. (in military medicine) a classification of casualties of war and other disasters according to the gravity of injuries, urgency of treatment and place of treatment. **2.** a process in which a group of patients is sorted according to their need for care. **3.** (in disaster medicine) a process in which a large group of patients is sorted so that care can be concentrated on those who are likely to survive.

triamcinolone acetonide, triamcinolone hexacetonide, corticosteroids used topically and systemically as anti-inflammatory agents in the treatment of dermatoses, stomatitis, lichen planus lesions and arthritis.

triamterene, a potassium-sparing diuretic used alone or with another diuretic in the treatment of oedema, hypertension and congestive heart failure.

triangular bandage, a square of cloth folded or cut into the shape of a triangle. It may be used as a sling, a cover or a thick pad to control bleeding.

triangular bone, the pyramidal carpal bone in the proximal row on the ulnar side of the wrist.

tribavirin, an aerosol antiviral drug used in the treatment of respiratory synctial virus (RSV) infections of the lower respiratory tract in infants and small children.

TRIC, abbreviation for trachoma inclusion conjunctivitis agent, which refers to *Chlamydia trachomatis,* the organism that causes both inclusion conjunctivitis and trachoma. See also **Chlamydia.**

tricarboxylic acid cycle. See **Krebs citric acid cycle.**

triceps brachii, a large muscle that extends the entire length of the dorsal surface of the humerus. It functions to extend the forearm and adduct the arm.

triceps reflex, a deep tendon reflex elicited by tapping sharply the triceps tendon proximal to the elbow, with the forearm in a relaxed position.

triceps skinfold, the thickness of a fold of skin around the triceps muscle. It is measured primarily to estimate the amount of subcutaneous fat.

triceps surae limp, an abnormal action in the walking or gait cycle. It is associated with a deficiency in the elevating and propulsive factors on the affected side of the body, especially a deficiency of the triceps surae. Such a deficiency prevents the triceps surae from raising the pelvis and carrying it forward during the walking cycle.

trichiasis, an abnormal inversion of the eyelashes that irritates the eyeball. It usually follows infection or inflammation.

trichinosis, infestation with the parasitic roundworm *Trichinella spiralis,* transmitted by eating raw or undercooked pork or bear meat. Early symptoms of infection include abdominal pain, nausea, fever and diarrhoea; later, muscle pain, tenderness, fatigue and eosinophilia are observed. Light infections may be asymptomatic.

trichloroethylene, a general anaesthetic, administered by mask with N_2O, used in dentistry, minor surgery and the first stages of labour.

trichobasalioma hyalinicum. See **cylindroma** def. 2.

trichoepithelioma, *pl.* **trichoepitheliomas, trichoepitheliomata,** a cutaneous tumour derived from the basal cells of the follicles of fine body hair.

trichoid, resembling a hair.

trichologia, an abnormal condition in which a person pulls out his or her own hair, usually seen only in delirium.

trichomonacide, an agent destructive to *Trichomonas vaginalis,* a parasitic protozoan flagellate that causes vaginitis, cystitis and urethritis. **trichomonacidal,** *adj.*

Trichomonas vaginalis, a motile protozoan parasite that causes vaginitis marked by a copious malodorous discharge and pruritus.

trichomoniasis, a vaginal infection caused by the protozoan *Trichomonas vaginalis*; it is characterized by itching, burning and frothy, pale yellow to green, malodorous vaginal discharge. In men, infection is usually asymptomatic but may be evidenced by a persistent or recurrent urethritis.

trichophytic granuloma. See **Majocchi's granuloma.**

Trichophyton, a genus of fungi that infects skin, hair and nails. See also **dermatomycosis, dermatophyte.**

trichostrongyliasis, infestation with *Trichostrongylus,* a genus of nematode worm.

Trichostrongylus, a genus of roundworm, some species of which are parasitic to humans, such as *Trichostrongylus orientalis.*

trichotillomania, a morbid impulse or desire to pull out one's hair, frequently seen in cases of severe mental deficiency and delirium. Also called **trichomania, hair pulling.** See also **trichologia. trichotillomanic, trichomanic,** *adj.*

trichuriasis, infestation with the roundworm *Trichuris trichiura.* The condition is usually asymptomatic, but heavy infestation may cause nausea, abdominal pain, diarrhoea, and occasionally anaemia and rectal prolapse.

Trichuris, a genus of parasitic roundworms, of which the species *Trichuris trichiura* infects the intestinal tract.

tricrotic pulse, an abnormal pulse that has three peaks of elevation on a sphygmogram, representing the pressure wave from the heart in systole followed by two pressure waves in diastole.

tricuspid, 1. of, or pertaining to, three points or cusps. 2. of, or pertaining to, the tricuspid valve of the heart.

tricuspid atresia, a congenital cardiac anomaly characterized by the absence of the tricuspid valve so that there is no opening between the right atrium and right ventricle. Clinical manifestations include severe cyanosis, dyspnoea, anoxia and signs of right-sided heart failure. Definitive diagnosis is made by cardiac catheterization.

tricuspid stenosis, narrowing or stricture of the tricuspid value. It is relatively uncommon and usually associated with lesions of other values caused by rheumatic fever.

Clinical characteristics include diastolic pressure gradient between the right atrium and ventricle, jugular vein distention, pulmonary congestion and, in severe cases, hepatic congestion and splenomegaly.

tricuspid valve, a valve with three main cusps situated between the right atrium and right ventricle of the heart. As the right and left ventricles relax during the diastole phase of the heartbeat, the tricuspid valve opens, allowing blood to flow into the ventricle. In the systole phase of the heartbeat, both blood-filled ventricles contract, pumping out their contents, while the tricuspid and mitral valves close to prevent any backflow.

tricyclic antidepressant. See **antidepressant.**

tricyclic compound, a chemical substance containing three rings in its molecular structure, especially a tricyclic antidepressant drug used in the treatment of reactive or endogenous depression.

trientine hydrochloride, an orally administered copper chelating agent, used in the treatment of Wilson's disease. It is not available commercially in the UK.

trifacial nerve. See **trigeminal nerve.**

trifluoperazine hydrochloride, a phenothiazine tranquilliser used in the treatment of anxiety, schizophrenia and other psychotic disorders, and as an antiemetic.

trigeminal nerve, either of the largest pair of cranial nerves, essential for the act of chewing, general sensibility of the face, and muscular sensibility of the obliquus superior.

trigeminal neuralgia, a neurological condition of the trigeminal facial nerve, characterized by paroxysms of flashing, stab-like pain radiating along the course of a branch of the nerve from the angle of the jaw. It is caused by degeneration of the nerve or pressure on it. Any of the three branches of the nerve may be affected. Neuralgia of the first branch results in pain around the eyes and over the forehead; neuralgia of the second branch leads to pain in the upper lip, nose and cheek; and neuralgia of the third branch causes pain on the side of the tongue and lower lip. The momentary bursts of pain recur in clusters lasting many seconds; paroxysmal episodes of the pains may last for hours.

trigeminal pulse, an abnormal pulse in which every third beat is absent.

trigeminy, 1. a grouping in threes. 2. a cardiac arrhythmia characterized by the occurrence of three heartbeats, a normal beat followed by two ectopic beats in rapid succession. **trigeminal,** *adj.*

triggered activity, rhythmic cardiac activity that results when a series of afterdepolarizations reach threshold potential.

triglyceride, a compound consisting of a fatty acid (oleic, palmitic or stearic) and glycerol. Triglycerides make up most animal and vegetable fats and are the principal lipids in the blood where they circulate, bound to a protein, and form high- and low-density lipoproteins.

trigone, 1. a triangle. **2.** the first three dominant cusps, considered collectively, of an upper molar.

trigone of the bladder. See **trigonum vesicae.**

trigonitis, inflammation of the trigone of the bladder, which often accompanies urethritis.

trigonum vesicae, a triangular area of the bladder between the opening of ureters and orifice of the urethra. Also called **trigone of the bladder.**

trihybrid, (in genetics) pertaining to, or describing, an individual, organism or strain that is heterozygous for three specific traits, being the offspring of parents differing in three specific gene pairs.

trihybrid cross, (in genetics) the mating of two individuals, organisms or strains that have different gene pairs which determine three specific traits, or in which three particular characteristics or gene loci are being followed.

trihydric alcohol, an alcohol containing three hydroxyl groups.

triiodothyronine (T3), a hormone that helps regulate growth and development, control metabolism and body temperature and, by a negative feedback system, inhibit the secretion of thyrotrophin by the pituitary.

trilaminar blastoderm, the stage of embryonic development in which all three of the primary germ layers, the ectoderm, mesoderm and entoderm, have formed.

trilostane, a synthetic steroid that inhibits the synthesis of adrenal steroids. It is used for the treatment of Cushing's syndrome and primary hyperaldosteronism.

trimalleolar fracture. See **Cotton's fracture.**

trimeprazine tartrate, a sedating antipruritic antihistamine. It is used in the treatment of pruritus and hypersensitivity reactions of the skin, and as an anaesthetic premedication.

trimester, one of the three periods of approximately 3 months into which pregnancy is divided.

trimethaphan camsylate, a ganglionic blocking agent used to produce controlled hypotension during surgery.

trimethoprim, an antibacterial inhibitor of bacterial dihydrofolate. It is used in the treatment of various infections, particularly of the urinary tract, middle ear and bronchi.

trimethoprim and sulphamethoxazole. See **co-trimoxazole.**

trimethylene. See **cyclopropane.**

trimipramine maleate, a sedative tricyclic antidepressant used in the treatment of depression, especially when accompanied by anxiety.

triple point, a situation in which a given substance may exist in solid, liquid and vapour forms at the same time. Every substance has a theoretical triple point, which depends on ideal conditions of temperature and pressure.

triple response, a triad of phenomena that occur in sequence after the intradermal injection of histamine. First, a red spot develops, spreading outwards for a few millimetres, reaching its maximal size within 1 minute and then turning to a bluish colour. Next, a brighter red flush of colour spreads slowly in an irregular flare around the original red spot. Finally, a wheal filled with fluid forms over the original spot.

triple sugar iron reaction, any one of several reactions seen in certain bacterial cultures growing on triple sugar iron agar, a culture medium used to aid in the identification of *Escherichia coli, Proteus, Salmonella, Shigella* and other pathogenic enteric bacteria.

triple X syndrome. See **XXX syndrome.**

triple-dye treatment, a therapy for burns in which three dyes, 6% gentian violet, 1% brilliant green and 0.1% acriflavin base, are applied.

triplet, 1. any one of three offspring born of the same gestation period during a single pregnancy. **2.** (in genetics) the unit of three consecutive bases in one polynucleotide chain of DNA or RNA that codes for a specific amino acid.

triploid (3n), 1. also **triploidic.** Of, or pertaining to, an individual, organism, strain or cell that has three complete sets of chromosomes. In humans, the triploid number is 69, found in rare cases of aborted or stillborn fetuses. **2.** such an individual, organism, strain or cell.

triploidy, the state or condition of having three complete sets of chromosomes.

tripodial symmelia, a fetal anomaly characterized by the fusion of the lower extremities and the presence of three feet.

triprolidine hydrochloride, an antihistamine used in the treatment of a variety of allergic conditions, including rhinitis, skin rash and pruritus.

trismus, a prolonged tonic spasm of the muscles of the jaw.

trisomy, a chromosomal aberration characterized by the presence of one more than the normal number of chromosomes in a diploid complement. In humans, the trisomic cell contains 47 chromosomes and is designated $2n + 1$. **trisomic,** *adj.*

trisomy 13, a congenital condition caused by the presence of an extra chromosome in the D group, predominantly chromosome 13, although in rare instances chromosome 14 or 15 may be present. It is characterized by multiple midline anomalies and CNS defects, including holoprosencephaly, microcephaly, myelomeningocele, microphthalmos and cleft lip and palate. Other features include severe mental deficiency, polydactyly, deafness, convulsions and abnormalities of the heart, viscera and genitalia.

trisomy 18, a congenital condition caused by the presence of an extra chromosome 18, characterized by severe mental deficiency and multiple deformities. Among the most common defects are scaphocephaly or other skull abnormalities, micrognathia, abnormal facies with low-set malformed ears and prominent occiput, cleft lip and palate, clenched fists with overlapping fingers, especially the index over the third finger, clubfeet and syndactyly. Ventricular septal defect, patent ductus arteriosus, atrial septal defect and renal anomalies are also common.

trisomy 21. See **Down's syndrome.**

trisomy 22, a congenital condition caused by the presence of an extra chromosome 22 in the G group, characterized by psychomotor deficiency and various developmental abnormalities. Common defects include microcephaly, micrognathia, hypotonia, hypertelorism, abnormal ears with preauricular tags or fistulas, and congenital heart disease. In partial trisomy 22, the extra chromosome is much smaller than the normal pair and causes coloboma of the iris or anal atresia, or both, in addition to other defects.

trisomy 8, a congenital condition associated with the presence of an extra chromosome 8 within the C group. Affected individuals are slender and of normal height, with a large asymmetrical head, prominent forehead, deep-set eyes, low-set prominent ears and thick lips. There is mild to severe mental and motor deficiency, often with delayed and poorly articulated speech. Skeletal anomalies and joint limitation, especially camptodactyly, may occur, and there are unusually deep palmar and plantar creases which are diagnostically significant. Most trisomy 8 individuals are mosaic.

trisomy C syndrome. See **trisomy 8.**

trisomy D syndrome. See **trisomy 13.**

trisomy E syndrome. See **trisomy 18.**

trisomy G syndrome. See **Down's syndrome.**

trisomy syndrome, any condition caused by the addition of an extra member to a normal pair of homologous autosomes or sex chromosomes, or by the translocation of a portion of one chromosome to another. Most trisomies occur as a result of complete or partial non-disjunction of the chromosomes during cell division.

tritium (3H), a low-level radioactive isotope of the hydrogen atom, used as a tracer.

tRNA, abbreviation for **transfer RNA.**

trocar, a sharp, pointed rod that fits inside a tube. It is used to pierce the skin and wall of a cavity or canal in the body, in order to aspirate fluids, instill a medication or solution, or guide the placement of a soft catheter. See also **cannula.**

trochanter, one of the two bony projections on the proximal end of the femur, serving for the attachment of various muscles.

trochlea, a pulley-shaped part or structure. **trochlear,** *adj.*

trochlear nerve, either of the smallest pair of cranial nerves, essential for eye movement and eye muscle sensibility.

trochlear notch of ulna, a large depression in the ulna, formed by the olecranon and coronoid processes, that articulates with the trochlea of the humerus.

trochoid joint. See **pivot joint.**

trolamine, a contraction for **triethanolamine.**

trombiculosis, an infestation with mites of the genus *Trombicula,* some species of which carry scrub typhus.

trophectoderm. See **trophoblast.**

trophic action, the stimulation of cell reproduction and enlargement, by nurturing and causing growth.

trophic fracture, a fracture resulting from the weakening of bone tissue caused by nutritional disturbances.

trophic hormones, hormones secreted by the adenohypophysis that stimulate target organs.

trophic ulcer, a decubitus ulcer caused by external trauma to a part of the body that is in poor condition. It results from disease, vascular insufficiency or loss of afferent nerve fibres.

trophoblast, the layer of tissue that forms the wall of blastocyst of placental mammals in the early stages of embryonic development. It functions in the implantation of the blastocyst in the uterine wall, and in supplying nutrients to the embryo. **trophoblastic,** *adj.*

trophoblastic cancer, a malignant disease of the uterus derived from chorionic epithelium, characterized by the production of high levels of human chorionic gonadotropin (HCG). The tumour may be an invasive hydatid mole (chorioadenoma destruens) formed by grossly enlarged, vesicular chorionic villi or a malignant uterine choriocarcinoma that arises from nonvillous chorionic epithelium. Initial symptoms are vaginal bleeding and a profuse, foul-smelling discharge; a persistent cough or haemoptysis signals pulmonary involvement. As the disease progresses, there may be frequent haemorrhage, weakness and emaciation.

trophotropic, pertaining to a combination of parasympathetic nervous system activity, somatic muscle relaxation and cortical beta rhythm synchronization, as in a resting or sleep state.

trophozoite, an immature amoeboid protozoon. When fully developed, a trophozoite may be identified as a schizont.

tropical acne, a form of acne caused or aggravated by high temperature and humidity. It is characterized by large nodules or pustules on the neck, back, upper arms and buttocks.

tropical medicine, the branch of medicine concerned with the diagnosis and treatment of diseases commonly occurring in tropical and subtropical regions of the world, generally between 30 degrees north and south of the equator.

tropical sprue, a malabsorption syndrome of unknown cause, endemic in the tropics and subtropics. It is characterized by abnormalities in the mucosa of the small intestine, resulting in protein malnutrition and multiple nutritional deficiencies often complicated by severe infection. Symptoms include diarrhoea, anorexia and weight loss. Megaloblastic anaemia may result from folic acid and vitamin B12 deficiency.

tropical typhus. See **scrub typhus.**

tropocollagen, fundamental units of collagen fibrils obtained by prolonged extraction of insoluble collagen with dilute acid.

tropomyosin, a protein component of sarcomere filaments; together with troponin, it regulates interactions of actin and myosin in muscle contractions.

troponin, a protein in the myocardial cell ultrastructure that modulates the interaction between actin and myosin molecules. See also tropomyosin.

Trousseau's sign {Armand Trousseau, French physician, b. 1801}, a test for latent tetany, in which carpal spasm is induced by inflating a sphygmomanometer cuff on the upper arm to a pressure exceeding systolic blood pressure for 3 minutes.

Trp, abbreviation for **tryptophan.**

true birth rate, the ratio of total births to the total female population of childbearing age, between 15 and 45 years of age.

true chondroma. See **enchondroma.**

true conjugate, a radiographic measurement of the distance from the upper margin of the symphysis pubis to the sacral promontory. It is usually 1.5 to 2.0 cm less than the diagonal conjugate.

true denticle, a calcified body composed of irregular dentine, found in the pulp chamber of a tooth.

true dwarf. See **primordial dwarf.**

true glottis. See **glottis.**

true neuroma, any neoplasm composed of nerve tissue.

true oxygen, the calculated concentration as either a percentage or a fraction, that when multiplied by the expiratory minute volume at STPD gives oxygen uptake.

true pelvis. See **pelvis.**

true rib. See **rib.**

true suture, an immovable fibrous joint of the skull, in which the edges of bones interlock along a series of processes and indentations.

true twins. See **monozygotic twins.**

true value, (in statistics) a value that is closely approximated by the definitive value and somewhat less closely by the reference value.

true vocal cord. See **vocal cord.**

truncal ataxia, loss of coordinated muscle movements for maintaining normal posture of the trunk.

truncal obesity, obesity that preferentially affects or is located in the trunk of the body, as opposed to the extremities.

truncus arteriosus, the embryonic arterial trunk that initially opens from both ventricles of the heart and later divides into the aorta and pulmonary trunk, the two portions separated by the bulbar septum.

trunk balance, the ability to maintain postural control of the trunk, including the shifting and bearing of weight on each side so as to free an extremity for a particular function. Weight shifting can involve righting, equilibrium and protective reactions. Head and neck control allows for dissociation of the shoulder and pelvic girdles from the trunk.

trunk incurvation reflex. See **Galant reflex.**

truss, an apparatus worn to prevent or retard the herniation of intestines or other organ through an opening in the abdominal wall.

trust, a risk-taking process whereby an individual's situation depends on the future behaviour of another person.

truth, a rule or statement that conforms to fact or reality.

Trypanosoma, a genus of parasitic organisms, several species of which can cause significant diseases in humans. Most *Trypanosoma* organisms live part of their lifecycle in insects and are transmitted to humans by insect bites.

Trypanosoma brucei gambiense. See **Gambian trypanosomiasis.**

trypanosomal infection. See **trypanosomiasis.**

trypanosome, any organism of the genus *Trypanosoma.* **trypanosomal,** *adj.*

trypanosomiasis, an infection by an organism of the *Trypanosoma* genus. Kinds of trypanosomiasis are **African trypanosomiasis.**

trypanosomicide, a drug destructive to trypanosomes, especially the species of the protozoan parasite transmitted to humans by various insect vectors that are com-

trypsin, crystallized, mon in Africa and Central and South America. **trypanosomicidal,** *adj.*

trypsin, crystallized, a proteolytic enzyme produced in the pancreas. It has been used as a debriding agent for open wounds and ulcers, and as an aid to digestion in various gastrointestinal disorders.

tryptophan (Trp), an amino acid essential for normal growth in infants and nitrogen balance in adults. Tryptophan is the precursor of several substances, including serotonin and niacin.

TSEM, abbreviation for **transmission scanning electron microscopy.**

tsetse fly, an insect of the genus *Glossina*, found in Africa, which carries the organisms of trypanosomiasis.

TSH, abbreviation for **thyroid stimulating hormone.**

TSH releasing factor. See **thyrotrophin releasing hormone.**

TSS, abbreviation for **toxic shock syndrome.**

tsutsugamushi disease. See **scrub typhus.**

TTP, abbreviation for **thrombotic thrombocytopenic purpura.**

tubal abortion, a condition of pregnancy in which an embryo, ectopically implanted, is expelled from the uterine tube into the peritoneal cavity. Tubal abortion is often accompanied by significant internal bleeding, causing acute abdominal and pelvic pain.

tubal dermoid cyst, a tumour derived from embryonal tissues, developing in an oviduct.

tubal ligation, one of several sterilization procedures in which both uterine tubes are blocked to prevent conception.

tubal pregnancy, an ectopic pregnancy in which the conceptus implants in the uterine tube. The most important predisposing factor is prior tubal injury. Pelvic infection, scarring and adhesions from surgery may result in damage that diminishes the motility of the tube. Transport of the ovum through the tube after fertilization is slowed, and implantation takes place before the conceptus reaches the uterine cavity.

tube, a hollow, cylindrical piece of equipment or structure of the body.

tube feeding, the administration of nutritionally balanced, liquefied foods through a tube inserted into the stomach or duodenum. The procedure is used after mouth or gastric surgery, in severe burns, paralysis or obstruction of the oesophagus, in severe cases of anorexia nervosa, for unconscious patients, for those who are unable to chew or swallow, and those who are unable to meet their nutritional requirements in another way.

tube gain, the overall electron gain of a photomultiplier tube, calculated as gn, where g is the dynode gain and n is the number of dynodes in the tube.

tubercle, 1. a nodule or small eminence, such as that on a bone. **2.** a nodule, especially an elevation of the skin that is larger than a papule, such as Morgagni's tubercles or the areolae of breasts. **3.** a small rounded nodule produced by infection with *Mycobacterium tuberculosis*, consisting of a grey translucent mass of small spheric cells surrounded by connective cells.

tuberculin purified protein derivative. See **purified protein derivative.**

tuberculin test, a test to determine past or present tuberculosis infection based on a positive skin reaction, using one of several methods. A purified protein derivative (PPD) of tubercle bacilli, called tuberculin, is introduced into the skin by scratch, puncture or intradermal injection. If a raised, red or hard zone forms surrounding the tuberculin test site, the person is said to be sensitive to tuberculin, and the test is positive. Kinds of tuberculin tests include **Heaf test, Mantoux test, Pirquet's test** and **tine test.**

tuberculin. See **tuberculin test, tuberculosis.**

tuberculoid leprosy. See **leprosy.**

tuberculoma, a rare tumour-like growth of tuberculous tissue in the CNS, characterized by symptoms of an expanding cerebral, cerebellar or spinal mass.

tuberculosis (TB), a chronic granulomatous infection caused by an acid-fast bacillus, *Mycobacterium tuberculosis*, generally transmitted by the inhalation or ingestion of infected droplets. It usually affects the lungs, although infection of other organ systems by different modes of transmission also occurs. Listlessness, vague chest pain, pleurisy, anorexia, fever and weight loss are early symptoms of pulmonary tuberculosis. Night sweats, pulmonary haemorrhage, expectoration of purulent sputum and dyspnoea develop as the disease progresses. The lung tissues react to the bacillus by producing protective cells that engulf the disease organism, forming tubercles. Untreated, the tubercles enlarge and merge to form larger tubercles that undergo caseation, eventually sloughing off into the lung cavities. Haemoptysis occurs as a result of cavitary spread. Physical examination reveals apical rales, amphoric bronchial sounds, decreased respiratory excursion and, in advanced cases, cyanosis.

tuberculosis vaccine. See **BCG vaccine.**

tuberculous spondylitis, a rare, grave form of tuberculosis caused by the invasion of Mycobacterium tuberculosis into the spinal vertebrae. The intervertebral disks may be destroyed, resulting in the collapse and wedging of affected vertebrae and the shortening and angulation of the spine.

tuberosity, an elevation or protuberance, especially of a bone.

tuberosity of the tibia, a large oblong elevation at the proximal end of the tibia that attaches to the ligament of the patella.

tuberous carcinoma, a scirrhous carcinoma of the skin, characterized by nodular projections.

tuberous sclerosis, a familial, neurocutaneous disease characterized by epilepsy, mental deterioration, adenoma sebaceum, nodules and sclerotic patches on the cerebral cortex, retinal tumours, depigmented leaf-shaped macules on the skin, tumours of the heart or kidneys and cerebral calcifications.

tuberous xanthoma. See **xanthoma tuberosum.**

tuboplasty, a surgical procedure in which severed or damaged uterine tubes are repaired.

tubular necrosis, the death of cells in the small tubules of kidneys, as a result of disease or injury.

tubule, a small tube, such as one of the collecting tubules in the kidneys, the seminiferous tubules of the testes, or Henle's tubules between the distal and proximal convoluted tubules. **tubular,** *adj.*

tuft fracture, fracture of any one of the distal phalanges.

tularaemia, an infectious disease of animals caused by the bacillus *Francisella (Pasteurella) tularensis,* which may be transmitted by insect vectors or direct contact. In humans, it is characterized by fever, headache and an ulcerated skin lesion with localized lymph node enlargement, or by eye infection, GI ulcerations or pneumonia, depending on the site of entry and response of the host.

tumoricide, a substance capable of destroying a tumour. **tumoricidal,** *adj.*

tumorigenesis, the process of initiating and promoting the development of a tumour. **tumourigenic,** *adj.*

tumour, 1. a swelling or enlargement occurring in inflammatory conditions. **2.** a new growth of tissue characterized by progressive, uncontrolled proliferation of cells. The tumour may be localized or invasive, benign or malignant.

tumour albus, a white swelling occurring in a tuberculous bone or joint.

tumour angiogenesis factor (TAF), a protein that stimulates the formation of blood vessels in cancers.

tumour marker, a substance in the body that is associated with the presence of a cancer.

tumour necrosis factor (TNF), a natural body protein, also produced synthetically, with anticancer effects. It is produced in the body in response to the presence of toxic substances, such as bacterial toxins.

tumour registry, a registry of data drawn from medical records on the incidence of cancers, cancer types and particular characteristics, treatment, and treatment outcomes of cancer patients.

tumour volume, a portion of an organ or tissue that includes both the tumour and adjacent areas of invasion.

tungsten (W), a metallic element. Its atomic number is 74 and its atomic weight is 183.85. It has the highest melting point of all metals, and is commonly used as a target material in x-ray tubes.

tunica, an enveloping coat or covering membrane.

tunica adventitia, the outer layer or coat of an artery or other tubular structure.

tunica intima, the membrane lining an artery.

tunica media, a muscular middle coat of an artery.

tunica vaginalis testis, the serous membrane surrounding the testis and epididymis.

tunica vasculosa bulbi. See **uvea.**

tuning fork, a small metal instrument consisting of a stem and two prongs, that produces a constant pitch when either prong is struck. It is used in auditory tests of nerve function and air and bone conduction.

tunnel vision, a defect in sight in which there is a great reduction in the peripheral field of vision, as if looking through a hollow tube or tunnel. The condition occurs in advanced chronic glaucoma.

TUR, abbreviation for **transurethral resection.**

turban tumour, a benign neoplasm consisting of multiple pink or maroon nodules that may cover the entire scalp and may also occur on the trunk and extremities.

turbidimetry, measurement of the turbidity (cloudiness) of a solution or suspension in which the amount of transmitted light is quantified with a spectrophotometer or estimated by visual comparison with solutions of known turbidity.

turbidity, a condition of light scattering in a liquid, resulting from the presence of suspended particles in the fluid.

turbinate, 1. of, or pertaining to, a scroll shape. **2.** the concha nasalis.

turgid, swollen, hard and congested, usually as a result of an accumulation of fluid. **turgor,** *n.*

turgor, the normal resiliency of skin, as a result of the outward pressure of cells and interstitial fluid. An evaluation of the skin turgor is an essential part of physical assessment.

turnbuckle cast, an orthopaedic device used to encase and immobilize the entire trunk, one arm to the elbow, and the opposite leg to the knee. It is constructed of plaster of paris or fibreglass, and incorporates hinges as part of its design in the treatment of scoliosis. The hinges are placed at the level of the apex of the curvature.

Turner's sign. See **Grey Turner's sign.**

Turner's syndrome {Henry H. Turner, American physician, b. 1892}, a chromosomal abnormality seen in about 1 in 3000 live female births, characterized by the absence of one X chromosome, congenital ovarian failure, genital hypoplasia, cardiovascular anomalies, dwarfism, short metacarpals, "shield chest" extosis of tibia, and underdeveloped breasts, uterus and vagina. Spatial disorientation and moderate degrees of learning disorders are common.

turricephaly. See **oxycephaly.**

TV, abbreviation for **tidal volume.**

TVL, abbreviation for **tenth value layer.**

tweezers, a kind of small spring forceps, used for removing unwanted hair

twelfth cranial nerve. See **hypoglossal nerve.**

twin, either of two offspring born of the same pregnancy, and developed from either a single ovum or two ova that were released from the ovary simultaneously and fertilized at the same time. The incidence of twin births is approximately 1 in 80 pregnancies. Kinds of twins include **conjoined twins, dizygotic twins, interlocked twins, monozygotic twins, Siamese twins** and **unequal twins.**

twinning, 1. the development of two or more fetuses during the same pregnancy, either spontaneously or through external intervention for experimental purposes in animals. **2.** the duplication of similar structures or parts by division.

two-way catheter, a catheter with a double lumen, one channel for injection of medication or fluids and the other for removal of fluid or specimens.

tyloma, aggregation of **hyperkeratotic skin.** See **callus.**

tympanic, of, or pertaining to, a structure that resonates when struck; drum-like, such as a **tympanic abdomen** that resonates on percussion because the intestines are distended with gas. **tympanum,** *pl.* **tympana,** *n.*

tympanic antrum, a relatively large, irregular cavity in the superior anterior portion of the mastoid process of the temporal bone, communicating with the mastoid air cells and lined by the extension of mucous membrane of the tympanic cavity.

tympanic cavity. See **middle ear.**

tympanic membrane, a thin, semitransparent membrane in the middle ear, that transmits sound vibrations to the internal ear by means of auditory ossicles. It is almost oval in form, and separates the tympanic cavity from the bottom of the external acoustic meatus.

tympanic reflex, the reflection of a beam of light shining on the eardrum. In a normal ear, a bright, wedge-shaped reflection is seen; its apex is at the end of the malleus and its base at the anterior inferior margin of the eardrum.

tympanoplasty, any of several operative

procedures on the eardrum or ossicles of the middle ear, designed to restore or improve hearing in patients with conductive deafness. These operations may be used to repair a perforated eardrum, for otosclerosis, and dislocation or necrosis of one of the small bones of the middle ear.

tympanotomy. See **myringotomy.**

tympanum. See **tympanic.**

Type A personality, a behaviour pattern associated with individuals who are highly competitive and work compulsively to meet deadlines. The behaviour also is associated with a higher than usual incidence of coronary heart disease.

Type B personality, a form of behaviour associated with persons who appear free of hostility and aggression, who lack a compulsion to meet deadlines, are not highly competitive at work and play, and have a lower risk of heart attack.

Type E personality, a term used to describe professional women who fit neither Type A nor Type B personality categories, but who have a marked sense of insecurity and strive to convince themselves that they are worthwhile.

type I diabetes mellitus. See **insulin-dependent diabetes mellitus.**

type I hyperlipidaemia. See **hyperlipidaemia type I.**

type I hypersensitivity. See **anaphylactic hypersensitivity.**

type II diabetes mellitus. See **non-insulindependent diabetes mellitus.**

type II hyperlipoproteinaemia. See **familial hypercholesterolaemia.**

type II hypersensitivity. See **cytotoxic hypersensitivity.**

type III hypersensitivity. See **immune complex hypersensitivity.**

type IV hypersensitivity. See **cell-mediated immune response.**

typhoid fever, a bacterial infection usually caused by *Salmonella typhi,* transmitted by contaminated milk, water or food. It is characterized by headache, delirium, cough, watery diarrhoea, rash and a high fever. Characteristic maculopapular rosy spots are scattered over the skin of the abdomen. Splenomegaly and leukopenia develop first. The disease is serious and may be fatal. Complications include intestinal haemorrhage or perforation and thrombophlebitis. Some people who recover from the disease continue to be carriers and excrete the organism, thus spreading the disease.

typhoid pellagra, a form of pellagra in which the symptoms also include continued high temperatures.

typhoid vaccine, a bacterial vaccine prepared from an inactivated, dried strain of *Salmonella typhi,* or from its capsular polysaccharide, or from a live attenuated strain of bacteria. It is used for the primary immunization of adults and children against typhoid fever. The dead vaccines are given by injection, and the live vaccines are given by mouth.

typhus, any of a group of acute infectious diseases caused by various species of *Rickettsia*. They are usually transmitted from infected rodents to humans by the bites of lice, fleas, mites or ticks. All these diseases are characterized by headache, chills, fever, malaise and a maculopapular rash. Kinds of typhus are epidemic typhus, murine typhus and scrub typhus. See also **Brill-Zinsser disease, Rocky Mountain spotted fever.**

typhus vaccine, any one of three vaccines, each of which is prepared for active immunization against one of the different rickettsial organisms that cause epidemic typhus, murine typhus or Brill-Zinsser disease.

typing, the process of ascertaining the classification of a specimen of blood, tissue or other substance.

Tyr, abbreviation for **tyrosine.**

tyramine, an amino acid synthesized in the body from the essential acid tyrosine. Tyramine stimulates the release of the catecholamines adrenaline and noradrenaline. People receiving monoamine oxidase inhibitors should avoid the ingestion of foods and beverages containing tyramine.

tyroma, *pl.* **tyromas, tyromata,** a new growth or nodule with a caseous or cheesy consistency.

tyromatosis, a process in which necrotic tissue is broken down and degenerates to a granular, amorphous, caseous mass.

tyrosine (Tyr), an amino acid synthesized in the body from the essential amino acid phenylalanine. Tyrosine is found in most proteins and is a precursor of melanin and several hormones, including adrenaline and thyroxine.

tyrosinaemia, 1. a benign, transient condition of the newborn, especially premature infants, in which an excessive amount of the amino acid tyrosine is found in the blood and urine. The disorder is caused by an abnormality in amino acid metabolism, which usually amounts to delayed development of the enzymes necessary to metabolize tyrosine. **2.** a hereditary disorder involving an inborn error of metabolism of the amino acid tyrosine. The condition is caused by an enzyme deficiency and results in liver failure or liver cirrhosis, renal tubular defects that can lead to renal ricketts and renal glycosuria, generalized aminoaciduria and mental deficiency.

tyrosinosis, a rare condition resulting from a defect in amino acid metabolism and characterized by the excretion of excessive amount of parahydroxyphenylpyruvic acid, an intermediate product of tyrosine, in the urine.

tyrosinurea, the presence of tyrosine in the urine.

Tzanck test {Arnault Tzanck, French dermatologist, b. 1886}, a microscopic examination of cellular material from skin lesions, to help diagnose certain vesicular diseases.

u, symbol sometimes used to stand for **micro-** (properly μ), as in "ul'" or "um", representing μ or μm.

U, **1.** abbreviation for unit. **2.** symbol for uranium.

UICC, abbreviation for **International Union Against Cancer, Union internacional contra el cancer, Union internationale contre le cancer, Unio internationalis contra cancrum** or **Unione internazionale contro il cancro.**

UKCC, abbreviation for **United Kingdom Central Council for Nursing, Midwifery and Health Visiting.**

UKCPA, abbreviation for **United Kingdom Clinical Pharmacy Association.**

ulcer, a circumscribed, crater-like lesion of the skin or mucous membrane, resulting from necrosis and accompanying some inflammatory, infectious or malignant processes. Kinds of ulcer include **decubitus ulcer, peptic ulcer** and **serpent ulcer.** **ulcerate,** *v.,* **ulcerative,** *adj.*

ulcerative blepharitis, a form of blepharitis in which a staphylococcal infection of the follicles of the eyelashes and glands of the eyelids results in sticky crusts forming on the lid margins. If the crusts are pulled off, the skin beneath bleeds. Tiny pustules develop in the follicles of the eyelashes and break down to form shallow ulcers.

ulcerative colitis, a chronic, episodic, inflammatory disease of the large intestine and rectum. It is characterized by profuse watery diarrhoea containing varying amounts of blood, mucus and pus. The attacks of diarrhoea are accompanied by tenesmus, severe abdominal pain, fever, chills, anaemia and weight loss. Children with the disease may suffer retarded physical growth. The debilitating symptoms often prevent persons with ulcerative colitis from continuing with the normal activities of daily living.

ulna, the bone on the medial or little finger side of the forearm, lying parallel with the radius. The ulna articulates with the humerus and radius.

ulnar artery, a large artery branching from the brachial artery, supplying muscles in the forearm, wrist, and hand. Arising near the elbow, it passes obliquely in a distal direction to become the superficial palmar arch.

nerve, one of the terminal branches of the brachial plexus that arises on each side from the medial cord of the plexus. It receives fibres from both cervical and thoracic nerve roots, and supplies the muscles and skin on the ulnar side of the forearm and hand. It can be easily palpated as the "funny bone" of the elbow.

ulocarcinoma, *pl.* **ulocarcinomas, ulocarcinomata,** any malignant neoplastic disease of the gums that is classified as a carcinoma.

ultimate strain, the strain at the point of failure.

ultimate stress, the highest load that can be sustained by a material at the point of failure.

ultracentrifuge, a high-speed centrifuge with a rotation rate fast enough to produce sedimentation of viruses, even in blood plasma.

ultradian, pertaining to a biorhythm that occurs in cycles of less than 24 hours.

ultrafiltrate, a solution that has passed through a special semipermeable ultrafilter membrane.

ultrafiltration, a type of filtration, sometimes conducted under pressure, through filters with very minute pores, as used by an artificial kidney. Ultrafiltration can separate large molecules from smaller molecules in body fluids.

ultramicroscopy. See **darkfield microscopy.**

ultrasonic cardiography. See **echocardiography.**

ultrasonic handpiece, a device for holding rotary instruments, such as drills, that permits rotational speeds of 100,000 to 300,000 rpm. It is used primarily for tooth cavity preparation.

ultrasonic nebulizer, a humidifier in which an electric current is used to produce high-frequency vibrations in a container of fluid. The vibrations break up the fluid into aerosol particles.

ultrasonography, the process of imaging deep structures of the body by measuring and recording the reflection of pulsed or continuous high-frequency sound waves.

ultrasound, soundwaves at the very high frequency of over 20,000 vibrations per second. Ultrasound has several medical applications, including fetal monitoring, imaging of internal organs and, at an extremely high frequency, the cleaning of dental and surgical instruments.

ultrasound imaging. See **ultrasonography.**

ultraviolet (UV), light beyond the range of human vision, at the short end of the spectrum, or that portion of the electromagnetic spectrum with wavelengths between 10 to 400 nm. It occurs naturally in sunlight; it burns and tans the skin and converts precursors in the skin to vitamin D. Ultraviolet lamps are used in the control of infectious, airborne bacteria and viruses, and in the treatment of psoriasis and other skin conditions. Black light is ultraviolet light used in fluoroscopy.

ultraviolet microscopy. See **fluorescent microscopy.**

ultraviolet radiation, a range of electromagnetic waves extending from the violet or short-wavelength end of the spectrum to the beginning of the x-ray spectrum. Near-ultraviolet radiation covers a range of wavelengths from 380 to 320 nm; middle-ultraviolet radiation covers a range from 320 to 280 nm; and far-ultraviolet radiation extends from 280 to about 10 nm. About 5% of the radiation from the sun is in the ultraviolet range, but little of this type of energy reaches the earth because much is absorbed by oxygen and ozone in the atmosphere. In medicine, ultraviolet radiation is used in the treatment of rickets and certain skin conditions. Milk and some other foods become activated with vitamin D when exposed to this type of energy.

umbilical, 1. of, or pertaining to, the umbilicus. **2.** of, or pertaining to, the umbilical cord.

umbilical catheterization, a procedure in which a radiopaque catheter is passed through an umbilical artery to provide a newborn infant with parenteral fluid, to obtain blood samples or both. It may also be passed through the umbilical vein for an exchange transfusion or emergency administration of drugs, fluids or volume expanders.

umbilical cord, a flexible structure connecting the umbilicus with the placenta in the gravid uterus, and giving passage to the umbilical arteries and vein. In the newborn, the umbilical cord is about 60 cm long and 3-5 cm in diameter.

umbilical duct. See **vitelline duct.**

umbilical fissure, a groove on the inferior surface of the liver that holds the ligamentum teres and separates the right and left lobes of the liver.

umbilical fistula, an abnormal passage from the umbilicus to the intestine, or more frequently to the remnant of the canal in the median umbilical ligament, that connects the fetal bladder with the allantois.

umbilical hernia, a soft, skin-covered protrusion of intestine and omentum through a weakness in the abdominal wall around the umbilicus.

umbilical region, the part of abdomen surrounding the umbilicus, in the middle zone between the right and left lateral regions.

umbilical vein, one of a pair of embryonic vessels that return the blood from the placenta and fuse to form a single trunk in the body stalk.

umbilical vesicle, a pear-shaped structure formed from the yolk sac at about the fourth week of prenatal development. It protrudes into the cavity of the chorion and connects to the developing embryo by the yolk stalk at the region of the future midgut.

umbilicus, the point on the abdomen at which the umbilical cord joined the fetal abdomen. In most adults it is marked by a depression; in some it is marked by a small protrusion of skin.

umbo, a landmark on the tympanic membrane created by the attachment of the membrane to the malleus.

uncal herniation, a condition in which the medial portion of the temporal lobe protrudes over the tentorial edge as a result of increased intracranial pressure. A dilated pupil on the side of herniation is a diagnostic sign of the disorder.

unciform bone. See **hamate bone.**

Uncinaria, a genus of nematode that causes hookworm in dogs, cats and other carnivores.

uncompensated gluteal gait. See **Trendelenburg gait.**

uncompetitive inhibitor, an enzymatic inhibitor that appears to bond only to the enzyme substrate complex and not to free enzyme molecules.

unconditioned response, an instinctive, unlearned reaction to a stimulus; one that occurs naturally and is not acquired by association and training.

unconscious, 1. being unaware of the surrounding environment; insensible; incapable of responding to sensory stimuli. **2.** (in psychiatry) the part of mental function in which thoughts, ideas, emotions or memories are beyond awareness and not subject to ready recall.

unconsciousness, a state of complete or partial unawareness or lack of response to sensory stimuli as a result of hypoxia, arising from respiratory insufficiency or shock; metabolic or chemical brain depressants, such as drugs, poisons, ketones or electrolyte imbalance; or a form of pathological condition of the brain, such as trauma, seizures, cerebral vasular accident, brain tumour or infection. Various degrees of unconsciousness can occur during stupor, fugue, catalepsy and dream states.

unction. See **ointment.**

undecenoic acid, an antifungal agent used in the treatment of athlete's foot and ringworm.

underdamping, (in cardiology) the transmission of all frequency components without a reduction in amplitude.

underdriving, a condition in artificial heart functioning in which there is insufficient compressed air during systole to eject the entire end diastolic volume of the ventricle.

underlying assumption, a set of rules one holds about oneself, others and the world.

underwater exercise, any physical activity performed in a pool or large bath where the buoyancy of water facilitates the movement of weak or injured muscles.

underwater seal, a seal formed by water allowed to flow over a tube that exits from the chest cavity of a patient. The water acts as a one-way valve and permits the outflow of air but denies the ingress of air.

underweight, less than normal in body weight after adjustment for height, body build and age.

undescended testis. See **cryptorchidism, monorchism.**

undifferentiated cell leukaemia. See **stem cell leukaemia.**

undifferentiated family ego mass, an emotional fusion in a family in which all members are similar in emotional expression.

undifferentiated malignant lymphoma, a lymphoid neoplasm containing many large stem cells that have large nuclei, small amounts of pale cytoplasm and borders that are not well defined.

undifferentiated schizophrenia. See **acute schizophrenia.**

undifferentiation, the lack or absence of normal cell differentiation into an identifiable cell type.

undisplaced fracture, a bone break in which cracks in the osseous tissue may radiate in several directions without the separation or displacement of fragmented sections.

undoing, the performance of a specific action intended to negate in part a previous action or communication. According to some psychologists, undoing is related to the magical thinking of childhood.

undulant fever. See **brucellosis.**

unequal cleavage, mitotic division of the fertilized ovum into blastomeres that are larger near the yolk portion of protoplasm, or vegetal pole, and smaller near the nucleus, or animal pole.

unequal twins, two non-joined fetuses born of the same pregnancy in which only one of the pair is fully formed, while the other shows various degrees of developmental defects.

ungual phalanx. See **distal phalanx.**

unguent. See **ointment.**

unguis. See **nail.**

uniaxial joint, a synovial joint in which movement is only in one axis, such as a pivot or hinge joint.

UNICEF, abbreviation for **United Nations International Children's Emergency Fund.**

unicellular reproduction, the formation of a new organism from a female egg that has not been fertilized; parthenogenesis.

unicentric blastoma. See **blastoma.**

unidirectional block, a pathological failure of cardiac impulse conduction in one direction while conduction is possible in the other direction.

unidose. See **unit dose.**

uniform reporting, the reporting of service and financial data by a hospital in conformance with prescribed standard definitions, to permit comparisons with other health facilities.

unilateral hypertrophy, enlargement of one side, or portion of one side, of the body.

unilateral long-leg spica cast, an orthopaedic cast applied to immobilize one leg and trunk of the body cranially as far as the nipple line.

unilateral neglect, a state in which an individual is perceptually unaware of and inattentive to one side of the body. Characteristics includes consistent inattention to stimuli on the affected side, inadequate self-care (as in positioning and/or safety precautions in regard to the affected side), absence of looking towards the affected side, and leaving food on the plate on the affected side.

unilateral paralysis. See **hemiplegia.**

uniovular, developing from a single ovum, as in monozygotic twins, as contrasted with dizygotic twins.

uniovular twins. See **monozygotic twins.**

unipolar depressive response, an affective disorder characterized only by symptoms of depression.

unipolar lead, **1.** an electrocardiographic conductor in which the exploring electrode is placed on the precordium or a limb while the indifferent electrode is in the central terminal. **2.** *informal,* a tracing produced by such a lead on an electrocardiograph.

unique radiolytic product, a product, such as a food substance, that has undergone chemical changes as a result of exposure to ionizing radiation.

UNISON, trade union association for hospital and government employees formed in 1993 from an amalgamation of NALGO, NUPE and COMSE.

unit (U), **1.** a single item. **2.** a quantity designated as a standard of measurement. **3.** an area of a hospital that is staffed and equipped for treatment of patients with a specific condition or other common characteristics.

unitary human conceptual framework, a complex theory in nursing that emphasizes the importance of holistic healthcare and an understanding of the human being in relation to the universal environment.

unit dose, a method of preparing medications in which individual doses of patient medications are prepared by the pharmacy and delivered in individual labelled packets to the patient's unit to be administered by the nurses on the ordered schedule. Also called **unidose.**

unit dose system, a system of drug distribution in which a portable cart containing a drawer for each patient's medications is prepared by the hospital pharmacy with a 24-hour supply of the medications.

United Kingdom Central Council for Nursing, Midwifery and Health Visiting (UKCC), maintains the professional register for all nurses in the United Kingdom, sets standards, and investigates complaints of bad practice.

United Kingdom Clinical Pharmacy Association (UKCPA), an organization involved in the education, training and professional development of pharmacists.

United Nations International Children's Emergency Fund (UNICEF), a fund established by the General Assembly of the United Nations in 1946, to aid children in devastated areas of the world.

unit of service, any individual, family, aggregate, organization or community given nursing care.

univalent, referring to a chemical valency of one, or the capacity of one atom of a chemical element to attract one atom of hydrogen or displace one atom of hydrogen.

univalent antiserum, antiserum which contains antibodies against a single antigen.

univalent reduction, a phenomenon during intracellular metabolism involving oxygen-reduction reactions in which superoxide radicals are produced.

universal cuff, an adaptive device worn on the hand to hold items such as utensils, shaver or pencil, allowing a patient with a weak grasp to increase participation in self-care activities.

universal donor, a person with blood of type O, Rh factor negative. Such blood may be used for emergency transfusion with minimal risk of incompatibility.

universalizability principle, a principle that an act is good if everyone should, in similar circumstances, perform the same act without exception.

universal qualifiers, (in neurolinguistic programming) the use of terms that give general impressions of limitations, such as all, common, every, only and never.

Unna's paste boot, a dressing for varicose ulcers formed by applying a layer of a gelatin-glycerin-zinc oxide paste to the leg, and then a spiral bandage covered with successive coats of paste to produce a rigid boot.

unresolved grief, a severe, chronic grief reaction in which a person does not complete the resolution stage of the grieving process.

unsaturated, 1. describing a solution that is capable of dissolving more of the solute; not saturated. **2.** also called **unsaturated hydrocarbon,** an organic compound in which two or more carbon atoms are united by double or triple valence bonds, as in unsaturated fatty acids.

unsaturated alcohol, an alcohol derived from an unsaturated hydrocarbon, such as an alkene or olefin.

unsaturated fatty acid, any of a number of glyceryl esters of certain organic acids, in which some of the atoms are joined by double or triple valence bonds. These bonds are easily split in chemical reactions and other substances are joined to them. Monounsaturated fatty acids have only one double or triple bond per molecule. Polyunsaturated fatty acids have more than one double or triple bond per molecule.

unsaturated hydrocarbon. See **unsaturated.**

unscrubbed team members, the members of a surgical team, including the anaesthetist and circulating nurse, who wear surgical attire but are not gowned or gloved and do not enter the sterile field.

unsocialized aggressive reaction, a behaviour disorder of childhood, characterized by overt and covert hostility, disobedience, physical and verbal aggression, vengefulness, quarrelsome behaviour and destructiveness, often manifested in acts such as lying, stealing, temper tantrums, vandalism and physical violence against others.

unstable, 1. in an excited or active state, such as an atom with a nucleus possessing excess energy **2.** easily broken down.

unstriated muscle. See **smooth muscle.**

upper extremity suspension, an orthopaedic procedure used in the treatment of bone fractures and correction of orthopaedic abnormalities of the upper limbs. Traction equipment is used, including metal frames, ropes and pulleys, aiming to relieve the weight of the upper limb involved rather than exert traction.

upper motor neuron paralysis, a brain or spinal cord injury or lesion, causing damage to the cell bodies or axons, or both, of the upper motor neurons which extend from the cerebral centres to the cells in the spinal column. Clinical manifestations include increased muscle tone and spasticity of the muscles involved, with little or no atrophy, hyperactive deep tendon reflexes, diminished or absent superficial reflexes, the presence of pathological reflexes such as Babinski's and Hoffmann's reflexes, and no local twitching of muscle groups.

upper respiratory infection. See **respiratory tract infection.**

upper respiratory tract, one of the two divisions of the respiratory system. The upper respiratory tract consists of the nose, nasal cavity, ethmoidal air cells, frontal sinuses, sphenoidal sinuses, maxillary sinus, larynx and trachea. The upper respiratory tract conducts air to and from the lungs, and filters, moistens and warms the air during each inspiration.

urachus, an epithelial tube connecting the

apex of the urinary bladder with the allantois. Its connective tissue forms the median umbilical ligament.

uraemia, the presence of excessive amounts of urea and other nitrogenous waste products in the blood, as occurs in renal failure.

uraemic frost, a pale, frost-like deposit of white crystals on the skin caused by kidney failure and uraemia. Urea compounds, and other waste products of metabolism that cannot be excreted by the kidneys into the urine, are excreted through the small superficial capillaries onto the surface of the skin where they collect.

uraemic gingivitis. See **nephritic gingivitis.**

uranium (U), a heavy, radioactive metallic element. Its atomic number is 92; its atomic weight is 238.03. Uranium is the heaviest of the natural elements.

urate, any salt of uric acid, such as sodium urate. Urates are found in the urine, blood and tophi or calcareous deposits in tissues. They may also be deposited as crystals in body joints.

urban typhus. See **murine typhus.**

urea, a systemic osmotic diuretic that has been used to reduce cerebrospinal and intraocular fluid pressure. It is also used topically as a hydrating agent in preparations for dry skin.

urea cycle, a series of enzymatic reactions by which ammonia is detoxified in the liver. In the series of steps for disposing of the ammonia molecule, a waste product of protein metabolism, five enzymatic reactions occur as NH_2 radicals are combined with carbon and oxygen atoms from carbon dioxide to form urea, which is excreted. The amino acid arginine is synthesized during the same process.

urea hydrogen peroxide, a topical antiinfective and cerulytic prescribed to soften impacted earwax.

Ureaplasma urealyticum, a sexually transmitted micro-organism that is a common inhabitant of the urogenital systems of men and women in whom infection is asymptomatic. Neonatal death, prematurity and perinatal morbidity are statistically associated with colonization of the chorionic surface of the placenta by *Ureaplasma urealyticum.*

ureter, one of a pair of tubes, about 30 cm long, that carry the urine from the kidney into the bladder. They are thick-walled, vary in diameter, and are divided into an abdominal portion and a pelvic portion. The ureter enters the bladder through an oblique tunnel that functions as a valve to prevent backflow of urine into the ureter when the bladder contracts. Connecting with the kidneys, the ureters expand into funnel-shaped renal pelves that branch into calyces, each calyx containing a renal papilla. Urine draining through renal tubules drops into the papillae, passes through the calyces and the pelvis

and down each ureter into the bladder. Urine is pumped through the ureters by peristaltic waves that occur an average of three times a minute. **ureteral,** *adj.*

ureteral dysfunction, a disturbance of the normal peristaltic flow of urine through a ureter, resulting from dysfunction of ureteral motor nerves.

ureteritis, an inflammatory condition of a ureter caused by infection or mechanic irritation of a stone.

ureterocele, a prolapse of the terminal portion of the ureter into the bladder. The condition may lead to obstruction of the flow of urine, hydronephrosis and loss of renal function.

ureterography, the radiographic imaging of a ureter, usually conducted as part of an examination of the urinary tract. The examination may involve injection of a radiopaque medium through a urinary catheter.

ureterosigmoidostomy, a surgical procedure in which a ureter is implanted in the sigmoid flexure of the intestinal tract.

ureterotomy, an incision into a ureter.

urethra, a small tubular structure that drains urine from the bladder. In women, it is about 3 cm long and lies directly behind the symphysis pubis, anterior to the vagina. In men, it is about 20 cm long and begins at the bladder, passes through the centre of the prostate gland, goes between two sheets of tissue connecting the pubic bones, and finally passes through the urinary meatus of the penis. In men, the urethra serves as a passage for semen during ejaculation, as well as a canal for urine during voiding.

urethral, of, or pertaining to, the urethra.

urethral papilla. See **papilla.**

urethral sphincter, the voluntary muscle at the neck of the bladder that relaxes so as to allow urination.

urethritis, an inflammatory condition of the urethra, characterized by dysuria. It is usually the result of an infection in the bladder or kidneys.

urethrocele, (in women) a herniation of the urethra. It is characterized by a protusion of a segment of the urethra and connective tissue surrounding it, into the anterior wall of the vagina.

urethography, radiographic visualization of the urethra following the introduction of a radiopaque contrast medium, usually via a catheter. **Micturating urethrography** visualizes the urinary bladder and urethra during micturition.

urethroplasty, a surgical procedure for the repair of a urethra, as in the correction of hypospadias.

urgency, a feeling of the need to void urine immediately.

URI, abbreviation for **upper respiratory infection.** See **respiratory tract infection.**

uric acid, a product of the metabolism of

protein present in the blood and excreted in the urine.

uricaciduria, a greater than normal amount of uric acid in the urine, often associated with urinary calculi or gout.

uricosuric drugs, drugs administered to increase the elimination of uric acid, and so prevent gout.

urinal, a plastic disposable or metal receptacle for collecting urine.

urinalysis, a physical, microscopic or chemical examination of urine. The specimen is physically examined for colour, turbidity, specific gravity and pH. It is then spun in a centrifuge, to allow collection of a small amount of sediment that is examined microscopically for blood cells, casts, crystals, pus and bacteria. Chemical analysis may be performed for the identification and quantification of any of a large number of substances, but most commonly for ketones, sugar, protein and blood.

urinary, of, or pertaining to, urine or formation of urine.

urinary bladder, the muscular membranous sac in the pelvis that stores urine for discharge through the urethra.

urinary calculus, a calculus formed in any part of the urinary tract. Calculi may be large enough to cause an obstruction in the flow of urine, or small enough to be passed with the urine. Kinds of urinary calculi are **renal calculus** and **vesicle calculus.**

urinary elimination, altered patterns, a disturbance in urine elimination. Characteristics include dysuria, urinary frequency, hesitancy, incontinence, nocturia and urgency of urination.

urinary frequency, a greater than normal frequency of the urge to void without an increase in the total daily volume of urine. The condition is characteristic of inflammation in the bladder or urethra, diminished bladder capacity or other structural abnormalities.

urinary hesitancy, a decrease in the force of the stream of urine, often with difficulty in beginning the flow. Hesitancy is usually the result of an obstruction or stricture between the bladder and urethral opening; in men, it may indicate an enlargement of the prostate gland; it may result from stenosis of the urethral opening.

urinary incontinence, involuntary passage of urine, with the failure of voluntary control over bladder and urethral sphincters.

urinary infection. See **urinary tract infection.**

urinary meatus, the external opening of the urethra.

urinary output, the total volume of urine excreted daily, normally between 700 and 2000 ml. Various metabolic and renal diseases may change the normal urinary output.

urinary retention, incomplete emptying of the bladder. Characteristics include bladder distention, small and infrequent voiding or absence of urine output, a sensation of bladder fullness, dribbling, residual urine, dysuria and overflow incontinence.

urinary system, all organs involved in the secretion and elimination of urine. These include the kidneys, ureters, bladder and urethra.

urinary system assessment, an evaluation of the condition and functioning of the kidneys, bladder, ureters and urethra, and an investigation of concurrent and previous disorders that may be factors in abnormalities in the urinary system. The patient is asked whether any of the following symptoms has occurred: dysuria; frequency or burning on urination; dribbling; a decreased urinary stream; nocturia; stress incontinence; headache; back pain; increased thirst. The colour, odour and amount of urine voided without a catheter, and with one in place, are determined. Diagnostic procedures may include cystoscopy, excretory and intravenous urography, renal angiography, retrograde studies and x-ray of the kidneys, ureters and bladder.

urinary tract, all organs and ducts involved in the secretion and elimination of urine from the body.

urinary tract infection (UTI), an infection of one or more structures in the urinary tract. Most of these infections are caused by gram-negative bacteria, most commonly *Escherichia coli* or species of *Klebsiella, Proteus, Pseudomonas* or *Enterobacter.* Urinary tract infection is usually characterized by urinary frequency, burning, pain with voiding and, if the infection is severe, visible blood and pus in the urine. Kinds of urinary tract infections include **cystitis, pyelonephritis** and **urethritis.**

urination, the act of passing urine.

urine, the fluid secreted by the kidneys, transported by the ureters, stored in the bladder and voided through the urethra. Normal urine is clear, straw-coloured, slightly acid, and has the characteristic odour of urea. Its normal constituents include water, urea, sodium chloride and potassium chloride, phosphates, uric acid, organic salts and the pigment urobilin.

urine osmolality, the osmotic pressure of urine. Normal values are 500 to 800 mOsm/L.

urine pH, the hydrogen ion concentration of urine, or a measure of its acidity or alkalinity. The normal pH values for urine are 4.6 to 8.0.

urine specific gravity, a measure of the degree of concentration of a sample of urine. The normal range of urine specific gravity is 1.002 to 1.030, depending on the patient's previous fluid intake, renal perfusion and renal function.

urinoma, *pl.* **urinoma, urinomata,** a cyst filled with urine.

urinometer, any device for determining the specific gravity of urine, including gravitometers and hydrometers.

urobilin, a brown pigment formed by the oxidation of urobilinogen, normally found in faeces and, in small amounts, in urine.

urobilinogen, a colourless compound formed in the intestine after the breakdown of bilirubin by bacteria. See also **urobilin.**

urogenital, of, or pertaining to, the urinary and reproductive systems. Also called **genitourinary.**

urogenital sinus, one of the elongated cavities, formed by the division of the cloaca in early embryonic development, into which open the ureter, mesonephric and paramesonephric ducts, and bladder.

urogenital system, the urinary and genital organs and associated structures that develop in the fetus to form the kidneys, ureters, bladder, urethra and genital structures of the male and female.

urography, a general term for the radiographic visualization of the urinary tract, using a radiopaque contrast medium. Types include **intravenous urography, retrograde pyelography, cystography.**

urokinase, an enzyme, produced in the kidney and found in urine, that is a potent plasminogen activator of the fibrinolytic system.

urolagnia, sexual stimulation gained from acts involving urine, such as watching people urinate or a desire to urinate on other persons.

urolithiasis. See **urinary calculus.**

urologist, a specialist in the practice of urology.

urology, the branch of medicine concerned with the study of the anatomy and physiology, disorders and care of the urinary tract in men and women, as well as of the male genital tract.

uromelus. See **sympus monopus.**

uropathy, any disease, or abnormal condition of any structure, of the urinary tract. **uropathic,** *adj.*

uroporphyria, a rare genetic disease characterized by excessive secretion of uroporphyrin in the urine, blistering dermatitis, photosensitivity, splenomegaly and haemolytic anaemia.

uroporphyrin, a porphyrin normally excreted in the urine in small amounts.

uroradiology, the radiological study of the urinary tract.

urorectal septum, a ridge of mesoderm covered with endoderm; in the early developing embryo, it divides the endodermal cloaca into the urogenital sinus and the rectum.

urostomy, the diversion of urine away from a diseased or defective bladder, through a surgically created opening, or stoma, in the skin.

ursodeoxycholic acid, a secondary bile salt. It is given by mouth to dissolve cholesterol gallstones.

urticaria, a pruritic skin eruption characterized by transient wheals of varying shapes and sizes, with well-defined erythematous margins and pale centres. It is caused by capillary dilatation in the dermis, resulting from the release of vasoactive mediators. **urticarial,** *adj.*

urticaria pigmentosa, an uncommon form of mastocytosis characterized by pigmented skin lesions that usually begin in infancy and become urticarial on mechanical or chemical irritation.

urushiol, a toxic resin in the sap of certain plants of the genus *Rhus*, such as poison ivy, poison oak and poison sumac. It produces allergic contact dermatitis in a number of people.

useful radiation, the portion of direct radiation that is permitted to pass from an x-ray tube housing through the tube head port, aperture or collimator. Also called **useful beam.**

user documentation. See **documentation.**

user-friendly, pertaining to computer hardware or software designed to assist the user by presenting operating information or instructions in a form that is familiar and easy to understand.

use test, a procedure used to identify offending allergens in foods, cosmetics or fabrics, by the systematic elimination and addition of specific items associated with the lifestyle of the patient involved.

U-shaped arch, a dental arch in which there is little difference in width between the first premolars and last molars, and the curve from canine to canine is abrupt and U-shaped.

uterine cancer, any malignancy of the uterus. It may be cervical cancer affecting the cervix, or endometrial cancer affecting the lining of the uterus.

uterine inertia, an abnormal relaxation of the uterus during labour.

uterine retroversion, a position of the uterus in which the body of the uterus is directed away from the midline, towards the back. Mild degrees of retroversion are common and have no clinical significance.

uterine tenaculum. See **tenaculum.**

uterine tube, one of a pair of ducts opening at one end into the uterus and at the other end into the peritoneal cavity, over the ovary. Each tube serves as the passage through which an ovum is carried to the uterus and through which spermatozoa move out towards the ovary.

uteritis. See **metritis.**

uteroglobulin. See **blastokinin.**

uterovesical. See **vesicouterine.**

uterus, the hollow, pear-shaped internal female organ of reproduction in which the fertilized ovum is implanted and the fetus develops, and from which the decidua of menses flows. Its anterior surface lies on the superior surface of the bladder. The uterus is composed of three layers: endometrium, myometrium and parametrium. The endometrium lines the uterus, and becomes thicker and more vascular in pregnancy and during the second-half of the menstrual cycle under the influence of the hormone progesterone. The myometrium is the muscular layer of the organ. The parametrium is the outermost layer of the uterus; it is composed of serous connective tissue and extends laterally into the broad ligament. During pregnancy, it can grow to many times its usual size, almost entirely by cellular hypertrophy. The uterus has two parts: a body and a cervix. The body extends from the fundus to the cervix, just above the isthmus. The cavity within the body is only a potential space. The walls of the body touch, unless the woman is pregnant. The cervix has a vaginal portion, protruding into the vagina, and a supravaginal portion at the juncture of the lower uterine segment.

uterus masculinis. See **prostatic utricle.**

UTI, abbreviation for **urinary tract infection.**

utilitarianism, a doctrine that the purpose of all action should be to bring about the greatest happiness for the greatest number of people, and that the value of anything is determined by its utility.

utricle, larger of two membranous pouches in the vestibule of the membranous labyrinth of the ear. It is an oblong structure that communicates with the semicircular ducts by five openings, and receives utricular filaments of the acoustic nerve.

utriculosaccular duct, a duct connecting the utricle with an endolymphatic duct of the membranous labyrinth.

uvea, the fibrous tunic beneath the sclera that includes the iris, ciliary body and choroid of the eye. **uveal,** *adj.*

uveitis, inflammation of the uveal tract of the eye, including the iris, ciliary body and choroid. It may be characterized by an irregularly shaped pupil, inflammation around the cornea, pus in the anterior chamber, opaque deposits on the cornea, pain and lacrimation.

uvula, *pl.* **uvulae,** the small, cone-shaped process, suspended in the mouth from the middle of the posterior border of the soft palate. **uvular,** *adj.*

uvulitis, inflammation of the uvula. Common causes are allergy and infection.

V, symbol for vanadium.

V, 1. symbol for **rate of gas flow.** 2. symbol for volt.

v, abbreviation for venous blood.

V deflection (HBE), a deflection on an electrocardiogram that represents ventricular activation.

VAC, an anticancer drug combination of vincristine, dactinomycin, and cyclophosphamide.

vaccination, any injection of attenuated micro-organisms, such as bacteria, viruses or rickettsiae, administered to induce immunity or reduce the effects of associated infectious diseases. **vaccinate,** *v.*

vaccine, a suspension of attenuated or killed micro-organisms, or extracts prepared from them, administered intradermally, intramuscularly, orally or subcutaneously, to induce active immunity to infectious disease.

vaccinia, an infectious disease of cattle caused by a poxvirus that may be transmitted to humans by direct contact or deliberate inoculation as a protection against smallpox. A pustule develops at the site of infection, usually followed by malaise and fever that last for several days. After 2 weeks the pustule becomes a crust that eventually drops off, leaving a scar.

vacuole, 1. a clear or fluid-filled space or cavity within a cell, as when a droplet of water is ingested by the cytoplasm. 2. a small space in the body enclosed by a membrane, usually containing fat, secretions or cellular debris. **vacuolar, vacuolated,** *adj.*

vacuum aspiration, a method of abortion in which the fetus and placenta are removed by suction to terminate an early pregnancy, up to the fourteenth week.

vagal, of, or pertaining to, the vagus nerve.

vagina, the part of the female genitalia that forms a canal from the orifice through the vestibule to the uterine cervix. It is behind the bladder and in front of the rectum. The canal is actually a potential space; the walls usually touch. The vagina widens from the vestibule upwards, and narrows towards the top, forming a curved vault around the protruding cervix. The vagina is lined with mucosa covering a layer of erectile tissue and muscle.

vagina bulbi. See **fascia bulbi.**

vaginal bleeding, an abnormal condition in which blood is passed from the vagina, other than during the menses. It may be caused by abnormalities of the uterus or cervix. The following terms are commonly used in describing the approximate amount of vaginal bleeding: **heavy vaginal bleeding,** which is greater than heaviest normal menstrual flow; **moderate vaginal bleeding,** which is equal to heaviest normal menstrual flow; **light vaginal bleeding,** which is less than heaviest normal menstrual flow; **vaginal staining,** which is a very light flow of blood, barely requiring the use of a sanitary towel or tampon; **vaginal spotting,** which is the vaginal passage of a few drops of blood; **bloody show,** which is an episode of light vaginal bleeding as often occurs in early labour, during labour, and particularly at the time of full dilatation of the cervix at the end of the first stage of labour.

vaginal cancer, a malignancy of the vagina occurring rarely as a primary neoplasm and more often as a secondary lesion or extension of vulvar, cervical, endometrial or ovarian cancer. Clear cell adenocarcinoma occurs in young women exposed in utero to diethylstilbestrol given to their mothers to prevent abortion. A predisposing factor is cervical carcinoma. Vaginal leukoplakia, erythematosis, erosion or granulation of the mucosa may prove to be carcinoma in situ. Symptoms of invasive lesions are postmenopausal bleeding, purulent discharge, pain and dysuria.

vaginal discharge, any discharge from the vagina. A clear or pearly-white discharge normal. The discharge is largely composed of secretions of the endocervical glands. Inflammatory conditions of the vagina and cervix often cause an increase in the discharge, which may have a foul odour and cause pruritus of the perineum and external genitalia.

vaginal fornix, a recess in the upper part of the vagina, caused by protrusion of the uterine cervix into the vagina.

vaginal instillation of medication, the instillation of a medicated cream, suppository or gel into the vagina, usually performed to treat a local infection of the vagina or uterine cervix.

vaginal jelly, a jelly-like product intended for vaginal application. It often contains a spermicide for use in conjunction with a contraceptive diaphragm or cervical cap. Some antibiotic medications are also supplied in the form of a vaginal jelly.

vaginal spotting, vaginal staining. See **vaginal bleeding.**

vaginismus, a psychophysiological genital

reaction of women, characterized by intense contraction of the perineal and paravaginal musculature tightly closing the vaginal introitus. It occurs in response to fear of painful intromission prior to coitus or pelvic examination. Vaginismus is considered abnormal if it occurs in the absence of genital lesions, and if it conflicts with a woman's desire to participate in coition or permit examination. However, it may be a normal or physiological response if painful genital conditions exist or forcible or premature intromission is anticipated.

vaginitis, an inflammation of the vaginal tissues, such as trichomonas vaginitis.

vagotomy, the cutting of certain branches of the vagus nerve, performed with gastric surgery, to reduce the amount of gastric acid secreted and lessen the chance of recurrence of a gastric ulcer. Because peristalsis will be diminished, an anastomosis of the stomach to the jejunum is done to assure proper emptying of the stomach.

vagotonus, an abnormal increase in the activity and effects of stimulation of the vagus nerve, especially bradycardia with decreased cardiac output, faintness and syncope.

vagovagal reflex, stimulation of the vagus nerve by a reflex in which irritation of the larynx or trachea results in slowing of the pulse rate.

vagueness, a communication pattern involving the use of global pronouns and loose associations that lead to ambiguity and confusion in communication.

vagus nerve, either of the longest pair of cranial nerves essential for speech, swallowing, and the sensibilities and functions of many parts of the body. The vagus nerves communicate through 13 main branches, connecting to four areas in the brain.

valence, 1. (in chemistry) a numeric expression of the capability of an element to combine chemically with atoms of hydrogen or their equivalent. A negative valence indicates the number of hydrogen atoms to which one atom of a chemical element can bond. A positive valence indicates the number of hydrogen atoms that one atom of a chemical element can displace. **2.** (in immunology) an expression of the number of antigen-binding sites for one molecule of any given antibody or the number of antibody-binding sites for any given antigen.

valence electron, any of the outermost orbiting electrons of an atom. They are responsible for the bonding of atoms into crystals, molecules and compounds.

valeric acid, an organic acid with a penetrating odour, found in the roots of *Valeriana officinalis.*

valgus, an abnormal position in which a part of a limb is bent or twisted outwards, away from the midline, as the heel of the foot in **talipes valgus.**

validation, 1. an agreement of the listener with certain elements of the patient's communication. **2.** The process of approving courses through a university.

validity, (in research) the extent to which a test measurement or other device measures what it is intended to measure. Kinds of validity include **content validity, current validity, construct validity, face validity** and **predictive validity.**

valine (Val), an essential amino acid needed for optimal growth in infants and for nitrogen equilibrium in adults.

vallecula, 1. any groove or furrow on the surface of an organ or structure. **2.** See vallecula epiglottica. **vallecular,** *adj.*

vallecula epiglottica, a furrow between the glossoepiglottic folds of each side of the posterior oropharynx. Also called *(informal)* vallecula.

vallecular dysphagia, difficulty or pain on swallowing, caused by inflammation of the vallecula epiglottica.

valley fever. See **coccidioidomycosis.**

valproate, an anticonvulsant used to treat all types of epilepsy.

valproic acid. See **valproate.**

Valsalva's manoeuvre {Antonio M. Valsalva, Italian surgeon, b. 1666}, any forced expiratory effort against a closed airway, as when an individual holds the breath and tightens the muscles in a concerted, strenuous effort to move a heavy object or to change position in bed. Most healthy individuals perform Valsalva's manoeuvres during normal daily activities, without any injurious consequences.

Valsalva's test {Antonio Valsalva}, a method for testing the patency of the eustachian tubes. With mouth and nose kept tightly closed, a forced expiratory effort is made; if the eustachian tubes are open, air will enter into the middle ear cavities.

value, a personal belief about the worth of a given idea or behaviour.

value clarification, a method whereby a person can discover his or her own values by assessing and determining what those personal values are and how they affect personal decision making.

value system, the accepted mode of conduct and the set of norms, goals and values binding any social group.

valve, a natural structure or artificial device in a passage or vessel that prevents reflux of the fluid contents passing through it. **valvular,** *adj.*

valve of Kerkring. See **circular fold.**

valve of lymphatics, one of the tiny semilunar structures in the vessels and trunks of the lymphatic system, that help regulate the flow of lymph and prevent venous blood from entering the system. There are no valves in the capillaries of the system, but there are many in the collecting vessels.

valvotomy, the incision into a valve, especially one in the heart, to correct a defect and allow proper opening and closure.

valvular heart disease, an acquired or congenital disorder of a cardiac valve. It is characterized by stenosis and obstructed blood flow, or valvular degeneration and regurgitation of blood. Diseases of aortic and mitral valves are most common and may be caused by congenital defects, bacterial endocarditis, syphilis or, most frequently, rheumatic fever. Valvular dysfunction results in changes in intracardiac pressure and pulmonary and peripheral circulation. It may lead to cardiac arrhythmia, heart failure and cardiogenic shock. Malaise, anorexia, embolism, pulmonary oedema and ventricular failure often accompany valvular heart disease. In moderate or severe **aortic stenosis,** pulse pressure is decreased; the carotid pulse is small and slow with a long upstroke, but the apical pulse may be strong and sustained during systole. The patient may experience anginal pain and syncope, and electrocardiography may show evidence of left ventricular hypertrophy, conduction defects or complete heart block. Characteristic signs of aortic regurgitation are dyspnoea, profuse sweating, flushed skin, pounding pulsations in neck arteries and a blowing heart murmur throughout diastole. The patient with **mitral stenosis** tires easily, is short of breath on exertion, may have paroxysmal nocturnal dyspnoea, and may develop haemoptysis and systemic embolism. Mitral regurgitation is typified by dyspnoea, fatigue, intolerance of exercise, heart palpitation and a large, laterally placed apical pulse. **Tricuspid stenosis** is relatively uncommon, usually associated with lesions in other valves resulting from rheumatic fever; in rare cases, it is caused by carcinoid heart disease or endomyocardial fibrosis. Characteristics of tricuspid stenosis are a diastolic pressure gradient between the right atrium and ventricle, jugular vein distention, pulmonary congestion and, in severe cases, hepatic congestion and splenomegaly. **Pulmonic stenosis** may cause the intraventricular septum to bulge into the right ventricular chamber, and regurgitation is a consequence of severe pulmonary hypertension.

valvular stenosis, a narrowing or constricture of any of the valves of the heart. The condition may result from a congenital defect or some disease process.

valvulitis, an inflammatory condition of a valve, especially a cardiac valve. Inflammatory changes in the aortic, mitral and tricuspid valves of the heart are most commonly caused by rheumatic fever and less frequently by bacterial endocarditis and syphilis.

VAMP, abbreviation for a combination drug regimen, used in the treatment of cancer containing three cytotoxic drugs (vincristine sulphate, methotrexate and mercaptopurine) and a corticosteroid (prednisolone).

van Bogaert's disease {Ludo van Bogaert 20th century Belgian physician}, a rare familial disorder of lipid metabolism in which the substance cholestanol is deposited in the nervous system, blood and connective tissue. Persons with the disease develop progressive ataxia and dementia, premature atherosclerosis, cataracts and xanthomas on the tendons.

Van de Graaff generator {Robert J. Van de Graaff, American physicist, b. 1901}, an electrostatic machine in which electronically charged particles build up a high potential on an insulated terminal. The generator is often used to inject particles into a larger accelerator.

Van Deemter's equation, an expression of a gas chromatography relationship between the height equivalent to the theoretical plate (HEPT) to the linear velocity of the carrier gas.

van den Bergh's test {Albert A. H. van den Bergh, Dutch physician, b. 1869}, a test for the presence of bilirubin in the blood serum. Blood is obtained from a patient who has fasted overnight, and the diluted serum is added to diazo reagent. A blue or violet colour indicates the presence of bilirubin.

van der Waals forces, weak attractive forces between neutral atoms and molecules. They occur because a fluctuating dipole moment in one molecule induces a dipole moment in another. The activity accounts for some deviation from Boyle's law at very low temperatures or very high pressures.

vanadium (V), a greyish metallic element. Its atomic number is 23 and its atomic weight is 50.942. Absorption of vanadium compounds results in a condition called vanadiumism, characterized by anaemia, conjunctivitis, pneumonitis and irritation of the respiratory tract.

vancomycin, a glycopeptide antibiotic used in the treatment of severe infections, particularly staphylococcal infections resistant to other antibiotics. It is not absorbed after oral administration, and is only given orally for the treatment of pseudomembranous colitis.

vanillylmandelic acid (VMA), a urinary metabolite of adrenaline and noradrenaline. A greater than normal amount of VMA is characteristic of phaeochromocytoma and neuroblastomas.

vapour pressure depression, a phenomenon in which the addition of a solute molecule to a solvent will decrease the amount of solvent in equilibrium between the vapour phase and the liquid phase.

variable behaviour, a response, activity or action that may be modified by individual experience. Compare **invariable behav-**

iour.

variable interval (VI) reinforcement, reinforcement that occurs after different lapses of time, following a response.

variable ratio (VR) reinforcement, reinforcement that occurs only sometimes, following a response.

variable region, the N-terminal portion of an immunoglobulin polypeptide chain whose amino acid sequence can change. The region includes the antigen combining site.

variable-performance oxygen delivery system. See **low-flow oxygen delivery system.**

variance, 1. (in statistics) a numerical representation of the dispersion of data around the mean in a given sample. It is represented by the square of the standard deviation, and is used principally in performing an analysis of variance. **2.** *non-technical,* the general range of a group of findings.

varicella zoster immunoglobulin (VZI), a passive immunizing agent, used for preventing or attenuating herpes zoster virus infection in immunosuppressed individuals who have been exposed to herpes zoster virus, or are at great risk of severe herpes zoster virus infection.

varicella zoster virus (VZV), a member of the herpesvirus family, which causes the diseases varicella (chickenpox) and herpes zoster (shingles). The virus has been isolated from vesicle fluid in chickenpox; it is highly contagious and may be spread by direct contact or droplets. Dried crusts of skin lesions do not contain active virus particles. Herpes zoster is produced by reactivation of latent varicella virus, usually several years after the initial infection.

varicella. See **chickenpox.**

varicelliform, resembling the rash of chickenpox.

varicocele, a dilatation of the pampiniform venous complex of the spermatic cord. The varicocele forms a soft, elastic swelling that can cause pain.

varicose, 1. (of a vein) exhibiting varicosis or a varicosity. **2.** abnormally and permanently distended, such as the bulging veins in some individuals.

varicose aneurysm, a blood-filled, sac-like projection that connects an artery and one or several veins, formed from a localized dilatation of the adjoining vessels.

varicose ulcer. See **stasis ulcer.**

varicose vein, a tortuous, dilated vein with incompetent valves. Causes include congenitally defective valves, thrombophlebitis, pregnancy and obesity. Varicose veins are common, especially in women. The saphenous veins of the legs are most often affected.

varicosis, a common condition characterized by one or more tortuous, abnormally dilated or varicose veins, usually in the legs

or lower trunk. Varicosis may be caused by congenital defects of the valves or walls of the veins, or by congestion and increased intraluminal pressure resulting from prolonged standing, poor posture, pregnancy, abdominal tumour or chronic systemic disease. Symptoms include pain and muscle cramps with a feeling of fullness and heaviness in the legs. Dilatation of superficial veins is often evident before the condition produces discomfort.

varicosity, 1. an abnormal condition, usually of a vein, characterized by swelling and tortuosity. **2.** a vein in this condition.

variegate, having characteristics that vary, especially in terms of colour.

variegate porphyria, an uncommon form of hepatic porphyria, characterized by skin lesions and photosensitivity. The condition may be congenital or acquired. See also **porphyria.**

variola, variola major. See **smallpox.**

variola minor. See **alastrim.**

varioloid, 1. resembling smallpox. **2.** a mild form of smallpox in a vaccinated person or one who has previously had the disease.

varix, *pl.* **varices, 1.** a tortuous, dilated vein. **2.** an enlarged, tortuous artery or a distended, twisting lymphatic.

varus, an abnormal position in which a part of a limb is turned inwards, toward the midline; for example, the heel and foot in **talipes varus.** Compare **valgus.**

vas, *pl.* **vasa,** any one of the several vessels of the body, especially those that convey blood, lymph or spermatozoa.

vas deferens, *pl.* **vasa deferentia,** the extension of the epididymis of the testis that ascends from the scrotum and joins the seminal vesicle to form the ejaculatory duct.

vascular, of, or pertaining to, a blood vessel.

vascular haemophilia. See **Von Willebrand's disease.**

vascular insufficiency, inadequate peripheral blood flow caused by occlusion of vessels with atherosclerotic plaques, thrombi or emboli, by damaged, diseased or intrinsically weak vascular walls, arteriovenous fistulas, haematological hypercoagulability or heavy smoking. Signs of vascular insufficiency include pale, cyanotic or mottled skin over the affected area, swelling of an extremity, absent or reduced tactile sensation, tingling, diminished sense of temperature, muscle pain, such as intermittent claudication in the calf and, in advanced disease, atrophy of muscles of the involved extremity.

vascular leiomyoma, a neoplasm that has developed from smooth muscle fibres of a blood vessel.

vascular spider. See **spider angioma.**

vascularization, the process by which body tissue becomes vascular and develops proliferating capillaries. It may be natural or induced by surgical techniques. **vascularize,** *v.*

vasculitis, an inflammatory condition of the blood vessels. It is characteristic of certain systemic diseases, or results from an allergic reaction. Kinds of vasculitis are **allergic vasculitis, necrotizing vasculitis** and **segmented hyalinizing vasculitis.**

vasectomy, a procedure for male sterilization, involving the bilateral surgical removal of a portion of the vas deferens. Vasectomy is most commonly performed as an office procedure using local anaesthesia.

vasoactive, (of a drug) tending to cause vasodilation or vasoconstriction.

vasoactive intestinal polypeptide (VIP), a hormone found in the pancreas, intestine and central nervous system. It is a member of the glucagon-secretin group of hormones and has a number of actions, including stimulation of insulin and glucagon release.

vasoconstriction, a narrowing of the lumen of any blood vessel, especially the arterioles and veins in the blood reservoirs of skin and abdominal viscera. It is accomplished by various mechanisms that together control blood pressure and distribution of blood throughout the body.

vasoconstrictor, 1. of, or pertaining to, a process, condition or substance that causes constriction of blood vessels. **2.** an agent that promotes vasoconstriction. Cold, fear, stress and nicotine are common exogenous vasoconstrictors. Internally secreted adrenaline and noradrenaline cause blood vessels to constrict by stimulating their adrenergic receptors.

vasodilatation, widening or distention of blood vessels, particularly arterioles, usually caused by nerve impulses or certain drugs that relax smooth muscle in the walls of blood vessels.

vasodilator, 1. a nerve or agent that causes dilatation of blood vessels. **2.** pertaining to the relaxation of smooth muscle of the vascular system. **3.** producing dilatation of blood vessels.

vasogenic shock, shock resulting from peripheral vascular dilatation produced by factors, such as toxins, that directly affect the blood vessels.

vasomotor, of, or pertaining to, the nerves and muscles that control the calibre of the lumen of blood vessels. Circularly arranged fibres of the muscles of arteries can contract, causing vasoconstriction; when they relax, they cause vasodilatation.

vasomotor centre, a collection of cell bodies in the medulla oblongata of the brain. It regulates or modulates blood pressure and cardiac function primarily via the autonomic nervous system.

vasomotor rhinitis, chronic rhinitis and nasal obstruction, in the absence of allergy or infection, characterized by sneezing, rhinorrhoea, nasal obstruction and vascular engorgement of the mucous membranes of the nose.

vasomotor system, the part of the nervous system that controls the constriction and dilatation of the blood vessels.

vasopressin. See **antidiuretic hormone.**

vasopressor. See **vasoconstrictor.**

vasospasm, a former term for **angiospasm.**

vasospastic, 1. relating to a spasmodic constriction of a blood vessel. **2.** any agent that produces spasms of the blood vessels.

vasospastic angina, an ischaemic myocardial chest pain caused by spasms of the coronary arteries. It has features that differ from exertional angina.

vasovagal syncope, a sudden loss of consciousness, resulting from cerebral ischaemia secondary to decreased cardiac output, peripheral vasodilation and bradycardia. The condition may be triggered by pain, fright or trauma, and may be accompanied by symptoms of nausea, pallor and perspiration.

vasovasostomy, a surgical procedure in which the function of the vas deferens on each side of the testes is restored, having been cut and ligated in a preceding vasectomy. The procedure is performed if a man wants to regain his fertility.

vastus intermedius, one of the four muscles of the quadriceps femoris, situated in the cente of the thigh. It functions with the other three muscles of the quadriceps to extend the leg.

vastus internus. See **vastus medialis.**

vastus lateralis, the largest of the four muscles of the quadriceps femoris, situated on the lateral side of the thigh. It functions to help extend the leg.

vastus medialis, one of the four muscles of the quadriceps femoris, situated in the medial portion of the thigh. It functions in combination with other parts of the quadriceps femoris to extend the leg.

Vater-Pacini corpuscles {Abraham Vater, German anatomist, b. 1684; Filippo Pacini, Italian anatomist, b. 1812}, kinesioceptors located in joint capsules and ligaments.

VC, abbreviation for **vital capacity.**

VD, abbreviation for **venereal disease.**

VDRL test, abbreviation for **Venereal Disease Research Laboratory test,** a serological flocculation test for syphilis. It is also positive in other treponemal diseases, such as yaws.

VDT, abbreviation for **video display terminal.**

VE, symbol for **volume expired in 1 minute.**

Ve, symbol for **expired volume.**

vector, 1. a quantity having direction and magnitude. It is usually depicted by a straight arrow, with its length representing magnitude and its head representing direction. **2.** a carrier, especially one that transmits disease. **A biological vector** is usually an arthropod in which the infecting organism completes part of its lifecycle. A **mechanical vector** transmits the infecting organism from one host to another but is not essential to the lifecycle of the parasite. **3**. a retrovirus that has been modified by alteration of its genetic component. Through recombinant DNA techniques, genes that cause harmful effects are removed and genes that mediate synthesis of essential enzymes are added. The vector can then be injected into a patient who suffers from an enzyme deficiency. **vector**, *v.*, **vectorial**, *adj.*

vecuronium bromide, an intravenous, non-depolarizing, neuromuscular blocking drug. It is used as an adjunct to general anaesthesia, to facilitate endotracheal intubation, and to relax skeletal muscles during surgery or mechanical ventilation.

vegan. a vegetarian whose diet excludes the use of all foods of animal origin.

veganism, the adherence to a strict vegetable diet, with the exclusion of all foods of animal origin.

vegetable albumin, albumin produced in plants.

vegetal pole, the relatively inactive part of the ovum protoplasm where the food yolk is situated, usually opposite the animal pole.

vegetarian, a person whose diet is restricted to foods of vegetable origin, including fruits, grains and nuts. Many vegetarians eat eggs and milk products but avoid all animal flesh. Kinds of vegetarians are **lacto-ovo-vegetarian, lacto-vegetarian, ovo-vegetarian** and **vegan.**

vegetarianism, the theory or practice of restricting the diet to food substances that are of vegetable origin.

vegetation, an abnormal growth of tissue around a valve, composed of fibrin, platelets and bacteria.

vegetative, 1. of, or pertaining to, nutrition and growth. **2.** of, or pertaining to, the plant kingdom. **3.** denoting involuntary function, as produced by the parasympathetic nervous system. **4.** resting, not active; denoting the stage of the cell cycle in which the cell is not replicating. **5.** leading a secluded, dull existence without social or intellectual activity. **6.** (in psychiatry) emotionally withdrawn and passive, as may occur in the depressive phase of bipolar disorder. **vegetate,** *v.*

vegetative nervous system. See autonomic nervous system.

vehicle, 1. an inert substance with which a medication is mixed to facilitate measurement and administration or application. **2.** any fluid or structure in the body that passively conveys a stimulus.

Veillon tube, a transparent tube whose ends are closed with removable stoppers, one cotton and one rubber. It is used for the laboratory growth of bacteriological cultures.

Veillonella {Adrien Veillon, French bacteriologist, b. 1864}, a genus of gram-negative anaerobic bacteria. The species *Veillonella parvula* is normally present in the alimentary tract, especially in the mouth.

vein, one of the many vessels that convey blood from the capillaries to the heart as part of the pulmonary venous system, the systemic venous network or the portal venous complex. Most of the veins in the body are systemic veins that convey blood from the whole body (except the lungs) to the right atrium of the heart. Each vein is a macroscopic structure enclosed in three layers of different kinds of tissue homologous with the layers of the heart. Deep veins course through the more internal parts of the body, and superficial veins lie near the surface where many of them can be seen through the skin. Veins have thinner coatings and are less elastic than arteries, and collapse when cut. They also contain semilunar valves at various intervals.

vein ligation and stripping, a surgical procedure consisting of the ligation of the saphenous vein and its removal from groin to ankle.

vein lumen, the central opening through which blood flows in a vein.

vein of Thebesius. See smallest cardiac vein.

veins of the vertebral column, the veins that drain blood from the vertebral column, adjacent muscles and meninges of the spinal cord.

velamentous insertion of the cord, a term to denote that umbilical cord vessels divide before reaching the placenta.

vellus hair. See lanugo.

velocity, the rate of change in the position of a body moving in a particular direction. Velocity along a straight line is linear velocity. Angular velocity is that of a body in circular motion.

velocity of growth, the rate of growth or change in growth measurements over a period of time.

velocity of ultrasound, the speed of ultrasound energy, measured in meters per second (m/sec), in a particular medium. The velocity varies from 331 m/sec in air, to 1450 m/sec in fat, 1570 m/sec in blood, and 4080 m/sec in the skull.

velocity spectrum rehabilitation, a rehabilitation programme that uses strength training at multiple speeds of movement, from slow to fast.

velopharyngeal closure, the blocking of any escape of air by the raising of the soft palate and contraction of the posterior pharyngeal wall.

velopharyngeal insufficiency, an abnormal condition resulting from a congenital defect in the structure of the velopharyngeal sphincter: Closure of the oral cavity beneath the nasal passages is not complete. Food may be regurgitated through the nose, and speech is impaired.

Velpeau's bandage {Alfred A. L. M. Velpeau, French surgeon, b. 1795}, a roller bandage that immobilizes the elbow and shoulder by holding the brachium against the side, and the flexed forearm on the chest.

vena cava, *pl.* **venae cavae,** one of two large veins returning blood from the peripheral circulation to the right atrium of the heart. **vena caval,** *adj.*

vena caval syndrome. See **supine hypotension.**

vena cavogram, a radiographic technique to visualize either the inferior or superior vena cava, following introduction of a radiopaque contrast medium into a selected vein.

vena comes, *pl.* **venae comites,** one of the deep paired veins that accompany the smaller arteries, one on each side of the artery. The three vessels are wrapped together in one sheath.

venereal, pertaining to, or caused by, sexual intercourse or genital contact.

venereal disease. See **sexually transmitted disease.**

venereal sore. See **chancre.**

venereal wart. See **condyloma acuminatum.**

venereology, the study of venereal diseases. **venereological,** *adj.*, **venereologist,** *n.*

venerupin poisoning, a potentially fatal form of shellfish poisoning that occurs from ingestion of oysters or clams contaminated with venerupin, a toxin that causes impaired liver functioning, GI distress and leukocytosis. The shellfish toxin occurs in waters around Japan.

venesection. See **phlebotomy.**

venipuncture, a technique in which a vein is punctured transcutaneously by a sharp, rigid stylet or cannula carrying a flexible plastic catheter, or by a steel needle attached to a syringe or catheter. The purpose of the procedure is to withdraw a specimen of blood, perform a phlebotomy, instill a medication, start an intravenous infusion, or inject a radiopaque substance for radiological examination of a part or system of the body.

venography, radiographic visualization of the venous drainage of a specific organ or site, following intravenous administration of a radiopaque contrast medium into a selected vessel. **venogram,** *n.*

venom, a toxic fluid substance secreted by some snakes, arthropods and other animals, and transmitted by their stings or bites.

venom extract therapy, the administration of antivenin as prophylaxis against the toxic effects of the bite of a specific poisonous snake or spider, or other venomous animal.

venom immunotherapy, the reduction of sensitivity to the bite of a venomous insect or animal, by the serial administration of gradually increasing amounts of the specific antigenic substance secreted by the insect or animal.

venotomy, the surgical opening of a vein.

venous, of, or pertaining to, a vein.

venous blood gas, the oxygen and carbon dioxide in venous blood, measured by various methods to assess the adequacy of oxygenation and ventilation and determine the acid-base status. The oxygen tension of venous blood normally averages 40 mm Hg; the dissolved oxygen averages 0.1% by volume, the total oxygen content 15.2%, and the oxygen saturation of venous haemoglobin 75%. The carbon dioxide tension normally averages 46 mm Hg, the dissolved carbon dioxide 2.9% by volume, and the total carbon dioxide content 50%. The normal average pH of venous plasma is 7.37.

venous hum, a continuous murmur heard on auscultation over the major veins at the base of the neck, particularly when the patient is anaemic, upright and looking to the contralateral side.

venous insufficiency, an abnormal circulatory condition characterized by decreased return of venous blood from the legs to the trunk of the body. Oedema is usually the first sign of the condition; pain, varicosities and ulceration may follow.

venous pressure, the stress exerted by circulating blood on the walls of veins, normally 60 to 120 mm of water in peripheral veins but elevated in congestive heart failure, acute or chronic constrictive pericarditis, and in venous obstruction caused by a clot or external pressure against a vein. Central venous pressure, normally 40 to 100 mm of water, is determined by inserting a catheter into a major vein and threading it through the superior vena cava to the right atrium. The catheter is attached by a three-way stopcock to a water manometer.

venous pulse, the pulse of a vein usually palpated over the internal or external jugular veins in the neck. The pulse in the jugular vein is taken to evaluate the pressure of the pulse and form of the pressure wave.

venous sinus, one of several sinuses that collect blood from the dura mater and drain it into the internal jugular vein. Each sinus is formed by the separation of the two layers of dura mater.

venous stasis, a disorder in which the normal flow of blood through a vein is slowed or halted.

venous stasis dermatitis. See **stasis dermatitis.**

venous thrombosis, a condition characterized by the presence of a clot in a vein in which the wall of the vessel is not inflamed. Pain, swelling and inflammation may follow if the vein is significantly occluded.

ventilate, 1. to provide with fresh air. **2.** to

provide the lungs with air from the atmosphere, and to aerate or oxygenate blood in the pulmonary capillaries. **3.** (in psychiatry) to open discussion of something; for example, to ventilate feelings.

ventilation, the process by which gases are moved into and out of the lungs. **ventilatory,** *adj.*

ventilation lung scan, a radionuclide imaging technique in which the patient inhales a radioactive gas while the lungs are scanned using a gamma camera.

ventilation perfusion defect, a disorder in which one or more areas of the lung receive oxygen but no blood, or blood but no oxygen.

ventilation/perfusion (V/Q) ratio, the ratio of pulmonary alveolar ventilation to pulmonary capillary perfusion. Both measured quantities are expressed in the same units.

ventilator, any of several devices used in respiratory therapy to provide assisted respiration and intensive positive pressure breathing. Kinds of ventilators are **pressure ventilator** and **volume ventilator.**

venting, (in intravenous therapy) a method for allowing air to enter the vacuum of the intravenous bottle and displace the intravenous solution as it flows out. Glass intravenous bottles are usually equipped with a venting tube attached to the primary IV tubing, or to a vent port incorporated with the bottle stopper.

ventral, of, or pertaining to, a position towards the abdomen; front; anterior.

ventral hernia. See **abdominal hernia.**

ventricle, a small cavity, such as one of the cavities filled with cerebrospinal fluid in the brain, or the right and left ventricles of the heart.

ventricular, of, or pertaining to, a ventricle.

ventricular aneurysm, a localized dilatation or saccular protrusion in the wall of the left ventricle, occurring most often after a myocardial infarction. Scar tissue is formed in response to the inflammatory changes of the infarction. This tissue weakens the myocardium, allowing its walls to bulge outwards when the ventricle contracts.

ventricular dysfunction, myocardial dysfunction within the ventricles that reflects abnormalities in contraction and wall motion.

ventricular extrasystole, an extrasystole arising from the ventricle.

ventricular fibrillation, a cardiac arrhythmia marked by rapid, disorganized depolarizations of the ventricular myocardium. The condition is characterized by a complete lack of organized electric impulse, conduction and ventricular contraction. Blood pressure falls to zero, resulting in unconsciousness. Death may occur within 4 minutes. Defibrillation and ventilation must be initiated immediately.

ventricular gallop, an abnormal cardiac rhythm in which a low-pitched extra heart sound (S3) is heard early in diastole on auscultation of the heart. When it is heard in an older person with heart disease, it indicates myocardial failure.

ventricular gradient, the algebraic sum of the areas within the QRS complex and within the T wave in the electrocardiogram.

ventricular hemiblock, an impulse blockage of only one division of the left bundle branch, such as an anterior superior or posterior inferior hemiblock.

ventricular septal defect (VSD), an abnormal opening in the septum separating the ventricles. It permits blood to flow from the left ventricle to the right ventricle, and recirculate through the pulmonary artery and lungs. It is the most common congenital heart defect.

ventricular tachycardia, tachycardia that usually originates in the ventricular Purkinje system.

ventriculoatrial shunt, a surgically created passage, consisting of plastic tubing and one-way valves, implanted between a cerebral ventricle and right atrium of the heart to drain excess cerebrospinal fluid from the brain in hydrocephalus.

ventriculocisternostomy, a surgical procedure performed to treat hydrocephalus. An opening is created that allows cerebrospinal fluid to drain through a shunt from the ventricles of the brain into the cisterna magna.

ventriculofallopian tube shunt, a surgical procedure with limited effectiveness for diverting cerebrospinal fluid into the peritoneal cavity. This procedure is used to correct both obstructive and communicating types of hydrocephalus.

ventriculography, 1. an imaging technique to visualize the ventricles of the heart. This is either a radiographic technique, following introduction of a radiopaque contrast medium, or radionuclide imaging, using radiolabelled red blood cells and a gamma camera. **2.** *(historical)* a radiographic technique to visualize the ventricles of the brain, usually following introduction of a radiolucent contrast medium such as air. **ventriculogram,** *n.*

ventriculoperitoneal shunt, a surgically created passageway, consisting of plastic tubing and one-way valves, between a cerebral ventricle and the peritoneum; it is performed for the draining of excess cerebrospinal fluid from the brain in hydrocephalus.

ventriculoperitoneostomy, a surgical procedure for temporarily diverting cerebrospinal fluid in hydrocephalus, usually in the newborn. In this procedure, a polyethylene tube is passed from the lateral ventricle subcutaneously down the dorsal spine, and is reinserted into the peritoneal cavity where the diverted fluid is absorbed.

ventriculopleural shunt, a surgical procedure for diverting cerebrospinal fluid from engorged ventricles in hydrocephalus, usually in the newborn. In this procedure, cerebrospinal fluid is diverted from the lateral ventricle into the pleural cavity.

ventriculostomy. See **ventriculocisternostomy.**

ventriculoureterostome, a surgical procedure for directing cerebrospinal fluid into the general circulation. It is performed in the treatment of hydrocephalus, usually in the newborn. In this procedure, a polyethylene tube is passed from the lateral ventricle down the dorsal spine subcutaneously to the twelfth rib; the tube is inserted through the paraspinal muscles into a ureter.

Venturi effect {Giovanni B. Venturi, Italian physicist, b. 1746}, a modification of the Bernoulli effect in which there is dilatation of a gas passage just beyond an obstruction or restriction. The principle is used in respiratory therapy equipment for mixing medical gases.

Venturi mask, a respiratory therapy face mask designed to allow entrained air to mix with oxygen, which is supplied through a jet at a fixed concentration.

venule, any one of the small blood vessels that gather blood from the capillary plexuses and anastomose to form the veins. **venular,** *adj.*

VEP, abbreviation for visual evoked potential.

veracity, a term that describes the obligation of healthcare professionals to be truthful in their interactions with patients and clients.

verapamil, a slow channel blocker or calcium ion antagonist. It is used for the treatment of angina pectoris, hypertension and cardiac arrhythmias.

Veratrum, a genus of poisonous herbs of the lily family. The dried rhizomes of the British and American hellebore provide alkaloids that are used as antihypertensive agents.

verbal aphasia. See **motor aphasia.**

verbal language, a culturally organized system of vocal sounds, communicating meaning between individuals.

vergence, movement of the two eyes in opposite directions.

verification, (in radiotherapy) a technique to check the planned treatment parameters for an individual patient, usually prior to commencement of the course.

vermicide, an agent that kills worms, particularly those in the intestine.

vermiform appendix, a worm-like, blunt process extending from the caecum. Its length varies from 8 to 16 cm, and its diameter is about 1 cm.

vermifuge, an agent that causes the evacuation of parasitic worms.

vermilion border, the external pinkish to red area of the upper and lower lips; it extends from the junction of the lips with the surrounding facial skin on the exterior, to the labial mucosa within the mouth.

vermis, 1. a worm. 2. a structure resembling a worm, such as the median lobe of the cerebellum. **vermiform,** *adj.*

vernal conjunctivitis, a chronic, bilateral form of conjunctivitis, thought to be allergic in origin. Most common symptoms include intense itching and crusting discharge.

Vernet's syndrome {Maurice Vernet, French neurologist, b. 1887}, a neurological disorder caused by injury to the ninth, tenth and eleventh cranial nerves as they pass through the jugular foramen when leaving the skull. The patient experiences dysphagia, the voice is nasal and hoarse, and there may be some loss of taste sensations.

Verneuil's neuroma. See **plexiform neuroma.**

vernix caseosa, a greyish-white, cheese-like substance, consisting of sebaceous gland secretions, lanugo and desquamated epithelial cells, that covers the skin of the fetus and newborn.

verruca, a benign, viral, warty skin lesion with a rough, papillomatous surface. It is caused by a common, contagious papovavirus. **verrucose, verrucous,** *adj.*

verruca plana, a small, slightly elevated, smooth, tan or flesh-coloured wart. It sometimes occurs in large numbers on the face, neck, back of the hands, wrists and knees, especially in children.

verruca senillis. See **basal cell papilloma.**

verruca vulgaris. See **verruca.**

verrucous carcinoma, a well-differentiated squamous cell neoplasm of the soft tissue of the oral cavity, larynx or genitalia. A slow-growing carcinoma, it tends to displace rather than invade surrounding tissue; it does not usually metastasize.

verrucous dermatitis, any skin rash with wart-like lesions.

verruga peruana. See **bartonellosis.**

version *rare,* the changing of position of the fetus in the uterus, usually done to facilitate delivery.

vertebra, *pl.* **vertebrae,** any one of the 33 bones of the spinal column, comprising the 7 cervical, 12 thoracic, 5 lumbar, 5 sacral and 4 coccygeal vertebrae. The vertebrae, with the exception of the first and second cervical vertebrae, are very similar and are composed of a body, an arch, a spinous process for muscle attachment, and pairs of pedicles and processes. The first cervical vertebra is called the atlas and has no vertebral body. The second cervical vertebra is called the axis and forms the pivot on which the atlas rotates, permitting the head to turn.

vertebral artery, each of two arteries branching from the subclavian arteries, arising deep in the neck from the cranial and dorsal subclavian surfaces. Each vertebral artery divides into two cervical and five cranial branches, supplying deep neck muscles, the spinal cord and spinal membranes, and the cerebellum.

vertebral body, the weight-supporting, solid, central portion of a vertebra. The pedicles of the arch project from its dorsolateral surfaces.

vertebral column, the flexible structure that forms the longitudinal axis of the skeleton. In the adult, it includes 26 vertebrae arranged in a straight line from the base of the skull to the coccyx. The vertebrae are separated by intervertebral disks. They provide attachment for various muscles, such as the iliocostalis thoracis and longissimus thoracis, which give the column strength and flexibility. In the adult, the five sacral and four coccygeal vertebrae fuse to form the sacrum and coccyx. The vertebral canal courses through the vertebral column and contains the spinal cord. The canal is formed by the posterior arches of the vertebrae.

vertex, 1. the top of the head; crown. 2. the apex or highest point of any structure.

vertex presentation, a fetal presentation in which the vertex of the fetus is the part nearest to the cervical os and can be expected to be born first. It is the most common presentation.

vertical angulation, (in dentistry) the measured angle within the vertical plane at which the central beam of an x-ray is projected relative to a reference in the horizontal or occlusal plane.

vertical plane. See **cardinal frontal plane.**

vertical resorption, a pattern of bone loss in which the alveolar bone adjacent to the affected tooth is destroyed without simultaneous crestal loss. See also **resorption.**

vertical transmission, the transfer of a disease, condition or trait from one generation to the next, either genetically or congenitally, such as the spread of an infection through breast milk or the placenta.

verticosubmental, a part of the skull used as a focal point for radiographic projection. It permits the central ray to pass from the vertex of the skull to its base.

vertigo. See **dizziness.**

very-low-density lipoprotein (VLDL), a plasma protein composed chiefly of triglycerides with small amounts of cholesterol, phospholipid and protein. It transports triglycerides primarily from the liver to peripheral sites in the tissues, for use or storage.

vesical fistula, an abnormal passage communicating with the urinary bladder.

vesical sphincter, a circular muscle surrounding the opening of the urinary bladder.

vesicant, a drug capable of causing tissue necrosis when extravasated.

vesicle, a small bladder or blister, such as a small, thin-walled, raised skin lesion containing clear fluid. **vesicular,** *adj.*

vesicle calculus, a concretion occurring in the bladder.

vesicle reflex, the sensation of a need to urinate when the bladder is moderately distended.

vesicoureteral reflux, an abnormal backflow of urine from the bladder to the ureter, resulting from a congenital defect, obstruction of the outlet of the bladder, or infection of the lower urinary tract. Reflux increases the hydrostatic pressure in the ureters and kidneys. The condition is characterized by abdominal or flank pain, enuresis, pyuria, haematuria, proteinuria and bacteriuria accompanied by persistent or recurrent urinary tract infections.

vesicouterine, of, or pertaining to, the bladder and uterus.

vesicular, pertaining to a blister-like condition.

vesicular appendix, a cystic structure on the fimbriated end of each of the uterine tubes. It represents a remnant of the mesonephric ducts.

vesicular breath sound, a normal sound of rustling or swishing heard with a stethoscope over the lung periphery. It is characteristically higher pitched during inspiration and fading rapidly during expiration.

vesicular mole. See **hydatid mole.**

vesiculitis, inflammation of any vesicle, particularly of the seminal vesicles.

vessel, any one of the many tubules throughout the body, that convey fluids such as blood and lymph. The main kinds of vessels are the arteries, veins and lymphatic vessels.

vestibular, of, or pertaining to, a vestibule, such as the vestibular portion of the mouth which lies between the cheeks and the teeth.

vestibular apparatus, the inner ear structures that are associated with the sense of balance and position. It includes the vestibule and semicircular canals.

vestibular function, the sense of balance.

vestibular gland, any one of four small glands, two on each side of the vaginal orifice. The vestibular glands secrete a lubricating substance.

vestibular toxicity, toxic effects (commonly of drugs) on the vestibule of the ear, resulting in dizziness, vertigo and loss of balance.

vestibular-bilateral disorder, a sensory integrative dysfunction characterized by shortened duration nystagmus, poor integration of the two sides of the body and brain, and difficulty in learning to read or compute. The disorder is caused by underreactive vestibular responses.

vestibule, a space or cavity that serves as the entrance to a passage, such as the vestibule of the vagina or vestibule of the ear.

vestibulo-ocular reflex, a normal reflex in which eye position compensates for movement of the head. It is induced by excitation of the vestibular apparatus.

vestibulocochlear nerve. See **auditory nerve.**

vestige, an imperfectly developed, relatively useless organ or other structure of the body that had a vital function at an earlier stage of life or in a more primitive form of life. **vestigial,** *adj.*

viable, capable of developing, growing and otherwise sustaining life, as a normal human fetus at 28 weeks of gestation. **viability,** *n.*

vial, a glass container with a metal-enclosed rubber seal.

vibration, a type of massage administered by quick tapping with the fingertips, alternating the fingers in a rhythmic manner, or by a mechanical device.

vibrio, any bacterium that is curved and motile, such as those belonging to the genus *Vibrio.* Cholera and several other epidemic forms of gastroenteritis are caused by members of the genus.

Vibrio cholerae, the species of comma-shaped, motile bacillus that is the cause of cholera.

vibrio gastroenteritis, an infectious disease acquired from contaminated seafood. It is characterized by nausea, vomiting, abdominal pain and diarrhoea, and is caused by *Vibrio parahaemolyticus.* Headache, mild fever and bloody stools may also be present.

Vibrio parahaemolyticus, a species of micro-organisms of the genus *Vibrio,* the causative agent in food poisoning associated with the ingestion of uncooked or under-cooked shellfish, especially crabs and shrimp. Thorough cooking of seafood prevents the infection, which causes watery diarrhoea, abdominal cramps, vomiting, headache, chills and fever.

vicarious liability, the liability of an individual or organization for acts of other people, usually employees.

vicarious menstruation, discharge of blood from a site other than the uterus at the time when the menstrual flow is normally expected. Such bleeding is usually caused by the increased capillary permeability that occurs during menstruation.

victimology, a psychological and psychiatric speciality which studies the experience of people who have been victims of disasters, accidents, combat, torture, rape, incest, violence, and other crimes and traumatic events. Interventions are required to prevent and treat the disability and psychological disorders associated with being a victim. See **survivor.**

vidarabine, an antiviral purine nucleoside, used systemically to treat herpes simplex encephalitis and locally to treat herpesvirus I keratoconjunctivitis and keratitis.

video display terminal (VDT), a cathode-ray tube device with a surface similar to a television screen, used in word processors, computer terminals and similar equipment.

villi. See **villus.**

villoma, *pl.* **villomas, villomata,** a villous neoplasm or papilloma, occurring chiefly in the bladder or rectum.

villous adenoma, a slow-growing, soft, spongy, potentially malignant papillary growth of the mucosa of the large intestine.

villous carcinoma, an epithelial tumour with several long, velvety, papillary outgrowths.

villous papilloma, a benign tumour with long, slender processes, usually occurring in the bladder, breast or a cerebral ventricle.

villus, *pl.* **villi,** one of the many tiny projections, barely visible to the naked eye, clustered over the entire mucous surface of the small intestine. The villi diffuse and transport fluids and nutrients. Each villus has a core of delicate areolar and reticular connective tissue supporting the epithelium, various capillaries and usually a single lymphatic lacteal that fills with milky white chyle during the digestion of a fatty meal. **villous,** *adj.*

vinblastine sulphate, a cytotoxic alkaloid used in the treatment of many malignant diseases, such as choriocarcinoma, testicular carcinoma, Hodgkin's disease and non-Hodgkin's lymphoma.

Vincent's angina, Vincent's infection. See **acute necrotizing gingivitis.**

vincristine sulphate, a cytotoxic alkaloid used in the treatment of many malignant diseases, such as leukaemia, neuroblastoma, lymphomas and sarcomas.

vindesine sulphate, a cytotoxic alkaloid used in the treatment of several cancers, including acute lymphoblastic leukaemia, breast cancer, malignant melanoma, lymphosarcoma and non-small-cell lung carcinoma.

vinegar acid. See **glacial acetic acid.**

violence, potential for: self-directed or directed at others, a state in which an individual experiences behaviours that can be physically harmful either to the self or to others. Defining characteristics of patients who are potentially violent include anxiety, fear of the self or other people, lack of verbal ability, complaining or demanding vocalization, provocative, argumentative or overreactive behaviour, poor self-esteem, psychological depression, a history of self-destructive behaviour, pacing, excitement, agitation or the possession of a weapon.

viosterol, synthetic vitamin D2 in an oil base.

VIP, 1. abbreviation for **vasoactive intestinal polypeptide. 2.** abbreviation for *very important person.*

vipoma, a type of pancreatic tumour that causes changes in secretion of vasoactive intestinal polypeptide (VIP). VIP causes dilatation of blood vessels throughout the body, as well as secretion of fluid and salt in the intestinal tract, resulting in diarrhoea.

viraemia, the presence of viruses in the blood.

viral disease. See **viral infection.**

viral gastroenteritis, an inflammation of the intestine caused by a virus. The symptoms usually include abdominal cramps, diarrhoea, nausea and vomiting.

viral hepatitis, a viral inflammatory disease of the liver, caused by one of the hepatitis viruses, A, B, or non-A, non-B. Transmission, speed of onset and probable course of the illness vary with the kind and strain of virus, but the characteristics of the disease and its treatment are the same. Viral hepatitis is marked by anorexia, malaise, headache, pain over the liver, fever, jaundice, clay-coloured stools, dark urine, nausea and vomiting, and diarrhoea. Severe infection, especially with hepatitis B virus, may be prolonged and result in tissue destruction, cirrhosis and chronic hepatitis, or in hepatic coma and death.

viral infection, any of the diseases caused by one of approximately 200 viruses pathogenic to humans. Some are the most communicable and dangerous diseases known; some cause mild and transient conditions that pass virtually unnoticed. If cells are damaged by the viral attack, disease ensues. The first step in the cycle, after entry into the body, is the attachment of the virus to a susceptible cell and cell's adsorption of the virus. This is followed by penetration of the viral nucleic acid into the parasitized cell. The dissembled virus at this point causes no symptoms and cannot be recovered from the cells in infectious form. The virus begins to mature within the cell and, carrying its own genetic information, begins to replicate, using chemical building blocks and energy available in the parasitized cell. The virus has now taken over the cell. After a variable period of time, masses of fully grown viruses appear, each able to survive outside the cell until more susceptible cells are found. In many viral diseases, including mumps, smallpox and measles, one attack confers permanent immunity. In others, immunity is short-lived. The incubation period for viral infection is short, the viruses do not circulate in the bloodstream, antibodies do not form, and most often immunity does not develop. See also specific viral infections.

viral pneumonia, pulmonary infection caused by a virus.

Virchow's node {Rudolf L. K. Virchow, German pathologist, b. 1821}, a firm supraclavicular lymph node, particularly on the left side, which enlarges to the extent that it is palpable.

virile, 1. of, pertaining to, or characteristic of an adult male; masculine; manly. **2.** possessing or exhibiting masculine strength, vigour,

force or energy. **3.** of, or pertaining to, the male sexual functions; capable of procreation. **virility,** *n.*

virilism, 1. See virilization. **2.** pseudohermaphroditism in a female. **3.** premature development of masculine characteristics in the male. Kinds of virilism are adrenal virilism and prosopopilary virilism.

virilization, a process in which secondary male sexual characteristics are acquired by a female, usually as a result of adrenal dysfunction or hormonal medication.

virion, a rudimentary virus particle with a central nucleoid surrounded by a protein sheath or capsid. The complete nucleocapsid with a nucleic acid core may constitute a complete virus, such as the adenoviruses and picornaviruses, or it may be surrounded by an envelope, as in the herpesviruses and myxoviruses. See also **capsid.**

virocytes, lymphocytes altered in appearance and staining, as seen in blood smears from patients with certain viral diseases.

viroid, a small, infective segment of nucleic acid, usually RNA. It is not translated, and is replicated by host cell enzymes. Viroids include segments that are complementary to introns and may bind to intron RNA.

virologist, a specialist in viruses and diseases caused by viruses.

virology, the study of viruses and viral diseases. **virological,** *adj.*

virucidal, pertaining to the destruction of viruses.

virucide, any agent that destroys or inactivates a virus. **virucidal,** *adj.*

virulence, the power of a micro-organism to produce disease.

virulent, of, or pertaining to, a very pathogenic or rapidly progressive condition.

virus, a minute parasitic micro-organism, much smaller than a bacterium, that, having no independent metabolic activity, may only replicate within a cell of a living plant or animal host. A virus consists of a core of nucleic acid (DNA or RNA), surrounded by a coat of antigenic protein which is sometimes enveloped by lipoprotein. The virus provides the genetic code for replication, and the host cell provides the necessary energy and raw materials. More than 200 viruses have been identified as being capable of causing disease in humans. Types include **adenovirus, arenavirus, enterovirus, herpesvirus** and **rhinovirus.** **viral,** *adj.*

virustatic, pertaining to the inhibition of growth and development of viruses, as distinguished from their destruction.

viscera, *sing.* **viscus,** the internal organs enclosed within a body cavity, primarily the abdominal organs.

visceral, of, or pertaining to, the viscera or internal organs in the abdominal cavity. Also **splanchnic.**

visceral afferent fibres, the nerve fibres of

the visceral nervous system. They receive stimuli and carry impulses towards the central nervous system and share the sensory ganglia of the cerebrospinal nerves with the somatic sensory fibres. Parts of the body with visceral afferents include the face, scalp, nose, mouth, descending colon, lungs, abdomen and rectum.

visceral larva migrans, infestation with parasitic larvae or *Toxocara,* or occasionally *Ascaris, Strongyloides* or other nematodes. See **toxocariasis.**

visceral leishmaniasis. See **kala-azar.**

visceral lymph node, a small, oval, nodular gland that filters lymph circulating in the lymphatic vessels of the thoracic, abdominal and pelvic viscera.

visceral nervous system, the visceral portion of the peripheral nervous system that comprises the whole complex of nerves, fibres, ganglia and plexuses by which impulses travel from the central nervous system to the viscera, and from the viscera to the central nervous system.

visceral pain, abdominal pain caused by any abnormal condition of the viscera. It is characteristically severe, diffuse and difficult to localize.

visceral peritoneum, one of two portions of the largest serous membrane in the body that invests the viscera. The free surface of the visceral peritoneum is a smooth layer of mesothelium, exuding a serous fluid that lubricates the viscera and allows them to glide freely against the wall of the abdominal cavity or over each other.

visceral pleura, the inner layer of pleura that is adjacent to the external lung tissue.

visceral protein status, the amount of protein that is contained in the internal organs.

viscid, sticky or glutinous. Also **viscous.**

viscometry, measurement of the viscosity of whole blood or plasma. It increases comparably with the ESR, and is preferable to ESR on stored specimen.

viscosity, pertaining to the quality of a sticky or gummy fluid, an effect caused by the adhesion of adjacent molecules.

viscous fermentation, the formation of viscous material in milk, urine and wine by the action of various bacilli.

viscus. See **viscera.**

visible light, the radiant energy in the electromagnetic spectrum that is visible to the human eye. The wavelengths cover a range of approximately 390 to 780 nm.

vision, the capacity for sight.

visit, 1. a meeting between a practitioner and a patient. The practitioner visits the patient in the hospital or at home; the patient visits the practitioner in the clinic or practice. **2.** (of a patient) to meet a practitioner so as to obtain professional services, or (of a practitioner) to see a patient or client so as to render a professional service.

visual, pertaining to the sense of sight.

visual accommodation, a process by which the eye adjusts and is able to focus, producing a sharp image at various changing distances from the object seen. The convexity of the anterior surface of the lens may be increased or decreased by contraction or relaxation of the ciliary muscle.

visual evoked potential (VEP), an evoked potential elicited by a repeatedly flashing light. High-risk infants are monitored with VEP to evaluate visual function.

visual field defect, one or more spots or defects in the vision that move with the eye, unlike a floater. This fixed defect is usually caused by damage to the retina or visual pathways, as by chorioretinitis, traumatic injury, macular degeneration, glaucoma or a vascular occlusion of the eye or brain.

visual memory, the ability to create an eidetic image of past visual experiences.

visual pathway, a pathway over which a visual sensation is transmitted from the retina to the brain. A pathway consists of an optic nerve, the fibres of an optic nerve travelling through or along the sides of the optic chiasm to the lateral geniculate body of the thalamus, and an optic tract terminating in an occipital lobe. Each optic nerve contains fibres from only one retina. The optic chiasm contains fibres from the nasal portions of the retinas of both eyes; these fibres cross to the opposite side of the brain at the optic chiasm.

visual purple. See **rhodopsin.**

visual-motor coordination, the ability to coordinate vision with the movements of the body or parts of the body.

visual-motor function, the ability to draw or copy forms or perform constructive tasks.

visualization, the conscious programming of desired change with positive images.

vital capacity (VC), a measurement of the amount of air that can be expelled slowly after a maximum inspiration, representing the greatest possible breathing capacity. The vital capacity equals the inspiratory reserve volume, plus the tidal volume, plus the expiratory reserve volume.

vital signs, the measurements of pulse rate, respiration rate and body temperature. Although not strictly a vital sign, blood pressure is also customarily included.

vital statistics, data relating to births or natality, deaths or mortality, marriages, health and disease or morbidity.

vitalograph, an instrument used for measuring vital capacity.

vitamin, an organic compound essential in small quantities for normal physiological and metabolic functioning of the body. With few exceptions, vitamins cannot be synthesized by the body and must be obtained from the diet or dietary supplements. No single food contains all the vitamins. Vitamin deficiency diseases produce specific symptoms, usually alleviated by the administration of the appropriate vitamin. Vitamins are classified according to their fat or water solubility, their physiological effects or their chemical structures, and they are designated by alphabetical letters and chemical or other specific names. The fat-soluble vitamins are A, D, E and K; the B complex and C vitamins are water-soluble.

vitamin A, a fat-soluble, solid terpene alcohol, essential for skeletal growth, maintenance of normal mucosal epithelium and visual acuity. It is derived from various carotenoids, mainly carotene, and is present in leafy green vegetables, yellow fruits and vegetables, the liver oils of cod and other fish, liver, milk, cheese, butter and egg yolk. Deficiency leads to atrophy of epithelial tissue resulting in keratomalacia, xerophthalmia, night blindness and lessened resistance to infection of mucous membranes.

vitamin B complex, 1. a group of water-soluble vitamins differing from each other structurally and in their biological effect. All of the B vitamins are found in large quantities in liver and yeast, and they are present separately or in combination in many foods. See also folic acid, and vitamins B1–B12. **2.** a pharmaceutical preparation containing a mixture of B vitamins.

vitamin B1. See **thiamine.**

vitamin B12. See **cyanocobalamin.**

vitamin B2. See **riboflavin.**

vitamin B6. See **pyridoxine.**

vitamin C. See **ascorbic acid.**

vitamin D, a fat-soluble vitamin, chemically related to the steroids. It is essential for the normal formation of bones and teeth, and for the absorption of calcium and phosphorus from the GI tract. Natural foods containing vitamin D are of animal origin and include saltwater fish, especially salmon, sardines and herring, organ meats, fish-liver oils and egg yolk. Deficiency results in rickets in children, osteomalacia, osteoporosis and osteodystrophy.

vitamin D-resistant rickets, a disease clinically similar to rickets but resistant to treatment with large doses of vitamin D. It is caused by a congenital defect in renal tubular reabsorption of phosphate, and is usually seen in men.

vitamin D2. See **calciferol.**

vitamin D3, an antirachitic, white, odourless, crystalline, unsaturated alcohol that is the predominant form of vitamin D of animal origin. It is found in most fish-liver oils, butter, brain and egg yolk. It is formed in the skin, fur and feathers of animals and birds exposed to sunlight or ultraviolet rays.

vitamin deficiency, a state or condition resulting from the lack of, or inability to use, one or more vitamins. The symptoms and manifestations of each deficiency vary depending on the specific function of the vitamin in promoting growth and development and maintaining body health.

vitamin E, any of the group of fat-soluble vitamins that consist of the tocopherols. They are essential for normal reproduction, muscle development, resistance of erythrocytes to haemolysis and various other biochemical functions. Vitamin E is an intracellular antioxidant and maintains the stability of polyunsaturated fatty acids and other fat-like substances, including vitamin A and hormones of the pituitary, adrenal and sex glands. The richest dietary sources are wheat germ, soybean, cottonseed, peanut and corn oils, margarine, whole raw seeds and nuts, soybeans, eggs, butter, liver, sweet potatoes and the leaves of many vegetables.

vitamin H. See **biotin.**

vitamin K, a group of fat-soluble vitamins known as quinones. They are essential for the synthesis of prothrombin in the liver and several related proteins involved in blood clotting. Vitamin K is widely distributed in foods, especially leafy green vegetables, pork liver, yogurt, egg yolk, kelp, alfalfa and fish-liver oils. It is synthesized by the bacterial flora of the GI tract. Deficiency results in hypoprothrombinaemia characterized by poor blood coagulation and haemorrhage, and usually occurs from inadequate absorption of the vitamin from the GI tract or the inability to use it in the liver.

vitamin K1. See **phytomenadione.**

vitamin K2, a pale-yellow, fat-soluble, crystalline vitamin of the vitamin K group, that is more unsaturated than vitamin K1 and slightly less active biologically. It is isolated from putrefied fish meal and synthesized by various bacteria in the GI tract. See also **vitamin K.**

vitamin P. See **bioflavonoid.**

vitellin, a phosphoprotein containing lecithin, found in the yolk of eggs. Also called **ovovitellin. vitelline,** *adj.*

vitelline artery, any of the embryonic arteries that circulate blood from the primitive aorta of the early developing embryo to the yolksac.

vitelline circulation, the circulation of blood and nutrients between the developing embryo and yolksac by way of the vitelline arteries and veins.

vitelline duct, (in embryology) the narrow channel connecting the yolksac with the intestine.

vitelline membrane, the delicate cytoplasmic membrane surrounding the ovum.

vitelline sac. See **yolk sac.**

vitelline sphere. See **morula.**

vitelline vein, any of the embryonic veins that return blood from the yolksac to the primitive heart of the early developing embryo.

vitellogenesis, the formation or production

of yolk. **vitellogenetic,** *adj.*

vitellus, the yolk of an ovum.

vitiligo, a benign, acquired skin disease of unknown cause, consisting of irregular patches of various sizes totally lacking in pigment and often having hyperpigmented borders. Exposed areas of skin are most often affected. **vitiliginous,** *adj.*

vitreous body. See **vitreous humour.**

vitreous cavity, the cavity posterior to the lens that contains the vitreous body and vitreous membrane. It is transected by the vestigial remnants of the hyaloid canal.

vitreous haemorrhage, haemorrhage into the vitreous humour of the eye.

vitreous humour, a transparent, semigelatinous substance contained in a thin hyoid membrane filling the cavity behind the crystalline lens of the eye.

vitreous membrane, a membrane that lines the posterior cavity of the eye and surrounds the vitreous body.

vitriol, oil of. See **sulphuric acid.**

vivax malaria. See **tertian malaria.**

viviparous, bearing living offspring rather than laying eggs, such as most mammals and some fishes and reptiles.

VLDL, abbreviation for **very-low-density lipoprotein.**

VMA, abbreviation for **vanillylmandelic acid.**

Vmax, the maximum rate of catalysis.

VO$_2$, symbol for **oxygen uptake.**

vocal cord, either of two strong bands of yellow elastic tissue in the larynx, enclosed by membranes called vocal folds and attached ventrally to the angle of the thyroid cartilage and dorsally to the vocal process of the arytenoid.

vocal cord nodule, a small, inflammatory or fibrous growth that develops on the vocal cords of people who constantly strain their voices.

vocal cues, a category of non-verbal communication that includes all noises and sounds that are extra-speech sounds.

vocal fremitus, the vibration of the chest wall as a person speaks or sings. It allows the person's voice to be heard by the examiner during auscultation of the chest with a stethoscope. Vocal fremitus is decreased in emphysema, pleural effusion, pulmonary oedema or bronchial obstruction.

voice, the acoustic component of speech that is normally produced by vibration of the vocal folds of the larynx.

voice box. See **larynx.**

void, to empty or evacuate, such as urine from the bladder.

volar, of, or pertaining to, the palm of the hand or sole of the foot.

volar ligament. See **retinaculum flexorum manus.**

volatile, (of a liquid) having the characteristics of boiling at a low temperature or evaporating at room temperature.

volatile solvent, an easily evaporated liquid capable of dissolving a substance.

volition, 1. the act, power or state of willing or choosing. **2.** the conscious impulse to perform or abstain from an act. **volitional,** *adj.*

Volkmann's canal {Alfred W. Volkmann, German physiologist, b. 1800}, any one of the small blood vessel canals connecting haversian canals in bone tissue.

Volkmann's contracture {Richard von Volkmann, German surgeon, b. 1830}, a serious, persistent flexion contraction of forearm and hand caused by ischaemia. A pressure or crushing injury in the region of the elbow usually precedes this condition, and pressure from a cast or tight bandage around the elbow are common causes.

Volkmann's splint {Richard von Volkmann}, a splint that supports and immobilizes the lower leg. It has a footpiece attached to two sides and extending from the foot to the knee, thus allowing ambulation.

volsella forceps, a kind of forceps having a small, sharp-pointed hook at the end of each blade.

volt (V) {Count Alessandro Volta, Italian physicist, b. 1745}, the unit of electric potential. One volt of potential difference exists between two points if one joule of work is performed in moving one coulomb of charge from one point to the other.

voltammetry, the measurement of an electric current as a function of potential.

voltmeter, an instrument, such as a galvanometer, that measures in volts the differences in potential between different points of an electric circuit.

volume (ATPS), abbreviation for **ATPS (ambient temperature, ambient pressure, saturated with water vapour)** conditions of a volume of gas. The conditions exist in a water-sealed spirograph or gasometer when the water temperature equals ambient temperature.

volume (BTPS), abbreviation for **BTPS (body temperature, ambient pressure, saturated with water vapour)** conditions of a volume of gas. For humans, normal respiratory tract temperature is measured at 37° C, the pressure as ambient pressure, and the partial pressure of water vapour at 37° C as 47 torr.

volume, the amount of space occupied by a body, expressed in cubic units.

volume control fluid chamber, any one of several types of transparent, plastic reservoirs with graduated volumetric markings, used to regulate the flow of intravenous solutions.

volume dose. See **integral dose.**

volume imaging, MRI imaging techniques in which MRI signals are gathered from the whole object volume to be imaged at once.

Several sequential plane imaging techniques can be generalized to volume imaging, at least in principle.

volume ventilator, a ventilator that delivers a predetermined volume of gas with each cycle.

volumetric flow rate, the rate at which a volume of fluid flows past a designated point, usually measured in litres per second.

voluntary, referring to an action or thought originated, undertaken, controlled or accomplished as a result of a person's free will or choice.

voluntary agency, a service agency legally controlled by volunteers rather than by owners or paid staff.

voluntary muscle. See **striated muscle.**

volunteer, a person who offers his or her services without pay.

volvulus, a twisting of the bowel on itself, causing intestinal obstruction. The condition is frequently the result of a prolapsed segment of mesentery, and occurs most often in the ileum, caecum, or the sigmoid portions of the bowel. If it is not corrected, the obstructed bowel becomes necrotic with resultant peritonitis and rupture of the bowel.

volvulus neonatorum, an intestinal obstruction in a newborn baby resulting from a twisting of the bowel, caused by malrotation or non-fixation of the colon. Typical symptoms include abdominal distention, persistent regurgitation often accompanied by faecal vomiting, and non-passage of stools.

vomer, the bone forming the posterior and inferior part of the nasal septum; it has two surfaces and four borders.

vomit, 1. to expel the contents of the stomach through the oesophagus and out of the mouth. **2.** the material expelled.

von Economo's encephalitis. See **epidemic encephalitis.**

von Gierke's disease {Edgar von Gierke, German pathologist, b. 1877}, a form of glycogen storage disease in which abnormally large amounts of glycogen are deposited in the liver and kidneys. The disorder is characterized by hypoglycaemia, ketoacidosis and hyperlipaemia.

von Hippel-Lindau disease. See **cerebroretinal angiomatosis.**

von Pirquet test. See **Pirquet's test.**

von Recklinghausen's disease. See **neurofibromatosis.**

von Willebrand's disease {Erick A. von Willebrand, Finnish physician, b. 1870}, an inherited disorder characterized by abnormally slow blood coagulation, spontaneous epistaxis and gingival bleeding, caused by a deficiency of factor VIII.

vortex, *pl.* **vortexes, vortices,** a whirlpool effect produced by the whirling of a more or less cylindrical mass of fluid (liquid or gas).

vox, voice, such as **vox cholerica,** the barely audible, hoarse voice of a patient in an advanced and severe case of cholera.

voxel, abbreviation for volume element, the three-dimensional version of a pixel.

voyeur, one whose sexual desire is gratified by the practice of voyeurism.

voyeurism, a psychosexual disorder in which a person derives sexual excitement and gratification from looking at the naked bodies and genital organs, or observing the sexual acts of others, especially from a secret vantage point.

vulnerable, being in a dangerous position or condition and thereby susceptible to being infected or injured.

vulnerable period, a short period in the cardiac cycle of the atria or ventricles, during which activation may result in tachycardia or fibrillation.

vulsella forceps. See **volsella forceps.**

vulva. See **pudendum.**

vulvectomy, the surgical removal of part or all of the tissues of the vulva, performed most frequently in the treatment of malignant or premalignant neoplastic disease. **Simple vulvectomy** includes the removal of the skin of labia minora, labia majora and clitoris. **Radical vulvectomy** involves excision of the labia majora, labia minora, clitoris, surrounding tissues and pelvic lymph nodes.

vulvocrural, of, or pertaining to, the vulva and thigh.

vulvovaginal, of, or pertaining to, the vulva and vagina.

vulvovaginitis, an inflammation of the vulva and vagina or the vulvovaginal glands.

VZV, abbreviation for varicella zoster virus.

W, symbol for **watt.**

w, the amount of energy required to ionize a molecule of air, as expressed by w = 33.85 eV/ion pair. This is an important quantity for radiation dosimetry, because it allows the extraction of dose from ionization measurements.

W chromosome and Z chromosome, the sex chromosomes of certain insects, birds and fishes. Females of such species are heterogametic and have one W and one Z chromosome, whereas males are homogametic and have two Z chromosomes. The ZZ-ZW system of nomenclature was chosen to differentiate the chromosomes from the XX-XY type, which occurs in humans and various other animals; the female is homogametic and the male is heterogametic.

W/cm², abbreviation for **watt per square centimetre.**

Wagner-Meissner corpuscle {Rudolf Wagner, German physiologist, b. 1805; Georg Meissner, German anatomist, b. 1829}, one of a number of small, special pressure-sensitive sensory end-organs in the corium of the hand and foot, the front of forearm, skin of the lips, mucous membrane of the tongue, palpebral conjunctiva and skin of the mammary papilla.

Wagstaffe's fracture {William Wagstaffe, English surgeon, b. 1834}, a fracture characterized by separation of the internal malleolus.

waking imagined analgesia (WIA), the pain relief experienced by a patient who employs the psychological technique, usually with the help of an attending nurse or a health care assistant, of concentrating on previous pleasant personal experiences that produced tranquillity. This technique is often effective in reducing mild to moderate pain.

Waldenström's disease. See **Perthes' disease.**

Waldenström's macroglobulinaemia. See **macroglobulinaemia.**

Waldeyer's ring {Heinrich W. G. von Waldeyer-Hartz, German anatomist, b. 1836}, the palatine, pharyngeal and lingual tonsils that encircle the pharynx.

walking frame, an extremely light, movable apparatus. approximately waist-high, made of metal tubing. It is used to aid a patient in walking, and has four widely placed, sturdy legs. The patient holds onto the walker and takes a step, then moves the walker forward and takes another step.

walking heel, a plastic or rubber heel placed in the sole of a leg cast to allow weight-bearing

walking pneumonia. See **mycoplasma pneumonia.**

wall, a limiting structure within the body, such as the wall of the abdominal, thoracic or pelvic cavities, or the wall of a cell.

wallerian degeneration {Augustus V. Waller, English physician, b. 1816}, the fatty degeneration of a nerve fibre after it has been severed from its cell body.

wander, 1. to move about purposelessly. **2.** to cause to move back and forth in an exploratory manner.

wandering goitre. See **diving goitre.**

Wangensteen apparatus {Owen H. Wagensteen, American surgeon, b. 1898}, a nasogastroduodenal catheter and a suction apparatus used for constant, gentle drainage and decompression of the stomach or duodenum.

Wangensteen tube {Owen H. Wagensteen}, the catheter portion of a Wangensteen apparatus.

war neurosis. See **combat fatigue, shell shock.**

ward sister, a nurse in charge of a ward or number of wards including the management of staff on the ward, the resources available and the overall care of patients in the ward.

warfarin poisoning {Wisconsin Alumni Research Foundation}, a toxic condition caused by the ingestion of warfarin, either accidentally in the form of a rodenticide or by overdose in its pharmacological anticoagulant form. The poison accumulates in the body and results in nosebleed, bruising, haematuria, melena and internal haemorrhage.

warfarin sodium, an oral anticoagulant used for the prophylaxis and treatment of thrombosis and embolism. It is also used as a rodenticide.

warm-blooded, having a relatively high and constant body temperature, such as the temperatures maintained by humans, other mammals and birds, despite changes in environmental temperatures. Heat is produced in the warm-blooded human body by the catabolism of foods in proportion to the amount of work performed by the body tissues. Heat is lost from the body by evaporation, radiation, conduction and convection. The average temperature of the healthy human is 37° C (98.6° F). The tolerance of the human body for change in its temperature is very small, and significant changes can have drastic, even fatal consequences.

wart. See **verruca.**

Warthin's tumour. See **papillary adenocystoma lymphomatosum.**

washout, the elimination or expulsion of one gas or volatile anaesthetic agent by the administration of another.

wasp, a slender, narrow-waisted hymenopteran insect with two pairs of membranous wings that are folded lengthwise when at rest, like parts of a fan. Many species of wasps may give painful stings, sometimes with severe results in hypersensitive persons.

Wassermann test {August P. von Wassermann, German bacteriologist, b. 1866}, a diagnostic blood test for syphilis, based on the complement fixation reaction.

wasted ventilation, the volume of air that ventilates the physiological dead space in a respiratory system.

wasting, a process of deterioration marked by weight loss and decreased physical vigour, appetite and mental activity.

watchfulness, continuous supervision provided either openly or unobtrusively as the situation indicates.

water (H_2O), a chemical compound, one molecule of which contains one atom of oxygen and two atoms of hydrogen. Almost three- quarters of the earth's surface is covered by water. Essential to life as it exists on this planet, water comprises more than 70% of living things. Pure water freezes at 0° C (32° F) and boils at 100° C (212° F) at sea level.

water intoxication, an increase in the volume of free water in the body, resulting in dilutional hyponatraemia.

water pollution, the contamination of lakes, rivers and streams by industrial or community sources of pollutants.

water trap. See **underwater seal.**

water-hammer pulse, a pulse associated with aortic regurgitation. It is characterized by a full, forcible impulse and immediate collapse, causing a jerking sensation.

waterborne, carried by water, such as a waterborne epidemic of typhoid fever.

Waterhouse-Friderichsen syndrome {Rupert Waterhouse, English physician, b. 1873; Carl Friderichsen, Danish physician, b. 1886}, overwhelming bacteraemia, characterized by the sudden onset of fever, cyanosis, petechiae and collapse from massive bilateral adrenal haemorrhage. The syndrome requires immediate emergency treatment, hospitalization and intensive care.

waters. See **amniotic fluid.**

watt {James Watt, Scottish engineer, b. 1736}, the unit of electric power in the SI system, where 1 watt is equal to 1 joule per second. One watt of power is dissipated when one ampere of current flows through a potential difference of one volt.

watt per square centimetre (W/cm^2), a unit of power density or intensity used in ultrasound.

wave, a periodic disturbance in which energy moves through a medium without permanently altering the constituents of the medium.

wavelength, the distance between a given point on one wave cycle and the corresponding point on the next successive wave cycle.

wax. See **cerumen.**

waxy flexibility. See **cerea flexibilitas.**

WBC, abbreviation for **white blood cell.** See **leukocyte.**

wean, 1. to train a child to give up breast feeding and accept other food in place of breast milk. Many children are ready for weaning during the second-half of their first year; some wean themselves. **2.** to withdraw a person from something on which he or she is dependent. **3.** to remove a patient gradually from dependency on mechanical ventilation.

wear-and-tear theory, a concept of the ageing process in which structural and functional changes associated with growing old are accelerated by abuse of the body and retarded with healthcare.

weaver's bottom, a form of bursitis affecting the ischial bursae of the hips of people whose work requires prolonged sitting in one position. Also called (obsolete) tailor's bottom.

web, a network of fibres forming a tissue or a membrane, such as the laryngeal web that spreads between the vocal cords.

web of causation, an interrelationship of multiple factors that contribute to the occurrence of a disease.

webbing, skinfolds connecting adjacent structures such as fingers or toes, or the neck from the acromion to the mastoid, associated with genetic abnormalities.

Weber (Wb), a unit of magnetic flux equal to m^{2}kg/s^{2}A.

Weber's tuning fork test, a method of assessing auditory acuity, especially useful in determining whether defective hearing in an ear is a conductive loss caused by a middle ear problem, or a sensorineural loss. The test is performed by placing the stem of a vibrating 256 Hz tuning fork in the centre of the person's forehead or the maxillary incisors. If hearing is normal, the loudness of the sound is equal in both ears.

Wechsler intelligence scales {David Wechsler, American psychologist, b. 1896}, a series of standardized tests designed to measure intelligence at several age levels, from preschool stage through to adulthood, by means of questions that examine general information, arrangement of pictures and objects, vocabulary, memory, reasoning and other abilities.

wedge angle, (in external beam radiotherapy) an angle through which the 50% isodose is turned as a result of inserting a wedge filter in the beam.

wedge filter, (in radiotherapy) a wedge-shaped metal device used to modify the percentage depth dose of an external radiation beam, by attenuating a greater proportion of the beam on one side than the other. Its purpose is to compensate for missing tissue, or to increase uniformity of an isodose distribution across a target volume.

wedge fracture, a fracture of vertebral structures with anterior compression.

wedge pressure, the capillary pressure in the left atrium, determined by measuring the pressure in a cardiac catheter wedged in the most distal segment of the pulmonary artery.

wedge resection, the surgical excision of part of an organ, such as a part of an ovary containing a cyst. The segment excised may be wedge-shaped.

weed. See **cannabis.**

weeping, 1. crying, lacrimating. **2.** oozing or exuding fluid, such as a sore or rash.

weeping lubrication, a form of hydrostatic lubrication in which the interstitial fluid of hydrated articular cartilage flows onto its surface when a load is applied.

Wegener's granulomatosis {F. Wegener, 20th century German pathologist}, an uncommon, chronic inflammatory process leading to the formation of nodules or tumour-like masses in the air passages, necrotizing vasculitis and glomerulonephritis. Symptoms, depending on the organs involved, may include sinus pain, a bloody, purulent nasal discharge, saddle-nose deformity, chest discomfort and cough, weakness, anorexia, weight loss and skin lesions.

weight, the force exerted on a body by the gravity of the earth. Weight is sometimes measured in units of force, such as newtons or poundals, but it is usually expressed in pounds or kilograms, as is mass.

weight holder, a metal, T-shaped bar that holds weights for traction.

weight per volume (W/V) solution, the relationship of a solute to a solvent, expressed as grams of solute per millilitre of the total solution. An example is 50 g of glucose in 1 L of water, considered a 5% W/V solution, even though it is not a true percent solution.

Weil's disease. See **leptospirosis.**

weismannism {August F. L. Weismann, German biologist, b. 1834}, the basic concepts of heredity and development as proposed by A. Weismann. These state that the vehicle of inheritance is the germ plasm, which is distinct from the somatoplasm, and that acquired characteristics cannot be inherited. **weismannian,** *adj., n.*

well baby clinic, periodic health supervision for infants and children to promote optimal physical, emotional and intellectual growth and development. Such healthcare measures include routine immunizations to prevent disease, screening procedures for early detection and treatment of illness, and parental guidance and instruction in proper nutrition, accident prevention, and specific care and rearing of the child at various stages of development.

well-being, 1. achievement of a good and satisfactory existence as defined by the individual. **2.** a dynamic state of health in which an individual progresses towards a higher level of functioning, achieving an optimal balance between internal and external environments.

well-differentiated lymphocytic malignant lymphoma, a lymphoid neoplasm characterized by the predominance of mature lymphocytes.

wen. See **pilar cyst.**

Wenckebach heart block. See **Mobitz I heart block.**

Wenckebach periodicity {Karel F. Wenckebach, Dutch-Austrian physician, b. 1864}, a form of second-degree atrioventricular block with a progressive beat-to-beat prolongation of the PR interval, finally resulting in a non-conducting P wave.

Werdnig-Hoffmann disease {Guido Werdnig, Austrian neurologist, b. 1862; Johann Hoffman, German neurologist, b. 1857}, a genetic disorder beginning in infancy or young childhood. It is characterized by progressive atrophy of the skeletal muscle, resulting from degeneration of cells in the anterior horn of the spinal cord and motor nuclei in the brainstem. Symptoms include congenital hypotonia, absence of stretch reflexes, flaccid paralysis especially of the trunk and limbs, absence of sucking ability, fasciculations of the tongue and sometimes other muscles, and often dysphagia.

Werlhof's disease. See **thrombocytopenic purpura.**

Wernicke's encephalopathy {Karl Wernicke, Polish neurologist, b. 1848}, an inflammatory, haemorrhagic, degenerative condition of the brain. The condition is characterized by double vision, involuntary and rapid movements of the eyes, lack of muscular coordination, and decreased mental function which may be mild or severe. Wernicke's encephalopathy is caused by a thiamine deficiency and is seen in association with chronic alcoholism.

West African sleeping sickness. See **Gambian trypanosomiasis.**

West nomogram, a nomogram used in estimating the body surface area. See also **nomogram.**

Westermark's sign, the absence of blood vessel markings beyond the location of a pulmonary embolism, as seen on a radiograph.

Western blot test, a laboratory blood test to detect the presence of antibodies to specific antigens. It is regarded as more precise than the enzyme-linked immunoabsorbent assay (ELISA), and is sometimes used to check the validity of ELISA tests.

wet cough. See **productive cough.**

wet dream. See **nocturnal emission.**

wet lung, an abnormal condition of the lungs, characterized by a persistent cough and rales at the lung bases. It occurs in workers exposed to pulmonary irritants.

wetting agent, a detergent, such as tyloxapol, used as a mucolytic in respiratory therapy.

Wharton's jelly {Thomas Wharton, English anatomist, b. 1614}, a gelatinous tissue that remains when the embryonic body stalk blends with the yolk sac within the umbilical cord.

wheal, an individual lesion of urticaria.

wheat weevil disease, a hypersensitivity pneumonitis caused by allergy to weevil particles found in wheat flour.

wheelchair, a mobile chair equipped with large wheels and brakes.

wheeze, 1. a form of rhonchus, characterized by a high-pitched musical quality. It is caused by a high-velocity flow of air through a narrowed airway, and is heard both during inspiration and expiration. **2.** to breathe with a wheeze.

whiplash injury *informal,* an injury to the cervical vertebrae or their supporting ligaments and muscles, marked by pain and stiffness. It usually results from sudden acceleration or deceleration, such as in a rearend car collision that causes violent back-and-forth movement of the head and neck.

Whipple's disease {George Hoyt Whipple, American pathologist, b. 1878}, a rare intestinal disease characterized by severe intestinal malabsorption, steatorrhoea, anaemia, weight loss, arthritis and arthralgia. Affected individuals are severely malnourished and have abdominal pain, chest pain and a chronic non-productive cough.

whipworm. See *Trichuris.*

whirlpool bath, immersion of the body or a part of the body in a tank of hot water agitated by a jet of equally hot water and air.

whispered pectoriloquy, the transmission of a whisper through the pulmonary structures, so that it is heard as normal audible speech on auscultation.

white blood cell. See **leukocyte.**

white cell *informal,* **white blood cell.** See also **leukocyte.**

white corpuscle. See **leukocyte.**

white damp. See **damp.**

white fibrocartilage, a mixture of tough, white, fibrous tissue and flexible cartilaginous tissue.

white gold, a gold alloy with a high content of palladium or platinum, used in some dental restorations such as prepared tooth cavities and gold crowns.

white matter. See **white substance.**

white substance, the tissue surrounding the grey substance of the spinal cord, consisting mainly of myelinated nerve fibres but also containing some unmyelinated nerve fibres, embedded in a spongy network of neuroglia. It is subdivided in each half of the spinal cord into three funiculi: the anterior, posterior and lateral white column. Each column subdivides into tracts that are closely associated in function.

white thrombus, 1. an aggregation of blood platelets, fibrin, clotting factors and cellular elements containing few or no erythrocytes. **2.** a thrombus comprised chiefly of white blood cells. **3.** a thrombus composed primarily of blood platelets and fibrin.

whitlow, an inflammation of the end of a finger or toe that results in suppuration. See also **felon.**

WHO, abbreviation for **World Health Organization.**

whole blood, blood that is unmodified except for the presence of an anticoagulant. It is used for transfusion.

whole body hyperthermia. See **systemic heating.**

whoop, a noisy spasm of inspiration that terminates a coughing paroxysm in cases of pertussis. It is caused by a sudden, sharp increase in tension on the vocal cords.

whooping cough. See **pertussis.**

whorl, a spiral turn, such as one of the turns of the cochlea or dermal ridges that form fingerprints.

Widal's test {Georges F. I. Widal, French physician, b. 1862}, an agglutination test used to aid in the diagnosis of salmonella infections, such as typhoid fever.

wide-angle glaucoma. See **glaucoma.**

wild-type gene, a normal or standard form of a gene, as contrasted with a mutant form.

will, 1. the mental faculty that enables a person consciously to choose or decide on a course of action. **2.** the act or process of exercising the power of choice. **3.** a wish, desire or deliberate intention. **4.** a disposition or attitude towards another person or others beings. **5.** determination or purpose; willfulness.

Willis' circle. See **circle of Willis.**

Willis' disease. See **diabetes mellitus.**

willow fracture. See **greenstick fracture.**

Wilms' tumour {Max Wilms, German surgeon, b. 1867}, a malignant tumour of the kidney, occurring in young children, before the fifth year of life in 75% of the cases. The most frequent early sign is hypertension, followed by the appearance of a palpable mass, pain and haematuria. The tumour, an embryonal adenomyosarcoma, is well encapsulated in the early stage, but may later extend into lymph nodes and the renal vein or vena cava, and metastasize to the lungs or other sites.

Wilson's disease {Samuel A. K. Wilson, English neurologist, b. 1877}, a rare, inherited disorder of copper metabolism, in which copper accumulates slowly in the liver and is then released and taken up in other parts of the body. Haemolysis occurs, followed by haemolytic anaemia as the copper accumulates in the red blood cells. Accumulation in the brain destroys certain tissues and may cause tremors, muscle rigidity, dysarthria and dementia. Kidney function is diminished and the liver becomes cirrhotic.

Winckel's disease. See **haemoglobinuria.**

wind chill, loss of heat from the body when it is exposed to wind of a given speed at a given temperature and humidity. The **wind chill index** is expressed in kilocalories per hour per square meter of skin surface. The **wind chill factor** is expressed in degrees Celsius or Fahrenheit as the effective temperature felt by a person exposed to the weather.

winding sheet, a shroud for wrapping a dead body.

windkessel effect, the stretching of the aorta during systole to accommodate the stroke volume of blood ejected. Energy that was stored propels this volume by recoil action into the peripheral artery tree during diastole.

window, 1. a surgically created opening in the surface of a structure or an anatomically present opening on the surface or between the chambers of a structure. **2.** a specific time period during which a phenomenon can be observed, a reaction monitored or a procedure initiated.

windowed, (of an orthopaedic cast) having an opening, especially to relieve pressure that may irritate and inflame the skin.

winged scapula, an outward prominence of the scapula, caused by disruption of its nerves or muscle weakness.

winter cough *non-technical,* a chronic condition characterized by a persistent cough precipitated by cold weather. See also **cough.**

winter itch, pruritus occurring in cold weather, in people with dry skin and particularly those suffering from atopic dermatitis.

wiry pulse, an abnormal pulse that is strong but small.

wisdom tooth, either of the last teeth on each side of the upper and lower jaw. These are third molars and are the last teeth to erupt, usually between 17 and 21 years of age. They often cause considerable pain, dental problems and the need for extraction.

wish fulfilment, 1. gratification of a desire. **2.** (in psychology) the satisfaction of a desire

or release of emotional tension through processes such as dreams, daydreams and neurotic symptoms. **3.** (in psychoanalysis) one of the primary motivations for dreams in which an unconscious desire or urge is given expression.

wishful thinking, the interpretation of facts or situations according to one's desires or wishes, rather than as they exist in reality. It tends to be used as an unconscious device to avoid painful or unpleasant feelings.

Wiskott-Aldrich syndrome {Alfred Wiskott, German paediatrician, b. 1898; Robert Anderson Aldrich, American paediatrician, b. 1917}, an immunodeficiency disorder inherited as a recessive, X-linked trait, characterized by thrombocytopenia, eczema, inadequate T and B cell function and an increased susceptibility to viral, bacterial and fungal infections and cancer.

witch hazel, 1. a shrub, *Hamamelis virginiana,* indigenous to North America, from which an astringent extract is derived. **2.** a solution comprised of the extract, alcohol and water, used as an astringent.

witch's milk, a milk-like substance secreted from the breast of the newborn, caused by circulating maternal lactating hormone.

withdrawal, a common response to physical danger or severe stress. It is characterized by a state of apathy, lethargy, depression, retreat into oneself and, in grave cases, catatonia and stupor.

withdrawal behaviour, the physical or psychological removal of oneself from a stressor.

withdrawal bleeding, the passage of blood from the uterus, associated with the shedding of endometrium that has been stimulated and maintained by the contraceptive pill.

withdrawal method, a contraceptive technique in coitus, wherein the penis is withdrawn from the vagina before ejaculation. Also called coitus interruptus.

withdrawal reflex. See **flexor withdrawal reflex.**

withdrawal symptoms, the unpleasant, sometimes life-threatening physiological changes that occur when some drugs are withdrawn after prolonged, regular use.

withdrawn behaviour, a condition in which there is a blunting of the emotions and a lack of social responsiveness.

witness, a person who is present and can testify that he or she has personally observed an event, such as the signing of a will or consent form.

Wittmaack-Ekbom syndrome. See **restless legs syndrome.**

wobble, an eccentric rotation that permits increased resolution of tomographic imaging devices composed of discrete detector systems.

Wolff-Chaikoff effect, the decreased formation and release of thyroid hormone in the presence of an excess of iodine.

Wolff-Parkinson-White syndrome {Louis Wolff, American physician, b. 1898; Sir John Parkinson, English cardiologist, b. 1885; Paul Dudley White, American cardiologist, b. 1886}, a disorder of atrioventricular conduction, characterized by two AV conduction pathways.

wolffian body. See **mesonephros.**

wolffian duct. See **mesonephric duct.**

wolfram. See **tungsten.**

Wolman's disease. See **cholesteryl ester storage disease.**

woman-year, (in statistics) 1 year in the reproductive life of a sexually active woman; a unit that represents 12 months of exposure to the possibility of pregnancy.

womb. See **uterus.**

wood alcohol. See **methanol.**

Wood's glass {Robert Williams Wood, American physicist, b. 1868}, a nickel oxide glass filter that holds back all light except a few violet rays of the visible spectrum and ultraviolet wavelengths of about 365 nm. It is used extensively to help diagnose fungal infections of the scalp, and erythrasma.

Wood's light {Robert Williams Wood}, an ultraviolet light of about 365 nm wavelength, used to diagnose certain scalp and skin diseases. The light causes hairs infected with a fungus, such as *tinea capitis,* to become brilliantly fluorescent.

wool fat, a fatty substance obtained from sheep's wool, and of which lanolin is a common chemical component.

woolsorter's disease, the pulmonary form of anthrax, given this name because it is an occupational hazard to those who handle sheep's wool. Early symptoms mimic influenza, but the patient soon develops high fever, respiratory distress and cyanosis.

word association test. See **association test.**

word association. See **controlled association.**

work simplification, the utilization of special equipment, ergonomics, functional planning and behaviour modification, to reduce the physical and psychological stresses of home maintenance for disabled persons or their family members.

work therapy, a therapeutic approach in which the client performs a useful activity or learns an occupation, as in occupational therapy.

work tolerance, the kind and amount of work that a physically or mentally ill person can or should perform.

working occlusion, the occlusal contacts of teeth on the side of the jaw towards which the mandible is moved.

working phase, (in psychology) the second stage of the nurse-patient relationship. During this stage, patients explore their experiences. Nurses assist patients by helping them to plan courses of action and try out the plans, and to begin to evaluate the effectiveness of their new behaviour.

working through, a process by which repressed feelings are released and reintegrated into the personality.

World Health Organization (WHO), an agency of the United Nations, affiliated with the Food and Agricultural Organization of the UN, International Atomic Energy Agency, International Labour Organization, Pan American Health Organization and UNESCO. The WHO is primarily concerned with worldwide or regional health problems, but in emergencies it is authorized to render local assistance on request. Its functions include furnishing technical assistance, stimulating and advancing epidemiological investigation of diseases, recommending health regulations, promoting cooperation among scientific and professional health groups, and providing information and support relating to health matters. Its headquarters are in Geneva, Switzerland.

worm, any of the soft-bodied, elongated invertebrates of the phyla *Annelida, Nemathelminthes* or *Platyhelminthes.* Kinds of worms that are parasitic for humans include **hookworm, pinworm** and **tapeworm.** See also **fluke, roundworm.**

wormian bone {Olaus Worm, Danish anatomist, b. 1588}, any of several tiny, smooth, segmented bones that are soft, moist and tepid to the touch. They are usually found as the serrated borders of sutures between the cranial bones.

worthlessness, a component of low self-esteem, characterized by feelings of uselessness and inability to contribute meaningfully to the well-being of others or to one's environment.

wound, 1. any physical injury involving a break in the skin, usually caused by an act or accident rather than a disease; for example, a gunshot wound. **2.** to cause an injury, especially one that breaks the skin.

wound irrigation, the rinsing of a wound or the cavity formed by a wound, using a medicated solution, water or antibiotic liquid preparation.

wound repair, restoration of the normal structure after an injury, especially of the skin.

Wright's stain {James H. Wright; American pathologist, b. 1869}, a stain containing methylene blue and eosin, used to colour blood specimens for microscopic examination, as for complete blood count, and particularly for malarial parasites.

wringing, a form of massage which involves lifting the tissues at right angles to the bone and applying a twist to enhance the stretching effect.

wrinkle test, a test for nerve function in the hand, by observing the presence of skin wrinkles after the hand has been placed in warm water for 20 to 30 minutes. Denervated skin does not wrinkle.

wrist joint. See **radiocarpal articulation.**

wrist. See **carpus.**

writer's cramp, a painful, involuntary contraction of the muscles of the hand when attempting to write.

wryneck. See **torticollis.**

Wuchereria {Otto Wucherer, German physician, b. 1820}, a genus of filarial worms found in warm, humid climates. *Wuchereria bancrofti*, transmitted by mosquitoes, is the cause of elephantiasis.

X chromosome, a sex chromosome that is present in both sexes in humans and many other species. It appears singly in the cells of normal males, and in duplicate in the cells of normal females. The chromosome is carried as a sex determinant by all female gametes and one-half of all male gametes.

X-inactivation theory. See Lyon hypothesis.

X-linked, pertaining to genes, or to the characteristics or conditions they transmit, that are carried on the X chromosome. Women may inherit the genes, but the recessive effects are usually masked by the normal dominant alleles carried on the second X chromosome. Compare Y-linked. X linkage, n.

X-linked dominant inheritance, a pattern of inheritance in which the transmission of a dominant gene on the X chromosome causes a characteristic to be manifested. All affected individuals have an affected parent. All of the daughters of an affected male are affected, but none of the sons. One-half of the sons and one-half of the daughters of an affected female are affected.

X-linked ichthyosis. See sex-linked ichthyosis.

X-linked inheritance, a pattern of inheritance in which the transmission of traits varies according to the sex of the person, because the genes on the X chromosome have no counterparts on the Y chromosome. The inheritance pattern may be recessive or dominant. Kinds of X-linked inheritance are X-linked dominant inheritance and X-linked recessive inheritance.

X-linked mucopolysaccharidosis. See Hunter's syndrome.

X-linked recessive inheritance, a pattern of inheritance in which transmission of an abnormal recessive gene on the X chromosome results in a carrier state in females and characteristics of the condition in males.

x-ray, 1. also called roentgen ray. Electromagnetic radiation of shorter wavelength than visible light. X-rays are produced when electrons, travelling at high speed, strike certain materials such as tungsten. They can penetrate most substances and are used to investigate the integrity of certain structures, to destroy diseased tissue for therapeutic purposes, and make photographic images for diagnostic purposes, as in radiography and fluoroscopy. Discrete x-rays are those with precisely fixed energies that are characteristic of differences between electron binding energies of a particular element. Tung-

sten, for example, has 15 different effective energies and no more, representing emissions from 5 different electron shells. 2. a radiograph made by projecting x-rays through organs or structures of the body onto a photographic plate. 3. to make a radiograph. x-ray, adj.

x-ray cassette, a light-tight device used in radiography for holding a sheet of x-ray film, and usually incorporating a set of intensifying screens. A grid cassette incorporates a secondary radiation grid to absorb scattered radiation.

x-ray fluoroscopy, real-time imaging using an x-ray source that projects through the patient onto an image intensifier.

x-ray microscope, a microscope that produces images by x-rays and records them on fine-grain film or projects them as enlargements.

x-ray pelvimetry, a radiographic technique to determine the dimensions of a woman's bony pelvis.

x-ray tube, an evacuated glass tube containing a filament in a cathode assembly which emits electrons when heated, and an anode, usually a rotating disc. When a large potential difference is applied between the cathode and anode, electrons are accelerated from the filament to the anode where they interact to produce x-rays and heat. The heat is dissipated by thermal radiation into the oil surrounding the x-ray tube. The x-rays passing through the window of the x-ray tube housing are collimated to form the x-ray beam.

X-tra densities, images on x-ray film caused by the presence of foreign objects, such as bullets or surgical clips, in the patient's body.

X-Y digitizer, a graphics input device that allows the motion of a cursor or pen to be transduced and fed into the computer as a series of X,Y coordinates.

xanthaemia. See carotenaemia.

xanthelasma, xanthelasma palpebrarum. See xanthoma palpebrarum.

xanthelasmatosis, a disseminated, generalized form of planar xanthoma frequently associated with reticuloendothelial disorders, especially multiple myeloma.

xanthine, a nitrogenous byproduct of the metabolism of nucleoproteins. It is normally found in the muscles, liver, spleen, pancreas and urine. xanthic, adj.

xanthine derivative, any one of the closely related alkaloids caffeine, theobromine or theophylline. They are found in plants widely distributed geographically, and are variously ingested as components in different beverages such as coffee, tea, cocoa and cola drinks. The xanthine derivatives or methylxanthines stimulate the CNS, produce diuresis and relax smooth muscles. They are used in the treatment of obstructive airways disease.

xanthinuria, 1. the presence of excessive quantities of xanthine in the urine. 2. a rare disorder of purine metabolism, resulting in the excretion of large amounts of xanthine in the urine because of the absence of an enzyme, xanthine oxidase, which is necessary in xanthine metabolism.

xanthochromia, a substance in cerebrospinal fluid that accounts for its yellow colouration. It is caused by the presence of haemoglobin breakdown products.

xanthochromic, having a yellowish colour, such as cerebrospinal fluid that contains blood or bile.

xanthogranuloma, *pl.* **xanthogranulomas, xanthogranulomata,** a tumour or nodule of granulation tissue containing lipid deposits. A kind of xanthogranuloma is **juvenile xanthogranuloma.**

xanthoma, *pl.* **xanthomas, xanthomata,** a benign, fatty, fibrous, yellowish plaque, nodule or tumour that develops in the subcutaneous layer of skin, often around tendons.

xanthoma disseminatum, a benign, chronic condition in which small orange or brown papules and nodules develop on several body surfaces.

xanthoma eruptivum. See **eruptive xanthoma.**

xanthoma multiplex. See **xanthoma disseminatum.**

xanthoma palpebrarum, a soft, yellow spot or plaque usually occurring in groups on the eyelids.

xanthoma planum. See **planar xanthoma.**

xanthoma striatum palmare, a yellow or orange flat plaque or slightly raised nodule, occurring in groups on the palms of the hands.

xanthoma tendinosum, a yellow or orange, elevated or flat, round papule or nodule. It occurs in clusters on tendons, especially the extensor tendons of the hands and feet of individuals with hereditary lipid storage disease.

xanthoma tuberosum, a yellow or orange, flat or elevated, round papule. It occurs in clusters on the skin of joints, especially elbows and knees, usually in individuals with a hereditary lipid storage disease.

xanthomasarcoma, *pl.* **xanthomasarcomas, xanthomasarcomata,** a giant cell sarcoma of the tendon sheaths and aponeuroses, containing xanthoma cells.

xanthomatosis, an abnormal condition in which there are deposits of yellowish fatty material in the skin, internal organs and reticuloendothelial system.

xanthopsia, an abnormal visual condition in which everything appears to have a yellow hue.

xanthosis, 1. a yellowish discolouration, sometimes seen in degenerating tissues of malignant diseases. 2. See **xanthomatosis.** 3. a reversible yellow discolouration of the skin, most commonly caused by the ingestion of large amounts of yellow vegetables containing carotene pigment.

xanthureic acid, a metabolite of tryptophan that occurs in normal urine and in elevated levels in patients with vitamin B6 deficiency.

Xe, symbol for **xenon.**

xenobiotic, pertaining to organic substances that are foreign to the body, such as drugs or organic poisons.

xenogeneic, 1. (in genetics) denoting individuals or cell types from different species and different genotypes. 2. (in transplantation biology) denoting tissues from different species that are therefore antigenically dissimilar. Also **heterologous.**

xenogenesis, 1. alternation of traits in successive generations; heterogenesis. 2. the theoretical production of offspring that are totally different from both parents. **xenogenetic, xenogenic,** *adj.*

xenograft, tissue from another species, used as a temporary graft in certain cases; for example, in treating a patient with severe burns where there is insufficient tissue from the patient, or tissue from a tissue bank is not available.

xenon (Xe), an inert, gaseous, non-metallic element. Its atomic number is 54 and its atomic weight is 131.30.

xenophobia, an anxiety disorder characterized by a pervasive, irrational fear or uneasiness in the presence of strangers, especially foreigners, or in new surroundings.

xeroderma, a chronic skin condition characterized by dryness and roughness.

xeroderma pigmentosum, a rare, inherited skin disease characterized by extreme sensitivity to ultraviolet light, exposure to which results in freckles, telangiectases, keratoses, papillomas, carcinoma and possibly melanoma. Keratitis and tumours developing on the eyelids and cornea may result in blindness.

xeromammogram, a radiographic image of the breast using xeroradiography.

xerophthalmia, a condition of dry and lustreless corneas and conjunctival areas, usually as a result of vitamin A deficiency; it is associated with night blindness.

xeroradiography, a radiographic imaging method in which the image is formed on a selenium-coated charged plate. Within areas exposed to x-rays, the charge dissipates leaving a pattern of charge which forms the latent image. The visible image is formed using charged powder fused into paper. **xerogram,** *n.*

xerosis. See **dry skin.**

xerostomia, dryness of the mouth caused by cessation of normal salivary secretion. The condition is a symptom of various diseases, such as diabetes, acute infections, hysteria and Sjögren's syndrome, and can be caused by paralysis of facial nerves.

xiphisternal articulation, the cartilaginous connection between the xiphoid process and body of the sternum.

xiphisternum. See **xiphoid process.**

xiphoid process, the smallest of three parts of the sternum, articulating caudally with the body of sternum and laterally with the seventh rib.

XO, (in genetics) the designation for the presence of only one sex chromosome; either the X or Y chromosome is missing so that each cell is monosomic and contains a total of 45 chromosomes.

XX, (in genetics) the designation for the normal sex chromosome complement in the human female.

XXX syndrome, a human sex chromosomal aberration characterized by the presence of three X chromosomes and two Barr bodies, instead of the normal XX complement, so that somatic cells contain a total of 47 chromosomes.

XXXX, XXXXX, (in genetics) the designation for an abnormal sex chromosome complement in the human female in which there are, respectively, four or five instead of the normal two X chromosomes, so that each somatic cell contains a total of 48 or 49 chromosomes.

XXXY, XXXXY, XXYY, (in genetics) the designation for an abnormal sex chromosome complement in the human male, in which there are more than the normal one X chromosome, resulting respectively in a total of 48, 49 or more chromosomes in each somatic cell.

XXY syndrome. See **Klinefelter's syndrome.**

XY, (in genetics) the designation for the normal sex chromosome complement in the human male.

xylitol, a sweet, crystalline pentahydroxy alcohol, obtained by the reduction of xylose and used as an artificial sweetener.

xylometazoline hydrochloride, an adrenergic vasoconstrictor used as a nose spray or drops in the treatment of nasal congestion in colds, hay fever, sinusitis and other upper respiratory allergies. It is also used as an ophthalmic vasoconstrictor.

XYY syndrome, the phenotypic manifestation of an extra Y chromosome, which tends to have a positive effect on height and may have a negative effect on mental and psychological development. However, the abnormality also occurs in normal males.

Y, symbol for **yttrium.**

yang, a polarized aspect of ch'i that is active or positive energy.

yaws, a non-venereal infection caused by the spirochaete *Treponema pertenue,* transmitted by direct contact and characterized by chronic ulcerating sores anywhere on the body, with eventual tissue and bone destruction leading to crippling if left untreated. All serological tests for syphilis may be positive in yaws.

Yb, symbol for **ytterbium.**

Y chromosome, a sex chromosome present only in the male, in humans and many other species. It appears singly in the normal male. It is carried as a sex determinant by one-half of the male gametes and none of the female gametes, is morphologically much smaller than the *Y* chromosome, and has genes associated with triggering the development and differentiation of male characteristics.

yeast, any unicellular, usually oval, nucleated fungus that reproduces by budding. *Candida albicans* is a kind of pathogenic yeast.

yellow card scheme, a reporting scheme organised by the committee on the safety of medicines, which enables medical practitioners to report suspected adverse reactions to drugs on post-paid, yellow cards. The data collected is used to identify safety problems with marketed medical products.

yellow cartilage, the most elastic of the three kinds of cartilage, consisting of elastic fibres in a flexible fibrous matrix. It is yellow and is located in various parts of the body, such as the external ear, auditory tube, epiglottis and larynx.

yellow fever, an acute arbovirus infection transmitted by mosquitoes. It is characterized by headache, fever, jaundice, vomiting and bleeding. There is no specific treatment, and mortality is approximately 5%. Recovery is followed by lifelong immunity.

yellow fever vaccine, a vaccine produced from live, attenuated, yellow fever virus, grown in chick embryos. It is used for active immunization against yellow fever.

yellow marrow. See **bone marrow.**

Yersinia arthritis {Alexandre E. J. Yersin, French bacteriologist, b. 1863}, a polyarticular inflammation occurring between a few days to 1 month after the onset of infection caused by *Yersinia enterocolitica* or *Y. pseudotuberculosis.* It usually persists longer than 1 month. Knees, ankles, toes, fingers and wrists are most often affected. The clinical presentation may mimic juvenile rheumatoid arthritis, rheumatic fever or Reiter's syndrome.

Yersinia pestis {Alexandre Yersin}, a small, gram-negative bacillus that causes plague. The primary host is the rat, but other small rodents also harbour the organism. Also called *Pasteurella pestis.*

Y fracture, a Y-shaped intercondylar fracture.

yin, a polarized aspect of ch'i that is passive or negative energy.

Y-linked, pertaining to genes, or to the characteristics or conditions they transmit, carried on the Y chromosome.

yoga (hatha), a discipline that focuses on the body's musculature, posture, breathing mechanisms and consciousness. The goal of yoga is attainment of physical and mental well-being.

yoghurt, a slightly acidic, semisolid, curdled milk preparation made from either whole or skimmed cow's, ewe' s or goat's milk and milk solids, by fermentation with organisms from the genus *Lactobacillus.*

yoke, a connector used to link small cylinders of medical gases, such as portable oxygen tanks, to respiratory equipment.

yolk, the nutritive material, rich in fats and proteins, contained in the ovum to supply nourishment to the developing embryo. In humans and most mammals, the yolk is absent or greatly diffused through the cell, because embryos absorb nutrients directly from the mother through the placenta.

yolk membrane. See **vitelline membrane.**

yolk sac, a structure that develops in the inner cell mass of the embryo and expands into a vesicle with a thick part that becomes the primitive gut and a thin part that grows into the cavity of the chorion. After supplying the nourishment for the embryo, the yolk sac usually disappears during the seventh week of pregnancy.

yolk sphere. See **morula.**

yolk stalk, the narrow duct connecting the yolk sac with the midgut of the embryo during the early stages of prenatal development.

Young's rule {Thomas Young, English physician, b. 1773}, a method for the calculation of the appropriate dose of a drug for a child 2 years of age or more, using the formula (age in years) ÷ (age + 12) x adult dose.

Y-plasty, a method of surgical revision of a scar, using a Y-shaped incision to reduce scar contractures.

Y-set, a device composed of plastic components, used for delivering intravenous fluids through a primary intravenous line connected to a combination drip chamberfilter section, from which two separate plastic tubes lead to fluid sources. The Y-set also includes three clamps, one for the primary intravenous line and one for each of the two separate tubes. It is often used to transfuse packed blood cells that must be diluted with saline solution to decrease their viscosity.

ytterbium (Yb), a rare earth metallic element. Its atomic number is 70 and its atomic weight is 173.04.

yttrium (Y), a scaly, greyish metallic element. Its atomic number is 39 and its atomic weight is 88.905. Radioactive isotopes of yttrium have been used in cancer therapy.

Z chromosome. See **W chromosome and Z chromosome.**

Z-plasty, a method of surgical revision of a scar or closure of a wound, using a Z-shaped incision to reduce contractures of the adjacent skin.

Zahorsky's disease. See **roseola infantum.**

ZEEP, abbreviation for **zero-end expiratory pressure.**

Zenker's diverticulum {Friedrich A. Zenker, German pathologist, b. 1825}, a circumscribed herniation of the mucous membrane of the pharynx as it joins the oesophagus. Food may become trapped in the diverticulum and may be aspirated.

zeranol, an oestrogenic substance used to fatten livestock. Consumption of beef from zeranol-treated cattle has been associated with precocious puberty in some boys and girls.

zero fluid balance, a state in which the amount of fluid intake is equal to the amount of fluid output.

zero order kinetics, a state at which the rate of an enzyme reaction is independent of the concentration of the substrate.

zero population growth, a situation in which there is no population increase during a given year, because the total of live births is equal to the total of deaths.

zero-end expiratory pressure (ZEEP), pressure that has returned to ambient or atmospheric pressure at the end of exhalation.

zeta potential, the potential produced by the effective charge of a macromolecule, usually measured at the boundary between what is moving in a solution with the macromolecule and the rest of the solution.

zeugmatography, another name for magnetic resonance imaging, suggesting the role of the gradient magnetic field in joining the rf magnetic field to a desired local spatial region through magnetic resonance.

zidovudine, an HIV virus inhibitor that interferes with DNA synthesis. It is used in the treatment of HIV infection, and was formerly called azidothymidine (AZT).

Ziehl-Neelsen test, {Franz Ziehl, German physician, b. 1859; Friedrich K. A. Neelsen, German pathologist, b. 1854}, one of the most widely used methods of acid-fast staining. It is commonly used in the microscopic examination of a smear of sputum suspected of containing *Mycobacterium tuberculosis.*

zinc (Zn), a bluish-white crystalline metal, commonly associated with lead ores. Its atomic number is 30a and its atomic weight is 65.38. Zinc is an essential nutrient in the body, and is used in numerous pharmaceuticals such as zinc oxide.

zinc deficiency, a condition resulting from insufficient amounts of zinc in the diet. It is characterized by abnormal fatigue, decreased alertness, a decrease in taste and odour sensitivity, poor appetite, retarded growth, delayed sexual maturity, prolonged healing of wounds, and susceptibility to infection and injury.

zinc gelatin, a topical protectant for varicosities and other lesions of the lower limbs.

zinc oxide, a topical protectant used for a wide range of minor skin irritations.

zinc oxide eugenol dental cement, a luting agent consisting of a powder that is essentially zinc oxide with strengtheners and accelerators, combined with a liquid that is basically eugenol.

zinc phosphate dental cement, a material for luting of dental inlays, crowns, bridges and orthodontic appliances, and for some temporary restorations of dentitions.

zinc salt poisoning, a toxic condition caused by the ingestion or inhalation of a zinc salt. Symptoms of ingestion include a burning sensation in the mouth and throat, vomiting diarrhoea, abdominal and chest pain and, in severe cases, shock and coma.

zinc sulphate, an ophthalmic astringent given in drops for nasal congestion or irritation of the eye. It is also applied topically in deodorants, given orally in tablets to promote healing, and used as a dietary supplement.

ZIP, abbreviation for *zoster immune plasma* See **chickenpox.**

zirconium (Zr), a steel-gray, tetravalent metallic element. Its atomic number is 40 and its atomic weight is 91.22.

Zn, symbol for **zinc.**

zoanthropy, the delusion that one has assumed the form and characteristics of an animal. **zoanthropic,** *adj.*

Zollinger-Ellison syndrome {Robert M. Zollinger, American surgeon, b. 1903 Edwin H. Ellison, American physician, b. 1918}, a condition characterized by severe peptic ulceration, gastric hypersecretion, elevated serum gastrin and gastrinoma of the pancreas or duodenum.

zona, *pl.* **zonae,** a zone or girdle-like segment of a rounded or spheric structure.

zona ciliaris. See **ciliary zone.**

zona fasciculata, the middle portion of the

adrenal cortex, which is the site of production of glucocorticoids and sex hormones.

zona glomerulosa, the outer portion of the adrenal cortex, where mineralocorticoids are produced.

zona pellucida, the thick, transparent, noncellular membrane that encloses the mammalian ovum. It is secreted by the ovum during its development in the ovary, and is retained until near the time of implantation.

zona radiata, a zona pellucida that has a striated appearance caused by radiating canals within the membrane.

zona reticularis, the innermost portion of the adrenal cortex, which borders on the adrenal medulla portion of the gland. It acts in consort with the zona fasciculata in producing various sex hormones and glucocorticoids.

zona striata. See **zona radiata.**

zonaesthesia, a painful sensation of constriction, as of a bandage bound too tightly, especially experienced around the waist or abdomen.

zone, an area with specific boundaries and characteristics, such as the epigastric, mesogastric or hypogastric zones of the abdomen. See also **zona.**

zone of equivalence, a region of an antibody-antigen reaction in which concentrations of both reactants are equal.

zone therapy, the treatment of a disorder by mechanical stimulation and counter-irritation of a body area in the same longitudinal zone as the affected organ or region.

zonula, *pl.* **zonulae,** a small zone.

zonula ciliaris, a ligament composed of straight fibrils radiating from the ciliary body of the eye to the crystalline lens, holding the lens in place and relaxing by the contraction of the ciliary muscle. Relaxation of the ligament allows the lens to become more convex.

zooerastia. See **bestiality.**

zoogenous, acquired from, or originating in, animals.

zoograft, tissue of an animal transplanted to a human, such as a heart valve from a pig to replace a damaged heart valve in a human.

zoology, the study of animal life.

zoomania, a psychopathological state characterized by an excessive fondness for, and preoccupation with, animals. **zoomaniac,** *n.*

zoonosis, a disease of animals that is transmissible to humans from its primary animal host. Some kinds of zoonoses are **equine encephalitis, leptospirosis, rabies** and **yellow fever.**

zooparasite, any parasitic animal organism. Kinds of zooparasites are **arthropods, protozoa** and **worms. zooparasitic,** *adj.*

zoopathology, th. study of diseases of animals.

zoophilia, 1. an abnormal fondness for animals. **2.** (in psychiatry) a psychosexual disorder in which sexual excitement and gratification are derived from the fondling of animals, or from the fantasy or act of engaging in sexual activity with animals. **zoophile,** *n.,* **zoophilic, zoophilous,** *adj.*

zoophobia, an anxiety disorder characterized by a persistent, irrational fear of animals, particularly dogs, snakes, insects and mice.

zoopsia, a visual hallucination of animals or insects, often occurring in delirium tremens.

zootoxin, a poisonous substance from an animal, such as the venom of snakes, spiders and scorpions. **zootoxic,** *adj.*

zoster. See **herpes zoster.**

zoster immunoglobulin. See **varicella zoster immunoglobulin.**

zosteriform, resembling the pocks seen in herpes zoster infection.

Zr, symbol for **zirconium.**

Zung Self-Rating Depression Scale, a "self-report test" of 20 negatively stated items, undertaken to determine the presence of depression.

zwitterion, an ion that has regions of both negative and positive charge. Amino acids, such as glycine, may act as zwitterions when in a neutral solution.

zygogenesis, 1. the formation of a zygote. **2.** reproduction by the union of gametes. **zygogenetic, zygogenic,** *adj.*

zygoma, 1. a long slender zygomatic process of the temporal bone. It arises from the lower part of the squamous portion of the temporal bone, passes forward to join the zygomatic bone, and forms part of the zygomatic arch. **2.** the zygomatic bone that forms the prominence of the cheek.

zygomatic bone, one of the pair of bones that forms the prominence of the cheek, the lower part of the orbit of the eye, and parts of the temporal and infratemporal fossae.

zygomatic head, See **zygomaticus minor.**

zygomaticus major, one of the 12 muscles of the mouth. It acts to draw the angle of the mouth up and back, in smiling or laughter.

zygomaticus minor, one of the 12 muscles of the mouth. It acts to deepen the nasolabial furrow in a sad facial expression.

zygomaxillare. See **key ridge.**

zygomycosis, an acute, often fulminant and sometimes fatal fungal infection, caused by a class of Phycomycetal water moulds; it is seen primarily in patients with chronic debilitating diseases. It begins with fever and pain, and discharge in the nose and paranasal sinuses that progresses to invade the eye and lower respiratory tract. The fungus may enter blood vessels and spread to the brain and other organs.

zygonema, the synaptic chromosome formation that occurs in the zygotene stage of the first meiotic prophase of gametogenesis. **zygonematic,** *adj.*

zygosis, a form of sexual reproduction in

unicellular organisms, consisting of the union of two cells and fusion of the nuclei. **zygotic,** *adj.*

zygosity, the characteristics or conditions of a zygote. The form occurs primarily as a suffix-combining form to denote genetic makeup, referring specifically to whether the paired alleles that determine a particular trait are identical (homozygosity) or different (heterozygosity).

zygospore, the spore resulting from the con-

jugation of two isogametes, as in certain fungi and algae.

zygote, (in embryology) the developing ovum from the time it is fertilized until it is implanted in the uterus as a blastocyst.

zygotene, the second stage in the first meiotic prophase of gametogenesis in which synapsis of homologous chromosomes occurs.

zymogenic cell. See **chief cell.**